Veterinary Pharmacology and Toxicology

Proceedings from the 2nd European Association for Veterinary Pharmacology and Toxicology held at Toulouse, 13th–17th September, 1982

EDITED BY

Yves Ruckebusch
Ecole Nationale Vétérinaire
23, chemin des Capelles
31076 Toulouse Cédex, France

Pierre-Louis Toutain
Pharmacologie-Toxicologie INRA
180, chemin de Tournefeuille
31300 Toulouse, France

Gary D. Koritz
College of Veterinary Medicine
University of Illinois
Urbana, Illinois 61801, USA

Published in the United States by

avi

AVI PUBLISHING COMPANY, INC.
Westport, Connecticut

First American Edition 1983

The AVI Publishing Company, Inc.
Westport, Connecticut

Published in UK by
MTP Press Limited
Falcon House
Cable Street
Lancaster, England

ISBN 0-87055-442-5

Printed in Great Britain

Contents

SECTION III NON-RUMINANT PHARMACOLOGY

SECTION V TOXICOLOGY

List of Contributors

W. M. ALLEN
Agricultural Research Council
Institute for Research on Animal Disease
Compton, Newbury, Berks. RG16 0NN
England

F. R. ALTHAUS
University of Zurich School
of Veterinary Medicine
Institute of Pharmacology and
Biochemistry
Winterthurerstrasse 260
8057 Zurich
Switzerland

A. ANADÓN
Department of Pharmacology
and Toxicology
Faculty of Veterinary Medicine
University of Leon
Leon, Spain

N. A. ANIS
Department of Physiology
Royal Veterinary College
London NW1 0TU, England

L.-E. APPELGREN
Department of Pharmacology
Faculty of Veterinary Medicine
The Swedish University of
Agricultural Science
Box 573, 75123 Uppsala, Sweden

Ph. ARCHIMBAULT
Virbac, BP 13
06201 Nice Cédex, France

B. ATTALI
Laboratoire de Pharmacologie et
de Toxicologie Fondamentales
CNRS, 205 route de Narbonne
31400 Toulouse, France

Y. AUDIGIER
Laboratoire de Pharmacologie et
de Toxicologie Fondamentales
CNRS, 205 route de Narbonne
31400 Toulouse, France

F. AWOUTERS
Department of Pharmacology
Janssen Pharmaceutica
B-2340 Beerse, Belgium

J. D. BAGGOT
School of Veterinary Medicine
University of California
Davis, California 95616, USA

F. M. BELPAIRE
J. F. & C. Heymans Institute of
Pharmacology
Faculty of Medicine, State University
Ghent, Belgium

S. C. BERRY
Department of Physiology
Royal Veterinary College
London NW1 0TU, England

J. BERTHE
Service Toxicologie
C. R. Clin-Midy
Rue de Prof. J. Blayac
34082 Montpellier Cédex, France

W. BEUTER
Institute of Pharmacology, Toxicology
and Pharmacy, University of Munich
Veterinärstrasse 13
D-8000 München 22, FRG

B. J. BLAAUBOER
Institute of Veterinary Pharmacology,
Pharmacy and Toxicology
State University of Utrecht
Biltstraat 172
3572 BP Utrecht, The Netherlands

LIST OF CONTRIBUTORS

J. C. BLANCHARD
Rhône-Poulenc Recherches
Centre Nicolas Grillet
13, quai Jules-Guesde
94400 Vitry-sur-Seine, France

A. BLÜTHGEN
Institute for Hygiene
Federal Dairy Research Centre
D-2300 Kiel, FRG

M. G. BOGAERT
J. F. & C. Heymans Institute
of Pharmacology
Faculty of Medicine, State University
Ghent, Belgium

J. A. BOGAN
Department of Veterinary Pharmacology
Veterinary Hospital, Bearsden Road
Glasgow G61 1QH, Scotland

J. BOISSEAU
Laboratoire National des Médicaments
Vétérinaires
Javené 35300 Fougères, France

R. BOIVIN
Laboratoire de Physiologie
École Nationale Vétérinaire de Lyon
Marcy L'Étoile
69260 Charbonnières-les-Bains, France

H. VAN DEN BOSSCHE
Department of Comparative Biochemistry
Janssen Pharmaceutica
B-2340 Beerse
Belgium

B. BOUR
INRA, Physiologie de la Reproduction
37380 Nouzilly, France

R. A. BRANDON
School of Veterinary Medicine
University of California
Davis, California 95616, USA

G. J. BROUWER
University Department of Anaesthesia
Royal Liverpool Hospital
Prescot Street, PO Box 147
Liverpool L69 3QX, England

L. BUENO
Station de Pharmacologie-Toxicologie
INRA, 180 chemin de Tournefeuille
31300 Toulouse, France

N. R. BURTON
Department of Physiology
Royal Veterinary College
London NW1 0TU, England

S. CHAKRABARTI
J. F. & C. Heymans Institute
of Pharmacology
Faculty of Medicine, State University
Ghent, Belgium

F. CHEVALIER
INRA, Physiologie de la Reproduction
37380 Nouzilly, France

J. CROS
Laboratoire de Pharmacologie et
de Toxicologie Fondamentales
CNRS, 205 route de Narbonne
31400 Toulouse, France

A. DAKKAK
Institut Agronomique et Vétérinaire
Hassan II, BP 6202
Rabat-Agdal, Maroc

R. DANTZER
Laboratoire de Neurobiologie
des Comportements
INRA, Université de Bordeaux II
146, rue Léo-Saignat
33076 Bordeaux Cédex, France

J. V. DAVIES
Department of Surgery
Royal Veterinary College
Hawkshead Lane, North Mymms
Hatfield, Herts., England

L. E. DAVIS
College of Veterinary Medicine
University of Illinois
Urbana, Illinois 61801, USA

P. DE BACKER
Veterinary Pharmacology and Toxicology
Faculty of Veterinary Medicine
Casinoplein 24, 9000 Ghent, Belgium

M. DEBACKERE
Veterinary Pharmacology and Toxicology
Faculty of Veterinary Medicine
Casinoplein 24, 9000 Ghent, Belgium

A. N. DEGRYSE
Department of Veterinary Pharmacology
Janssen Pharmaceutica
B-2340 Beerse, Belgium

P. DELATOUR
Laboratoire de Biochimie
École Nationale Vétérinaire de Lyon
69260 Charbonnières, France

A. DE RICK
Department of Small Animal Medicine
Faculty of Veterinary Medicine
State University, Ghent, Belgium

L. DESPLENTER
Janssen Pharmaceutica
Turnhautseweg 30
2340 Beerse, Belgium

C. J. DI CUOLLO
Smith Kline Animal Health Products
1600 Paoli Pike
West Chester, Pennsylvania 19380
USA

P. H. DILOV
Veterinary Medical Faculty
Higher Institute of Zootechnics
and Veterinary Medicine
62 D. Blagoev Str.
Stara Zagora-6000, Bulgaria

G. DOST
Hoechst AG
Abteilung für Veterinärmedizin
Forschung, Postfach 800320
623 Frankfurt am Main 90, FRG

C. F. DRAKE
Agriculture Research Council
Institute for Research on Animal
Disease
Compton, Newbury, Berks RG16 0NN
England

D. DROUMEV
Department of Pharmacology
Veterinary Medical Faculty
62, D. Blagoev. Str.
Stara Zagora-6000, Bulgaria

C. DUMONTEIL
Sica, BP 202
12, rue des Beaux-Soleils
95520 Osny, France

R. H. DUNLOP
University of Minnesota, Twin Cities
College of Veterinary Medicine
1971 Commonwealth Avenue
St. Paul, Minnesota 55108, USA

S. EDMISTON
California Department of Food
and Agriculture
1220 N Street
Sacramento, California 95814, USA

B. ENRIQUEZ
Ecole Nationale Vétérinaire
7, avenue du Général-de-Gaulle
94700 Maisons Alfort, France

J. ESPINASSE
Ecole Nationale Vétérinaire d'Alfort
7, avenue du Général de Gaulle
94704 Maisons Alfort, France

P. EYRE
Pharmacology Laboratory
Department of Biomedical Sciences
University of Guelph
Guelph, Ontario, Canada N1G 2WI

T. B. FARVER
Department of Epidemiology
and Public Health
School of Veterinary Medicine
University of California
Davis, California 95616, USA

J. FIORAMONTI
Laboratoire de Physiologie
Ewe Nationale Vétérinaire
23 chemin des Capelles
31076 Toulouse Cédex, France

S. M. FREE
Smith Kline Animal Health Products
1600 Paoli Pike
West Chester, Pennsylvania 19380
USA

H.-H. FREY
Laboratory of Pharmacology-Toxicology
School of Veterinary Medicine
Free University Berlin
Berlin West, FRG

L. G. FRIEDLANDER
Department of Veterinary Physiology
and Pharmacology
College of Veterinary Medicine
Texas A & M University
College Station, Texas 77843, USA

LIST OF CONTRIBUTORS

C. FRIIS
Royal Veterinary and Agricultural University
Department of Pharmacology and Toxicology
13, Bülowsvej, KD-1870
Copenhagen V, Denmark

P. GALTIER
Station de Pharmacologie-Toxicologie
INRA
180, chemin de Tournefeuille
31300 Toulouse, France

R. C. GARG
Veterinary Physiology and Pharmacology
School of Veterinary Medicine
Tuskegee Institute, Al. 36088, USA

E. L. GERRING
Department of Surgery
Royal Veterinary College
Hawkshead Lane, North Mymms
Hatfield, Herts., England

O. GLARDON
Veterinär-Medizinische
Klinik de Universität
Zürich
Winterthurerstrasse, 260
Ch-8057 Zurich, Switzerland

P. GORSE
Laboratoire d'Etudes et de Recherches
Economiques sur les Industries
Agricoles et Alimentaires
MIN, BP 333
94153 Rungis Cédex, France

C. GOUARDÈRES
Laboratoire de Pharmacologie et de Toxicologie Fondamentales
CNRS, 205 route de Narbonne
31400 Toulouse, France

M. VAN GRAFT
Institute of Veterinary Pharmacology, Pharmacy and Toxicology
State University of Utrecht
Bilstraat 172
3572 BP Utrecht, The Netherlands

P. M. HEADLEY
Department of Physiology
Royal Veterinary College
London NW1 0TU, England

R. D. HEDDE
Smith Kline Animal Health Products
1600 Paoli Pike
West Chester, Pennsylvania 19380
USA

W. HEESCHEN
Institute for Hygiene
Federal Dairy Research Centre
D-2300 Kiel, FRG

R. C. HERSCHLER
Syntex Research
3401 Hillview Avenue
Palo Alto, California 94022, USA

G. R. HEWETT
Beecham Pharmaceuticals
Research Division
Walton Oats, Dorking Road
Tadworth, Surrey KT20 7NT
England

C. J. HILLIDGE
Department of Physiology
Royal Veterinary College
Hawkshead Lane, North Mymms
Hatfield, Herts., England

N. M. HONHOLD
Department of Physiology
Royal Veterinary College
London NW1 0TU, England

J. HRDLICKA
Department of Veterinary Pathology and Public Health
University of Queensland
St. Lucia, 4067 Brisbane, Australia

J. M. HUNTER
University of Liverpool
Leahurst, Neston Wirral L64 7TE
England

L. P. JAGER
CDI, PO Box 65
82000 AB Lelystad, The Netherlands

P. JAUSSAUD
Ecole Nationale Vétérinaire
69260 Charbonnières-les-Bains
France

W. L. JENKINS
Department of Veterinary Physiology and Pharmacology
College of Veterinary Medicine
Texas A & M University
College Station, Texas 77843, USA

R. S. JONES
The University Department of Anaesthesia
Royal Hospital, Prescot Street
Liverpool L7 8XP, England

J. P. JOUANY
Laboratoire de la Digestion des Ruminants
CRZV de Theix
63122 Ceyrat, France

D. JOURBINEV
Research Institute of Cattle Breed and Sheep Breed
Stara Zagora-6000, Bulgaria

L. JULOU
Rhône-Poulenc Recherches
Centre Nicolas Grillet
13, quai Jules-Guesde
94400 Vitry-sur-Seine, France

T. JUSZKIEWICZ
Department of Pharmacology and Toxicology
Veterinary Research Institute
Al. Partyzantow 57
24-100 Pulawy, Poland

G. KECK
Ecole Nationale Vétérinaire
Marcy l'Etoile
69260 Charbonnières-les-Bains
France

J. S. KENT
Syntex Research
3401 Hillview Avenue
Palo Alto, California 94022, USA

O. KERN
Boehringer-Ingelheim Vetmedica GmbH
6507 Ingelheim, FRG

M. KESSABI
Institut Agronomique et Vétérinaire
Hassan II, BP 6202
Rabat-Agdal, Maroc

G. D. KORITZ
College of Veterinary Medicine
University of Illinois
Urbana, Illinois 61801, USA

F. W. VAN DER KREEK
Ministerie van Volksgezondheid en Milieuhygiëne, Postbus 439
2260 AK Leidschendam
The Netherlands

P. LACROIX
Centre de Recherches SOBIO
35760 St-Grégoire, France

J. LE BARS
Station de Pharmacologie-Toxicologie
INRA
180, chemin de Tournefeuille
31300 Toulouse, France

J. S. LEE
Department of Veterinary Pathology and Public Health
University of Queensland
St. Lucia, 4067 Brisbane, Australia

P. LEES
Department of Physiology
Royal Veterinary College
Hawkshead Lane, North Mymms
Hatfield, Herts., England

A. LIEBISCH
Tierärztliche Hochschule
Bünteweg 17
D-3000 Hannover 71, RFA

P. LINÉE
Centre de Recherches SOBIO
35760 St-Grégoire, France

M. LOBRY
Ministère de l'Agriculture
Direction de la Qualité
44–46, boulevard de Grenelle
75732 Paris Cédex, France

D. LODGE
Department of Physiology
Royal Veterinary College
London NW1 0TU, England

G. LORGUE
Ecole Nationale Vétérinaire
Marcy l'Etoile
69260 Charbonnières-les-Bains
France

K. MADDY
California Department of Food and Agriculture
1220 N Street, Sacramento
California 95814, USA

S. E. MARRINER
Department of Veterinary Pharmacology
Veterinary Hospital, Bearsden Road
Glasgow G61 1QH, Scotland

D. MATTHEEUWS
Department of Small Animal Medicine
Faculty of Veterinary Medicine
State University, Ghent, Belgium

H. MAZARGUIL
Laboratoire de Pharmacologie et
le Toxicologie Fondamentales
CNRS, 205 route de Narbonne
31400 Toulouse, France

G. MAZUÉ
Service Toxicologie
C. R. Clin-Midy
Rue de Prof. J. Blayac
34082 Montpellier Cédex, France

N. McHARDY
Department of Biochemical Parasitology
Wellcome Research Laboratory
Beckenham, Kent, England

M. J. MEREDITH
Department of Physiology and
Animal Husbandry
The Royal Veterinary College
Field Station, North Mymms
Hatfield, Herts., England

A. S. J. P. A. M. VAN MIERT
Institute of Veterinary Pharmacology,
Pharmacy and Toxicology
Bilstraat 172, 3572 BP Utrecht
The Netherlands

G. MILHAUD
Ecole Nationale Vétérinaire
7, avenue du Général-de-Gaulle
94700 Maisons Alfort, France

P. R. MOORE
Agricultural Research Council
Institute for Research on Animal Disease
Compton, Newbury, Berks. RG16 0NN
England

J. P. MORETAIN
Laboratoire National des Médicaments
Vétérinaires
Javené 35300 Fougères, France

P. NIELSEN
Department of Pharmacology
and Toxicology
Royal Veterinary and Agricultural
University, Copenhagen, Denmark

C. J. E. NIEMEGEERS
Department of Pharmacology
Janssen Pharmaceutica
B-2340 Beerse, Belgium

J. C. NG
Department of Veterinary Pathology
and Public Health
University of Queensland
St. Lucia, 4067 Brisbane, Australia

J. VAN NOORDWIJK
RIV
Bilthoven
The Netherlands

L. OOMS
Department of Veterinary Pharmacology
Janssen Pharmaceutica
B-2340 Beerse, Belgium

F. OSDOIT
Ecole Nationale Vétérinaire
7, avenue du Général-de-Gaulle
94704 Maisons-Alfort, France

E. PALMER
Physiologie de la Reproduction
INRA
37380 Nouzilly, France

R. C. PARISH
Smith Kline Animal Health Products
1600 Paoli Pike
West Chester, Pennsylvania 19380
USA

D. PASHOV
Department of Pharmacology
Veterinary Medical Faculty
62, D. Blagoev Str.
Stara Zagora-6000, Bulgaria

A. PETKOV
Department of Physiology
Faculty of Zootechnics
Stara Zagora-6000, Bulgaria

L. P. PHANEUF
Department d'Anatomie et
Physiologie Animales
Faculté de Médecine Vétérinaire
de l'Université de Montréal
Saint-Hyacinthe
Qué., Canada J2S 7C6

R. W. PHILLIPS
Department of Physiology
and Biophysics
Colorado State University
Fort Collins, Colorado 80523, USA

L. PINAULT
Service de Pharmacie-Toxicologie
École Nationale Vétérinaire de Nantes
BP 527, 44026 Nantes Cédex, France

J. D. POWERS
Department of Veterinary Physiology
and Pharmacology
The Ohio State University
1900 Coffey Road
Columbus, Ohio 43210, USA

T. E. POWERS
Department of Veterinary Physiology
and Pharmacology
The Ohio State University
1900 Coffey Road
Columbus, Ohio 43210, USA

R. QUACH
Smith Kline Animal Health Products
1600 Paoli Pike
West Chester, Pennsylvania 19380
USA

F. RASMUSSEN
Department of Pharmacology
and Toxicology
Royal Veterinary and Agricultural
University, Copenhagen, Denmark

J. P. RAYNAUD
Rhone-Merieux (IST)
4, chemin du Calquet, BP 31–38
31026 Toulouse Cédex, France

R. REICHE
Laboratory of Pharmacology-Toxicology
School of Veterinary Medicine
Free University Berlin
Berlin West, FRG

L. RENAULT
Laboratoire Vétérinaire Sanders
17, quai de l'Industrie
91200 Athis-Mons, France

P. RICHEZ
Service Toxicologie
C. R. Clin-Midy
Rue du Prof. J. Blayac
34082 Montpellier Cédex, France

F. RIVIÈRE
Ecole Nationale Vétérinaire
7, avenue du Général-de-Gaule
94700 Maisons Alfort, France

V. ROUSSEV
Department of Physiology
Faculty of Zootechnics
Stara Zagora-6000, Bulgaria

Y. RUCKEBUSCH
Laboratoire de Physiologie
Ecole Nationale Vétérinaire
23, chemin des Capelles
31076 Toulouse Cédex, France

W. SAMBETH
Hoechst AG
Abteilung für Veterinärmedizinische
Forschung, Postfach 800320
623 Frankfurt am Main 80, FRG

B. V. SANSOM
Agricultural Research Council
Institute for Research on Animal Disease
Compton, Newbury, Berks. RG16 0NN
England

H. SCHILL
Boehringer-Ingelheim GmbH
6507 Ingelheim, FRG

A. SCHMID
Institute of Pharmacology, Toxicology
and Pharmacy
University of München
Veterinärstrasse 13
D-8000 München 22, RFG

A. J. H. SCHOTMAN
Department of Large Animal Medicine
State University of Utrecht
3572 BP Utrecht
The Netherlands

A. A. SEAWRIGHT
Department of Veterinary Pathology
and Public Health
University of Queensland
St. Lucia, 4067 Brisbane, Australia

A. J. M. SEEGERS
Pharmacy de Riet Wietelweg 1
5981 TG Helden, The Netherlands

J. SENAUD
Biologie Comparée des Protistes
LA CNRS n° 138
Université de Clermont II, Les Cézeaux
BP 45, 63170 Aubière, France

LIST OF CONTRIBUTORS

L. SERRANO
Department of Physiology
Royal Veterinary College
Hawkshead Lane, North Mymms
Hatfield, Herts., England

L. SHOR
Smith Kline Animal Health Products
1600 Paoli Pike, West Chester
Pennsylvania 19380, USA

C. R. SHORT
Department of Veterinary Physiology
School of Veterinary Medicine
Louisiana State University
Baton Rouge, Louisiana 70803, USA

S. L. SPURLOCK
Department of Veterinary Physiology
and Pharmacology
The Ohio State University
1900 Coffey Road
Columbus, Ohio 43210, USA

E. P. STEFFEY
Department of Veterinary
Medical Surgery
School of Veterinary Medicine
University of California
Davis, California 95616, USA

P. THIVEND
Laboratoire de la Digestion
des Ruminants, IRNA
CNRZ de Theix
63110 Beaumont, France

R. V. TOMLINSON
Syntex Research
3401 Hillview Avenue
Palo Alto, California 94022, USA

P. L. TOUTAIN
Station de Pharmacologie-Toxicologie
INRA, 180 chemin de Tournefeuille
31300 Toulouse, France

J. E. UTTING
University of Liverpool
Leahurst, Neston Wirral L64 7TE
England

O. VAINIO
Farmos Group Ltd Research Centre
PO Box 425, 20101 Turku 10, Finland

K. J. VARMA
Department of Veterinary Physiology
and Pharmacology
The Ohio State University
1900 Coffey Road
Columbus, Ohio 43210, USA

J. H. M. VERHEIJDEN
Department of Herd Health and
Ambulatory Clinic
State University of Utrecht
3572 BP Utrecht
The Netherlands

A. E. WATERMAN
Department of Pharmacology
Medical School
Bristol BS8 1TD, England

J. WELLINGS
California Department of Food
and Agriculture
1220 N Street
Sacramento, California 95814, USA

D. C. WEST
Department of Physiology
Royal Veterinary College
London NW1 0TU, England

J. I. D. WILKINSON
Lilly Research Centre Ltd.
Erl Wood Manor, Windlesham
Surrey GU20 6PH, England

G. M. WILLIAMS
Naylor Dana Institute for
Disease Prevention
American Health Foundation
One Dana Road, Valhalla
New York 10595, USA

M. WOLINER
Department of Epidemiology
and Public Health
School of Veterinary Medicine
University of California
Davis, California 95616, USA

D. ZWART
Institute of Veterinary Tropical
and Protozoan Diseases
State University of Utrecht
3572 BP Utrecht
The Netherlands

Preface and Acknowledgements

The Second Congress of the European Association for Veterinary Pharmacology and Toxicology (EAVPT) was held from 13th to 17th September 1982 at the quiet setting of the National Veterinary School of Toulouse. The meeting was organized by Dr Y. Ruckebusch and the Scientific Programme Committee consisting of Dr M. Debackere (Belgium), Dr J. Espinasse (France), Dr R. Faustini (Italy), Dr. H. Frey (FRG), Dr P. Lees (UK) and Dr F. Sanz (Spain), in close co-operation with the organizing local committee comprising the staff members from the host institutions (ENV: Ecole Nationale Vétérinaire, INRA: Institut National de la Recherche Agronomique, and IST: Institut de Sérothérapie de Toulouse).

The programme covered the fields of perinatal pharmacology and toxicology, comparative pharmacolgy and toxicology, pharmacokinetics and drug therapy, pharmacological methods and new animal models. Five sessions (out of nine) were devoted to the ruminant, hence the sections of the Proceedings: (1) Developmental pharmacology, (2) Ruminant pharmacology, (3) Non-ruminant pharmacology, (4) Pharmacological methods, and (5) Toxicology. The week's plan was for series of lectures presented during the days with evenings free for two workshops and informal discussion of posters and presentations. On the last day a series of demonstrations* was presented simultaneously at the INRA, IST and in the Departments of Veterinary Physiology and Pharmacology and of Large Animal Clinic of the ENV.

A congress book of near 500 pages (no. 8 of the series 'Les Colloques de l'INRA') which provided abstracts of the lectures and full texts corresponding to the 64 poster presentations and 16 demonstrations was distributed to more than 300 participants from 36 countries. This book ('Pharmacologie et Toxicologie Vétérinaires, 1982', ISBN – 85340-439-0) is still available from the Service des Publications de l'INRA, Route de Saint-Cyr, 78000 Versailles, France.

The programme of the congress started out with the official opening by Dr Lautié (ENV) and Dr Mauléon (INRA). Dr van Miert commemorated Dr Yoxall, the President of the Association. Highlights of the Congress were the assessment of carcinogenic properties of veterinary drugs, the clinical utility of pharmacokinetics as well as the use of levamisole in neonatal disease of calves, or the slow release formulation of fenprostalene. The words to be remembered in pharmacotherapy for the next decade are: detomidine, etomidate, metoclopramide, atracurium, augmentin, and ketanserin. A detailed account about these new drugs will be found in the Proceedings.

The Proceedings which contain 64 reports invited by the EAVPT Scientific Committee and two workshops have been prepared with the help of my colleagues Dr Toutain and Dr Koritz (on leave from USA) and of various referees. I would like to thank especially two of them, Prof. Phaneuf, Editor of the Canadian Veterinary Journal, who spent several days after the Congress at Toulouse, and Prof. Lees, Co-editor of the Journal of Veterinary Pharmacology and Therapeutics for his preparation of the workshop on anaesthesia.

At the closing dinner, provided courtesy of Dr Terré (Director of IST), the dean of the ENVT (Dr Lautié) discussed the input of the Congress upon veterinary pharmacology, toxicology and pharmacotherapy. On behalf of the non-European countries, Dr Short (USA) spontaneously expressed recognition of the meeting as a success: thanks to the early sponsorships of the Institut National de la Recherche Agronomique (Dr J. Poly), the Direction Générale de l'Enseignement et de la Recherche (Dr M. Gervais) and the Mission Interministérielle de l'Information Scientifique et Technique (Dr B. Cassen) who made this possible.

On behalf of the Scientific Committee, I would like to express also my appreciation to the Conseil Général de la Haute-Garonne, le Crédit Agricole, la Ville de Toulouse, and the firms listed below for special financial support: Boehringer-Ingelheim, *Reims*, Clin-Midy, *Montpellier*, Elanco (Div. Vét. of Eli Lilly), *Saint-Cloud*, Pierre Fabre (Centre de Recherches), *Castres*, Licotal (Div. Vét. of Wellcome), *Paris*, Madaus, *Köln*, Pfizer Int., *Orsay*, Specia (Rhone-Poulenc), *Paris*, Sanofi Santé Animale, *St-Jean-la Ruelle*, Institut de Sérothérapie, *Toulouse* and Vétoquinol, *Lure*.

Y. Ruckebusch

*– New computerized system for the evaluation of drug effect on digestive motility.
- Use of echography in the mare.
- Specific drug responses of the uterine cervix in the conscious ewe.
- Mass spectrometric identification of chloramphenicol traces in animal tissues.
- Use of analogue computer in the calculation of rate constants.
- Broncho-alveolar sampling in cattle.
- Serum production by plasmaphresis (horse).
- Bottle-pack system for filling of drugs.
- Production of bacterias and toxoids.

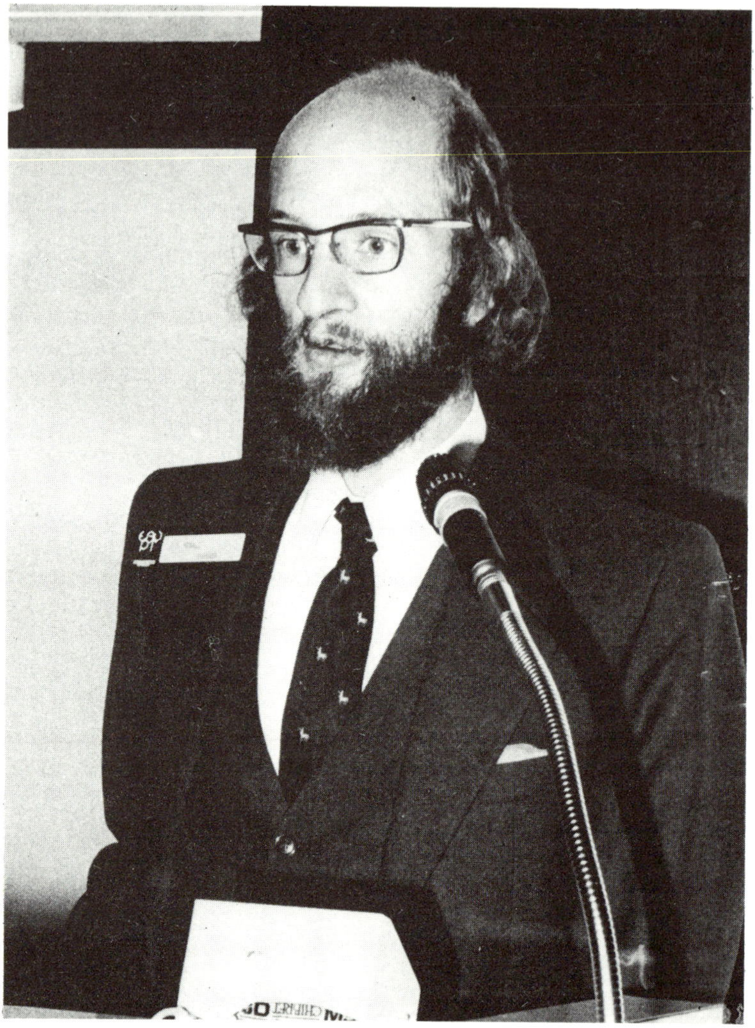

A. T. YOXALL 1949–1982

Co-founder and editor of the *Journal of Veterinary Pharmacology and Therapeutics*, co-editor of *The Pharmacological Basis of Small Animal Medicine* and *The Physiological Basis of Small Animal Medicine*, Andrew Yoxall will long be remembered for the energy with which he pursued the organizational advancement of the discipline of veterinary pharmacology in the UK and in Europe, and as a catalyst in the emergence of clinical pharmacology as a recognized entity in veterinary medicine.

In Appreciation of Andrew Thomas Yoxall

MA, Vet MB, MRCVS, DVA

A. S. J. P. A. M. van Miert and P. Lees

Dr A. T. Yoxall, president of our Society, first secretary of the Association for Veterinary Clinical Pharmacology and Therapeutics in the UK, co-founder and co-editor of the *Journal of Veterinary Pharmacology and Therapeutics*, died quite unexpectedly on January 5, 1982 in Balderton near Newark, where he ran his own practice. His tragically early death, at the age of 33, was a real shock for all his colleagues and friends in the UK, Europe and the United States. As vice-president, I am not the right person for the presentation of a balanced account of Dr A. T. Yoxall's many contributions to our profession, but it is clear that they were both considerable and distinctive. This short contribution is a tribute to a clinician who was highly dedicated to veterinary clinical pharmacology and therapeutics. He was a bright young student, an easy learner with an active interest in physiology, pharmacology and veterinary medicine. After qualifying from the Cambridge School in 1972, he pursued, at Cambridge, postgraduate studies which led to the Royal College Diploma in Veterinary Anaesthesia. It is in the field of veterinary clinical pharmacology, however, that he made a profound and lasting impact. As a teacher, clinician, editor and author he contributed more than anyone within so short a span. He demonstrated that he could complete work, write about it clearly and simply, and publish it. He was co-author of several texts including *The Pharmacological Basis of Small Animal Medicine* and *The Physiological Basis of Small Animal Medicine*. It was to his vision and seemingly limitless reserves of energy, that the AVCPT was founded in the UK. Moreover, he supported us with the creation of EAVPT. He approached colleagues with youthful enthusiasm and with the unshakable belief that free exchange of ideas and experiences among individuals from different backgrounds and different countries enables us to move forward step by step.

As part of the Biocentennial celebrations of the 'Tierärztliche Hochschule', veterinary pharmacologists from all over Europe met in Hannover in June 1978 to exchange views on the proposed foundation of a European Association for Veterinary Pharmacology and Toxicology. During that meeting the Association was formally founded and Dr Yoxall was elected as first president of EAVPT. In his address to the audience, he expressed his hope that a pleasant and productive programme of active work would ensue, with co-operation between schools, universities, research institutes and pharmaceutical industries. In discussing the purposes of the *Journal of Veterinary Pharmacology and Therapeutics*, he stressed the aim to give an identity and coherence to a movement which has resulted in the almost simultaneous creation of associations for veterinary pharmacology in the UK, USA and Europe. 'It is hoped', he said, 'that the Journal will improve co-ordination and communication among pharmacologists and veterinary clinicians; it is designed for the publication of topics relating both to the clinical aspects of veterinary pharmacology, and to fundamental pharmacological topics of veterinary relevance'. He was worried about the schism between 'scientific' pharmacology and veterinary clinical medicine. I recall some quotations from editorials with which he addressed the readers of the Journal: 'Veterinary clinicians have had to devise their own advances in surgery, radiology, anaesthesia, clinical pathology, preventive medicine, and other clinical disciplines, whilst the rapid transition of veterinary therapeutics from *materia medica* to a branch of pharmacology has taken place within 'pure science' laboratories and within the establishments of the pharmaceutical industries'.

Andrew Yoxall was an active participant in the first EAVPT congress which was held at Woudschoten Conference Centre in Zeist in September 1979; he was the sole organizer of the first International Conference on Veterinary Pharmacology, Therapeutics and Toxicology, held in Cambridge in July 1980 and prepared at that time with Dr Ruckebusch the programme of the Second EAVPT Congress specially devoted to the ruminant species. It is not for me to judge the success or otherwise of these meetings, not least because the success of any meeting must be judged by each individual in terms of the benefits that he hoped to obtain from attending the meeting, and the extent to which these hopes were fulfilled. One clear benefit that did arise from these conferences, however, was the possibility to contact other workers. Most participants did gain some benefit from personal contacts, and did come away with some sense of stimulation.

In January 1981, Andrew Yoxall wrote me a letter in which he requested to be relieved of his task as president of EAVPT and also of his editorship of the *Journal of Veterinary Pharmacology and Therapeutics*. A protracted illness had forced him to give up many of his professional duties.

Dr Andrew Yoxall was a tireless worker, often overcommitted, but always dedicated to the discipline covered by the umbrella title of 'Veterinary Pharmacology, Therapeutics and Toxicology'. He perhaps accomplished more in a few short years than many do in a lifetime and will be sadly missed by his many friends and colleagues.

It is fitting that Andrew Yoxall and his outstanding contribution to veterinary pharmacology be both remembered and honoured by this Congress.

Section I
Developmental Pharmacology

1
Perinatal pharmacology in ruminant models

Y. Ruckebusch

The primary physiological concern of the newborn is simply to survive[35]. This is achieved only by the onset of a vast air–blood interface for gas exchange, the separation of pulmonary and systemic circulations, the maintenance of body heat which supplies the energetic cost for moving, and the development of immune responsiveness.

Use of drugs during pregnancy[27] may produce adverse effects on the neuroendocrine factors during fetal development, and on the potential for functional adjustments at birth. The intensity of pharmacological effects depends on the magnitude of their pharmacodynamic actions on the fetus, and the extent of fetal exposure to the drug administered to the mother[45].

The chronic pregnant ewe model has been widely used to study the disposition and elimination of drugs in the ovine maternal–fetal unit by serial determinations over time during the last weeks prior to birth[10]. Relevant data are scant on the pharmacological effect of reversibly-acting drugs on fetal development and postnatal behaviour[3].

The objective of this chapter is to show the pregnant ewe model as a tool to stress the key points of fetal growth and functional adjustments at birth susceptible to be involved in expected drug effects. It may be a way to bridge the gap between specialized disciplines concerned with developmental physiology and pharmacology.

FETAL GROWTH AND BIRTH WEIGHT

A positive relationship between neonatal mortality, the major form of reproductive loss in ruminants, and *birth weight* below the breed norms, has been recognized for many years (Figure 1.1). The birth weight of lambs, unlike that of human infants, is very sensitive to the level of maternal nutrition and to heat stress in the last third of pregnancy. In both cases, the weight of cotyledons is reduced. Hence, the idea has arisen of the surgical removal of

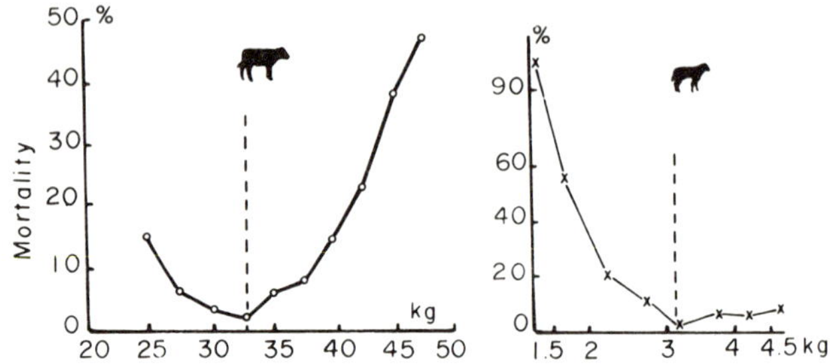

Figure 1.1 Relationship between birth weight and mortality. The mortality reached 15% in intrauterine growth retarded calves weighing 25 kg. Difficulties at birth are involved in the mortality of large size neonates. In growth-retarded lambs, the percentage of mortality is related to the birth weight with 40% for 2 kg v. 5% for 3 kg

cotyledons prior to conception in order to reduce fetal growth[1]. That the *placenta* may limit fetal growth, particularly near term, is supported by (1) the high degree of association of fetal and placental weight in sheep (4.5 : 0.5 kg with a correlation coefficient of 0.84 between animals at 146–149 days of gestational age), (2) the intrauterine growth retardation obtained by surgically reducing the number of caruncles prior to conception, and (3) the occurrence during the last weeks of pregnancy of infectious abortions as a result of placental insufficiency. Hypotrophy has also been obtained by uterine artery ligation[50] or by introduction of emboli into the maternal cotyledonary circulation[9]. The ovine uterine blood flow increases from 0.5 ml/min per g placenta at 80 days gestation to approximately 3 ml/min per g placenta near term. The estimated growth rate during the last 30 days of pregnancy is 70 g per day and 3.7 times faster after birth[26].

Maternal nutrition

The sensitivity of the fetus to *maternal nutrition* is linked to the supply of glucose to the utero-placental mass, which consumes two-thirds of the glucose and produces about 50% of the CO_2. Relative to weight, the placental glucose utilization rate is 35 times the maternal rate and 10 times the fetal glucose consumption rate[4], hence the strong influence of the size of placenta on birth weight (Figure 1.2). A decrease of fetal growth rate by 40% occurs within 3 days of severe maternal underfeeding during the last 60–70 days of pregnancy. Change in birth weight is negligible when ewes are fed again after 9–16 days of undernutrition. In contrast, refeeding after 21 days has reduced growth rate of the fetus, suggesting the occurrence of a factor limiting the utilization of substrates by the fetus[26].

Low fetal growth rate is paralleled at birth by physical weakness. Thyroid and thymus glands are particularly small, and the emergency reservoir of blood in the spleen, blood glucose, the size of the liver and hepatic energy reserves are reduced. Lower thermal insulation at birth is related to the ratio of surface area to mass, e.g. it is 0.12 m^2/kg in a 1 kg lamb, and 0.07 m^2/kg

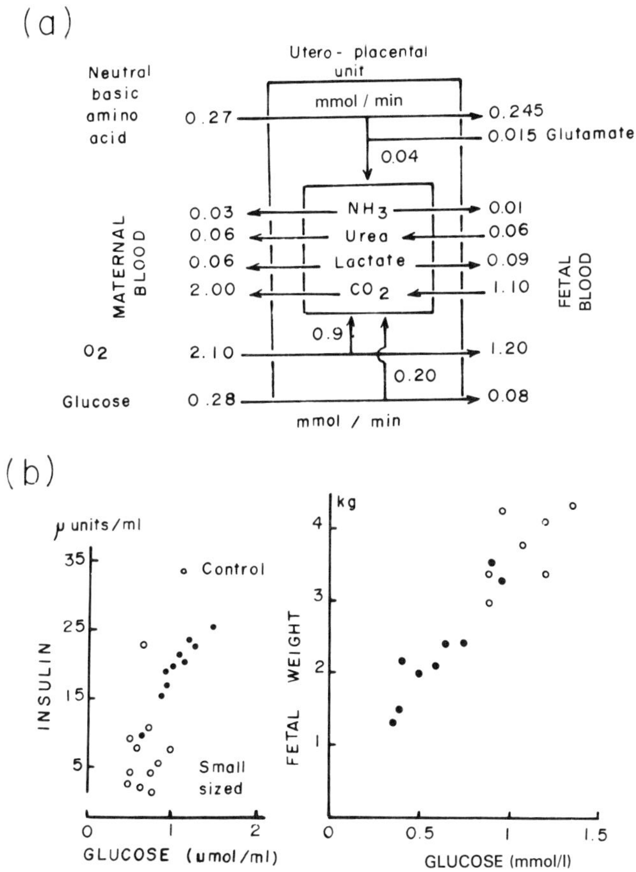

Figure 1.2 (a) Fluxes of substrates into and out of the utero-placental unit of sheep near term, in nitrogen mEq/min for amino acids, and in mmol/min for other substrates[4]. (b) Relationship between mean plasma insulin concentration and mean plasma glucose in control (•) and small size fetuses (o)[36], and between body weight at birth and glycaemia[1] in large (o) and small size fetuses(•)

in a lamb. A tendency to hypothermia is usual as the maximum metabolism approximates 20 W/kg body weight.

The quest for *hormones* involved in fetal growth strongly implicates insulin rather than pituitary hormones. The concentration of circulating hormones in small fetuses (60% of control weight) is much lower for insulin (and prolactin) than in the controls and is accompanied by hypoglycaemia[37] and poor pancreatic β cell growth[14]. It may be that the primary limitation to growth is a reduced transport of glucose to the fetus that in turn keeps the plasma insulin concentration low. A common feature of growth retardation after birth is also hypoglycaemia, suggesting a lowered postnatal glycogenolysis and a decreased capacity for gluconeogenesis.

Fetal thyroidectomy

Fetal thyroidectomy in the latter half of pregnancy affects the viability of the newborn which fails to establish normal breathing and dies soon after birth. It also retards growth, e.g. a mean body weight with 144 days gestation of 2.34 ± 0.09 kg vs. 3.5 ± 0.07 kg in the control[19,31]. As in hypothyroidism[21], long bones are shorter than in the control animals due to a lack of ossification in the epiphyseal centres. However, an earlier effect of thyroidectomy is apparent since reduction of the size has been recorded with fetal thyroidectomy between 50 and 60 days gestational age[25]. Total body length was less than 50 cm, and hydroencephaly and arthrogryposis developed in three out of 36 operated lambs.

Substantial reduction in amniotic fluid volume, pulmonary hypoplasia, microcephaly and reduction in weight rather than in size, has also been observed after bilateral nephrectomy between 105 and 125 days of gestation[47]. In addition, the transplacental gradients of ionized calcium and inorganic phosphate in favour of the fetus disappeared after nephrectomy. The endocrine changes which follow nephrectomy are similar to those described in children with chronic renal failure, with a significant elevation of (1) the placental lactogen levels in the plasma, and (2) the somatomedins and their binding proteins. These proteins may limit the movement of somatomedins across the blood–brain barrier, thereby explaining growth retardation despite high levels of somatomedin-like activity[5].

Effects of perinatal drugs

Major aspects of perinatal pharmacology linked to fetal growth and birth weight which must be stressed in ruminants are: (1) the use of antithyroid drugs which readily cross the placenta with subsequent inhibition of the thyroid–pituitary axis, and (2) the lower therapeutic and toxic thresholds of many drugs in the low birth weight neonate. Adverse effects are to be expected with all drugs involved in: carbohydrate metabolism of the feto–placental unit, blood flow to the utero–placental mass, fetal iodine uptake even at the stage which coincides with the phase of neuroblast multiplication, and renal functions (involved in calcium and phosphate homeostasis). The timing and duration of the insult may be of importance when considering the heavy nutritional demands during the last third of gestation.

FUNCTIONAL ADJUSTMENTS AT BIRTH

Functional deficits at birth and alterations in postnatal developmental behaviour (lack of vitality, weak calf syndrome) may result from many disturbances. The development of the central nervous system (CNS), the altered maturation of the lung, the effective closure of the special vascular channels of the fetus (foramen ovale, ductus venosus and ductus arteriosus), the differentiation of the gut, and the development of the thermoregulatory, inflammatory and immune systems may be impaired.

CNS development

During the last decade, to gain insight into fetal CNS development as term approaches, research has studied fetal respiratory and body movements (Figure 1.3), and the differentiation of the different states of sleep (high voltage slow activity, HVSA and low voltage fast activity, LVFA) and wakefulness (AW)[39]. The percentage of time the fetus spends near term in the HVSA state is 53% and 41.4% for the LVFA state, but no more than 5.6% in the AW state. The monosynaptic reflex induced by electric stimulation of the fibular nerve is enhanced during both LVFA and AW *in utero* as after birth[20]. Accordingly, all substances able to cross the placenta and to reach the fetus at an effective dose, such as pethidine, acepromazine, and thiopentone, disrupt the fetal sleep cycles[41] or, like 5-HTP, modify breathing movements[34].

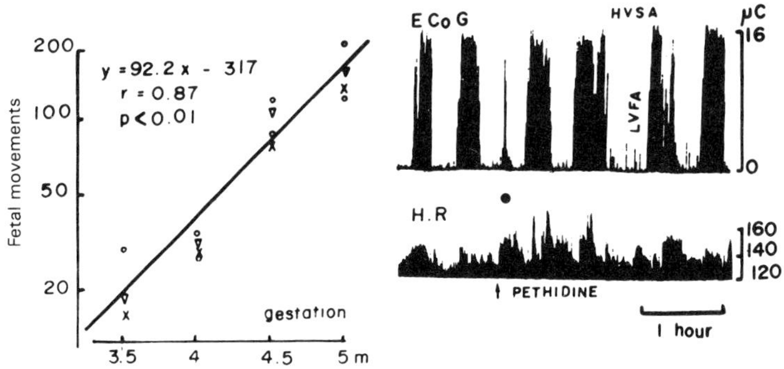

Figure 1.3 Increased kinesis expressed as the log of gross movements per day as term approaches in four fetal lambs. These movements correspond to periods of low voltage fast activity (LVFA or NREM sleep) which alternate with periods of high voltage slow activity (HVSA or REM sleep). A short-lived synchronization of the electrocorticogram (•) without changes in heart rate (HR) indicated the placental passage of pethidine (meperidine) injected intravenously to the mother at the dosage of 1 mg/kg at the time of a period of fetal LVFA[10]

The extent to which such transient pharmacological effects produce more persistent changes in a developing brain is important. Postnatal changes, including altered locomotor activity, growth retardation and susceptibility to audiogenic siezures, have been observed with the drugs listed in Table 1.1, in

Table 1.1 Alterations of postnatal development and behaviour[5]

Adrenaline	Imipramine	Pimozide
Alcohol	Iproniazid	Propoxyphene
Amphetamine	Isocarboxazid	Reserpine
Cannabinol	Meprobamate	Salicylate
Chlorpromazine	Morphine	Sex steroids
Corticosteroids	Penfluridol	Sodium bromide
Cytotoxics	Pentobarbital	Somatotrophin
Fenfluramine	Phenobarbital	Thyroxine
Haloperidol	Phenytoin	Vitamin A

relation with cortical synaptogenesis (somatotrophin, thyroxin), with DNA synthesis (corticosteroids), and with sexual differentiation of the brain (sex steroids). For salicylate and vitamin A, the nature of their interactions with the CNS to produce behavioural abnormalities is poorly understood[3]. Brain and behavioural defects due to maternal hyperthermia and maternal diabetes have also been reported[18]. Possible influences of drugs on postnatal behaviour might be overestimated, however, since low birthweight lambs are inadequately groomed, cool quickly, show delayed standing sucking times, and have a reduced chance of survival[2]. An approach could be the study of longterm effects of drugs on the fetal sleep and wakefulness states of organization.

Onset of breathing

During the final minutes of lambing, the expansion of the lungs leads to a marked fall in pulmonary vascular resistance with subsequent increase in pulmonary blood flow and functional closure of the foramen ovale. Separation of the pulmonary and systemic circulation is then obtained by closure of the ductus arteriosus (Figure 1.4). The degree of hypoxia required to initiate the first gasp is modulated by the pCO_2. Increase in arterial pO_2 initiates the closure of the ductus arteriosus, but asphyxia may lead to its re-opening. Only 4–5 min of anoxia are compatible with survival in species born in a mature state[15].

Surface active substance (surfactant) is a prerequisite to lung maturation; its deficiency leads to the respiratory distress syndrome (RDS). Cortisol stimulates the synthesis of surfactant, and adrenaline its release together with resorption of alveolar fluid[53]. The near-term fetal lamb is fully capable of manifesting a profound catecholamine response to hypoxaemia, noradrenaline being the predominant component. A decrease from 23 to 12 in fetal carotid arterial pO_2 with bradycardia and systemic arterial hypertension produced by umbilical cord constriction is accompanied by an exponential increase in catecholamine concentrations from 250 to 2000 pg/ml[22]. However, study of the response to KCN infusion suggests a postnatal maturation of the O_2 sensitive chemoreceptors in the first 10 days of life in newborn lambs[7]. The study of factors able to modify breathing *in utero* suggest that endogenous opioid peptides could participate in the physiological suppression of breathing in fetal life[30]. At birth, the presence of fluid in the upper respiratory airways inhibits ventilation (see Thermoregulatory responses).

Neonatal pharmacology can be summed up into four major points.

(1) The necessity of early oxygenotherapy. In the dog and cat, born in a relative immature state, up to 15 min may elapse between hysterotomy and delivery. In the bovine fetus only 4 min of anoxia (compression or rupture of the umbilical cord) are compatible with survival (Figure 1.5). A concomitant feature of anoxia is the release of meconium and staining of the skin[15].

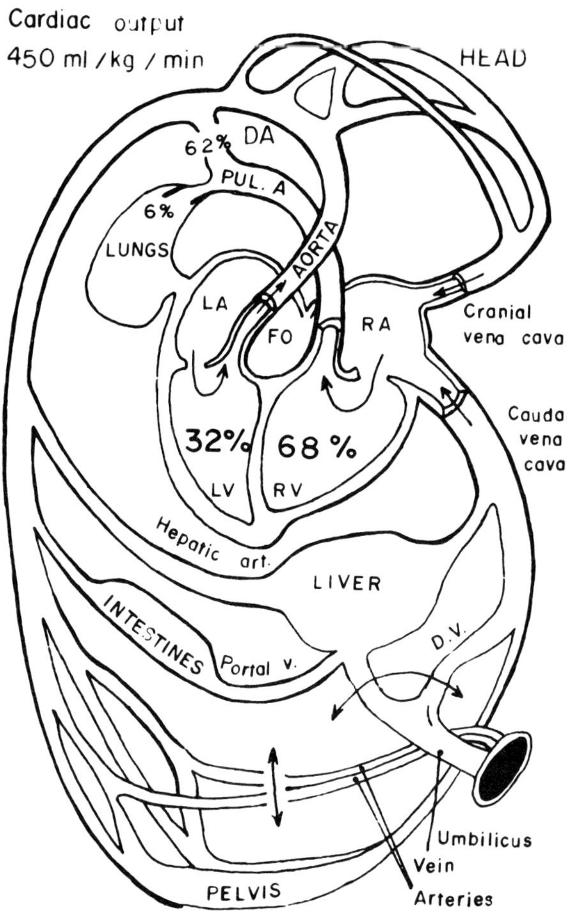

Figure 1.4 Diagram of the circulation in the fetal lamb with the channels involved in the shunt of the umbilical blood flow through the liver (ductus venosus, D.V.), in the shunt of 62% of the right ventricle output towards the descending aorta (ductus arteriosus, D.A.), and of a part (26%) of the inferior vena cava towards the left auricle (foramen ovale, F.O.)

(2) The adverse effect of pCO_2 in the re-opening of the ductus arteriosus and thus the necessity to stimulate breathing to maintain the separation of the pulmonary and systemic circulation by the so-called analeptics.

(3) The relevance of opiate antagonists in stimulating the central control of respiratory movements[8]. Naloxone invariably stimulates breathing in apnoeic fetuses and facilitates the fetal breathing response to CO_2 as expressed by a decreased CO_2 threshold and by an increased fetal sensitivity of CO_2. Since naloxone influences both threshold and sensitivity to CO_2, whereas somatic stimulation affects threshold alone, these effects of naloxone might be caused by displacement of endogenous opioids from their natural receptor sites[30].

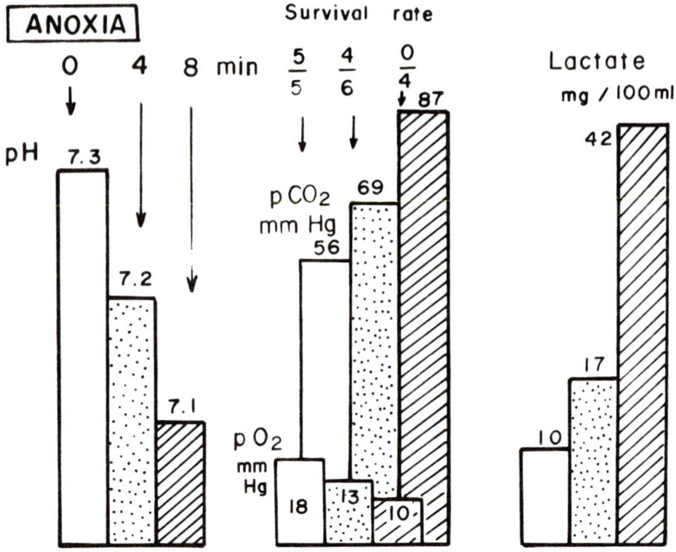

Figure 1.5 Survival rate (4/6 and 0/4) after clamping the umbilical cord during 4 and 8 min and blood gas (pO_2 and pCO_2) and lactate levels of the umbilical blood in 15 calves near term[15]

(4) The possible role for serotoninergic pathways in the maturation of the ventilatory control. *In utero*, several long periods of breathing lasting up to 14 h have occurred following an infusion of 5-HTP (30 mg/kg) when the fetus was made hypoxic for 5–15 min 2 days after the infusion (by giving the ewe a mixture of 9% O_2 and 3% CO_2 in nitrogen to breathe from a plastic bag tied over the head). The fall in fetal PO_2, which in normal fetuses would be associated with arrest of breathing, is then accompanied by pronounced stimulation[34].

Fetal and neonatal circulation

In the fetus, the work of the right ventricle, ejecting two thirds of the combined ventricular output, exceeds that of the left ventricle. The fetal body receives about half of the combined ventricular output (225 ml/kg per min), the remaining being distributed to the umbilical–placental circulation with 6% to the lungs (Figure 1.4). Following their transfer across the placenta, drugs enter the umbilical vein and must pass the liver prior to reaching the inferior vena cava or fetal right heart. Negligible hepatic drug metabolism and/or bypass from the liver via the ductus venosus may be of major significance in increasing the concentration of pharmacologically active material presented directly to the fetal heart and central nervous system. For example, a slow infusion of propranolol (1 mg/kg over 10 min) has produced peak plasma concentrations of 2 μg/ml in the ewe and 0.8 μg/ml in the fetus, but the duration of β blockade is 3 h in the pregnant ewe vs. 8–10 h in the fetus[24].

In the neonate, the low-resistance umbilical-placental circulation is altered and the cardiac output of about 450 ml/kg per min is no longer a combined ventricular output. The abrupt decrease of blood flow and blood pressure in the umbilical sinus causes the orifice of the ductus venosus to retract and narrow, resulting in functional closure of the vascular shunt. In addition, a selective effect of noradrenalin at birth is possible[52]. Permanent structural closure, consisting of connective tissue deposition within the entire lumen of the ductus, starts within days after birth and is completed by 1–3 months of age[16]. The O_2 consumption which is about 5–6 ml/min per kg for a blood flow to the body of about 225 ml/kg per min in the fetus rises to 16–18 ml/min per kg, the blood flow becoming nearly twice that before birth (figure 1.6). The percentage of fetal haemoglobin which is 80% in the immediate postnatal period drops to 40% by 3 weeks and it is almost completely replaced by adult haemoglobin by about 8 weeks after birth. The effect of this change is to shift the O_2 equilibration curve of the blood towards the right (Figure 1.6), hence a higher quantity of O_2 can be delivered to the tissues for O_2 tension between 5.3 and 13.3 kPa[34]. The blood volume is strongly correlated with body weight: 116 ml/kg in the feto-placental unit (50 ml/kg for [^{51}Cr]red cell) and 81 ml/kg (30 ml/kg for red cell) in the newborn[33]. In the latter a high resting cardiac output results in a decreased reserve response to volume loading and in the tolerance of a left to right shunt of small magnitude. A frequent phenomenon which accompanies low birth weight seems to be anaemia[17]. While the neonate responds like the adult with tachycardia and increased cardiac output to hypoxia, the fetal lamb develops bradycardia with a fall in the combined ventricular output corresponding to a redistribution of the circulation (umbilical-placental blood flow is maintained, but blood flow to the fetal body is reduced). A reduction of total cardiac output associated with bradycardia is also recorded in acute fetal haemorrhage and in severe maternal stress. In these cases, both placental and body blood flows are reduced. Such fetal cardiac responses have occurred near term despite fully developed plasma catecholamine responses[22]. Recently, the reactivity to autonomic agonists after chemical sympathectomy using 6-hydroxydopamine (1 ml/kg followed 12 h later by a weekly dose of 20 ml/kg) has shown a minor role for the α adrenergic system to maintain the resting tone of peripheral circulation in the fetus and neonate: the supersensitivity of fetal circulation to acetylcholine and isoproterenol is secondary to changes in the pulmonary vascular bed[46]. In the emergency state of hypoxia the role of the α-adrenergic system becomes predominant[36].

At least three of the therapeutic considerations in relation to perinatal cardiovascular adjustments deserve attention:

(1) The fetal ductus seems to be kept patent by a relaxant prostaglandin, probably PGE[44]. The persistence of a left to right shunt after birth may be reduced by prostaglandin synthetase blockade by indomethacin (1.9–2.5 mg/kg).

(2) The haemolysis and anaemia in low birthweight lamb are possibly related to erythrocyte membrane or enzyme defects. In this case, no rise in 2,3-diphosphoglycerate blood level occurs within 10 days after

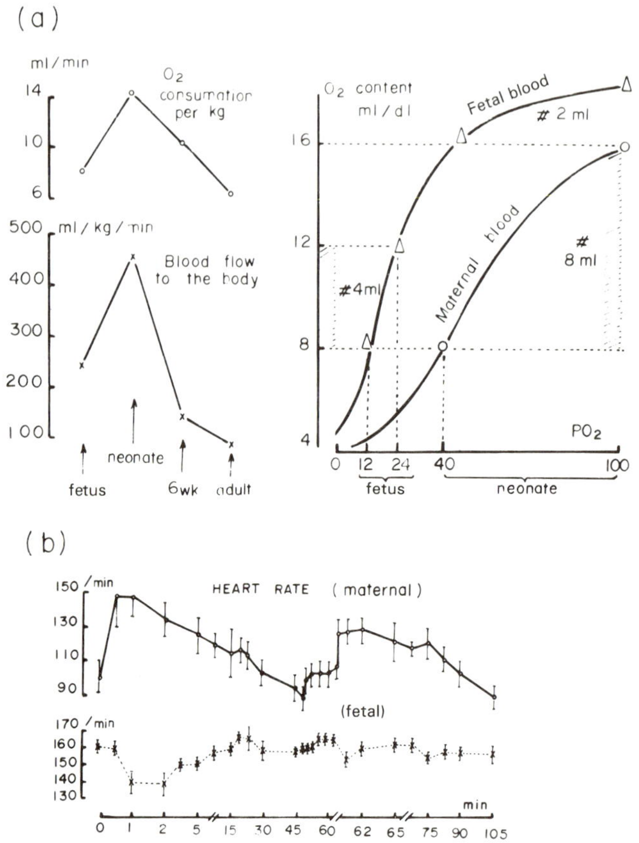

Figure 1.6 (a) At birth, the cardiac output rises to about 480 ml/min per kg of body weight during the first week after birth and the O_2 consumption increases from 6 ml to 14 ml/min per kg. The cardiac output in relation to body weight falls to levels of 320 and 160 ml/min per kg by 3 and 6 weeks, after birth[41]. Oxygen equilibration curves for fetal and maternal blood show that the delivery is only 4 ml/dl of O_2 when the pO_2 decreases from 24 to 12 in the fetus (•) and 8 ml/dl of O_2 when the pO_2 decreases from 100 to 40 in the neonate (○). For similar pO_2 levels, blood with fetal haemoglobin would provide only one fourth the amount of O_2 (▲). (b) Fetal bradycardia in response to maternal stress induced by painful stimuli (application of rubber-covered clamp to the ewe's ear lobe for 15 min) and its suppression following the intravenous administration of 0.2 ml/kg of diazepam to the ewe[29]

birth[32]. The therapeutic usefulness of α-tocopherol requires further investigations.

(3) The transient decrease in fetal heart and oxygenation occurs in response to a major reduction in uterine blood flow during maternal stress. Substances other than autonomic antagonists seem to be indicated. Among the sedatives, diazepam has been found to be able to prevent both maternal tachycardia and fetal bradycardia following severe stressful conditions[29] (Figure 1.6).

Digestion and absorption during development

In the fetal lamb, stimulation of the perioral region at 0.8 of term is accompanied by gastric filling, a phenomenon which seems to correspond to daily swallowing of 60–400 ml of amniotic fluid and full development of the bovine intestinal mucosa. No motor activity of the small bowel is detected before 40 and 90 days of fetal life in dogs and sheep, respectively, thus

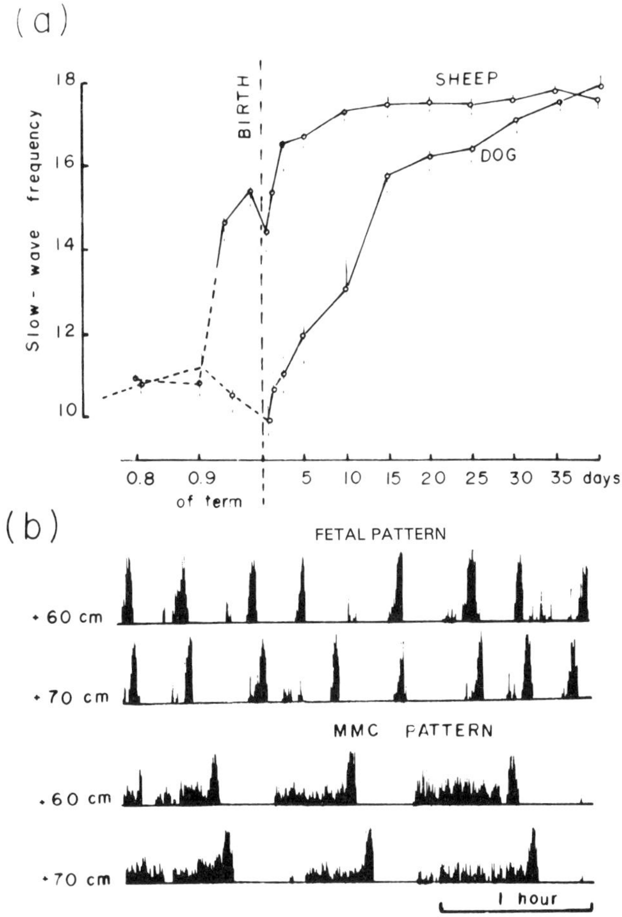

Figure 1.7 (a) Ontogenesis of the slow wave activity of the proximal jejunum in fetal and newborn dogs and sheep. Broken lines indicate intermittent presence of slow waves. They were always present (solid lines) by 0.9 of term in the fetal lamb. In the dog, slow-wave frequency remained low and their presence intermittent until birth[6]. (b) Fetal and MMC (adult) patterns of spiking activity. Unorganized spiking activity was converted in the fetal lamb at 0.8 of term to a fetal pattern characterized by cyclic 3–4 min periods of regular spiking occurring at 10–20 min intervals and propagated along a short intestinal segment. The MMC pattern which corresponds to myoelectric complexes, occurred during the last 10 days of fetal life. In dogs, the fetal pattern was recorded from 5 days before to 15 days after birth.

suggesting that movement of contents prior to these times, if any, must depend on a pressure gradient rather than on intestinal motility. In both dogs and sheep, a progressive increase in the incidence of slow waves is recorded before the increased duration of spiking activity[40]. A striking feature is that birth is not accompanied by acute changes in the motor profile because the fetal pattern persists 10–15 days after birth in the dog, whereas in sheep typical MMCs were detected from 5 to 10 days prior to birth[6]. The patterns seen in the last third of fetal life are seemingly related to the functions of mixing and absorption but not expulsion of the intestinal contents (Figure 1.7).

The passage of meconium-stained amniotic fluid during parturition is a sign of potential fetal distress. Meconium-stained fluid noted at the time of rupture of the fetal membranes and thick meconium passed at this time suggest fetal asphyxia, hence the effects of low pO_2 on the propulsion of digestive contents.

Major changes in intestinal absorption occur at birth in ungulates since they are part of a unique group of mammals which deliver young that are agammaglobulinaemic; thus the newborn is dependent upon colostrum, not only for nutrients, but also for antibodies[28]. Changes in gut growth, motility and gut enzyme activities, together with dramatic adjustments in intermediary metabolism, may be induced by intermittent enteral feeding. Small quantities of food in the gut seem to be the trigger for the gut hormonal surges of motilin, neurotensin and GIP. Phasic changes in enteroglucagon, gastrin and secretin also occur following feeding, but progressively decrease with postnatal age. Among the factors affecting the duration of the transfer of intact proteins, a possible shortening factor might be cortisone whereas starvation prolongs the period of protein absorption[43].

Since depriving non-sucking neonates from colostrum could have permanent consequences in terms of lack of trophic hormonal stimulation of the gut mucosa, the recommended administration of small quantities of colostrum to improve their resistance to infectious diseases might also have special significance for adaptation to extra-uterine nutrition[11].

A final consideration is the ingestion of milk containing drugs, most often antimicrobial, by nursing offspring. Although ruminants have considerable excretory competence, fetal intoxication can occur in the absence of signs by the mother.

Thermoregulatory responses

The neonatal lamb is equipped with adequate defense mechanisms against decreasing body temperature to the cold ambient air below thermal neutrality when released from immersion. The O_2 consumption increases almost threefold during the first 24 h after birth. A rise in the general level of sympathetic activity in arterial pO_2 and in blood flow and in tone of skeletal muscles may contribute to this phenomenon. The principal metabolic fuel, i.e. carbohydrate from the liver (20%) and skeletal muscles, changes progressively to free fatty acids. The reserves of fat at birth are relatively small and in the sheep the rate of transfer of long-chain free fatty acids across the syndesmochorial placenta is very low. However, on the basis of the triglyceride contents of milk (6.2%), it can be calculated that about 2.1 g of linoleic acid is secreted daily by the ewe and that, in one day of postnatal life, the sucking lamb ingests more essential fatty acids than it accumulates during the whole of fetal development.

The state of total immersion of the fetus in its warm amniotic fluid environment strongly inhibits its respiration[13]. The respiratory ability of a tracheotomized lamb, subjected to cord occlusion and immersed, was compromised so severely that survival did not occur. The role of a cool vs. warm environment is demonstrated by the production of greater ventilatory depression by immersion in a warm water bath (Figure 1.8). Similar ventilatory depression is observed when water is introduced retrogradely into the trachea and nasopharynx.

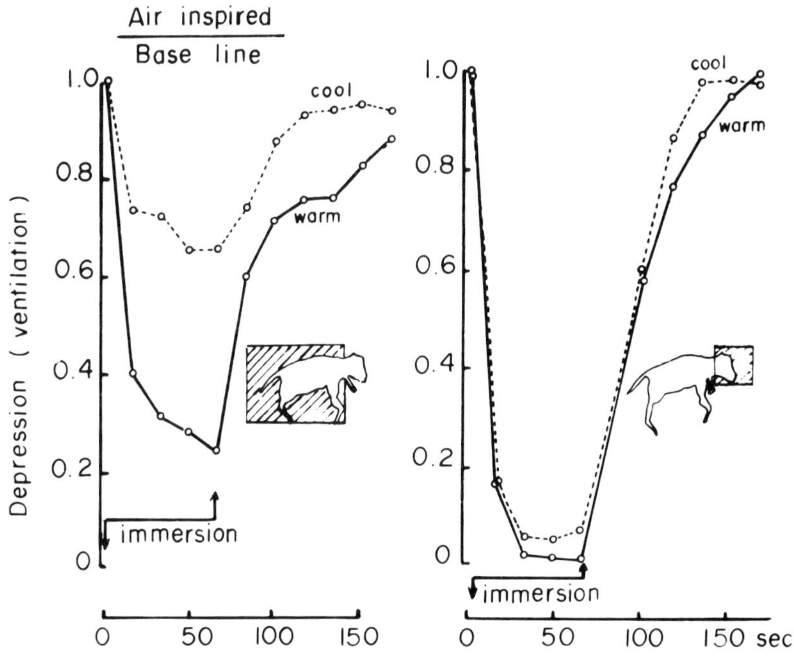

Figure 1.8 Effect of immersion of a lamb 10 min after delivered by hysterotomy and with a baseline minute volume of 2020 ml in either warm (39–40 °C) or cool (23–24 °C) water decreased the ratio of air inspired to the baseline with a more rapid recovery from the respiratory depression when emerging from cool water. The immersion of the head alone shows more marked depression

The implications of such observations are that:

(1) The maintenance of adequate respiration at birth outweighs any advantage of conservation of heat.
(2) Endotracheal intubation in respiratory distress is less important than the removal of fluid in the upper respiratory passages.

Ontology of inflammatory and immune responses

The importance of inflammation as a fetal defense mechanism is largely unknown. Inflammatory processes in the ruminant fetus occur in a variety of infectious diseases, and the responses of a fetus to a particular agent differ from the responses of the adult. In most instances, the fetal response involves primarily monocytes and macrophages, while the adult response is predominantly a polymorphonuclear leukocyte reaction. Neutrophils and monocytes are observed in peripheral blood as early as 58–60 days of gestation, but constitute only 3–8% of the total white blood cell count until 135 days of gestation. Two weeks before birth, neutrophil numbers increase dramatically, but these cells lack lysosomal esterase and lipase enzyme activity until shortly before birth. The earliest fetal responses have been to bacteriophage at 41 days, ferritin at day 46, chicken erythrocytes at 58 days, and graft rejection at 76 days. The factors influencing the immune responses are to be considered during pregnancy and postmortem.

(1) A variety of factors operating during pregnancy and in the immediate perinatal period may influence the immune capabilities of the conceptus. They include maternal-fetal hormones and passive transfer of immunity to the newborn. An important role of oestrogen in the maternal system is to facilitate the selective transport of IgG and complement into colostral secretions. The lymphopenia, due to elevated corticosteroids at birth, could contribute to the extreme susceptibility of the newborn to infectious agents.

(2) The mammary gland is part of the local immune system since, among the important immunological ingredients in colostrum for the newborn, large quantities of IgG_1 are selectively transported into colostrum. The other immunoglobulins IgM_2, IgA, IgG_2 are in the same relative quantities as found in serum. Successful transfer of colostrum to the newborn and its subsequent absorption seem to involve a variety of factors[11]. Organ weight/bodyweight ratios of all lymphoid organs except the thymus are highest in the fetus or young animals after which they decrease (somewhat irregularly) with age[23].

Modulation of immunity is accomplished by a wide variety of substances including microbial, biological, and pharmacological agents – roughly divided into immunosuppressants and immunostimulants. For example, levamisole, which enhances the protective effect of vaccines against virulent species of *Brucella*, seems to have an effect similar to the thymic hormones used to restore immune responsiveness. Of importance is that glucocorticoids fail to inhibit the absorption of colostral antibody from the gut, except in the case of too young a gestational age at the time of parturition[38].

THE PREGNANT EWE MODEL

Criteria that should be used in evaluating the pharmacological effect and relative safety of a drug for a fetus are the amount of fetal uptake after an intravenous bolus, and the ratio of the steady state drug concentration in the fetus to that in the mother.

Fetal drug elimination

In the chronic pregnant ewe model, the fetal urine is excreted into the amniotic sac via the urethra, and into the allantoic sac via the urachus. Thus indirect evidence for renal clearance of drugs can be obtained by the presence of drug in these fluids or by cannulation of the bladder of the fetal lamb (Figure 1.9). For example, pethidine is detectable in allantoic fluid as early as 3 min after its administration and is not found in amniotic fluid until 30 min after injection. A final route of drug elimination from the fetal compartment is diffusion across the chorio-allantoic membrane[45].

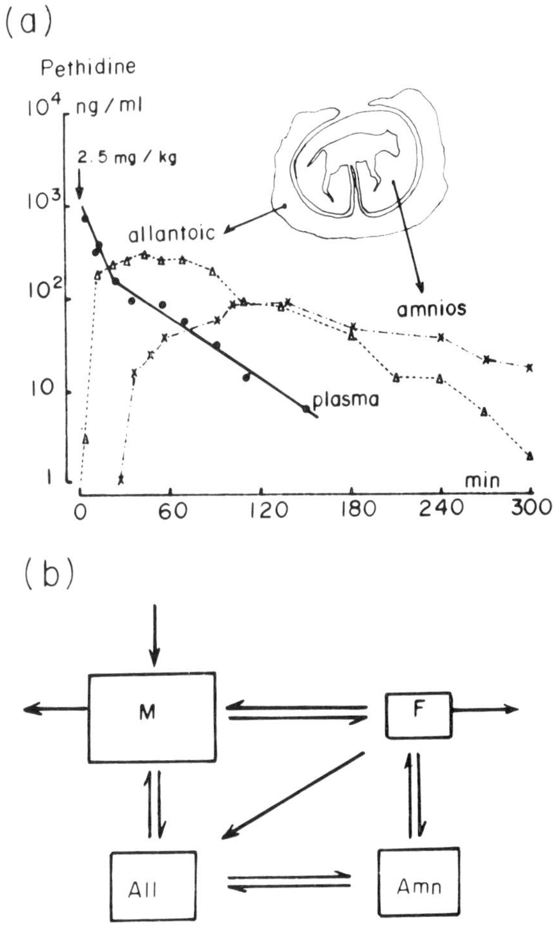

Figure 1.9 (a) Semi-logarithmic plot of data obtained in a pregnant ewe with fetal bladder catheterization following intravenous injection of pethidine (meperidine) (2.5 mg/kg). (b) The cumulative urinary excretion of pethidine by the fetus supports a pharmacokinetic model where the disposition of pethidine can be described by a four-compartment open model with elimination from both maternal and fetal compartments after exchange between the amniotic and allantoic fluid[45]

Maternal-fetal drug distribution

The rate of distribution of a drug to fetal tissues may not be uniform, hence the pharmacokinetic necessity of a fetal peripheral compartment[49]. For example, there is little correlation between the incidence of neonatal respiratory depression and the concentration of pethidine in fetal blood. The time-course of pethidine concentration in the brain, as estimated by measuring the arterio-venous concentration difference across the fetal brain, indicates, in the chronic pregnant ewe model, a time lag between peak plasma and peak brain concentration. In addition, the brain peak concentration was 3–4 times greater after i.v. than i.m. administration and occurred within 60 min for i.v. instead of 25 min for i.m.[44].

The distribution of drugs between ewe and fetus at steady state always shows a fetal/maternal concentration ratio of less than one (Table 1.2). Drug

Table 1.2 Ratio of fetal drug concentration to maternal concentration[3]

Negligible binding in both fetus and mother
Morphine = 0.13
Antipyrine = 0.90
Lesser binding in the fetus
Methadone = 0.15 (90 day)
Meperidine = 0.30
Similar binding in both fetus and mother
Methadone = 0.18 (near term)
Acetylsalicylic acid = 0.22
Dexamethasone = 0.67
Indomethacin = 0.28
Lidocaine = 0.76

binding in plasma is usually less in the fetus than in the mother, and cannot account for the concentration gradient. Both fetal and placental drug clearance are involved. The steady state compartmental method which requires maternal and fetal isotope labelled drug infusions shows that the blood clearance rate of aldosterone was 98 l/h or 41 ml/kg per min in the pregnant ewe and 24 l/h in the fetus. A small percentage (4%) of the maternal production rate of aldosterone is due to the fetus and 29% of the fetal production rate is assumed by the maternal compartment. The liver blood flow (46 ml/kg per min) seems the main determinant of the clearance in the sheep and also in the fetus for which the liver blood flow is approximately 124 ml/min per kg[51].

Fetal responses to autonomic drugs

The pregnant ewe model has been one of the earliest used to demonstrate the small and transient blood pressure responses of the fetus to autonomic agents compared to that of the mother[48]. Intravenous administration of progressively increasing doses of noradrenaline has produced a rise in the arterial pressure and a fall in the heart rate in the fetus, neonate, and adult. The bradycardia is most likely related to baroreceptor stimulation produced by the rise in pressure. The changes produced by a given dose are significantly greater in the adult and neonate than in the fetus. Taking the effect of 0.4 μg/kg as an example, the average pressure rise is 25% in the fetus, 37% in the neonate and 50% in the adult (Figure 1.10).

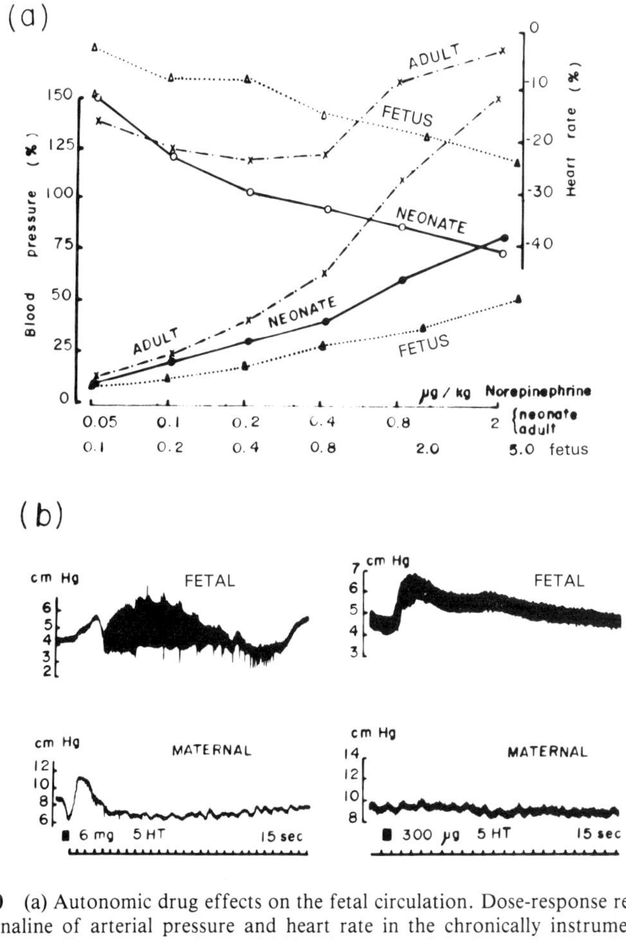

Figure 1.10 (a) Autonomic drug effects on the fetal circulation. Dose-response relationships to noradrenaline of arterial pressure and heart rate in the chronically instrumented fetus, neonate and adult[46]. (b) Changes in arterial blood pressure of the fetus after the administration of serotonin (100 μg/kg) in the mother and in the fetus. Note the more sustained responsiveness of the fetus to the maternal administration of serotonin. Preparation under chloralose anaesthesia[48]

The pregnant ewe model has been also used to detect the amount of autonomic agents which reach the fetal circulatory system. For example, similar fetal hypotension and bradycardia follow the maternal blood pressure changes after the injection of 10 μg/kg of adrenaline and of 5 μg/kg of acetylcholine (after injection of physostigmine, 100 μg/kg) in the ewe. Of interest is the comparison of the changes in fetal arterial pressure which are more marked after the maternal administration of 100 μg/kg of serotonin than after the same dosage to the fetus (Figure 1.10). In addition, the model could be useful in detecting the role played by some systems in emergency situations. For example, hypoxaemia causes a redistribution of cardiac output with an increase in blood flow to some organs (brain, heart, adrenal glands), no change in blood flow to the placenta, and a decrease in blood flow to organs like lungs, kidney, spleen, gut, and somatic muscles. This redistribution is by an increase in the vascular resistances of some organs and a decrease in others; the net effect is to augment systemic arterial blood pressure. The effect of α adrenergic blockade, minimal during normal oxygenation, allows increases in blood flow to the brain, the heart and placenta to occur without a change in cardiac output. Blocking with phenoxybenzamine during hypoxia decreased the calculated vascular resistances of the gut, spleen, liver, and lungs, demonstrating that α-adrenergic activity was necessary to maintain vasoconstriction and shift blood flow away from these organs[36].

Finally, the pregnant ewe model has furnished the most complete information on specific drugs

(1) For the study of an appropriate route of administration,
(2) For the selection and design of safer and more effective dosage regimens during pregnancy, and
(3) For the evidence of hormonal factors involved in their activity[12,37,47].

CONCLUSION

Pregnancy is a dynamic process with rapid growth of a fetal compartment. If a pregnant subject, be it animal or man, is exposed to pharmacologically active chemicals, one can assume that the compounds will also reach the conceptus. However, the rate and the extent of both transfer and pharmacological toxic effects vary depending upon the gestational period.

Birth brings about dramatic physiological changes in the internal environment which can be modified by pharmacologically active chemicals.

The relevant questions that arise concern the nature of the effects of drugs on the increasing metabolic needs of the rapidly growing fetus and the homeostatic mechanisms which began to operate at birth. Clinicians should be provided with enough data to permit rational use of innocuous drugs in both pregnant and newborn animals. A more positive approach is that of therapeutical intervention in late pregnancy to prevent impairment of immune and other regulatory systems at birth. This includes exposure of the neonate to drugs transferred through the placenta and the mammary gland during the perinatal period.

References

1. Alexander, G. (1964). Studies on the placenta of the sheep (*Ovis aries L.*). Placental size. *J. Reprod. Fertil.*, **7**, 289–305; Effect of reduction in the number of caruncles. *Ibid.*, 307–22

2. Bareham, J. R. (1976). The behaviour of lambs on the first day after birth. *Br. Vet. J.*, **132**, 152–62
3. Barlow, S. M. (1982). Drugs in pregnancy. *Trends Pharm. Sci.*, **3**, 251–6
4. Battaglia, F. C. and Meschia, G. (1981). Foetal and placental metabolisms: their interrelationship and impact upon maternal metabolism. *Proc. Nutr. Soc.*, **40**, 99–113
5. Brinsmead, M. W., Waters, M. J. and Thorburn, G. D. (1980). Increase in placental lactogen and somatomedins after fetal nephrectomy. *J. Dev. Physiol.*, **2**, 205–18
6. Bueno, L. and Ruckebusch, Y. (1979). Perinatal development of intestinal myoelectrical activity in dogs and sheep. *Am. J. Physiol.*, **237**, E61–7
7. Bureau, M. A. and Begin, R. (1982). Postnatal maturation of the respiratory response to O_2 in awake newborn lambs. *J. Appl. Physiol.*, **52**, 428–33
8. Chernick, V. and Craig, R. J. (1982). Naloxone reverses neonatal depression caused by fetal asphyxia. *Science*, **216**, 1252–4
9. Creasy, R. K., Barrett, C. T., De Swift, M. *et al.* (1972). Experimental intrauterine growth retardations in the sheep. *Am. J. Obstet. Gynecol.*, **112**, 566–73
10. Dancis, J. and Hwang, J. C. (1974). *Perinatal Pharmacology: Problems and Priorities*. p. 128. (New York: Raven Press)
11. Dardillat, C. (1982). Comment obtenir des veaux résistants. *Bull. Techn. C.R.Z.V. Theix, I.N.R.A.*, **47**, 37–45
12. Davicco, M. J., Lefaivre, J. and Bartlet, J. P. (1982). Plasma iodothyronine levels in lambs during the perinatal period: influence of thyrotropin injection. *Reprod. Nutr. Dev.*, **22**, 557–68
13. Dawes, G. S. and Bost, J. (1977). Homéostasie périnatale du milieu intérieur. Symposium on The Maintenance of the Internal Environment in the Foetus and Newborn in Domestic Animals, Lyon. *Ann. Rech. Vét.*, **8**, 343–501
14. De Prins, F. A. and Van Assche, A. (1982). Intra-uterine growth retardation and development of endocrine pancreas in the experimental rat. *Biol. Neonate*, **41**, 16–21
15. Dufty, J. H. and Sloss, V. (1977). Anoxia in the bovine foetus. *Aust. Vet. J.*, **53**, 262–7
16. Edelstone, D. I. (1980). Regulation of blood flow through the ductus venosus. *J. Dev. Physiol.*, **2**, 219–38
17. Fisher, E. W. (1980). Neonatal survival. *Br. Vet. J.*, **136**, 585–89
18. Hetzel, B. S. and Smith, R. M. (1981). *Fetal Brain Disorders*. (Amsterdam: Elsevier Biomedical Press)
19. Hopkins, P. S. and Thorburn, G. D. (1972). The effects of fetal thyroidectomy on the development of the ovine fetus. *J. Endocrinol.*, **54**, 55–66
20. Ioffe, S., Jansen, A. H., Russell, B. J. *et al.* (1980). Sleep, wakefulness and the monosynaptic reflex in fetal and newborn lambs. *Pflügers Arch.*, **388**, 149–57
21. Lascelles, A. K. and Setchell, B. P. (1959). Hypothyroidism in sheep. *Aust. J. Biol.*, **12**, 445–65
22. Lewis, A. B., Evans, W. N. and Sischo, W. (1982). Plasma catecholamine responses to hypoxemia in fetal lambs. *Biol. Neonate*, **41**, 115–22
23. Lubis, I., Ladds, P. W. and Reilly, L. R. (1982). Age associated morphological changes in the lymphoid system of tropical cattle. *Res. Vet. Sci.*, **32**, 270–7
24. Marshall, A. W., Mihaly, G. W., Smallwood, R. A. *et al.* (1981). Foetal hepatic function: the disposition of propranolol in the pregnant sheep. *Res. Commun. Chem. Pathol. Pharmacol.*, **32**, 3–26
25. McIntosh, G. H. (1978). Foetal thyroidectomy and hydranencephaly in lambs. *Aust. Vet. J.*, **54**, 408–9
26. Mellor, D. J. and Murray, L. (1982). Effects on the rate of increase in fetal girth of refeeding ewes after short periods of severe nutrition during late pregnancy. *Res. Vet. Sci.*, **32**, 377–82
27. Mirkin, B. L. (1976). *Perinatal Pharmacology and Therapeutics*. (New York: Academic Press).
28. Molla, A. (1978). Immunoglobulin levels in calves fed colostrum by stomach tube. *Vet. Rec.*, **103**, 377–80
29. Morishima, H. O., Sakuma, K., Bruce, S. L. *et al.* (1980). The effect of diazepam on maternal and fetal stress responses in the sheep. *Dev. Pharmacol. Ther.*, **1**, 364–71
30. Moss, I. R. and Scarpelli, E. M. (1979). Generation and regulation of breathing *in utero*: fetal CO_2 response test. *J. Appl. Physiol.*, **47**, 527–31

31. Nathanielsz, P. W., Silver, M. and Comline, R. S. (1973). Plasma triiodothyronine concentration in the foetal and newborn lamb. *J. Endocrinol.*, **58,** 683–4
32. Noble, N. A., Cabalum, T. C., Nathanielsz, P. W. *et al.* (1982). Erythrocyte enzymes in sheep: comparison of activity in fetal, newborn, maternal and nonpregnant ewe erythrocytes. *Biol. Neonate*, **41,** 161–71
33. Pipkin, B. and Kirkpatrick, S. M. L. (1973). The blood volumes of fetal and newborn sheep. *Q. J. Exp. Physiol.*, **58,** 181–8
34. Quilligan, E. J., Clewlow, F., Johnston, B. M. *et al.* (1981). Effect of 5-hydroxytryptophan on electrocortical activity and breathing movements of fetal sheep. *Am. J. Obstet. Gynecol.*, **141,** 271–5
35. Randall, G. C. B. (1978). Perinatal mortality: some problems of adaptation at birth. *Adv. Vet. Sci. Comp. Med.*, **22,** 53–81
36. Reuss, L., Parer, J. T., Harris, J. L. *et al.* (1982). Hemodynamic effects of adrenergic blockade during hypoxia in fetal sheep. *Am. J. Obstet. Gynecol.*, **142,** 410–15
37. Robinson, J. S., Hart, I. P., Kingston, E. J. *et al.* (1980). Studies on the growth of the foetal sheep. The effect of reduction of placental size on hormone concentration in foetal lambs. *J. Dev. Physiol.*, **2,** 239–48
38. Roth, J. A. and Kaeberle, M. L. (1982). Effect of glucocorticoids on the bovine immune system. *J. Am. Vet. Med. Assoc.*, **180,** 894–901
39. Ruckebusch, Y. (1972). Development of sleep and wakefulness in the foetal lamb. *Electroenceph. Clin. Neurophysiol.*, **32,** 119–25
40. Ruckebusch, Y. and Grivel, M. L. (1974). A technique for long-term studies of the electrical activity of the gut in the foetus and neonate. In Daniel, E. *et al.* (eds.) *Proceedings of the 4th International Symposium on Gastrointestinal Motility, Banff*, pp. 428–34. (Vancouver: Mitchell Press)
41. Ruckebusch, Y., Gaujoux, M. and Eghbali, B. (1976). Placental transfer of CNS depressants in sheep. *Eur. J. Pharmacol.*, **37,** 193–6
42. Rudolph, A. M. and Heymann, M. A. (1979). Developmental considerations in cardiac failure. *Les Colloques de l'INSERM*, **89,** 235–44
43. Scott, G. H., Marx, D. B., Menefee, B. E. *et al.* (1979). Colostral immunoglobulin transfer in calves. I. Period of absorption. *J. Dairy Sci.*, **62,** 1632–8
44. Starling, M. B., Neutze, J. M. and Elliott, R. B. (1978). Effect of prostaglandins and some methyl derivatives on the ductus arteriosus. In Coceani, F. and Olley, P. M. (eds.) *Prostaglandins and Perinatal Medicine. Advances in Prostaglandin and Thromboxane Research.* Vol. IV, pp. 335–43. (New York: Raven Press)
45. Szeto, H. H. (1982). Pharmacokinetics in the ovine maternal-fetal unit. *Ann. Rev. Pharmacol. Toxicol.*, **22,** 221–43
46. Tabsch, K., Nuwayhid, B., Murad, S. *et al.* (1982). Circulatory effects of chemical sympathectomy in fetal, neonatal and adult sheep. *Am. J. Physiol.*, **243,** 113–32
47. Thorburn, G. D. (1974). The role of the thyroid gland and kidneys in fetal growth. In *Size at Birth, Ciba Foundation Symposium 27.* pp. 185–200. (North Holland: Elsevier Excerpta Medica)
48. Vauthier, G. (1964). Etude expérimentale du passage de quelques substances à effet pharmacodynamique de la mère au foetus. *Thèse Doct. Vét.*, Paris
49. Welsch, F. (1972). Placental transfer and fetal uptake of drugs. *J. Vet. Pharmacol. Ther.*, **5,** 91–104
50. Wigglesworth, J. S. (1964). Experimental growth retardation in the foetal rat. *J. Pathol. Bact.*, **88,** 1–13
51. Wintour, E. M., Coghlan, J. P., Hardy, K. J. *et al.* (1980). Placental transfer of aldosterone in the sheep. *J. Endocrinol.*, **86,** 305–10
52. Zink, J. and Van Petten, G. R. (1980). The effect of norepinephrine on blood flow through the fetal liver and ductus venosus. *Am. J. Obstet. Gynecol.*, **137,** 71–7
53. Zachman, R. D. and Farrell, P. M. (1982). Use of prenatal corticosteroids. In Farrell, P. M. (ed.) *Lung Development*. Vol. II, pp. 297–302. (New York: Academic Press)

2
Placental transfer of drugs in ruminant animals

L. E. Davis and G. D. Koritz

The exchange of drugs and other xenobiotics between the maternal circulation and the conceptus is of clinical significance because of possible adverse effects of these chemical on development and function of the fetus *in utero*. Following fertilization, the gestational period can be divided into three unequal segments of differing pharmacological significance: (1) the period from fertilization to implantation of the blastocyst, (2) implantation to the end of metamorphosis, and (3) period of growth. These periods comprise the following respective proportions of the gestation period: 12%, 4% and 84% in the cow; 10%, 11% and 79% in the doe and ewe. The transfer of drugs and the potential consequences of exposure of the conceptus will differ depending on the stage of pregnancy in which administration takes place. Exposure of the blastocyst to toxic materials prior to implantation will cause death of the conceptus and termination of pregnancy. After implantation, the embryo develops and organogenesis takes place. It is during this time that the embryo is most vulnerable to teratogenic effects. After metamorphosis has been completed the fetus grows in size and the fetal organs become functional. In the latter three-quarters of pregnancy, drugs entering the fetal circulation may exert effects on maturation of the nervous system, withdrawal of the umbilical hernia and a few other aspects of organ development. The primary effects, however, are as pharmacological agents acting on placental or fetal functions. The purpose of this chapter is to discuss the processes by which xenobiotics enter the female genital tract and fetus.

PREIMPLANTATION

The ovum is fertilized in the segment of the oviduct nearest the ovary and proceeds to divide as it passes, floating in intraductal fluid, through the duct toward the uterus. This sojourn lasts for 4 days. During this time drugs can diffuse from capillaries in the wall of the oviduct into the intraductal fluid.

This fluid has a pH higher than that of blood plasma[25]. Acidic drugs attain higher concentrations and basic drugs lower concentrations in this fluid than in plasma due to ion trapping[16]. Highly polar compounds and drugs which are highly bound to serum albumin would be excluded by the epithelium and endometrium. Caffeine, nicotine, thiopental, DDT and isoniazid attained concentrations in the luminal fluid which were 50% greater than their concentrations in blood plasma of pregnant rabbits[30]. Al-Guedawy *et al.*[4] were able to measure concentrations of gentamicin in the lumen of the bovine uterus within 15–30 min following intramuscular injection (4 mg/kg) of the drug. We observed that oxytetracycline administered intravenously attained concentrations in the wall of the uterus of the cow which were equivalent to plasma concentrations[15]. Drugs present in luminal fluids can diffuse into the developing zygote or blastocyst during migration and early implantation. This corresponds with the period of time during which much of embryonic development takes place in ruminant animals. In the cow, implantation occurs at 35 days post-oestrus while the end of the embryonic period is 30 days and the end of metamorphosis is 45 days; while the corresponding times for the ewe and doe are 15, 21 and 32 days, respectively[17]. The uptake of drugs by the blastocyst has been studied[21]. Caffeine, nicotine, DDT, barbital, thiopental, isoniazid, antipyrine, sulphanilamide, thalidomide and salicylate were taken up rapidly by rabbits' blastocysts. Compounds which exceeded 60 000 molecular weight did not penetrate the blastocyst. Rates of penetration of the blastocyst were a function of the lipid solubility of the drugs.

PLACENTAL TRANSFER

On about the 35th day of pregnancy in the cow and 15th day in the ewe and doe, the trophoblast attaches to the maternal caruncles and placentomes are formed[22]. There are 30–80 cotyledons forming attachments to the caruncles of ruminant animals. The placentation of ruminant animals is of the syndesmochorial type which means that there are five tissue layers separating the maternal and fetal blood. These are the maternal endothelium and connective tissue and the fetal trophoblast, connective tissue, and endothelium[6]. The maternal and fetal capillaries are intermingled in the placentomes in close apposition[31] which permits exchange of gases, nutrients, hormones, waste products and xenobiotics.

The placentomes are continually changing during pregnancy and reach their maximum weight halfway through gestation (Table 2.1). During the latter half of pregnancy they decline in weight up to term[8]. These morphological changes are accompanied by increasing permeability of the membranes separating the maternal and fetal circulations. This apparently is associated with a decrease in thickness of the trophoblastic epithelium with aging of the placenta[26]. The placentomes are complex structures which serve as endocrine organs and as a means of protecting the internal milieu of the growing fetus. By maintaining a differential permeability to salts and nutrients the placenta maintains osmotic equilibrium. This is accompanied by a potential gradient of 30 mV across the placentome (the fetal circulation

Table 2.1 Changes in weights of the fetus, cotyledons and membranes during the last half of pregnancy in sheep (mean ± SE). From reference 18

Gestation age (days)	*Number*	*Fetus* (kg)	*Cotyledons* (g)	*Membranes* (g)
86–98	21	0.65	562 ± 25	125 ± 7
110–127	23	2.29	409 ± 23	167 ± 13
130–143	30	3.54	402 ± 9	224 ± 11

is negative)[18]. This could serve to limit migration of drug anions into the fetal circulation (e.g. heparin).

Most drugs are weak electrolytes of moderate molecular weight (600–800). As with other membranes of the body, drugs traverse the placental membranes by simple diffusion. Thus, permeability to drugs is determined by lipid solubility, ionization state and molecular size of the drug; placental blood flow; placental metabolism of drugs; and aging of the

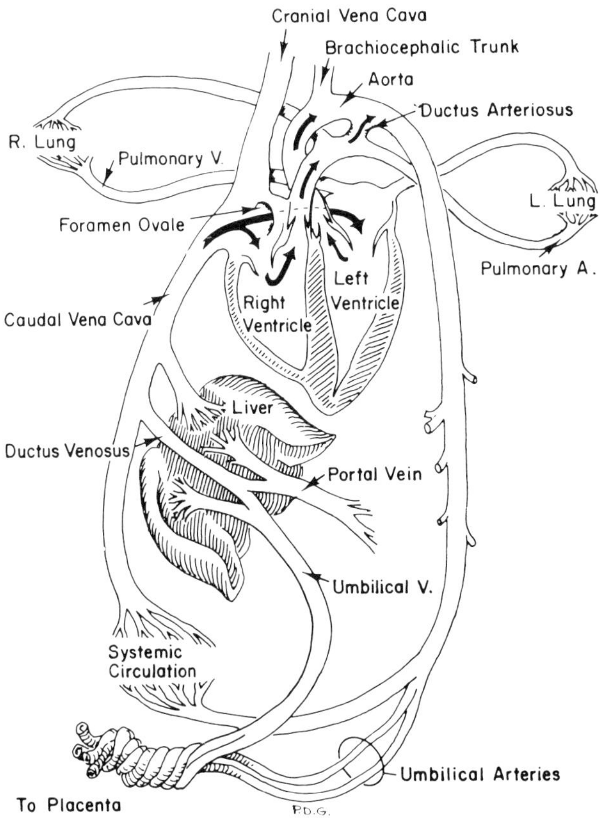

Figure 2.1 Circulatory system of the fetal goat

placentomes[26]. Blood flow to the uterus of sheep at term was observed to be within the range of 186–260 ml/min[7]. Ahlquist found that epinephrine, norepinephrine, pitressin, and pitocin decreased blood flow to the pregnant uterus of the bitch and phenoxybenzamine, tolazoline, histamine, pentobarbital and acetylcholine caused vasodilation[2]. These effects were confirmed in the ewe[1]. For lipid soluble drugs, exchange between the maternal and fetal blood would be expected to be flow-limited rather than diffusion-limited.

After drugs enter the umbilical vein they are distributed in the fetus (Figure 2.1). 60–85% of the blood flow in the umbilical vein enters the portal vein while 15–40% passes through the ductus venosus into the vena cava[26]. Thus, the fetal liver may be exposed to large amounts of drug following entry into the fetal circulation. The blood enters the right heart and 46% passes through the foramen ovale, 35% goes through the ductus arteriosus into the aorta and only 10% perfuses the fetal lungs[19]. The distribution of drugs to specific tissues or organs of ruminant animals is unknown.

The fetus grows within an environment in which it is surrounded by amniotic fluid. The fluid is formed during the latter half of gestation by fetal elimination of hypotonic urine[3]. The fluid is swallowed by the fetus and absorbed from the intestinal tract. Drugs could enter the amniotic fluid via the fetal circulation and renal excretion or by diffusion from the amniotic membrane into the fluid. Substances in amniotic fluid could enter the fetus by intestinal absorption or by diffusion through the fetal skin. These relationships are uncertain at this time.

STUDIES OF PLACENTAL TRANSFER IN GOATS

Most studies of placental transfer of drugs have been conducted by sampling from maternal artery and umbilical vein during caesarotomy in women, by studying perfused isolated placentas and studying placental sections *in vitro*. When one attempts to relate pharmacokinetic data obtained from sampling the maternal blood after bolus doses to the time-course of drug concentrations in the fetal circulation, the problem becomes extraordinarily complex. However, if one maintains constant drug concentrations in the maternal circulation and measures changes in concentration in the fetal circulation one should be able to determine relative permeability characteristics of the placenta by evaluating the equation

$$Pt = \ln\left(1 - \frac{C_1}{C_2 R}\right)$$

at various times (Pt = the permeability coefficient for the drug, C_1 = concentration in fetal blood, C_2 = concentration in maternal blood and R = the ratio of drug concentration in fetal blood to that in maternal blood at the steady state)[29].

In order to use this approach we developed a technique for placing catheters in the vena cava of fetuses of goats and into the amnionic fluid *in utero*[5]. The catheters were exteriorized through the abdominal wall. Eight

Table 2.2 Pharmacokinetic parameters for several drugs studied in pregnant goats

Drug	p*Ka*	*Dose* (mg/kg)	β (h^{-1})	$T_{1/2\beta}$ (h)	*Ri* ($mg\,kg^{-1}\,h^{-1}$)	*Pt*
Sulphanilamide	1.04	150	0.154	4.5	23	0.70
Salicylate	3.0	44	0.984	0.7	43	0.75
Pentobarbital	8.1	22	0.889	0.78	19.7	—
Phenylbutazone	4.4	33	0.037	19.0	1.2	—
Antipyrine	1.4	110	0.347	2.0	38	0.76
Thiocyanate	—	20	0.043	16.0	0.9	0.39
Diazoxide	—	5	0.058	12.0	2.9	—

drugs were studied: sulphanilamide, chlorpromazine, pentobarbital, salicylate, phenylbutazone, diazoxide, antipyrine and thiocyanate. In order to calculate infusion rates to maintain constant drug concentrations in the maternal plasma we first determined values for pharmacokinetic parameters in does. These results are shown in Table 2.2. The dose of each drug listed was administered to pregnant does at about 110–115 days of gestation and the drug was infused at a constant rate into the jugular vein of the doe (Figure 2.2). Samples were collected simultaneously, at periodic intervals, from the opposite jugular vein, the fetal vena cava and the amniotic fluid.

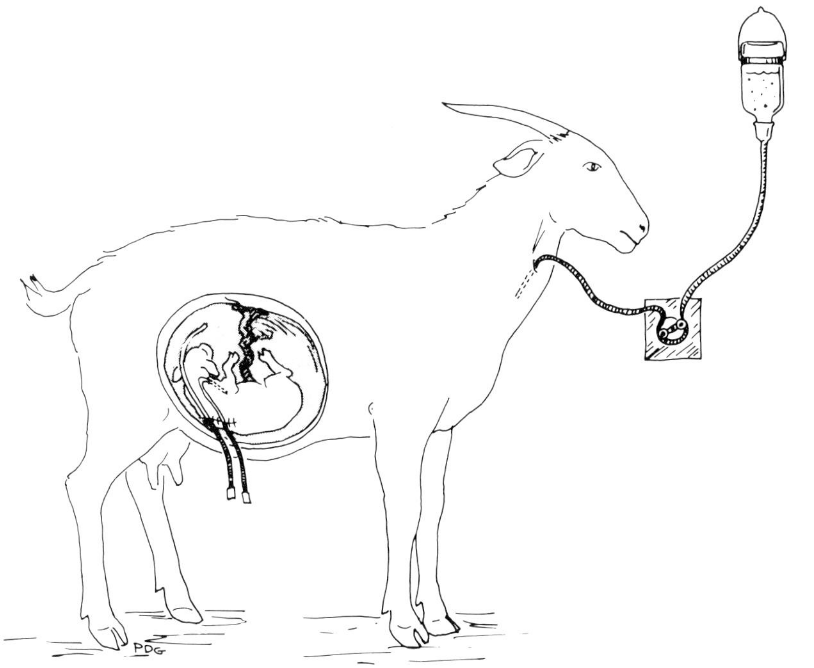

Figure 2.2 Arrangements for the study of placental transfer of drugs in the goat

The results of experiments with salicylate infused into six pregnant does for a period of 2h are shown in Figure 2.3. Concentrations of salicylate increased rapidly in fetal blood and amniotic fluid with concentrations in the amniotic fluid exceeding those in fetal blood throughout the period of study. Following cessation of drug administration the maternal plasma concentrations declined more slowly than would be expected from the preliminary data following a single bolus dose. The difference between maternal and fetal concentrations at equilibrium might be explained on the basis of differential protein binding. The extent of salicylate binding to plasma proteins in maternal blood was $72.2 \pm 2.8\%$ and in the fetal blood was $50.4 \pm 1.9\%$[9].

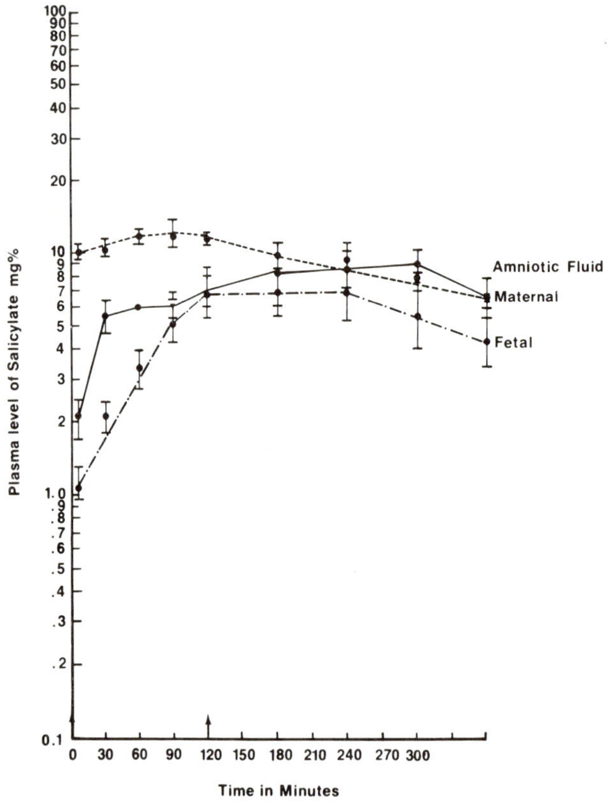

Figure 2.3 Concentrations of salicylate in maternal blood, fetal blood and amniotic fluid. The points are mean ± SE values from six does

Experiments with sulphanilamide were performed in four does. The results are shown in Figure 2.4. The drug was infused for a period of 4h. In this case we observed different relationships than in the case of salicylate. Equilibration occurred at about 90–120 min with the plateau in concentration in amniotic fluid lagging behind that seen in the fetal blood. The concentration in amniotic fluid persisted somewhat while the maternal and fetal blood

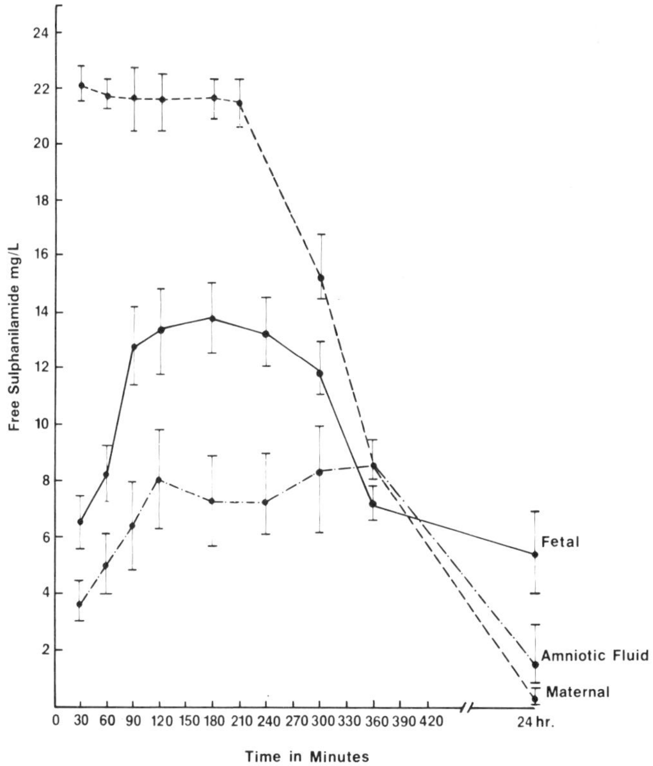

Figure 2.4 Concentrations of sulphanilamide in maternal blood, fetal blood and amniotic fluid. The values are mean ± SE values from four does

concentrations were declining. The ratios observed[11] at 120 min were fetal : maternal 0.62, amniotic fluid : fetal 0.65 and amniotic fluid : maternal 0.36.

Pentobarbital was studied in ten does and the results are shown in Figure 2.5. The drug was infused for 60 min because of short halflife in the goat and its prominent pharmacological effect on the doe. Concentrations in fetal blood increased more rapidly than those in the amniotic fluid during the infusion period. Following infusion, while the maternal and fetal blood concentrations were falling, the concentration of pentobarbital continued to increase in the amniotic fluid and remained high at 24 h. During the infusion of pentobarbital, the maternal and fetal electrocardiograms were monitored. The doe developed bradycardia and the fetus had tachycardia which persisted for 4 h following termination of the infusion. The ratios of concentrations at 60 min were similar to those observed for sulphanilamide and were[12]: fetal : maternal 0.56, amniotic fluid : fetus 0.62 and amniotic fluid : maternal 0.35.

Phenylbutazone was studied in six does and the drug was infused for 2 h. This is a drug which has a long halflife in the goat in contrast to salicylate or

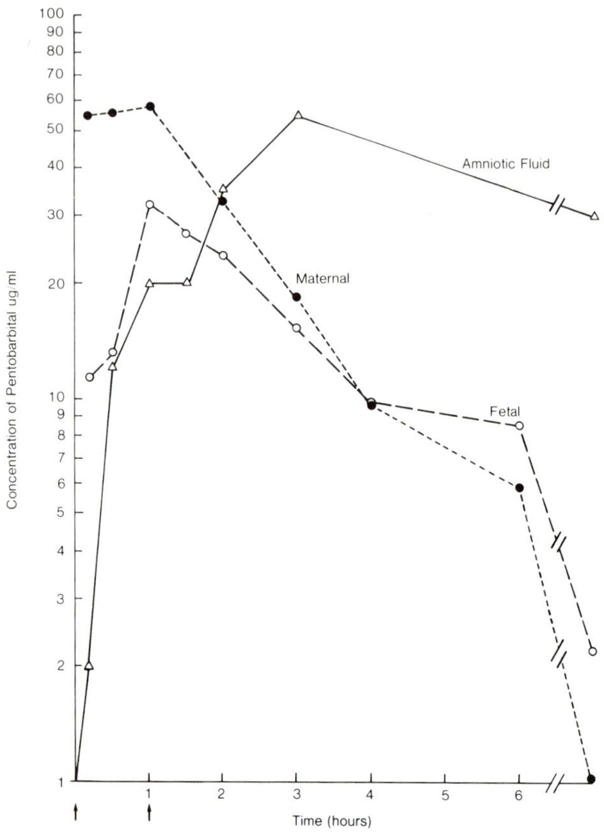

Figure 2.5 Concentrations of pentobarbital in maternal blood, fetal blood and amniotic fluid. The values are the means from ten animals

pentobarbital (see Table 2.2). Concentrations of phenylbutazone increased rapidly in fetal blood and attained equilibrium at 30 min (Figure 2.6). The drug continued to accumulate in the amniotic fluid for 2 h after cessation of infusion, then slowly declined over the next 2 days. The concentration of drug remained high in the fetus at 48 h. The ratios at the end of infusion were[12]: fetal : maternal 0.55, amniotic fluid : fetus 1.1, amniotic fluid : maternal 0.61.

Antipyrine is a pyrazolon-derivative similar to phenylbutazone except that it has a very low extent of binding to plasma proteins. It was infused for a 4 h period and the results appear in Figure 2.7. Equilibrium between the maternal and fetal blood occurred rapidly (30 min). After termination of the infusion, concentrations in the fetus declined more slowly than those in maternal blood. The concentrations in amniotic fluid were more erratic. After an apparent equilibrium during the first hour, concentrations increased and remained higher than those in maternal or fetal blood after the infusion was terminated. Concentration ratios[13] at 60 min were: fetal : maternal 0.61, amniotic fluid : fetal 0.61, and amniotic fluid : maternal 0.37.

Thiocyanate is an ion which is commonly employed to estimate the volume of the extracellular space. It was studied in six animals following a single dose of 20 mg/kg. Concentrations were not measured in the amniotic fluid. The results are shown in Figure 2.8. Concentrations were attained rapidly in fetal blood and remained fairly constant for 8 h but the fetal concentrations were only about 16% of those in the doe. Throughout the study the fetal : maternal ratio increased continuously because of the declining concentration in maternal blood[13].

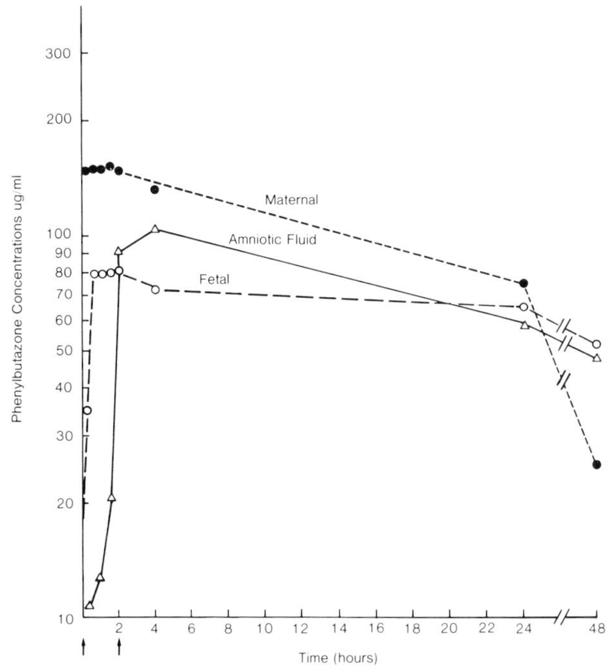

Figure 2.6 Concentrations of phenylbutazone in maternal blood, fetal blood and amniotic fluid. The values are the means from six animals

Two other studies which were performed involved the intravenous administration of chlorpromazine (4.4 mg/kg) to seven does as a bolus and diazoxide administered intravenously to seven ewes (5 mg/kg), every 8 h for 4 days. These were of interest because of the widespread use of phenothiazine derivatives in veterinary practice and diazoxide is an antihypertensive drug which also inhibits insulin-release in insulinoma which would make the information useful relative to pregnant women. The concentrations of chlorpromazine are shown in Table 2.3 and the results for diazoxide are shown in Figure 2.9. Concentrations of chlorpromazine disappeared rapidly from

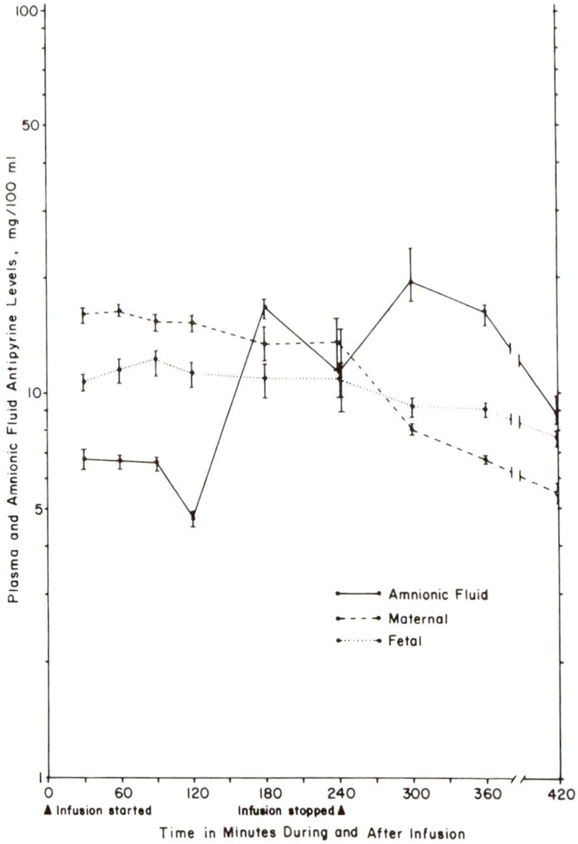

Figure 2.7 Concentrations of antipyrine in maternal blood, fetal blood and amniotic fluid. The values are the mean ± SE from six animals

the maternal and fetal blood plasma but persisted in the amniotic fluid and tissues of the doe and fetus[12]. Diazoxide concentrations were maintained at fairly constant values in maternal and fetal blood throughout the treatment period[10].

IMPLICATIONS TO VETERINARY THERAPEUTICS

There is probably no aspect of drug therapy in veterinary medicine which is surrounded by greater uncertainty than the administration of drugs to female animals following breeding. If at all possible, it is prudent to avoid drug treatment for the first 45 days following breeding in cow and for the first month in ewes or does. These periods comprise the time during which the conceptus is most vulnerable to lethal or teratogenic effects of chemicals.

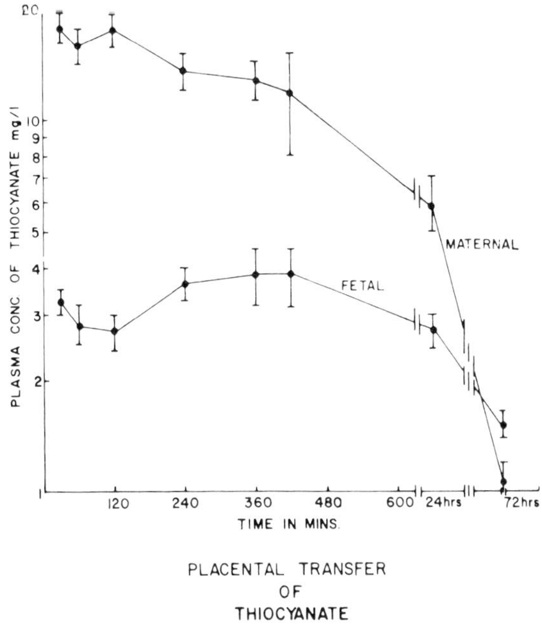

Figure 2.8 Concentrations of thiocyanate in maternal and fetal blood. Values are mean ± SE from six animals

Table 2.3 Concentration of chlorpromazine (μg/ml) in various tissues of goats following administration of an intravenous bolus (4.4 mg/kg) to seven pregnant does[12]

	Time (min)							
Tissue	0	10	30	60	90	120	150	24 h
Maternal blood	0	1.9	1.7	0.8	trace	trace	trace	ND
Fetal blood	0	0.7	0.8	0.5	trace	trace	trace	ND
Amniotic fluid	0	0.1	0.5	0.9	1.1	1.2	2.2	ND
Maternal liver								1.1
Maternal kidney								0.9
Maternal heart								0.6
Maternal brain								0.4
Fetal liver								0.9*
Fetal kidney								0.8*
Fetal heart								0.8*
Fetal brain								0.3*

* Three fetuses were aborted

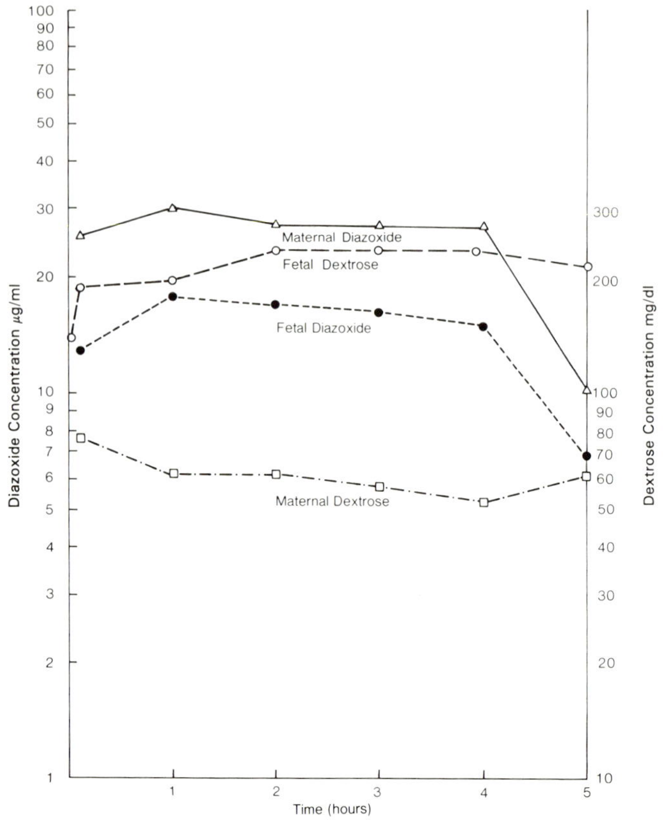

Figure 2.9 Concentrations of diazoxide and dextrose in maternal and fetal blood. Each point is the mean value from seven ewes

Later in pregnancy, the principal hazard is tissue toxicity in the fetus or adverse effects related to alterations in function within the fetus or placenta. Both alpha and beta adrenergic receptors are present in the fetal lamb by the middle of gestation. Injection of isproterenol, epinephrine, levarterenol or methoxamine into the fetal circulation will elicit characteristic cardiovascular effects and norepinephrine is known to cause constriction of the ductus arteriosus and ductus venosus[27]. Cholinergic receptors, acetylcholine and acetylcholinesterase are present in embryos at a very early stage which antedates the innervation of developing tissues[23]. ACTH, vasopressin, renin and angiotensin are all present in the fetus by the middle of gestation and appreciable quantities of prostaglandins are present[28]. Drugs which modify their functions could be deleterious to the fetus. Prostaglandin E_1 constricts the umbilical–placental blood vessels, dilates the pulmonary vasculature and maintains the patency of the ductus arteriosus. Indomethacin will induce closure of the ductus[14], an effect which could be deleterious to the fetus *in utero*. The fetal thyroid gland may be affected by drugs administered to the dam during the last half of gestation. Neonatal goitre may be produced by iodides, methimazole, propylthiouracil, chlorpromazine, lithium, phenylbutazone, sulphonamides, theophylline, and radioactive iodine[24]. The goitre may result in neonatal respiratory distress, difficult delivery or mental retardation of the offspring.

In usual circumstances, drugs are administered in discrete doses at periodic intervals, so the concentrations in maternal blood rise and fall during the interval and the fetus may not experience exposure to high drug concentrations. Rapid biotransformation and excretion of a drug from the maternal blood prevents the attainment of steady-state concentrations of the drug in the fetus. Higher proportions of the maternal cardiac output perfuse the liver and kidneys than pass through the uterine vasculature during pregnancy. This would tend to protect the fetus from being exposed to more than a small fraction of the drug dose.

In our studies we had the opportunity to observe what happens when this is not the case. When the drug concentrations were maintained constant in the maternal blood an inordinate incidence of adverse effects on the fetus was observed. Three fetal deaths occurred among the seven does given chlorpromazine. Histopathological study revealed major liver damage in these fetuses. During the study the fetal heart rate increased markedly for 7 h following administration of the drug. In the study of phenylbutazone, two kids had signs of renal insufficiency following birth. These animals were sacrificed and examined. Sections of the kidneys, which were swollen, revealed swelling of the glomeruli and polymorphonuclear cellular infiltration of the interstitium. Diazoxide had no effect on the ewes, but caused a marked hyperglycaemia in the fetus within 30 min of administration of the drug to the ewe. Lambs were either aborted or died by the fifth day following delivery. At necropsy tissues were collected and examined histologically. The cells of the pancreatic islets had degenerated and one lamb had bilateral cataracts and complete fibrosis of the gastrocnemius and popliteus muscles.

Clinical situations in which these observations might be relevant are renal insufficiency in the pregnant patient, presence of hepatic disease or microsomal enzyme inhibitors or the administration of drugs having exceptionally long halflives in the ruminant animal. Phenylbutazone might be of concern within this context. Its halflife in sheep and goats is 19 h and in the cow[20] is 32–61 h. The drug has not had widespread use in these species so it is not possible to evaluate whether its use in pregnant ruminant animals might be contraindicated. It is probable that under normal conditions of clinical use, most drugs which have been approved for use in ruminant animals are safe to use for treatment during pregnancy. Still the veterinarian should be conservative about using drugs in pregnant animals and remain alert to the possibility of adverse effects on the fetus.

References

1. Adams, F. H., Assali, N., Cushman, M. and Westersten, A. (1961). Interrelationships of maternal and fetal circulations. I. Flow-pressure responses to vasoactive drugs in sheep. *Pediatrics*, **27**, 627–35

2. Ahlquist, R. P. (1950). The actions of various drugs on the arterial blood flow of the pregnant canine uterus. *J. Am. Pharm. Assoc.*, **39**, 370–3
3. Alexander, D. P., Nixon, D. A., Widdas, W. F. and Wohlzogen, F. X. (1958). Gestational variations in the composition of the foetal fluids and foetal urine in the sheep. *J. Physiol.*, **140**, 1–13
4. Al-Guedawy, S., Davis, C. A., Davis, L. E., Whitmore, H. L. and Gustafsson, B. K. (1982). Disposition of gentamicin in blood and uterine fluid. *J. Vet. Pharmacol. Ther.*, in press
5. Almond, C. H., Boulos, B. M., Davis, L. E. and Mackenzie, J. W. (1970). New surgical technique for studying placental transfer of drugs *in vivo*. *J. Surg. Res.*, **10**, 7–11
6. Amoroso, E. C. (1952). Placentation. In Parkes, A. S. (ed.) *Marshall's Physiology of Reproduction*. 3rd edn, Vol. 2, pp. 127–311. (London: Longmans, Green and Co.)
7. Assali, N. S., Dasgupta, K., Kolin, A. and Holmes, L. (1958). Measurement of uterine blood flow and uterine metabolism. *Am. J. Physiol.*, **195**, 614–20
8. Barcroft, J. (1946). *Researches on Pre-natal Life*. (Oxford: Blackwell Scientific Publications)
9. Boulos, B. M., Almond, C. H., Davis, L. E. and Hammer, M. (1972). Placental transfer of salicylate under constant maternal blood levels. *Arch. Int. Pharmacodyn. Ther.*, **196**, 357–62
10. Boulos, B. M., Davis, L. E., Almond, C. H. and Jackson, R. L. (1971). Placental transfer of diazoxide and its hazardous effect on the newborn. *J. Clin. Pharmacol.*, **11**, 206–10
11. Boulos, B. M., Davis, L. E., Almond, C. H. and Sirtori, C. R. (1971). Placental transfer of sulfanilamide as determined at constant drug concentrations in the maternal blood. *Arch. Int. Pharmacodyn. Ther.*, **193**, 61–7
12. Boulos, B. M., Davis, L. E., Larks, S. D., Larks, G. G., Sirtori, C. R. and Almond, C. H. (1971). Placental transfer of chlorpromazine, pentobarbital and phenylbutazone with fetal electrocardiographic changes as determined by direct lead tracing. *Arch. Int. Pharmacodyn. Ther.*, **194**, 403–14
13. Boulos, B. M., Hanna, F., Davis, L. E. and Almond, C. H. (1973). Placental transfer of antipyrine and thiocyanate and their use in determining maternal and fetal body fluids in a maintained pregnancy. *Arch. Int. Pharmacodyn. Ther.*, **201**, 42–51
14. Brash, A. R., Hickey, D. E., Graham, T. P., Stahlman, M. T., Oates, J. A. and Cotton, R. B. (1981). Pharmacokinetics of indomethacin in the neonate. Relation of plasma indomethacin levels to response of the ductus areteriosus. *N. Engl. J. Med.*, **305**, 67–72
15. Bretzlaff, K. N., Ott, R. S., Koritz, G. D., Lock, T. F., Bevill, R. F., Shawley, R. V., Gustafsson, B. K. and Davis, L. E. (1982). Distribution of oxytetracycline in the genital tract of cows. *Am. J. Vet. Res.*, **43**, 12–16
16. Connor, E. A. and Miller, J. W. (1973). The distribution of selected substances into rat uterine luminal fluid. *J. Pharmacol. Exp. Ther.*, **184**, 291–8
17. Davis, L. E. and Stanton, H. C. (1980). Drug therapy during pregnancy and the neonatal period. In Morrow, D. A. (ed.) *Current Therapy in Theriogenology*. pp. 46–57. (Philadelphia: W. B. Saunders)
18. Dawes, G. S. (1968). *Foetal and Neonatal Physiology*. p. 27. (Chicago: Yearbook Medical Publishers)
19. Dawes, G. S., Mott, J. C. and Widdicombe, J. G. (1954). The foetal circulation in the lamb. *J. Physiol.*, **126**, 563–87
20. Eberhardson, B., Olsson, G., Appelgren, L. and Jacobsson, S. (1979). Pharmacokinetic studies of phenybutazone in cattle. *J. Vet. Pharmacol. Ther.*, **2**, 31–7
21. Fabro, S. and Sieber, S. M. (1969). *The Foeto-Placental Unit*. International Congress Series, No. 183, p. 313. (Amsterdam: Excerpta Medica Found.)
22. Greenstein, J. A. and Foley, R. C. (1958). Early embryology of the cow. I. Gastrula and primitive streak stages. *J. Dairy Sci.*, **50**, 409–21
23. Karczman, A. G. (1963). Ontogenesis of cholinesterases. In Koelle, G. B. (ed.) *Handbuch der Experimentellen Pharmakologie*. Vol. 15, p. 129. (Berlin: Springer-Verlag)
24. Martin, E. W., Alexander, S. F., Hassan, W. E. Jr. and Farage, D. J. (1971). *Hazards of Medication*. p. 278. (Philadelphia: Lippincott)
25. McLachlan, J. A., Sieber, S. M., Cowherd, C. M., Straw, J. A. and Fabro, S. (1970). The pH values of the uterine secretions and preimplantation blastocyst of the rabbit. *Fertil. Steril.*, **21**, 84–7

26. Mirkin, B. L. (1973). Drug distribution in pregnancy. In Boreus, L. O. (ed.) *Fetal Pharmacology*. pp. 1–27. (New York: Raven Press)
27. Owman, C., Aronson, S., Gennser, G. and Sjöberg, N. O. (1973). Histochemical and pharmacological evidence of amine mechanisms in human vascular shunts. In Boreus, L. O. (ed.) *Fetal Pharmacology*. p. 179. (New York: Raven Press)
28. Rudolph, A. M. (1977). Homeostasis of the fetal circulation and the part played by hormones. *Ann. Rech. Vét.*, **8**, 405–12
29. Schanker, L. S. (1962). Passage of drugs across body membranes. *Pharmacol. Rev.*, **14**, 501–30
30. Sieber, S. M. and Fabro, S. (1971). Identification of drugs in the preimplantation blastocysts and in the plasma, uterine secretion and urine of the pregnant rabbit. *J. Pharmacol. Exp. Ther.*, **176**, 65–75
31. Steven, D. H. (1966). Further observations on placental circulation in the sheep. *J. Physiol.*, **183**, 13–15

3
Drug disposition in the fetus

L.-E. Appelgren

The fetotoxic and teratogenic properties of several drugs and other substances have been extensively studied in small experimental animals. The mechanisms behind the effects caused by these agents are not always known. Distribution studies, e.g. using whole body autoradiography, is one route which together with many others may finally lead to a better understanding of the influence of chemicals on fetal development.

Reviews of the distribution of drugs and other substances in the fetus have recently been published, but they are almost entirely confined to small experimental animals[23,45,49]. Data on the distribution of drugs in the fetuses of ruminants rarely occur in the literature and therefore most data presented here will be from other species. Attempts to apply these data to the ruminant fetus will, however, be made when specific teratological and/or other effects on the fetus have been reported for ruminants.

This review is mainly confined to results obtained from whole body autoradiographic studies of pregnant experimental animals. The following groups of drugs and other compounds have been selected since they may have significance for ruminants:

(1) Environmental contaminants (polybrominated biphenyls (PBB), polychlorinated biphenyls (PCB), DDT, fluorine, toxic plants),
(2) Mycotoxins (aflatoxin, ochratoxin, zearalenone),
(3) Hormones (gestagens, corticosteroids),
(4) Vitamins and trace elements (Vitamins A and B_{12}, Zn, Se).

(For other substances the reader is referred to the extensive review articles mentioned previously[23,45,49].)

ENVIRONMENTAL CONTAMINANTS

Autoradiographic studies of PCB[20], PBB and DDT have shown that these substances are selectively localized in the fetal adrenal cortex (Figure 3.1). An uptake of these substances in the adrenal cortex may indicate a risk for an interference in steroid production as has been shown for diphenylethenes which inhibit Δ^5-3β-OH steroid dehydrogenase in the corpora lutea as well as in the adrenal cortex[3,4]. It is a known fact that disturbances of the hypothalamic-pituitary-adrenal cortex-axis may cause a defect in the mechanism for the termination of normal pregnancy in ewes and cows[35,51] and that glucocorticoids from fetal adrenals cause the induction of oestrogen synthesis from progesterone[42]. It is, therefore, very tempting to correlate the uptake of [^{14}C]PBB in the adrenal cortex of mice fetuses with the reported prolonged pregnancy in cows accidentally exposed to Fire Master in which the used polybrominated biphenyl is a major component[25].

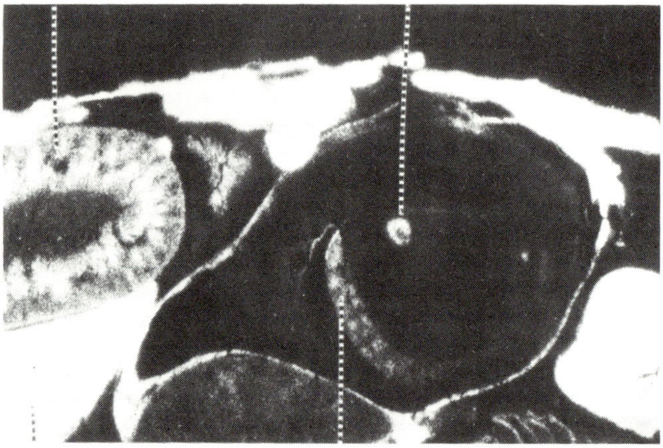

Figure 3.1 Detail of a whole body autoradiogram of a mouse in late pregnancy (17 days) 24 h after i.v. injection of [^{14}C]hexachlorobiphenyl showing the selective uptake of radioactivity in the fetal adrenal cortex[20]

Autoradiography using ^{18}F in pregnant mice has shown that although the fluoride ion passes poorly to the fetus, it is selectively accumulated in the mineralized hard tissue[7]. Fluorine can be expected also to pass the placental barrier in ruminants. The environmental pollution of fluorine is a reality in some industrial areas[21] and fluorosis in cows can therefore be expected to affect dental and skeletal development in the fetuses.

No autoradiographic or other distribution studies on the alkaloids from *Veratrum californicum* have been found. These alkaloids are known to cause prolonged gestation and malformations (hypophysial aplasia and thyroid, adrenal and gonadal hypoplasia) in the ovine species[35]. The structures of some of the teratogenic alkaloids in *V. californicum* have been determined to be 11-deoxyjervine, jervine and cycloposine[36].

MYCOTOXINS

The fetotoxic and teratogenic properties of the mycotoxins aflatoxin B_1, ochratoxin A and zearalenone have been studied in different species[12, 13, 24, 29, 38, 39]. The risk of fetal disturbances in the ruminant species from mycotoxins ingested by the mother is not known, but field observations of pancreatic hypoplasia in calves from cows that had been fed aflatoxin-contaminated feed have been reported[51]. Our findings using whole body autoradiography of pregnant mice after injection of labelled mycotoxins[8, 9, 11] indicate what should be looked for when analysing cases of abortions and malformations in ruminants where aflatoxin B_1, ochratoxin A and zearalenone might be involved. After injection of [^{14}C]aflatoxin in mice in late pregnancy[11], a pronounced uptake of ^{14}C was seen in the pigmented layer of the eye (Figure 3.2). The pigment affinity of [^{14}C]aflatoxin does not seem to be as irreversible as that of chloroquine[37], known to cause damage in the eye. In addition, a rather high concentration of radioactive material was found in the nasal mucosae of the fetuses (Figure 3.2). In the fetal liver and kidney, however, no radioactivity was found although these organs had taken up considerable amounts of the radioactivity in the dams and are known target organs for aflatoxin B_1-toxicity[10].

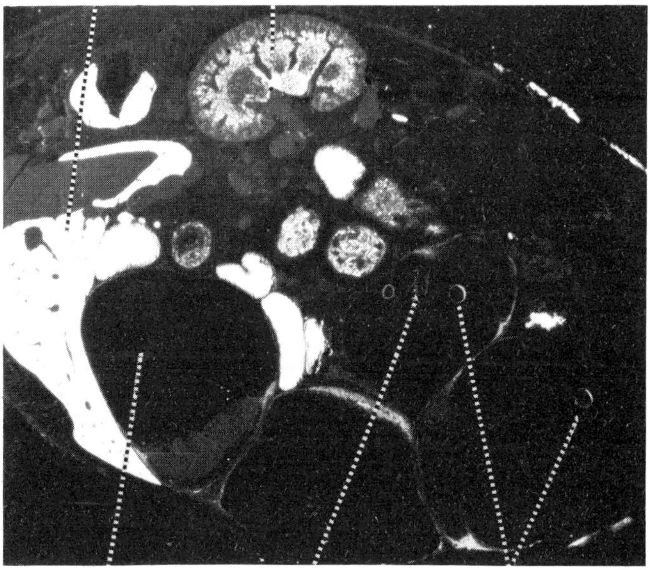

Figure 3.2 Detail of whole body autoradiogram of a mouse in late pregnancy (17 days) 20 min after i.v. injection of [^{14}C]aflatoxin. Note the high concentration of ^{14}C in the pigment layers of the fetal eyes[11]

When [^{14}C]ochratoxin was injected in 9 day pregnant mice, the radioactivity concentration in the uterine wall was higher than that of the blood and still higher concentrations were seen in the ectoplacental cone and in some fetal structures most likely corresponding to the allantois and the gut (Figure 3.3). The corresponding 10 day pregnant animal showed lower concentrations in the uterine wall and placental structures, but in some fetuses a high concentration of ^{14}C could be detected in allantois. 17 days after conception, the concentration was very low in the fetuses, indicating that very small amounts of radioactivity passed the placental barrier. When the corresponding sections were studied under ultraviolet light, the blue fluorescence

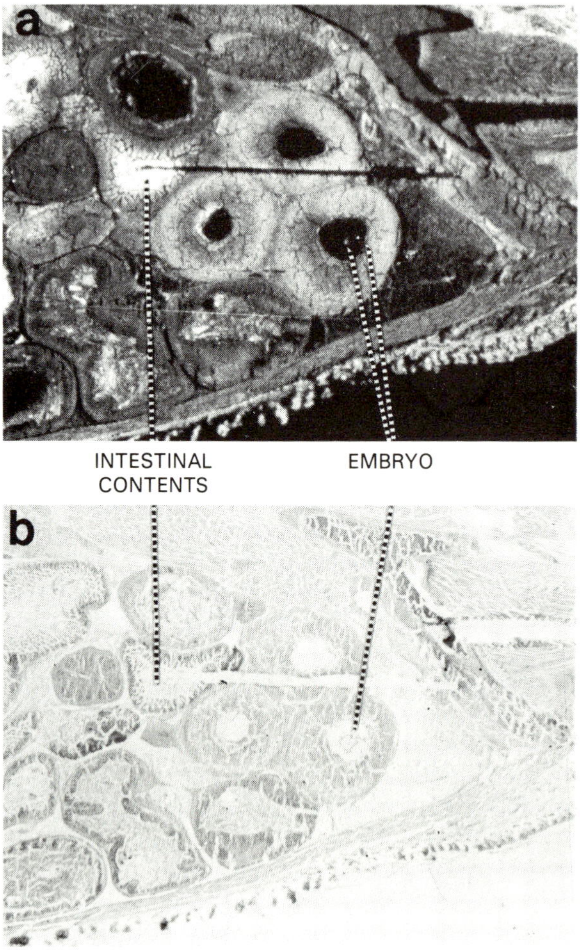

Figure 3.3 Details of whole body autoradiogram (a) and corresponding section (b) of a 9 day pregnant mouse 20 min after i.v. injection of [^{14}C]ochratoxin. Note the radioactivity in the ectoplacental cone and in the embryo[8]

of ochratoxin showed the same pattern in the pregnant uterus and embryo/fetus as was shown by autoradiography[8]. The distribution pattern of labelled ochratoxin seems to be similar to the distribution patterns of cadmium and trypan blue in mice. These substances were taken up by the visceral yolk sac and the embryonic endoderm up to the time of closure of the vitelline duct at about 9 days after the conception but not in the fetuses in late gestation[23]. According to Dencker[22] an accumulation of teratogens in the (gut) endoderm could explain a disturbed interaction between the ectoderm and endoderm, and later between the neuroepithelium and the gut, causing, e.g. exencephaly. Exencephaly was the most frequent malformation registered when ochratoxin was given on day 8 and 9 and not later[13].

When [^{3}H]zearalenone was given to mice in different gestation states specific localization was found in oestrogen target organs of the dams but in the fetuses radioactivity was found only in late pregnancy, mainly in the kidney, bile and connective tissue[9]. In the 8, 9 and 10 day pregnant animals, no radioactivity was registered in specific embryonic tissues, but in the placental tissue and uterine fluid[9]. Remarkably, there was an accumulation of radioactivity in the follicular fluid in the ovaries of the adult mice; it is tempting to correlate this to reports that zearalenone causes malfunction of the ovary in sows and that the oocyte dies in the Graafian follicle[46,48].

It must be remembered that the radioactivity registered by the autoradiograms does not necessarily show the injected compound unchanged. Synthesis of aflatoxin B_1 by incubation of *Aspergillus flavus* in the presence of sodium-[1-^{14}C]acetate yields ring-labelled aflatoxin B_1[18,31]. This means that the major metabolites known to be formed in the body of mammals would still be labelled. Thus, the radioactivity in our autoradiograms most probably represents the unchanged compound and/or its major metabolites

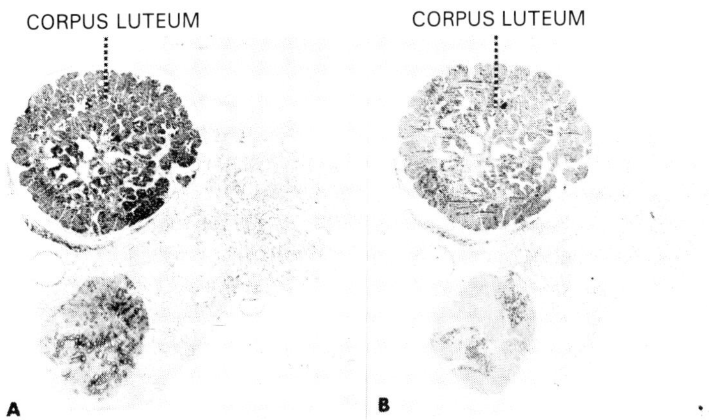

Figure 3.4 Sections from an ovary from a non-pregnant cow showing the Δ^5-3β-hydroxysteroid dehydrogenase activity using pregnenolone as a substrate. **B** shows the inhibitory effect on enzyme activity of medroxyprogesterone added to the incubation medium. **A** is the corresponding control section[5]

with the ring structure intact. Regarding ochratoxin, radiochromatographic investigations[8] have shown that the radioactivity in the fetuses corresponds to the reference substance [^{14}C]ochratoxin A. [^{3}H]zearalenone, on the other hand, was extensively metabolized and, according to our radiochromatography studies, only minute amounts represented unchanged zearalenone in the mouse fetuses[9].

The differences observed regarding the distribution of ochratoxin and zearalenone are reflected in the teratogenic effects of the two substances; ochratoxin caused malformations to high extent on day 8 and 9 but no such effects were registered when zearalenone was administered during these pregnancy stages[12]. A protective effect of zearalenone against ochratoxin-induced malformations has also been demonstrated[50], but this effect can only be correlated to the distribution of [^{3}H]zearalenone and/or its metabolites in uterine and placental tissues[9]. The protective effect of zearalenone seems to be caused by its oestrogenic properties, since equipotent doses of diethylstilboestrol had the same protective effect against ochratoxin induced malformations[50].

HORMONES

[^{14}C]4-progesterone accumulates in the human fetal adrenal cortex[17] where it probably is used as a precursor for steroidogenesis. It is also found in fetal testes, pituitary, parts of the brain, thyroid and thymus[17].

Synthetic gestagen compounds have been used both as oral contraceptives and for oestrus synchronization in cattle. The hypothalamic-pituitary system is regarded as the main target for the contraceptive action of the gestagens, but also the ovaries, oviducts, uterus and cervix should be considered. The local effects of gestagens on the ovaries might be due to impaired steroid synthesis. This is supported by the large accumulation of medroxyprogesterone and chlormadinone[6] in the corpora lutea of mice and the ability of medroxyprogesterone to decrease enzyme activity in these structures in mice ovaries as well as in bovine ovaries[5] (Figure 3.4). Also, in the adrenal cortex of the mother as well as of the fetus an accumulation of these gestagens was shown[6]. Medroxyprogesterone has been shown also to interfere with the steroid synthesis in the adrenals.

Weak oestrogenic compounds, diphenyl derivatives, were also shown to be selectively localized in the ovarian corpora lutea[27] where they were found to interfere with progesterone formation[3,4]. The small amount which penetrated into the fetus localized mainly in the adrenal cortex. The natural oestrogen, oestradiol, showed a marked fetal accumulation while the placental passage of diethylstilboestrol was partially blocked[16,43].

Natural and synthetic corticosteroids have also been shown to penetrate into the fetuses of mice[26] and sheep[1,14]. A synthetic corticosteroid (Draco 371/28) has been shown to be localized selectively in the fetal adrenal cortex of the mouse, but the risk for disturbance of the adrenal cortex of the ruminant fetus is probably unimportant compared to the abortive effect of corticosteroids in these species.

VITAMINS AND TRACE ELEMENTS

Vitamin A has been studied from a teratological point of view since an excess or a deficit are both known to produce malformations. In the early mouse embryo, vitamin A (retinyl acetate) was found to be localized in neuroepithelial tissues (parts of the brain, spinal cord and retina) and its metabolite retinoic acid showed an even higher uptake than vitamin A in the neuroepithelium[23]. Both vitamin A and retinoic acid are known to participate in the synthesis of glycoproteins and overproduction as well as underproduction of these substances may be hazardous for normal embryonic development[23]. Data on the concentrations of vitamin A in the fetuses of cows (blood serum and liver) have shown that they were significantly lower than in the blood serum and liver tissue of cows[47].

[^{60}Co]vitamin B_{12} accumulates in the mouse fetus more than a hundred-fold after an initial high concentration in the placenta if a low dose is given to the mother[44]. There seems to be an active transport process mediated via carriers or receptors; this placental 'pump' is saturable and the transport is depressed by vitamin B_{12} analogues[45]. In the bovine species there seems to be no risk of vitamin B_{12} deficiency as long as the cobalt content of the feed is sufficient[51]. Disturbances of normal pregnancy are reported (abortion) when cobalt is missing in the feed[51]. Fetal damage may also be caused by a disturbance of the mechanism for transport of vitamin B_{12} to the fetus.

Zinc has been shown to be required for normal fetal development and severe malformations are reported under deficiency conditions[32]. It is transferred rapidly to the fetus and accumulated in all the embryonic structures of mice and hamsters, especially in the neuroepithelium[22]. In the late fetuses of mice the liver and skeleton showed[22] a high uptake of ^{65}Zn which can be compared with reports of high contents of ^{65}Zn in the liver and bone of sheep fetuses[30]. According to the same author[30], no fetal skeletal

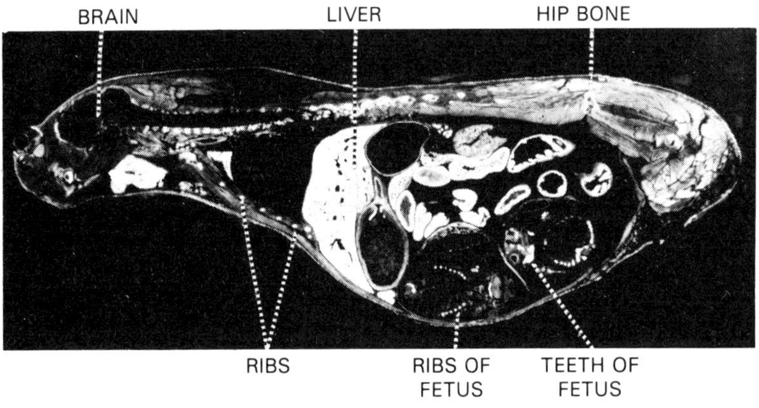

Figure 3.5 Whole body fluorogram from a pregnant mouse 5 h after i.v. injection of demethylchlortetracycline. Light areas indicate the yellow fluorescence of the tetracycline compound. Note the high concentrations in both the fetal and maternal skeleton[19]

malformations associated with zinc deficiency have yet, however, been observed in the ruminant fetus.

Selenium has been reported to cause malformations of the extremities and eyes of lambs whose mothers had been kept on seleniferous pastures[15], but it is well-known that if ewes and cows receive their selenium supply in therapeutic doses, it will provide protection against muscle degeneration in the lambs and calves[30]. Autoradiography in mice of [^{75}Se]sodium selenite and [^{75}Se]selenomethionine[28, 33] showed that more selenium was transported through the placenta when the organic compound was administered. Also, the distribution within the fetuses differed when the different compounds were given. The organic selenium reached the highest concentration in the fetal pancreas while the inorganic selenium was mainly confined to the liver. Also in sheep, a larger amount of selenium was transmitted through the placenta when [^{75}Se] was given as selenomethionine than when it was given as sodium selenite[34].

CONCLUSIONS

It is apparent from the examples given that some drugs have been found to accumulate in specific fetal tissues where they caused certain damage. Fluorine and tetracycline[2] (Figure 3.5) which are known to cause enamel spots, are localized selectively in the fetal hard tissues and especially in the developing teeth. In other cases, however, substances known to be teratogenic or fetotoxic are not found specifically in the embryo or fetus but in the visceral yolk sac or chorioallantoic placenta, perhaps causing disturbance of the nutrition of the fetus. It is important to consider that the species differences which we know from drug metabolism and pharmacokinetic studies can result in different concentrations of drugs and active metabolites and thus change the action on the fetus. Also, differences in placentation should be considered. The specific findings on drug distribution in the fetus/embryo of small experimental animals can, however, as mentioned earlier, indicate what we should look for when analysing cases of abortion and malformation in the ruminant species.

References

1. Anderson, D. F., Stock, M. K. and Rankin, J. H. G. (1979). Placental transfer of dexamethasone in near-term sheep. *J. Dev. Physiol.*, **1**, 431–6
2. André, T. (1956). Studies on the distribution of tritium-labelled dihydrostreptomycin and tetracycline in the body. *Acta Radiol. Suppl.*, **142**, 1–89
3. Appelgren, L.-E. (1967). Sites of steroid hormone formation. Autoradiographic studies using labelled precursors. *Acta Physiol. Scand. Suppl.*, **301**, 1–108
4. Appelgren, L.-E. (1969). Histochemical demonstration of drug interference with progesterone synthesis. *J. Reprod. Fert.*, **19**, 185–6
5. Appelgren, L.-E. (1969). Interference with progesterone synthesis of some antifertility compounds as shown by histochemistry. Presented at the *2nd European Congress on Sterility*, October 8–11, Dubrovnik, Yugoslavia

6. Appelgren, L.-E. (1972). Distribution of labelled chlormadinone acetate in mice. Abstract No. 47 of volunteer papers. Presented at the *Fifth International Congress on Pharmacology*, July 23–28, San Francisco, California
7. Appelgren, L.-E., Ericsson, Y. and Ullberg, S. (1961). A comparison of the distribution of radioactive fluorine and calcium by use of double-isotope autoradiography. *Acta Physiol. Scand.*, **53**, 339–47
8. Appelgren, L.-E. and Arora, R. G. (1982). Distribution studies of ^{14}C-labelled aflatoxin B_1 and ochratoxin A in pregnant mice. In *Proceedings of International Conference on Veterinary Pharmacology, Toxicology and Therapeutics*, Cambridge, England, 1980. To be published in *Vet. Res. Comm.*
9. Appelgren, L.-E., Arora, R. G. and Larsson, P. (1982). Autoradiographic studies of ^{3}H-zearalenone in mice. *Toxicology*, **25**, 243–53
10. Arora, R. G. (1981). Enhanced susceptibility of weanling mice to aflatoxin B_1 toxicity. *Acta Pathol. Microbiol. Scand.*, Sect. A, **89**, 303–8
11. Arora, R. G., Appelgren, L.-E. and Bergman, A. (1978). Distribution of [^{14}C]-labelled aflatoxin B_1 in mice. *Acta Pharmacol. Toxicol.*, **43**, 273–9
12. Arora, R. G., Frölén, H. and Nilsson, A. (1981). Interference of mycotoxins with prenatal development of the mouse. I. Influence of aflatoxin B_1, ochratoxin A and zearalenone. *Acta Vet. Scand.*, **22**, 524–34
13. Arora, R. G. and Frölén, H. (1981). Interference of mycotoxins with prenatal development of the mouse. II. Ochratoxin A induced teratogenic effects in relation to the dose and stage of gestation. *Acta Vet. Scand.*, **22**, 535–52
14. Bayard, F., Louvet, J. P., Ruckebusch, Y. *et al.* (1972). Transplacental passage of dexamethasone in sheep. *J. Endocrinol.*, **54**, 349–50
15. Beath, O. A., Eppson, H. F., Gilbert, C. S. *et al.* (1939). Poisonous plants and livestock poisoning. *Bull. Wyo. Agric. Exptl. Stn.*, **231**, 1–104
16. Bengtsson, G. and Ullberg, S. (1963). The autoradiographic distribution pattern after administration of diethylstilboestrol compared with that of natural oestrogens. *Acta Endocrinol. (Kbh.)*, **43**, 561–70
17. Bengtsson, G., Ullberg, S., Wiquist, N., *et al.* (1964). Autoradiographic studies on previable human foetuses perfused with radioactive steroids. I. Distribution of radioactive material following perfusion of progesterone-4-^{14}C. *Acta Endocrinol. (Kbh.)*, **46**, 544–51
18. Biollaz, M., Buchi, G. and Milne, G. (1970). The biosynthesis of the aflatoxins. *J. Am. Chem. Soc.*, **92**, 1035–43
19. Blomquist, L. and Hanngren, Å. (1966). Fluorescence technique applied to whole body sections for distribution studies of tetracyclines. *Biochem. Pharmacol.*, **15**, 215–19
20. Brandt, I. (1977). Tissue localization of polychlorinated biphenyls. Chemical structure related to pattern of distribution. *Acta Pharmacol. Toxicol.*, **40** (Suppl. II), 1–108
21. Debackere, M. (1980). Poisoning of domestic animals as an indication of environmental pollution. In Van Miert, A. S. *et al.* (eds.) *Trends in Veterinary Pharmacology and Toxicology*. pp. 314–20. (Amsterdam: Elsevier)
22. Dencker, L. (1976). Tissue localization of some teratogens at early and late gestation related to fetal effects. *Acta Pharmacol. Toxicol.*, **39** (Suppl. I), 1–131
23. Dencker, L. (1979). Embryonic-fetal localization of drugs and nutrients. In Persaud, T. V. N. (ed.) *Advances in the Study of Birth Defects*. Vol. I, pp. 1–18. (Lancaster: MTP Press)
24. DiPaolo, J. A., Elis, J. and Erwin, H. (1967). Teratogenic response by hamsters, rats and mice to aflatoxin B_1. *Nature (London)*, **215**, 638–9
25. Getty, S. M., Rickert, D. E. and Trapp, A. L. (1977). Polybrominated biphenyl (PBB) toxicosis: an environmental accident. *CRC Crit. Rev. Environ. Control*, **7**, 309–23
26. Hanngren, Å., Hansson, E., Sjöstrand, S. E. *et al.* (1964). Autoradiographic distribution studies with ^{14}C-cortisone and ^{14}C-cortisol. *Acta Endocrinol. (Kbh.)*, **47**, 95–104
27. Hanngren, Å., Einer. Jensen, N. and Ullberg, S. (1965). Specific uptake in corpora lutea of a non-steroid substance with anti-gestagenic properties. *Nature (London)*, **208**, 461–2
28. Hansson, E. and Jacobsson, S. O. (1966). Uptake of [^{75}Se]selenomethionine in the tissues of the mouse studied by whole-body autoradiography. *Biochim. Biophys. Acta*, **115**, 285–93
29. Hayes, A. W., Hood, R. D. and Lee, H. L. (1974). Teratogenic effects of ochratoxin A in mice. *Teratology*, **9**, 93–7

30. Hidiroglou, M. (1980). Trace elements in the fetal and neonate ruminant: a review. *Can. Vet. J.*, **21**, 328–35
31. Hsieh, D. P. H. and Mateles, R. I. (1970). The relative contribution of acetate and glucose to aflatoxin biosynthesis. *Biochim. Biophys. Acta*, **208**, 482–6
32. Hurley, L. S. and Swenerton, H. (1966). Congential malformations resulting from zinc deficiency in rats. *Proc. Soc. Exp. Biol. Med.*, **123**, 692–6
33. Jacobsson, S. O. and Hansson, E. (1965). Distribution of selenium in mice studied by whole body autoradiography after injection of Se^{75}-sodium selenite. *Acta Vet. Scand.*, **6**, 287–98
34. Jacobsson, S. O. and Oksanen, H. E. (1966). The placental transmission of selenium in sheep. *Acta Vet. Scand.*, **7**, 66–76
35. Van Kampen, K. R. and Ellis, L. C. (1972). Prolonged gestation in ewes ingesting *Veratrum californicum*: morphological changes and steroid biosynthesis in the endocrine organs of cyclopic lambs. *J. Endocrinol.*, **52**, 549–60
36. Keeler, R. F. (1969). Teratogenic compounds of *Veratrum californicum* (Durand). VII. The structure of the glycosidic alkaloid cycloposine. *Steroids*, **13**, 579–88
37. Lindquist, N. G. and Ullberg, S. (1972). The melanin affinity of chloroquine and chlorpromazine studied by whole body autoradiography. *Acta Pharmacol. Toxicol.*, **31** (Suppl. II), 1–32
38. Moré, J. and Galtier, P. (1974). Toxicité de l'ochratoxine A. I. Effet embryotoxique et tératogène chez le rat. *Ann. Rech. Vét.*, **5**, 167–78
39. Patterson, D. S. P., Roberts, B. A. and Small, B. J. (1976). Metabolism of ochratoxins A and B in the pig during early pregnancy and the accumulation in body tissues of ochratoxin A only. *Fd. Cosmet. Toxicol.*, **14**, 439–42
40. Schmidt, R. E. and Panciera, R. J. (1980). Effects of aflatoxin on pregnant hamsters and hamster foetuses. *J. Comp. Pathol.*, **90**, 339–47
41. Stabenfeldt, G. H., Edqvist, L.-E. and Drost, M. (1975). Endocrine changes during normal and prolonged bovine pregnancy. *Acta Endocrinol. (Kbh.) Suppl.*, **199**, 385
42. Steele, P. A., Flint, A. P. F. and Turnball, A. C. (1976). Activity of steroid C-17,20-lyase in the ovine placenta: effect of exposure to foetal glucocorticoid. *J. Endocrinol.*, **69**, 239–46
43. Ullberg, S. and Bengtsson, G. (1963). Autoradiographic distribution studies with natural oestrogens. *Acta Endocrinol. (Kbh.)*, **43**, 75–86
44. Ullberg, S., Kristoffersson, H., Flodh, H. *et al.* (1967). Placental passage and fetal accumulation of labelled vitamin B_{12} in the mouse. *Arch. Int. Pharmacodyn. Thér.*, **167**, 431–49
45. Ullberg, S., Dencker, L. and Danielsson, B. (1982). The distribution of drugs and other agents in the foetus. In Snell, K. (ed.) *Developmental Toxicology*. pp. 123–163. (London: Croom Helm)
46. Ványi, A., Széky, A. and Romváryné, S. E. (1974). Fusariotoxicoses. V. The effect of F_2 toxin on the sexual activity of female swine. *Magyar Allat. Lapja*, **11**, 723–30
47. Vlček, Z., Nedbálková, J., Svobodová, R. *et al.* (1980). Vitamin A in the blood serum, liver, corpora lutea, placentomas, and fetal fluids of cows, and in the blood serum and liver of their fetuses in the latter third of pregnancy. *Acta Vet. Brno.*, **49**, 37–44
48. Volintir, V., Popescu, I., Jivănescu, I. *et al.* (1971). Aspects of stachybotryotoxicosis and fusariotoxicosis in swine. *Rev. Zootech. Med. Vet.*, **21**, 68–78
49. Waddell, W. J. and Marlowe, G. C. (1976). Disposition of drugs in the fetus. In Mirkin, B. L. (ed.) *Perinatal Pharmacology and Therapeutics*. pp. 119–268. (New York: Academic Press)
50. Arora, R.G., Frölén, H. and Fellner-Feldegg, H. (1983). (Accepted for publication.) (*Fd. Chem. Toxicol.*)
51. Rosenberger, G., Dirksen, G., Gründer, H. D. *et al.* (1970). *Krankheiten des Rindes*. pp. 1–1390. (Berlin and Hamburg: Verlag Paul Parey)

4
Drug disposition in the newborn

R. Reiche

During the prenatal period drug actions on the fetus are nearly always undesired effects of the medication to the mother. In contrast, drug effects on the newborn organism are of high therapeutic interest since many diseases occur during early postnatal life which make drug treatment mandatory. Drug therapy of the neonate is often accompanied by adverse drug effects which may be due to its higher sensitivity to drugs but more often to differences in drug disposition[1]. Thus it is necessary to gain knowledge of the pharmacokinetics of drugs during this period of life in order to obtain a pharmacological basis of drug treatment.

Most of the physiological changes dealing with drug disposition in the neonatal period are of functional nature. Thus, the limited metabolic and excretory capacity of drug elimination leads to a prolongation of halflives of drugs during the first weeks of life. Furthermore, the reduced degree of binding to plasma proteins, the relative volumes of body fluid compartments and the permeability of the blood–brain barrier influence the distribution of the drug and sensitivity to the effects. Moreover, gross anatomical alterations are involved such as in the case of ruminants in which the development of the rumen influences the extent of drug absorption.

It is well-known fact that in newborn animals there is a deficiency in certain drug-metabolizing enzymes in liver microsomes. The immaturity of the enzyme system after birth includes nearly all oxidative and reductive reactions and the conjugation to glucuronic acid[10,15]. The activity of these enzymes rapidly increases with age and in small rodents the enzyme activities reach the level of the adult at 3–4 weeks of age[3,16].

A review of the literature about the elimination pattern of drugs in newborn and adult large animals shows, in general, a prolonged elimination time in the newborn animal. Only a limited number of studies have been undertaken in which drug-metabolizing capacity was determined by measuring plasma halflives of drugs administered to newborn calves.

The elimination halflives of different drugs in newborn calves and adult cattle are summarized in Table 4.1. In the neonatal ruminant mainly antibiotic and chemotherapeutic agents were studied. The age of the calves was

Table 4.1 Elimination halflives ($t_{1/2}$) of different drugs in newborn calves and cows

Drugs	*Calves* *Age* (weeks)	$t_{1/2}$ (h)	*Cows* $t_{1/2}$ (h)	*References*
Penicillin G	5–7	2.5	0.7	26, 27
Gentamicin	4–5	3.9	1.9	28, 29
Oxytetracycline	5–7	10.0	4.1	27, 28
Chloramphenicol	5–7	9.0	3.5	27, 30
Ampicillin	2–6	1.7	1.2	26, 31
Amoxycillin	2–6	1.6	1.3	31, 32
Streptomycin	5–7	3.0	2.0	27, 33
Kanamycin	2–4	2.2–2.7	3.5	34, 35

in the range of 2–7 weeks of life. In comparison to adult cattle, the halflives in calves of penicillin G, gentamicin, oxytetracycline and chloramphenicol were increased by a factor of 2–3.5. On the other hand, the halflives of ampicillin, amoxycillin and streptomycin were only slightly prolonged and in the case of kanamycin the halflife was even shorter in the newborn.

Similar findings were noted in newborn piglets (Table 4.2). The halflives of sulfadimethoxine and sulphadimidine were significantly prolonged in piglets and a more marked prolongation was observed for chloramphenicol and hexobarbital.

There is a wide variation in the ability to metabolize different drugs in newborn calves and piglets. It should not be concluded, therefore, that all metabolic pathways are deficient to the same degree. However, these pronounced differences make it necessary to find a dosage regimen only on the basis of individual evaluation of each drug in each species.

In recent experiments in our laboratory, the pharmacokinetics of chloramphenicol during the initial weeks of life were studied until values valid for adult cattle had been reached[20]. It was demonstrated that the pharmacokinetics of chloramphenicol in calves depends on age, at least during the first weeks of life. After intravenous injection, the halflife of the drug was nearly 15 h on the first day of life, and then fell rather rapidly to an average of 6.5 h on day 7. Further decline of the elimination halflife proceeded more slowly

Table 4.2 Elimination halflives ($t_{1/2}$) of different drugs in newborn piglets and growing pigs (8–12 weeks of life)

Drugs	*Piglets* *Age* (days)	$t_{1/2}$ (h)	*Pigs* $t_{1/2}$ (h)	*References*
Sulfadimethoxine	7–14	16.1	9.4	9
Sulphadimidine	1–2	12.9	9.1	10
Chloramphenicol	1–2	6.1	0.8	10
Hexobarbital	1–2	5.0	1.7	10

to 5.5 h at the age of 3 weeks. Even at the age of 10–12 weeks there remained a slight difference from the values obtained in adult animals (4.2 h vs. 4.8 h). The results seem to predominantly reflect a lack of or at least a deficiency in the ability to form the glucuronide of chloramphenicol which is the main metabolite. Thus, one could suggest that the ability of calves to form glucuronides develops mainly during the first 3 weeks of age.

Similar results were obtained by other groups in *in vitro* studies with liver homogenates of pigs at different ages[25,26]. In these studies the development of enzyme activity appeared to be most rapid during the first 3–4 weeks after birth and reached a plateau between 4 and 6 weeks of life. *In vivo* pharmacokinetic studies support the assumption that the age-related change in the enzyme activities occurred in the immediate postnatal period up to an age of 3–4 weeks[22,27]. Thereafter only slight differences from adult values would be expected.

It seems remarkable that the rate of development of liver enzyme systems in large animals like calves and piglets equals that of small rodents. Therefore, it is possible that this pattern is universal among all mammalian species, regardless of such factors as the size of the species and the maturation time and normal life span of the animal.

For drug therapy of the newborn, the delayed metabolism deserves special consideration if drugs are given which are inactive *per se* and must be converted into the biologically active form throughout the body.

In our laboratory, newborn calves and adult cattle were injected intravenously with chloramphenicol as the monosuccinate which has to be hydrolysed in order to release free chloramphenicol[20]. It was demonstrated that the rate at which the monosuccinate was hydrolysed to free chloramphenicol was age-dependent. The halflife of the intact ester fell from 33 min on the first day of life to 14 min in adult cattle. Free chloramphenicol, on the other hand, reached its maximum concentration 2–3 h after the injection of the ester in newborn calves, whereas the peak occurred in less than 15 min in cows.

It must therefore be taken into account that the time at which therapeutic concentrations are reached could be somewhat delayed in newborn animals if inactive drug forms were given.

In contrast, the risk of drug overdosage in the postnatal period may be enhanced if drugs are administered which are eliminated in a dose-related manner. An example of such a drug is the antiepileptic phenytoin. The dose-dependent elimination of phenytoin is apparent at high plasma concentrations, because a genetically determined saturation phenomenon inhibits the drug's metabolism. In the neonatal animal this saturation may occur at lower concentrations because of the immaturity of the liver enzyme systems. In order to test this possibility we studied the pharmacokinetics of phenytoin in newborn calves and cows[11].

It can be seen from the individual curves in Figure 4.1 that in a newborn calf, after the intravenous injection of 10 mg/kg phenytoin, a plateau was reached which lasted for nearly 2 days, whereas in the adult animal the plasma concentrations declined rapidly after injection. Even at the dose of 5 mg/kg the plateau lasted for 1½ days in a newborn calf before plasma

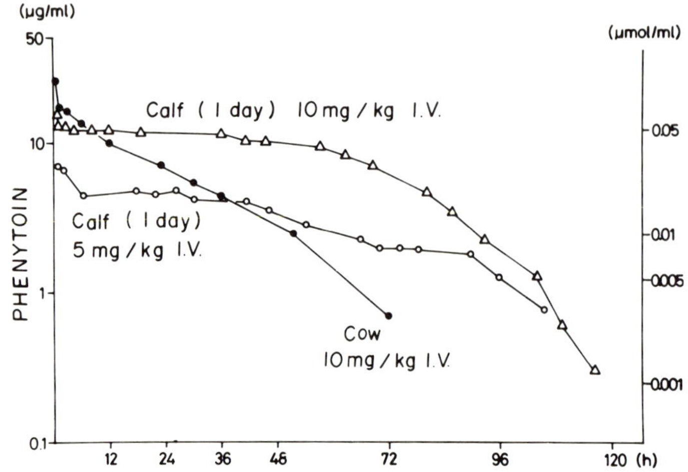

Fig. 4.1 Plasma concentrations of phenytoin after intravenous administration of 5 and 10 mg/kg (0.02 and 0.04 mmol/kg) in a newborn calf at an age of 1 day and in a cow

concentrations began to decrease. Thus, it could be concluded that a subsequent drug injection during the first 2–3 days after the initial dose of phenytoin would elevate the plasma level to toxic concentrations.

Next to metabolic degradation, renal excretory capacity is decisive for the termination of drug action. In most mammalian species, renal functions are limited in the postnatal period[2,11,12]. This leads to augmented and prolonged drug levels. In contrast to other newborn animals, the neonatal calf has efficient renal function[4,5], therefore, excretory function of the kidney should only play a minor role for age-related changes in drug disposition in the newborn calf.

Besides elimination, drug disposition is influenced by changes in body composition in the growing animal. In cattle, the total body water declines from 74% of body weight in newborns to 58% in adults. In contrast, in the same period of time the fat content increases from 2.8% to nearly 18% of body weight. In addition, differences in the compartmentalization of total body water must be considered. There is a decrease with age of the extracellular fluid volume which parallels the decline of the total body water, whereas the proportion of intracellular water remains constant[9,14,18]. Thus, changes in water and fat content of the body may cause age-dependent differences in drug distribution.

For example, the apparent volume of distribution of sulphadimidine in pigs and chloramphenicol in cattle decreases from 80% in newborns to 60% of body weight in adults, which probably reflects the decline of total body water[20,27]. Furthermore, the volume of distribution of sulfadimethoxine in pigs and Na-salicylate in pigs, dogs and cats ranged from 30% to nearly 50% of body weight in newborn animals and from 20% to more than 30% in adults suggesting that these drugs distribute mainly in extracellular fluid[6,7,22]. In contrast, the distribution of hexobarbital in pigs slightly increases with age[27]. Taking into account that hexobarbital is partly concentrated in the body fat, the age-related increase in fat content explains the observed difference.

Generally, this specific pattern of body composition results in a greater volume of distribution with correspondingly low plasma levels in the neonatal animal.

Besides differences in body composition, the distribution of drugs depends on the extent of plasma protein binding. In newborns there is a greater fraction of free drug available for distribution due to lower binding to plasma proteins[17,20]. This is certainly one of the reasons for stronger effects or even side-effects of drugs in the neonate. For instance, in the case of centrally active agents the lower binding results in higher brain concentrations and this effect is intensified by the underdevelopment of the blood–brain barrier[1].

Finally, the oral absorption of drugs in ruminants deserves special consideration. The characteristics of digestive physiology in adult ruminants limit the absorption of certain drugs, but newborn ruminants are functionally monogastric in the first weeks of life. Thus, drug absorption may be comparable with non-ruminants. This offers the chance to administer drugs via the oral route which is often impossible at a later age.

When acetylsalicylic acid and chloramphenicol were administered orally to calves at different ages, the maximum plasma concentrations attained differed markedly. With doses recommended for monogastric mammals and man, near therapeutic plasma concentrations can be reached during the first week of life, but during the following weeks these concentrations decline rapidly paralleling the development of the ruminant stomach[8,24]. The reason for the reduced rate of absorption in older calves is either an inactivation by ruminal content or a change of the pH gradients between plasma and gastrointestinal fluid[1,28].

In conclusion, drug disposition in the newborn differs markedly from adults and therefore special therapeutic implications should be considered. In general, when quantitative data are not available, the initial dose may be increased, especially in the case of antibiotics, with respect to the greater volume of distribution. On the other hand, since drug elimination is delayed, a larger dose interval should be used or the maintenance dose should be decreased to avoid accumulation. These general recommendations should be considered for the first 3–4 weeks of life. Thereafter the dose for adults may be given per unit of body weight.

References

1. Baggot, J. D. (1977). *Principles of Drug Disposition in Domestic Animals*. (Philadelphia, London, Toronto: W. B. Saunders)
2. Bräulich, H. (1974). In Ankermann, H. (ed.) *Entwicklungspharmakologie*. (Stuttgart: Gustav Fischer Verlag)
3. Brown, A. K., Zuelzer, W. W. and Burnett, H. H. (1958). Studies on the neonatal development of the glucoronide conjugating system. *J. Clin. Invest.*, **37**, 332–40
4. Dalton, R. G. (1968). Renal function in neonatal calves: urea clearance. *Br. Vet. J.*, **124**, 451–9
5. Dalton, R. G. (1968). Renal function in neonatal calves: inulin, thiosulphate and para-amino-hippuric acid clearance. *Br. Vet. J.*, **124**, 498–502

6. Davis, L. E. and Westfall, B. A. (1972). Species differences in biotransformation and excretion of salicylate. *Am. J. Vet. Res.*, **33**, 1253–62
7. Davis, L. E., Westfall, B. A. and Short, C. R. (1973). Biotransformation and pharmacokinetics of salicylate in newborn animals. *Am. J. Vet. Res.*, **34**, 1105–8
8. De Backer, P., Debackere, M. and De Corte-Baeten, K. (1978). Plasma levels of chloramphenicol after oral administration in calves during the first weeks of life. *J. Vet. Pharmacol. Ther.*, **1**, 135–40
9. Ellenberger, H. B., Newlander, J. A. and Jones, C. H. (1950). Composition of the bodies of dairy cattle. *Vermont Agric. Exp. Stn. Bull.*, **558**, 1–66
10. Fouts, J. R. and Adamson, R. H. (1959). Drug metabolism in the newborn rabbit. *Science*, **129**, 897–8
11. Friis, C. (1979). Postnatal development of renal function in piglets: glomerular filtration rate, clearance of PAH and PAH extraction. *Biol. Neonate*, **35**, 180–7
12. Friis, C. (1981). Postnatal development of renal function in piglets: changes in excretory pattern of sulphachlorpyridazine. *Acta Pharmacol. Toxicol.*, **48**, 409–17
13. Hammond, P. B. (1953). Dihydrostreptomycin dose-serum level relationships in cattle. *J. Am. Vet. Med. Assoc.*, **122**, 203–6
14. Hix, E. L., Underbjerg, G. K. L. and Hughes, J. S. (1959). The body fluids of ruminants and their simultaneous determination. *Am. J. Vet. Res.*, **20**, 184–91
15. Jondorf, W. R., Maickel, R. P. and Brodie, B. B. (1958). Inability of newborn mice and guinea pigs to metabolize drugs. *Biochem. Pharmacol.*, **1**, 352–4
16. Kato, R., Vassanelli, P., Frontino, G. *et al.* (1964). Variation in the activity of liver microsomal drug-metabolizing enzymes in rats in relation to the age. *Biochem. Pharmacol.*, **13**, 1037–51
17. Kurz, H., Mauser-Ganshorn, A. and Stickel, H. H. (1977). Differences in the binding of drugs to plasma proteins from newborn and adult man. *Eur. J. Clin. Pharmacol.*, **11**, 463–72
18. Payne, E., Ryley, J. W. and Gartner, R. J. W. (1967). Plasma, blood and extracellular fluid volumes in grazing Hereford cattle. *Res. Vet. Sci.*, **8**, 20–6
19. Pilloud, M. (1973). Pharmacokinetics, plasma protein binding and dosage of chloramphenicol in cattle and horses. *Res. Vet. Sci.*, **15**, 231–8
20. Reiche, R., Mülling, M. and Frey, H.-H. (1980). Pharmacokinetics of chloramphenicol in calves during the first weeks of life. *J. Vet. Pharmacol. Ther.*, **3**, 95–106
21. Reiche, R., Mülling, M. and Frey, H.-H. (1982). In preparation
22. Righter, H. F., Showalter, D. H. and Teske, R. H. (1979). Pharmacokinetic study of sulfadimethoxine depletion in suckling and growing pigs. *Am. J. Vet. Res.*, **40**, 713–15
23. Rutgers, L. J. E., van Miert, A. S. J. P. A. M., Nouws, J. F. M. *et al.* (1980). Effect of the injection site on the bioavailability of amoxycillin trihydrate in dairy cows. *J. Vet. Pharmacol. Ther.*, **3**, 125–32
24. Sechserova, M., Sechser, T., Raskova, H. *et al.* (1979). Ontogenic drug studies in calves. 1. Age dependent salicylate levels and metabolism. *Arzneimitt. Forsch.*, **29**, 650–1
25. Short, C. R. and Davis, L. E. (1970). Perinatal development of drug-metabolizing enzyme activity in swine. *J. Pharmacol. Exp. Ther.*, **174**, 185–96
26. Short, C. R. and Stith, R. D. (1973). Perinatal development of hepatic microsomal mixed function oxidase activity in swine. *Biochem. Pharmacol.*, **22**, 1309–19
27. Svendsen, O. (1976). Pharmacokinetics of hexobarbital, sulphadimidine and chloramphenicol in neonatal and young pigs. *Acta Vet. Scand.*, **17**, 1–14
28. Theodorides, V. J., Dicuollo, C. J., Guarini, J. R. *et al.* (1968). Serum concentration of chloramphenicol after intraruminal and intra-abomasal administration in sheep. *Am. J. Vet. Res.*, **29**, 643–5
29. Ziv, G. (1977). Comparative clinical pharmacology of amikacin and kanamycin in dairy calves. *Am. J. Vet. Res.*, **38**, 337–40
30. Ziv, G. and Sulman, F. G. (1974). Distribution of aminoglycoside antibiotics in blood and milk. *Res. Vet. Sci.*, **17**, 68–74
31. Ziv, G. and Sulman, F. G. (1974). Analysis of pharmacokinetic properties of nine tetracycline analogues in dairy cows and ewes. *Am. J. Vet. Res.*, **35**, 1197–200
32. Ziv, G., Nouws, J. F. M., Groothuis, D. G. *et al.* (1977). Oral absorption and bioavailability of ampicillin derivatives in calves. *Am. J. Vet. Res.*, **38**, 1007–13

33. Ziv, G., Shani, J. and Sulman, F. G. (1973). Pharmacokinetic evaluation of penicillin and cephalosporin derivatives in serum and milk of lactating cows and ewes. *Am. J. Vet. Res.*, **34**, 1561–5
34. Ziv, G., Nouws, J. F. M. and van Ginneken, C. A. M. (1982). The pharmacokinetics and tissue levels of polymycin B, colistin and gentamycin in calves. *J. Vet. Pharmacol. Ther.*, **5**, 45–58
35. Ziv, G., Wanner, M. and Nicolet, J. (1982). Distribution of penicillin G, dihydrostreptomycin, oxytetracycline, and chloramphenicol in serum and subcutaneous chamber fluids. *J. Vet. Pharmacol. Ther.*, **5**, 59–69

5
Postnatal development of renal function in goats

C. Friis

It is well established that the efficiency of the kidney is lower in newborn than in adult animals. In the newborn, renal blood flow and glomerular filtration rate (GFR) are low, concentrating and acidifying functions are restricted and the capacity to secrete organic compounds is limited[11]. However, the level of maturity in renal function at birth varies widely from one species to another. In most laboratory animals such as rats[12], rabbits[16], and dogs[14] the functional values increase several times from birth to adulthood, whereas relatively small rises are reported for infants[6], pigs[8] and sheep[3,1]. The aim of the present study was to extend our knowledge of renal maturation to a second ruminant, the goat.

METHODS

Clearance of inulin (GFR) and clearance of *p*-aminohippurate (PAH) were measured in nine unanaesthetized female goats ranging in age from 1 to 78 days. The animals were studied serially at two or three different ages. After a subcutaneous administration of inulin (200 mg/kg) and PAH (120 mg/kg), an equilibration period of 50 min was allowed before three 20- or 30-min urine samples were collected through a Foley catheter. Blood samples were obtained from the jugular vein 5 min before the midpoint of each urine collection period to correct for urinary dead space.

Six kids aged 2–82 days and one adult goat were subjected to renal PAH extraction studies. The animals were anaesthetized with sodium pentobarbital (25 mg/kg i.v.) and prepared surgically for the study as described previously[8]. A priming dose of inulin (40 mg/kg) and PAH (30–60 mg/kg) was administered followed by constant infusion of inulin (0.6 mg kg^{-1} min^{-1}) and PAH (0.4–1.0 mg kg^{-1} min^{-1}) in physiological saline at a rate of 0.2–0.5 ml/min. After an equilibration period of 30 min three 20-min urine samples were collected. At the midpoint of each period arterial and renal venous blood samples were obtained simultaneously. Systemic arterial blood pressure was monitored continuously by means of a Statham transducer P 23 AA.

Urine and plasma were analysed for inulin by the hexokinase method[21] and for PAH by the method of Bratton and Marshall[4].

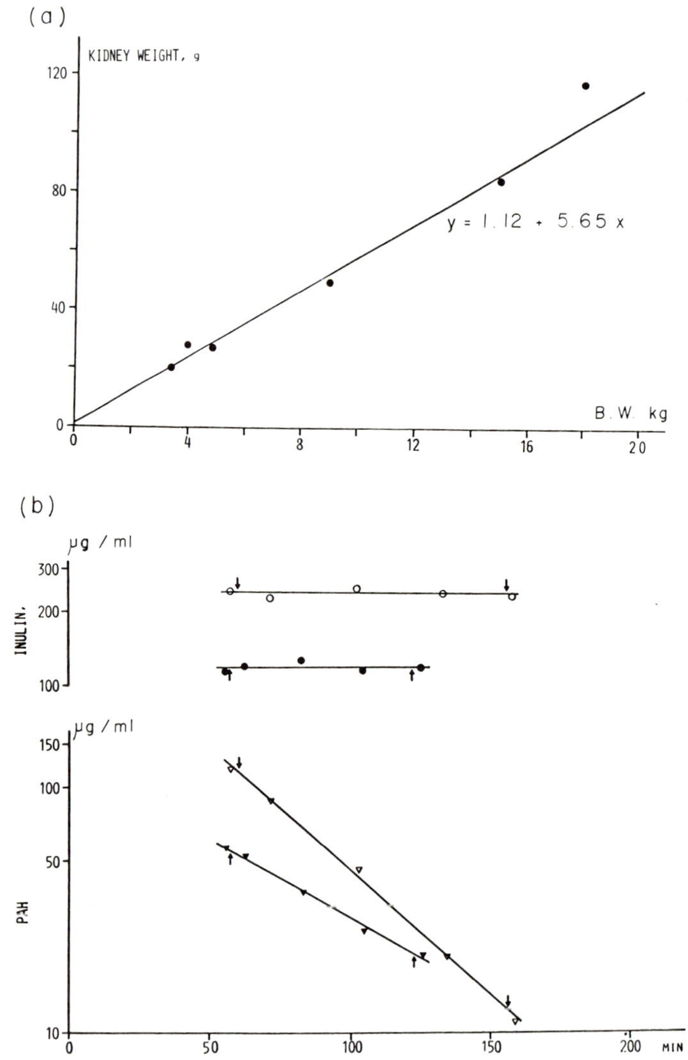

Figure 5.1 (a) Kidney weight as a function of body weight during the neonatal period in the goat. (b) Plasma concentrations of inulin and PAH, after subcutaneous administration, plotted on a semilogarithmic scale. ○, ▽: 1 day old goat; ●, ▼: 66 day old goat. The arrows indicate the period during which clearance measurements were performed

RESULTS

Relationship between kidney weight and body weight

The kidney weight and body weight were closely correlated over the age range studied ($r = 0.97$, $p < 0.001$) (Figure 5.1 (a)). In order to present the results per gram of kidney, the kidney weight was calculated for each subject using the equation:

$$\text{Kidney wt. (g)} = 1.12 + 5.65 \times \text{body wt (kg)}$$

Glomerular filtration rate and clearance of PAH in unanaesthetized goats

As illustrated in Figure 5.1 (b) the subcutaneous administration of inulin caused a constant plasma concentration during the urine collection periods. Glomerular filtration rate (GFR) increased slightly from birth to 2 weeks of age whether comparisons were made on basis of body weight or kidney weight (Table 5.1). At 2 weeks GFR was similar to that found at 10 weeks suggesting that the mature level was reached during the first 2 weeks of life.

The absorption of PAH was rapid with maximal plasma concentration obtained within 20–30 min following injection. Accordingly, the plasma PAH concentration declined during the experiments (Figure 5.1 (b)). Clearance of PAH (C_{PAH}) per kg body weight or per g kidney weight increased twofold from birth to adult level attained at 2 weeks (Table 5.1).

As a consequence of the more pronounced increase in C_{PAH} than in GFR the ratio C_{PAH}/GFR increased with age (Table 5.1). (The ratio was calculated for each subject.)

Table 5.1 Glomerular filtration rate (GFR) and PAH clearance (C_{PAH}) in unanaesthetized goats aged 1–78 days (mean ± SD)

Age	*Body wt.*	*GFR*		*C_{PAH}*		*C_{PAH}*
		$ml\ min^{-1} kg^{-1}$	$ml\ min^{-1} g^{-1}$	$ml\ min^{-1} kg^{-1}$	$ml\ min^{-1} g^{-1}$	———
days	kg	*Body wt.*	*Kidney wt.*	*Body wt.*	*Kidney wt.*	*GFR*
1-3 $N = 5$	2.6 ± 0.4	2.1 ± 0.6	0.35 ± 0.09	5.5 ± 0.5	0.90 ± 0.08	2.76 ± 0.82
14–20 $N = 5$	4.9 ± 0.8	3.3 ± 0.2	0.56 ± 0.04	10.2 ± 0.8	1.74 ± 0.14	3.15 ± 0.36
64-78 $N = 9$	12.5 ± 1.0	2.8 ± 0.5	0.48 ± 0.09	12.8 ± 2.9	2.22 ± 0.51	4.66 ± 0.90

PAH extraction and renal blood flow in anaesthetized goats

Renal PAH extraction (E_{PAH}) appeared to increase with age in parallel with C_{PAH}, reaching the mature value within the first 2 weeks of life (Table 5.2). In general, the values for GFR and C_{PAH} measured simultaneously with E_{PAH} were a little lower than those found in unanaesthetized goats (Tables 5.1 and 5.2).

Table 5.2 Renal PAH extraction (E_{PAH}) and renal blood flow (RBF) in anaesthetized goats of different age

Age days	*Body wt.* kg	*GFR* $ml\,min^{-1}g^{-1}$ *Kidney wt.*	C_{PAH} $ml\,min^{-1}g^{-1}$ *Kidney wt.*	E_{PAH}	*RBF* $ml\,min^{-1}g^{-1}$ *Kidney wt.*	*FF* *F*	*MAP* mmHg
2	3.4	0.39	0.62	0.42	2.25	0.26	65
16	4.0	0.43	1.03	0.84	1.89	0.35	115
16	4.8	0.49	1.49	0.87	2.52	0.29	90
36	9.0	0.47	1.43	0.71	2.89	0.23	100
74	18.0	0.33	1.50	0.68	4.03	0.15	105
82	17.0	0.33	1.06	0.62	2.83	0.20	120
adult	20.0	0.41	1.89	0.88	3.12	0.19	135

Renal blood flow (RBF) was calculated by applying the formula:

$$RBF = (C_{PAH}/E_{PAH})/(1 - \text{venous haematocrit})$$

RBF related to kidney weight tended to increase with age (Table 5.2)

Mean arterial blood pressure (MABP) was markedly lower at birth than found after the 2nd postnatal week (Table 5.2).

The fraction of plasma filtered (FF), measured as $GFR/(C_{PAH}/E_{PAH})$ varied from 0.26 to 0.35 during an early postnatal age and from 0.15 to 0.20 at the end of the period under study.

DISCUSSION

The observed maturational changes in GFR, C_{PAH}, and E_{PAH} in goats are compared with those previously reported for various species in Table 5.3. The rise in GFR corrected for kidney weight in goats corresponds well with findings in sheep[2] and cattle[10,20] but is somewhat smaller than that observed in pigs[8] and much smaller than those seen in dogs[14], rabbits[16], and rats[12]. The different levels of maturity in GFR at birth may partially be attributed to the different degree of anatomical development between species. In sheep[22] and cattle[5] the formation of new nephrons terminates during fetal life, whereas it continues until 3 weeks after birth in pigs[9], dogs[13], rabbits[19], and rats[17]. No study has been published on the anatomical development of the goat kidney. Several factors including enlargement of the filtering area[15,18], changes in the permeability of the filtering membrane[14], increases in effective filtration pressure[24] and glomerular blood flow[2,3] are considered to contribute to the development in GFR. In the newborn sheep the glomerular blood flow appears to be the main determinant of the rise in GFR[2,22].

During the early postnatal period, the filtration fraction increases in dogs[14] and rats[12], while it remains constant in infants[6] and pigs[8]. The few experiments in the present study do not allow any conclusions to be drawn concerning the age-related change in the filtration fraction in goats. However, the data seem to present a conflict in that the filtration fraction declines after the renal functions have reached adulthood. This paradox may partly be explained by the variation in E_{PAH}.

Table 5.3 Postnatal development of glomerular filtration rate (inulin clearance), clearance of PAH and PAH extraction in various species

Species	*Age* days	*GFR* ml min^{-1}kg^{-1} *Body wt.*	ml min^{-1}g^{-1} *Kidney wt.*	C_{PAH} ml min^{-1}kg^{-1} *Body wt.*	ml min^{-1}g^{-1} *Kidney wt.*	E_{PAH}	*Reference*
Rat	1–3	0.3	0.04	2.6	0.36	0.21	12
	16–18	2.0	0.33	5.6	0.94	0.74	
Rabbit	10	0.3	0.04	1.2	0.15	0.29	16
	28	1.6	0.31	5.1	0.96	0.72	
Dog	2–8	1.5	0.18	1.8	0.22	0.23	14
	60–77	5.0	0.90	12.4	2.21	0.77	
Pig	1–3	2.2	0.27	8.4	1.02	0.75	8
	56–79	3.0	0.59	8.7	1.72	0.87	
Goat	1–3	2.1	0.35	5.5	0.90	0.42	Friis
	64–78	2.8	0.48	12.8	2.22	0.73	
Sheep	2–4	2.7*	0.32*	5.5†	—	—	*2
	53–79	2.6*	0.54*	12.7†	—	—	†1
Cattle	1–3	1.8	0.47	6.2	1.61	—	10
	adult	1.8	0.87	—	—	—	20

As for GFR the age-related increases in C_{PAH} and E_{PAH} are less pronounced in goats than found in dogs[14], rabbits[16], and rats[12]. Factors considered to account for the developmental changes in C_{PAH} and E_{PAH} include increases in tubular mass[12,23], intrinsic transport capacity[11,23], and peritubular blood supply[7]. Recently, Evan *et al.*[7] have shown that the young puppy kidney does not possess peritubular capillaries, but instead sinusoidal vessels that connect directly to the venous system. This creates a shunt in that the blood flow from the efferent arteriole would be directed into the venous system, thus bypassing the proximal tubule. Accordingly, only a small load of PAH may reach the developing proximal tubule, resulting in a low secretory rate and subsequently a low extraction ratio.

The age-related increase in the ratio C_{PAH}/GFR observed in the present study indicates a greater postnatal rise in the tubular than in the glomerular function. This increase may be related to the above mentioned change in intrarenal vascular structure as well as to a demonstrated morphological imbalance between glomerular and tubular growth[13,22].

In summary, the present study demonstrates a postnatal rise in GFR, C_{PAH} and E_{PAH} in goats. Mature values are reached within the first 2 weeks of life. The observed changes agree well with findings in other ruminants but are less pronounced than those seen in most laboratory animals.

References

1. Alexander, D. P. and Nixon, D. A. (1962). Plasma clearance of *p*-aminohippuric acid by the kidney of faetal, neonatal and adult sheep. *Nature (London)*, **194**, 483–4
2. Aperia, A., Broberger, O. and Herin, P. (1974). Maturational changes in glomerular perfusion rate and glomerular filtration rate in lambs. *Pediatr. Res.*, **8**, 758–65

3. Aperia, A. and Herin, P. (1975). Development of glomerular perfusion rate and nephron filtration rate in rats 17–60 days old. *Am. J. Physiol.*, **228,** 1319–25
4. Bratton, A. C. and Marshall, E. K., Jr. (1939). A new coupling component for sulfanilamide determination. *J. Biol. Chem.*, **128,** 537–50
5. Cade-Treyer, D. and Tsuji, S. (1975). *In vitro* culture of the proximal tubule of the bovine nephron. *Cell Tissue Res.*, **163,** 15
6. Calcagno, P. L. and Rubin, M. I. (1963). Renal extraction of *para*-aminohippurate in infants and children. *J. Clin. Invest.*, **42,** 1632–9
7. Evan, A. P., Jr., Stoeckel, J. A., Loemker, V. and Baker, J. T. (1979). Development of the intrarenal vascular system of the puppy kidney. *Anat. Rec.*, **194,** 187–200
8. Friis, C. (1979). Postnatal development of renal function in piglets: glomerular filtration rate, clearance of PAH and PAH extraction. *Biol. Neonate*, **35,** 180–7
9. Friis, C. (1980). Postnatal development of the pig kidney: ultrastructure of the glomerulus and the proximal tubule. *J. Anat.*, **130,** 513–26
10. Friis, C. Unpublished
11. Hook, J. B. and Bailie, M. D. (1979). Perinatal renal pharmacology. *Ann. Rev. Pharmacol. Toxicol.*, **19,** 491–509
12. Horster, M. and Lewy, J. E. (1970). Filtration fraction and extraction of PAH during neonatal period in the rat. *Am. J. Physiol.*, **219,** 1061–5
13. Horster, M., Kemler, B. J. and Valtin, H. (1971). Intracortical distribution of number and volume of glomeruli during postnatal maturation in the dog. *J. Clin. Invest.*, **50,** 796–800
14. Horster, M. and Valtin, H. (1971). Postnatal development of the renal function: micropuncture and clearance studies in the dog. *J. Clin. Invest.*, **50,** 779–95
15. John, E., Goldsmith, D. I. and Spitzer, A. (1981). Quantitative changes in the canine glomerular vasculature during development: physiologic implications. *Kidney Int.*, **20,** 223–9
16. Kaplan, M. R. and Lewy, J. E. (1978). Stimulation of *p*-aminohippurate extraction in the maturing rabbit kidney. *Pediatr. Res.*, **12,** 834–7
17. Larsson, L. (1975). The ultrastructure of the developing proximal tubule in the rat kidney. *J. Ultrastruct. Res.*, **51,** 119–39
18. Larsson, L. and Maunsbach, A. B. (1980). The ultrastructural development of the glomerular filtration barrier in the rat kidney: a morphometric analysis. *J. Ultrastruct. Res.*, **72,** 392–406
19. Perey, D. Y. E., Herdman, R. C. and Good, R. A. (1967). Polycystic renal disease: new experimental model. *Science*, **158,** 494–6
20. Poulsen, E. (1957). Renal clearance in the cow. *Royal Veterinary and Agricultural College, Copenhagen, Yearbook*. pp. 97–126.
21. Renschler, H. E. (1963). Die Anwendung enzymatischer Methoden zur Bestimmung von Inulin. *Klin. Wochenschr.*, **41,** 615–18
22. Robillard, J. E., Weismann, D. N. and Herin, P. (1981). Ontogeny of single glomerular perfusion rate in fetal and newborn lambs. *Pediatr. Res.*, **15,** 1248–55
23. Schwartz, G. J., Goldsmith, D. I. and Fine, L. G. (1978). *p*-Aminohippurate transport in the proximal straight tubule: Development and substrate stimulation. *Pediatr. Res.*, **12,** 793–6
24. Spitzer, A. and Edelmann, C. M., Jr. (1971). Maturational changes in pressure gradients for glomerular filtration. *Am. J. Physiol.*, **221,** 1431–5

6
Developmental patterns of penicillin G excretion

C. R. Short

The old adage reminding us that 'the newborn infant is more than a miniature version of the adult' is never more important than when considering drug therapy. Indeed, during the immediate postnatal period, the infant is biochemically, physiologically and microbiologically distinct from the adult of its species. Since drug therapy is designed to manipulate biochemistry, physiology, or flora, it is not unexpected that the approach to treatment of disease in the newborn has unique features.

Almost all drugs, or their metabolites, are removed from the body to some extent via renal excretion. The mechanisms operative in renal excretion are glomerular filtration, active proximal tubular secretion, and passive tubular reabsorption. Since the fetus produces only very small amounts of urine, if any (depending on species), it is obvious that profound changes take place at birth. Of particular interest are the (a) increase in renal plasma flow, (b) functional development of glomeruli, (c) the maturation of active secretory processes in the proximal tubule and an increase in tubular mass, and (d) changes in urinary pH which affect the reabsorbability of drugs in the lower nephron. These processes change at different rates in different species, as do the elimination profiles of most drugs that have been studied to date.

Since many antibiotics are eliminated primarily via renal excretion, it is apparent that there may be substantial age-related changes in halflife for these agents in the early postnatal period. Very few studies, however, have examined the pharmacokinetics of antibiotics in the newborn, particularly the offspring of domestic agricultural species. Two recent papers[16,24] have reported marked age-related changes in chloramphenicol halflives in the pig and calf, respectively. Both of these groups observed marked declines in halflife during the first week, with smaller decreases in the ensuing weeks. Since chloramphenicol is also extensively metabolized, principally by glucuronidation, the rate of maturity of this function (and biliary excretion) in the liver will influence these changes in halflife.

In order to evaluate the influence of renal maturation on excretion, we have chosen to study the developmental pharmacokinetics of penicillin G. This antibiotic is rapidly excreted via active tubular secretion in the adult. Thus, its excretion would be affected as much as that of any antibiotic by deficiencies in the newborn kidney. These studies were conducted in the pig because it has a very marked deficiency in hepatic drug metabolizing mechanisms at birth[19,20,21], and we were interested in whether or not the active renal acidic secretory system developed in parallel with drug metabolism. We have also studied the calf, because of its precocious development of inulin and *p*-aminohippuric acid (PAH) clearances[6], which suggest a very rapid development of renal function.

ANATOMICAL DEVELOPMENT

Numerous studies have described the morphological character of the rat kidney at birth, and its development over the first several weeks of life. Postnatal nephrogenesis has been found to be a marked feature of the rat kidney[3]. The number of nephrons tripled between birth and 28 days. The peripheral neogenic zone developed slowly with age and did not appear to contain functional nephron units at birth. Many of the proximal tubules, even of the inner cortex, were characterized by poorly developed microvillae. At birth, the glomeruli of the rat are in various stages of formation, and the tubular system is likewise not fully formed[4]. The brush border of the proximal tubules is very poorly developed and the loop of Henle is weakly differentiated. Renal papillae are short, and the collecting tubules are few in number. The mitochondria of the proximal tubule are round rather than elongated, as in the adult, and they do not have the basal orientation characteristic of the adult. We have confirmed the embryonic state of the rat kidney at birth by scanning and transmission electron microscopy[22].

The kidney of the rabbit has been shown also to be quite immature at birth, from a morphological standpoint[10]. The kidney of man, however, has been reported to be highly differentiated at birth[7,8,15,26], and it is well known that the human fetus produces urine as early as the mid-trimester. It is also well established that the full-term human infant possesses a full complement of glomeruli, and that the number of nephrons does not increase after birth. Indeed, the presence of a subcapsular neogenic zone is indicative of prematurity of the newborn[15]. There is, instead, a considerable increase in tubular tissue and tubular volume in each nephron[8] with age. The proximal tubules in the full-term infant are small in relation to their corresponding glomeruli, and glomerulotubular balance develops over a period of several months. There is also a decrease in the heterogeneity of glomerulotubular units, which is quite prominent at birth[7].

We have examined the morphological development of pig kidney for comparison with man and the rat, which are at opposite extremes with regard to the extent of neogenesis after birth. It is apparent that the pig is more similar to man, although there is a distinct subcapsular neogenic zone in the newborn piglet, which is evident for at least 3 weeks.

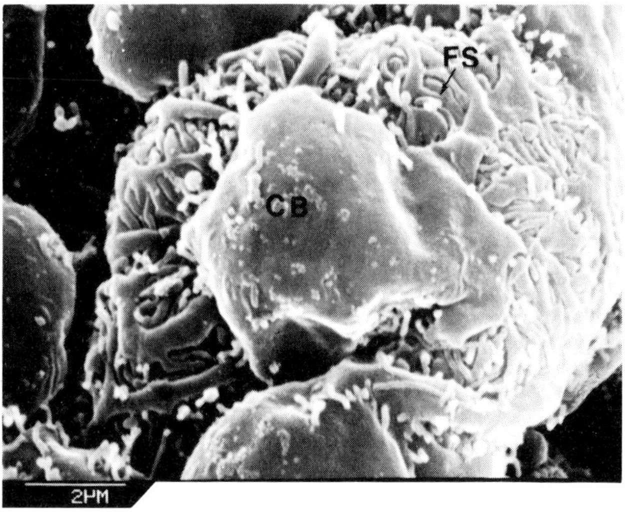

Figure 6.1 Scanning electron micrograph of a glomerulus of a 12–24 h old pig. Kidney was perfused with 4% formal–1% gluteraldehyde solution, dehydrated in an alcohol series, critical point dried, and sputter coated with gold-palladium alloy. High magnification provides an evaluation of podocyte cell body (CB) and filtration slit (FS)

The glomeruli of the inner cortex are considerably larger and contain more podocytes on the first day than those of the rat. Higher magnification (Figure 6.1) provides an evaluation of the degree of podocytic branching, which is also more advanced than in most glomeruli of the rat. While not all cells show

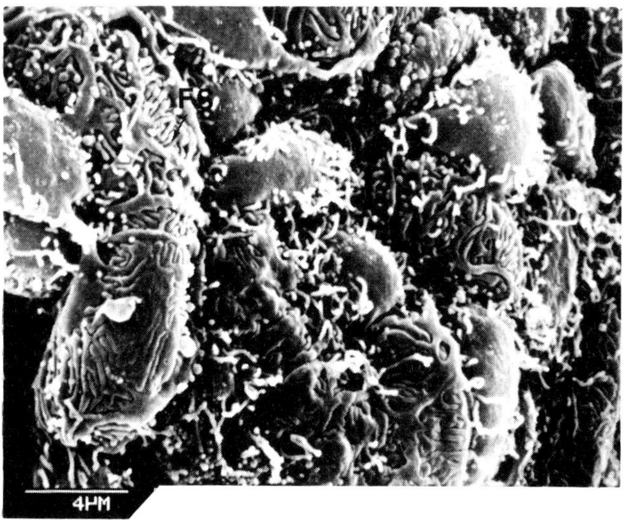

Figure 6.2 Glomerulus of a 4 day old pig. Specimen prepared as described above illustrating extensive interdigitation of podocytic feet. Filtration slits (FS)

this degree of differentiation, filtration slits surrounding the glomerular capillaries are evident. Figure 6.2 shows a higher degree of organization at 4 days of age. Under high magnification, primary, secondary and tertiary branches are observed on nearly all podocyte cell bodies. Between 4 and 21 days (the oldest age examined) it was difficult to distinguish morphological differences in glomerular structure by scanning electron microscopy.

Transmission microscopy, however, reveals that the endothelial cells of the capillary vasculature within the glomerulus have not yet developed a lumenal character (Figure 6.3). While the podocytic feet are observed attached to the basilar lamina, forming filtration slits, there are few clear fenestrations on

(a)

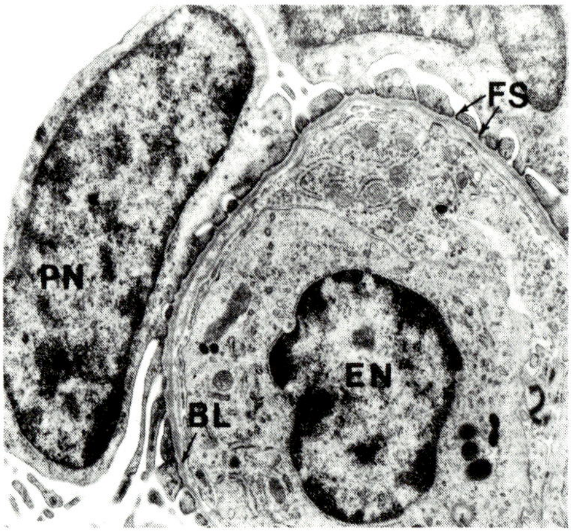

(b)

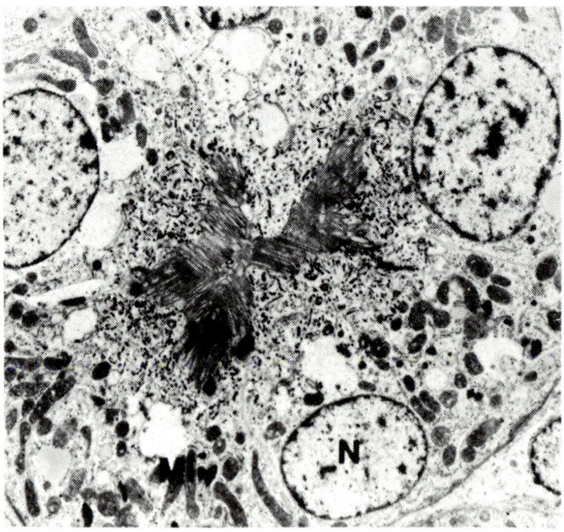

Figure 6.3 Transmission electron micrograph of a portion of a glomerulus within the inner renal cortex of a 12–24 h old pig. (a) Kidney was perfused, osmicated, dehydrated and embedded in Epon/Araldite resin. Podocyte nucleus (PN), filtration slits (FS), basilar lamina (BL), endothelial cell nucleus (EN) (×4900). (b) Cross-section of a proximal tubule from the inner renal cortex. Nucleus of tubular epithelial cell (N), microvillae (Mv), mitochondria (Mi) (×3100)

the capillary side of the membrane. Moreover, the nucleus and cytoplasm of the cell fill the intracellular space, and there is little or no lumen present. There was very little heterogeneity in the degree of endothelial cell immaturity within any single glomerulus examined. Larger lumens were observed in other glomeruli, but in no case was a typically mature endothelial cell observed. By 3 weeks of age, nearly all glomerular capillaries in the inner cortex are of characteristic adult morphology.

The proximal tubular segment of the typical nephron from the pig also appears to be more mature than that of the rat. A prominent 'brush border' of microvillae is present in nearly all cross-sections, and can even be observed under light microscopy. As seen in Figure 6.3, the nuclei also have a basilar orientation, and the mitochondria are numerous and elongated as in the mature kidney. By 4 days of age, however, the cells lining the tubule clearly show more organization, increased nuclear density, and increased membrane development. By 3 weeks of age, a more obvious tubular lumen is evident.

To summarize, the kidney of the newborn pig is, from a morphological point of view, much more mature than that of the rat, but shows structural characteristics which would suggest functional immaturity. Particularly striking is the lack of capillary endothelial cell differentiation, and it is tempting to propose that the postnatal decrease in renal resistance observed in the pig[9] is at least partly a function of increase in endothelial cell lumen.

FUNCTIONAL STUDIES

Two commonly studied parameters of renal function are the measurement of inulin clearance and the clearance of *para*-aminohippuric acid (PAH). The former is useful as an estimate of glomerular filtration rate (GFR), while the latter provides an estimate of active tubular secretion and effective renal plasma flow. Clinical studies[18] in human infants indicate that GFR increases rapidly in the newborn human infant, reaching the normal adult range of values within 5–10 days after birth when calculated on the basis of cell mass. Rapid increases in mannitol clearance (C_m) per unit surface area are observed over the first 2 weeks of life[26]. However, marked species differences in the rate of GFR increase, as measured by inulin clearance (C_{IN}), have been reported. The rat at 1 day of age is reported to have a very low GFR compared to the dog[11], the sheep[1], and the cow[6]. The calf, in particular, is reported to increase C_{IN} very rapidly, achieving an essentially mature filtration rate by the second day after birth. Comparable data has not been found in the literature for the pig.

PAH clearance (C_{PAH}), likewise, varies among species in their postnatal development. In contrast to the relatively rapid increase in C_{IN} in human infants, tubular secretory activity (C_{PAH}) increases slowly, and does not fall within the adult human range of values for at least 1 month of age[18]. A relatively slow increase in C_{PAH} is reported[26] compared to C_m.

Indeed, the filtration fraction (C_m/C_{PAH}) decreased slowly during the first few months after birth. The maximal tubular excretory capacity (Tm_{PAH}) increased slowly for approximately 30 weeks. The C_{PAH}/Tm_{PAH} ratio fell rapidly to a value which did not change from that point to 2 years of age, suggesting a proportional increase in renal blood flow accompanying development of the tubules. The initially high values could be explained by an anatomic imbalance between glomerular and tubular development, the former being favoured by a disproportionally large glomerular surface or increased glomerular pressure. The imbalance might also be caused by a decreased PAH extraction ratio[5].

In the human infant, the apparent anatomical imbalance between glomerular and tubular development probably explains the rapid increase in filtration rate, relative to body surface area, and the slower development of tubular excretory function and effective renal plasma flow. Once again, however, substantial species variations are apparent, as studies in the rat, dog, sheep and cow have shown developmental profiles similar to those for C_{IN} in these species. The most rapid increase in C_{PAH} has been reported in the calf[6] where adult values are observed by the second day after birth. The only data available on the pig[25] indicates that PAH excretion is limited to the proximal tubule in both the neonate and the adult.

Renal blood flow has been measured as a function of postnatal age in the pig, and found to increase over 18 fold in the first 45 days of life[9]. To avoid the possibility of lower PAH extraction efficiency in the newborn pig, the flow was measured with scandium-96 nuclide microspheres. A 7.2 fold increase in cardiac output was calculated over this period, and an 86% drop in renal vascular resistance, which together could largely account for the increase in renal flow.

Another method which has been developed to study the active tubular secretion of organic acids is the renal cortex slice-binding experiment. This *in vitro* assay measures renal cortical slice uptake of an acidic substrate, such as PAH or penicillin, or a base, which is commonly tetraethylammonium (TEA). The inference made is that binding occurs to a transport protein, and may be an index of the activity of the acidic or basic secretory mechanisms in the proximal tubule. For example, it has been shown that the binding of both PAH and TEA increased over the first several weeks after birth in the dog[17]. Studies in the pig show that with both substrates, binding increases with age in the subcapsular cortex, but remains fairly constant in the deeper cortex. This is reasonable to expect if there is some degree of nephrogenesis occurring during the first several weeks in the pig. The exact meaning of these studies is, however, difficult to define, as binding of PAH was shown to be higher in the near-term fetal pup than at birth. A similar finding was reported in rabbits[14], and mitigates against a correlation between binding and active secretion.

EXCRETION OF PENICILLINS

Deficiencies in filtration and tubular secretion at birth would be expected to cause prolonged elimination of most antibiotics. If effective renal plasma flow is low at birth, one would expect that the excretion of penicillin would also be reduced, as it is actively secreted by the proximal tubule in the same manner as PAH. Several studies in the human infant indicate that this is the case, i.e. that the clearance of penicillin roughly parallels C_{PAH} during the first 2–3 months after birth. Comparing clearances of penicillin G in premature infants and children, it was found that the infants, which weighed approximately 2.3 kg and were 4–8 days old, had clearances of about 10 ml/min compared to almost 400 ml/min in children aged 8.5–11.6 years[2]. Corrected for surface area (1.73 m^2), the difference became 102 ml/min vs. 596 ml/min. Penicillin clearance is correlated with prematurity and postnatal age and much lower clearances are reported in infants weighing less than 2.0 kg who are less than 7 days of age than those over 2 kg and over 1 week old[12]. Similar findings have been reported for the semi-synthetic penicillins, and the reader is referred to a review[13] for further details on human clinical studies.

Although penicillin has been a standard for bacterial therapy in the newborn for several decades, there have been no discrete pharmacokinetic analyses reported in any species which have described the developmental changes in penicillin G clearance.

A pharmacokinetic analysis of penicillin G excretion in the newborn pig, and in 5, 10 and 15 day old pigs is presented in Table 6.1. In this study, Na penicillin G was injected intravenously (4545 IU/kg) and plasma samples were drawn at varying intervals from 5 to 100 min postinjection. Plasma was

Table 6.1 Summary of $T_{1/2\beta}$ and body clearance values (Cl_B) for penicillin G injected intravenously at a dose of 4400 IU/kg in pigs of the Landrace breed of either sex and in male calves of the Holstein breed

	Parameter	Units	AGE 12–24 h	5 d	10 d	15 d
PIGS	*one compartment*					
	$T_{1/2\beta}$	min	25.5	22.3	20.2*	21.4
	CL_B	ml/min/kg	2.08	2.50	3.61*	3.17*
	two compartment					
	$T_{1/2\beta}$	min	47.42	28.1	25.7	25.7
	CL_B	ml/min/kg	1.71	2.06	3.47*	3.23*
CALVES	$T_{1/2\beta}$	min	29.7	25.7	27.6	23.5
	CL_B	ml/min/kg	2.98	4.83	3.11	4.65*

* ≠ from 12-24 h at $P \leq 0.05$

analysed for penicillin by the cylinder plate method, using *Sarcinia lutea* as the test organism. Data were analysed by a least-squares non-linear method.

Data for all pigs appeared to fit a two-compartment model in the 12–24 h old animals, but a gradual shift to a one-compartment profile was noted with age. For this reason, data are presented which represent both one- and two-compartment analysis. By one-compartment analysis, there was a significant decrease in the $T_{1/2\beta}$ between the day of birth and 10 days after birth. This was also reflected by an increase in body clearance, which had increased by 75% at 10 days of age.

By two-compartment analysis, there were no significant changes in $T_{1/2\beta}$, even though the newborn pigs had a higher mean value (and a high variability). Clearance values increased by 10 and 15 days, as in one-compartment analysis, and had doubled by 10 days.

Even though it is possible to observe a significantly deficient Cl_B for penicillin on the day of birth, the newborn pig must be credited with a highly efficient mechanism for excreting penicillin. In spite of the appearance of glomerular capillary cells and the previously mentioned report that effective renal blood flow increases 18 fold in 45 days, there is obviously enough renal capillary flow to present penicillin to an active and relatively mature tubular penicillin secreting mechanism. One other interpretation that must be considered, and may play a partial role, is that very low plasma albumin levels, characteristic of the newborn pig[23], may allow a much higher fraction of penicillin to be filtered (because of lower fractional plasma protein binding).

We have recently conducted a similar study in the calf. As noted above, it is known that C_{IN} and C_{PAH} develop very rapidly after birth, or at least that adult range values are apparent by the second day in this species. Our preliminary studies indicate that the calf kidney is more mature than that of the pig on the day it is born, in that there is little or no subcapsular neogenic zone. We anticipated that the newborn calf would be capable of excreting penicillin, and as seen in Table 6.1, we were essentially correct. The $T_{1/2\beta}$ did not change significantly over the 15 days of the study, although clearance values were higher by the 5th (and 15th) days of age.

CONCLUSIONS

The kidney of the pig has a high degree of morphological maturity at birth, but still undergoes considerable glomerular development, and probably an increase in tubular mass. It is known that large increases in renal blood flow occur over a period of 1–2 months, and that part of this increase results from reduced renal resistance. In spite of these developmental changes, however, the newborn pig has a remarkable ability to excrete penicillin, as does the neonatal calf. While we have not attempted to measure age-related changes in the tubular maxima for penicillin, the elimination rate constants for a therapeutic dose of the drug approach those of the adult very soon after birth in the pig and calf.

It is tempting to attribute this maturity to the efficiency of the proximal tubular secreting mechanisms, but this interpretation cannot be substantiated at present. In the pig, it is quite possible that low plasma albumin levels play some role. Additionally, competition studies (as with probenecid) would be necessary to relate changes in plasma decay to the active proximal tubular secretory mechanism known to exist in the adult.

References

1. Alexander, D. P. and Nixon, D. A. (1962). Plasma clearance of *p*-aminohippuric acid and inulin by the kidneys of foetal, neonatal and adult sheep. *Nature (London)*, **194**, 483–4
2. Barnett, H. L., McNamara, H., Shultz, S. *et al.* (1949). Renal clearances of sodium penicillin G, procaine penicillin G, and inulin in infants and children. *Pediatrics*, **3**, 418–22
3. Baxter, J. S. and Yoffey, J. M. (1947). The post-natal development of renal tubules in the rat. *Anatomy*, **82**, 189–97
4. Bogomolova, N. A. (1965). Age changes in kidney of White rat. *Arkh. Anat. Gistol. Embriol.*, **48**, T295–9
5. Calcagno, P. L. and Rubin, M. I. (1963). Renal extraction of *para*-aminohippurate in infants and children. *J. Clin. Invest.*, **42,**, 1632–9
6. Dalton, R. G. (1968). Renal function in neonatal calves: inulin, thiosulfate and PAH clearance. *Br. Vet. J.*, **124**, 489–98
7. Edelmann, C. M. (1966). Maturation of the neonatal kidney. *Proc. Int. Congr. Nephrol.*, Washington, **3**, 1–12
8. Fetterman, G. H., Shuplock, N. A., Philipp, F. J. *et al.* (1965). The growth and maturation of human glomeruli and proximal convolutions from term to adulthood. *Pediatrics*, **35**, 601–19
9. Gruskin, A. G., Edelmann, C. M. and Yaun, S. (1970). Maturational changes in renal blood flow in piglets. *Pediatr. Res.*, **4**, 7–13
10. Hirsch, G. H., Cowan, D. F. and Hook, J. B. (1971). Histological changes in normal and drug-induced development of renal PAH transport. *Proc. Soc. Exp. Biol. Med.*, **137**, 116–21
11. Horster, M. and Valtin, H. (1971). Postnatal development of renal function: micropuncture and clearance studies in the dog. *J. Clin. Invest.*, **50**, 779–95
12. McCraken, G. H., Ginsburg, C. and Chrane, D. F. (1973). Clinical pharmacology of penicillin in newborn infants. *J. Pediatr.*, **82**, 692–8
13. McCraken, G. H. and Nelson, J. D. (1977). Antimicrobial therapy for newborns. In *Monographs in Neonatology*. (New York: Grune and Stratton)
14. New, N., McNamara, H. and Kretchmer, N. (1959). Accumulation of *para*-aminohippurate by slices of kidney from rabbits of various ages. *Proc. Soc. Exp. Biol. Med.*, **102**, 558–60
15. Potter, E. L. and Thierstein, S. T. (1943). Glomerular development in the kidney as an index of fetal maturity. *J. Pediatr.*, **22**, 695–706
16. Reiche, R., Mulling, M. and Frey, H. H. (1980). Pharmacokinetics of chloramphenicol in calves during the first weeks of life. *J. Vet. Pharmacol. Ther.*, **3**, 95–106
17. Rennick, B., Hamilton, B. and Evans, R. (1961). Development of renal tubular transports of TEA and PAH in the puppy and piglet. *Am. J. Physiol.*, **201**, 743–6
18. Schreiter, G. (1966). Neue physiologische und klinische Aspekt der Nieren-Funktion bei Frudgeborenen. *Dtsch. Gesundh. Wesen.*, **21**, 433–41
19. Short, C. R. and Davis, L. E. (1970). Postnatal development of drug metabolizing enzyme activity in swine. *J. Pharmacol. Exp. Ther.*, **174**, 185–96
20. Short, C. R., Kinden, D. A. and Stith, R. (1976). Fetal and neonatal development of the microsomal monooxygenase system. *Drug Metab. Rev.*, **5**, 1–42
21. Short, C. R. and Stith, R. (1973). Perinatal development of hepatic mixed function oxidase activity in swine. *Biochem. Pharmacol.*, **22**, 1309–19
22. Short, C. R. (1980). Drug elimination in the newborn animal. *Proc. Symp. Vet. Pharmacol. Ther.*, Philadelphia, **2**, 81–99
23. Short, C. R. and Tumbleson, M. E. (1973). Binding of drugs to plasma proteins of swine during the perinatal period. *Toxicol. Appl. Pharmacol.*, **24**, 612–24
24. Svendsen, O. (1976). Pharmacokinetics of hexobarbital, sulfadimidine and chloramphenicol in neonatal and young pigs. *Acta Vet. Scand.*, **17**, 1–14

25. Vogh, B. and Cassin, S. (1966). Stop flow analysis of renal function in newborn and maturing swine. *Biol. Neonate*, **10,** 153–65
26. West, J. R., Smith, H. W. and Chasis, H. (1948). Glomerular filtration rate, effective renal blood flow, and maximal tubular excretory capacity in infancy. *J. Pediatr.*, **32,** 10–18

7 Drug effects during development and carcinogenicity

G. M. Williams

Animals in early developmental stages differ substantially from their mature counterparts in susceptibility to the adverse effects of xenobiotics. In the response to some agents that require biotransformation for activity, developing animals can be more resistant than adults because of undeveloped xenobiotic biotransformation enzyme systems. More often, developing animals are more sensitive to adverse effects because of one or more of several characteristics, including undeveloped xenobiotic detoxification enzyme systems, vulnerability of replicating cells to injury, susceptibility of regulatory systems to modulation and susceptibility of systems concerned with differentiated function.

Perinatal exposure of animals to chemicals can produce adverse effects specific to the developing animal including malformation and permanent enzyme and endocrine modulation. Other perinatal adverse effects which also occur in mature animals are physiological disturbances, a variety of toxic effects including perturbations of the immune and endocrine systems, behavioural disorders, and cancer.

The response of the developing animal to drugs is a complex function of the drug-recipient interactions, the biological effects of the drug and the developmental status of the organism.

PERINATAL XENOBIOTIC INTERACTIONS

The interactions of xenobiotics with developing animals are determined by the same factors that influence interactions in mature animals. These consist principally of the type of exposure, absorption, distribution, biotransformation and excretion of the chemical. The contribution of each of these factors to xenobiotic effects in developing animals has special characteristics.

Xenobiotic exposures and absorption

The nature of xenobiotic exposures differ during three distinct states of development – *in utero*, postnatal preweaning and postweaning develop ment. *In utero* exposures to xenobiotics result from exposure of the mother and are dependent upon placental transfer of the compound or products of maternal metabolism. During the neonatal period, ingestion is the main route of exposure to xenobiotics.

Most xenobiotics absorbed by pregnant females rapidly traverse the placenta of various species[5, 21] in spite of the fact that species differ markedly in the structure of the placenta[6]. For example, in pigs and horses, the epitheliochorial-type placenta possesses the maximum six tissue layers separating maternal and fetal blood, while in rodents and primates, the absence of the three maternal layers in the haemochorial-type placenta permits maternal blood to bathe the chorion directly.

The movement of xenobiotics across the placenta occurs primarily by diffusion, although it has an active transport system for concentrating molecules in the fetus[5]. In particular lipid-soluble compounds, hormones and most drugs are readily transferred across the placenta by this mechan ism[1, 5]. Thus, the major rate-limiting factor in placental transfer seems to be blood flow to the placenta[5].

The placenta possesses many types of xenobiotic biotransformation enzymes[9], particularly those involved in oxidation reactions. Biotransformation of a compound by maternal or placental enzyme systems to polar conjugates retards placental transfer, but placental biotransformation does not constitute a significant impediment to passage of xenobiotics[9].

Maternal-fetal pharmacokinetics have been studied mainly in the pregnant ewe[21] because of the relatively large size of the fetal lamb. Xenobiotics are carried from the placenta to the fetus by the umbilical vein and as much as 50% of this blood flow is distributed to the fetal liver while the remainder is shunted systemically. For most drugs that have been studied, transfer to the fetus is very rapid, but under steady state conditions, the fetal concen tration is lower than the maternal[21].

Following birth, exposures of the developing animal can occur as a result of transfer in maternal milk or by direct exposure. A variety of xenobiotics have been found to be carried in milk[12, 13]. The composition of milk differs between species[12] and accordingly, exposures of neonates to xenobiotics by this route are probably different.

For xenobiotics that are ingested by postnatal animals, the extent of absorption from the gastrointestinal tract determines the systemic exposure. Certain factors may affect absorption during developmental stages. In newborns, the gastric acidity is often not as high (or the pH not as low) as in adults, which permits bacterial colonization, and thus the presence of bacterial enzymes such as nitroreductases, or azo dye reductase, capable of metabolizing appropriate substrates leading to products whose absorption in the small intestine may differ from that of the parent compound. Absorption of xenobiotics in the gastrointestinal tract could presumably be different in newborns as a consequence of distinct metabolism by bacterial or intestinal enzymes, but this has not been documented.

Exposures to xenobiotics during postweaning development are direct and similar to those of mature animals. For exposures by the oral route, absorption is more similar to that of adults than is absorption in newborns because of more advanced development. However, significant species' differences in absorption are well established. For example, an oral dose of the simple polar compound nitrilotriacetic acid, a chelating agent, is absorbed by 80% in dogs, 70% in rats and 23% in rabbits[17].

Xenobiotic disposition

In the passage of xenobiotics from the umbilical vein or intestine to the systemic circulation, they may be biotransformed (see below) by the liver or intestinal epithelium, liver and lung, respectively, resulting in presystemic elimination. This 'first pass' effect reduces bioavailability. The disposition of the fraction of a xenobiotic that gains access to systemic circulation is further determined by tissue distribution, biotransformation and excretion.

The initial systemic distribution of a xenobiotic reflects cardiac output and regional blood flow. A second phase of distribution is determined by subsequent diffusion of the chemical into tissues. Accumulation in tissues is further affected by factors such as pH gradients, partitioning into fat, and binding to intracellular constituents.

Tissue distribution of xenobiotics has been elegantly studied by the technique of whole body autoradiography developed by Ullberg and coworkers[1]. Using this approach, a variety of patterns of distribution have been observed, mainly in the fetal mouse. For example, the antibiotic benzyl penicillin is uniformly distributed in fetal tissues whereas thiouracil, a thyrostatic agent which has been used to promote growth in cattle, sheep and swine, shows marked accumulation in the thyroid. The protozoacide, chloroquine, is accumulated in the uvea of the eye of pigmented mice[24].

Xenobiotic biotransformation

The biotransformation of xenobiotics in tissues is carried out by a variety of enzymes depending upon the nature of the substrate. The reactions performed on xenobiotics can be categorized into two types (Table 7.1), phase I reactions in which the substrate is altered and phase II reactions in which a specific group is conjugated to the substrate, often producing a product with a sizeable increase in molecular weight and polarity or hydrophilicity. Liver has the greatest capacity for xenobiotic biotransformation[26], but kidney[26], lung[11], the gastrointestinal epithelium[7]and intestinal bacterial flora[20] are also involved.

Xenobiotic biotransformation in developing organisms is distinctly different from that of mature animals because of undeveloped enzyme systems[1, 10, 16]. The fetus develops xenobiotic biotransformation capability early in gestation; in the human fetal liver it is present by the first trimester[10]. Generally, most organ enzyme activities are lower in fetuses and newborns than in mature animals. However, some organ activities, such as liver uridine

Table 7.1 Major pathways of enzyme-catalysed xenobiotic biotransformation reactions in mammals

Phase I reactions

(1) Oxidation
- (a) Mono-oxygenation
  - (i) Cytochrome P-450-dependent
  - (ii) Flavoprotein-dependent
- (b) Dehydrogenation
- (c) Other oxidation reactions
  - (i) Monoamine oxidation
  - (ii) Cyclooxygenase (endoperoxide synthetase)

(2) Reduction
- (a) Azo linkages
- (b) Nitro groups
- (c) Carbonyl groups

(3) Hydrolysis
- (a) Carboxylic acid esters
- (b) Amides–peptides
- (c) Sulphate esters
- (d) Glycoside esters
- (e) Epoxides

Phase II reactions

(1) Conjugation
- (a) Glycosylation
  - (i) Glucuronide formation
  - (ii) Riboside formation
  - (iii) Glucoside formation
  - (iv) *N*-Acetylaminoglycoside formation
  - (v) Xyloside formation
- (b) Acylation
  - (i) Acetylation
  - (ii) Amino acid conjugation
- (c) Sulphation
- (d) Glutathione conjugation
- (e) Methylation

diphosphoglucuronyltransferase, which functions in biotransformation to form water-soluble glucuronic acid conjugates, show a marked increase following birth with eventual decline to lower yet substantial adult levels[15].

Biotransformation activities are similar in neonates of both sexes, but with puberty in rats, sexual differentiation occurs in the activities of several types of enzymes[14, 15]. The sex differences in some of these enzyme activities have been eliminated by hypophysectomy[15], which taken together with the expression of sex differences at puberty, suggests that control mediated by the pituitary-hypothalamic axis is programmed during early development. The development of this sex-dependent differentiation in domestic animals has not been determined.

The effect of enzymatic biotransformation on tissue-xenobiotic interactions depends upon whether the xenobiotic is active as the parent compound or requires biotransformation to an active metabolite. For compounds that are active in their parent form, biotransformation usually produces an inactive metabolite(s). For this type of agent, undeveloped enzyme systems would permit greater persistence of the active compound, enhancing the biological effects. In contrast, xenobiotics that require biotransformation for activity may display less action in developing animals because of undeveloped enzyme systems. In many instances, however, both types of metabolism occur and it is the ratio of activation/detoxification, which can differ with age and between species, that determines the biological effect. Thus, the relative rate of development of type I enzyme systems including those concerned with biochemical activation reactions, and of type II enzyme systems, most often related to conjugation and hence detoxification, is important. For many substrates, activation systems develop earlier, accounting for the fact that newborn animals are often exquisitely sensitive to adverse drug effects.

Xenobiotic excretion

Excretion of xenobiotics occurs in the fetus by diffusion into the maternal blood bathing the placenta or by renal clearance. For reverse transfer of xenobiotics from the fetal to the maternal compartment, the same factors that determine fetal uptake (see above) govern excretion.

Chemicals cleared by the fetal kidneys are excreted in the urine and thence into the amniotic fluid. In the neonate, and by inference in the prenate, renal blood flow, and glomerular filtration rate are low and the capacity to excrete organic compounds is limited[8]. Thus, organic anions, such as penicillin, are poorly excreted. Because of low renal transport, newborns display resistance to the nephrotoxicity of the antibiotic cephaloridine[28]. Interestingly, renal organic anion extraction can be stimulated by exposure to substrates for transport. Such stimulation then enhances the nephrotoxicity of cephaloridine.

In postnatal animals, xenobiotics or their metabolites are excreted primarily by the kidneys into urine or by the liver into bile. Excretion is qualitatively similar to that in mature animals although quantitative differences exist, both for renal clearance as noted and liver clearance, primarily as a consequence of immature mechanisms for excretion. As a generalization, for compounds with a molecular weight of more than 350, the predominant pathway is in the bile in rabbits and probably larger species, whereas compounds with lower molecular weights are preferentially excreted in urine. However, substantial species differences exist[16].

For compounds that are excreted in the bile as conjugates that can be split by bacterial enzymes (sulphate esters, glucuronides, bile acid conjugates), the liberated aglycone is partially or totally reabsorbed. Further liver-mediated metabolism (enterohepatic cycle) then occurs.

PERINATAL RESPONSES TO XENOBIOTICS

The response of a developing animal to a xenobiotic is a complex function of the xenobiotic–animal interactions discussed above, the biological effects of the xenobiotic, and the developmental status of the animal. Of particular importance during development is the rate of cell proliferation in growing tissues. Cells that are actively dividing are generally more susceptible than resting cells to the toxic effects of xenobiotics. Thus, developing animals can display either reduced or enhanced responses to xenobiotics depending upon the contribution of several factors.

Two responses which are specific or enhanced in developing animals are, respectively, permanent enzyme and endocrine system modulation and carcinogenesis.

Permanent enzyme modulation (imprinting)

Imprinting or programming of enzyme activity is a form of permanent modulation of enzyme activity that results from neonatal exposure to hormones or homonally active agents. This effect was first delineated by Einarsson *et al.*[3] for sexual differentiation of hepatic steroid metabolism. Subsequently, imprinting of drug metabolizing enzymes was described[14].

The imprinting effect produced by hormones is manifested only in postpubertal animals when sexual differentiation of enzyme activities (see above) occurs. For enzyme activities that are normally higher in adult males than in females, such as uridinediphosphoglucuronyl-transferase and many oxidative activities, neonatal exposure of males to hormones such as diethylstilboestrol or testosterone abolishes sexual differentiation (Table 7.2).

Table 7.2 Effects of neonatal diethylstilboestrol or testosterone proprionate on the sexual differentiation of rat hepatic enzymes

	Adult male/female specific activity ratios		
Enzyme	*Control*	*Neonatal diethylstilboestrol*	*Neonatal testosterone*
Ethylmorphine demethylase	4.2	1.3	1.6
Cytochrome P-450	1.1	1.0	1.0
Uridinediphosphoglucuronyl transferase	1.9	1.2	1.4

Adapted from Lucier[15]

Exposure of newborn rats to hormones alters their response later in life to carcinogens that are biotransformed in the liver[27]. Also prenatal or neonatal exposure of animals to oestrogens and hormones generally produces a disturbance in the hypothalamo-pituitary axis resulting in persistent oestrogenic stimulation[2,4] such that animals are more suceptible to carcinogenic effects in hormonally-responsive organs later in life[19].

Perinatal carcinogenesis

The transplacental induction of tumours and the sensitivity of neonatal and infant animals to carcinogens is well documented[18,22,23]. The features of perinatal carcinogenesis are summarized in Table 7.3.

Table 7.3 Features of perinatal carcinogenesis

(1) No known carcinogen is active exclusively in the fetus or neonate.

(2) The sensitivity of the fetus or neonate varies from 100 times that of the adult to considerably less.

(3) Low perinatal susceptibility often results from low biotransformation in the fetus or neonate.

(4) Virtually no transplacental carcinogens are dependent upon maternal or placental biotransformation for their activity.

(5) Most tumours produced by perinatal exposure to carcinogens are histologically identical to tumours occurring in adults.

For chemicals that require metabolic activation in order to exert their carcinogenic effects[26], undeveloped xenobiotic biotransformation enzyme systems can render younger animals resistant or at least with low sensitivity[23]. Nevertheless, many carcinogens are active transplacentally (Table 7.4) and in the neonatal period. Some of these, including urethane which was used as an anaesthetic in veterinary medicine, diethylnitrosamine and polycyclic aromatic hydrocarbons such as benzo(a)pyrene, are more carcinogenic with perinatal exposures than in adults. Importantly, all transplacental carcinogens except diethylstilboestrol and all carcinogens that are more active in neonates than adults are of the type that damage DNA and hence are referred to as genotoxic[25].

Table 7.4 Chemical carcinogens active with prenatal exposure

Alkylating agents
Diethyl sulphate
Dimethyl sulphate
Methyl methanesulphonate
1,3-Propane sultone

Aromatic amines
o-Aminoazotoluene
Benzidine
3,3′-Dichlorobenzidine

Polycyclic aromatic hydrocarbons
Benzo(a)pyrene
7,12-Dimethylbenz(a)anthracene
3-Methylcholanthrene

Nitrosamines
Nitrosodiethylamine
Nitrosodimethylamine

Nitrosamides
Ethylnitrosobiuret
Ethylnitrosourea
Ethylnitrosourethane
Methylnitrosourea
Methylnitrosourethane
n-Propylnitrosourea

Triazines
Diethyltriazine
1-Phenyl-3,3-diethyltriazine
1-Phenyl-3,3-dimethyltriazine
1-Pyridil-3,3-diethyltriazine

Others
Aflatoxin B_1
Azoethane
Azoxyethane
Azoxymethane
Crude cycad material (Methylazoxymethanol)
1,2-Diethylhydrazine
1-Methyl-2-benzylhydrazine
N-Isopropyl-α-(2-methyl-hydrazino)-*p*-toluamide HCl (Procarbazine, Natulan)
Elasiomycin
4-Nitroquinoline-1-oxide
Safrole
Urethane

Hormone
Diethylstilboestrol

Adapted from Tomatis *et al.*[22]

The greater susceptibility of perinatal tissues to genotoxic carcinogens is largely due to the high rates of cell replication during development. The DNA damage produced by genotoxic carcinogens can be repaired, but if it is not and the cell replicates using the damaged DNA for a template, permanent alterations in DNA result. These genetic alterations appear to lead to neoplastic conversion of the cell. The higher rates of cell proliferation in growing animals allow less opportunity for repair of DNA damage in dividing cells and therefore increase the probability that a cell with damaged DNA will replicate and give rise to an abnormal progeny.

A different type of transplacental carcinogen is the hormonally-active substance diethylstilboestrol (DES), which produces adenosis and vaginal cancer in experimental animals and humans[18]. DES is non-genotoxic and the restriction of its carcinogenic effects to hormonally responsive tissues suggests that hormonal effects underly its carcinogenicity. The appearance of DES-induced tumours at puberty may indicate abnormal functioning of the endocrine system due to imprinting (see above) thereby leading to the expression of neoplasia in cells altered by the *in utero* exposure.

CONCLUSIONS

A variety of characteristics render the developing organism different from its mature counterpart in its response to drugs. These can result in adverse effects such as permanent alteration of differentiated systems or increased susceptibility to cancer. Thus, the special hazards of drugs in developing organisms necessitate careful consideration of their use.

References

1. Boreus, L. O. (ed.) (1973). *Fetal Pharmacology*. (New York: Raven Press)
2. Dun, T. B. and Green, A. W. (1963). Cysts of the epididymis, cancer of the cervix, granular cell myoblastoma, and other lesions after estrogen injection in newborn mice. *J. Natl. Cancer Inst.*, **31**, 425–55
3. Einarson, K., Gustafsson, J. and Stenberg, A. (1973). Neonatal imprinting of liver microsomal hydroxylation and reduction of steroids. *J. Biol. Chem.*, **248**, 4987–97
4. Forsberg, J. G. (1974). Induction of condition leading to cancer in the genital tract by estrogen during the differentiation phase of the genital epithelium. *Adv. Biosci.*, **13**, 139–51
5. Green, T. P., O'Dea, R. F. and Mirkin, B. L. (1979). Determinants of drug disposition and effect in the fetus. *Ann. Rev. Pharmacol. Toxicol.*, **19**, 285–322
6. Hafez, E. S. E. (ed.) (1970). *Reproduction and Breeding Techniques for Laboratory Animals*. (Philadelphia: Lea and Febiger)
7. Hartiala, K. (1973). Metabolism of hormones, drugs and other substances by the gut. - *Physiol. Rev.*, **53**, 496–534
8. Hook, J. B. and Bailie, M. D. (1979). Perinatal renal pharmacology. *Ann. Rev. Pharmacol. Toxicol.*, **19**, 491–509
9. Juchau, M. R. (1980). Drug biotransformation in the placenta. *Pharmac. Ther.*, **8**, 501–24
10. Juchau, M. R., Chao, S. T. and Omiecinski, C. J. (1980). Drug metabolism by the human fetus. *Clin. Pharmacokinet.*, **5**, 320–39
11. Junod, A. F. and de Haller, R. (eds.) (1975). *Lung Metabolism*. (New York: Academic Press)

12. Kirchgessner, M., Friesecke, H. and Koch, G. (1967). *Nutrition and the Composition of Milk*. (Philadelphia and Toronto: J. B. Lippincott)
13. Knowles, J. A. (1965). Excretion of drugs in milk – a review. *Pediatr. Pharmacol. Ther.*, **66**, 1068–82
14. Lucier, G. W., Lui, E. M. K. and Lamartiniere, C. A. (1979). Metabolic activation/deactivation reactions during perinatal development. *Environ. Health Perspect.*, **29**, 7–16
15. Lucier, G. W. (1976). Perinatal development of conjugative enzyme systems. *Environ. Health Perspect.*, **18**, 25–34.
16. La Du, B. N., Mandel, H. G. and Way, C. L. (eds.) (1971). *Fundamentals of Drug Metabolism and Drug Disposition*. (Baltimore: Williams and Wilkins)
17. Michael, W. R. and Wakim, J. W. (1971). Metabolism of nitrilotriacetic acid (NTA). *Toxicol. Appl. Pharmacol.*, **18**, 407–16
18. Rice, J. M. (ed.) (1979). *Perinatal Carcinogenesis*. National Cancer Institute Monograph 51, US Department of Health Education and Welfare
19. Rustia, M. and Shubik, P. (1979). Effects of transplacental exposure to diethylstilbestrol on carcinogenic susceptibility during postnatal life in hamster. *Cancer Res.*, **39**, 4636–44
20. Scheline, R. R. (1973). Metabolism of foreign compounds by gastrointestinal microorganisms. *Pharmacol. Rev.*, **25**, 451–523
21. Szeto, H. H. (1982). Pharmacokinetics in the ovine maternal-fetal unit. *Ann. Rev. Pharmacol. Toxicol.*, **22**, 221–43
22. Tomatis, L., Turusov, V. and Guibbert, D. (1972). Prenatal exposure to chemical carcinogens. In Nakahara, W., Takayama, S., Sugimura, T. *et al.* (eds.) *Topics in Chemical Carcinogenesis*. pp. 445–61. (Baltimore: University Park Press)
23. Toth, B. (1968). A critical review of experiments in chemical carcinogenesis using newborn animals. *Cancer Res.*, **28**, 727–38
24. Ullberg, S., Lindquist, N. G. and Sjostrand, S. E. (1970). Accumulation of chorioretinotoxic drugs in the foetal eye. *Nature (London)*, **227**, 1257–8
25. Weisburger, J. H. and Williams, G. M. (1980). Chemical carcinogens. In Amdur, M. O., Doull, J. and Klaassen, C. D. (eds.) *Toxicology, The Basic Science of Poisons*. 2nd Edn., pp. 84–138. (New York: Macmillan)
26. Weisburger, J. H. and Williams, G. M. (1982). Metabolism of chemical carcinogens. In Becker, F. F. (ed.) *Cancer: A Comprehensive Treatise*. 2nd Edn., pp. 241–333. (New York: Plenum Press).
27. Weisburger, E. K., Yamamoto, R. S., Glass, R. M., Grantham, P. H. and Weisburger, J. H. (1968). Effect of neonatal androgen and estrogen injection on liver tumor induction by *N*-hydroxy-*N*-2-fluorenylacetamide and on the metabolism of the carcinogen in rats. *Endocrinology*, **82**, 685–92
28. Wold, J. S. and Turnipseed, S. A. (1978). Age-dependent renal accumulation of cephaloridine in the rabbit. *Drug Metab. Dispos.*, **6**, 87–90

7 APPENDIX
Assessment of carcinogenic properties of veterinary drugs

Domestic animals are clearly susceptible to the carcinogenic effects of chemicals, as shown by the production of experimental cancer in dogs and rabbits and the development of bladder cancer in cows consuming bracken fern. Also, tumours are regularly found in meat-producing animals[3,7,8] in spite of the fact that they are slaughtered at a young age. Nevertheless, the potential carcinogenicity to recipient animals of veterinary drugs does not appear to be the subject of regulatory concern, at least in the United States, probably because of the generally short durations of usage of drugs in domestic animals relative to their lifetime or to their maintenance prior to slaughter. Situations exist, however, such as the administration of drugs to long-lived household pets or to experimental animals being used to assess the effects of other agents, where carcinogenic effects could be manifested.

The major concern regarding the potential carcinogenicity of veterinary drugs involves residues in consumable tissues of food-producing animals. In the United States, under the Federal Food, Drug and Cosmetic Act, the Food and Drug Administration (FDA) is charged with determining whether a compound to be given to food-producing animals may be carcinogenic and whether its use may leave carcinogenic residues in edible tissues. The regulations that were proposed by the FDA in 1979 to establish the criteria by which data on carcinogenicity would be collected generally required lengthy data collection. This was perceived to be unnecessary for certain drugs and, therefore, revised guidelines were proposed in 1982[2].

The new guidelines (Table 7.5) utilize a 'decision-tree approach' for the determination of whether a sponsored compound should be evaluated as a carcinogen. These guidelines correspond closely to the first steps in the Decision Point Approach (DPA) (Table 7.6) proposed by Weisburger and Williams in 1978[11] for evaluating chemical carcinogens. The major difference is that the FDA guidelines do not include limited *in vivo* bioassays as a step intermediate between *in vitro* short-term tests and chronic bioassay. The validity of such assays is well established[18], in addition to which they provide a means of reducing the costs of testing and the use of experimental animals. Therefore, the decision point approach to carcinogen testing is

Table 7.5 1982 Food and drug administration factors for assessment of potential carcinogenic significance

Compounds are assigned to four categories A–D reflecting increasing carcinogenic potential of veterinary drugs based upon:

(1) Chemical structure,
(2) Data from short-term genetic toxicity tests,
(3) Other biological, physiological or pharmacological data,
(4) Data from subchronic or chronic feeding studies.

Food and Drug Administration, Federal Register, **47**, 4972–7, 1982

Table 7.6 The decision point approach for evaluation of carcinogens or promoters

A. Structure of chemical

B. Battery of *in vitro* short-term tests
   (1) Hepatocyte DNA repair,
   (2) Bacterial mutagenesis,
   (3) Mammalian cell mutagenesis,
   (4) Mammalian cell chromosome effects,
   (5) Mammalian cell transformation (optional).

C. Panel of limited *in vivo* bioassays
   (1) Induction of altered foci in rodent liver,
   (2) Skin tumour induction in mice,
   (3) Lung tumour induction in mice,
   (4) Breast cancer induction in rats,
   (5) Tests for promoting effects.

D. Chronic bioassay

E. Final evaluation

recommended as a means of effectively and reliably evaluating the carcinogenicity of veterinary drugs.

THE DECISION POINT APPROACH TO CARCINOGEN TESTING

The DPA involves five sequential steps in the evaluation of the potential carcinogenicity of chemicals (Table 7.6) which take into account new advances in chemical carcinogenesis. Of prime importance is the concept that chemicals can increase the tumour incidence in treated animals, and thus be called carcinogenic, by several distinct mechanisms, each with different theoretical and practical consequences[14].

Briefly, carcinogens can be divided into two principal categories, genotoxic and epigenetic[12]. Genotoxic carcinogens are those with the capacity, either in their parent form or following biotransformation, to operate as reactive species and to damage DNA. Such carcinogens are active in genetic toxicity tests. Epigenetic carcinogens do not form electrophilic reactants or damage DNA. Rather, they operate by a variety of indirect mechanisms, including chronic toxicity, solid state effects, hormonal effects, immunosuppression and cocarcinogenic or promoting effects. Thus, carcinogens can be classified mechanistically (Table 7.7).

This concept of diverse mechanisms of action of carcinogens is addressed in the DPA in two ways:

Table 7.7 Classes of carcinogenic chemical

Type of agent	*Mode of action*	*Example*
Genotoxic		
(1) Activation-independent	Electrophile, interacts with DNA	Ethylene imine
(2) Activation-dependent	Requires conversion through biotransformation by host to type 1	Vinyl chloride, benzo(a)pyrene 2-naphthylamine, dimethylnitrosamine
(3a) Inorganic	Interact with DNA	Hydrazine, nickel, chromium
Epigenetic		
(3b) Inorganic	Not directly genotoxic, leads to changes in DNA by selective alteration in fidelity of DNA replication	
(4) Cytotoxic	Chronic tissue injury	Nitrilotriacetic acid
(5) Solid-state material	Mechanism unknown; usually affects only mesenchymal cells and tissues; physical form vital	Polymer or metal foils, asbestos
(6) Hormonally-active	Alters endocrine system balances and differentiation; often acts as promoter	Oestradiol, diethylstilboestrol
(7) Immunosuppressor	Mainly stimulates 'virally induced', transplanted, or neoplasms	Azathioprine
(8) Cocarcinogen	Enhances effect of type 1 or type 2 agent when given at the same time. May modify conversion of type 2 to type 2	Phorbol esters, pyrene, catechol, ethanol, *n*-dodecane, SO_2
(9) Promoter	Enhances effect of type 1 or type 2 agent when given subsequently	Phorbol esters, phenol, anthralin, bile acids, tryptophan metabolites, saccharin

Based on Weisburger and Williams[12]

(1) Genotoxic carcinogens are identified by effects in a battery of short-term tests for genetic effects. In addition, *in vitro* systems are becoming available to identify agents that operate via epigenetic mechanisms.
(2) A stepwise approach to testing provides a guide to minimal testing, but with the recognition that all forms of subchronic testing may not detect chemicals that can induce tumours in animals under specific conditions upon chronic administration.

The battery of short-term tests utilized in the DPA may either eliminate the need for further testing of the chemical or enable the verification of carcinogenic potential in one of four limited *in vivo* bioassays for genotoxic carcinogens. Thus, the DPA is a systematic stepwise approach to the reliable evaluation of the potential carcinogenicity of chemicals which provides a framework in which to minimize and optimize the necessary testing and, at the same time, develop an understanding of the mechanism of action of a test chemical.

A. Structure of chemical

The evaluation starts with assessment of structure/activity relationships. Present knowledge permits prediction of formation of possible electrophilic intermediates with fair success within certain structural classes. In addition, substituents that block carcinogenicity have been identified. Structure also provides a guide to the selection of the most appropriate limited *in vivo* bioassay at stage C and should eventually be similarly useful in selecting *in vitro* short-term tests at stage B.

B. *In vitro* short-term tests

A battery of *in vitro* tests is recommended since, as a consequence of the complexities of metabolism and mechanism of action of chemical carcinogens, no single test has detected all genotoxic carcinogens. Moreover, with positive results in tests that are complementary in their metabolic parameters or endpoints, strong supporting evidence of carcinogenic potential is obtained.

An essential component of the battery is a microbial mutagenesis test since such tests have been the most sensitive, effective and readily performed screening tests thus far. The *Salmonella*/microsome test of Ames (see Haroun and Ames, ref. 9) is the most widely used.

Mutagenesis of mammalian cells is also part of the battery because it is a sensitive endpoint like bacterial mutagenesis, but involves the more highly organized eucaryotic genome. Appropriate tests include assays for mutagencsis at the hypoxanthine-guanine phosphoribosyl transferase locus in V79 or CHO cells (see Hsie in ref. 17) and mutagenesis at the thymidine kinase locus in mouse lymphoma cells (see Clive in ref. 17).

Tests for DNA damage provide direct evidence that a chemical can alter genetic material. Indicators of DNA damage that have been proposed include DNA binding, DNA fragmentation, inhibition of DNA synthesis, and DNA repair. Of these, DNA repair is a specific response to DNA damage that is simple to measure and, unlike DNA fragmentation and inhibition of DNA synthesis, cannot be produced by general toxicity. Thus, a DNA repair test provides an endpoint of high specificity and biological significance. The system of Williams (see Williams in ref. 9 and in ref. 17) which assesses DNA repair in freshly isolated hepatocytes offers a test with intact cell metabolism in the cell type with the broadest capability for xenobiotic biotransformation.

A chromosomal test is included to detect effects at the highest level of genetic organization. Such tests, however, may respond to non-genotoxic agents through effects on DNA replication, chromosome separation, etc. Sister chromatid exchange (SCE) can be readily monitored and is therefore recommended for a chromosomal level test. The best validated system at present is that using CHO cells (see Wolff in ref. 9).

Cell transformation is considered for inclusion in the battery because this alteration may be directly relevant to carcinogenesis. The correlation between production of transformation and carcinogenicity of chemicals appears to be good in several systems[6], but transformation assays are difficult and less widely available that the other systems described. Therefore, at present the performance of the first four tests is recommended with the use of a transformation assay only if the battery results require amplification.

Decision point 1

Completion of the six steps (A plus B, 1–5) provides a basis for primary decision making. If definite evidence of genotoxicity in more than one test has been obtained, a chemical is highly suspect of carcinogenicity. In particular, because of the complementary nature of the biotransformation and the endpoints in the mutagenesis test of Ames and the DNA repair test of Williams, positive results in both systems provide strong and possibly certain evidence of carcinogenicity. Since there is some redundancy between bacterial and mammalian mutagenicity, these two systems support rather than extend the significance of positive results. An agent that is DNA damaging, mutagenic, and clastogenic is virtually certain to be carcinogenic and, regardless, represents an unequivocal toxic hazard.

On the other hand, genotoxicity found in only one test requires interpretation with caution. For example, mutagenicity has been obtained in bacteria with compounds such as flavones having phenolic structures. *In vivo*, such compounds are conjugated and excreted readily and thus far have not been carcinogenic. Similarly, positive results only for mammalian mutagenesis or SCE must be interpreted with caution. On the other hand, evidence of DNA damage in the hepatocyte/DNA repair test strongly indicates covalent binding to DNA, an established property of carcinogens. Any positive results in the *in vitro* battery can be extended through limited *in vivo* bioassays (stage C).

A wide variety of structurally different organic chemicals capable of forming reactive electrophiles are readily detected in genetic toxicity tests. Other substances, such as solid state materials, possibly some metal ions, hormones, and promoters, are negative in such tests and appear to operate by indirect and complex mechanisms.

Most promoters are effective mainly on one tissue and thus require specialized protocols for detection. Potential promoters can be detected through newly developed *in vitro* systems (Trosko *et al.* in ref. 9) or *in vivo* by exposure to animals pretreated with a limited amount of a genotoxic carcinogen for a specific target organ (stage C).

If the results in the battery of short-term tests yield no indication of genotoxicity, the priority for further testing depends on two criteria: (1) the structure and known physiological properties (e.g. hormone) of the material, and (2) the potential human exposure. If substantial human exposure is likely, careful consideration should be given to the necessity for additional testing. The chemical structure and the properties of the material provide guidance on the proper course of action.

C. Limited *in vivo* bioassays

This stage of testing is designed to yield further evidence of the potential carcinogenicity of chemicals with limited or equivocal evidence of genotoxicity, without the necessity of undertaking a costly and time-consuming chronic bioassay.

The limited *in vivo* tests recommended[18] are those that will provide definitive evidence of carcinogenicity, including cocarcinogenicity and promotion, in a relatively short period (i.e. 30 weeks or less). Unlike the *in vitro* tests, these are not applied as a battery, but rather are used selectively according to the information available on the specific properties of the chemical. An important feature of limited bioassays is that positive results are definitely significant, but negative results cannot be taken as evidence of lack of carcinogenicity.

(1) Altered foci induction in rodent liver. In rats several distinct hepatocellular lesions, altered foci and hyperplastic (neoplastic) nodules precede the development of hepatocellular carcinomas. The earliest appearing of these, the altered focus, can be visualized by sensitive histochemical techniques, including reactions for the enzymes γ-glutamyl transpeptidase, glucose-6-phosphatase, adenosine triphosphatase, and resistance to iron accumulation. Thus, the rapid production of foci and nodules has been used for carcinogen screening. The sensitivity of this approach for detecting genotoxins can be enhanced by subsequent administration of a tumour promoter such as phenobarbital.

Since the number of 'preneoplastic' liver lesions produced by a carcinogen is very great relative to the eventual numbers of tumours, only small numbers of animals are required. Moreover, this approach, unlike others to be described, can be applied to any species. Also, the release of γ-glutamyl transpeptidase from foci into the serum provides a facile means of monitoring hepatocarcinogenic effects.

(2) Skin tumour induction in mice. The carcinogenicity of a limited number of chemicals and crude products can be revealed readily upon continuous application to the skin of mice, producing papillomas or carcinomas, or upon subcutaneous injection, yielding sarcomas. Activity as initiating agents can be rapidly revealed by the concurrent or sequential application of a promoter such as phorbol ester.

(3) Pulmonary tumour induction in mice. Certain mouse strains, especially the A/Heston and related strains such as A/J, are extremely sensitive to the induction of lung tumours by chemicals. The test must be conducted with young mice to avoid the complication of the high incidence of spontaneous tumours that develops later in life. Results are expressed as the percentage of animals with tumours compared to controls, and the multiplicity of tumours is an additional parameter indicative of potency.

(4) Breast cancer induction in female Sprague-Dawley rats. Certain classes of chemicals rapidly induce cancer in the mammary gland of young, female Sprague-Dawley rats. These animals are most sensitive to the effects of carcinogens with exposure at about 55 days of age. Multiplicity of tumours is an additional parameter of potency.

(5) Assays for promoters. In addition to providing evidence of carcinogenicity, limited *in vivo* bioassays can be adapted to specifically test for promoting substances. For this purpose, small doses of a genotoxic carcinogen active at specific target organs, such as skin, breast, colon, urinary bladder, or liver, are applied, followed by the test substance. The liver of certain commonly used mouse strains reacts as if it already has an abnormal genome, and thus responds positively to promoters for liver carcinogenesis.

Decision point 2

Positive results in two of the limited *in vivo* bioassays are considered unequivocal evidence of carcinogenicity. Also, positive results in two or more of the *in vitro* tests reliably indicating genotoxicity, together with a definite positive result in a limited *in vivo* bioassay, would indicate potential carcinogenicity. Positive results in only one *in vitro* test and/or one *in vivo* test must be considered equivocal.

The demonstration of promoting activity in any of the modified assays in the absence of genotoxicity indicates a specific type of hazard of the chemical, deserving investigation as an epigenetic phenomenon.

D. Chronic bioassay

The DPA reserves a chronic bioassay as a last resort for confirming questionable results in the more limited testing. Chronic bioassay would also be applied for compounds that are inactive in the preceding stages but where extensive human exposure is likely.

The requirements for the conduct of a chronic bioassay have been established over a number of years[4]. In addition, however, testing should include approaches to develop data on possible carcinogenicity through epigenetic mechanisms. Also, multispecies and dose response data are most important to permit the results to be realistically applied to human risk assessment. The elimination of unnecessary chronic testing of many chemicals by application of the DPA makes more extensive testing of suspected epigenetic agents economically feasible.

E. Decision point 3 or final evaluation

Chronic bioassays as an endpoint in the DPA should yield definitive data on carcinogenicity. The production of tumours in high yield in multiple organs and with a short latency is indicative of a genotoxic effect, whereas a low yield of tumours in select organs, particularly only liver, kidney or endocrine glands, after lifetime exposure, suggests an epigenetic basis for the oncogenicity.

Nonetheless, the results of the *in vitro* short-term tests must be taken into account for an assessment of mechanisms of action and risk extrapolation to humans. Thus, convincing positive results in the *in vitro* tests together with documented *in vivo* carcinogenicity permits classification of the chemical as a genotoxic carcinogen. Such a chemical would be regarded as a qualitative carcinogenic hazard[13].

In the absence of convincing evidence for genotoxicity of a chemical but, nonetheless, indication of carcinogenicity in certain animal bioassays, it is possible that the chemical is an epigenetic carcinogen. The reliability of this conclusion depends upon the relevance of the *in vitro* tests. For example, the failure of some stable organochlorine pesticides to show genotoxic properties in the same liver cell systems as the *in vivo* target cell for these agents is a powerful argument for an epigenetic mechanism of action[16]. The nature of the epigenetic mechanisms are poorly understood, but are probably distinct for different classes of carcinogens and may involve chronic tissue injury, immunosuppressive effects, hormonal imbalances, stimulation of cell proliferation, release of existing altered cells from growth control, or processes not yet known. In any case, most types of agents acting via epigenetic mechanisms have carcinogenic characteristics different from genotoxins[19]. Thus, these types of agents, in contrast to genotoxic carcinogens, may represent only quantitative hazards to humans and, with information from appropriate toxicological dose-response studies, safe levels of exposure may be formulated[13, 19].

APPLICATION OF DECISION POINT APPROACH TO EVALUATION OF VETERINARY DRUGS

The DPA is a systematic process for evaluation of the carcinogenicity of any type of chemical. Moreover, since the DPA provides mechanistic data for human risk assessment, it is highly appropriate for evaluation of veterinary drugs where the major concern is secondary human exposure.

Among drugs used in food-producing animals, hormonally-active compounds which increase body weight and compounds to combat microbial infections and parasitic infestations are widely used. An important example is diethylstilboestrol (DES), a synthetic oestrogen which has been used as a feed additive for cattle and sheep.

DES possesses a stilbene double bond and, therefore, has been suggested to be capable of forming a reactive species that could damage DNA[5]. DES has been reported to produce genetic effects in some systems, but is inactive in most *in vitro* tests[1]. According to the mechanistic concepts underlying the DPA (i.e. the classification of carcinogens detailed in Table 7.7), a non-genotoxic agent with hormonal activity would have to be evaluated for the possibility of production of tumours by a hormonal mechanism. Evidence does exist that hormonal effects are the basis for the carcinogenicity of DES both in animals and in humans[15]. For example, with chronic exposure to adult mice, DES produces mammary tumours only in mice carrying the mammary tumour virus. Thus, its hormonal effects may exert a promoting action on the mammary gland that facilitates the development of tumours from cells initiated by the virus. Likewise, with high level exposure to neonates, tissue changes are produced in the hormonally-sensitive vaginal epithelium. Neoplasia, similar to that in humans exposed *in utero*, occurs only later in life when alterations produced in the endocrine system during development may play a role. Therefore, the lack of convincing genotoxicity in the battery and the dependence of carcinogenicity upon hormonal effects permits the conclusion that DES is a type of epigenetic carcinogen that requires a risk evaluation distinct from that of genotoxic carcinogens.

For hormonal substances there is a definite threshold below which they do not perturb the endocrine system and hence are not carcinogenic. No evidence exists that DES residues in food would result in the sustained levels in adults or the extremely high levels in fetuses required for carcinogenicity. Therefore, the data base provided for in the DPA, and the understanding of the mechanisms of carcinogenesis that are integral to it, lead to the conclusion that trace residues of DES in food do not represent a carcinogenic hazard to humans. Similarly, other hormonal agents used in food-producing animals such as trenbolone, zeranol and sex steroids hormones, can be ascertained not to pose a threat to human health.

Several quinoxaline-type compounds are used for growth promotion and the treatment of enteric diseases in swine. One of these, quinoxaline-1,4-dioxide, produces liver and nasal tumours in rats[10]. Therefore, two others, carbadox and olaquindox, were tested in the *Salmonella*/microsome test and hepatocyte/DNA repair test. Both compounds were positive (Table 7.8). Thus, as recommended in the DPA, they should be considered as potential carcinogens. Moreover, since a structurally related compound is an established carcinogen, support is added to this conclusion from structural considerations. Regarding risk evaluation, these agents are carcinogens of the genotoxic type, and therefore, they must be presumed to be a hazard at any significant level of exposure.

Table 7.8 Genotoxicity of quinoxalines

	Salmonella/*microsome*					*Hepatocyte/*
	TA 100	*TA 1535*	*TA 98*	*TA 1537*	*TA 1538*	*DNA repair*
Carbadox	+	–	+	+	–	+
Olaquindox	+	–	+	–	–	+

Carbadox is rapidly metabolized to several compounds including quinoxaline-2-carboxylic acid which is the most persistent residue. Quinoxaline-2-carboxylic acid is therefore designated as the marker substance with a regulatory level of 30 μg/kg. Thus, an individual consuming 100 g of pork might ingest 3 μg or less than 0.06 μg/kg body weight. Tucker[10] observed carcinogenicity of quinoxaline 1,4-dioxide at 10 mg/kg body weight continuously, but not at 1 mg/kg. Given this rather steep dose-response curve, potential episodic exposures from residues representing less than 0.001% of the carcinogenic dose would appear not to represent a hazard. However, exposure of individuals engaged in feed preparation would require a different evaluation.

CONCLUSIONS

The DPA for carcinogen testing is applicable to the evaluation of veterinary drugs and is compatible with FDA guidelines in the United States.

Using the data base that would be acquired under the DPA and the interpretations derived from the mechanistic concepts incorporated into the DPA, non-genotoxic hormonal substances used for growth promotion are seen not to represent a human carcinogenic hazard whereas human exposure to genotoxic veterinary drugs must be minimized.

References

1. Clayson, D. L., Jansen, J. D., Rosenkranz, H., Upton, A. C. and Williams, G. M. Report of ICPEMC task group on the differentiation between genotoxic and nongenotoxic carcinogens. In preparation
2. Food and Drug Administration (1982). Chemical compounds in food-producing animals; availability of criteria for guide lines. *Fed. Register*, **47**, 4972–7
3. Hayashi, M., Ishihara, Y., Nishio, O., Tatematsu, M., Makino, M. and Asai, T. (1980). Histopathological observations of spontaneous tumors in slaughtered-animals (73 cases). *Nagoya Med. J.*, **24**, 163–76
4. International Agency for Research on Cancer (1980). Long-term and short-term screening assays for carcinogens: a critical appraisal. *IARC*, Lyon
5. Metzler, M. (1976). Metabolic activation of carcinogenic diethylstilbestrol in rodents and humans. *J. Toxicol. Environ. Health*, **1** (Suppl.), 21–35
6. Mishra, N., Dunkel, V. and Mehlman, M. (eds.) (1981). Advances in Modern Environmental Toxicology. Vol. 1. (Princeton: Senate Press)
7. Moulton, J. E. (1978). *Tumors in Domestic Animals*. (Berkeley and Los Angeles: University of California Press)
8. Smith, H. A. and Jones, T. C. (eds.) (1961). *Veterinary Pathology*. (Philadelphia: Lea and Febiger)
9. Stich, H. F. and San, R. H. C. (eds.) (1981). Short-Term Tests for Chemical Carcinogens. (New York: Springer-Verlag)
10. Tucker, M. J. (1975). Carcinogenic action of quinoxaline 1,4-dioxide in rats. *J. Natl. Cancer Inst.*, **55**, 137–45
11. Weisburger, J. H. and Williams, G. M. (1978). Decision point approach to carcinogen testing. In Asher, I. M. and Zervos, C. (eds.) *Structural Correlates of Carcinogenesis and Mutagenesis*. pp. 45–52. (FDA Rockville: The Office of Science)
12. Weisburger, J. H. and Williams, G. M. (1980). Chemical carcinogens. In Doull, J., Klaasen, C. D. and Amdur, M. O. (eds.) *Toxicology, The Basic Science of Poisons*. 2nd Edn, pp. 84–138. (New York: Macmillan)
13. Weisburger, J. H. and Williams, G. M. (1981). Basic requirements for health risk analysis: the decision point approach for systematic carcinogen testing. In *Proceedings of the Third Life Sciences Symposium on Health Risk Analysis*. pp. 249–71. (Philadelphia: Franklin Press)
14. Weisburger, J. H. and Williams, G. M. (1981). Carcinogen testing. Current problems and new approaches. *Science*, **214**, 401–7
15. Weisburger, J. H. and Williams, G. M. (1982). Metabolism of chemical carcinogens. In Becker, F. F. (ed.) *Cancer: A Comprehensive Treatise*. 2nd Edn, pp. 241–333. (New York: Plenum Press)
16. Williams, G. M. (1981). Liver carcinogenesis: the role for some chemicals of an epigenetic mechanism of liver tumor promotion involving modification of the cell membrane. *Food Cosmetics Toxicol.*, **19**, 577–83
17. Williams, G. M., Kroes, R., Waaijers, H. W. and van de Poll, K. W. (eds.) (1980). *The Predictive Value of Short-Term Screening Tests in Carcinogenicity Evaluation*. (New York: Elsevier/North-Holland)

18. Williams, G. M. and Weisburger, J. H. (1981). Systematic carcinogen testing through the decision point approach. *Ann. Rev. Pharmacol. Toxicol.*, **21**, 393–416
19. Williams, G. M. and Weisburger, J. H. (1982). Risk assessment of dietary carcinogens and tumor promoters. In Campbell, C. and Schottenfeld, D. (eds.) *Diet and Cancer; from Basic Research to Policy Implications*. (A. R. Liss). In press

8
Chemical induced teratogenesis

P. Delatour

Teratology, a descriptive science until the 19th century, has entered an experimental phase, with pharmacological as well as biochemical approaches[1]. Many substances are teratogenic for man (thalidomide, aminopterin, diphenylhydantoin) and laboratory animals. Teratological accidents in domestic animals reported since 1960 have not been from genopathic origin but rather induced by drugs or food factors.

This chapter aims to demonstrate not only the diversity of incriminated substances, and the species most sensitive, but mainly to illustrate the basic laws of chemical teratogenesis in domestic animals. The main factors influencing embryotoxic induction include (1) species sensitivity, (2) low amplitude of the teratogenic stimulus, (3) concept of the critical period, (4) effect of single dosage, and (5) distinction between general and specific teratogens.

SPECIES SENSITIVITY

The degree of sensitivity among animal species is not identical; some are even refractory. Parbendazole is teratogenic in sheep[14,15,19,21] but not in pigs[10]; oxfendazole is also teratogenic in sheep[4], but not for cattle[16]. Griseofulvin is active in cats[8,11,20] but does not seem teratogenic in dogs.

THE LOW AMPLITUDE OF THE TERATOGENIC STIMULUS

By definition, the ideal teratogenic agent is a substance which causes deviations from the normal course of embryonic development without affecting the health of the mother. The range of dosages at which the agent is effective is such that it does not harm the adult, e.g. parbendazole is a teratogen in sheep between 30 and 60 mg/kg whereas the maximum tolerated dosage in adults is 1000 mg/kg. For thalidomide, the corresponding figures[3,13] are 30 and 1500 mg/kg respectively. There is a very narrow margin between the posology which is teratogenic and that which is embryolethal. The optimal teratogenic dosage is often one which induces a moderate embryolethal effect, e.g. for dogs, the teratogenic incidence of thalidomide is unnoticeable at 500 mg/kg[18], very weak 'in some cases' at 400 mg/kg[17], of 26% at 100–200 mg/kg[23], and finally of 37% at 30 mg/kg[3]. At high dosages the embryolethal effect may cover the teratogenic effect or limit its expression by provoking the death of the sensitive embryos.

CONCEPT OF THE CRITICAL PERIOD

Studies have shown that the teratogenic effect occurs only during organogenesis. At the initial stages corresponding to the 'refractory period' the embryo expresses an all-or-nothing response to the aggression of the toxic substance: embryolethality or a process of 'regulation' will occur giving rise to normal further development. In the latter stages of histogenesis or 'fetal period' the opposite occurs, malformations of dys- or aplastic type are no longer possible and only functional troubles of tissular differentiation appear. Table 8.1 lists data concerning experimental teratology.

Table 8.1 Implantation and teratogenic periods during the pregnancy of species of laboratory and veterinary interest

Animal species	*Implantation period* (day)	*Teratogenic period* (day)	*Length of pregnancy* (days)
Mouse	5	5–15	21
Rat	5	5–15	22
Rabbit	7	8–16	29
Cat	13	5–20	55–63
Dog	17	8–25	55–70
Pig	15	10–24	115
Sheep	15–16	10–25	148

The data shows a long and delayed period in the histological and structural differentiation of the reproductive organs and the nervous system. For instance, trichlorfon in the pig is responsible for an ataxia syndrome, when administered between day 45 and day 63 of pregnancy[12]. It should be pointed out that, contrary to what has been shown for laboratory animals, the teratogenic period does not always occur after implantation, e.g. albendazole causes exencephaly in sheep on day 12, thalidomide is active in the dog[3] between day 8 and 20, 10-methyl-folic acid is teratogenic in the cat[22] between day 5 and day 11, and cyclopamine from *Veratrum californicum* is teratogenic on day 14 in the sheep[2].

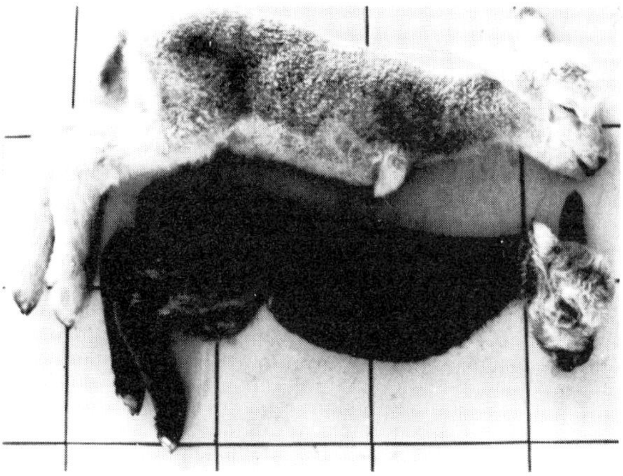

Figure 8.1 Thoracic amelia in the sheep; cambendazole, single oral dose of 75 mg/kg, on day 21 of pregnancy

EFFECT OF SINGLE DOSAGE

It is understood from the laws of embryology that teratogenesis is a form of acute toxicity since it can appear after a single administration of drug (Figure 8.1). Within the critical period the preliminary form of the different organs does not develop synchronously and the nature of the abnormality produced depends on the timing of the treatment. This concept is called the 'teratological calendar'. This calendar had been established for humans through epidemiological research, and for laboratory animals through experiment. For domestic animals, our knowledge is limited in this respect. The teratological calendar for sheep is given in Table 8.2.

Severe abnormalities happen in the early teratogenic stage (head and face, day 12–17; spinal column, day 16–21) whereas the less important malformations occur at later stages (limb distortions, day 22–25). In the case of cambendazole, taking into account the halflife in blood and the value of the maximum no-effect level, it can be confirmed that thoracic amelia occurs on

Table 8.2 Teratological calendar of the sheep

Day 12	Exencephaly (albendazole)
Day 14	Cyclopia (*V. californicum*)
Day 16	Microphthalmia, fused vertebrae (parbendazole)
Day 17	Hare-lip, uterus aplasia, fused ribs, eye lids defects (oxfendazole)
Day 21	Thoracic amelia, kidney ectopia, scoliosis (cambendazole)
Day 22	Dysmelia (parbendazole)
Day 24	Arthrogryposis (parbendazole)

day 21 in the sheep after about 18 h of drug stimulation, i.e. 1/200 of the length of the embryofetal development in this species, or 1/20 of the teratogenic period.

DISTINCTION BETWEEN GENERAL AND SPECIFIC TERATOGENS

This distinction[1] is a limitation in the concept of the teratological calendar. The general agent harms all sensitive organs, and produces a variety of damages. The specific agent has a precise target and strikes with an all-or-nothing response depending on chronological considerations. For instance, in sheep and rats, parbendazole, cambendazole and albendazole act as general teratogens whereas cyclopamine produces a specific effect on day 14 but is not effective at any other period[2].

ROLE OF METABOLISM

This concept is not related specifically to chemical teratogenesis but to general pharmacology. It explains why, among anthelmintics from the benzimidazole family, fenbendazole and oxibendazole are not teratogenic, whereas parbendazole, mebendazole, oxfendazole and albendazole are. The latter are teratogenic in themselves or indirectly by a metabolite which by its nature and kinetics is responsible for the effect. It is also true for febantel[6,7].

These facts may eventually explain the different degree of sensitivity among inter-species. Thalidomide is active in mice, rabbits, monkeys, dogs, pigs and humans but not in rats. It has been recently demonstrated[9] that the mechanism of the teratogenic action of this compound implies the microsomal creation of an arene oxide reactive metabolite. This latter compound is produced from samples of monkey and rabbit liver but not from those of rats. Nevertheless, in the present state of our knowledge, these observations do not take into account all the experimental evidence available. For instance, in the case of albendazole, the metabolism in cattle coincides with that in sheep although the bovines are refractory to the teratogenic effect.

In fact, if we disregard the horse for which we lack embryological information and teratological data, it would appear that the basic laws of embryotoxic induction defined for laboratory animals are also applicable for domestic animals. This new concept helps us to make more prudent use of incriminated drugs and improve prevention for similar manifestations seen in vegetable toxins and inducible drugs as well.

References

1. Ancel, P. (1950). La Chimiotératogénèse. *Doin Ed.*, Paris
2. Binns, W., Shupe, J. L., Keeler, R. F. *et al.* (1965). Chronologic evaluation of teratogenicity in sheep fed *Veratrum californicum. Am. J. Vet. Med. Assoc.*, **147**, 839–42
3. Delatour, P., Dams, R. and Favre-Tissot, M. (1965). Thalidomide: embryopathies chez le chien. *Thérapie*, **20**, 573–89

4. Delatour, P., Debroye, J., Lorgue, G. *et al.* (1977). Embryotoxicité expérimentale de l'oxfendazole chez le rat et le mouton. *Rec. Méd. Vét.*, **153**, 639–45
5. Delatour, P., Lorgue, G., Courtot, D. *et al.* (1975). Embryotoxicité expérimentale du cambendazole chez le mouton. *Bull. Soc. Sci. Vét. Méd. Comp. Lyon*, **77**, 197–203
6. Delatour, P. (1980). Some aspects of the teratogenicity of veterinary drugs. Paper presented at the *International Conference on Veterinary Pharmacology, Toxicology and Therapy*, Cambridge
7. Delatour, P., Daudon, M., Garnier, F. *et al.* (1982). Relation métabolisme-toxicité du fébantel chez le rat et le mouton. *Ann. Rech. Vét.*, **13**, 163–70
8. Gillitch, A. (1972). Griseofulvine, a possible teratogen. *Can. Vet. J.*, **13**, 244
9. Gordon, G. B., Spielberg, S. P., Blake, D. A. *et al.* (1981). Thalidomide teratogenesis: evidence for a toxic arene oxide metabolite. *Proc. Nat. Acad. Sci. USA*, **78**, 2545–8
10. Hancock, N. A. and Poulter, D. A. L. (1974). The effects of parbendazole on reproduction in sheep and other animals. *Cornell Vet.*, **64** (Suppl.), 92–6
11. Klein, M. F. and Beale, J. R. (1972). Griseofulvine: a teratogenic study. *Science*, **175**, 1483–4
12. Knox, B., Askaa, J., Basse, A. *et al.* (1978). Congenital ataxia and tremor with cerebellar hypoplasia in piglets born by sows treated with Neguvon vet. (metrifonate, trichlorfon) during pregnancy. *Nord. Vet. Med.*, **30**, 538–45
13. Kunz, W., Keller, H. and Mückter, H. (1956). *N*-Phthalyl-glutaminsäure-imid. Experimentelle Untersuchungen an einem neuen synthetischen Produkt mit sedativen Eigenschaften. *Arzneim. Forsch.*, **6**, 426–39
14. Lapras, M., Deschanel, J. P., Delatour, P. *et al.* (1973). Accidents tératologiques chez le mouton après administration de parbendazole. *Bull. Soc. Sci. Vét. Méd. Comp. Lyon*, **75**, 53–60
15. Middleton, M. D., Plant, J. W., Walker, C. E. *et al.* (1974). The effects of methyl 5(6)-butyl-2-benzimidazole carbamate (parbendazole) on reproduction in sheep and other animals: teratological studies in ewes in Australia. *Cornell Vet.*, **64** (Suppl.), 56–68
16. Piercy, D. W. T., Reynolds, J. and Brown, P. R. M. (1979). Reproductive safety studies on oxfendazole in sheep and cattle. *Br. Vet. J.*, **135**, 405–10
17. Riemschneider, R. and Brockmeyer, K. (1963). Teratogene Wirksamkeit organischer Verbindung. Weitere Thalidomid-Versuche. *Az. Naturforsch.*, **186**, 584–5
18. Roberjot, G. (1966). De l'utilisation de la chienne en vue de la recherche du pouvoir tératogène d'un médicament. *Communic. Symp. Int. sur les Animaux de Lab.*, Lyon. pp. 221–6
19. Saunders, L. Z., Shone, D. K., Philip, J. R. *et al.* (1974). The effects of methyl 5(6)-butyl-2-benzimidazole carbamate (parbendazole) on reproduction in sheep and other animals: malformation in newborn lambs. *Cornell Vet.*, **64** (Suppl.), 7–41
20. Scott, F. W., de la Hunta, A., Schultz, R. D. *et al.* (1975). Teratogenesis in cats associated with griseofulvin therapy. *Teratology*, **11**, 79–86.
21. Szabo, K. T., Miller, C. R. and Scott, G. C. (1974). The effects of methyl 5(6)-butyl-2-benzimidazole carbamate (parbendazole) on reproduction in sheep and other animals: teratological study in ewes in the United States. *Cornell Vet.*, **64** (Suppl.), 41–55
22. Tuchmann-Duplessis, H. and Lefebvres-Boisselot, J. (1957). Les effets tératogènes de l'acide 10-méthyl-folique chez la chatte. *C.R. Soc. Biol.*, **151**, 2005–8
23. Weidman, W. H., Young, H. H. and Zollman, P. E. (1963). The effects of thalidomide on the unborn puppy. *Staff Meet. Mayo Clin.*, **38**, 518–22

9
Levamisole as an immunomodulator in the prevention of neonatal disease

L. Desplenter

Disease in newborn calves is mainly of enteric origin. Both morbidity and mortality of calves with diarrhoea have been related to low postcolostral serum immunoglobulin concentration. The IgM is considered as the principal immunoglobulin giving immune protection against enteric disease. Enhanced susceptibility to infection can result from agammaglobulinaemia or hypogammaglobulinaemia, defective cellular immune responses, disorders of complement metabolism and functional defects in the phagocytic cell.

Levamisole (Figure 9.1), an anthelmintic used world-wide in man and animals, has proved to act as an immunomodulator in experimental models and in a number of selected human and animal immunodeficiencies with related pathology. These properties have been extensively reviewed[4,12,21]. The studies on its application in veterinary practice, and specially in bovine practice, have been partly reviewed[6,15].

Levamisole modulates the immune function at 2–3 mg/kg of body weight, in contrast to the greater anthelmintic dosage. When administered in amounts above the immunotherapeutic dose, levamisole may even suppress immune function. Intermittent treatment is more efficient than continuous treatment in restoring the immune responsiveness.

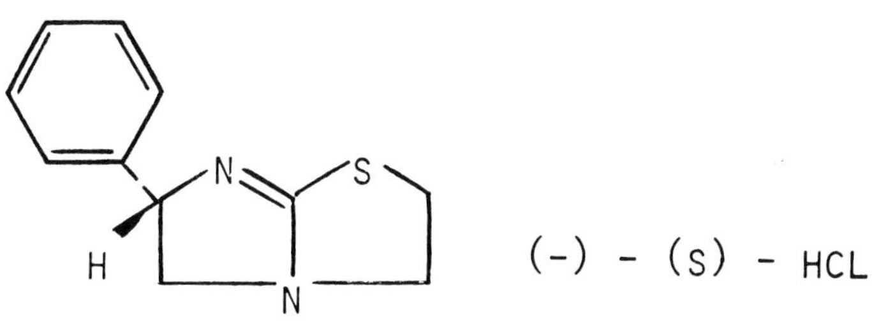

Figure 9.1 Structure of levamisole

In vitro and *in vivo* levamisole is able to restore to normal the major functions of effector cells of the cell-mediated immune response. There is evidence that the maturation of granulocytes and of precursor cells into functioning T-lymphocytes is induced *in vivo* but not *in vitro*. Levamisole also induces a serum factor which, when transferred into untreated animals, mimics the effect of levamisole on immune functions.

The restoration to normal of the major functions of the effector cells involved in cell-mediated immune responses is most pronounced and consistent in compromised hosts, whose T-lymphocytes or phagocyte functions are below normal. Usually an adequate immune response is not increased. The B-lymphocyte activity is not directly stimulated: the proliferative response to mitogens is not increased and there is no direct effect on antibody production. The evidence of the maturation of T-lymphocytes and granulocytes is provided by the experiments in nude and thymectomized mice.

The serum factor, induced by levamisole, is a dialysable factor and seems not to be a complement factor or a levamisole metabolite. It is not found in animals that fail to respond to levamisole, or in untreated animals. Serum from levamisole-treated rabbits or mice mimics the effect of levamisole on immune functions, when injected in untreated animals. In summary, the regulation of the cell mediated immune function by levamisole, directly or by release of a serum factor, is dual:

(1) Restoration of effector functions of peripheral T-lymphocytes and phagocytes.
(2) Stimulation of precursor T-lymphocytes into mature T-cells.

The accumulated data suggest that levamisole behaves physiologically as a thymomimetic agent on the cellular arm of the immune system. The biochemical mechanism of action remains a matter of speculation. The various mechanisms by which levamisole might act are not mutually exclusive and it is still not clear which are the more important mechanisms for its therapeutic actions.

However, one should keep in mind that the responses to levamisole are not always predictable, even if it is used in appropriate conditions. For example, there are responders and non-responders in every animal species, experimental model or disease tested. The responsiveness of mice to levamisole seems to be related to the ability to produce a serum factor. In addition, there are variables such as immune repulsion by pathogens or humoral blocking factors, which may inhibit responsiveness to the drug.

The therapeutic potential of levamisole as immunomodulator in human medicine has been well defined. It is used in combination with vaccinations and has been proven to have a favourable effect in recurrent and chronic infections. Important indications are also its application in inflammatory diseases, such as rheumatoid arthritis, and in cancer patients[18].

In veterinary medicine, levamisole has been used as immunomodulator in nearly all animal species for a variety of indications. The results, described in the reported experiments, are fluctuating between highly favourable and no effect. In cattle, for example, protective effects have been obtained in the prevention or reduction of complications associated with shipping fever[11,23].

An increase in resistance to re-infection or challenge with parasites, such as *Trichostrongylus axei* and *Dictyocaulus viviparus*, has also been reported when the primary infection had been eliminated by levamisole treatment[9,16–17]. The potentiating effects of levamisole in combination with antiviral vaccination or the increase in resistance to viral challenge are rather variable, depending on the method applied for evaluation of the trials. In cattle, experiments with infectious bovine rhinotracheitis[10,14], herpes[2,3] and foot-and-mouth disease virus[20] have been reported. The anti-Brucella agglutinin titres have[1] or have not[5] increased after levamisole treatment, while favourable results have been obtained when immunodeficient cattle were used in the experiments[13].

The largest experience with levamisole in cattle, including the highest number of animals, has been the treatment of cattle during the last stage of pregnancy. This treatment results in the prevention or reduction in the incidence of clinical postpartum mastitis and endometritis[6,8,19]. Trials in Belgium to confirm this effect have not been successful (Symoens and Tuyttens: personal communication).

The most consistent results have been obtained and reported in the prevention of neonatal disease, morbidity and mortality in newborn calves after treatment of the pregnant cows with levamisole[7,8,22]. The experiments on calf mortality are summarized in Table 9.1. The cattle farms involved in these trials are selected farms with a known history of high calf mortality, in spite of the routine use of electrolytes and antibiotics. The mortality is reduced from 13.1% in 987 control calves to 2.3% in 657 calves from levamisole-treated cows. Levamisole treatment in these pregnant cows is an i.m. injection at 2.5 mg/kg or a 'pour-on' application at 5 mg/kg once weekly during 4 consecutive weeks before parturition.

In experiment 4 not only was mortality recorded, but also the number of diseased calves (Table 9.2) and the duration of their disease (Table 9.3). In the control group of 369 calves, 50.9% were ill during one or more days,

Table 9.1 Prevention of calf mortality by pretreatment of pregnant cows with levamisole

Experiment	*Investigator*	*Treatment*	*Calves* Born	Died
1	Tamarin	Control	20	4
		Levamisole	20	0
2	Flesh	Control	32	8
		Levamisole	16	0
3	Marsboom	Control	117	7
		Levamisole	104	2
4	Marsboom	Control	369	8
		Levamisole	323	2
5	Antoine	Control	70	8
		Levamisole	69	5
6	Flesh	Control	379	94
		Levamisole	125	6
	Total	Control	987	129
		Levamisole	657	15

Table 9.2 Number of diseased calves (Experiment 4)

Cow treatment	*Total number of calves*	*Number of diseased calves*	%	p-*value*
Placebo	369	188	50.9	0.001
Levamisole	323	104	32.2	

Table 9.3 Duration of disease (Experiment 4)

Days of disease	*Control (188 calves) number of calves*	%	*Levamisole (104 calves) number of calves*	%	p-*value*
1	51	27.1	38	36.5	n.s.
2	40	21.3	30	28.8	n.s.
3	97	51.6	36	34.6	0.007

compared to 32.2% in the 323 calves from treated cows. Analysed in function of the duration of illness, the number of calves that were sick for 1 or 2 days was similar in both groups, but the number of animals that were sick for 3 days or more was significantly higher in the control group.

In order to evaluate the possibility of establishing a profile on the immune status of the animals, some samples were taken in experiments 4 and 5 to determine the immunoglobulin levels in serum and colostrum or the metabolic activity of the lymphocytes in calves. In experiment 4, lymphocytes from six control calves and six calves from treated cows were incubated with Con A, PWM or PHA. After determination of the glucose consumption in the cultures, no difference between these two groups was observed. By means of the zinc sulphate turbidity test, the total immune globulin level was determined in the serum of 12 control and 12 treated cows and in the serum of 13 control calves and 13 calves from treated cows. No statistical difference was obtained between the cows or the calves of the two groups. By the same method the increase in serum immunoglobulin level before and after colostrum uptake was compared in six control calves and six calves from treated cows. The increase was comparable in both groups. The same results have been obtained by comparing IgG, IgM and IgA in the serum and IgG in the colostrum of control and treated cows (Nelkin: personal communication). In experiment 5, Antoine (personal communication, 1979) compared the albumin, total protein, α, β and γ globulins in the colostrum of treated ($n = 39$) and control ($n = 44$) cows. A statistical difference was not observed for any of these parameters.

This means that with this limited number of samples and determinations, it is impossible to provide an explanation for the observed clinical effects. From the experience in the human medicine, we learn that the effects observed with levamisole are reproducible only if populations of patients are studied. Usually, there is no correlation between clinical improvement and restoration of immune functions, as measured by the current parameters. This statement is confirmed in veterinary medicine by the experiments reported here.

References

1. Arnault, G. (1981). Note à propos de la production des anticorps immédiats après vaccination des génisses avec le B-19. Influence de quelques facteurs intercurrents. *Bull. Soc. Vét. Prat.*, **65**, 439–61
2. Babiuk, L. A. and Misra, V. (1981). Levamisole and bovine immunity: *in vitro* and *in vivo* effects on immune responses to herpes virus immunization. *Can. J. Microbiol.*, **27**, 1312–19
3. Babiuk, L. A. and Misra, V. (1982). Effect of levamisole in immune responses to bovine herpes virus. *Am. J. Vet. Res.*, **43**, 1349–54
4. Brunner, C. and Muscoplat, C. (1980). Immunomodulatory effects of levamisole. *J. Am. Vet. Med. Assoc.*, **176**, 1159–62
5. De Diego, A., Carillo, C. and Trumper, S. (1974). Influencia de los antiparasitarios sistemicos sobre las aglutininas antibrucelicas. *Gac. Vet.*, **36**, 164–70 and 584–8
6. Espinasse, J. (1980). Immunostimulation par le lévamisole en clinique vétérinaire. *Cah. Méd. Vét.*, **49**, 5–13
7. Flesh, J., Ovadia, H. and Nelken, D. (1977). Prevention of calf mortality by pretreatment of pregnant cows with levamisole. *Refuah Vet.*, **34**, 97–8
8. Flesh, J., Harel, W. and Nelken, D. (1982). Immunopotentiating effect of levamisole in the prevention of bovine mastitis, fetal death and endometritis. *Vet. Rec.*, **111**, 56–7
9. Herlich, H. (1978). Resistance dynamics of calves to infection with *Trichostrongylus axei*. *Vet. Parasitol.*, **4**, 153–60
10. Irwin, M. R., Holmberg, C. A., Knight, H. D. *et al.* (1976). Effects of vaccination against I.B.R. and simultaneous administration of levamisole on primary humoral responses in calves. *Am. J. Vet. Res.*, **37**, 223–6
11. Irwin, M. R., Melendy, D. R. and Hutcheson, D. P. (1980). Reduced morbidity associated with shipping fever pneumonia in levamisole phosphate-treated feedlot cattle. *Southwest. Vet.*, **33**, 45–9
12. Janssen, P. A. J. (1976). The levamisole story. In Jucker, E. (ed.) *Progress Research*. Vol. 20, pp. 347–83. (Basel: Birhäuser)
13. Kaneene, J. M. B., Okino, F. C., Anderson, R. K. *et al.* (1981). Levamisole potentiation of antigen specific lymphocyte blastogenic response to *Brucella abortus* exposed but non-responsive cattle. *Vet. Immunol. Immunopathol.*, **2**, 75–85
14. Lejan, C. and Asso, J. (1981). Induction of an interferon activity in the nasal mucus of calves by administration of inactivated I.B.R. virus and levamisole. *Vet. Med. Anim. Sci.*, **12**, 283–92
15. Lucas, T. E. (1977). Levamisole as an experimental immunomodulating agent. In *Proceedings of the 10th Annual Convention of the American Association of Bovine Practition*. pp. 103–5
16. Oakley, G. A. (1980). The comparative efficacy of levamisole and diethylcarbamazine citrate against *Dictyocaulus viviparus* infection in cattle. *Vet. Rec.*, **107**, 166–70
17. Oakley, G. A. (1981). Protection developed against reinfection by *Dictyocaulus viviparus* following anthelmintic treatment of a one-day-old primary infection in cattle. *Vet. Rec.*, **109**, 485–7
18. Oakley, G. A. (1982). Comparison of protection against lungworm infection between levamisole-treated and vaccinated calves. *Vet. Rec.*, **111**, 28–31
19. Ovadia, H., Flesh, J. and Nelken, D. (1978). Prevention of bovine mastitis by treatment with levamisole. *Israel J. Med. Sci.*, **14**, 394–6
20. Schmied, L. M. and Rosenbusch, C. (1973). Effectos del levamisole sobre el indice de sueroproteccion en privacunation antiaftosa. *Rev. Med. Vet*, **54**, 467–71
21. Symoens, J., de Cree, J., van Bever, W. *et al.* (1979). Levamisole. In Goldberg, N. E. (ed.) *Pharmacological and Biochemical Properties of Drug Substances*. Vol. 2, pp. 407–64. (Washington: Acad. Pharm. Assoc.)
22. Symoens, J. (1980). Potential and limitations of immunotherapy. In Van Miert, A. S. *et al.*(eds.) *Trends in Veterinary Pharmacology and Toxicology*. pp. 90–6. (Amsterdam: Elsevier Scientific)
23. Ziprin, R. L., Steel, E. G., Petersen, H. D. *et al.* (1980). Hematologic study of effects of levamisole on stressed cattle. *Am. J. Vet. Res.*, **41**, 1884–5

10
Development and prophylaxis of anaemia in calves and lambs

P. H. Dilov

Certain changes take place in the composition and volume of the blood of newborn animals that are of species- and age-specific character and that are most clearly expressed during the perinatal period. Most important are the changes in the red blood cells. The content of haemoglobin in the blood of newborn pigs is greater than 10–11 g/100 ml and this drops to about 9 g/100 ml in the course of the first 24 h. According to Furugouri *et al.*[6], this decrease is due to dilution of the blood resulting from the absorption of colostrum. The haemoglobin content in the blood of the newborn calves is 12.5–13.5 g/100 ml, the erythrocyte count is $8.1\text{–}8.9 \times 10^6$ per mm^3 and the haematocrit is 38–40%[7,13]. These all decline in the course of the following 2 weeks. Gürtler *et al.*[8] observed a decrease in the blood iron in calves of the German Black-and-White breed from $159 \pm 52\,\mu g/100$ ml to $69 \pm 25\,\mu g/100$ ml in the course of the first 96 h after birth. The erythrocytes in pigs at birth contain less fetal haemoglobin (11.1 g/100 ml) and more adult type haemoglobin. At the 6th hour following birth the level of fetal haemoglobin drops to 6.7 g/100 ml and on the 3rd day to 3.3 g/100 ml[12]. The erythrocytes in calves and lambs at birth contain only fetal haemoglobin which is replaced by adult haemoglobin by the 9th and the 2nd week, respectively[15].

According to Shalm[14], calves are considered anaemic when the haemoglobin content drops below 8 g/100 ml and the erythrocyte count is less than 5×10^6 per mm^3, according to Bünger *et al.*[3] when the haemoglobin content is below 10.5 g/100 ml and the haematocrit below 33.5%. Bremmer and Dolgarno[1] established a decrease in plasma iron to $20\,\mu g/100$ ml to denote anaemia in calves. According to most authors, anaemia in calves is hypochromic and microcytic[9,11] and is related primarily to iron deficiency[2,7]. Hyperchromic anaemia in newborn calves suffering from gastroenteritis of non-specific aetiology has also been described[15]. Anaemic animals have a reduced resistance to respiratory and gastrointestinal diseases, poorly utilize feed and their growth is arrested[4,17]. Under the conditions of extensive animal breeding, however, anaemia in calves and lambs does not constitute a serious veterinary problem.

We have made it our aim to carry out investigations on the following:

(1) Ontogenetic changes in the blood of calves born on dairy farms of the industrial type;
(2) Species differences in the absorption and metabolism of the ferrodextran complex (calves and lambs); and
(3) Prophylaxis and therapy of anaemia (calves and lambs).

ONTOGENETIC CHANGES IN THE BLOOD OF CALVES

Investigations have been carried out on 17 dairy farms of the industrial type with a total of 788 calves of up to 30 days of age and of the following breeds: Black-and-White, Simmenthal, and Bulgarian Brown and their crosses. Calves born in the winter–spring and summer–autumn months have been taken from every dairy farm. Changes in the blood have been followed with regard to the content of haemoglobin (as cyanmethaemoglobin), the iron in the serum (after Ramzi's method), the erythrocyte and leukocyte counts (by the camera method or with a computer) and the haematocrit (by means of a microcentrifuge or with a computer). The significance of the differences has been determined by the Student–Fisher's test.

It has been ascertained that anaemia in sucking calves based upon blood haemoglobin content is a comparatively common disease with an incidence of 28.1% during the winter–spring months and 19.4% during the summer–autumn months. Higher haemoglobin and haematocrit values were observed during the summer–autumn months (9.81 ± 0.40 g/100 ml and 41.9 ± 1.8 g/100 ml respectively); the differences, however, were not significant. The same trend was observed in serum iron concentrations ($137 \pm 7.6\,\mu$g/100 ml vs. $123 \pm 8.41\,\mu$g/100 ml). There was no significant difference in the erythrocyte count in the blood of calves born during the two mentioned periods. The number of leukocytes was significantly higher ($p < 0.001$) in calves born in the winter–spring months (8137 ± 504 vs. 6579 ± 369 per mm^3). However, there were no significant differences in the haematological values of the female vs. male calves as has been reported by some authors[9]. Certain breed differences, however, have been found. The calves of the Simmenthal breed and crosses in comparison with the Black-and-White breed and Bulgarian Brown calves and their crosses showed significantly lower values of haemoglobin, erythrocytes and haematocrit. It is known that there are breed differences with respect to blood haemoglobin content. Subphysiological values for haemoglobin and erythrocytes were observed in calves of the Simmenthal breed and their crosses born in the winter–spring months (47.9% with haemoglobin below 8 g and 36.7% with erythrocytes below 5×10^6 per mm^3). Comparatively frequent cases of anaemia were observed in twin calves which were about 50% of the calves studied and in calves born to dams giving birth for the first time (about 40% and 20%, respectively). In regard to the calving season and the breed, changes occurred in the haemoglobin and less considerable changes occurred in the erythrocyte count, haematocrit and blood iron concentration.

A comparative high percentage of the day-old calves showed subphysiological values for hacmoglobin and for the remaining values but to an insignificant degree. The percentage of such animals rose in the following 7 days, then dropped. Vajda *et al.*[16] reported that anaemia was more frequently observed in calves within 14 days after birth. An interesting finding is that calves were very often born with anaemia. Furugouri[6] also mentions a congenital iron deficiency anaemia in calves.

These haematological investigations showed that anaemia in newborn calves exists, although it is less pronounced than anaemia in pigs. It is likely that the anaemia aggravates gastrointestinal and respiratory diseases, thus affecting the economics of cattle breeding. It should be duly considered, and regular prophylactic and therapeutic measures should be taken.

In contrast to pigs, calves were often born with hypochromaemia, sideropenia and erythropenia which did not progress significantly within the following 2–3 weeks. On the contrary, as the calves begin comparatively early consumption of starter mixtures and hay, and as their rate of weight gain decreases, an improvement in the haematological values without treatment is sometimes observed. On the other hand, the changes in the blood under the influence of therapeutic drugs take place more slowly than in pigs. The concept put forward by some authors[6,8], that factors influencing the fetal development of calves do affect the presence of anaemia, is confirmed; however, studies on this particular question are insufficient.

SPECIES-SPECIFIC DIFFERENCES IN IRON RESORPTION AND METABOLISM

Using ^{59}Fe and some other methods, we determined that Dextrofer-100 S.E.A. Pharmachim, containing 100 mg Fe^{3+}/ml) was well absorbed following i.m. administration to calves and lambs. In calves, peak levels of sideraemia were reached at the 8th and 12th hour and at the 24th and 48th hour in lambs. Radioactive iron appeared in the blood of calves and lambs at the 1st hour (Figure 10.1). Until the 24th hour, radioactivity was found primarily within the blood plasma and later it entered the erythrocytes. In calves on the 5th and 10th day, the highest levels of radioactive iron were found in the liver and spleen (the percentage difference was insignificant). No radioactivity was found in the heart and kidneys. In lambs, the highest radioactivity was observed in the spleen with lower levels in the liver, heart and kidneys.

There is, however, a species-specific peculiarity in the absorption and distribution of iron in calves and lambs treated with Dextrofer-100. It is known[10] and we have also demonstrated[3,5] that pigs treated i.m. with Feridextran complexes store a higher percentage of iron in the liver and a considerably lower percentage in the spleen. Both in calves and pigs, we found more iron in the reticuloendothelial organs on the 5th day after treatment, while in lambs considerably more iron was found on the 10th day. The difference in iron metabolism after i.m. injection of Feridextran preparations in pigs, lambs and calves is most likely due to physiological peculiarities and to the need for iron.

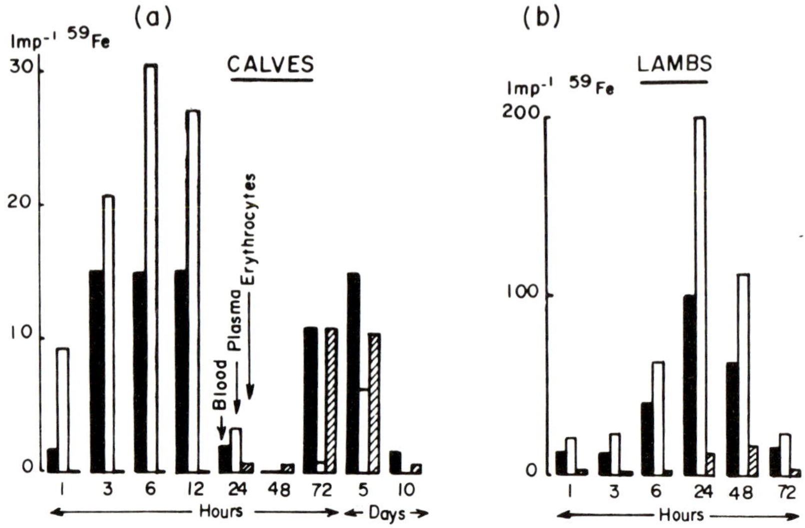

Figure 10.1 Dynamics of ^{59}Fe in the blood of calves (a) and lambs (b)

PROPHYLAXIS AND THERAPY OF ANAEMIA

The following preparations were used in the tests: Dextrofer-100, Dextrofer-100 with B_{12} (R & D Dept., Chemical and Pharmaceutical Works, Troyan, SED Pharmachim) containing 100 mg Fe^{3+} plus 80 μg cyanocobalamin per ml; Ferizin (laboratory batches) containing Feridextran, zinc and some vitamins; Biofer (laboratory batches) containing Feridextran, bovine γ-globulin, copper sulfuricum cobalto-chloride, cyanocobalamin and protein hydrolysate; Antianemin, a vitamin mineral premix; ferrisulphate containing 8% iron; iron glycerophosphate containing 10% iron; and Sucsal (IST, France).

Studies were carried out with pregnant cows and newborn calves. The content of haemoglobin and iron in the blood (by the bethophenanthroline method and with Boehringer's tests), the erythrocyte and leukocyte count (by means of a computer) and the haematocrit were followed up in the calves born by 23 cows treated 15–25 days before calving with the preparation Ferizin injected i.m. with 20 ml twice at an interval of 5 days, and in another 15 non-treated cows (controls).

A favourable but insignificant trend was observed with regard to the blood content of haemoglobin and iron, erythrocyte and leukocyte counts and haematocrit in the calves from cows treated with Ferizin when pregnant (Figure 10.2(a)). In five of the calves (30.3%) born by the control dams, the iron content was below 80 μg/100 ml; in six of the calves (26.3%) born by treated dams, it was also below 80 μg/100 ml which made us believe that in cows, as in sows, as shown by a number of authors, the placental transport of iron is limited.

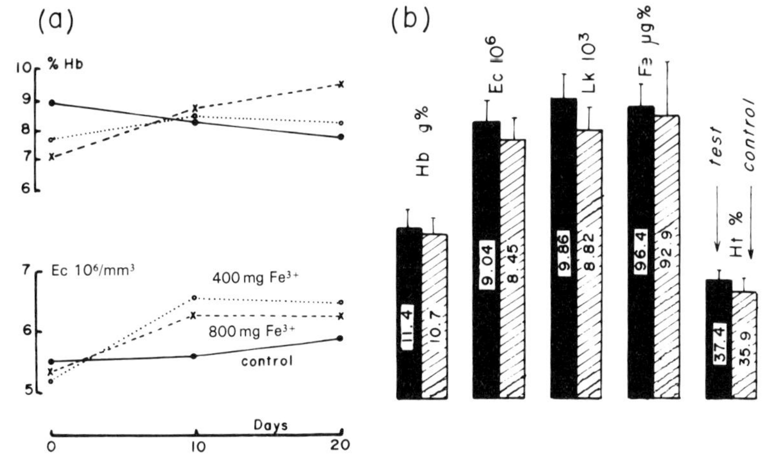

Figure 10.2 (a) Changes in haemoglobin and erythrocyte content in calves treated with Dextrofer-100. (b) Calves born from dams treated with Ferizin and not treated (control)

The erythropoietic effect of Dextrofer-100 was tested on calves up to 20 days of age with ascertained anaemia. The preparation was injected at 400 and 800 mg Fe^{3+}. The greatest number of the calves were born by dams giving birth for the first time and not adequately fed during pregnancy (food-beet, maize silage, and concentrate feed and straw without hay).

Data in Figure 10.2 (b) show that before Dextrofer-100 administration, subphysiological levels for haemoglobin and erythrocytes were ascertained in the blood of the test animals. A number of young erythrocytes (polychromasia) and, in individual animals, reticulocytes were found.

Increased haemoglobin content and erythrocyte count were noted following the injection of the preparation (haemoglobin was more favourably influenced by the 800 mg Fe^{3+}), while in the control animals during the 20 days of observation, haemoglobin and erythrocytes either declined or remained at the same level. Almost all calves on the farm were affected with enteritis during the first days after birth. Among the calves treated additionally (30–40 calves) for prophylactic purposes with Dextrofer-100 (in a dose of 800 ml Fe^{3+}), not so many cases of enteritis were reported or the reported cases were mild and the calves developed favourably.

In 33 calves aged up to 7 days (Black-and-White breed and crosses), the antianaemic effect of Dextrofer-100 and Sucsal was studied. The changes in the haemoglobin content, erythrocyte count, serum iron level, and iron-binding capacity (by the method of Ramsay) were followed for 30 days. Dextrofer-100 in a dose of 8 ml (800 mg Fe^{3+}) was injected i.m. in seven of the calves; 16 calves were treated simultaneously with Dextrofer-100 at the same dose and Sucsal i.m. at a dose of 100 ml; ten of the calves were used as controls. Calves with anaemia were selected for the trial; almost all of them were suffering from gastrointestinal diseases in varying forms.

Dextrofer-100 increased the quantity of haemoglobin, the erythrocyte count and the level of iron in comparison to the control calves (Figure 10.3).

On the 15th day, the effect produced in the test animals treated with a combination of Dextrofer-100 and Sucsal was not better than the effect in those treated with Dextrofer-100 only. On the 30th day, however, the effect with regard to haemoglobin and the erythrocyte and leukocyte counts was better in the calves treated with Dextrofer-100 and Sucsal.

The influence of Biofer was followed on the blood composition of 21 calves of the Black-and-White breed and crosses up to 10 days of age. Biofer in a dose of 0.6 ml/kg body weight (20 mg Fe^{3+}/kg body weight) was injected i.m. in seven calves. Dextrofer-100 at 0.2 ml/kg body weight (20 mg Fe^{3+}/kg) was injected in seven other calves; and the remaining seven calves were used as controls. Higher levels for haemoglobin, haematocrit, erythrocytes and leukocytes (counted by a computer) and growth rate were reported on the 30th day for the calves treated with Biofer, and the lowest levels were reported for the control animals (Figure 10.3). The content of serum iron was lower in the calves treated with Biofer, while there was no significant difference in the total protein content. We referred the better effect of Biofer to the introduction of copper, vitamins B_{12} and B_6, and normal bovine γ-globulin together with iron. Good results were obtained in Czechoslovakia through the application of a similar preparation[16].

The effects of the application of 3 g of iron glycerophosphate mixed with the milk and given twice daily for 9 consecutive days or 6 days with interruption were compared with the effects obtained after the i.m. administration

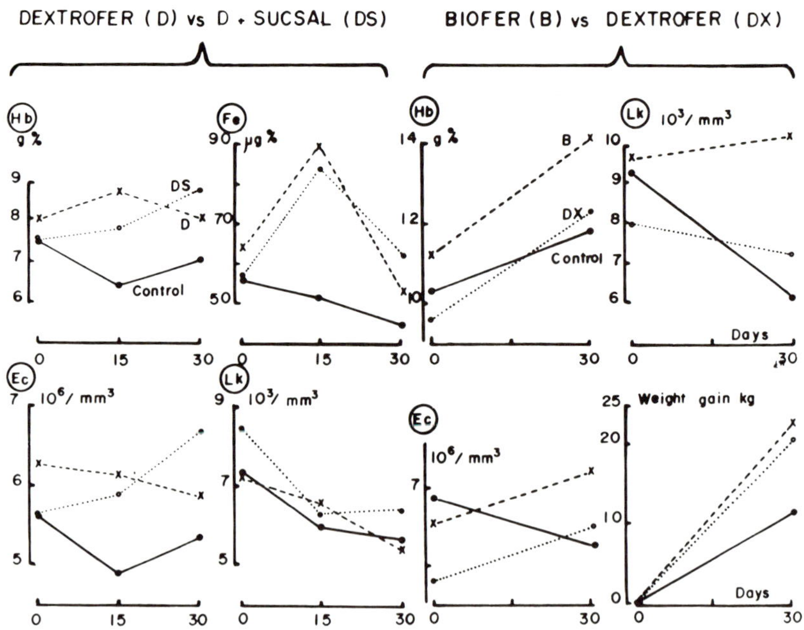

Figure 10.3 Changes in the blood of calves treated with 8 ml/kg Dextrofer-100 (D) vs. Dextrofer-100 (8 ml i.m.) plus Sucsal (100 ml i.v.) (DS), and 0.2 mg/kg body weight i.m. Dextrofer-100 (DX) vs. 10.6 mg/kg Biofer (B)

of Dextrofer-100 and Biofer. Iron glycerophosphate mixed well with the milk and was consumed readily by the calves, but the results were less satisfactory than those obtained with the i.m. preparations.

Iron suphate mixed with the milk was not readily consumed by the calves. Therefore, it was excluded from the test.

Antianemin (trace element and vitamin premix) combined with the milk was readily consumed by the calves, but its effect on the blood morphological composition was insignificant.

These investigations suggest that iron-containing drugs produce a favourable effect on the red blood cell picture in calves; this effect was better when the drugs were combined with other trace elements, vitamins and amino-acids. The drugs administered parenterally proved to be more useful as the effect occurred earlier than that of the oral drugs. Treatment *per os* was effective when suitable iron polysaccharide complexes were given in the first hours after birth; for this purpose Ursoferan-150 is recommended[16]. Of course, it must be taken into consideration that in the first weeks after birth calves usually suffer from inflammation of the intestinal mucous membrane, which reduces to a great extent the absorption of oral drugs.

According to our observations, anaemia in 10–15% of the calves was not adequately influenced by the application of iron preparations only.

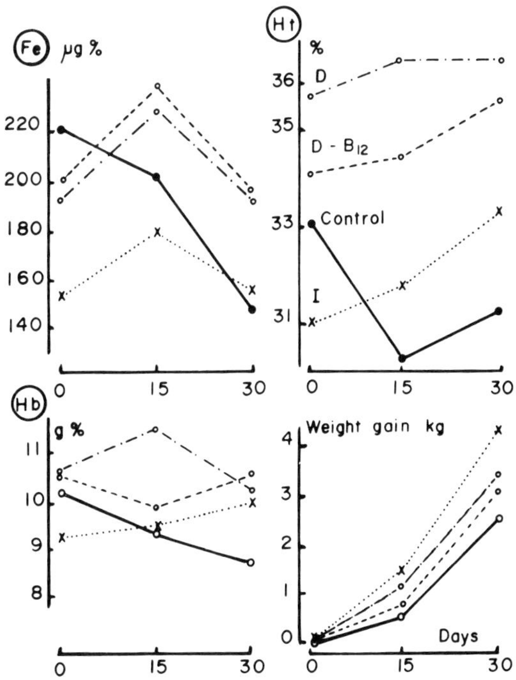

Figure 10.4 Changes in the blood of lambs treated with iron glycerophosphate 1 g/l milk (I), Dextrofer-100 0.7 ml/kg body weight i.m. (D), Dextrofer-100 with B_{12} 0.7 ml/kg body weight i.m. (D–B_{12}), and control

Observations were also made on the changes in the blood of twin lambs of both sexes (Black-faced Pleven breed and crosses) weaned in the first 3–5 days after birth and given milk replacer and starter mixtures. The study was done with 72 lambs divided into four groups of 18 lambs each (Figure 10.4). Haemoglobin, haematocrit, erythrocyte and leukocyte count, iron concentration, and the weight and growth rate of the test and control animals were determined twice at intervals of 15 days.

The results show that the animals not treated with iron preparations suffered from anaemia and required iron therapy. There was no significant difference in the effect produced by Dextrofer-100 and that of Dextrofer-100 with B_{12}. Good results in lambs were obtained from the administration of iron glycerophosphate (1 g/l of milk replacer in the course of the entire period) both with regard to blood composition and growth rate.

Hypochromaemia gradually occurred in the early-weaned lambs fed milk replacer. This hypochromaemia could be successfully overcome by adding iron glycerophosphate to the milk replacer or by injecting Ferodextran complexes.

CONCLUSIONS

Newborn calves on farms of the industrial type are very often affected with anaemia which is observed more frequently in twin calves, calves born by dams giving birth for the first time, and in the calves from 2 to 7 days of age. A comparatively higher percentage of anaemia occurs in calves on the 1st day following birth. With regard to haematological values in the calves, there are no differences between sexes but certain differences are reported between breeds.

Administered i.m. to calves (800–1200 mg Fe^{3+}) and to lambs (50–70 mg Fe^{3+}), Dextrofer-100 is quickly absorbed and included in the erythrocytes as early as the 24th hour. The iron stored in the liver and spleen of calves is approximately equal (expressed in terms of percentage); in lambs a higher quantity of iron (per gram of fresh tissue) is deposited in the spleen.

The administration of Ferizin to pregnant cows produces an insufficient effect on the erythropoiesis of newborn calves.

Dextrofer-100 injected i.m. in calves in doses of 800–1000 mg Fe^{3+} improves erythropoiesis. The influence is more favourable when combined with i.v. injection of Sucsal or with bovine γ-globulin, copper, cobalt and vitamins B_{12} and B_6 (Biofer).

Iron glycerophosphate, copper sulphate and a mineral–vitamin premix (Antianemin) given orally mixed with milk are slightly effective in the prophylaxis and therapy of anaemia in newborn calves.

Lambs weaned in the first 3–4 days after birth and fed milk replacer without trace elements develop anaemia, which is favourably influenced by the oral administration of iron glycerophosphate or the i.m. injection of Dextrofer-100.

References

1. Bremner, I. and Dolgarno, A. C. (1973). Iron metabolism in the veal calf. The availability of different iron compounds. *Br. J. Nutr.*, **29**, 229–43
2. Bremner, I. and Dolgarno, A. C. (1973). Iron metabolism in the veal calf. Iron requirements and the effect of copper supplementation. *Br. J. Nutr.*, **30**, 61–76
3. Dilov, P. (1976). Pharmacological properties and biologic standardization of iron-dextran preparations. *PhD in Veterinary Science*, Veterinary Medicine Faculty, Sofia
4. Dilov, P. and Vrigazov, A. (1975). Iron-dextran preparations in the prophylaxis of anemia in calves. *Vet. Collect.*, **5**, 34–8
5. Dilov, P. and Vrigazov, A. (1978). Comparative pharmacokinetic investigations about oral administration of iron-dextran preparations in piglets. *Vet. Sci.*, **15**, 68–76
6. Furugouri, K. (1978). Effect of nutrient deficiencies in animals: iron. *C.R.C. Handbook Series Nutr. Food*, **2**, 256–85
7. Gartner, K. J. W., Ryley, J. W. and Beattie, A. W. (1966). Variations of blood constituents in grazing Hereford cattle. *Res. Vet. Sci.*, **7**, 424–34
8. Gürtler, H., Wohlfarch, E., Bünger, U., Drekopf, E. and Liebaug, E. (1981–82). On the application of Urzoferan preparations to pigs and calves. *Medicamentum (Germed.)*, special vet. issue, 20
9. Hallemond, K. and Sprietsma, J. (1979). Is de anemie bij het mestkalf normochroom of hypochroom. *Tijdschr. Diergeneesk.*, **104**, 543–9
10. Lalov, H. and Antonov, S. (1963). Über den Eisengehalt in dem Lymphknoten von Saufferkeln nach Injektion von Eisen-Dextran. *Berliner u. Münchener tierärztl. Wochenschr.*, **76**, 27–30
11. Panichi, G. (1970). Cosiderazioni sull'anemia ferropriva e sull'ipercheratosi linguale del vitello. *Vet. (Milano)*, **19**, 187–95
12. Radeff, T., Lalov, H., Savov, A., Boukoureshtliev, A., Antonov, S. and Boukoureshtlieva, A. D. (1962). Absorption and distribution of the iron in pigs after parenteral application of iron-containing preparations. *News NIINBZ*, **2**, 5–20
13. Scheidegger, H. R. (1973). Veränderungen des roten Blutbildes und der Serumeisen-Konzentration bei Simentaler Kälbern. *Schw. Arch. Tierheilk.*, **115**, 483–97
14. Shalm, O. W. (1972). Differential diagnosis of anemia in cattle. *J. Am. Vet. Med. Assoc.*, **161**, 1269–75
15. Tumanova, E. I. and Strigin, A. P. (1978). Impozil influence on the hemopoiesa in calves healthy and suffering from anemia. *Trans. Moscow Vet. Acad.*, **99**, 112–14
16. Vajda, V., Slanina, L. and Lehocky, J. (1981). Profylaxia a terapia anemie u teliat. *Biol. Chem. Vet. (Praha)*, **17**, 271–8
17. Vovenko, E. N. and Puzureva, N. (1978). Feroglucin prophylaxis of dyspepsia in calves. *Veterinarya*, **4**, 90

11
Oral fluid therapy: some concepts on osmolality, electrolytes and energy

R. W. Phillips

In veterinary medicine, a principal requirement for fluid therapy is in the treatment of neonatal diarrhoeal diseases. Restoration and maintenance of fluid and electrolyte balance, as well as energy support, are necessary considerations. Effective fluid replacement therapy for diarrhoeic neonates should fulfil several basic needs. First, the dehydration must be reversed and adequate fluid input provided to compensate for normal body water turnover plus increased fecal losses. From the standpoint of the animal's requirement, the best therapeutic approach would be a continuous fluid input at a rate equal to body losses, a condition best provided by continuous intravenous administration[24, 58]. This is not a practical approach under many conditions. In some situations subcutaneous fluid administration can also be effective in providing a sustained fluid input, as subcutaneous fluids are slowly absorbed over a period of several hours[6].

Currently, the major emphasis on fluid and electrolyte therapy for diarrhoeic calves is focused on the use of oral fluids. A principle basis for this approach is the outstanding success of oral glucose electrolyte therapies for the treatment of *Vibrio cholera* diarrhoea in humans. Associated with this beneficial effect is the recognition that the mechanism by which *Escherichia coli* enterotoxin induces diarrhoea is analogous to the mechanisms of *V. cholera* as well as other enterotoxigenic bacteria. Increased secretory activity is responsible for the diarrhoea, yet absorption may continue and even be increased[3, 8, 33, 57]. However, the general assumption, that during diarrhoea absorption is normal or increased as is seen with many bacterial diarrhoeas[18], may be fallacious when considering the spectrum of diarrhoeal aetiologies. There is also speculation regarding the role of motility in diarrhoea[47]. Both increased motility, as with parasympathetic stimulation or flaccid paralysis, creating an open tube, can conceivably cause more rapid transit and diarrhoea. Malabsorption of sugars and lipids are well recognized in diarrhoeal diseases[43]. It could be anticipated that viral diseases which cause significant changes in both individual epithelial cells and in villus morphology[7, 33, 45, 46, 59] would be associated with inhibited absorptive capacity. Most evidence supports the thesis that decreased absorption is the basis for viral diarrhoeas[1,7,26,31].

The use of oral antibiotics has been linked to malabsorption syndromes (diarrhoea) in domestic and laboratory animals, and in man. Several of these antibiotics are commonly used in veterinary medicine as prophylaxis or therapy of neonatal diarrhoeas. For example, oral chloramphenicol in calves can cause a malabsorptive diarrhoea with villus atrophy and epithelial cell dysfunction[39,42]. When malabsorption causes the diarrhoea, particularly if glucose absorption is limited[31], then oral therapies will be ineffective, and may actually exacerbate the diarrhoea by providing an increased supply of energy-rich substrate for bacteria, particularly in the large intestine. A secondary consequence of bacterial fermentation is the creation of excessive osmolality in the lower bowel. A number of the antibiotic-induced malabsorption syndromes in humans are associated with colonic overgrowth of *Clostridium difficile* and other Gram-positive enterotoxigenic organisms[20].

DIARRHOEAL LOSSES AND IMBALANCES

Therapy composition should be based on several factors, a major one being the extent of fluid and electrolyte loss. It can be considered that, regardless of the route of administration, diarrhoeic animals that require fluid, electrolyte and energy support will have the same requirements. As animals become diarrhoeic they also become dehydrated. It is not uncommon to find that neonatal calves have lost 6–12% of their body fluids. Therefore, therapeutic provision of large quantities of water is necessary. Water losses are not evenly distributed through body water pools[35]. The greatest loss is from the extracellular fluid (ECF) and blood volume is most severely depleted[28,36,38]. Blood volume may be decreased as much as 50% causing peripheral vasoconstriction and hypovolaemic shock. The rest of the ECF is also decreased but not to the same extent[38]. Only small changes are seen in the intracellular water pool, and it may in fact be increased in volume[38], presumably due to decreased cellular metabolism and cellular swelling[55]. The ionic composition of oral fluid replacement therapy should, therefore, be designed to approximate the composition of the ECF[35]. This approach is necessary so that crystalloids will remain after energy substrates are utilized, otherwise there will not be sufficient water retention.

Significant fecal losses of sodium, potassium, chloride and bicarbonate occur during diarrhoea[27,33,34,49,50]. Routine clinical assessment of electrolyte status is dependent on measurement of plasma or serum ion concentrations but these values are not necessarily indicative of fecal losses. Further, they may give false impressions of whole body electrolytes. This is particularly true for potassium which may be significantly increased in the blood, reaching cardiotoxic levels[19,29,30,35,41,52], yet a whole body potassium deficit occurs during diarrhoea (Figure 11.1)[19,28,52]. Potassium accumulation in extracellular fluids is a complex phenomenon associated with developing acidosis and cellular energy imbalances. Fecal bicarbonate loss, accumulation of lactic acid in the blood, and decreased renal function are all

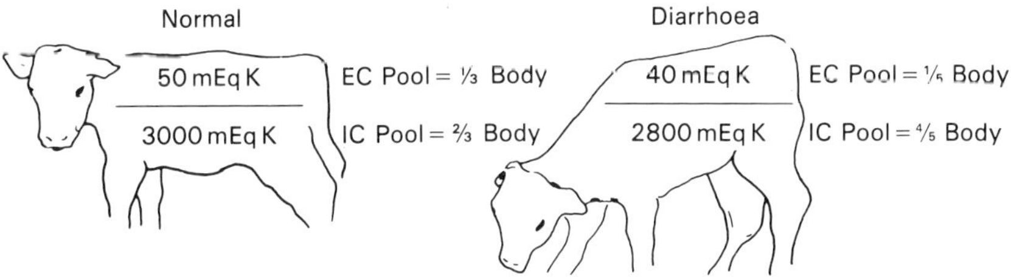

Figure 11.1 Changes in extracellular fluid (EC) and intracellular fluid (IC) potassium pools as a result of diarrhoea. Both pools decrease in total potassium content but the EC change is masked by an increase in plasma potassium concentration.

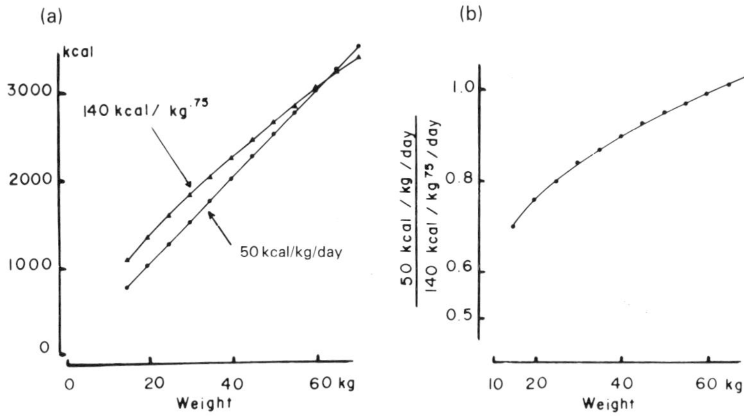

Figure 11.2 (a) Maintenance energy required as a function of increasing body size from 15 to 70 kg using metabolic body size (140 kcal/kg$^{.75}$) and straight line method (50 kcal kg^{-1} day^{-1}) from ref. 27, 37. (b) Effectiveness of the straight line (50 kcal kg^{-1} day^{-1}) method of energy provision as a percentage of metabolic body size determination of energy requirements. In smaller animals (15 kg), only 70% of maintenance is provided. At approximately 60 kg, they are equivalent

involved. Potassium–hydrogen ion shifts occur across cellular membranes and the decrease in intracellular potassium with a resultant increase in extracellular potassium cause myocardial and skeletal muscle dysfunction[19, 28, 29, 55]. There is a whole body potassium deficit, but an increase in potassium concentration in the vascular pool[19, 28]. Since the volume of the vascular pool is decreased due to extracellular dehydration, the total plasma potassium content as well as intracellular potassium content are often diminished (Figure 11.1).

The metabolic rate of neonatal calves for maintenance, without growth or consideration of febrile-induced metabolic increases, may be calculated as a function of body weight (W). Using Kleiber's general formula for metabolic body size for maintenance, metabolic requirement may be calculated (Figure 11.2 (a)). Maintenance[27] (kcal/day) equals $140 \times W/kg^{.75}$. Data from Alexander *et al.*[2] indicate that the resting metabolic rate of growing calves less than one week of age is 2213 kcal/day, while using the Kleiber formula (140 kcal/kg$^{.75}$) for these same calves it would be 2226 kcal/day. Both estimates are adjusted to a 40 kg calf. An alternative, simple, but less accurate, estimate of metabolic rate is also shown in Figure 11.2 based on a straight line derivation of 50 kcal/kg which is a reasonable approximation in the size range of neonatal calves[37]. Figure 11.2 (b) is a plot of the straight line method as a ratio with metabolic body size requirements. The straight line method underestimates in smaller animals. Both methods would underestimate actual metabolic rate or dietary energy requirements in rapidly growing or febrile calves.

During diarrhoea many animals have a decrease in food intake, a decreased net absorptive function, and an increase in metabolism associated with fever. In neonates these are potentially more serious manifestations as they have relatively meagre energy reserves. Only about 1.8% of the body weight of neonatal calves is adipose tissue and a significant proportion of that is brown adipose tissue (BAT)[2]. BAT is helpful in maintaining normal body temperature in neonates but is not an effective source of free fatty acids (FFA) for general body metabolism. Neonatal calves do not have high levels of circulating FFA except in the peripartum period[14]. Also, plasma FFA are not increased in diarrhoeic calves with hypoglycaemia due either to the low reserves or an inability to mobilize[15].

In severely diarrhoeic calves, hypoglycaemia and lactic acidosis are an almost constant finding[11,15,40,49]. Hypoglycaemia and lactic acidosis are also pathognomic signs of endotoxaemia[23]. Similar blood levels of glucose lactate and potassium are seen in diarrhoeic and in endotoxaemic calves[11,15,35,38,40,49,51]. These similarities have led to the tenet that diarrhoeal damage to the intestinal epithelial barrier allows both bacteria and endotoxin to enter the bloodstream in increased quantities and that endotoxaemia is a common sequelae to diarrhoea. The hypoglycaemia, hyperlactataemia and hyperkalaemia seen in diarrhoeic neonates may represent a combination of altered epithelial transport and developing endotoxic-septic shock. However, the relative role of each dysfunction is now known.

During diarrhoea, dehydration occurs with the greatest losses from the extracellular pool. Acidosis is seen due to bicarbonate loss and increased lactate levels, hypoglycaemia is common and major losses of Na, Cl and K occur. Intracellular-extracellular potassium imbalance may become severe resulting in reduced resting membrane potential, altered cardiac and general muscular function[35].

INTESTINAL FUNCTION

Some current concepts of normal gastrointestinal function are a helpful prelude to developing a basis for oral therapy. The intestine is a major transport system in that absorption and secretion are continually occurring across the mucosal epithelial barrier. Enterocytes are formed in the crypts and move rapidly up the villi, particularly in young animals. In calves, the lifespan of an epithelial cell, from formation in the crypt to sloughing at the tip[32], is about 48 h. Intestinal epithelial cells have several functions. They serve as the barrier limiting entry of organisms and toxins and as the barrier preventing loss of body substance. In the small intestine this barrier is somewhat leaky, as water and some solutes can pass in a paracellular manner. The junctional complexes between epithelial cells are functionally important structures. They are similar to a fence, in that they serve as a barrier; to a gate, in that they allow certain substances to pass; and to a bridge in that adjacent cells may interact directly via gap junctions[17]. Like any barrier, it is not absolute, and normally some bacteria and bacterial toxins enter the portal blood[25]. During diarrhoea, significant changes in the integrity of the barrier permit the loss of fluids and body constituents, an increase in the gate function. Also, with barrier modification, it is easier for intestinal micro-organisms and toxins to enter the body at an increased rate, a decreased fence function. This may lead to septicaemia and endotoxaemia with potentially lethal consequences.

Most absorption occurs in the small intestine, and intestinal epithelial cells transport many nutrients. For this discussion, nutrients will include water, electrolytes and energy-yielding substrates such as carbohydrates, amino acids and lipids. Absorptive transport is primarily via the more mature cells near the villus tip which also have the greatest degree of contact with intestinal contents.

The villus, with its vessels and surrounding absorptive epithelial cells, is the functional unit of the small intestine. The vessels are arranged so that a countercurrent flow pattern is established[22]. The central arteriole in each villus is like a fountain and sprays capillaries which descend toward the base of the villus adjacent to the epithelial cells (Figure 11.3)[48]. Absorbed nutrients enter descending capillaries causing an increase in osmolality. The diffusion pattern is such that water leaves the arterioles and enters capillaries and absorbed nutrients diffuse from capillaries to arterioles. Together these effects create an increasing concentration gradient in the ascending arteriole and increased osmolality at the villus tip[22]. During active absorption, this gradient may reach an osmolality of 600 mOsm or roughly twice body fluid osmolality. An additional osmotic gradient develops between epithelial cells when they are absorbing, which aids solute flux to the capillaries. These two osmolar gradients are believed to enhance nutrient absorption.

During absorption, nutrients cross the microvillus brush border, enter the cytoplasm and leave via the lateral cellular membrane. The mechanisms involved are similar for glucose, galactose, amino acids and short peptides, although peptides are hydrolysed in the epithelial cell. Glucose transport has been most extensively studied and will be used as an example[31]. A microvillus membrane receptor binds both sodium and glucose. They enter the epithelial cell together based on the sodium diffusion potential. These cells, like others, have only a minimal intracellular Na^+ concentration, and a constant diffusion gradient exists for sodium to move from the intestine into the epithelial cell. Electrochemical neutrality is maintained by cotransport of a negative ion, generally Cl^- or HCO_3^-. Sodium is then pumped by active transport into the lateral intercellular space below the junctional barrier. Again, the anion follows, maintaining electrochemical neutrality. Glucose is believed to

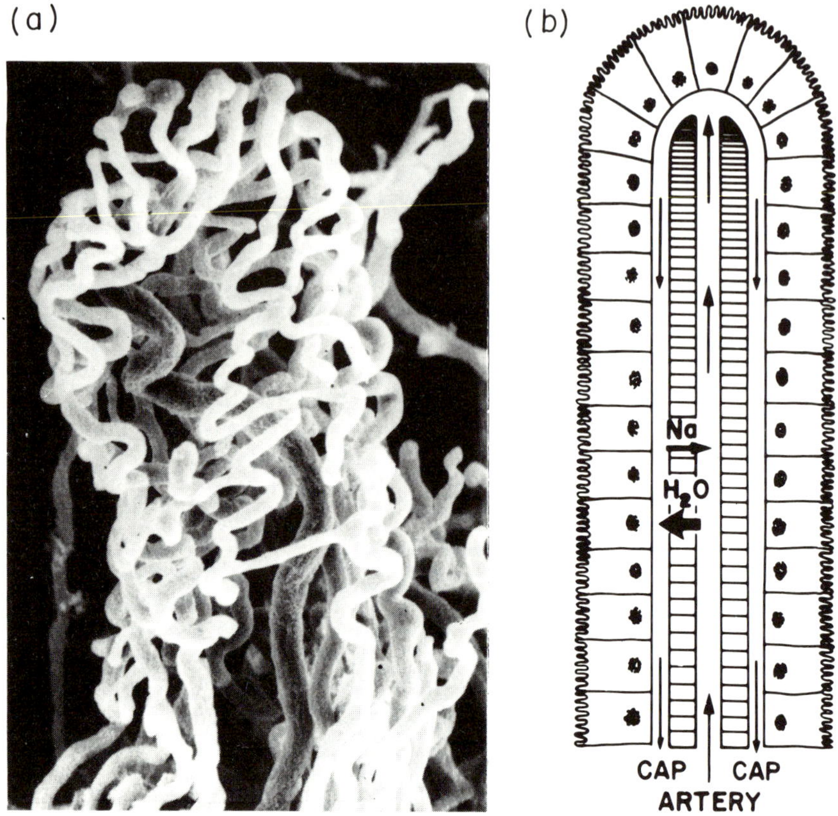

Figure 11.3 (a) The villus vascular network is such that a central arteriole ascends to the tip and branches into a 'spray' of capillaries which descend toward the base of the villus creating a countercurrent flow system ×350. (b) The villus countercurrent multiplier system is depicted. During absorption there is net water diffusion from the ascending arteriole to the descending capillary. Some solute diffuses in the opposite direction. The result is an increasing osmotic gradient at the villus tip (modified from ref. 22)

diffuse out with minimal metabolism occurring during the absorptive process. Sodium, anion and glucose increase in concentration in the lateral intercellular space causing a concomitant increase in osmolality. Water diffusion follows both from the cell and also by paracellular movement across the leaky junctional complex directly from the intestine. Figure 11.4 represents resting and absorbing intestinal epithelial cells in relation to both transepithelial and vascular fluxes[21, 22]. Osmolality in the lateral intercellular space at the apex of the cell near the villus tip would normally achieve the highest intestinal osmolality. The continuing solute and solvent movement into the lateral space near the apex of the cell causes a flow from apex to base carrying the absorptive products[17, 21]. In the lamina propria at the base of the cell, absorptive products diffuse into the descending capillary network and help develop the villus countercurrent osmolar gradient system[22]. As depicted in Figure

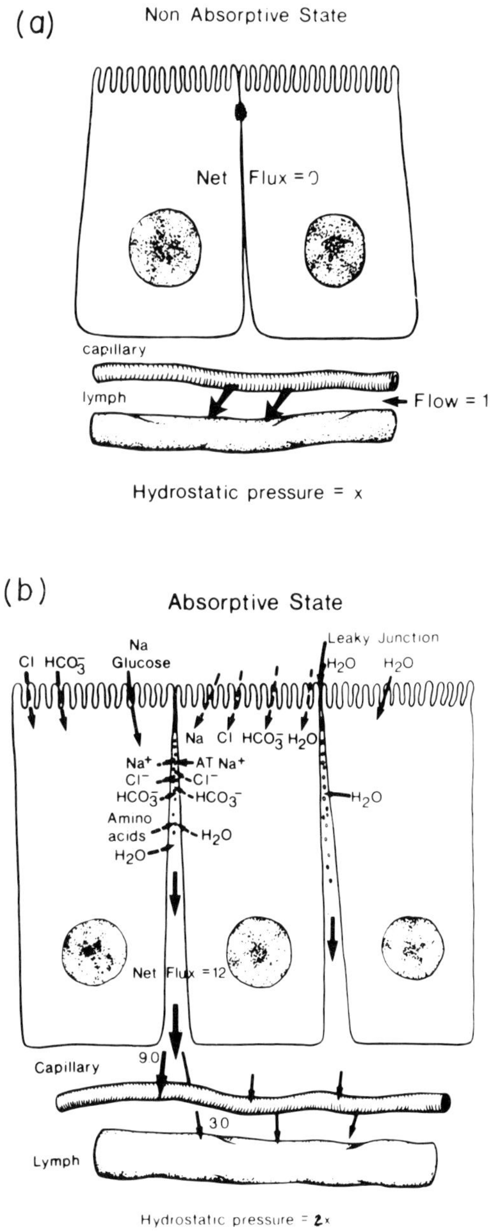

Figure 11.4 (a) In a resting intestinal epithelial cell, there is no net absorptive cellular flux. The lateral intercellular space is collapsed. Lymph flow is present due to capillary leakage. (b) In active intestinal epithelial cells, net absorption causes a solute and solvent flow from cell apex to base. There is net uptake by capillaries, and due to increased hydrostatic pressure, an increase in lymph formation (modified from ref. 21)

11.4 (b), absorption across the epithelial cells also increases tissue hydrostatic pressure and lymphatic flow. The input of absorbed lipid and chylomicrons (not shown) would additionally increase lymphatic flow.

THE CALF

In the normal calf, nutrient presentation to the intestine and subsequent absorption rate is controlled in large part by gastric emptying. Bell and Razig[4,5] have studied factors modifying abomasal emptying in calves. They found that highly hypertonic pure solutions of electrolytes or carbohydrates will delay emptying. Their data indicates that maximal gastric emptying of NaCl and $NaHCO_3$ solutions in calves occurs at an osmolality of 400–600 mOsm/l (Figure 11.5), well above body fluid osmolality (290 mOsm/l), but similar to the villus vascular osmolality previously presented[4,5]. In a study with young adult pigs it was found that duodenal osmolar equilibration of fluid diets ranging from 250 to 700 mOsm/l was at 450–500 mOsm/l with declining osmolality further down the intestine[12].

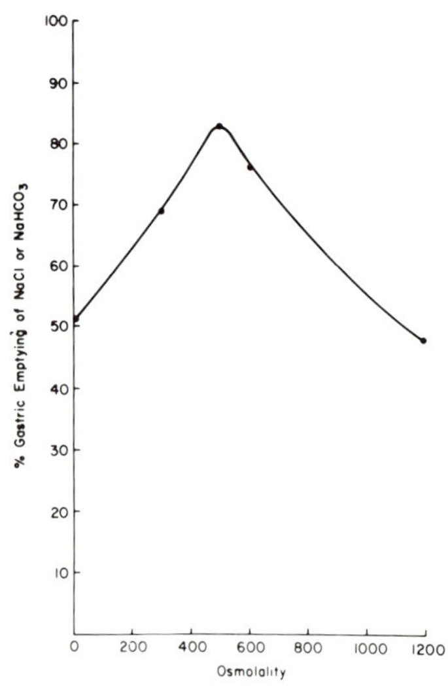

Figure 11.5 The effect of varying osmolality of NaCl or $NaHCO_3$ on rate of abomosal emptying (calculated from refs. 4, 5).

Although gastric emptying may be slower with a hypertonic glucose-electrolyte solution, more total carbohydrate is provided to the small intestine over a longer period[4,5]. Rapid gastric emptying may not be of benefit; in fact, one is tempted to ask why it should be considered beneficial, if a sustained fluid input to the absorptive surface of the small intestine is a valid therapeutic goal. Delayed gastric emptying by feeding hypertonic solutions would also provide more total nutrients and energy, if tonicity is increased

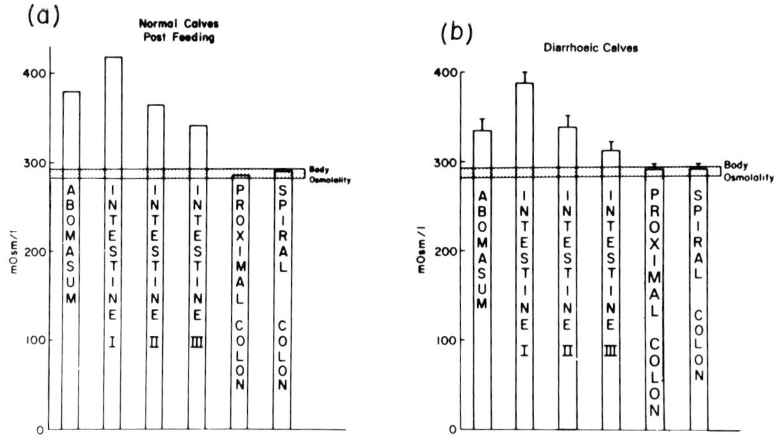

Figure 11.6 (a) Intestinal osmolality of normal calves 6 h after a milk meal. (b) Intestinal osmolality of diarrhoeic calves 6 h after a milk meal (modified from ref. 56)

by adding energy-yielding absorbable nutrients. In another study, the addition of 80 mOsm/l of NaCl to a 10% glucose solution enhanced glucose absorptive rate in calves, yet increased osmolality from 555 to 715 mOsm/l[13]. Cow's milk is an isosmotic fluid when secreted. During digestion, the breakdown of milk protein and lactose causes an increase in luminal osmolality. 6 h following milk ingestion by normal or diarrhoeic calves, upper small intestine osmolality was greater than blood osmolality (Figure 11.6 (a), (b))[56]. Finally, it has been reported that increasing the dry matter content of calves' diets, which presumably increased gastrointestinal osmolality, resulted in a decreased incidence of diarrhoea[44].

Based on the absorption rates of glucose following either oral glucose or lactose administration and calculated rates of glucose transport[8,9,54], the small intestine in the normal calf can absorb larger quantities of glucose and presumably amino acids than are presented by most oral therapies. Further, to achieve a necessary provision of energy substrates to the young calf, the most appropriate approach physiologically is to have a slow constant provision of nutrients from the stomach.

Two conclusions can be made:

(1) During absorption, the environment of the upper small intestine, both contents and mucosa, is hyperosmotic compared to body fluids, and hyperosmolar gradients which develop during absorption are normal and beneficial to the absorptive process.

(2) The rate of gastric emptying is in part controlled by gastric and intestinal osmolality, and increased osmolality of ingested fluid will provide a prolonged input to the intestines.

ORAL FLUID THERAPY

The use of fluid therapy during diarrhoea represents a combination of replacement and maintenance. Replacement fulfils the need to reverse the dehydration and ion losses. The quantity administered is based on the estimated degree of dehydration. For instance, a 40 kg calf that was 10% dehydrated would require 4 l of fluid. In addition, if diarrhoea is still present, daily net loss must be considered. It may range from negligible quantities to 7.5% of body weight/day, which can result in a 3 l daily loss in a 40 kg calf. Fluid required for replacement plus maintenance for 3 sizes of calves with varying degrees of initial dehydration and a continuing loss of 50 ml/kg daily is plotted in Figure 11.7. If dehydration is cured the required volume will be less on succeeding days.

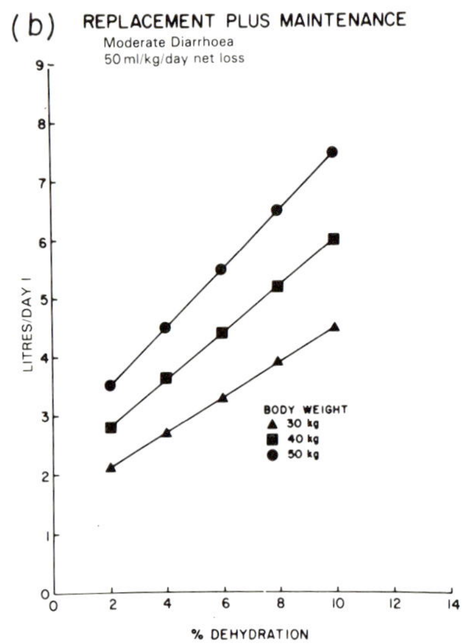

Figure 11.7 Daily fluid requirements for a calf with moderate fluid loss

Many of the oral therapies currently on the market in Europe and in the United States have been formulated on the hypothesis that it is desirable for such solutions to be reasonably isosmotic with regard to body fluids. The basis for this view is that hyperosmotic fluids will remove water from the body by increasing gastrointestinal secretory activity. In my opinion, this is fallacious and has resulted in the preparation of a great many products that provide only minimal energy input (Figure 11.8). This figure presents the available energy nutrient source in a number of products currently being marketed in Britain, France and the United States. Table 11.1 lists the osmolality, volume and total energy provision of a number of oral therapies. With the exception of one product (Suradavo), mean osmolality was 348 mmol. The majority provide sufficient water to combat dehydration if used at the manufacture's maximum recommended level (Table 11.1). The greatest

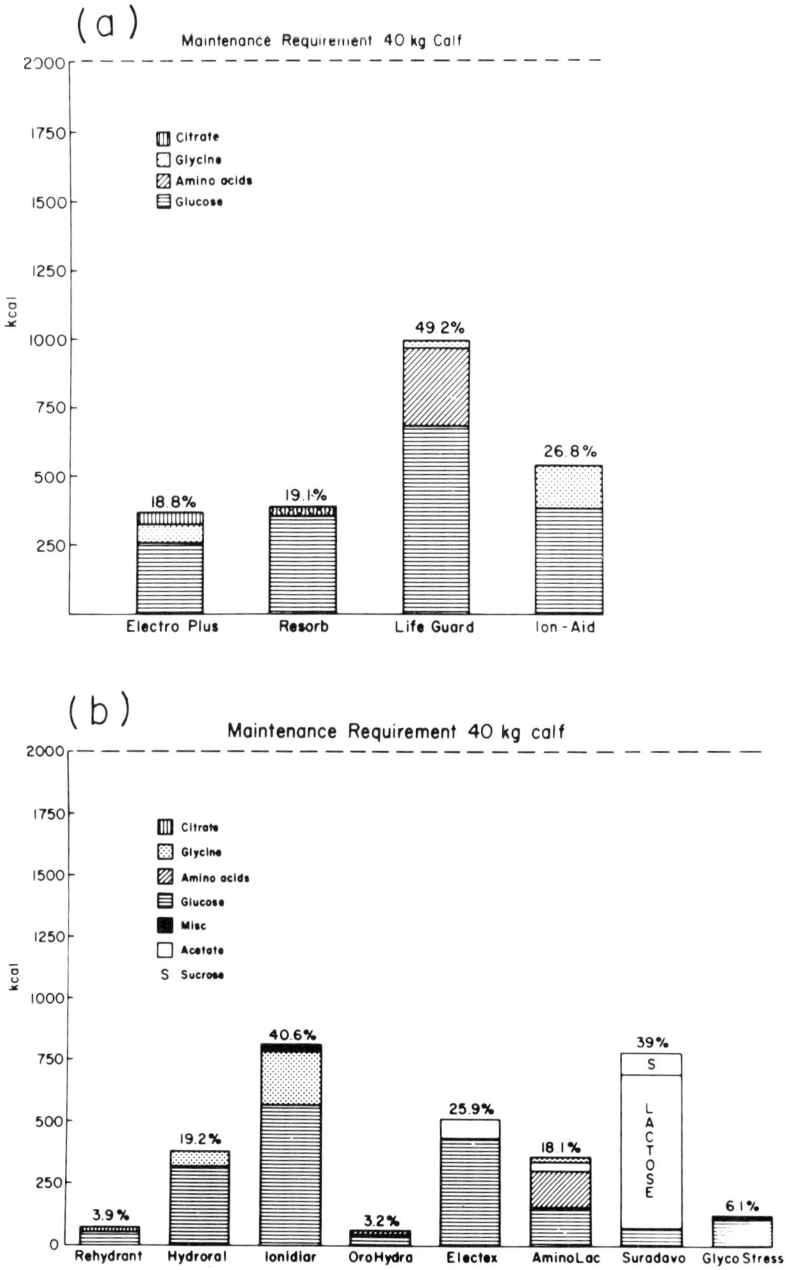

Figure 11.8 A summation of maximum energy yield by substrate from several commercial therapies currently marketed in Britain and the United States (a) and in France (b). Resorb is also marketed as Lectade and Biodiet. The minimal maintenance requirement of neonatal calves is listed at the top and the percentage of maintenance provided

Table 11.1 A comparison of osmolality, volume and energy content of some oral therapies available in Britain, France and the United States

Product	*Country*	*Osmolality* (mOsm/l)	*Volume** (ml/day)	*Energy content* (kcal/day*)
Aminolac	France	160	8000	362
Electex	France	318	6000	518
Glycostress	France	290	3000	122
Hydroral	France	352	4000	384
Ionidiar	France	482	6000	811
Orohydra	France	256	4000	64
Rehydrant 2412	France	305	800	78
Suradavo	France	2284	1500	780
Electroplus A	USA	323	6000	387
Ionaid	USA, Britain	515	3784	536
Lifeguard	USA	490	5676	984
Resorb†	USA	390	4000	382

* Maximum dosage per calf/day or per 40 kg calf/day
† Also sold in Britain (Lectade) and France (Biodiet)
Osmolality and energy content have been calculated from label ingredients. Energy content is based on the manufacturer's maximum recommended dosing schedule

deficit is in energy provision. Even using a conservative maintenance estimate for a 40 kg calf of 2000 kcal kg^{-1} day^{-1} vs. the calculated and measured values of over 2200 kcal kg^{-1} day^{-1}, the highest energy provision (Life Guard) provides only 49% of required energy (Figure 11.8).

A word of caution regarding oral therapy – the gastrointestinal tract may not be capable of absorbing when villus atrophy has occurred[33] and the villus countercurrent flow system is destroyed, not when there are changes in epithelial cell transport function[1,42,43]. The use of oral therapies during a malabsorptive diarrhoea may exacerbate the problem by providing an additional growth media to intestinal microbes. However, the assumption that oral fluids are of benefit is sound, as general clinical results indicate that most diarrhoeic neonates can absorb significant quantities of nutrients from the gastrointestinal tract. The final question is what should be included in therapies? From a theoretical standpoint, several points may be considered.

(1) Absorbability,
(2) Fluid maintenance
(3) Ion replacement
 (a) Na^+, K^+
 (b) Cl^-, HCO_3^-,
(4) Acid–base correction HCO_3^- or bicarbonate equivalent, such as acetate, citrate, or l-lactate, and
(5) Energy maintenance with glucose, amino acids, lipids.

On the basis of fecal losses and changes in the size of the ECF pool, the fluid should be essentially an ECF replacement, i.e. it should contain sodium at 120–140 mEq/l, chloride at 30–40 mEq less than sodium, and either bicarbonate or a bicarbonate equivalent such as acetate, citrate or lactate.

Both acetate and citrate can be recommended as they can be more readily utilized than lactate which is an isomeric mixture, one half of which d-lactate is poorly utilized. Further, the diarrhoeic calf is often suffering from hyperlactataemia with a decreased lactate utilization rate[11]. Reports have been published of the beneficial effect of both acetate[16] and citrate[9, 10] on intestinal absorption rates in calves. Studies on optimal concentrations of either ion are not available. However, the rationale for their inclusion seems valid, if they are present in sufficient quantities. For instance, provision of 4 g of Na acetate to a 40 kg calf would only yield an increase of 2–3 mEq of HCO_3^- if every molecule of carbon was converted to HCO_3^-. It is more likely that one half as much could be gained, i.e. one HCO_3^-/Na^+. This quantity would not materially affect acid–base status and HCO_3^- deficit. Similar calculations can be made for citrate or lactate but they contain even less sodium and are potentially less efficient sources of bicarbonate buffer on a gram basis.

Potassium should be present to restore whole body potassium deficits as hyperkalaemia is corrected. An available energy supply in the form of glucose is an important component for several reasons. Diarrhoeic calves are hypoglycaemic, glucose is readily absorbed in most cases, and following absorption, glucose will facilitate movement of potassium into cells, correcting the hyperkalaemia. Other carbohydrate sources may be of less value. Neonatal calves do not have sucrase nor significant quantities of maltase in the brush border[53] so that sucrose and maltose will not be digested and absorbed[13]. Their inclusion is of negligible value. Lactose would seem to be a logical choice but lactase in the brush border is a particularly fragile enzyme and it tends to be severely diminished in activity in many diarrhoeal diseases. Therefore, glucose appears to be the carbohydrate of choice for inclusion in therapies.

Glycine has also been shown to stimulate overall intestinal absorption of sodium and water, and in addition may provide a protein-sparing effect by increasing available amino nitrogen. Lipids could be considered of possible benefit due to their high energy content. However, lipids are less stable and little information seems available on their absorbability during diarrhoeal diseases.

In conclusion, it is my thesis that (1) most available oral therapies for diarrhoea are woefully inadequate in energy, (2) that undue attention has been given to providing isosmotic fluids, and (3) finally, based on these conclusions, more effective oral therapies can be provided for diarrhoeic neonates, particularly calves.

References

1. Abel, J. H., Phillips, R. W. and Lewis, L. D. (1972). Intestinal mucosae enzymatic and histochemical changes during infectious diarrhea in calves. *Am. J. Dig. Dis.*, **17**, 423–9
2. Alexander, G., Bennett, J. W. and Gemmell, R. T. (1975). Brown adipose tissue in the newborn calf (*Bos. Taurus*). *J. Physiol.*, **244**, 223–34
3. Argenzio, R. A. (1978). Physiology of diarrhea – large intestine. *J. Am. Vet. Med. Ass.*, **173**, 667–72
4. Bell, F. R. and Razig, S. A. D. (1973). Gastric emptying and secretion in the milk-fed calf. *J. Physiol.*, **228**, 499–511

5. Bell, F. R. and Razig, S. A. D. (1973). The effect of some molecules and ions on gastric function in the milk-fed calf. *J. Physiol.*, **228**, 513–26
6. Buck, D. and Phillips, R. W. (Unpublished observations)
7. Butler, D. G., Gall, D. G., Kelly, M. H. and Hamilton, J. R. (1974). Transmissible gastroenteritis: mechanisms responsible for diarrhea in an acute viral enteritis in piglets. *J. Clin. Invest.*, **53**, 1336–42
8. Bywater, R. J. (1970). Some effects of *E. coli* enterotoxin on net fluid, glucose and electrolyte transfer in calf small intestine. *J. Comp. Pathol.*, **80**, 565–73
9. Bywater, R. J. (1977). Evaluation of an oral glucose-glycine-electrolyte formulation and amoxicillin for treatment of diarrhea in calves. *Am. J. Vet. Res.*, **38**, 1983–7
10. Bywater, R. J. (1980). Comparison between milk deprivation and oral rehydration with a glucose-glycerine-electrolyte formulation in diarrhoeic and transported calves. *Vet. Rec.*, **107**, 549–51
11. Case, G. L., Phillips, R. W. and Cleek, J. L. (1980). Lactic acid and glucose metabolism in healthy, lactic acid infused and diarrhoeic calves. *Am. J. Vet. Res.*, **41**, 1035–8
12. Case, G. L., Lewis, L. D., Phillips, R. W. and Cleek, J. L. (1981). Effects of osmolality of liquid nutrient diets on meal passage and nutrient absorption in Yucatan miniature swine. *Am. J. Clin. Nutr.*, **34**, 1868–78
13. Cleek, J. L., Phillips, R. W. and Johnson B. D. (1979). Availability of oral carbohydrates in neonatal calves. *J. Am. Vet. Med. Assoc.*, **134**, 373–7
14. Demigné, C. and Remesy, C. (1979). Fetal and postnatal metabolism in the calf. *Ann. Biol. Anim. Biochem. Biophys.*, **19**, 159–65
15. Demigné, C. and Rémesy, C. (1979). Evolution of the postnatal metabolism in the healthy or diarrhoeic calf. *Ann. Rech. Vet.*, **20**, 12–31
16. Demigné, C., Remesy, C., Chartier, F. and LeFaivre, J. (1981). Effect of acetate or chloride anions on intestinal absorption of water and solutes in the calf. *Am. J. Vet. Res.*, **42**, 1356–9
17. Diamond, J. M. (1977). The epithelial junction: bridge, gate and fence. *The Physiologist.*, **20**, 10–18
18. Donaldson, R. M., Jr. (1967). Role of enteric microorganisms in malabsorption. *Fed. Proc.*, **26**, 1426–31
19. Fisher, E. W. (1971). Hydrogen ion and electrolyte disturbances in neonatal calf diarrhea. *Ann. NY Acad. Sci.*, **176**, 223–30
20. George, W. L., Rolfe, R. D. and Finegold, S. M. (1980). Treatment and prevention of antimicrobial agent-induced colitis and diarrhea. *Gastroenterology*, **79**, 366–72
21. Granger, D. N. (1981). Intestinal microcirculation and transmucosal fluid transport. *Am. J. Physiol.*, **240**, G343–9
22. Hallback, D. A., Hulten, L., Jodal, M., Lindhagen, J. and Lundgren, O. (1978). Evidence for the existence of a countercurrent exchanger in the small intestine in man. *Gastroenterology*, **74**, 683–890
23. Hinshaw, L. B. (1976). Concise review: the role of glucose in endotoxic shock. *Circ. Shock*, **3**, 1–10
24. Hoffsis, G. F., Gingerich, D. A., Sherman, D. M. and Bruner, R. R. (1977). Total intravenous feeding of calves. *J. AM. Vet. Med. Assoc.*, **171**, 67–70
25. Jacob, A. I., Goldberg, P. K., Bloom, N., Degenshein, G. A. and Kozinn, P. J. (1977). Endotoxin and bacteria in portal blood. *Gastroenterology*, **72**, 1268–970
26. Kerzner, B., Kelly, M. H., Gall, D. G., Butler, D. G. and Hamilton, J. R. (1977). Transmissible gastroenteritis: sodium transport and the intestinal epithelium during the course of viral enteritis. *Gastroenterology*, **72**, 457–61
27. Kleiber, M. (1961). *The Fire of Life.* (Newark: Wiley and Sons)
28. Lewis, L. D. and Phillips, R. W. (1972). Water and electrolyte losses in neonatal calves with acute diarrhea – a complete balance study. *Cornell Vet.*, **62**, 596–607
29. Lewis, L. D. and Phillips, R. W. (1978). Pathophysiologic changes due to coronavirus-induced diarrhea in the calf. *J. Am. Vet. Med. Assoc.*, **173**, 636–42
30. Lewis, L. D. and Phillips, R. W. (1973). Diarrheic induced changes in intracellular and extracellular ion concentrations in neonatal calves. *Ann Rech. Vet.*, **4**, 99–111
31. McClung, H. J., Butler, D. G., Kerzner, B., Gall, D. G. and Hamilton, J. R. (1976). Transmissible gastroenteritis: mucosal ion transport in acute viral enteritis. *Gastroenterology*, **70**, 1091–5

32. Moon, H. W. and Joel, D. D. (1975). Epithelial cell migration in the small intestine of sheep and calves. *Am. J. Vet. Res.*, **36**, 187–9
33. Moon, H. W. (1978). Mechanisms in the pathogenesis of diarrhea: a review. *J. Am. Vet. Med. Assoc.*, **172**, 443–8
34. Mitchell, A. R. (1974). Body fluids and diarrhoea: dynamics of dysfunction. *Vet. Rec.*, **94**, 311–15
35. Phillips, R. W. (1983). Water and electrolyte imbalances in diarrhea. In Woodard, J. C. and Bouss, M. (eds.) *Comparative Aspects of Nutritional and Metabolic Diseases.* pp. 61–72. (Boca Raton, Fla.: CRC Press Inc.)
36. Phillips, R. W., Lewis, L. D. and Knox, K. L. (1971). Alterations in body water turnover and distribution in neonatal calves with acute diarrhea. *Ann. NY Acad. Sci.*, **176**, 231–43
37. Phillips, R. W. and Lewis, L. D. (1972). Milk replacers: evaluation and use. *Bovine Pract.*, **7**, 28–33
38. Phillips, R. W. and Lewis, L. D. (1973). Viral induced changes in intestinal transport and resultant body fluid alterations in neonatal calves. *Ann. Rech. Vet.*, **4**, 87–98
39. Phillips, R. W., Huffman, E. M., Cleek, J. L. and Clark, C. H. (1982). The effect of oral chloramphenicol in neonatal calves. In *Proceedings of 2nd Congress European de Pharmacologie et Toxicologie Veterinaires.* Toulouse, September
40. Phillips, R. W. and Case, G. L. (1980). Altered metabolism, acute shock, and therapeutic response in a calf with severe coronavirus-induced diarrhea. *Am. J. Vet. Res.*, **41**, 1039–44
41. Radostits, O. M. (1975). Treatment and control of neonatal diarrhea in calves. *J. Dairy Sci.*, **58**, 464–70
42. Rollin, R., Levine, K., Mero, L. N., Morita, M. and Phillips, R. W. (1982). Structural and functional changes seen in chloramphenicol-induced malabsorption in calves. In *Proceedings of XII World Congress on Diseases of Cattle.* In press
43. Rosenberg, I. H., Solomons, N. W. and Schneider, R. E. (1977). Malabsorption associated with diarrhea and intestinal infections. *Am. J. Clin. Nutr.*, **30**, 1248–53
44. Stiles, R. P., Grieve, D. G., Butler, D. G. and Willoughby, R. A. (1974). Effects of fluid intake level and dry matter concentration on the incidence of scours in milk replacer-fed calves. *Can. J. Anim. Sci.*, **54**, 73–8
45. Storz, J., Collier, J. R., Eugster, A. K. and Altera, K. P. (1971). Intestinal bacterial changes in chlamydia-induced primary enteritis of newborn calves. *Ann. NY Acad. Sci.*, **176**, 162–75
46. Storz, J., Doughri, A. M. and Hajer, I. (1978). Coronaviral morphogenesis and ultrastructural changes in intestinal infections of calves. *J. Am. Vet. Med. Assoc.*, **173**, 633–5
47. Summers, R. W. (1981). Role of motility in infectious diarrhea. *Gastroenterology*, **80**, 1070–1
48. Swan, K. G., Spees, E. K., Reynolds, D. G., Kerr, J. C. and Zinner, M. J. (1978). Microvascular architecture of anthropoid primate intestine. *Circ. Shock*, **5**, 375–82
49. Tennant, B., Harrold, D. and Reina-Guerra, M. (1968). Hypoglycemia in neonatal calves associated with acute diarrhea. *Cornell Vet.*, **58**, 136–46
50. Tennant, B., Harrold, D. and Reina-Guerra, M. (1972). Physiologic and metabolic factors in the pathogenesis of neonatal enteric infection in calves. *J. Am. Vet. Med. Assoc.*, **161**, 993–1007
51. Tennant, B., Reina-Guerra, M. and Harrold, D. (1973). Metabolic response of calves following acute experimental endotoxemia. *Ann. Rech. Vet.*, **4**, 135–47
52. Tennant, B., Ward, D. E., Braun, R. K., Hunt, E. L. and Baldwin, B. H. (1978). Clincical management and control of neonatal enteric infections of calves. *J. Am. Vet. Med. Assoc.*, **173**, 654–69
53. Toofanian, F., Hill, F. W. G. and Kidder, D. E. (1973). The mucosal disaccharidases in the small intestine of the calf. *Ann. Rech. Vet.*, **4**, 57–69
54. Toofanian, F. (1976). Small intestinal infusion studies in the calf. *Br. Vet. J.*, **132**, 215–20
55. Trump, B. F., Croker, B. P., Jr. and Mergner, W. L. (1971). The role of energy metabolism, ion and water in the pathogenesis of cell injury. In Richter, G. W. and Scarpelli, D. G. (eds.) *Cell Membranes, Biological and Pathological Aspects.* pp. 84–128. (Baltimore: Williams & Wilkins)
56. Ward, D. E. (1976). Pathophysiology of enteric calibaccilosis in the intact neonatal calf. *PhD Thesis*, Cornell University

57. Whipp, S. C. (1978). Physiology of diarrhea – small intestines. *J. Am. Vet. Med. Assoc.*, **173**, 662–6
58. Willoughby, R. A. and Butler, D. G. (1967). An apparatus for the continuous administration of fluid and electrolytes in large animals. *Can. Vet. J.*, **3**, 70–4
59. Woode, G. N., Smith, C. and Dennis, M. J. (1978). Intestinal damage in rotavirus infected calves assessed by *D*-xylose malabsorption. *Vet. Rec.*, **102**, 340–1

Section II
Ruminant Pharmacology

12
Drug bioavailability in the developing ruminant

P. de Backer and M. G. Bogaert

Respiratory and gastrointestinal infections as well as systemic infections are common in newborn and developing animals. In fact, immunodeficiency makes the young animal more susceptible to disease, so there is often a need for drug administration in the newborn and the young animal. Antibiotics and chemotherapeutics will often have to be given[10,47].

Increasing information about the fate of drugs in general, and also about the bioavailability of drugs after oral administration during the early stages of life, has become available in man[21,22,28,29,38]. It is known that the reduced gastric acid secretion and the delayed gastric emptying, which are present in the newborn human, influence drug absorption. For example, the oral bioavailability of acid-labile drugs, such as benzylpenicillin and ampicillin, is increased[19,37]. Other factors affecting drug absorption in young humans are the immaturity of the biliary function, the colonization rate of the intestine by the microbial flora, the high level of β-glucoronidase activity in the newborn intestine, differences in blood perfusion of the gastrointestinal tract, etc.

In view of the complex postnatal development of the gastrointestinal tract in ruminants, one certainly expects also in these species differences in absorption of drugs in the early age period as compared to adult life. Experimental data in this field are scarce. In this review the data we have found in the literature about bioavailability in the developing ruminant will be summarized, with emphasis on our own data. This is preceded by a short discussion of the mechanisms underlying the change of absorption with age.

Following oral administration in ruminants or in other species, most drugs are absorbed through the membranes by passive, non-ionic diffusion. Active transport mechanisms or carrier-mediated transport, which are of great importance for the absorption of many ions, are only of very limited importance. Presystemic drug elimination or the so-called first pass extraction can influence the bioavailability of many drugs. The important factors which can influence drug absorption are listed. All of them show age-dependent changes: anatomy of the gastrointestinal tract and structure of epithelium, pH, gastrointestinal motility, blood circulation in gut wall and splanchnic area, presence and localization of metabolic enzymes and establishment of an intensive microbial population.

ANATOMY

At birth, in lambs as in calves, all features of the adult ruminant digestive tract are present, but in a juvenile state[43]. The forestomachs are relatively non-functional and are underdeveloped compared with the abomasum. After birth, however, the rumen has the fastest growth rate, followed in that order by reticulum, omasum and abomasum, and, at about 8 weeks of age for lambs and 12 weeks for calves, the relative proportion of the four parts of the stomach reach adult values. From a morphological point of view a relatively adult[44] rumen function in ruminants is obtained at 8–12 weeks postpartum. It was found that there was a great difference in anatomical development of the reticulo-rumen between milk-fed and roughage-fed calves[16,39]. The postnatal rumen development has been divided into three periods: the non-ruminant phase from birth to 3 weeks of age, the transition phase from 3 to 8 weeks of age, and the adult phase from 8 weeks on [26,45].

With the increase in volume, there is also a large augmentation of surface area which is mainly brought about by development of the papillae. In calves at birth the ruminoreticular papillae are less than 1 mm. With the ingestion of solid food they reach the adult size and form by 8 weeks of age[25,27].

This development of the ruminal papillae is related to the ability of producing free fatty acids[40]. The large number of fully developed papillae with an intensive blood and lymph supply is very favourable for absorption. It was believed previously that the squamous, stratified epithelium of the reticulo-rumen precluded intensive absorption[8]. Now it is generally accepted that the forestomach wall offers little resistance to the passage of most molecules[14].

pH CHANGES

It is clear that pH changes in the gastrointestinal tract affect non-ionic diffusion of some drugs. In adult animals the pH of the rumen is usually in the range of 5.5–6.5, while in 3 week old calves a pH between 6.0 and 8.0 is recorded in the reticulo-rumen[1]. In the abomasum too, large pH fluctuations can be registered during post-natal development: at birth the abomasal pH is 7.5, but on intake of colostrum or milk it drops immediately to 4.0[18]. During the following 2 weeks, with the increase of pepsin activity, the abomasal pH falls gradually to 2, with temporary rises on ingestion of milk substitute. On change to solid food only, the average pH of the abomasum[23] is 3.6.

MOTILITY

Another important factor which influences gastrointestinal absorption of drugs is the motility of the gastrointestinal tract, more particularly of the reticulo-rumen[32]. In newborn calves movements of the forestomachs are not registered in the first 2 weeks of life. At 3 weeks of age slight movement of the reticulum followed by slow movement of the rumen is noticed. Only at 6 weeks of age, and solely in roughage-fed calves, active diphasic contraction of the reticulum and strong movement of the rumen have been noticed[1]. It is obvious that the contents of the rumino-reticulum of the neonatal and young ruminant are very poorly stirred. A lack of propulsive activity in the forestomachs will also enhance the rate of transfer of endogenous and exogenous substances to the omasum, abomasum and duodenum and will affect the absorption and bioavailability of most drugs.

In adult ruminants, as in developing animals, it is possible to influence the absorption of drugs by changing the gastrointestinal motility with atropine[32,42].

BLOOD FLOW

In the first weeks of life an important increase in blood flow in ruminal veins and portal vein, favouring a faster absorption, was noticed[13].

MICROBIAL POPULATION

The establishment of an intensive microbial population in the forestomachs during the first weeks of postnatal development also influences the absorption of certain drugs. Indeed, metabolization of drugs by the gastrointestinal flora is possible; moreover, since there is a shortage of hydrogen acceptors during the anaerobic fermentations in the rumen, reduction of orally-administered substances can occur. All this can result in an important presystemic drug elimination.

PUBLISHED STUDIES

Several studies about plasma concentrations after oral administration and absorption in the newborn and young ruminant have been published[6,7,12,17,20,24,34–36,42,48–52]. However, conclusions about the evolution of absorption and the bioavailability of drugs in function of age have been drawn only in a few studies.

Sulphadoxine and trimethoprim

In one study the plasma concentrations of sulphadoxine after oral administration were followed in 1 day old, 2 weeks old and in adult goats[31]. In

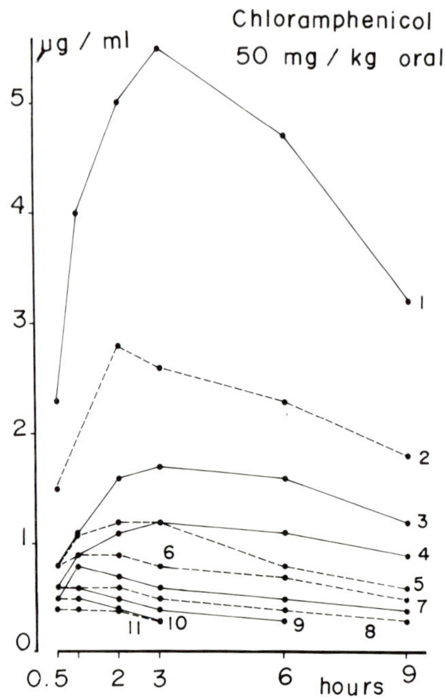

Figure 12.1 Plasma concentrations in function of time after oral administration of chloramphenicol, 50 mg/kg, in a calf at weeks 1–11 after birth

newborn kids the drug was very slowly absorbed. The absorption rate increased with age and at 8 weeks it reached the adult value. The faster absorption was not thought to be related to a change in pH of the gastrointestinal tract but was mainly due to an increase of blood flow in the intestinal tract. The elimination rate for sulphadoxine was lowest in newborn kids and increased with age.

In the same experiment, the authors studied the disposition of trimethoprim. Oral administration of equal doses of the chemotherapeutic (20 mg/kg) to kids and goats of different ages resulted in lower plasma concentration of trimethoprim in the older age groups than in newborn kids. In the adult goats the plasma concentrations of trimethoprim were extremely low. A possible explanation is the development of metabolism in the liver of the older goats, with a first pass effect. From *in vitro* experimental results degradation of trimethoprim in ruminal fluid has been found possible.

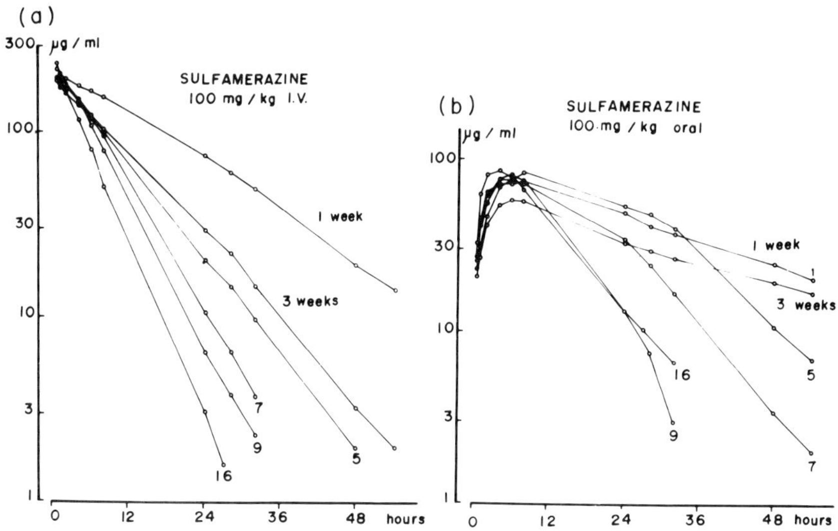

Figure 12.2 Plasma concentrations in function of time after intravenous (a) and oral (b) administration of sulfamerazine, 100 mg/kg, in a lamb at weeks 1, 3, 5, 7, 9, and 16 after birth

Chloramphenicol

The influence of age on the oral absorption of chloramphenicol in calves was studied, because in adult ruminants with a fully developed rumen function, it is reported that no plasma levels could be detected following oral administration of the antibiotic[9,11,41] while in monogastric animals adequate levels are achieved[15,46]. Once weekly an oral dose of 50 mg/kg of the drug was given from the first until the 11th week of life[4,5]. The plasma concentrations of chloramphenicol obtained in one calf are shown in Figure 12.1. The highest plasma levels were obtained in the first week of life but even then a therapeutic level (5 µg/ml) was only obtained for a few hours. As the calves became older, much lower plasma concentrations were obtained. It is suggested that this evolution is probably due as well to the anatomical development of the forestomachs as to the gradual appearance of the microbial fauna and flora.

Sulfamerazine

The pharmacokinetics and bioavailability of sulfamerazine and antipyrine have been studied in lambs[3]. Lambs were treated repeatedly from birth until the 16th week of life, intravenously or orally with sulfamerazine at a dosage of 100 mg/kg. In some animals sulfamerazine was given intravenously in order to better understand the complex absorption problems.

In Figure 12.2(a) the time course of sulfamerazine plasma concentrations after intravenous administration of 100 mg/kg in one lamb at different times after birth is shown. An age-dependent evolution of the curve was noticed in all animals. The older the animal, the faster the elimination of sulfamerazine. Halflife, distribution volume and clearance of the drug after intravenous administration in function of age were determined and are shown in Table 12.1. A long elimination halflife and a low clearance were found in the first week of birth. This is in accordance with the known immaturity of liver and kidney function in newborn and young animals.

Table 12.1 Pharmacokinetic parameters of sulfamerazine after intravenous administration of 100 mg/kg in lambs in function of age ($n=8$)

Week	$t_{1/2}$ (h)	V_d (l/kg)	*Cl* (ml kg^{-1}h^{-1})
1	11.3 (9.0–13.9)	0.50 (0.43–0.60)	31 (22–38)
3	8.1 (7.1–8.8)	0.40 (0.30–0.50)	34 (24–41)
5	7.3 (6.1–9.1)	0.39 (0.30–0.47)	38 (28–51)
7	6.2 (5.3–7.4)	0.39 (0.36–0.48)	45 (34–55)
9	5.5 (4.1–6.6)	0.40 (0.36–0.47)	57 (42–79)
16	5.1 (3.8–6.7)	0.41 (0.36–0.44)	66 (50–83)

Mean values and ranges are given

The clearance increased and the halflife then decreased gradually until the 9th week. The values obtained at 9 and 16 weeks were not different from those found in adult animals[2]. The volume of distribution was high in the first week, decreased in the next weeks and remained constant afterwards, an evaluation which can be partly explained by the changes in plasma binding of sulfamerazine. Indeed, in the newborn, plasma binding of the drug was lowest, but increased together with the albumin concentration in function of age (Table 12.2).

Table 12.2 Percentage plasma binding of sulfamerazine and albumin concentration in lambs in function of age ($n=8$)

Week	*Binding* %	*Albumin concentration* g/l
1	38.2 (10.6–55.1)	23.6 (22.2–25.3)
3	55.6 (44.7–65.5)	26.3 (23.0–31.1)
5	58.7 (42.6–68.2)	29.0 (24.4–32.1)
7	64.3 (60.8–70.4)	32.5 (28.8–36.4)
9	64.9 (60.9–71.7)	32.1 (30.3–34.9)
16	60.1 (58.0–64.9)	27.9 (24.5–32.0)

Mean values and ranges are given

In nine lambs, the same drug was administered orally at weeks 1, 2, 3, 5, 7, 9 and 16 after birth at a dose of 100 mg/kg. A semilogarithmic plot of sulfamerazine concentrations vs. time after oral administration in one lamb is shown in Figure 12.2(b). Here too, a pronounced change was seen in function of age. A very slow decline in the plasma concentration in the first and third week of life was found in all animals. From the 5th week on, a marked change in the shape of the curve appeared.

No attempt was made to calculate kinetic parameters after oral administration as it was not possible to distinguish between absorption, distribution and elimination phases. However, it is clear from the shape of the oral curves that these profound changes with age cannot be explained solely by a slower elimination but are also caused by changing absorption. Many factors such as a delayed gastric emptying, a not yet developed mucosal surface, a limited blood flow to and in the gastrointestinal tract, infavourable pH gradients, etc. could be proposed as possible causes.

In order to study this problem further, antipyrine was administered orally in the same animals (18 mg/kg). No suggestion of an age-dependent evolution of the absorption after oral administration was found for antipyrine. Therefore, it is obvious that the evolution of absorption in function of age seen for sulfamerazine is not a general feature for all drugs.

CONCLUSION

In conclusion, it can be said that there is a lack of information about the oral bioavailability of drugs in the developing ruminant. Anatomical and physiological changes in the gastrointestinal tract during postnatal development certainly affect the absorption of pharmacological substances as shown by the scarce studies performed.

It is necessary to carry out kinetic and bioavailability studies for each drug for each period of life in order to find an accurate and correct dosage regimen.

References

1. Asai, T. (1973). *Jpn. J. Vet. Sci.*, **35**, 239–52
2. de Backer, P., Belpaire, F. M., Debackere, M. *et al.* (1981). *Zbl. Vet. Med. A.*, **28**, 468–74
3. de Backer, P., Belpaire, F. M., Bogaert, M. G. *et al.* (1982). *Am. J. Vet. Res.*, **43**, 174–5
4. de Backer, P., Debackere, M. and de Corte-Baeten, K. (1978). *J. Vet. Pharmacol. Ther.*, **1**, 135–40
5. de Backer, P. and Debackere, M. (1979). *J. Vet. Pharmacol. Ther.*, **2**, 195–202
6. Barcroft, J., McAnally, R. A. and Phillipson, A. T. (1944). *J. Exp. Biol.*, **20**, 132–3
7. Bourne, D. W. A., Bevill, R. F. and Sharma, R. H. (1977). *Am. J. Vet. Res.*, **38**, 967–72
8. Colin, G. (1886). *Traité de Physiologie Comparée des Animaux.* Vol. 2, p. 102. (Paris: Baillière)
9. de Corte-Baeten, K. and Debackere, M. (1975). *Zbl. Vet. Med.*, **22**, 704–12
10. Davis, L. E. (1979). *J. Am. Vet. Med. Assoc.*, 246–7
11. Davis, L. E., Neff, C. A., Baggot, J. D. *et al.* (1972). *Am. J. Vet. Res.*, **33**, 2259–66
12. Dobson, A. (1967). *Fed. Proc.*, **26**, 994–1000
13. Dobson, A. and Phillipson, A. T. (1956). *J. Physiol.*, **133**, 76
14. Dobson, A. and Phillipson, A. T. (1968). In *Handbook of Physiology.* pp. 2761–74. (Baltimore: Williams & Wilkins)
15. English, P. B. and Withy, D. (1959). *Austr. Vet. J.*, **35**, 187–93
16. Flatt, W. P., Warner, R. G. and Loosli, J. K. (1959). Memoir 361, Agricultural experiment station, Cornell University
17. Hayashi, M., Bourne, D. W. A., Bevill, R. F. *et al.* (1979). *Am. J. Vet. Res.*, **40**, 1578–82

18. Hill, K. J. (1968). Abomasal function. In *Handbook of Physiology*. p. 2747. (Baltimore: Williams and Wilkins)
19. Huang, N. N. and High, R. H. (1953). *J. Pediat.*, **42**, 657–68
20. Huffman, E. M., Clark, C. H., Olson, J. D. *et al.* (1981). *J. Vet. Pharmacol. Ther.*, **4**, 225–31
21. Jaffe, S. J. and Danish, M. (1978). *Drug Metab. Rev.*, **8**, 303–18
22. Jaffe, S. J. and Juchau, M. R. (1974). *Ann. Rev. Pharmacol.*, **14**, 219–38
23. Juhasz, B., Szegedi, B. and Keresztes, M. (1976). *Acta Vet. Acad. Sci. Hung.*, **26**, 281–95
24. Lapka, R., Urbanova, Z., Kobrylka, B. *et al.* (1978). *Drug Metab. Disp.*, **6**, 637–39
25. Lauwers, H. (1973). Morfologische bijdrage tot de kennis van het resorberend vermogen van rundervoormagen. *Aggregaatsthesis*, Rijks Universiteit Gent
26. Leat, W. M. F. (1970). In Phillipson, A. T. (ed.) *Physiology of Digestion and Metabolism in the Ruminant*. pp. 211–22. (Newcastle-upon-Tyne: Oriel Press)
27. McGilliard, A. D. and Jacobson, N. L. (1965). In Dougherty, R. W. (ed.) *Physiology of Digestion in the Ruminant*. (London: Butterworth)
28. Morselli, P. L. (1976). *Drug Disposition during Development*. (New York: Spectrum Publications INC)
29. Morselli, P. L., Franco-Morselli, R. and Bossi, L. (1980). *Clin. Pharmacokinetics*, **5**, 485–527
30. Morselli, P. L. and Olive, G. (1978). *Drug Measurement and Drug Effects in Laboratory Health Science*. (Basel: Karger)
31. Nielsen, P., Romvary, A. and Rasmussen, F. (1978). *J. Vet. Pharmacol. Ther.*, **1**, 37–46
32. Nimmo, W. S. (1981). In Presscott, and Nimmo, W. S. (eds.) *Drug Absorption*. pp. 11–20. (Lancaster: MTP Press)
33. Oyaert, W., Quin, J. I. and Clark, R. (1951). *Onderstepoort J. Vet. Res.*, **25**, 59
34. Righter, H. F., Showalter, D. H. and Teske, R. H. (1979). *J. Vet. Pharmacol. Ther.*, **2**, 203–8
35. Sechserova, M., Sechser, T., Raskova, H. *et al.* (1979). *Arzneim-Forsch./Drug. Res.*, **29**, 650–1
36. Sechserova, M., Sechser, T., Raskova, H. *et al.* (1979). *Arzneim-Forsch./Drug Res.*, **29**, 804–7
37. Silverio, J. and Poole, J. W. (1973). *Pediatrics*, **51**, 578–80
38. Stevenson, I. H., Salem, S. A. M., O'Malley, K., *et al.* (1981). *Drug Absorption*. pp. 253–61. (Lancaster: MTP Press)
39. Tamate, H. (1957). *Tohoku J. Agric. Res.*, **8**, 65
40. Tamate, H., McGilliard, A. D., Jacobson, N. L. *et al.* (1962). *J. Dairy Sci.*, **45**, 408
41. Theodorides, V. J., Di Cuollo, C. J., Guarini, J. R. *et al.* (1968). *Am. J. Vet. Res.*, **29**, 643–5
42. Thompson, S. M. R. and Black, W. D. (1978). *Can. J. Comp. Med.*, **42**, 255–9
43. Trautmann, A. (1932). *Arch. Tierernähr. Tierz.*, **7**, 400
44. Wardrop, I. D. and Coombe, J. B. (1960). *J. Agric. Sci. Camb.*, **54**, 140
45. Wardrop, I. D. and Coombe, J. B. (1961). *Aust. J. Agric. Res.*, **12**, 661
46. Watson, A. D. J. (1974). *Res. Vet. Sci.*, **16**, 147–51
47. Wilkinson, P. J. (1982). *J. Antimicrob. Chemother.*, **9**, 21–9
48. Wooley, J. L., Sigel, C. W. and Wels, C. M. (1980). *Life Sci.*, **27**, 1819–26
49. Woolley, J. L. and Sigel, C. W. (1982). *Am. J. Vet. Res.*, **43**, 768–74
50. Ziv, G., Nouws, J. F. M. and van Ginncken, C. A. M. (1982). *J. Vet. Pharmacol. Ther.*, **5**, 45–58
51. Ziv, G., Nouws, J. F. M., Groothuis, D. G. *et al.* (1977). *Am. J. Vet. Res.*, **38**, 1007–13
52. Ziv, G., Wanner, M. and Nicolet, J. (1980). *J. Vet. Pharmacol. Ther.*, **3**, 87–94

13
Oral antibacterial therapy in pre- and postweaning calves

W. L. Jenkins and L. G. Friedlander

A variety of primary and secondary microbial infections are known to occur in young calves prior to weaning[4]. This is especially true during the neonatal period[29]. Specific and non-specific bacterial diseases are often precipitated by a complexity of predisposing causes, mainly of managemental and nutritional nature[25]. However, primary viral infections are also frequently responsible for secondary bacterial invasion. The inadequate immunocompetence so often encountered in very young calves adds an extra dimension to the pathogenesis of many of the disease syndromes that commonly occur at this age[27,31]. For convenience, the most prominent diseases in young calves may be divided into the bacterial septicaemias and the diarrhoea-respiratory disease syndromes. The septicaemic diseases usually occur soon after birth and may be caused by many genera of bacteria but the most common are *Escherichia*, *Salmonella*, *Corynebacteria*, *Klebsiella*, *Proteus* and *Streptococcus.* Bacterial and/or viral induced diarrhoea-respiratory disease syndromes are the most prevalent causes of preweaning calf losses. Many different agents are involved in the pathogenesis of diarrhoeal disease in the calf. Bacterial causes include enteropathogenic *Escherichia coli* (colibacillosis), *Salmonella typhimurium*, *Salmonella dublin* and other *Salmonella spp.* (Salmonellosis), occasionally other genera and *Chlamydia spp.* Viral agents associated with pneumonenteritis include adenovirus, parvovirus, coronavirus, rotavirus, enterovirus, bovine virus diarrhoea and infectious bovine rhinotracheitis.

During the postweaning period respiratory diseases are more common than gastrointestinal infections and usually result from stress-associated management and handling procedures that impair the immune competence of the calves. The bovine respiratory disease complex or shipping fever best exemplifies this particular problem[10]. In these cases a primary viral infection (such as infectious bovine rhinotracheitis, parainfluenza type 3, adenoviruses, rhinovirus or bovine viral diarrhoea) commonly produces a pablum favourable for secondary bacterial invasion (such as by *Pasteurella haemolytica*, *Pasteurella multocida*, *Corynebacterium pyogenes*, *Haemophilus somnus*, *Myocoplasma spp.* or *Chlamydia spp.*)[20].

Several preventative and therapeutic approaches are usually instituted in order to control these destructive bacterial infections, that are capable of substantially limiting the productivity and economic viability of veal or feeder operations. Of great importance amongst these measures is the use of antibacterial agents which are administered either orally or parenterally for both prophylactic and therapeutic purposes[28].

During the past 25 years this procedure has become a routine component of many intensive calf-rearing and feedlot enterprises throughout the world. Yet several questions remain unanswered regarding the ultimate benefit of what would seem to be a logical approach to restricting infectious disease losses in pre- and postweaning calves. It must also be noted that the employment of antimicrobial agents for these purposes is distinct from their use as 'feed additives' which are routinely included in rations at low levels to promote growth. Considerable controversy still exists with regard to the potential hazards associated with this latter practice[5,33] but the issues are beyond the scope of this discussion except to note that several classes of antimicrobial agents are used for both purposes, though at substantially different dosage rates.

An array of antimicrobial compounds have been used to combat bacterial infections in both pre- and postweaning calves. Those that may be administered orally and which either are, or might be used in the future, include the following: (1) penicillins (ampicillin, amoxycillin), (2) cephalosporins and cephamycins (cephalexin, cefachlor, cephamycin C), (3) aminocyclitols (streptomycin, neomycin, framycetin, paromomycin, gentamicin, kanamycin, apramycin, spectinomycin), (4) tetracyclines (oxytetracycline, chlortetracycline, tetracycline), (5) chloramphenicol, (6) macrolides (erythromycin, tylosin, carbomycin), (7) polypeptides (bacitracin, polymyxin B, colistin), (8) sulfonamides (sulfamethazine, sulfabromomethazine, sulfadiazine, sulphathiazole, sulfadimethoxine, sulfaethoxypyridazine, sulfachloropyridazine and others), (9) potentiated sulfonamides (cotrimoxazole, cotrimazine), (10) nitrofurans (furazolidone, nifuraldezone), and (11) quinoxalines (carbadox) and quinolines (iodochlorhydroxyquin).

Several of these antibacterial agents are primarily indicated to prevent or control gastrointestinal infections, whereas others are administered because of their systemic disposition. They are also used either alone or in combinations of two or even three agents.

In the United States between 40 and 50% of the total antibiotics sold (about 11.2 million kg in 1980) are given to animals either as feed additives or for medical reasons. As is well known, this whole scenario has enjoyed considerable scrutiny by regulatory agencies in many countries and great concern is expressed periodically about the indiscriminate use of antibiotics in the animal food sector by the veterinary profession. To date only a few substantiated reports of serious potential hazards have emerged[18,23] and the debate on the risk ratio: benefit ratio continues unabated. Perhaps it is only right that the issue remains controversial, since the currently available evidence remains somewhat equivocal.

There are obvious concerns about the misuse of antibacterial agents in calves and it behoves us as veterinary pharmacologists to pay attention to what is happening in the field so that we too can contribute to the resolution of this particularly difficult problem. Antibacterial therapy needs to be rational in order to be acceptable and defensible. Based on this tenet, there are a number of considerations that are of special concern when antimicrobials are administered to calves for either prophylactic or therapeutic reasons. A few selected features will be briefly emphasized here, recognizing at the outset that there is a notable paucity of specific information. This is a deficiency which needs to be rectified as soon as possible, since recent public statements such as, 'The overuse of antibiotics, including their use in livestock, is now a worldwide health problem', are becoming more and more frequent and need to be either validated or discredited.

SELECTED PHARMACOTHERAPEUTIC FEATURES

There are a number of factors which will determine in large measure the success or failure of the use of chemotherapeutic agents in calves to control or eliminate bacterial infections. A few of these will be briefly reviewed in order to emphasize some of the difficulties associated with this particular field of veterinary medicine.

Clinical diagnosis

An accurate clinical diagnosis is the basis of sound therapeutics. Fortunately, the septicaemic, enteric and pulmonary disease syndromes which occur in calves are fairly easily recognized clinically but great care should be taken always to clearly define the disease process. It is particularly important to establish the physiopathological changes and any secondary complications that occur. Septicaemia and endotoxaemia produce notable cardiovascular responses as well as inhibition of rumino-reticular motility in older calves[11]. The diarrhoeal syndromes lead to dehydration, acid–base and electrolyte derangements and ultimately to cardiovascular collapse[25]. Pneumonic conditions principally lead to hypoxaemic responses and acid–base disorders. In every instance, renal and/or hepatic involvement may also occur as a secondary complication. The disturbed biochemical profiles which are associated with these disease syndromes are quite well established[4]. Clearly, many of these pathological components of the disease process are capable of modifying the disposition and elimination kinetics of the antibacterial agents that may be administered orally. This should always be borne in mind when examining sick calves and when deciding on an appropriate therapeutic regimen even though little specific information is available.

Aetiological diagnosis

A definitive bacteriological diagnosis, though the ideal, is not always attainable, especially when *E. coli* is incriminated as the possible causative organism. Often the aetiological diagnosis remains presumptive even after the isolation and identification of a potential pathogen has taken place. In addition, the possibility of a polymicrobial infection has to be considered in many cases. Antibacterial sensitivity tests are proving to be of greater clinical use, as many of the early difficulties experienced with these techniques have been overcome. The modal minimal inhibitory concentration values (MIC) for many members of specifically susceptible bacterial populations are now available[17] and can serve as the basis for antibiotic dosage schedules, recognizing that many physiological and pharmacological characteristics may have to be taken into account. Even minimal antibiotic concentration values (MAC) are becoming available for those agents that possess residual effects (on susceptible bacteria) at subminimal inhibitory concentrations.

Selection of antibacterial agents

Many factors govern the selection of the most appropriate antibacterial agent or agents to be used to control disease episodes. These considerations have been reviewed by Hjerpe and Routen[13], Burrows[7], Amstutz[2], Radostits[26] and Tennant *et al.*[32]. Only a few of special note will be covered here.

An accurate clinical and bacteriological diagnosis together with a sensitivity test would be the ideal determinant of antibiotic selection, as was mentioned earlier. However, surprising differences between *in vivo* responses and *in vitro* results may and do occur for a multitude of reasons.

The virulence of the pathogen, together with the acuteness of the infection and the physiopathological changes that occur as a result of the disease process, will also influence the choice of antimicrobial agents. Their intrinsic modes of action and whether they produce bacteriostatic, bactericidal or bacteriolytic effects may also have direct bearing on a case. The latter effects often depend in large measure on the concentration of the drug at the site of infection.

In addition, the disposition and fate of any orally administered antibacterial need to be taken into account. This area, until recently, had enjoyed little attention in cattle and the guidelines followed were often very arbitrary. However, recent contributions have at last provided some of the data necessary to place antibacterial therapy in pre- and postweaning calves on a much sounder basis[9,11,35].

Finally, the potential toxicities and side-effects associated with the array of antibacterial agents listed earlier and used in calves need to be taken into account, especially in relation to the disease process present.

Selection of dosage schedules

There are no single optimal dosage rates for any given antibacterial. There are simply too many variables such as age, host resistance, bacterial virulence, bacterial sensitivity, the site of infection and, especially, the disease process with the lesions that are present. The nutritional status and diet may also play a role.

The aspect which will be emphasized here is that of the influence of the pathological changes which occur on the kinetic fate of orally administered agents. The majority of proposed dosage schedules are invariably determined on pharmacokinetic data obtained from normal animals and, in the case of the antimicrobial agents, on known MIC values for various pathogenic micro-organisms. However, there is ever accruing evidence to suggest that disease processes and associated physiopathological responses may markedly alter the disposition and elimination kinetics of antibiotics and other antimicrobial agents, such as the sulfonamides. Examples include fever and endotoxaemia[11], enteritis and diarrhoea[1], rumino-reticular atony[11], pneumonia[34], and renal disease[8]. Until further evidence is available, dosage regimens should be adjusted accordingly or plasma levels monitored in order to control the dosage schedule.

It must be added that the bioavailability of a particular agent may also vary with the diet[35] or with age, in the specific case of chloramphenicol[9].

Special concerns

There are a number of special considerations which should be borne in mind when antibacterial agents are administered orally – either alone or in combination with others.

The combined use of antibiotics always produces the potential for interaction between such agents and synergism, additive effects, antagonism or indifference may result. Once again, so many factors may play a role that only a few instances of interaction are clearly documented and general guidelines are all that are available at this time[17].

Colonization and suprainfection by opportunistic pathogens are a major detriment to antibacterial therapy. The alteration of the host's endogenous flora by broad spectrum antibacterial agents, or combinations thereof, and the subsequent emergence of resistant pathogenic organisms, is a clinical phenomenon now being more frequently recognized. Antibiotic-induced enterocolitis in the human caused by *Clostridium difficile* best exemplifies this particular problem. How prevalent suprainfection is in treated diarrhoeic calves remains obscure.

Reinfection or clinical relapses may also occur if the instituted therapeutic regimen is inadequate.

The final special consideration to be emphasized here concerns the very real problem of plasmid-mediated or transmissible antibiotic resistance[30]. The potential hazards associated with the use of antimicrobial agents in calves at either therapeutic or at subtherapeutic levels in feed have enjoyed a great deal of attention in the past[5, 33] and continue to do so as more and more instances are reported where identical antibiotic resistance patterns are encountered in isolates from both calves and humans who have been in contact with the animals[23]. Although the number of confirmed clinical cases is still fairly limited, the fact is that the issue remains one of concern. It is difficult to theorize on a risk: benefit ratio at this time simply because insufficient definitive data is available. However, it is at least necessary that the application of these antibacterial agents in veal and feeder calves be reasonable and rational to prevent the widespread dissemination of R-factor-bearing resistant strains of bacteria.

Supportive therapy

There is now ample evidence to suggest that the success or failure of treating specific or undifferentiated diarrhoeic syndromes in calves often depends only in small measure on the oral use of antibacterial agents[16,25]. In fact, it is possible that oral antibiotic therapy may well be detrimental if opportunistic pathogens emerge as a result of suprainfection.

The physiopathological features of many of the enteric diseases of calves, and especially of acute colibacillosis due to enterotoxin-producing strains of *E. coli*, have been established[8,25]. Consequently, a rational therapeutic regimen has become possible with several innovative concepts added in recent years. It is beyond the scope of this presentation to review all of the aspects of the treatment of neonatal diarrhoea and several pharmacotherapeutic concepts will simply be outlined[8,15,16]: (1) fluid and electrolyte replacement, (2) antimicrobial therapy – as anti-infective or as anti-adhesive agents, (3) intestinal adsorbents and protectants, (4) antisecretory agents, (5) non-steroidal anti-inflammatory drugs, (6) modulators of intestinal motility such as anticholinergic agents and opiate derivatives, and (7) hyperalimentation and nutritional support.

Supportive treatment for the bovine respiratory disease complex is less well-established, although bronchodilator agents and mucolytics have been employed at times. The correction of fluid, electrolyte and acid–base disturbances is important in these cases as is the treatment of the secondary rumino-reticular atony which frequently occurs. The use of corticosteroids is probably contraindicated since they appear to prolong the course of the disease and the incidence of relapses is often higher following corticosteroid administration. This issue, however, remains controversial. Once again it must be noted that the success rate of treating pneumonic calves with antibacterial agents, especially by the oral route, is not always great, and frequently this procedure simply prolongs the course of the disease with the ultimate mortality rate not being significantly different from that in untreated cases.

Immune competence

The success or failure of antibacterial therapy may depend in large measure on the efficiency of affected calves' defence mechanisms. This is particularly true for the bacteriostatic agents and for bactericidal agents present at subinhibitory concentrations. This is an often neglected consideration when sick calves are treated with antibacterial agents and may well explain in part the limited success often attained when managing enteric and/or pneumonic syndromes[4,25].

The increased susceptibility of neonatal calves to infectious agents is a well-recognized clinical phenomenon but the reasons for this vulnerability have not been fully elucidated. Hypogammaglobulinaemia has been incriminated as an important contributing factor. Newborn calves have very low levels of immunoglobulin and passive immunity is acquired by absorption of immunoglobulins from ingested colostrum[6]. The most frequent cause of hypogammaglobulinaemia is failure of passive transfer of maternal immunoglobulins.

Other differences in host defence factors of the calf, as compared to adult cattle, have been reported. The newborn calf does not possess the capacity to mount an active humoral immune response to all antigens that are responded to by older animals[24]. Cellular immune functions may also be depressed in the calf as compared to the adult. Finally, the components of the complement system have been found to be low in the neonatal calf[27].

A large number of psychological and somatic stressors are imposed on feeder calves from the time of separation from their dams until they are satisfactorily on feed in a lot. These stressors include weaning, castration, dehorning, vaccination, deworming, spraying, rigorous handling, use of persuaders, mixing of groups, overcrowding, transportation, exhaustion, lack of feed and water, unfamiliar feed, inadequate nutrition, parasitism, digestive disturbances, change of environment, exposure to inclement weather, temperature extremes and, finally, subclinical bacterial and viral infections. Preliminary evidence suggests that host defence factors and especially pulmonary protective mechanisms are jeopardized under these conditions. Thus, the development of infectious pneumonic syndromes in feeder calves should not be unexpected[10].

There appear to be complex interactions between host defence mechanisms, antibiotics and infective micro-organisms and this area is currently enjoying some attention. For example, tetracyclines readily penetrate macrophages and leukocytes and may inhibit chemotaxis[3]. In addition, many antibacterial agents penetrate alveolar macrophages quite readily, with erythromycin and particularly clindamycin attaining remarkably high concentrations within these cells when compared with extracellular antibiotic levels[14]. Enhanced activity of leukocytes against pretreated bacteria also has been recognized recently[19].

Tissue residues

Clearly, an inherent problem associated with the administration of antibacterial agents to calves is the possibility of residues in the meat. Current evidence seems to indicate that there have been few major human health problems to date[12] but the monitoring of meat for xenobiotic residues is required by regulating agencies throughout the world. If residues are found, serious economic sanctions may follow at great cost to the livestock producer. Fortunately, the application of pharmacokinetics to this problem is gradually making it possible to estimate and project drug withdrawal intervals in food-producing animals[21]. In addition, withdrawal times and limitations for use of certifiable antibacterials in food-producing animals are usually legally defined by Public Health regulatory authorities.

Nevertheless, much additional quantitative information is still required in order to avoid the contamination of meat products intended for human consumption. Once again the presence of disease processes can substantially alter the normally accepted withdrawal times, as was demonstrated by Nouws and Ziv[22] in nephrotic animals.

CONCLUSIONS

It is evident from this general review of selected features of oral antibacterial therapy in pre- and postweaning calves, that many pharmacological aspects still require considerable investigation. The issues are complex and have implications beyond the realm of veterinary medicine alone. It has become imperative to resolve these issues and to establish a rational basis for the oral treatment and control of bacterial infections in calves.

References

1. Ahrens, F. A. (1978). Influence of enteritis on pharmacodynamics. *J. Am. Vet. Med. Assoc.*, **173,** 673–4
2. Amstutz, H. E. (1979). Recent findings in respiratory diseases of cattle. In *Proceedings of 27th Annual Pfizer Research Conference.* pp. 122–40.
3. Belsheim, J., Gnarpe, H. and Persson, S. (1979). Tetracyclines and host defense mechanisms interference with leukocyte chemotaxis. *Scand. J. Infect. Dis.*, **11,** 141–5
4. Blood, D. C., Henderson, J. A. and Radostits, O. M. (1979). *Veterinary Medicine A Textbook of the Diseases of Cattle, Sheep, Pigs and Horses.* (Philadelphia: Lea and Febiger)
5. Braude, R. (1981). Antibiotics as feed additives for livestock. In Ninet, L., Bost, P. E., Bouanchaud, D. H. and Florent, J. (eds.) *The Future of Antibiotherapy and Antibiotic Research.* pp. 169–182. (London: Academic Press)
6. Buntain, B. J. and Silman, I. E. (1980). Controlled studies of various treatments for neonatal calf diarrhoea in calves of known immunoglobulin levels. *Vet. Rec.*, **107,** 245–8
7. Burrows, G. E. (1980). Therapeutic considerations in the use of antibacterials. *Bovine Practit.*, **15,** 99–102
8. Bywater, R. J. (1976). Pathogenesis and treatment of *Escherichia coli* infections in calves. *J. S. Afr. Vet. Assoc.*, **47,** 193–5
9. de Backer, P., Debackere, M. and de Corte-Baeten, K. (1978). Plasma levels of chloramphenicol after oral administration in calves during the first weeks of life. *J. Vet. Pharmacol. Ther.*, **1,** 135–40
10. Dyer, R. M. (1982). The bovine respiratory disease complex: a complex interaction of host, environmental and infectious factors. *Compendium of Continuing Education.* Vol. 4, No. 7 S296–307
11. Groothuis, D. G., VanMiert, A. S. J. P. A. M., Ziv, G. *et al.* (1978). Effects of experimental *Escherichia coli* endotoxemia on ampicillin: amoxycillin blood levels after oral and parenteral administration in calves. *J. Vet. Pharmacol. Ther.*, **1,** 81–4
12. Hewitt, W. L. (1975). Clinical implications of the presence of drug residues in food. *Fed. Proc.*, **34,** 202–4
13. Hjerpe, C. A. and Routen, T. A. (1976). Practical and theoretical considerations concerning treatment of bacterial pneumonia in feedlot cattle, with special reference to antimicrobial therapy. In *Proceedings of the Annual Convention American Association of Bovine Practitioners.* Vol. 9, pp. 97–140

14. Johnson, J. D., Hand, W. L., Francis, J. B. *et al.* (1980). Antibiotic uptake by alveolar macrophages. *J. Lab. Clin. Med.*, **95**, 429–39
15. Larvor, P. (1979). Treatment of the newborn calf. In Hoffmann, B., Mason, I. L. and Schmidt, J. (eds.) *Calving Problems and Early Viability of the Calf.* pp. 539–50. (The Hague: Martinus Nijhoff)
16. Lewis, L. D. and Phillips, R. W. (1979). Treatment of the calf with diarrhoea. *Vet. Clin. N. Am.: Large Anim. Pract.*, **1**, 395–409
17. Lorian, V. (Ed.). (1980). *Antibiotics in Laboratory Medicine.* (Baltimore: Williams and Wilkins)
18. Lyons, R. W., Samples, C. L., DeSilva, H. N., Ross, K. A., Julian, E. M. and Checko, P. J. (1980). An epidemic of resistant *Salmonella* in a nursery. *J. Am. Vet. Med. Assoc.*, **243**, 546–7
19. McDonald, P. J., Wetherall, B. L. and Pruul, H. (1981). Postantibiotic leukocyte enhancement: increased susceptibility of bacteria pretreated with antibiotics to activity of leukocytes. *Rev. Infec. Dis.*, **3**, 38–44
20. McKercher, D. G. (1979). Disease incidence and epidemiology - the situation in the USA. In Martin, W. B. (ed.) *Respiratory Diseases of Cattle.* pp. 71–83. (The Hague: Martinus Nijhoff)
21. Mercer, H. D. (1978). The practical applications of pharmacokinetics in veterinary medicine. In *Proceedings, First Symp. on Vet. Pharmacol. and Therapeutics.* pp. 47–74. (Amsterdam: Elsevier)
22. Nouws, J. F. M. and Ziv. G. (1978). Pre-slaughter withdrawal times for drugs in dairy cows. *J. Vet. Pharmacol. Ther.*, **1**, 47–56
23. O'Brien, T. F., Hopkins, J. D., Gilleece, E. S. *et al.* (1982). Molecular epidemiology of antibiotic resistance in *Salmonella* from animals and human beings in the United States. *N. Engl. J. Med.*, **307**, 1–6
24. Osburn, B. I., Stabenfeldt, G. H., Ardans, A. A. *et al.* (1974). Perinatal immunity in calves. *J. Am. Vet. Med. Assoc.*, **164**, 295–8
25. Radostits, O. M. (1981). Neonatal diarrhea in ruminants (calves, lambs, and kids). In *Current Veterinary Therapy Food Animal Practice.* Howard, J. L. (ed.) pp. 116–26. (Philadelphia: W. B. Saunders)
26. Radostits, O. M., Rhodes, C. S., Mitchell, M. E. *et al.* (1975). A clinical evaluation of antimicrobial agents and temporary starvation in the treatment of acute undifferentiated diarrhea in newborn calves. *Can. Vet. J.*, **16**, 219–27
27. Renshaw, H. W., Allert, C. C., Richards, A. B. *et al.* (1980). Classical and alternate complement pathway activity in sera from colostrum-fed calves during the initial three days after birth. In *Proceedings Third Int. Symp. Neonatal Diarrhea.* Vol. 3, pp. 161–71
28. Ruckebusch, Y. (1981). Antimicrobial drugs in veterinary medicine. In Ninet, L., Bost, P. E., Borianchaud, D. H. and Florent, J. (eds.) *The Future of Antibiotherapy and Antibiotic Research.* pp. 141–67. (London: Academic Press)
29. Rutter, J. M. (ed.) (1975). *Perinatal Ill Health in Calves.* (Newbury, Berkshire: Simpsons)
30. Sonnenschein, V. B. (1980). Grundlagen und Bedeutung der Antibiotikaresistenz von Bakterien. *Dtsche. Tierärztl. Wschr.*, **87**, 299–303
31. Stott, G. H. (1980). Immunoglobulin absorption in calf neonates with special considerations of stress. *J. Dairy Sci.*, **63**, 681–8
32. Tennant, B., Ward, D. E., Braun, R. K. *et al.* (1978). Clinical management and control of neonatal enteric infections of calves. *J. Am. Vet. Med. Assoc.*, **173**, 654–61
33. VanHouweling, C. D. and Gainer, J. H. (1978). Public health concerns relative to the use of subtherapeutic levels of antibiotics in animal feeds. *J. Anim. Sci.*, **46**, 1413–24
34. Young, J. K. (1973). Blood sulfonamide levels in feedlot cattle with respiratory disease. *Mod. Vet. Pract.*, **54**, 21–2
35. Ziv, G., Nouws, J. F. M., Groothius, D. G. *et al.* (1977). Oral absorption and bioavailability of ampicillin derivatives in calves. *Am. J. Vet. Res.*, **38**, 1007–13

14
Influence of ruminant gastrointestinal physiology on the pharmacokinetics of drugs in dosage forms administered orally

G. D. Koritz

The complexity of the ruminant digestive tract in comparison to that of the monogastric animal creates unique problems and opportunities as concerns the absorption of drugs administered orally. Bioavailability studies and the construction of pharmacokinetic models provide information concerning the fate of a drug administered orally to a ruminant animal but provide little comprehension of the factors which influence drug absorption. Such insight is provided by an understanding of the physiology of the ruminant, particularly of its gastrointestinal tract.

BIOAVAILABILITY OF DRUGS ADMINISTERED ORALLY

Following oral administration of a solid drug formulation such as a bolus, the processes leading directly to absorption of the drug are those of disintegration of the formulation, followed by dissolution of the drug particles released from the formulation in the enteric fluids. A number of competing mechanisms may lead to non-absorption or destruction of the drug in the ruminant digestive system and thereby reduce the amount of drug ultimately available for absorption. These processes are subject to modification by the physiological state of the gastrointestinal tract.

Disintegration of a solid dosage form following its oral administration may be controlled to a variable extent by the physical and chemical characteristics of substances other than the drug in the formulation, for seldom is a drug administered to an animal as a single chemical entity. Included in most formulations are not only the biologically-active drug ingredient but also inactive ingredients known as vehicles or excipients. These substances include various fillers, binding agents, lubricants, protectants and coatings which may perform a number of functions, the most important of which is the control of the site and rate of dosage form disintegration. A dosage form may be designed to disintegrate in a segment of the digestive tract in which degradation of a particular drug is minimal, thus increasing the amount of drug available for absorption. Through control of the rate of dosage form disintegration, the rate that the drug is ultimately absorbed may be influenced, as well as the subsequent duration and intensity of the drug's biological effect(s).

Drug particles released by disintegration of the dosage form generally must dissolve next in the enteric fluids in order to be absorbed into the blood. Dissolution is influenced by the chemical and physical properties of the drug and the solvent, i.e. the enteric fluids. Important drug characteristics include the salt form, crystalline structure, particle size, pK_a, and both lipid and aqueous solubilites. Drug absorption occurs primarily by passive diffusion of the drug in solution from the aqueous environment of the enteric fluids through the lipid phase of the cell membranes of the digestive tract mucosa. Thus, both the aqueous and lipid solubilities of the drug influence its absorption.

The principle physiological factors which modify the aforementioned processes are gastrointestinal motility, pH, surface area and reactivity, i.e. chemical, enzymatic, and microbiological. Physiological modification of drug absorption will be considered in more detail later.

All of the previously mentioned processes may vary drug bioavailability, i.e. the rate and extent to which the active drug ingredient is absorbed from the formulation and becomes available at the site of drug action[14]. If the rate of drug absorption is slow, then effective blood concentrations of the drug may not be attained, even if the extent of absorption is complete. Conversely, if the fraction of an oral dose of drug absorbed is small then effective blood concentrations may never be realized, regardless of the rapidity of drug absorption. Figure 14.1 illustrates the importance of variable bioavailability

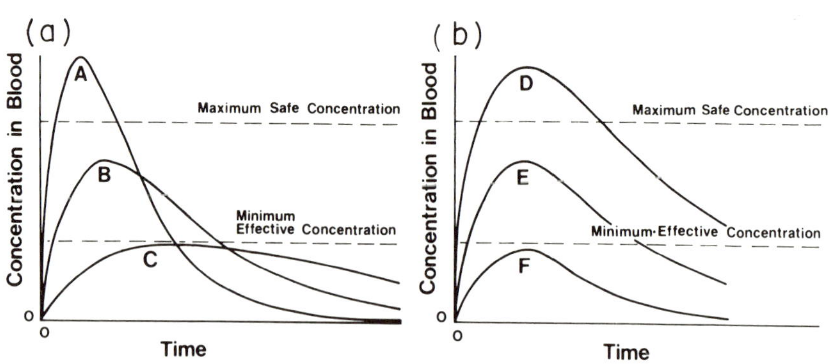

Figure 14.1 (a) Influence of rate of absorption (A > B > C) on blood concentrations from three drug formulations which are absorbed to the same extent. (b) Influence of extent of absorption (D > E > F) on blood concentrations from three drug formulations which are absorbed at the same rate

upon the safety and efficacy of six hypothetical oral drug products which contain identical amounts of the same drug but differ in formulation; physiological effects are assumed to be constant[25]. As shown in Figure 14.1, the maximum safe drug concentration was exceeded by formulations A and D whereas formulations C and F failed to produce effective blood concentrations.

Two methods are commonly used to determine drug bioavailability. These employ the principles that the area under a blood concentration vs. time curve and the amount of drug excreted in urine are both proportional to the amount of drug absorbed. The ratio of the test formulation to the standard formulation of the area under the blood concentration vs. time curves or of the urinary drug recoveries determined, following equivalent doses of each formulation in the same subject, provides an index of the drug's bioavailability. When both the test and standard formulations are administered orally, the relative bioavailability is calculated. Comparison of an orally administered test formulation with the intravenously injected, and therefore completely absorbed, drug provides the absolute bioavailability of, or fraction of the dose absorbed from, the test formulation. The rate of drug absorption from an oral dosage form is represented by the time required to produce the peak blood concentration. Pharmacokinetic analysis of blood drug concentration vs. time data may be used to estimate rate constants for the process(es) involved in the absorption of the drug. Practical application of these concepts is well presented in an article concerning the absorption of sulphamethazine as a solution, fast-release bolus, and sustained-release bolus administered to cattle[3].

RUMINANT GASTROINTESTINAL PHYSIOLOGY AND DRUG ABSORPTION

The uniqueness of the ruminant digestive tract resides in the evolutionary development of a series of three chambers, the rumen, reticulum, and omasum, anterior to the true stomach, the abomasum. This anatomical and physiological evolutionary adaptation allows the ruminant to thrive upon products of the fermentation of cellulose-rich forages by commensalite micro-organisms living within the rumino-reticular fluids. The environment of the anterior ruminant digestive tract is thus very different from that of the monogastric animals. Frequently, this accounts for the often dramatic differences observed between ruminants and monogastrics in the oral absorption of drugs.

The rumino-reticulum is usually the first enteric chamber encountered by an orally administered drug. However, ingested fluids may partially bypass the rumino-reticulum to enter the abomasum via the omasum following closure of the reticular groove, a reflex especially well developed in the nursing ruminant but inconsistently active in the adult. Thus, variable portions of a drug solution administered orally may become divided between the rumino-reticulum and abomasum, resulting in a complex absorption process which may then contribute to unpredictable drug efficacy. Studies conducted with meclofenamic acid[7,26] and febendazole[24,27], administered orally or directly into the rumen or abomasum, have contributed a great deal to an appreciation of the significance of reflex closure of the reticular groove as a factor influencing drug absorption and efficacy.

The rumino-reticulum is not fully developed in the immature ruminant in either relative volume or microbial activity. Since dilution of a drug in the large fluid volume of the functional rumen and drug degradation by rumen microflora both lead to decreased efficiency of drug absorption, it follows that some drugs administered orally to ruminants would show dramatic changes in both rate and extent of absorption between the time of birth and the maturation of rumen function at 2–3 months of age. An appreciation of the importance of this phenomena in regard to the absorption of drugs by ruminants of various ages and the research conducted to elucidate the mechanisms involved is best obtained by reviewing the excellent series of papers investigating the fate of chloramphenicol administered orally to ruminants[9–13,37,39].

The functionally mature rumino-reticulum is essentially a fermentation vat, the contents of which are bathed in copious alkaline saliva which acts to buffer the acidic byproducts of microbial metabolism and maintain a slightly acidic pH of 5.5–6.5 within the broth[15]. The contents are relatively poorly stirred by rhythmic contractions of the rumino-reticular musculature, which results in stratification of the ingesta with the less dense material in the upper layers in the rumen and the heavier material in the lower layers and in the reticulum. Periodically, small amounts of ingesta are regurgitated for further mastication which results in a reduction in forage fibre size and a more thorough mixing with saliva. The rate at which the ingesta flows into the next enteric chamber, the omasum, is governed by fibre size and density with the more rapid transit times exhibited by small, lighter fibres. The flow rate of polyethylene glycol, a water soluble marker, from the rumino-reticulum to the omasum in adult sheep[35] is about 380–460 ml/h. If one assumes a rumen volume of 4 l, this corresponds to a fractional rate of emptying halflife of 7 h. The rumino-reticular retention of particles is longer. Particles with a density of 1.2 g/cm^3 and a volume of 20–30 ml exhibited the shortest retention time in the cow[35]. More details concerning these and other aspects of ruminant physiology may be found in the texts by Church[6] and by Ruckebusch and Thivend[36].

The rumino-reticular environment does not favour drug absorption, although drugs of sufficient lipid solubility do traverse the stratified squamous epithelium of the mucosa by passive, non-ionic diffusion[1,8,15,22,23,38]. As mentioned previously, the large fluid volume of the chamber causes dilution of the drug, thus lowering the concentration gradient between the rumen liquor and blood, which weakens the driving force for drug diffusion. The drug may bind to the ingested forage or be destroyed by rumen microbes[34], thereby further lowering its concentration. The slow mixing of the ingesta may prolong the disintegration of a solid dosage form and thus retard the rate at which the solubilized drug fraction comes into contact with the absorptive surface of the ruminal mucosa. Finally, if the pH within the rumino-reticulum is not conducive to non-ionic diffusion of the drug, the rate of flow to a more favourable pH in the lower digestive tract may further slow the rate of drug absorption.

The influence of the rate of rumino-reticular flow on drug absorption has been impressively demonstrated by the oral administration of sulphamethazine to sheep in the presence and absence of an intravenous infusion of atropine[4]. Atropinic inhibition of rumino-reticular motility and, thus, of flow to the more favourable sites for sulphamethazine absorption in the abomasum and small intestine, resulted in peak sulphamethazine blood concentrations of only one quarter of those observed in the control animals. Therapeutic blood concentrations of sulphamethazine (greater than 5 mg/100 ml) were maintained for 30 h in the control animals by a single oral dose of sulphamethazine at 214 mg/kg but were never attained by the animals which had also received atropine.

The limited capacity of the omasum results in a short retention time for material passing from the rumino-reticulum to the abomasum. The omasum appears to further reduce particulate size of the ingesta and to expel fluid from the ingesta by compression within its leaf-like mucosal folds. The pH of the omasum is slightly more acidic than that of the rumino-reticulum. The stratified squamous epithelium of the omasal mucosa readily absorbs water, small ions and nutrients[5], but no information is available concerning the absorption of drugs.

The abomasum or true stomach secretes a solution of pepsin and hydrochloric acid of pH 1.0–1.3, which results in a pH of 2–3 within the abomasal contents[29]. Digestion and absorption of some nutrients occurs within the abomasum. Unlike the monogastric animals, onward flow to the small intestine is relatively continuous. Maximal flow occurs during food intake then decreases soon after feeding to gradually increase to maximum again at the time of the subsequent feeding. Although continuous over the long-term, flow from the abomasum into the duodenum actually occurs in gushes of 30–40 ml in sheep with an average flow[29] of 400 ml/h. If one assumes an average fluid volume of 400 ml for the abomasum, this flow rate corresponds to an emptying halflife of 0.7 h.

A number of studies have indicated good absorption of drugs introduced directly into the abomasum. Quite likely, this represents drug absorption from both the abomasum and small intestine, considering the rapid rate of abomasal emptying. Many of these studies were conducted with the primary intention of investigating either the role of reticular groove closure in directing some fraction of an orally administered drug solution past the rumen to the abomasum, as with meclofenamic acid[7,26], or the degradative effect of rumen microflora on drugs such as chloramphenicol[10,11,13,39].

Large volumes of digesta can be transported by the small intestine. Duodenal flow tends to be variable but continuous while that of the ileum is intermittent. In adult sheep, duodenal flow rate varies from about 200 to 800 ml/h depending upon the nature of the diet and frequency of feeding[6]. Flow rate then decreases progressively with distance aborally from the pylorus as fluid is absorbed from the digesta. Particulate matter is transported from the pylorus to the large intestine in 2–4.5 h.

The pH of the intestinal contents increases gradually from about 2.7 at the pylorus to 7.5 in the ileum[6]. Alkalinization of the acidic digesta from the abomasum is achieved by both pancreatic and intestinal secretions.

It is anticipated that drug absorption from the abomasum and small intestine of ruminants would be similar to that observed in monogastric animals. The acidic environment of the stomach favours the absorption of drugs which are weak acids. The nearly neutral pH of the intestine favours the absorption of weakly basic drugs, while its tremendous surface area is conducive to the absorption of all drugs of sufficient lipid solubility.

PHYSIOLOGICAL-COMPARTMENTAL PHARMACOKINETIC MODEL OF RUMINANT DRUG ABSORPTION

The various types of pharmacokinetic models (empirical, compartmental and physiological) as well as their relative advantages and disadvantages have recently been reviewed[40]. Such models have been used to describe the pharmacokinetics of orally administered drugs and gastrointestinal flow indicator substances in ruminants. Currently, a promising approach to the pharmacokinetic analysis of drugs administered orally to ruminants utilizes a combination of the physiological (gastrointestinal flow) and compartmental (drug disposition) models.

The conceptual basis for a physiological-compartmental pharmacokinetic model to study the absorption of drugs administered orally to ruminants has been presented previously[17]. Expansion of these concepts and inclusion of average gastrointestinal pH values[32] resulted in the model shown in Figure 14.2(a).

In this model, the flow of the liquid phase of the digesta and thus of an orally administered drug in aqueous solution is determined with an indigestible, unabsorbed marker such as chromium ethylenediamine tetra-acetic acid (Cr-EDTA)[16, 18] or polyethylene glycol[19–21]. The drug and marker may be administered orally or into specific enteric compartments by means of surgically introduced fistulae. Samples of digesta obtained from these fistulae allow the determination of regional pH and drug and marker concentrations as a function of time. Pharmacokinetic analysis of these concentration data then provides values for compartmental volumes and for rate constants describing the disappearance of drug from the enteric compartments by absorption (k_a), destruction (k_d), or flow to the next region (k_r, k_o, k_{ab}, k_e). Diffusion of the drug into the digestive tract from the blood (central compartment) is studied by administering the drug intravenously and then measuring its concentrations in both blood and digesta. Greater complexity is added to the model if the drug is subject to first-pass metabolism or biliary recycling.

A number of these concepts have recently been applied in a study of the pharmacokinetics of fenbendazole and thiabendazole administered intraruminally to cattle simultaneously with Cr-EDTA to measure digesta flow rates[33]. Models such as this are especially useful when gastrointestinal flow is a critical determinant of drug efficacy as is the case with the benzimidazole anthelmintics. In the future, similar models may predict the effect of

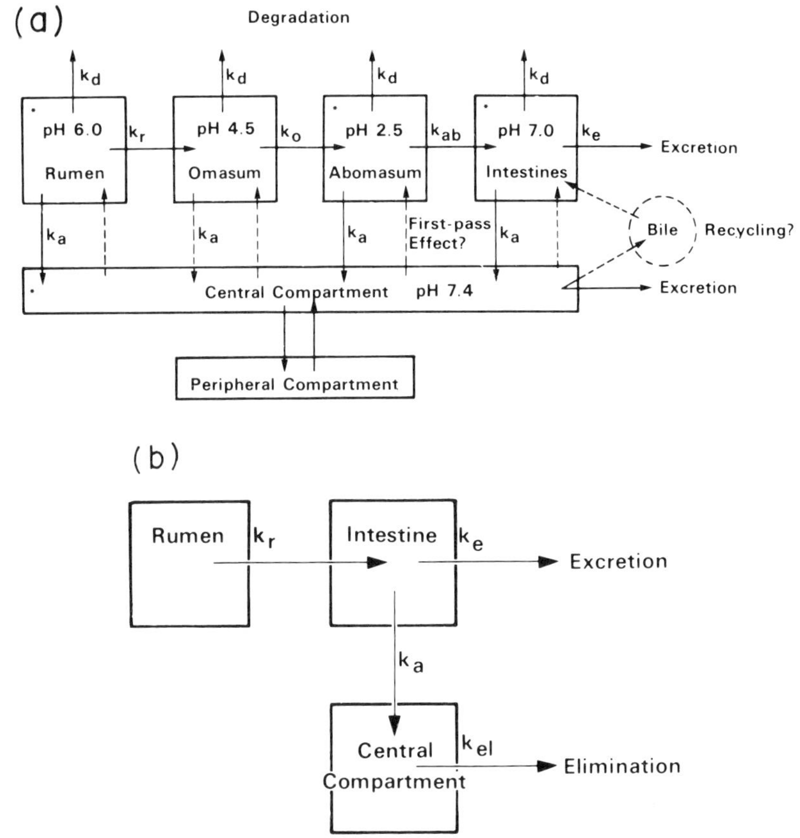

Figure 14.2 (a) Physiological-compartmental pharmacokinetic model of ruminant drug absorption. (b) Simplified model of ruminant drug absorption

decreased gastrointestinal motility (as occurs with fever in the ruminant[41] on dosage form dissolution and subsequent drug absorption.

Depending upon the characteristics of the drug and the purposes for which the pharmacokinetic model is intended, some of the rate constants (depicted by dashed lines) and compartments in Figure 14.2 may not be required. In pharmacokinetic analysis, it is generally accepted that the simplest model which adequately explains the data is the 'best' model. For instance, if it is established that (1) ruminal emptying rate is monoexponential and slower than that of the omasum and abomasum, (2) drug degradation does not occur within the gastrointestinal tract, (3) drug absorption occurs only within the intestine, (4) drug diffusion from plasma to enteric fluids is negligible, (5) first-pass metabolism and biliary recycling of drug do not occur, and (6) drug disappearance following intravenous administration is monoexponential, then the model in Figure 14.2(a) may be simplified to that in Figure 14.2(b).

In this model, flow from the rumen (k_r) to the intestine is determined by intraruminal administration of an unabsorbable marker compound followed by pharmacokinetic analysis of the compound's rate of disappearance from the rumen. The absorption and elimination rate constants (k_a and k_{el}, respectively) are derived from analysis of drug concentrations in the central compartment (blood). Unabsorbed drug is excreted in the faeces (k_e) and absorbed drug is eliminated from the central compartment by metabolism and excretion. The total of the amounts of unchanged drug and its metabolites recovered from the excreta should be equal to the dose administered.

A study recently completed by myself but not yet subjected to pharmacokinetic analysis, illustrates many of these concepts. Six mature non-pregnant ewes were administered single doses of prednisolone on separate days by different routes. Prednisolone succinate was given intravenously at 0.64 mg/kg and into the duodenum via a surgically implanted 0.2 mm diameter cannula at 2.56 mg/kg (equivalent to 0.5 and 2.0 mg/kg, respectively, as prednisolone); an aqueous suspension of finely ground tablets of prednisolone was administered into both the fistulated rumen and abomasum at 2.0 mg/kg.

The results of these experiments are summarized in Figure 14.3 (a). By comparison of the areas (corrected for dosage) under the plasma drug concentration curves of the enteral doses to the intravenous dose, the absolute bioavailability of prednisolone administered into the rumen, abomasum and duodenum was estimated to be 5%, 21% and 20%, respectively. Apparently, prednisolone was extensively metabolized and/or sequestered in the rumen and to a lesser extent in the abomasum and small intestine. Metabolic degradation of the drug by the liver (first-pass effect) may have occurred as well.

The influence of digesta flow rates from one gastrointestinal compartment to the next is clearly demonstrated in Figure 14.3 (b). In the rumen, prednisolone is diluted by the large fluid volume, probably degraded in or bound to the ingesta and allowed to flow only slowly toward the more favourable site of drug absorption in the small intestine. The role of rumen flow rate in controlling the intestinal absorption of prednisolone and its subsequent elimination (i.e. 'flip-flop' model) is supported by the flow of polyethylene glycol from the rumen which parallels prednisolone disappearance from plasma. The net result of these effects was that the administration of prednisolone into the rumen at 2.0 mg/kg resulted in low drug plasma concentrations with a broad peak of about 15 ng/ml betwen 1.5 and 3 h.

Following the abomasal administration of prednisolone at 2.0 mg/kg, an abrupt peak plasma concentration of 151 ng/ml was observed at 1.0 h (Figure 14.4 (a)), while duodenal administration of an equivalent dosage of prednisolone succinate resulted in an even sharper and earlier peak of 318 ng/ml at 15 min. Since the bioavailability of prednisolone was essentially the same by either the abomasal or duodenal route and since the peak plasma concentration following abomasal administration was later and lower than that following duodenal administration, this suggests that the small intestine was the most efficient site for prednisolone absorption. The role of abomasal emptying in presenting prednisolone to the small intestine for absorption is supported by Figure 14.4 (b). The flow from the abomasum, as indicated by the abrupt decline in polyethylene glycol concentrations, occurred with such rapidity as to quickly present a large fraction of the abomasal dose of

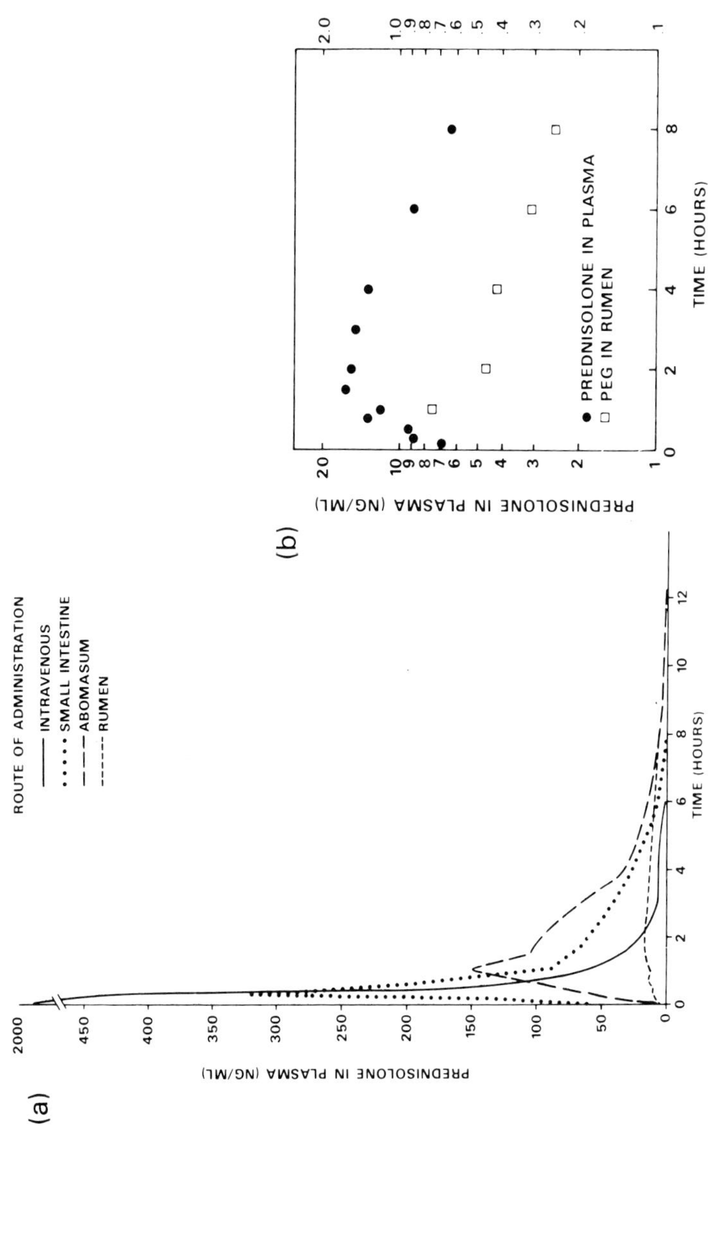

Figure 14.3 (a) Mean plasma concentrations of prednisolone in six sheep following the intravenous and duodenal administration of prednisolone succinate at 0.64 and 2.56 mg/kg, respectively (equivalent to 0.5 and 2.0 mg/kg as prednisolone) and the ruminal and abomasal administration of prednisolone at 2.0 mg/kg. (b) Semilogarithmic plot of mean plasma concentrations of prednisolone in six sheep following the ruminal administration of prednisolone at 2.0 mg/kg and of mean ruminal concentrations of 0.2 g/kg polyethylene glycol (PEG)

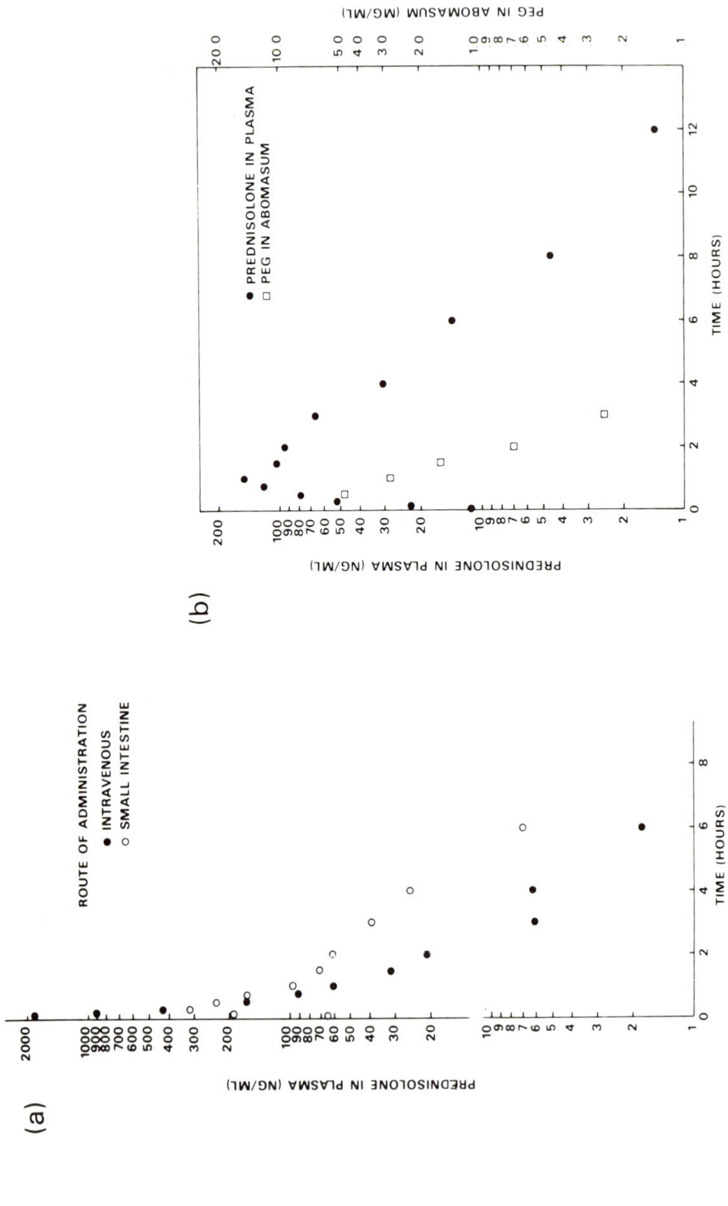

Figure 14.4 (a) Semilogarithmic plot of mean plasma concentrations of prednisolone in six sheep following the intravenous and duodenal administration of prednisolone succinate at 0.64 mg/kg and 2.56 mg/kg, respectively (equivalent to 0.5 and 2.0 mg/kg as prednisolone). (b) Mean plasma concentrations of prednisolone in six sheep following the abomasal administration of prednisolone at 2.0 mg/kg and of mean abomasal concentrations of polyethyleneglycol (PEG) following its simultaneous administration at 0.1 g/kg

prednisolone to the small intestine where its subsequent rapid absorption occurred. In fact, intestinal absorption of prednisolone was so rapid following duodenal administration that a drug distribution phase is discernable in the plasma data and the drug elimination phase parallels that of the intravenous dose.

Pharmacokinetic analysis of the data represented by Figures 14.3 and 14.4 will probably result in a physiological compartmental model of complexity intermediate to the models in Figures 14.2 and 14.3. The rather low bioavailability of prednisolone from all segments of the digestive tract suggests that this drug is a poor candidate for the design of a special oral dosage formulation for use in ruminants.

ORAL DOSAGE FORMS DESIGNED FOR RUMINANTS

Because the rumen functions as a large reservoir anterior to the abomasum and small intestine which are the more important sites for drug absorption, several possibilities exist for the manufacture of special oral dosage forms for use in ruminants[31]. Formulations which provide prolonged release of drug, either from boluses or pellets of zero buoyancy or from devices which lodge temporarily in the rumen, are suitable for drugs which are resistant to or intended to act upon the ruminal microflora and for which persistent drug concentrations are desirable[32]. Cobalt boluses for the prevention of cobalt deficiency and sulphonamide boluses for the treatment of bovine bacterial pneumonia are two examples of such products. On the other hand, it may be desirable to prevent release of the drug in the rumen to avoid drug degradation by the microflora as with chloramphenicol[32, 34] or, alternatively, to prevent deleterious effects on the microflora by the drug as with the penicillins and sulphonamides[28, 34]. Various dosage form coatings have been developed which can protect a drug from microbial degradation in the rumen and subsequently release the drug in either the abomasum or small intestine[30, 32]. Further discussion of the objectives and design of oral drug formulations for the provision of optimized drug delivery may be found in a recent review[2].

CONCLUSIONS

Adequate comprehension of the fate of drugs administered orally to ruminants requires that both physiological and pharmacokinetic factors be considered. Appropriately designed studies can provide drug concentrations in plasma and enteric fluids as well as ingesta flow rates from one enteric region to another. Physiological compartmental modelling of these data should then provide for an improved understanding of ruminant drug absorption and give insight to the means to improve the absorption of some drugs through the design and administration of special oral dosage forms.

References

1. Austin, F. H. (1967). Absorption, distribution and excretion of sulfonamides in ruminants. *Fed. Proc.*, **26**, 1001–5
2. Banker, G. S. and Sharma, V. E. (1981). Advances in controlled gastrointestinal absorption. In *Drug Absorption*. Chap. 19, pp. 194–204. (Lancaster: MTP Press)
3. Bevill, R. F., Dittert, L. W. and Bourne, D. W. A. (1977). Disposition of sulfonamides in food-producing animals. IV. Pharmacokinetics of sulfamethazine in cattle following administration of an intravenous dose and three oral dosage forms. *J. Pharm. Sci.*, **66**, 619–23
4. Bischop, C. R., Janzen, R. E., Landals, D. C. *et al.* (1973). Effect of rumen stasis on sulfamethazine blood levels after oral administration in sheep. *Can. Vet. J.*, **14**, 269–71
5. Buéno, L. (1975). Les fonctions motrices et digestives du feuillet. *Thèse Sci.*, Université Paul Sabatier, Toulouse. pp. 1–206
6. Church, D. C. (1975). *Digestive Physiology and Nutrition of Ruminants*. Vol. 1, 2nd edn., pp. 1–350. (Corvallis, Oregon: O & B Books)
7. Cooke, R. G. and Nicholson, T. (1981). The reticular groove and drug absorption. *J. Vet. Pharmacol. Ther.*, **4**, 311–3
8. Davis, L. E. and Jenkins, W. L. (1974). Some considerations regarding drug therapy in ruminant animals. *Bov. Pract.*, **9**, 57–80
9. Davis, L. E., Neff, C. A., Baggot, J. D. *et al.* (1972). Pharmacokinetics of chloramphenicol in domesticated animals. *Am. J. Vet. Res.*, **33**, 2259–66
10. DeBacker, P. and Debackere, M. (1979). Comparative study of chloramphenicol absorption after oral, intraruminal and intra-abomasal administration. *J. Vet. Pharmacol. Ther.*, **2**, 195–202
11. DeBacker, P., Debackere, M. and DeCorte-Baeten, K. (1978). Plasma levels of chloramphenicol after oral administration in calves during the first weeks of life. *J. Vet. Pharmacol. Ther.*, **1**, 135–40
12. DeCorte-Baeten, K. and Debackere, M. (1975). Chloramphenicol plasma levels in horses, cattle and sheep after oral and intramuscular administration. *Zbl. Vet. Med. A*, **22**, 704–12
13. DeCorte-Baeten, K. and Debackere, M. (1978). The nonabsorption of chloramphenicol after oral administration in adult ruminants: a tentative explanation from *in vitro* studies. *J. Vet. Pharmacol. Ther.*, **1**, 129–34
14. Dittert, L. W. and DiSanto, A. R. (1978). The bioavailability of drug products, a background review for the practitioner. In *The Bioavailability of Drug Products*. pp. 9–20. (Washington, DC: Am. Pharm. Assoc.)
15. Dobson, A. (1967). Physiological peculiarities of the ruminant relevant to drug distribution. *Fed. Proc.*, **26**, 994–1000
16. Downes, A. M. and McDonald, I. W. (1964). The chromium-51 complex of ethylenediamine tetra-acetic acid as a soluble rumen marker. *Br. J. Nutr.*, **18**, 153–62
17. Dresback, D. S. (1978). Ruminant g.i. dynamics: effect on pharmacokinetics of oral dosage forms. In Monkhouse, D. C. (ed.) *Animal Health Products: Design and Evaluation*. Chap. 3, pp. 22–31. (Washington, DC: Am. Pharm. Assoc., Acad. Pharm. Sci.)
18. Faichney, G. J. (1975). The use of markers to partition digestion within the gastrointestinal tract of ruminants. In McDonald, I. W. and Warner, A. C. I. (eds.) *Digestion and Metabolism in the Ruminants*. pp. 227–91. (Armidale: University of New England Publishing Unit)
19. Hyden, S. (1955). A turbidimetric method for the determination of higher polyethylene glycols in biological materials. *Kungl. Lant. Ann.*, **22**, 139–45
20. Hyden, S. (1956). The recovery of polyethylene glycol after passage through the digestive tract. *Kungl. Lant. Ann.*, **22**, 410–24
21. Hyden, S. (1961). Determination of the amount of fluid in the reticulorumen of the sheep and its rate of passage to the omasum. *Kungl. Lant. Ann.*, **27**, 51–79.
22. Jenkins, W. L. and Davis, L. E. (1975). A method for the *in vitro* study of drug transfer across ruminal epithelium. *J. S. Afr. Vet. Assoc.*, **46**, 153–60
23. Jenkins, W. L., Davis, L. E. and Boulos, B. M. (1975). Transfer of drugs across the ruminal wall in goats. *Am. J. Vet. Res.*, **36**, 1771–76

24. Kelly, J. D., Hall, C. A., Whitlock, H. V. *et al.* (1977). The effect of route of administration on the anthelmintic efficacy of benzamidazole anthelmintics in sheep infected with strains of *Haemonchus contortus* and *Trichostrongylus colubriformis* resistant or susceptible to thiabendazole. *Res. Vet. Sci.*, **22**, 161–8
25. Koritz, G. D. (1980). Bioequivalence of drug products. *J. Am. Vet. Med. Assoc.*, **177**, 279–81
26. Marriner, S. and Bogan, J. A. (1979). The influence of the rumen on the absorption of drugs: studies using meclofenamic acid administered by various routes to sheep and cattle. *J. Vet. Pharmacol. Ther.*, **2**, 109–15
27. McEwan, A. D. and Oakley, G. A. (1978). Anthelmintics and closure of the oesophageal groove in cattle. *Vet. Rec.*, **102**, 314–5
28. O'Connor, J. J., Myers, G. S., Jr., Maplesden, D. C. *et al.* (1970). Chemical additives in rumen fermentations: *in vitro* effects of various drugs on rumen volatile fatty acids and protozoa. *J. Anim. Sci.*, **30**, 812–8
29. Phillipson, A. T. (1975). Ruminant digestion. In Swenson, M. J. (ed.) *Duke's Physiology of Domestic Animals.* 8th Edn., pp. 424–81. (Ithaca, NY: Cornell University Press)
30. Phillipson, A. T. (1972). The protection of dietary compounds from rumen fermentations. *Proc. Nutr. Soc.*, **31**, 159–64
31. Pope, D. G. (1978). Animal health specialized delivery systems. In Monkhouse, D. C. (ed.) *Animal Health Products: Design and Evaluation.* Chap. 6, pp. 78–114. (Washington, DC: Am. Pharm. Assoc., Acad. Pharm. Sci.)
32. Pope, D. G. (1975). Factors to be considered in the formulation of pharmaceuticals for oral administration to ruminant animals. *Aust. J. Pharm. Sci.*, **NS4**, 65–78
33. Prichard, R. K., Steel, J. W. and Hennessy, D. R. (1978). Fenbendazole and thiabendazole in cattle: partition of gastrointestinal absorption and pharmacokinetic behavior. *J. Vet. Pharmacol. Ther.*, **4**, 295–304
34. Prins, R. A. (1978). Nutritional impact of intestinal drug–microbe interactions. In Hathcock, J. N. (ed.) *Nutrition and Drug Interrelations.* Chap. 7, pp. 189–251. (New York: Academic Press)
35. Ruckebusch, Y., Buéno, L. and Fioramonti, J. (1981). *La Mécanique Digestive chez les Mammifères.* Institut National de la Recherche Agronomique, Masson, Paris, 63
36. Ruckebusch, Y. and Thivend, P. (eds.) (1980). *Digestive Physiology and Metabolism in Ruminants.* pp. 1–798. (Lancaster: MTP Press)
37. Sisodia, C. S., Dunlop, R. H., Gupta, V. S. *et al.* (1973). A pharmacologic study of chloramphenicol in cattle. *Am. J. Vet. Res.*, **34**, 1147–51
38. Stowe, C. M. (1967). Comparative therapeutics in large domestic animals. *Fed. Proc.*, **26**, 1244–6
39. Theodorides, V. J., DiCuollo, C. J., Guarini, J. R. *et al.* (1968). Serum concentrations of chloramphenicol after intraruminal and intra-abomasal administration in sheep. *Am. J. Vet. Res.*, **29**, 643–5
40. Tucker, G. T. (1981). Emperical vs. compartmental vs. physiological models. In Breimer, D. D. and Speiser, P. (eds.) *Topics in Pharmaceutical Sciences.* pp. 33–48. (Amsterdam: Elsevier/North-Holland Biomedical Press)
41. Van Miert, A. S. J. P. A. M. (1980). Fever and gastric function. In Lipton, J. M. (ed.) *Fever.* pp. 57–70. (New York: Raven Press)

15
Ruminal influences on drug action

R. H. Dunlop

Oral administration of drugs to ruminant animals has had a chequered history. It might be summed up as having involved a lot of speculative uncontrolled clinical use and little science. As a result, there has been little evidence of efficacy, a substantial incidence of iatrogenic disease added as a tax on any pre-existing ailments, and a considerable amount of ineffectual waste. Consequently, it is a thankless task to review the current status of the pharmacology of drugs entering the rumen. It is more important to focus on the nature of the biological systems that interact with chemicals introduced to the rumen so that some relevant principles can be identified. Above all, it is necessary to stress the urgency of the need for more sophisticated pharmacological research in diseased animals followed by properly designed clinical trials on drugs for oral use in ruminants.

There are two sides to the coin of drug administration into the rumen: one is the effect of the forestomachs on the drug and its bioavailability, the other is the effect of the drug on the various facets of these complex components of the ruminant 'ecosystem'. A further complication that must be addressed is the impact of disease states on the subtleties of these functions. The failure of the veterinary profession to identify the need for quantitative clinical pharmacology long ago is one of the mysteries of professional evolution. While great contributions were being made to the study of anatomical, pathological, physiological, microbiological and parasitological science and to clinical diagnosis, the discipline of clinical pharmacology or scientific therapeutics failed to develop. Thus veterinary science failed to keep pace with the industrial production of new products utilizing the great progress in organic and synthetic chemistry. The new discipline, long overdue, is slowly emerging at last and this Congress is a healthy sign of the change. It is no consolation that our sister profession, that restricts its concerns to a single species, has been similarly delinquent about clinical pharmacology until recently.

Another area where inadequate attention has been paid to pathophysiological changes and scientific evaluation is the art of formulation which aims to dispense the drug or drugs into a dosage form that is convenient to administer and effective in meeting pharmacokinetic criteria while avoiding side-effects such as toxicity or local irritation. Nevertheless, a great deal of ingenuity has been applied to formulation manipulation during the last decade to achieve protection from degradation or graded release of a drug. This field, largely in the domain of industrial research and development, has been reviewed[45]. More recent developments have been largely in the field of sustained release of anthelmintics[5], sulfonamides[45], bloat preventatives[33] or nutrients[44].

THE RETICULO-RUMEN (RR) SYSTEM

For absorption of a drug into the bloodstream to occur from any site of its introduction into the body, a concentration gradient must exist for the drug between that site and the local extracellular fluid. Also, it must be able to penetrate any structural barriers in between.

An immediate problem confronting a drug administered orally to a ruminant for systemic effect is the very large volume of the contents of the reticulo-rumen as a proportion of total body weight. It cannot, therefore, avoid being 'disguised by dilution'[15].

In addition, the relatively slow and inefficient system of mixing the rumen contents by the co-ordinated motility of the RR causes delays in attaining uniform concentrations of a drug throughout the multiphasic ingesta. Sampling errors are unavoidable during the first hour or so after administration. Any subsequent additions of feed, water or saliva compound the problem while the intermittent outflow of aliquots of the liquid ingesta to the omasum further complicates the system. When the effects of the periodic processes of regurgitation and eructation are allowed for as well, it becomes understandable that those working on ruminant pharmacokinetics have preferred to avoid the mathematical modelling of the influence of the RR system. It is, in fact, a theoretician's nightmare.

Some of the features of the RR system as they pertain to the study of drugs introduced to it are illustrated in Figure 15.1. Although this system is familiar to the physiologist, its complexity is alarming to the pharmacologist since the figure is a gross over-simplification. It does not indicate the diversity of metabolic processes that occur in the microbial inhabitants. It does not even illustrate gross differences among these organisms such as protozoa, bacteria and fungi, let alone the wide range of species represented in each of these classes. Similarly, it does not indicate the complex neural and humoral systems that regulate and co-ordinate the functions of the overall system. It gives no indication of diurnal variations related to food intake or rumination or of changes related to dietary alterations, starvation, stress, disease or drug administration. However, it should be emphasized that the well-being of a ruminant animal derives in the first instance from the function to which the majority of its activity is committed, namely the filling and processing of the forestomach contents. Any proposed formulation of drugs to be administered into this system must be assessed with an evaluation of the possibility of a detrimental effect on its function.

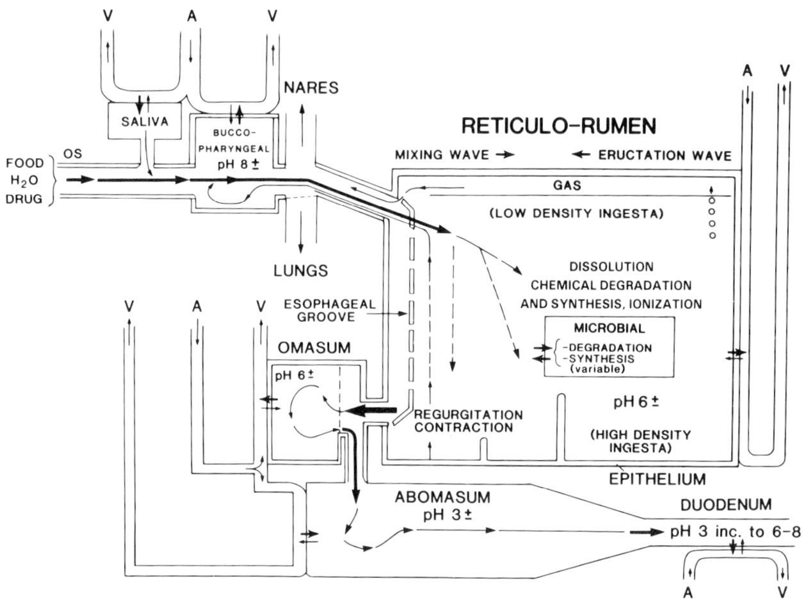

Figure 15.1 Diagram representing the main features of the reticulo-rumen system that may influence bioavailability of a drug

THE FATE OF DRUGS INTRODUCED TO THE RR

Distribution of drug following administration

Drugs can be administered to the rumen in liquid form, such as solutions or suspensions, as additions to the feed or water, or in solid form as tablets, boluses, capsules or specialized delivery devices. Each of these dosage forms leads to different sites of arrival in the rumen and variable distribution patterns result.

It has been pointed out that liquids containing drugs arrive in greater concentration in the reticulum and adjacent areas[43]. Consequently, a disproportionate amount may pass through the reticulo-omasal orifice before mixing can occur. This allows part of the dose to escape ruminal degradation and to present early for intestinal absorption. This process can be maximized if the oesophageal groove can be induced to close prior to drug swallowing, as occurs with milk bypassing the rumen in the sucking calf. Pretreatment with atropine can be used to increase the chance of deposition of a dense bolus, magnet or sustained-release device onto the floor of the reticulum.

Dissolution of drugs given in solid form

During a study in normal cows fitted with a rumen fistula[3] potential ruminatoric drugs were identified. Among them, tartar emetic (antimony potassium tartrate) was reported to be an effective stimulant of both the frequency and amplitude of reticulo-rumen contractions. This information was extrapolated by some pharmaceutical companies to yield the assumption that a bolus of tartar emetic would be effective as a stimulant to restore motility in a static or sluggish rumen. It appears that they proceeded to the formulation and marketing stage without further research or clinical trials. For convenience of administration, some of the companies utilized a compacted bolus form that could be readily given by a balling gun.

The author happened to observe the consequences of administering a single bolus containing 45% of tartar emetic (20 g) to a fistulated cow that had been engorged on grain 4 days previously. The reticulo-rumen was completely static. The day after the bolus was given, the atony persisted. Manual examination via the fistula detected the bolus on the floor of the anterior dorsal sac. A circumscribed lesion several inches in diameter was palpated in the wall of the rumen beneath and around the bolus. Despite attempts to treat the animal, it died in a few days. The necropsy revealed necrosis and severe inflammation with thrombosis of the wall. This finding led to a research study[50] that showed that tartar emetic in bolus form caused phlegmonous gastritis in four out of four calves whose reticulo-rumen had been rendered static by prior starvation (36 h) and dosing with atropine sulphate intramuscularly. The stasis was maintained for 6 h by additional doses of atropine as required. Two calves treated identically except for the omission of atropine sustained their rumen motility and suffered no apparent ill-effects. Lesions similar to those seen in the engorgement case and other retrospective cases were observed in the ventral area of either the reticulum or the anterior dorsal sac of the rumen depending upon where the bolus had lodged.

The iatrogenic implications are obvious. Tartar emetic is soluble in water about 1:12 and is extremely irritating to tissues. It is interesting to note that Amadon's original report[3] indicated that tartar emetic depressed the frequency of RR motility when applied directly to the surface of the epithelium. It was shown that the ruminatoric effect involved a lag time of about 90 min after oral administration as a drench because it required delivery of the drug to the abomasum leading to reflex stimulation of RR motility. Toxic signs were described. Generous dilution of a dose of 90–150 grains was recommended to 'reduce the degree of irritation within the reticulum and facilitate passage of the drug solution into the abomasum'. Alas, this sound advice went unheeded.

Evaluation of local irritation in the static reticulo-rumen should be carried out for every product administered in solid form. If normal mixing contractions are present, irritation is unlikely to occur. Controlled rates of release are often desired and great strides have been made in this area recently. Drugs and trace nutrients formulated in prolonged-release boluses or pellets have been made utilizing a variety of materials and techniques[45]. The goal of sustained bioavailability over a desired time period requires developmental research. More complex hinged devices have been developed that spring open to prevent regurgitation after a sealing adhesive has been dissolved or digested. These have been used to attain chronic delivery of surfactants to effect control of foaming as a means to preventing bloat[33] but the technique can be applied to other drugs such as anthelmintics[5].

Absorption of drugs from the RR

After the issue of whether or not absorption of the volatile fatty acids (VFA) did occur through the lining skin of the rumen had been settled, definitive experiments were performed to explain the relationship between rate of absorption and physical chemical factors[14]. The latter included ionization as a function of pH, molecular size and concentration gradients. This elegant work set the stage for modern theories of absorption from the gastrointestinal tract that are applicable to most nutrients and drugs[21]. It demonstrated that acetic, propionic and butyric acids are absorbed rapidly from the closed RR in the unionized acidic form and more slowly in the ionized form accompanied by a cation. The sodium salts are absorbed at rates in inverse relationship to their molecular size. In all cases absorption of VFA occurred down a concentration gradient for the molecular species.

Study of the absorption of drugs from the rumen has not attracted a large following. The difficulty of maintaining physiological conditions in such a complex organ, while avoiding errors due to inflow or outflow of material via the cardia or the reticulo-omasal orifice, has plagued this field of experimentation. This problem was addressed by inserting balloons into these two orifices in goats, supplemented by a suction catheter in the oesophagus to safeguard against salivary contamination[28]. Rapid continuous mixing was achieved by a peristaltic pump and extracorporeal plastic tubing. Bidirectional transfer of drugs across the rumen wall using this system was reported later[29]. The data on absorption indicated that the rate of absorption from the rumen was dependent on the concentration of the unionized form of the compound; this in turn was dependent upon the concentration and pK_a of the drug and upon the pH of the medium in the rumen. Direct evidence for the absorption of the ionized forms was not obtained in this study. When the same drugs were infused intravenously at a rate designed to sustain a steady state concentration in the plasma, transfer into the rumen liquid could be measured. Using several different pH values in the rumen so that the possibility of ion-trapping could be evaluated, clear evidence was obtained to support this concept. Both pentobarbital and salicylate (weak acids) concentrations in the rumen rose to exceed plasma levels when the rumen pH was higher than that of the plasma, while an even more marked relative increase occurred with the weak base, quinine, when the rumen contents were more acidic than plasma. The principles underlying the partitioning of acidic and basic drugs between plasma and rumen contents or saliva have been illustrated[16].

An alternative system for studying absorption from the rumen of the cow was developed[17]. It involved the insertion of a small tyre inner tube under the cranial and caudal pillars to isolate the ventral sac of the rumen for absorption trials[20]. This model was used to study the absorption and exchange of water across the epithelium with tritiated water as a marker. It was found that water transfer was greater when the rumen contents were either hypotonic or hypertonic (Figure 15.2). Very large changes in mucosal bloodflow occurred with large departures from isotonicity in the rumen. Further studies[18] indicated that solute absorption changed dramatically

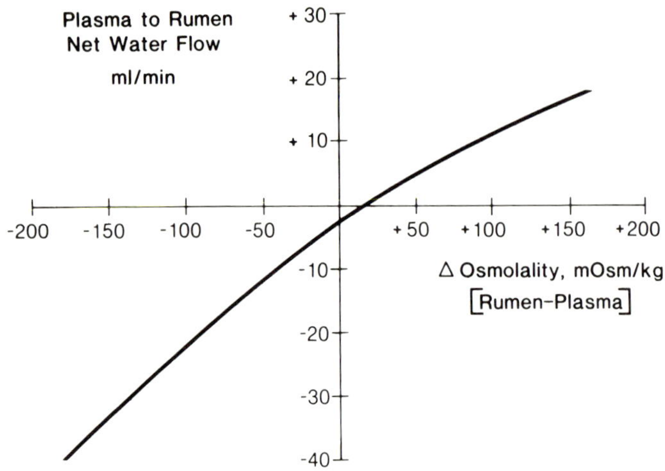

Figure 15.2 Bidirectional movement of water as a function of the osmolality of bovine rumen contents. Redrawn from ref. 18

when the rumen contents were over 30–40 mmol/kg hypertonic to plasma. Even chromium ethylenediamene tetra-acetic acid (Cr-EDTA) became absorbable under these conditions (Figure 15.3). It was suggested that the increased permeability might be attributable to opening of the tight junctions existing between the epithelial cells of the outer layer beneath the desquamating cells[49].

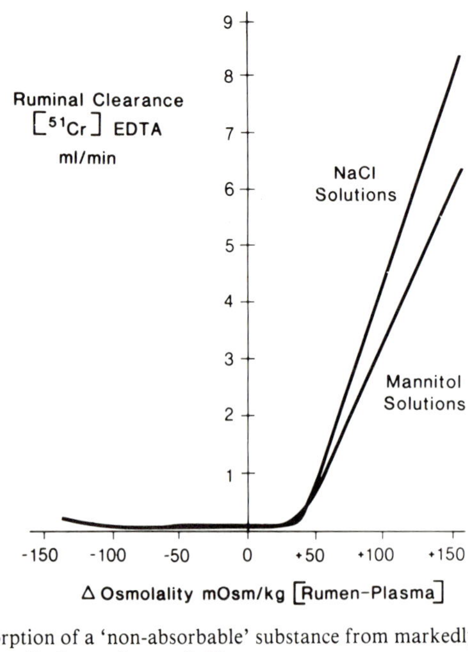

Figure 15.3 Absorption of a 'non-absorbable' substance from markedly hypertonic solutions in the bovine rumen. Redrawn from ref. 17

It is not clear whether or not this phenomenon is of significance in practical drug usage, but it should be tested because hypertonic conditions arise after feeding and may become extreme in lactic acidosis when histopathological changes are observed in the epithelium[2]. It was reported that thiamine was not absorbed from pH 6.8 buffered solutions in the ovine rumen having osmolalities over the range 240–360 mmol/l[26].

The importance of differentiating between absorption from the fore-stomachs and from the intestine has been stressed[43].

The bloodflow to the RR mucosa is an important variable that should influence the rate of absorption of drugs from the reticulo-rumen. Recent studies have reported the dramatic effect of feeding on foregut bloodflow in sheep using the injection of 15-micron radioactive microspheres into the left ventricle, followed by measurement of bloodflow by the reference organ technique (Table 15.1)[19]. This interesting finding will influence future drug absorption studies. Using a similar technique, a dramatic reduction in mucosal bloodflow was seen after infusion of adrenaline or noradrenaline into the jugular vein[40] at about $10\,\mu g\,kg^{-1}\,min^{-1}$.

Table 15.1 The effect of feeding and digestion on portal bloodflow and its foregut contribution in sheep. Data from ref. 19

	Portal blood flow (ml/g)	*Foregut contribution* (%)
Prefeeding	2.83	20.9
Feeding	2.76	26.2
2 h post-prandial	3.30	46.0
4 h post-prandial	2.81	37.3

Although several investigators have established the permeability of the salivary gland[48] and the rumen wall to the unionized forms of weak acids and bases, there is much less certainty about the passage of ionized molecules except for the lower volatile fatty acids and other small molecules. An interesting example is the base, histamine, which has two pK_a values, 5.97 and 9.80. The resulting ionization states are illustrated in Figure 15.4, along with the proportions of each form at selected pH values. Introduction of a solution containing polyethylene glycol 4000 (PEG) as a marker with histamine in a buffered medium at pH 3.9 to the empty rumen allowed the question of the absorption of ionized histamine to be investigated in a cow fitted with a rumen fistula. Figure 15.5 indicates that there was no evidence for absorption of histamine under these conditions in which most of its molecules were in the doubly charged form with a small proportion having a single charge and virtually none uncharged. The shape of the curve of declining concentrations of both PEG and histamine is attributable to outflow of rumen contents and replacement by saliva and any ingested water. Exchanges of water across the rumen wall could have contributed.

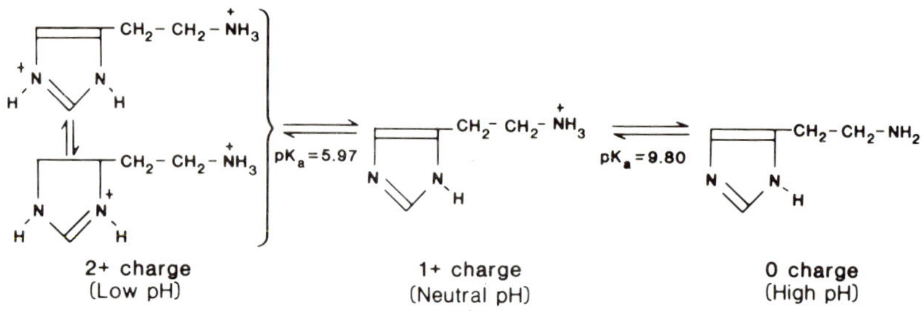

Theoretical Distribution of Ionization Forms with pH

pH	% 2+ form	% 1+ form	% 0 form	examples
4.0	**98.9**	**1.1**	**0.0**	**Abomasum; Rumen in Grain Overload**
7.0	**8.5**	**91.5**	**~ 0.0**	**Normal Rumen; Intestine; Plasma**
9.0	**0.0**	**86.3**	**13.7**	**Rumen in Urea Poisoning; Buccal Cavity; Intestine; Antacid Therapy.**

General Equation:

$$\text{\% of Base Ionized} = \frac{100}{1 + \text{Antilog}\,(\text{pH}-\text{p}K_a)}$$

Figure 15.4 Ionization states of histamine as a function of pH with examples of situations where selected pH values might occur

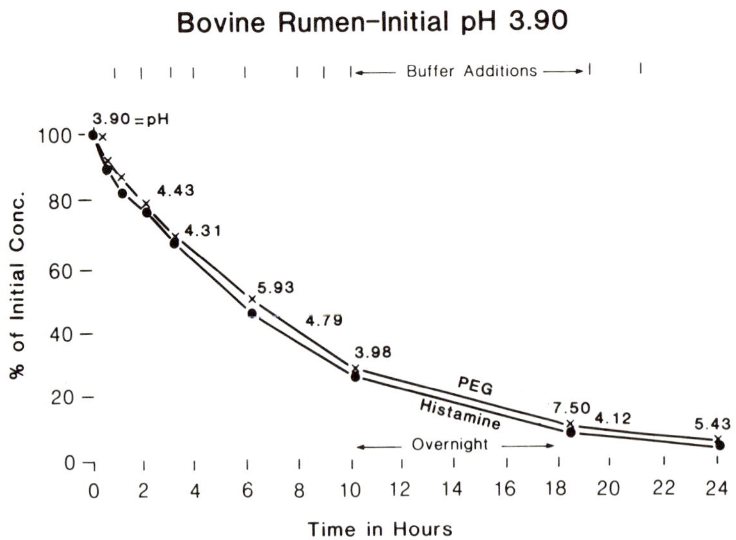

Figure 15.5 Non-absorption of histamine from acidic solution in the bovine rumen; starting concentrations PEG 4000 4 mg/ml, histamine free base equivalent 100 μg/ml

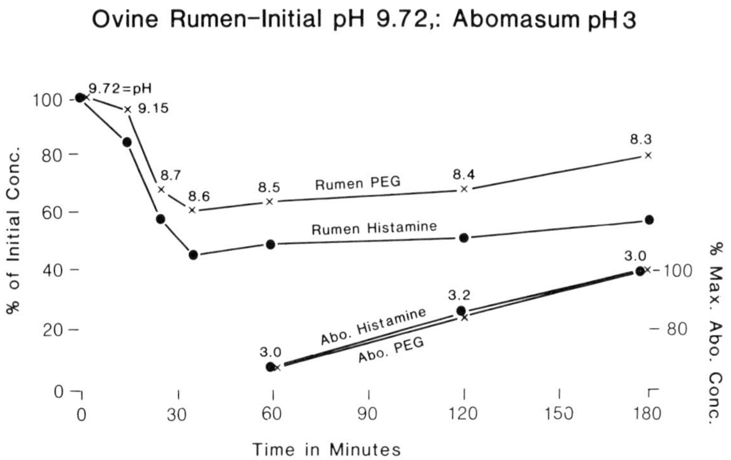

Figure 15.6 Absorption of histamine from alkaline solution in the bovine rumen; non-absorption from the acidic abomasum; starting concentrations as for Figure 15.5

A similar experiment with a sheep fitted with ruminal and abomasal fistulas involved use of a histamine–PEG solution buffered to a starting pH of 9.72. Figure 15.6 shows that clear evidence was obtained of absorption by the faster decline of the histamine concentration than that of PEG. The flattening of the concentration curves suggests that salivation and rumen motility may have been arrested or that the water absorption rate may have increased. Even at the high pH range maintained in the rumen (8.3–9.7) in this experiment, the majority of the histamine molecules would have carried a single charge but a significant proportion of unionized base would have been present to account for the absorption. Unfortunately, rumen volume at the end of the experiment and rumen motility were not measured. Transfer to abomasum did occur and it continued after the levelling of the rumen concentration curves. Abomasal pH was about 3 and no absorption seemed to occur under these conditions from this organ. The solutions used in these experiments were isotonic at the start. It would be interesting to see if absorption of ionized forms could be achieved from hypertonic solutions.

The effect of bypassing the rumen by means of stimulating the oesophageal groove has been studied with controversial results[4, 12, 46]. In general, it appears that such bypass techniques move a drug through the gastrointestinal tract more rapidly. They may even have the opposite of the desired effect of greater efficacy, as in the case of benzimidazole anthelmintics which were reported to be more effective if given into the rumen than to the omasum because of the longer exposure of worms to the drug[46], especially in cases where nematodes have developed resistance to the drug.

Other studies comparing oral and parenteral administration in ruminants have encompassed lithium[37], acetylsalicylic acid[22], phenylbutazone[6] and meclofenamic acid[35].

One aspect of absorption of substances in rumen ingesta, that does not seem to have been investigated, is the bucco-pharyngeal site during rumination. Since the pH of the oropharyngeal secretions is over 8, a completely different environment exists from that in the rumen which may have a concentration of hydrogen ion over one hundred times greater. Consequently, the possibility of absorption of bases that would not be absorbed from the rumen exists and should be examined. Also, the venous blood draining this region would not go via the liver so it would pass to the tissues without hepatic metabolism.

Volume turnover in the rumen

The halftime for emptying the RR by outflow through the reticulo-omasal orifice is about 5–7 h for the liquid component of the ingesta in mature cattle having normal motility. Much higher values are observed for the roughage component and after starvation or stasis. This dynamic process has been the source of uncertainty about the site of absorption based on concentration curves alone. A soluble drug introduced to the rumen may be deposited in the reticulum. Part of the dose may pass rapidly to the omasum, abomasum and small intestine. This allows rapid absorption to occur, initiating a rapid rise in plasma concentration. The remainder passes back into the rumen, slowly mixing with the ingesta via the mixing cycles. This portion is passed to the omasum more gradually, because it will be dispersed in the large rumen volume (over 40 l in a cow), with each outflow through the reticulo-omasal orifice. Consequently, curves of concentration of a drug in the rumen liquor with time must be interpreted very cautiously. Its plasma concentration may have arisen from intestinal rather than ruminal absorption. Experiments comparing drug concentration to that of a non-absorbable marker are essential to determine whether or not ruminal absorption occurred. The effect of gastrointestinal hormones on motility and outflow is important[41].

Whereas therapeutic drugs are administered to diseased animals and since sick animals frequently exhibit ruminal stasis, the pharmacokinetics of oral remedies can change dramatically in illness. Examples have been reported by several authors[7,27,42]. Typically, the plasma concentration is much lower when the rumen is atonic. Several factors may contribute to this change. A very marked reduction in rumen outflow rate occurred when atony was present[1]. In one cow that experienced spontaneous rumen stasis, estimated outflow rate dropped from 10.4 l/h to about 3 l/h. Although the authors were concerned that their technique overestimated outflow by as much as 58%, it is likely that the proportional change may be appropriate. Flow fell to 28% of the control value. This would have a very dramatic effect on the pharmacokinetics of a drug in the system, particularly if the site of absorption was the intestine rather than the rumen.

Another factor that may contribute to the reduced absorption is a likely reduction in mucosal blood flow, although this has not been measured during atonic states. If absorption normally occurs from the reticulo-rumen, other effects of stasis include failure to provide mechanical mixing in the diffusion layer at the surface of the mucosa along with loss of movement of the papillae, changes in the pH, temperature and osmolality of the medium, alteration of microbial activity, cessation of rumination, and changes in inflow of feed, water and saliva. Absorption also varies quite markedly with changes in the diet and in starvation[11,27]. The outcome may depend upon whether or not the drug is absorbable from the rumen and changes in rumen pH.

Sulfonamides are widely used by oral administration in ruminants. Several studies have reported on their pharmacokinetics[32,38,45,51] and the effects of rumen stasis[7,42] but there have been very few reports on efficacious or detrimental effects[25]. A better situation exists with respect to anthelmintics and where efficacy is more readily measurable. Levamisole[8] and benzimidazole anthelmintics[23] have received special attention.

Microbial metabolism of drugs

The microbiota of the rumen is very complex and includes protozoa, bacteria, yeasts and moulds. There are several groups of protozoa. Attempts have been made to create defaunated animals by using detergents to destroy all the protozoa. The different protozoal species vary in their sensitivity to these agents which are also toxic for the host. The wetting agents tested in sheep have included dioctyl sodium sulphosuccinate and nonyl phenol ethoxylates (Terics). An alternative approach has involved emptying the rumen and disinfecting the wall with formaldehyde 0.15% wt./vol. Comparison of these approaches[34] indicated that it is difficult both to attain complete defaunation and to maintain the defaunated state. Deaths occurred in all three treatments with rumenitis and nephritis leading to electrolyte imbalance and dehydration occurring in the detergent-treated animals. It would be very valuable to have a dependable defaunated model so that the contribution of protozoal metabolism to pharmacokinetics could be evaluated. Better results were obtained with certain alkanates, particularly sodium lauryl diethoxy sulphate, than with Terics. A large increase in propionate concentration occurred at the expense of acetate[9]. It is interesting to note that the propionate-enhancing drug, monensin, is also toxic to protozoa[24]. Since protozoa returned in a few days after a single treatment with alkanates, the authors saw a need for a slow release device to maintain a near-defaunated state for metabolic studies. This model awaits adoption for studies of drug metabolism. The well-known inactivation of chloramphenicol by reduction of its nitro group to an arylamine has been shown to be attributable to the protozoa[13].

The bacteria in the rumen populate three identifiably distinct environments, the rumen liquor, the solid particles and the epithelial wall where they are tenaciously adherent. Many different species can inhabit these various components of the system. Although there is a large literature on the effect of drugs on the digestion of nutrients in the rumen, there is very little published work on the metabolism of drugs by rumen bacteria. Defaunation and selective removal of bacterial species would be a useful technique for such studies. Alternatively, the use of gnotobiotes inoculated with selected strains of microbes would be valuable.

The wall-adherent bacteria in calves can be severely depleted by starvation for 3 days with or without antibiotics (clindamycin and gentamicin) added to the rumen solution[10]. This reduction in attached bacteria is accompanied by severe depression of the urease activity of the rumen wall and desquamation of epithelial cells. This system allows the distinguishing of tissue activity from bacterial activity. It may also provide a clue to one mechanism of a detrimental effect of certain chemotherapeutic agents in the rumen that can be monitored. The ability to differentiate between microbial and epithelial effects on drug metabolism would be a valuable tool.

The bacteria associated with the particulate matter include the cellulolytic bacteria. Some of these adhere to the plant cells. Their role in drug metabolism does not appear to have been studied selectively. Because fibrous particulate matter has a long retention time in the rumen, these bacteria presumably persist there longer than those in the fluid component of the ingesta.

Most studies that have been carried out on ruminal metabolism of drugs have involved sampling the rumen liquor. *In vitro* studies also have tended to be based on such samples. Consequently, an incomplete picture of the rumen microbiota's effect on chemical compounds results. Most of the studies of microbial metabolism of drugs in the rumen have involved chemotherapeutic agents and potential toxicants. Newer technology, such as high pressure liquid chromatography, is making possible more specific assay of drugs and their metabolites. Pathways can be checked by isotope studies. A recent study of the pharmacokinetics of albendazole and its major metabolites, the sulphoxide and the sulphone, in sheep is one example[36]. It was interesting to note that, although the parent compound was barely detectable in the plasma, substantial concentrations of the two major metabolites were found after oral administration of albendazole.

The rumen bacteria are capable of a very wide range of biochemical transformations. Drugs entering the system may have a profound effect on digestive and nutritional processes. This field has been reviewed thoroughly[47].

Some recent developments relevant to the understanding and control of detrimental nutritional disorders are worth noting. One is the identification of skatole (3-methyl indole or 3MI) formed from L-tryptophane in the rumen as a probable participant in the pathogenesis of 'fog fever' or acute bovine pulmonary oedema and emphysema[52]. Cattle grazing aftermath or 'foggage' and other lush feeds form 3MI in the rumen. It is said to be absorbed and passed to the lung where further metabolism by mixed function oxidase leads to pneumotoxicity, presumably mediated via reactive intermediates. The 3MI is covalently bound in the lung preferentially. Prevention by reducing conversion of tryptophane to skatole in the rumen has been achieved experimentally using monensin orally[39].

The problem of nitrate toxicity in cattle involves ingestion of large amounts of nitrate in a single feed. The nitrate is reduced rapidly to nitrite in the rumen. The latter is absorbed and reacts with blood to form methaemoglobin. Although adaptation to high nitrate intakes does occur, losses from nitrite intoxication are important. A new approach to controlling the problem has been proposed and tested[31]. It was found that significant inhibition of nitrate reductase in the rumen could be attained with orally administered sodium tungstate at up to 6.6 mg of tungsten per kg body weight. Whether or not there are toxic side-effects involving other divalent cations or enzymes needs further study. Nevertheless, this work is another indication of application of biochemical knowledge to pharmacological ends. The overall goal is to take the risk out of hazardous nutritional situations. Further studies of this type are required in such conditions as urea poisoning that involves ammonia toxicity and lactic acidosis.

A major challenge to the use of low level antibiotics as feed additives to improve productive performance has arisen from the concern about its implications for the spread of transferable antibiotic resistance among bacteria in the digestive tract. A recent review of the evolution of antibiotic resistance gene function evaluates current theories of persistence of resistant strains[30]. Since such strains have a profound influence on the metabolic fate or the efficacy of antimicrobial compounds, the topic has considerable relevance to the practical use of oral drugs in ruminants and the development of policies governing such use.

Chemical reactions in the rumen

Because of the large array of chemicals present in the rumen liquor, many chemical reactions may occur that do not involve micro-organisms directly. One example of this type is the appearance of thiaminase I in the rumen because of its presence in the feed or as an enzyme formed by bacteria that escapes to the rumen fluid. This enzyme is a tranferase that requires amine bases as cosubstrates, such as pyridine. It destroys thiamine and forms a new derivative of pyrimidine after the thiazole moiety has been removed. The product may be an antithiamine compound depending on the nature of the exchanged base. In any event this process renders the animal deficient in thiamine. This can lead to the clinical disease, polioencephalomalacia. The pharmacological implication is that it would be virtually useless to administer thiamine orally. It would be necessary either to deploy an inhibitor of thiaminase I first or to use physiologically effective compounds related to thiamine that are resistant to destruction by the enzyme, such as thiamine propyl disulphide or thiamine tetrahydrofurfuryl disulphide.

Concerns about efficacy

The study of bioavailability of drugs introduced to the rumen is a question of pharmacokinetics. However, in the zeal to generate tidy mathematical models of such a system, the ultimate reason for giving the drug often gets overlooked. It is notoriously easy to be misled by clinical impressions and quantitative clinical trials are essential to determine if the medication has any value on the one hand or a possible detrimental effect on the other.

Table 15.2 Oral treatment of experimental grain engorgement in sheep; all treatments initiated 24 h after dosing with ground barley 35 or 40 gm/kg

Oral treatments		*No.*	*Survivors*	*% Survival*
Untreated controls		12	4	33.3
Antacids				
$NaHCO_3$	1–2 g/kg × 3	12	3	25.0
$Mg(OH)_2$	1.1 g/kg	8	2	25.0
$CaCO_3$	1.9 g/kg	3	2	66.7
NH_4OH	1.5–3 g × 6	8	3	37.5
Antibiotics				
Penicillin V	1.5–3 g × 3	9	1	11.1
Tetracycline	44 mg/kg × 2	4	0	0.0
Chloromycetin	1–2 gm × 1	6	5	83.3
Miscellaneous				
Mineral Oil	about 1 l × 2	2	0	0.0
Creolin	0.2 ml/kg	4	0	0.0
'Anamas'†	21.3 g	3	0	0.0
Surgical				
Rumenotomy + fresh ingesta		4	3*	75.0
Prophylaxis				
Penicillin V with the grain	1.5 g	1	1	100.0

*The fatal case had surgery at 30 h instead of 24.
†Commercial preparation containing aminopyrine, pyrocatechol, MgO, Na formaldehyde sulphoxylate and charcoal.

In conclusion, one example that may illustrate the magnitude of the problem in the rumen setting is offered. A standardized model of ruminant lactic acidosis due to grain engorgement was developed. A variety of treatments was tested in this model, including several combinations of oral and systemic pharmacological approaches based on what appeared to be tenable hypotheses. Pulling out all of the cases where oral medicaton were involved, gave the results presented in Table 15.2. The trial was of the nature of a large scale screening exercise seeking clues to effective therapy. The animals received 35 or 40 gm/kg of ground barley by stomach tube as a slurry. Treatment was commenced at exactly 24 h after loading with grain. In crude terms of survival vs. death, the only dependable treatments were (1) rumenotomy with removal and replacement of the ingesta, and (2) oral chloramphenicol. Calcium carbonate deserved further evaluation. However, a closer look revealed that the rumenotomy animals recovered rapidly and fully (except for the one in which surgery was delayed 6 h) while the chloramphenicol-treated animals were inappetant and unthrifty for several weeks.

The lesson in this frustrating study lies in the fact that many of the products were in common use in clinical practice. Some were selected for use in the trial because of the testimony to their value given by practitioners. Some are still in widespread use. It is possible that some of the products used may be effective if given earlier in the condition. The conclusion should be that, at least until better evidence is available, emptying the reticulo-rumen and insertion of some fresh ingesta is the only treatment in which one can have confidence in a severe case. How many other formulations in common use for oral administration need similar evaluation? It is perhaps fortunate that the functional forestomach complex is remarkably resistant to chemical insults. When dysfunction is present, however, it becomes vulnerable and special care must be exercised before introducing medications that might be handled safely by a normal animal.

References

1. Aafjes, J. H. and Nijhof, J. K. (1968). Measurement of flow through the cow's rumen by continuous infusion of a marker. *Tijdschr. Diergeneesk.*, **93**, 16–27
2. Ahrens, F. A. (1967). Histamine, lactic acid, and hypertonicity as factors in the development of rumenitis in cattle. *Am. J. Vet. Res.*, **28**, 1335–42
3. Amadon, R. S. (1930). An experimental study of drugs stimulating the motility of the ruminant stomach. *J. Am. Vet. Med. Assoc.*, **76**, 65–74
4. Anderson, N. (1979). Reticular groove activity and anthelmintic efficacy of fenbendazole. *Vict. Vet. Proc.*, **37**, 42
5. Anderson, N., Laby, R. H., Prichard, R. K. *et al.* (1980). Controlled release of anthelmintic drugs: a new concept for prevention of helminthosis in sheep. *Res. Vet. Sci.*, **29**, 333–41
6. de Backer, P., Braeckman, R., Belpaire, F. *et al.* (1980). Bioavailability and pharmacokinetics of phenylbutazone in the cow. *J. Vet. Pharmacol. Ther.*, **3**, 29–33
7. Bischop, C. R., Janzen, R. E., Landals, D. C. *et al.* (1973). Effects of rumen stasis on sulfamethazine blood levels after oral administration in sheep. *Can. Vet. J.*, **14**, 269–71
8. Bogan, J. A., Marriner, S. E. and Galbraith, E. A. (1982). Pharmacokinetics of levamisole in sheep. *Res. Vet. Sci.*, **32**, 124–6
9. Burggraaf, W. and Leng, R. A. (1980). Antiprotozoal effects of surfacant detergents in the rumen of sheep. *N. Z. J. Agr. Res.*, **23**, 287–91
10. Cheng, K.-J., Bailey, C. B. M., Hironaka, R. *et al.* (1979). A technique for depletion of bacteria adherent to the epithelium of the bovine rumen. *Can. J. Anim. Sci.*, **59**, 207–9
11. Clark, R. and Wessels, J. J. (1952). The influences of the nature of the diet and of starvation on the concentration curve of sulphanilamide in the blood of sheep after oral dosing. *Onderstepoort J. Vet. Res.*, **25**, 75–83
12. Cooke, R. G. and Nicholson, T. (1981). The reticular groove and drug absorption. *J. Vet. Pharmacol. Ther.*, **4**, 311-3
13. de Corte-Baeten, K. and Debackere, M. (1978). The non-absorption of chloramphenicol after oral administration in adult ruminants: a tentative explanation from *in vitro* studies. *J. Vet. Pharmacol. Ther.*, **1**, 129–34
14. Danielli, J. F., Hitchcock, M. W. S., Marshall, R. A. *et al.* (1945). The mechanism of absorption from the rumen as exemplified by the behaviour of acetic, propionic and butyric acids. *J. Exp. Biol.*, **22**, 75–84
15. Davis, L. E. and Jenkins, W. L. (1974). Some considerations regarding drug therapy in ruminant animals. *Bov. Practitioner*, **9**, 57–60 and 80
16. Dobson, A. (1967). Physiological peculiarities of the ruminant relevant to drug distribution. *Fed. Proc.*, **26**, 994–1000
17. Dobson, A., Sellers, A. F. and Gatewood, V. H. (1976). Absorption and exchange of water across rumen epithelium. *Am. J. Physiol.*, **231**, 1588–94
18. Dobson, A., Sellers, A. F. and Gatewood, V. H. (1976). Dependence of Cr-EDTA absorption from the rumen on luminal osmotic pressure. *Am. J. Physiol.*, **231**, 1595–1600
19. Dobson, A., Comline, R. S. and Barnes, R. D. (1981). The components of hepatic portal flow during feeding. Report on the *XVI Conference on Rumen Function.* p. 11. (Washington, DC: CSRS, USDA)

20. Dobson, A., Sellers, A. F. and Shaw, G. T. (1970). Absorption of water from isolated ventral sac of rumen of the cow. *J. Appl. Physiol.*, **28**, 100–4
21. Dresbach, D. S. (1978). Ruminant GI dynamics – effect on pharmacokinetics of oral dosage forms. In Monkhouse, D. C. (ed.) *Animal Health Products: Design and Evaluation.* pp. 22–31. (Washington, DC: *Am. Pharm. Assoc.*)
22. Gingerich, D. A. Baggot, J. D. and Yeary, R. A. (1975). Pharmacokinetics and dosage of aspirin in cattle. *J. Am. Vet. Med. Assoc.*, **167**, 945–8
23. Hennessy, D. R. and Prichard, R. K. (1981). The role of absorbed drug in the efficacy of oxfendazole against gastrointestinal nematodes. *Vet. Res. Commun.*, **5**, 45–9
24. Hino, T. (1981). Action of monensin on rumen protozoa. *Jap. J. Zootech. Sci.*, **52**, 191
25. Hjerpe, C. A. and Routen, T. A. (1976). Practical and theoretical considerations concerning treatment of bacterial pneumonia in feedlot cattle, with special reference to antimicrobic therapy. In Williams, E. I. (ed.) *Proceedings of the 9th Annual Conference of the American Association of Bovine Practitioners.* pp. 97–140. (Stillwater, Okla.: AABP)
26. Höller, H., Buchkop, K. and Breves, G. (1979). Untersuchungen zur Passage von Thiamin (vit. B_1) durch die Pansenewand von Schafen in vivo. *Zbl. Vet. Med. B.*, **26**, 841–6
27. Jenkins, W. L. (1969). Studies on the effects of the intraruminal administration of sulphadimidine to adult sheep. *J. S. Afr. Vet. Med. Assoc.*, **40**, 159–78
28. Jenkins, W. L. and Davis, L. E. (1970). An approach for the study of drug distribution across ruminal epithelium *in vitro*. *J. S. Afr. Vet. Med. Assoc.*, **41**, 325–7
29. Jenkins, W. L., Davis, L. E. and Boulos, B. M. (1975). Transfer of drugs across the ruminal wall in goats. *Am. J. Vet. Res.*, **36**, 1771–6
30. Koch, A. L. (1981). Evolution of antibiotic resistance gene function. *Microbiol. Rev.*, **45**, 355–78
31. Korzeniowski, A., Geurink, J. H. and Kemp, A. (1981). Nitrate poisoning in cattle. 6. Tungsten (Wolfram) as a prophylactic against nitrate-nitrite intoxication in ruminants. *Neth. J. Agric. Sci.*, **29**, 37–47
32. Koritz, G. D., Bourne, D. W. A., Dittert, L. W. *et al.* (1977). Disposition of sulfonamides in food-producing animals: pharmacokinetics of sulfathiazole in sheep. *Am. J. Vet. Res.*, **38**, 979–82
33. Laby, R. H. (1975). Surface active agents in the rumen. In McDonald, I. W. and Warner, A. C. I. (eds.) *Digestion and Metabolism in the Ruminant.* pp. 537–50. (Armidale, Australia: Univ. of New England Publ.)
34. Lovelock, L. K. A., Buchanan-Smith, J. G. and Forsberg, C. W. (1982). Difficulties in defaunation of the ovine rumen. *Can. J. Anim. Sci.*, **62**, 299–303
35. Marriner, S. and Bogan, J. A. (1979). The influence of the rumen on the absorption of drugs: studies using meclofenamic acid administered by various routes to sheep and cattle. *J. Vet. Pharmacol. Ther.*, **2**, 109–15
36. Marriner, S. E., Bogan, J. A. and Vandaele, W. (1981). Comparison of the pharmacokinetics of albendazole and its major metabolites after oral administration of albendazole as a suspension and as a paste formulation in sheep. *Zbl. Vet. Med. B.*, **28**, 19–26
37. Mormede, P. and Ledoux, J-M. (1980). Pharmacokinetics of lithium in sheep. *J. Vet. Pharmacol. Ther.*, **3**, 169–76
38. Nielsen, P., Romvary, A. and Rasmussen, R. (1978). Sulphadoxine and trimethoprin in goats and cows: absorption fraction, half-lives and the degrading effect of the ruminal flora. *J. Vet. Pharmacol. Ther.*, **1**, 37–46
39. Nocerini, M. R., Carlson, J. R., Breeze, R. G. *et al.* (1981). Effect of dose and tissue glutathione concentrations on *in vivo* covalent binding and 3-methylindole-induced lung injury in goats. Report of *XVI Conference on Rumen Function.* p. 5. (Washington, DC: CSRS, USDA)
40. Olowookorun, M. D. (1980). Blood flow in the various compartments of the goat stomach. *Res. Vet. Sci.*, **28**, 254–5
41. Onapito, S. J., Donawick, W. J. and Merritt, A. M. (1978). Effect of gastrin on emptying and composition of digesta of the omasum of sheep. *Am. J. Vet. Res.*, **39**, 1455–8
42. Oyaert, W., Quin, J. I. and Clark, R. (1951). Studies on the alimentary tract of the Merino sheep in South Africa. XIX. The influence of sulphanilamide on the activity of the ruminal flora of sheep and cattle. *Onderstepoort J. Vet. Res.*, **25**, 59–65

43. Phillipson, A. T. (1967). Comments on absorption in ruminants. In Cafruny, E. J. (ed.) *Proceedings of Int. Symp. on Comp. Pharmacol. Fed. Proc.* pp. 1006–7. (Bethesda: FASEB)
44. Pope, D. G. (1975). Factors to be considered in the formulation of pharmaceuticals for oral administration to ruminant animals. *Aust. J. Pharm. Sci.*, **NS4,** 65–78
45. Pope, D. G. (1978). Animal health specialized delivery systems. In Monkhouse, D. C. (ed.) *Animal Health Products: Design and Evaluation.* pp. 78–114. (Washington, DC: *Am. Pharmaceut. Assoc.*)
46. Prichard, R. K. (1980). Host influences on the efficacy of benzimidazole anthelmintics. In Van den Bossche, H. (ed.) *The Host Invader Interplay.* Janssen Research Foundation. pp. 731–4. (Amsterdam: Elsevier)
47. Prins, R. A. (1978). Nutritional impact of intestinal drug – microbe interactions. In Hathcock, J. N. and Coon, J. (eds.) *Nutrition and Drug Interrelations.* Chap. 7, pp. 189–251. (New York: Academic Press)
48. Rasmussen, R. (1964). Salivary excretion of sulfonamides and barbiturates by cows and goats. *Acta Pharmacol. Toxicol.*, **21,** 11–19
49. Steven, D. H. and Marshall, A. B. (1970). Organization of the rumen epithelium. In Phillipson, A. T. (ed.) *Physiology of Digestion and Metabolism in the Ruminant.* pp. 80–100. (Newcastle Upon Tyne: Oriel)
50. Stevens, C. E., Hammond, P. B. and Nielsen, N. O. (1959). Phlegmonous gastritis in cattle resulting from ruminatoric doses of tartar emetic. *J. Am. Vet. Med. Assoc.*, **134,** 323–7
51. Wooley, J. L. and Sigel, C. W. (1982). Development of pharmacokinetic models for sulfonamides in food animals: metabolic depletion profile of sulfadiazine in the calf. *Am. J. Vet. Res.*, **43,** 768–74
52. Yokoyama, M. T. and Carlson, J. R. (1974). Dissimilation of tryptophan and related indolic compounds by ruminal microorganisms *in vitro. Appl Microbiol.*, **27,** 540–8

16
Recent developments in the treatment of metabolic diseases

W. M. Allen, B. F. Sansom, C. F. Drake and P. R. Moore

The classical metabolic diseases are non-infectious diseases such as milk fever, hypomagnesaemia and ketosis. Recently the fatty liver syndrome[26] has been shown to be associated with these conditions and also with several other periparturient problems such as mastitis, retained placenta and infertility. In addition, there are many metabolic diseases caused by nutritional deficiencies of either the major or the trace mineral elements. In the past few years new ideas or methods have been introduced for the treatment of all these diseases. The purpose of this paper is to review these recent advances.

MILK FEVER

The incidence of milk fever appears to be continuing to rise as the productivity of the dairy cow increases; by 1975 the annual incidence in the UK had risen to 9% whereas in 1960 it had been only 4%[17,23]. Therapy has not changed substantially[23] but there has been progress in preventive methods based largely upon new knowledge of vitamin D metabolism and the identification of predisposing factors[25].

The concentration in plasma of the most active metabolite of vitamin D, 1,25 dihydroxycholecalciferol ($1,25(OH)_2D_3$), increases when there is a low calcium concentration in the diet during pregnancy. Unfortunately, the increase only occurs when the daily calcium intake is below 25–30 g and such a diet is impractical for use on farms. However, under experimental conditions, when the daily intake of calcium was less than 25–30 g, the efficiency of calcium uptake from the intestine increased and so also did the mobilization of calcium from body stores. Both processes helped to prevent hypocalcaemia at the time of parturition. Recently, the effect of using diets containing low phosphorus concentrations was investigated[15]. Such diets also prevent hypocalcaemia and the authors suggested that, rather than acting via increased $1,25(OH)_2D_3$ synthesis, the low phosphorus diet increased the local binding of the hormone to the gut wall and increased the efficiency of absorption of calcium.

When the metabolites and analogues of vitamin D had been identified and synthesized, their potential for preventing milk fever could be assessed. These compounds include cholecalciferol (D_3); its 25-hydroxylated metabolite (25-OH D_3); a synthetic analogue of this natural compound (1α-OH D_3) and the dihydroxylated metabolite ($1,25(OH)_2D_3$) which is physiologically the most active compound. The use of all of these substances is made difficult by the need to treat cows before calving and the uncertainty of predicting parturition accurately. Nevertheless, all the compounds have been tested and the evidence suggests that in terms of efficiency and cost 1α-OH D_3 is the best available for preventing milk fever.

It is considered that $100\,\mu g$ 1α-OH D_3 protects cows against milk fever if administered within 12 h of calving, but that larger doses are less effective[11]. It is reported that injections of $350\,\mu g$ 1α-OH D_3, provided that they were administered more than 24 h before calving, prevented all cases of milk fever[4]. However, in more extensive trials which involved several hundred animals, it was concluded that $500\,\mu g$ 1α-OH D_3 administered more than 24 h before calving, resulted in at best a 75% decrease in the incidence of milk fever[8,27]. Although $1,25(OH)_2D_3$ is the most active metabolite of vitamin D it appears to be less efficient than 1α-OH D_3 for milk fever prophylaxis because a single injection has a more short-lived effect[6].

Cholecalciferol (D_3) is now considered to be of limited value as a preventive and has been shown[19] to be slower in action and less efficient than 1α-OH D_3[19]. The dose required (10^7 units – 250 mg) is much greater than the doses of the other compounds and a recent report has suggested that in pregnant animals only slightly larger doses may be associated with irreversible toxic changes, principally metastatic calcification[18].

In addition to the effects of dietary calcium and the relationship between vitamin D metabolism and milk fever, there are other factors which affect the likelihood of milk fever occurring[12]. One of the most important is the magnesium status of the pregnant animal[7]. Subclinical hypomagnesaemia (approx. 0.5–0.85 mmol Mg/1) decreases the ability of a cow to mobilize calcium in response to hypocalcaemia and thus prejudices her ability to adapt successfully to the greatly increased calcium requirements at the start of lactation. It is therefore important to ensure that pregnant cows receive an adequate intake of magnesium so that the concentration of magnesium in blood does not decrease. The maintenance of normomagnesaemia is especially difficult when the dry cows are at pasture and relying solely on a diet of grass. To avoid the difficulty of feeding a concentrate rich in magnesium, systems using medicated drinking water have recently been developed. Sufficient magnesium acetate is added to the water troughs so that, provided the weather is dry and no other water supplies are accessible, each animal is provided with up to 20 g Mg/day. Rumen 'bullets' have also been devised but they can carry only small amounts of magnesium and it is released only slowly (approx. 1–3 g/day); furthermore, they may be regurgitated and lost soon after administration.

ACUTE AND CHRONIC HYPOMAGNESAEMIA

Hypomagnesaemia can also be sufficiently severe to cause a clinical disease which can be difficult to treat in its acute stages and difficult to prevent thereafter by maintaining an adequate intake of magnesium. In beef animals supplementation may be provided from magnesium rich blocks laid on the pasture as well as by the methods already discussed, but there have been few other recent developments. The acute disease can be precipitated by stress, usually in the form of sudden adverse weather or transient starvation. It is therefore important, especially in beef animals, to ensure that they receive an adequate energy intake and are not subjected to short periods of starvation or exposed to adverse weather conditions.

KETOSIS AND FATTY LIVER (OR FAT MOBILIZATION) SYNDROME

The realization that a fatty liver (>20% fat in the hepatocytes) predisposes dairy cattle to a number of periparturient diseases including ketosis and infertility has underlined the importance of feeding appropriate diets throughout the complete reproductive cycle[26]. During pregnancy, particularly, the energy intake must be adequate for, but not exceed, the animals' requirements because if the cow is too fat before and at calving she is more likely to develop fatty liver.

Table 16.1 The effect of body condition 4 weeks prepartum upon fatty liver, metabolic diseases, fertility and milk yield

	Controls	*Affected*
Body condition score 4 weeks before calving	2.72	3.94
Mean % fat in liver cells 2 weeks postpartum	15.2	30.8
Diseases (no. of cases)		
ketosis	2	5
mastitis	1	3
milk fever	1	2
Number of days calving to 1st oestrus	36.8	42.7
Milk yield (kg) in first 84 days of lactation	2567	2323

Data from ref. 26

Cows which store too much fat during pregnancy may begin to mobilize these fat depots during late pregnancy and mobilize them even more rapidly at the start of lactation. As a result, fat accumulates in all the rapidly metabolizing tissues, especially the liver, kidney and muscle; because of this wide tissue distribution the term 'fatty liver' may be too restrictive. Fat accumulates because the fat input into the tissues increases and because the tissues use less fat. Therapeutic methods have aimed therefore to increase the rate at which the affected tissues, especially the liver, catabolize fat. The compounds which have been used for this purpose have also been tried prophylactically. They include nicotinic acid (niacin), biotin and methionine, all of which can be supplied as feed additives, and provided that the latter is protected from degradation in the rumen. Unfortunately, the initial results from prophylactic feeding trials do not appear promising. The most successful method of preventing 'fatty liver' is to maintain pregnant animals in good but not fat body condition. The animal's appetite (and therefore dry matter intake) then remains high around the time of parturition and increases rapidly thereafter, minimizing the need for the body stores to be mobilized.

TRACE ELEMENTS

The most important essential trace elements are copper, selenium, cobalt and iodine. The successful prevention and treatment of diseases associated with a deficiency of these trace elements still present a challenge because of the world-wide extent of the deficiencies and the variety of extensive husbandry systems which frequently use extremely low stocking densities. In the case of severe and acute deficiencies of copper and selenium, parenteral injections of a supplement probably remain the best method for restoring normal mineral concentrations in the deficient animals' tissues[1]. However, several new methods for prevention and treatment have recently been introduced for when supplementation is required throughout the grazing season.

One of these methods, the addition of the element to the drinking water, has already been described for supplementation with magnesium (as a solution of its acetate). More recently, compressed pellets, each containing one trace element, have been designed for addition to drinking water troughs. The solubility of the contained element is controlled so that the animals drinking the water should be provided approximately with their daily needs. However, the theoretical advantages do not always seem to be borne out in practice. Copper-containing tablets failed to prevent the onset of hypocupraemia in cattle[10]. The tablets, which cannot be used in galvanized water tanks, disintegrated and formed a copper-containing sludge on the bottom of the water tank. The copper content of the water never exceeded 0.2 mg Cu/l although the tablets were designed to provide between 2.5 and 5 mg Cu/l water. Similar conclusions have also been reported but the manufacturers now claim to have improved the solubility of their copper pellets[20].

In the case of pellets containing selenium it is reported[5] that they could provide up to 3 mg selenium per cow per day from water containing up to 0.074 mg Se/l. Observations suggest that selenium tablets added to the drinking water of dairy cows may be of some value. However, their effect on GSH-Px activities in blood was apparently so short-lived after the tablets had been removed from the troughs, even though the biological halflife of selenium is known to be of the order of 1–3 months, that these conclusions should be treated with caution.

It is also reported that similar pellets containing cobalt failed to prevent a decline of vitamin B_{12} concentrations in the plasma of calves[20]. However, B_{12} concentrations increased in calves which were supplied with water to which cobalt had been added by means of a proportioning device. This device can also be used for other trace elements.

With the 'Rowett Water Proportioning Device', it is claimed that the addition of between 2.5 and 5 mg Cu/l of drinking water is as effective as repeated injections of copper in preventing hypocupraemia in suckler cows and growing heifers[13].

Unfortunately, this method of utilizing the water supply to act as a carrier for trace elements has major disadvantages. It can be effective only when the animals receive water from the treated source alone. If they have access to extraneous or natural sources of supply the method is virtually useless. Similarly, the efficacy of the method depends on the climate; high rainfall reduces voluntary water intake and makes it impossible to predict trace element intake.

Continuous release of the trace element directly into the digestive tract would overcome these difficulties and methods of administering some trace elements as long-lived ruminal boluses or bullets have been devised. The method has most commonly been applied to cobalt, administered as a bullet which contains 30% cobalt oxide with iron grit. This has been proved to be effective both for therapy and for the longterm prevention of cobalt deficiency in sheep. Unfortunately, the bullets do not appear to be as effective in cattle. Our evidence suggests that the release of cobalt decreases substantially after the bullet has been in the rumen for a short time, possibly because of surface coating (Figure 16.1). Bullets containing 5% selenium also

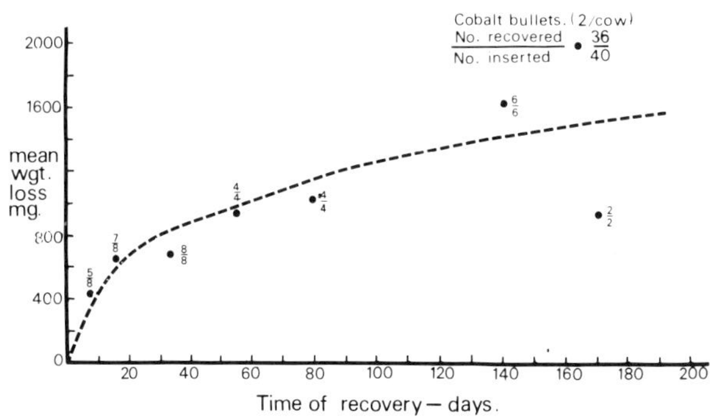

Figure. 16.1 Weight loss in the rumen of cobalt bullets

dispersed in iron grit have been developed also for longterm prevention of selenium deficiency[16] but they, too, decline in solubility with time. This behaviour has been ascribed[24] to the use of certain sizes of selenium particles or grains, particularly those less than 10 μm. It is claimed that an effective rate of release of selenium could be maintained provided that the selenium grains were larger than 10 μm, and that the optimum grain size was of the order of 35–40 μm. However, there are no field trial data available to support this claim.

Material of a quite different physical form has been used to provide animals with longterm oral supplements of copper. After oral administration copper oxide wire or needles lodge at sites either in the fore-stomachs or abomasum[9]. They dissolve slowly and some of the released copper is absorbed by the normal physiological processes. They can be recovered from the sites of retention for several weeks after dosing and during this period the reserves of copper in the liver, the principal storage organ, increase. The copper stored in the liver then acts as a depot from which copper can be slowly released to maintain normal concentrations of copper in the blood during periods when the animal may be receiving an inadequate copper intake. They have been used most frequently in sheep but they are also effective in cattle. Administration of 25 g of oxidized copper wire to cows and calves has prevented the development of hypocupraemia for up to 33 weeks thereafter[14]. It is demonstrated that 4 g of copper oxide needles administered to ewes during the first half of pregnancy protect their lambs from sway-back[29]. Two grams of copper oxide needles administered to lambs provided sufficient copper to prevent the development of hypocupraemia until the lambs were weaned[28].

All methods for providing supplements of copper, cobalt or selenium so far discussed supplement the animal's requirements for periods of only a few weeks to a few months. Methods to provide adequate supplements for at least the length of the grazing season in the temperate zones still need to be developed. Soluble glasses provide a type of physical system which could provide controlled longterm supplementation. These soluble controlled release glasses (CRG) are phosphate glasses into which many minerals and trace elements can be incorporated, including sodium, potassium, magnesium, copper, selenium, cobalt, zinc and iodine.

Copper and selenium containing CRG have been developed for use as subcutaneous implants. Selenium-containing implants will slowly release selenium over a period of 7 months without deleterious effect[3], whereas similar copper-containing CRG unfortunately produce unacceptable local tissue reactions. Nevertheless, copper containing CRG have been developed for subcutaneous use which are at least as effective in preventing copper deficiency as other available therapeutic preparations[1,22].

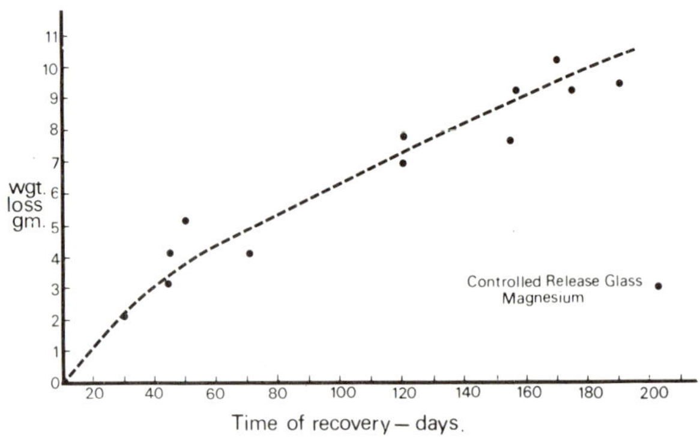

Figure 16.2 Weight loss of magnesium CRG in the rumen of cattle

For the simple and practical prevention of copper and cobalt deficiencies CRG used as rumen boluses have greater potential[2]. CRG boluses continue to release their trace element constituents at an almost uniform rate, dependent upon surface area, for longer than 6 months. Copper-containing CRG with four different rates of solubility have dissolved approximately linearly for 190 days when suspended in dacron bags in the rumen of steers[21]. Figure 16.2 shows the rate of dissolution of a magnesium-containing CRG over a similar period. Twelve boluses were administered and all were recovered at slaughter up to 190 days after dosing.

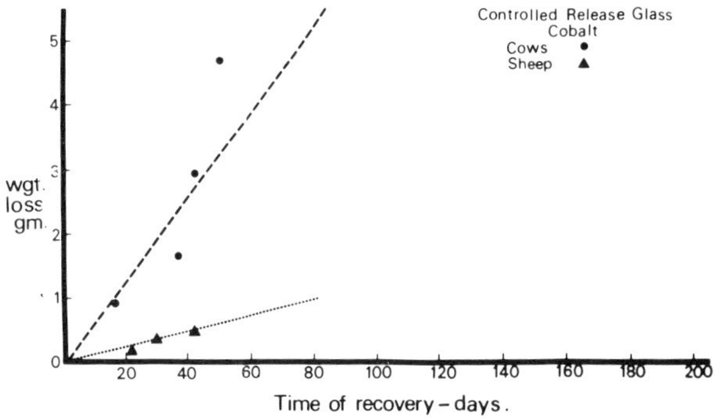

Figure 16.3 Weight loss of cobalt CRG in the rumen of sheep and cows

CRG containing cobalt also dissolve at a linear rate (Figure 16.3), and recently boluses weighing approximately 65 g have been shown to release between 0.8 and 1.6 mg Co/day for at least 50 days, a quantity sufficient to satisfy the requirements of growing and adult cattle. Smaller boluses would provide enough cobalt for sheep.

These initial experiments with CRG as a source of trace elements suggest that they do not suffer from the disadvantages of either arrested dissolution or the development of insoluble surface coatings. They may, like the metallic magnesium boluses, be liable to regurgitation from the reticulo-rumen but in the experiments so far conducted more than 90% of the glass boluses administered have been recovered after periods of up to 190 days. The mass and density of the boluses appear to have surprisingly little influence on their probability of retention. All the glasses administered have a density only slightly greater than 2.5, and it has therefore been considered unnecessary to interfere with the composition by adding material of high density. Boluses weighing only between 5 and 6 g have also been recovered up to 134 days after dosing.

CONCLUSION

The productivity of farm livestock in terms of milk and meat output continues to increase and, in consequence, the stresses imposed upon the animals and their nutritional requirements also increase. The likelihood of imbalances between input and output will therefore rise and metabolic diseases will be an increasingly important cause of losses unless new methods of treatment and prevention can be developed. In this paper we have shown that significant progress has been made during the past decade. However, while the main objective of agriculture remains to increase productivity, it will continue to be essential to develop new, better and more practical methods for preventing metabolic diseases.

References

1. Allen, W. M. and Moore, P. R. (1982). Parenteral methods of trace element supplementation. In *Proceedings of British Veterinary Association/BSAP Symposium*, York, July 31–Aug. 1. In press
2. Allen, W. M., Moore, P. R., Mallinson, C.B. *et al.* (1981). Slow release methods for trace element supplementation. In *Proceedings of Association for Veterinary Clinical Pharmacology and Therapeutics*. Guildford University, December 17–18. In press
3. Allen, W. M., Moore, P. R. and Sansom, B. F. (1982). Controlled release glasses for selenium supplementation. In *Trace Element Metabolism in Man and Animals*. pp. 195–8. (New York: Springer Verlag)
4. Bar, A. and Sachs, M. (1980). Observations on the use of 1α-hydroxycholecalciferol in the prevention of bovine parturient paresis. *Vet. Rec.*, **106**, 529–32
5. Blowey, R. W. (1982). Primary evaluation of water soluble selenium tablets in the treatment of selenium deficiency in dairy cattle. *Vet. Rec.*, **110**, 477
6. Capen, C. C., Hoffsis, G. F. and Norman, A. W. (1977). Dose response of 1:25 dihydroxycholecalciferol on serum calcium and phosphorus, urine electrolytes and hydroxyproline excretion in cattle. In *Proceedings of Third Workshop on Vitamin D*. Asilomar, California. Vol. 3, pp. 565–7. (Berlin: P. de Gruyter)
7. Contreras, P. A., Manston, R. and Sansom, B. F. (1982). Calcium mobilisation in hypomagnesaemic cattle. *Res. Vet. Sci.*, **33**, 10–16
8. Davies, D. C., Allen, W. M., Hoare, M. N. *et al.* (1978). A field trial of 1α-hydroxycholecalciferol (1α-OH D_3) in the prevention of milk fever. *Vet. Rec.*, **102**, 440–2
9. Dewey, D. W. (1977). An effective method for the administration of trace amounts of copper to ruminants. *Search*, **8**, 326–7
10. Farmer, P. (1982). The use of copper tablets to supplement the copper status of cattle grazing teart pastures. In *Proceedings of British Veterinary Association/BSAP Symposium*, York, July 31–Aug. 1. In press
11. Gast, D. R., Marquardt, J. P., Jorgensen, N. A. *et al.* (1977). Efficacy and safety of 1α-hydroxyvitamin D for prevention of parturient paresis. *J. Dairy Sci.*, **60**, 1910–20
12. Harris, D. J. (1981). Factors predisposing to parturient paresis. *Aust. Vet. J.*, **57**, 357–61
13. Humphries, W. R., McPherson, A. and Farmer, P. E. (1982). Drinking water as a carrier for trace elements for cattle. In *Proceedings of British Veterinary Association/BSAP Symposium*, York, July 31–Aug. 1. In press
14. Judson, G. J., Dewey, D. W., McFarlane, J. D. *et al.* (1982). Oxidised copper wire for oral copper therapy in cattle. In Gawthorne, J. M., Howell, J. McC. and White, C. L. (eds.) *Trace Element Metabolism in Man and Animals*. pp. 187–9. (New York: Springer Verlag)
15. Kichura, T. S., Horst, R. L., Beitz, D. C. *et al.* (1982). Relationship between pre-partal dietary calcium and phosphorus, vitamin D metabolism, and parturient paresis in cows. *J. Nutr.*, **112**, 480–7
16. Kuchel, R. E. and Buckley, R. A. (1969). The provision of selenium to sheep by means of a heavy pellet. *Aust. J. Agric. Res.*, **20**, 1099–107
17. Leech, F. B., Davies, M. E., McCrae, W. D. *et al.* (1960). *Disease Wastage and Husbandry in the British Dairy Herd. Report of the National Survey 1958–59*. (London: HMSO)
18. Littledike, E. T. and Horst, R. L. (1982). Vitamin D_3 toxicity in dairy cows. *J. Dairy Sci.*, **65**, 749–59

19. McMurray, C. H., Rice, D. A. and McBride, P. S. (1980). Milk fever controls: comparison of 1α and vitamin D_3 in conjunction with induced parturition. *Vet. Rec.*, **107**, 188–91
20. McPherson, A. (1982). Oral methods for trace element supplementation. In *Proceedings of British Veterinary Association/BSAP Symposium*, York, July 31–Aug. 1. In press
21. Moore, P. R. and Drake, C. F. (1982). Controlled release glass as a source of trace minerals for grazing animals. (This volume)
22. Moore, P. R., Hall, G. A., Sansom, B. F. *et al.* (1982). The use of copper-containing controlled release glass for systemic supplementation of sheep with Cu. *Proc. Nutr. Soc.*, **41**, 84A
23. Mullen, P. A. (1975). Clinical and biochemical responses to the treatment of milk fever. *Vet. Rec.*, **97**, 87–92
24. Peter, D. W., Hunter, R. A. and Hudson, D. R. (1982). Optimum Se grain size for selenium pellets. In *Trace Element Metabolism in Man and Animals.* pp. 218–21. (New York: Springer-Verlag)
25. Sansom, B. F. (1977). The use of vitamin D metabolites and analogues for the prevention of milk fever in cattle. *Vet. Sci. Commun.*, **1**, 323–35
26. Treacher, R. J., Reid, I. M. and Roberts, C. J. (1981). The effect of body condition at calving on the development of fatty liver and metabolic disease. In *Proceedings of BSAP Winter Meeting*, Paper 30
27. Vagg, M. J., Allen, W. M., Davies, D. C. *et al.* (1981). A field trial to determine the efficacy of two doses of 1α-hydroxycholecalciferol in the prevention of milk fever. *Vet. Rec.*, **109**, 273–5
28. Whitelaw, A., Armstrong, R. H., Evans, C. C. *et al.* (1980). Effects of oral administration of copper oxide needles to hypocupraemic sheep. *Vet. Rec.*, **107**, 87–8
29. Whitelaw, A., Fawcett, A. R. and McDonald, A. J. (1982). Cupric oxide needles in the prevention of swayback. *Vet. Rec.*, **110**, 522

17
Drug excretion by the mammary gland

J. Boisseau and J. P. Moretain

The chief aim of the legislation concerning veterinary pharmacy is to protect the consumer's health against the hazards of drug residues, which may contaminate the foods of animal origin. Pharmacokinetic studies performed in normal conditions cannot take into account all the particular situations to which a veterinarian may be confronted. A good knowledge of the various parameters likely to influence the mammary excretion of veterinary drugs is required by (1) the manufacturer of veterinary drugs to improve his dosage forms, and by (2) the veterinary practitioner to fix withdrawal times according to the particular cases he has on hand.

Both literature data and personal results on the parameters likely to influence the elimination of antibiotics into the milk will be presented, taking into account factors depending on the drug, the treatment and the animal.

DRUG FORMULATION

Active ingredient

It is obvious that the physicochemical properties of the active ingredient determine its elimination through the mammary gland. The capacity of a drug to pass into the milk depends on its ability to penetrate the mammary parenchyma by going through a biological membrane, the basic membrane of the secretory cell of the mammary gland, which is in close contact with the blood capillaries perfusing the gland[3,7]. The drug passage from blood to milk might be explained by a mechanism of non-ionic passive diffusion which depends on the percentage of ionization in the serum as well as in milk, lipid solubility, percentage of binding to plasma proteins and molecular weight.

It is generally admitted that the non-ionic passive diffusion chiefly accounts for the capability of an antibiotic to pass the blood–milk barrier. This ability is all the greater if the molecular weight is low, the solubility in lipids high, the drug ionized and unbound to serum proteins.

Table 17.1 Influence of the ionization of drugs on their mammary excretion with theoretical vs. experimental concentration[7]

Drugs	pK_a	*Milk/serum concentration ratio* Theoretical	*Experimental*
Acids			
Sulphanilamide	10.4	1.00	0.97
Sulphapyridine	8.4	0.94	0.86
Pentobarbital	8.0	0.9	1.1
Sulphadimidine	7.4	0.51	0.59
Sulphathiazole	7.1	0.37	0.35
Sulphadiazine	6.5	0.28	0.21
Sulphadimethoxine	6.0	0.19	0.20
Sulphacetamide	5.4	0.13	0.08
PAH acid	3.8	0.25	0.28
Salicylic acid	3.0	0.36	0.35
Penicillin	2.7	0.16	0.25
Bases			
Urea	0.2	1.00	1.00
Antipyrine	1.4	1.00	1.00
Creatinine	3.6	1.00	0.92
Aminopyrine	5.0	1.00	1.10
Lincomycin	7.6	2.8	3.9
Trimethoprim	7.6	3.9	3.7
Ephedrine	9.6	7.9	7.9

Many experiments performed on several drugs having acid or base pK_a have confirmed this hypothesis[3, 7]. However, it is not possible to discard the eventuality for some drugs of an active mechanism of secretion. Such a mechanism of secretion would thus, as in the case of PAH acid, explain the high ratio of milk/plasma concentration and the decrease of this ratio when plasma concentration increases[6].

Among the factors involved in the process of non-ionic passive diffusion, the percentage of ionization of the drug in the serum has to be considered. The compounds reacting as highly ionized acids in the plasma diffuse less easily in the milk than compounds reacting as weak bases. The ratio of concentrations of antibiotics in the ultrafiltrates of the milk and the serum is less than 1 for acid compounds and greater than 1 for macrolides

Table 17.2 Percentage of recovery of the given dose of parenterally-administered antibiotics

Antibiotics	pK_a	%
Penicillin	2.8	0.010
Amoxycillin	2.8–7.2	0.004
Ampicillin	2.8–7.2	0.002
Tylosin	7.1	0.5
Spiramycin	8.2	6.0
Dihydrostreptomycin	8.8	0.15
Colistin	10.0	0.20
Chloramphenicol	—	0.07
Oxytetracycline	—	0.3
Tetracycline	—	0.3

(Table 17.1). In the same manner, the percentage of recovery in the milk of the parenteral administered dose is higher for antibiotics acting as weak bases than for antibiotics acting as weak acids (Table 17.2).

The lipid solubility of drugs influences their mammary excretion by determining their capacity to pass through the biological membranes. For example, in the case of compounds having very similar pK_a, such as macrolides, aminoglycosides and colistin, a low lipid solubility leads to a limited mammary excretion and, consequently, to a low percentage of recovery in the milk. Experimental results are related to those expected from the application of the concept of non-ionic passive diffusion, for drugs having a high or moderate lipid solubility. When the lipid solubility is low, the mammary excretion is still lower than that anticipated (Table 17.3).

Since the non-protein-bound plasma fraction is likely to diffuse, it is necessary to ascertain the role of this parameter. The results compiled in Table 17.4 show a limited influence. No significant differences between the concentration and the percentage of recovery in the milk occurred for

Table 17.3 Influence of the lipid solubility of drugs on their mammary excretion[12]. (mod – moderate; h – high; l – low)

Drugs	pK_a	*Solubility*	*Milk/serum concentration ratio* *Theoretical*	*Experimental*
Acids				
Sulphanilamide	10.4	mod	1.00	0.97
Sulphapyridine	8.4	mod	0.94	0.86
Sulphamethazine	7.4	mod	0.51	0.59
Sulphadiazine	6.5	mod	0.28	0.21
Sulphadimethoxine	6.0	h	0.19	0.20
Sulphacetamide	5.4	l	0.13	0.08
Penicillin G	2.8	mod	0.16	0.20
Penicillin V	2.8	mod	0.16	0.22
Cloxacillin	2.8	h	0.16	0.22
Ampicillin	2.8–7.2	h	0.26	0.26
Amoxycillin	2.8–7.2	h	0.26	0.26
Cephaloride	3.4	mod	0.25	0.26
Cephaloglycin	4.9	h	0.30	0.33
Cephacetril	2.4	mod	0.12	0.15
Rifampicin	7.9	h	0.85	1.10
Novobiocin	4.3	h	0.30	0.33
Bases				
Penethamate	8.5	h	5.7	6.1
Neomycin	8.3	l	7.5	0.5
Colistin	10.0	l	8.0	0.3
Erythromycin	8.8	h	6.2	8.5
Tylosin	7.1	h	5.0	4.5
Spiramycin	8.2	h	4.8	4.6
Lincomycin	7.6	h	4.2	4.4
Chloramphenicol (alcohol)	—	h	1.0	1.0
Tetracyclines (amphoteric)	—	mod	0.4–0.8	0.6–1.4

Table 17.4 Relation between the rate of binding to plasma proteins, the lipid solubility (octanol/water partition), the concentration ratio milk/serum and recovery (%) of antibiotics[12]

Antibiotic	*Unbound* %	*Oct./H_2O coeff.*	*Milk/serum concentration*	*Recovery* (%) *Theoretical*	*Experimental*
Penicillin G	66	58	0.20	0.16	0.20
Penicillin V	20	102	0.20	0.16	0.22
Ampicillin	86	150	0.26	0.26	0.26
Cloxacillin	24	275	0.20	0.16	0.22
Neomycin	50	weak	0.4–0.6	7.5	0.5
Kanamycin	96	weak	0.6–0.8	7.5	0.5
Oxytetracycline	77	25	0.75	0.4–0.8	0.6–1.4
Tetracycline	64	36	1.25	0.4–0.8	0.6–1.4
Doxycycline	9.8	430	1.53	0.4–0.8	0.6–1.4

antibiotics with different rates of plasma protein binding but with close ionization and lipid solubility characteristics.

Vehicle

Since the nature of the vehicle is related to that of the active ingredient, it is therefore difficult to assess these two parameters separately. Both factors may interfere with the bioavailability of active ingredients and, consequently, influence the absorption rate of the drug at the site of injection and thus influence the plasma drug concentration and indirectly the milk drug concentration.

When colistin sulphate and colistin methane sulphonate are administered at the same dosage of 25 000 IU/kg, the mammary excretion of the first one differs from that of the second by (1) a longer withdrawal time (four milkings instead of two), (2) a higher maximum concentration in the milk (4.2 IU/ml instead of 1.74 IU/ml), and (3) a higher percentage of recovery of the administered dose (0.18% instead of 0.10%).

The influence of a sustained release salt on the elimination of an antibiotic in the milk is illustrated by the comparison of aqueous suspensions of procaine penicillin and benzathine penicillin. The duration of excretion of the latter persists for 34 milkings vs. eight milkings for the procaine penicillin.

The part played by the nature of the vehicle may be important. With glycerol-formal and glycols in aqueous vehicles, the excretion of oxytetracycline is of similar duration but the percentage of recovery is higher (0.40% vs. 0.23%) and thus the maximal concentration of the antibiotic in the milk reaches 1.14 parts/10^6 vs. 0.56 parts/10^6 with glycerol-formal.

When an oily vehicle was substituted for an aqueous one the duration of excretion of procaine penicillin was lengthened by one milking[1]. For an equal dosage (5 mg/kg), the replacement of an aqueous vehicle by an oily one had the following effects: the withdrawal time of tetracycline was lengthened (13 vs. five milkings), the maximum concentration in the milk decreased (0.31 vs. 1.24 parts/10^6, and the percentage of recovery of the administered dose declined (0.20% vs. 0.44%). By the intramammary route, the persistence of mastitis and drying-off formations in the udder also depends on the vehicle used in formulation.

TREATMENT

Dosage

The persistence of antibiotics increases when the administered dose augments. When the dosage of procaine penicillin was doubled (6×10^6 IU instead of 3 per cow), the withdrawal time[1] was increased by 33%. A similar study carried out with benzathine penicillin in an aqueous solution (20 000 IU/kg daily vs. 10 000) showed that the duration of excretion was nearly doubled (31 instead of 21 milkings).

For oxytetracycline as an aqueous solution, dosages of 5, 10 and 20 mg/kg require withdrawal times of four, six and ten milkings respectively. The maximal concentration of oxytetracycline in the milk was 0.75 parts/10^6 for 5 mg kg^{-1} day^{-1} and 1.85 parts/10^6 for 10 mg kg^{-1} day^{-1} (unpublished data). Similar results were obtained with neomycin[8].

Duration

Repeated administration of procaine penicillin in either an aqueous or an oily vehicle did not modify the duration of elimination of the antibiotic in the milk[10]. Our own results confirm the limited influence of this parameter on the excretion of antibiotics by the mammary gland. For example, the administration of an oxytetracycline formulation as an aqueous solution at a dose of 10 mg/kg for 1, 2 or 3 days, did not affect the duration of excretion of this antibiotic into the milk, the percentage of recovery (0.41%, 0.40% and 0.33%) and the maximal concentration in the milk (1.73, 1.79 and 1.57 parts/10^6.

However, an injection after 24 h of 10 000 IU/kg of benzathine penicillin as an oily suspension increases the withdrawal time by 50% (21 vs. 15 milkings).

It is thus possible to conclude that repeated parenteral administrations do not affect the mammary elimination of antibiotics so far as the absorption and plasma clearance are fairly quick. In contrast, the administration of sustained release drugs may prolong the duration of the elimination into the milk.

Route of administration

The route of administration directly influences the bioavailability of a veterinary drug and consequently the plasma concentration and the concentration in the milk.

The comparison of the elimination of antibiotics by the intramuscular and intramammary routes shows (Table 17.5) that, except for tetracycline, the

Table 17.5 Percentage of recovery during the withdrawal time indicated by number of milkings from the administered dose of antibiotics via the intramuscular (i.m.) and intramammary (i.ma.) routes

Antibiotic		*Dosage*	*Milkings number*	*Recovery %*	*Max. conc. parts/10⁶*
Penicillin procaine	i.m.	20×10^6 IU	7–8	0.01	0.17
	i.ma.	400×10^6 IU	6	15	86.1
Tetracycline	i.m.	3 g	11	0.30	0.22
	i.ma.	2.5 g	5	47	57.2
Dihydrostreptomycin	i.m.	20 g	2	0.1	1.3
	i.ma.	1.5 g	5	34	51.8
Colistin	i.m.	37.5×10^6 IU	4	0.18	4.5
	i.ma.	0.5×10^6 IU	3	20.9	25.8
Chloramphenicol	i.m.	8 g	1	0.08	0.9
	i.ma.	2 g	1	1.1	2.2

duration of elimination into the milk is nearly the same or higher when the antibiotic is administered by the intramammary route, even if the dose is lower[8]. However, the percentage of recovery, which depends on the drug formulation and the functional stage of the udder, differs with a ratio of 1500 for penicillin, 345 for dihydrostreptomycin, 150 for tetracycline, 100 for colistin and 10 for chloramphenicol. Similarly, the ratio of maximal concentration of antibiotics in the milk following intramammary vs. intramuscular administrations is 500 for penicillin, 260 for tetracycline, 40 for dihydrostreptomycin, 6 for colistin and 3 for chloramphenicol. The low percentage of recovery of chloramphenicol after intramammary injection (1.1% vs. 15 and 47% for other antibiotics) indicates a good resorption by the mammary gland, as already observed[5].

A high percentage of recovery after intramammary administration corresponds to a concentration of antibiotics hazardous for public health and the milk industry, especially for the manufacturing of yoghurts (Table 17.6).

The use of other criteria would provide a more sensitive detection of the impairment.

Table 17.6 Hazards for the milk industry. Maximum concentrations of antibiotics subsequent to the administration by the intramammary route, minimum concentration of antibiotics impairing the manufacture of yoghurts (IU/ml and parts/10^6)[4] and number of litres of milk to be discarded after contamination by a 10 litres milking

Antibiotic	*Maximum concentration*	*Minimum concentration*	*Litres*
Penicillin	86 IU/ml	0.01 IU/ml	86 000
Erythromycin	40 ppm	0.01 ppm	40 000
Tetracycline	57 ppm	0.1 ppm	5 700
Dihydrostreptomycin	52 ppm	1 ppm	520
Chloramphenicol	2 ppm	1 ppm	20

ANIMAL

Few studies have been devoted to the comparison of drug excretion in the main species bred for milk. The percentages of recovery were 0.016% and 0.012% for neomycin, 0.012% and 0.015% for kanamycin, for cows and ewes respectively[11]. Pharmacokinetic studies of penicillins and cephalosporins confirm the small difference between the two species. Nevertheless, data remain too fragmentary to allow any extrapolation from one species to another.

Following an *intramammary* application, a high milk yield is accompanied by a quicker elimination for penicillins and aminoglycosides[2]. As far as penicillin, dihydrostreptomycin, neomycin and tetracyclines are concerned, it seems that the functional stage of the udder is of importance (8.1%) regarding the absorption. For example, in the drying-off period, the absorption is slow but in the first postparturient months much faster absorption results in shorter persistence in the udder. The results obtained under laboratory conditions for penicillin, cloxacillin, dihydrostreptomycin, neomycin, tetracycline, chlortetracycline, chloramphenicol, colistin and bacitracin, do not suggest an influence of milk yield on either the duration of elimination or on the percentage of recovery.

After a *parenteral* administration, the influence of milk is well evidenced (Table 17.7). The results confirm those of Rasmussen on the influence of milk yield on the concentration of antibiotics[7]. The concentrations of a

Table 17.7 Influence of the milk yield on the quantity of antibiotics excreted by the mammary gland

Antibiotic	*Milk* (litres)	*Recovery* (%)	*Increase* (%)
Penicillin	11	0.011	
	18	0.016	+45
Ampicillin	8	0.003	
	14	0.007	+130
Dihydrostreptomycin	12	0.080	
	18	0.175	+120
Oxytetracycline	7.5	0.28	
	11	0.37	+30
Chloramphenicol	7	0.065	
	13	0.110	+70
Tylosin	8.5	0.37	
	14	0.91	+145
Spiramycin	9.5	5.4	
	16	10.1	+90
Colistin sulphate	6.5	0.17	
	11.5	0.24	+41
Colistin methane sulphonate	11.5	0.075	
	15.1	0.110	+46

parenterally administered sulphonamide are, however, the same in the milkings of quarters containing 45, 85, 150, or 3200 ml of milk. The quick and bidirectional diffusion between plasma and milk together with the important vascular perfusion of a lactating udder might explain the lack of effect of the level of milk yield on the drug concentration[13].

The influence of a *pathological state* on the mammary excretion of drugs is of paramount importance, since many pharmacokinetic studies are carried out on healthy animals while drugs are used in diseases when more or less impairment of functions is involved in the fate of drugs. The modifications of intestinal resorption and biliary or renal excretion will not be studied here. In spite of their importance for the assessment of the elimination of antibiotics into the milk and the determination of withdrawal times, they do not seem to affect the mechanism of mammary excretion but the persistence of residues due to the modification of plasma concentration–time curve. It must be noted, however, that for some antibiotics (cephalexin, lincomycin, clindamycin and chloramphenicol), a decrease in plasma concentrations may augment for these products the rate of passage through the biological membranes[11]. In contrast, the exchanges between the mammary gland and the blood are severely impaired in the case of *mastitis*. During udder inflammation the functional integrity of the lipoid barrier may be temporarily deranged, leading to an accelerated leakage of drugs into the circulatory system. It was also proved that the rate of binding of most antibiotics to milk proteins (benzylpenicillin, tetracycline and chloramphenicol) rose from 10% in normal milk to 25% in the milk of the mastitis case, a value near to the rate of plasma protein binding (32–37%) of these substances[13].

In addition, the change in *the pH of milk* varying from 6.6 for a normal milk to 7.4 in the case of mastitis affects the non-ionic passive diffusion of antibiotics. However, this variation will not influence the antibiotics which have an acid-type, such as those belonging to the lactam group, since their pK_a are far from this range of pH. Both van Os *et al.*[9] in the cow and Ziv *et al.*[14] in the ewe have recorded a small lengthening of the withdrawal time in the case of mastitis. For several penicillins injected intramuscularly to healthy and unhealthy animals, no significant differences were recorded in the percentages of recovery in milk and in the ratio of concentrations in both serum and milk. In contrast, the mammary excretion of weak bases such as macrolides which have a pK_a between 7 and 9 is severely impaired. These products, which are usually weakly ionized in the plasma (pH 7.4), diffuse easily into the udder because of their high lipid solubility. The accumulation of some antibiotics in the udder is related to a limited back diffusion. For example, clindamycin (a macrolide-related antibiotic), tylosin and erythromycin diffuse back easily but not spiramycin which is highly protein-bound. Thus, only spiramycin accumulates in milk.

As shown in Table 17.8 the ratio of the areas under the curve in serum and milk has an average growth for most antibiotics. Accordingly, the percentage of recovery of the administered dose in the milk decreases. In contrast, the mammary excretion of aminoglycosides and colistin, which behave as weak bases, is unmodified because of their low solubility in lipids and hence poor ability to penetrate the mammary gland. Finally, amphoteric or non-ionized

Table 17.8 Pharmacokinetic parameters for antibiotics administered by the intramammary route to healthy and mastitic cows[12]

Antibiotic	*AUC*	*Milk Serum*	*Recovery (%)*	
	normal	*mastitis*	*normal*	*mastitis*
Penicillin G	20	5	0.001	0.001
Cloxacillin	15	55	0.001	0.001
Ampicillin	3	3	0.08	0.10
Cephaloridine	5	4	0.001	0.001
Streptomycin	25	15	0.001	0.001
Neomycin	30	20	0.02	0.02
Kanamycin	10	8	0.02	0.03
Gentamicin	15	8	0.006	0.01
Colistin	8	3	0.001	0.001
Erythromycin	0.1	0.4	3.80	2.20
Tylosin	0.3	0.5	2.60	1.40
Spiramycin	0.2	0.4	6.80	2.40
Lincomycin	0.3	0.5	1.40	0.80
Chloramphenicol	2	2	0.10	0.10
Oxytetracycline	3	2	0.07	0.08
Doxycycline	2	2	0.15	0.15

antibiotics are not affected by the modification of the milk pH and thus their mammary excretion is not impaired.

CONCLUSIONS

The above results show that the process of non-ionic passive diffusion explains the major part of the mechanism of drug mammary excretion.

The elimination of antibiotics into the milk depends firstly on the nature of the formulation. The percentage of ionization and lipid solubility are predominant regarding the rate of plasma and milk bindings. The penetration of parenteral drug formulations into the mammary gland by passive diffusion depends on their blood concentration and any modification in their bioavailability alters their mammary excretion. In the case of a sustained release, the elimination is linked to the nature of the salt of the active ingredient and to the vehicle composition.

An increase in the dosage regimen generally increases both the withdrawal times and the maximal concentration of antibiotics in milk while repetition of treatment modifies only slightly the mechanism of mammary excretion. The intramammary administration of drugs leads to high concentrations, hence serious hazards to the public health and the milk industry. The volume of milk seems to exert an influence but on the overall quantity of antibiotics eliminated in the milk. In contrast, the duration of elimination and the drug concentration in the milk after parenteral application are not modified.

The mechanism of mammary excretion is largely influenced by the pathological states of the body as well as of the udder. The smaller difference of pH between the milk and plasma in the case of mastitis reduces the concentration of macrolides by ion entrapment, an example of the influence of the ionization rate of the antibiotics on their bidirectional non-ionic passive diffusion between blood and milk.

References

1. Blobel, H. and Burch, C. W. (1960). Concentrations of penicillin in milk of cows following intramuscular administration. *J. Am. Vet. Med. Assoc.*, **136**, 477–80
2. Mercer, H. D., Geleta, J. N., Schultz, E. J. *et al.* (1970). Milk out rates for antibiotics in intramammary infusion products used in the treatment of bovine mastitis: relationship of somatic cells counts, milk production level and drug vehicle. *Am. J. Vet. Res.*, **31**, 1549–60
3. Miller, G. E., Banerjee, N. C. and Stowe, C. M. (1967). Diffusion of certain weak organic acids and bases across the bovine mammary gland membrane after systemic administration. *J. Pharmacol. Exp. Ther.*, **157**, 245–53
4. Mourot, D. and Loussouarn, S. (1981). Sensibilité des ferments lactiques aux antibiotiques utilisés en médecine vétérinaire. *Rec. Méd. Vét.*, **157**, 175–7
5. Nouws, J. F. M. and Ziv, G. (1982). Pharmacological aspects of chloramphenicol administration by the intramammary route to lactating dairy cows. *Vet. Q.*, **4**, 23–31
6. Rasmussen, F. (1969). Active mammary excretion of N4 acetylated p. aminohippuric acid. *Acta Vet. Scand.*, **10**, 193–4
7. Rasmussen, F. (1971). Excretion of drugs by milk. In Brodie, B. B. and Gilette, J. R. (eds.) *Handbook of Experimental Pharmacology*. Vol. 28, pp. 390–402. (Berlin: Springer)
8. Siddique, J. H., Loken, K. I. and Hoyt, H. H. (1965). Concentrations of neomycine, dihydrostreptomycine and polymyxine in milk after intramuscular or intramammary administration. *J. Am. Vet. Med. Assoc.*, **146**, 594–9
9. van Os, J. L., Buitelaarj, W. and Goudswaard, J. (1974). Intramuscular treatment of bovine mastitis with various penicillin. Penicillin concentration in the milk. *Tijdschr. Diergeneesk.*, **99**, 114–22
10. Wright, W. W. and Harold, L. C. (1960). Antibiotic residues in milk. *J. Am. Vet. Med. Assoc.*, **137**, 525–33
11. Ziv, G. and Sulman, F. G. (1972). Binding of antibiotics to bovine and ovine serum. *Antimicrob. Agents Chemother.*, **2**, 206–13
12. Ziv, G., Gordin, S., Bachar, G. *et al.* (1973). Concentration and persistence of antibiotics in milk following intramammary infusion in cows. *Refuah Vet.*, **30**, 85–100
13. Ziv, G., Bogine, E., Shoni, J. and Sulman, F. G. (1974). Penetration of radioactive labelled antibiotics from blood serum into milk in normal and mastitic ewes. *Ann. Rech. Vet.*, **5**, 15–28

18
Pharmacology of uterine motility and relaxation

O. Kern and H. Schill

Uterine motor activity is regulated in particular by hormonal mechanisms, but neural or neurohormonal mechanisms are also involved. A selective effect on these mechanisms can be achieved by the exogenous administration of substances with a pharmacodynamic action.

MOTOR ACTIVITY IN THE OESTRUS CYCLE

The response of the myometrium to exogenous or endogenous pharmacodynamic stimuli is largely dependent on whether oestrogens or progesterone predominate. Up to the pro-oestrus period no or only ineffectual uterine contractions are observed. As oestrogen production increases, pronounced uterine contractions begin, first from the oviduct towards the cervix, and then from the cervix towards the oviduct depending upon the ratio of oestrogen to progesterone. The contractions may be inhibited by adrenaline and increased by oxytocin[30]. Figure 18.1 shows electromyograms as examples of the influence of hormonal status on uterine motility and the effect of oxytocin[23].

During the oestrous cycle, sheep exhibit similar motor activity of the uterus and Fallopian tubes to that of cattle[25], and the threshold response to oxytocin during oestrus is reduced to one tenth of that found during the dioestrus period[24].

MOTOR ACTIVITY AND UTERINE RESPONSE DURING PREGNANCY

Progesterone inhibits the readiness of the smooth musculature of the uterus to contract (protection of pregnancy). This changes when the progesterone level exhibits a rapid decrease (from about 36 h) while oestrogens increase (from approximately the tenth day) before delivery.

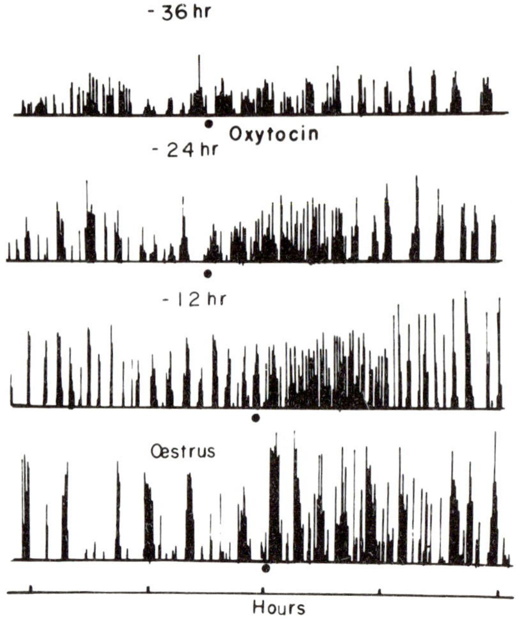

Figure 18.1 Integrated records of uterine activity and effects of oxytocin in the cow. The short phases seen 24 h before oestrus are progressively replaced by prolonged phases of activity during oestrus. Their strength and number are doubled following injection of oxytocin (from ref. 23)

For example, in the rat the ability of the uterus to react to oxytocin exhibits a very sharp increase shortly before delivery, reaching one thousand times that found during pregnancy[15].

The results of numerous investigations in different animal species and in man support the view that α- and β-receptors are present in the uterus, and also that the relationship of these to each other is species-specific (Review in ref. 18). For example, in isolated strips of muscle from non-pregnant uteri and those in the early stages of pregnancy, a functional predominance of β-receptors was observed in the cow, and of α-receptors in the mare. In later pregnancy, β-receptors predominate in both species[19].

Experiments in rabbits demonstrate the effect of sex hormones. Administration of oestrogen brings about a pronounced increase in the number of α-receptors but only a slight increase in β-receptors. Subsequent treatment with progesterone reverses these changes[22].

PERINATAL MOTOR ACTIVITY

In ruminants, labour is initiated when the secretion of fetal adrenocortical hormones commences. In cattle and goats, fetal corticosteroids stimulate the synthesis of $PGF_{2\alpha}$ in the chorion and endometrium, which abolishes the protective effect of progesterone by luteolysis of the corpus luteum of pregnancy; in sheep this takes place due to the sharp increase in oestrogens shortly before delivery[26].

Prepartum changes in the sex hormone status enable the uterus to react adequately to oxytocin. In cattle (as in horses, sheep and goats), the oxytocin plasma level does not increase until second stage labour, as soon as the fetus enters the cervix and vagina[9]. As a result of stimulation of the dorsal pressure receptors by the fetal head, a reflex increase in oxytocin release occurs (Ferguson reflex). This brings about an increase in uterine contractions, which have been initiated previously by other mechanisms.

During labour, four receptors are of considerable pharmacotherapeutic importance[16]: oxytocin, prostaglandin and α-adrenergic receptors for stimulation of motor activity, and β-adrenergic receptors for inhibition of motor activity.

The β-adrenergic agents which bring about tocolysis (relaxation of the myometrium) have recently gained increasing importance in veterinary medicine[14,16]. Their effect on the uterus and interactions with ecbolic substances will therefore be examined in greater detail.

For uterine smooth muscle relaxation, β-adrenergic agents which principally affect β_2-receptors are required, so that the undesirable cardiac (β_1) effect remains insignificant in comparison to the desired tocolytic effect[10]. N-AB 365 (clenbuterol, Planipart®) is a new specific β_2-adrenergic agent of this type.

In the following discussion, some pharmacological and clinical effects will be demonstrated, mainly by using this substance as an example.

PHARMACOLOGICAL BASIS OF TOCOLYSIS

At the time of a normal delivery the uterus is oestrogen-dominated. The effect of a β-adrenergic agent on the uterus which is contracting under the influence of oestrogen and oxytocin is therefore important. β-adrenergic agents, given beforehand, antagonize oxytocin-induced spasm of the isolated uterine horn of the rat in oestrus. In this type of comparative study with other substances (isoprenaline, orciprenaline, salbutamol), N-AB 365 has been shown to have a superior effect. In addition, after a single immersion of uterine tissue in an organ bath, N-AB 365 was found to be 'difficult to flush out'. This indicates pronounced binding of the substance to the β_2-receptors of the uterine musculature, thus suggesting a prolonged duration of action[8].

Using the same experimental model, N-AB 365 was also found to be far superior to other substances as an inhibitor of uterine motility. The mean minimum concentration (ng/ml) of the substance which brings about complete inhibition of spontaneous motility of the rat uterus *in vitro* was 3.9 ± 3.5 for clenbuterol vs. 59.2 ± 34.1 for ritodrine and 142.8 ± 65.8 for isoxsuprine[20].

Another feature of N-AB 365, besides its prolonged duration of action, is its extremely good absorption following oral administration[8] (Table 18.1).

However, the antagonistic effect of N-AB 365 on oxytocin is not absolute. The degree of this effect is dependent on the relationship between the relative

Table 18.1 Effect on inhibition of oxytocin-induced spasm of the rat uterus in oestrus (from ref. 8)

	Intravenous ED_{50} (μg/kg)	*Intraduodenal* ED_{50} (μg/kg)
Clenbuterol	7.0	7.0
Isoprenaline	0.9	2347
Orciprenaline	29.6	9600
Salbutamol	5.3	840

doses of oxytocin and N-AB 365. This was also confirmed when it was used in cattle (see below).

TOCOLYTIC EFFECT OF N-AB 365 IN CATTLE

Intramuscular or oral doses of between 200 and 400 μg/animal are used to abolish uterine activity during parturition in cattle (equivalent to about 0.3–0.4 to 0.6–0.8 μg N-AB 365/kg body weight). From the point of view of side-effects, these doses are harmless, even when given intravenously[1,4]. Following a dose of 0.6 μg/kg, transitory cardiovascular effects were observed only in the e.c.g. These were of no quantitative clinical importance even after 1.5 μg/kg, so that no clinical effect on the heart or circulation was apparent.

The duration of the tocolytic effect during parturition is dependent on the dose and on the position of the fetus. It can be prolonged by repeated administration, if the next dose is given when uterine contractions recommence[1]. Depending on the position of the fetus at the time of injection, delivery was completed after an average of 4–7.25 h (200 μg) or an average of 7.5–12.7 h (400 μg). Following doses of 2× and 3×200 μg/animal, parturition was not completed for 14.2 and 19 h respectively. It was also observed that during abolition of uterine activity with N-AB 365, purely passive dilation of the cervical canal continued. In two cases in which four doses of 400 μg were given orally at intervals of 10–14 h, delivery was delayed to such an extent that it took place spontaneously 53 and 53.5 h after the first treatment. After abolition of uterine activity the animals began to eat and ruminate again.

After a dose of 300 μg N-AB 365/cow, given intramuscularly when the cervix was 2–4 cm dilated, uterine contractions were suppressed for about 8 h and delivery was delayed by approximately 5.5 h compared with the controls[5] (Table 18.2).

Tocographic investigations were performed using pressure detectors and electrodes implanted in the myometrium of seven cattle during labour in which expulsive contractions had already started. Shortly after a single intravenous administration of 150–300 μg N-AB 365, an initial decrease in the frequency of contractions occurred, followed by their complete cessation[32]. Abolition of uterine activity persisted for at least 3.25 h, despite intravenous administration (Figure 18.2). Dilation of the cervix continued during tocolysis.

Table 18.2 Retardation of delivery by intramuscular administration of 300 μg N-AB 365/cow, in relation to the stage of labour (from ref. 5)

Stage of dilation	*N-AB 365 per animal*	*No. of animals*	*Interval between examination and completion of parturition Mean ± Range* (h)
Control			
cervix 3 cm		10	2.72 (±0.7)
cervix 4 cm		10	2.63 (±0.55)
rupture of membranes		10	2.25 (±0.18)
Treated			
cervix 2 cm	300 μg	5	8.1 (±0.58)
cervix 3 cm	300 μg	20	8.07 (±0.9)
cervix 4 cm	300 μg	21	7.92 (±0.92)
calf in cervical canal	300 μg	8	6.23 (±1.65)

The results from Italy[5] were confirmed by a study carried out in Ireland[11] in 100 treated and 55 control cows (Table 18.3). If treatment was given at the time when the cervix was dilated to the width of the whole hand, delivery took place at an average of at least 5.2 h later in the treated animals than in the controls. If parts of the fetus had already passed through the cervix, an average delay of only about 2 h occurred.

Several clinical investigators attempted to avoid night-time deliveries by means of a double administration. The cows were treated with 400 μg and 200 μg N-AB 365 intramuscularly or orally[6], or with 2×400 μg N-AB 365 orally[2], at an interval of 4 h (at about 18.00 and 22.00 hours), if the stockman

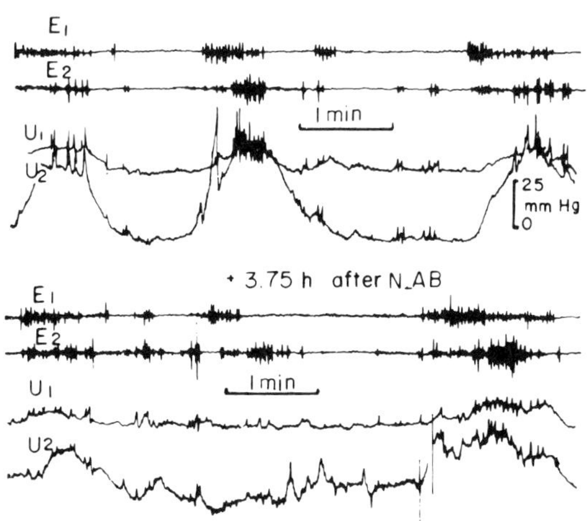

Figure 18.2 Electrical (E) and mechanical (U) activity of the myometrium during second stage labour (above) and subsequent complete cessation of contractions (below). Recordings taken before and 3.75 h after i.v. injection of 300 μg N-AB 365 (from ref. 32)

Table 18.3 Retardation of delivery in cows by intramuscular treatment with 300 μg N-AB 365/animal, in relation to the stage of labour (from ref. 11)

Dilation of cervix	*No. of animals (*treated)*	*Av. interval from exam./treatment to delivery* (h)	*Range of deviation* (h)	*Difference in mean values between treated animals and controls* (h)
2 fingers	32*	23.4	5–43	+9.8
	11	13.6	4.5–25.5	—
3–4 fingers	40*	14.2	4–25	+7.5
	12	6.7	1–17.5	—
whole hand	19*	9.9	2.5–31.5	+5.2
	16	4.7	1–9	—
fetus partway through cervix	9*	5.2	1–13	+1.9
	16	3.3	1–6	—

believed that delivery was to be expected during the following night. The majority of the animals calved after 06.00 hours the next morning.

An even better result was achieved using a single intramuscular injection of 300 μg N-AB 365 at between 23.00 and 24.00 hours[11]. The injection was given if, judging by the external signs of imminent parturition, the stockman expected delivery to take place during the next 12 h. Only one out of 127 treated animals calved sooner than 7 h after treatment (at 05.30 hours), and only three animals calved between 06.00 and 07.00 hours. Nine animals did not calve after the first injection; they were treated a second time 24–96 h later.

Several authors[2,6,12,31] agreed that deliveries were easier after tocolysis, and one investigator[21] also reported a reduction in the duration of the second stage.

A favourable secondary finding on farms with a very high percentage of non-infectious retained placenta (30–60%) was obtained after administration of N-AB 365, namely spontaneous delivery of the placenta in 20 animals[2] and a reduction in the incidence of retained placenta to 5% in about 100 animals[29].

The clinical use of N-AB 365 for the relaxation of the uterus in obstetrics and in embryo transfer will not be presented herein.

ANTAGONISM TO OXYTOCIN

The interaction of N-AB 365 and oxytocin at the time of delivery is dependent on which substance at what dose first reaches its maximum effect, and at what point afterwards and at what dose the second substance is administered (Figure 18.3). Given 25 min after 300 μg N-AB 365, 20 IU oxytocin does not result in the re-establishment of contractions[27]. Given 1 h after 300 μg N-AB 365, 60 IU oxytocin brings about renewed contractions 15–20 min later[3].

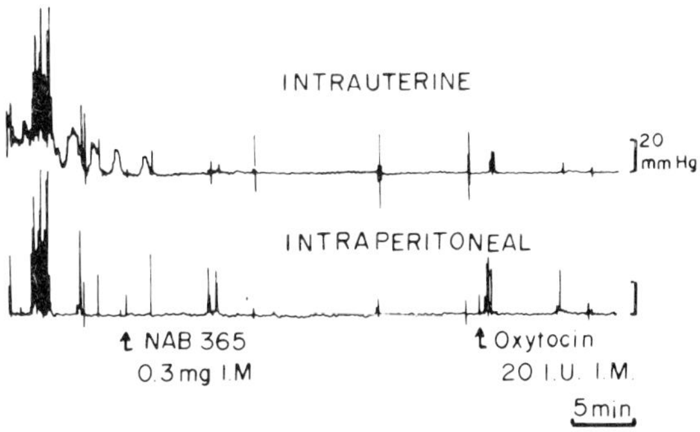

Figure 18.3 Pressure recordings during the first stage of labour in a cow showing the effect of N-AB 365 blocking uterine contractions and the lack of response to oxytocin (from ref. 27)

Oxytocin is ineffective when given shortly after the full effect of N-AB 365 is established. It increasingly regains its efficacy the later it is given after the time of administration of N-AB 365. If normal doses of oxytocin are given towards the end of tocolysis, they are sufficient to increase uterine contractions. Conversely, an oxytocin injection given immediately beforehand can prevent, or at least diminish[32], the effect of N-AB 365.

ANTAGONISM TO PROSTAGLANDIN $F_{2\alpha}$

According to results obtained in human medicine, β_2-adrenergic agents bring about dose-dependent partial or total inhibition of uterine contractions in women, even in labour or abortion induced by $PGF_{2\alpha}$. The tocolytic effect extends both to the basal tone and to the intensity and frequency of contractions of the myometrium[13, 17]. Similar reactions are expected in cows, but no experimental results using N-AB 365 are so far available.

ANTAGONISM TO β-ADRENERGIC BLOCKING AGENTS

β-adrenergic blocking agents are substances which prevent the effect of β-sympathomimetics on β-adrenergic receptors. The mechanism of action is based on competitive displacement[10]. Thus, the relative dose of the substances with opposing effects is of great importance as shown by the following example using isoproterenol (isoprenaline) and propranolol in the rat uterus *in situ*[7] (Figure 18.4).

In laboratory tests in the rat uterus *in situ*, the tocolytic effect of 10 μg N-AB 365/kg was abolished by various β-adrenergic blocking agents. (ED_{50} doses: propranolol, 6.6; pindolol, 1.8; toliprolol, 29.0 μg/kg intravenously[8].)

The tocolytic effect of N-AB 365 can be overridden in pregnant women also, by propranolol for example[28].

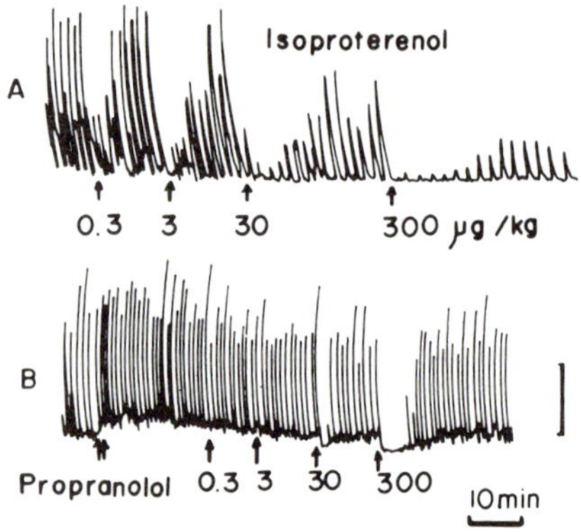

Figure 18.4 Effects of 0.3, 3, 30 and 300 μg/kg of isoproterenol in the absence (A) and in the presence (B) of an adrenergic β-blocker (1.5 mg/kg of propranolol) on the rat uterus *in situ* (from ref. 7)

Thus, it also may be possible in cattle to overcome the tocolysis due to N-AB 365 by using a suitable β-adrenergic blocking agent. However, bunitrolol, for example, does not appear to be suitable for this, either in cattle or in sheep or pigs[32].

ANTAGONISTIC EFFECT OF ERGOT ALKALOIDS

The form of administration of ergot alkaloids may be of particular importance. Investigations in ten cows in which caesarean section was performed after intramuscular administration of 300 μg N-AB 365 showed the following results. When 5 mg methylergometrine were injected into the uterine musculature at several sites, following delivery of the fetus and suture of the uterus (45–105 min after Planipart), local contractions were observed in the injection area within 15 min. Within 20 min, contraction of the pregnant uterine horn and, in eight cases, of the whole uterus was observed[3].

In contrast, no increase in contractility was achieved following parenteral administration of ergometrine maleate (5–20 mg) in 12 cows during the postpartum period (1st–14th day after parturition)[31]. No abolition of the effect of Planipart can therefore be expected following parenteral administration of ergometrine.

References

1. Arbeiter, K. and Thurnher, M. (1977). Über die Wirkung des Sympathikomimetikums Planipart[R] (N-AB 365) auf den Geburtsablauf beim Rind. *Tierärztl. Umschau*, **32**, 423–7
2. Arbeiter, K. and Holler, W. (1980). Zur protrahierten und induzierten Geburt beim Rind. In *11th International Congress on Diseases of Cattle*, Tel Aviv, Oct. 20–23. Vol. 2, pp. 1070–80. (Haifa: Bregman Press)
3. Arbeiter, K. (1980). Personal communication
4. Ballarini, G. and Zannetti, G. (1977). Klinisch-pharmakologische Befunde bei der Anwendung des beta-2-Mimetikums Clenbuterol beim Rind. *Clin. Vet.*, **100**, 671–6
5. Ballarini, G. (1978). Erste Untersuchungen zur klinischen Pharmakologie und zur pharmakologischen Tokolyse mit dem β-Mimetikum N-AB 365 (Planipart[R]) bei Kühen. *Tierärztl. Umschau*, **33**, 421–7

6. Ballarini, G. (1980). Suppression chez les bovins des mises bas nocturnes au moyen de deux applications du tocolytique N-AB 365 (Planipart). In *11th International Congress on Diseases of Cattle*, Tel Aviv, Oct. 20–23. Vol. 2, pp. 1081–6. (Haifa: Bregman Press)
7. Ban, T. (1974). A quantitative study on the effects of isoproterenol and beta-adrenergic blocking agents in the rat uterus *in situ*. *Arzneim.-Forsch.*, **24**, 179–81
8. Engelhardt, G. (1976). Pharmakologisches Wirkungsprofil von N-AB 365 (Clenbuterol), einem neuen Broncholytikum mit einer selektiven Wirkung auf die adrenergen β_2-Rezeptoren. *Arzneim.-Forsch.*, **26**, 1404–20
9. Fitzpatrick, R. J. (1966). The posterior pituitary gland and the female reproductive tract. In Harris, G. W. and Donovan, B. T. (eds.) *The Pituitary Gland.* (London: Butterworth)
10. Forth, W., Henschler, D. and Rummel, W. (1975). *Allgemeine und spezielle Pharmakologie und Toxikologie.* (Zürich: Verlag Bibliographisches Institut AG)
11. Greene, H. J. (1981). Clinical study of the use of Clenbuterol for postponing parturition in cows. *Vet. Rec.*, **109**, 283–5
12. Grunert, E. and Verhülsdonk, M. (1980). Untersuchungen über die verzögerung des Geburtstermins beim Rind durch das β_2-Mimetikum Planipart[R]. In *11th International Congress on Diseases of Cattle*, Tel Aviv, Oct. 20–23. Vol. 2, pp. 1087–97. (Haifa: Bregman Press)
13. Herberger, J., Steyer, M., Poleska, W. *et al.* (1976). Inhibition of prostaglandin-induced labor at term and prostaglandin-induced abortion in first trimester pregnancies. In *8th World Congress—Gynecology and Obstetrics*, Mexico, Oct. 17–22. Excerpta Medica 123, Abstract 252
14. Kern, O. (1977). Tierärztliche Nutzung jüngerer Ergebnisse der Pharmaforschung für Biotechnik und Therapie am Beispiel des Clenbuterol (N-AB 365). *Tierärztl. Umschau*, **32**, 245–53
15. Kuriyama, H. and Suzuki, H. (1976). Effects of prostaglandin E_2 and oxytocin in the electrical activity of hormone-treated and pregnant rat myometria. *J. Physiol.*, **260**, 335–49
16. Lehmann, H. D. (1978). Pharmakologie und Uterusmotorik. *Prakt. Tierärzt*, **59**, 930–8
17. Lindmark, G., Melander, S., Nilsson, B. A. *et al.* (1973). Inhibition of prostaglandin induced uterine activity in the second trimester of pregnancy by β-mimetic adrenergic agents. *Prostaglandins*, **3**, 481–9
18. Miller, J. W. (1967). Adrenergic receptors in the myometrium. *Ann. NY Acad. Sci.*, **139**, 788–98
19. Mitolo-Chieppa, D., Minoia, P., Renna, G. *et al.* (1977). α- und β-Rezeptoren der Uterusmuskulatur von Rind und Pferd. *Atti Soc. Ital. Sci. Vet.*, **31**, 443–4
20. Mitolo-Chieppa, D., Lograno, M. D., Carratù, R. *et al.* (1979). Tokolytische Wirksamkeit des Clenbuterol am Rattenuterus *in vitro*. *Riv. Farmacol. Ter.*, **10**, 259–63
21. Rice, L. E. (1981). Personal communication
22. Roberts, J. M., Insel, P. A., Goldfien, R. D. *et al.* (1977). α-adrenoreceptors but no β-adrenoreceptors increase in rabbit with oestrogen. *Nature (London)*, **270**, 624–5
23. Ruckebusch, Y. and Bayard, F. (1975). Motility of the oviduct and uterus of the cow during the oestrus cycle. *J. Reprod. Fert.*, **43**, 23–32
24. Ruckebusch, Y. and Pichot, D. (1975). Effects of adrenergic drugs on sheep oviduct motility. *Eur. J. Pharmacol.*, **33**, 193–6
25. Ruckebusch, Y. and Babapour, V. (1976). La motricité utéro-tubaire au cours du cycle oestral chez les ruminants. *Rev. Méd. Vét.*, **127**, 431–45
26. Rüsse, M. W. and Grunert, E. (1976). In Rosenberg, G. and Tillmann, H. (eds.) *Tiergeburtshilfe*. p. 126. (Berlin and Hamburg: Verlag Paul Parey)
27. Welch, R. A. S. (1979). Personal communication
28. Zahn, V. and Krumbachner, G. (1981). Clenbuterol – a long term uterine relaxant. *J. Perinat. Med.*, **9**, 96–100
29. Zebracki, A. (1980). Personal communication
30. Zerobin, K. (1976). In Scheunert, A., Trautmann, A. (eds.) *Lehrbuch der Veterinär-Physiologie*. pp. 748. (Berlin and Hamburg: Verlag Paul Parey)
31. Zerobin, K. (1980). Die uterusmotorischen Abläufe während Geburt und Puerperium beim Rind und deren Beeinflußbarkeit. In *11th International Congress on Diseases of Cattle*, Tel Aviv, Oct. 20–23. Vol. 2, pp. 1156–64. (Haifa: Bregman Press)
32. Zerobin, K. and Kündig, H. (1980). The control of myometrial functions during parturition with a β_2-mimetic compound, Planipart. *Theriogenology*, **14**, 21–35

19
New prostaglandins: present studies and future

R. C. Herschler, J. S. Kent and R. V. Tomlinson

The primary use of prostaglandin $F_{2\alpha}$ and its analogues is as luteolytic agents in cattle, sheep, goats and swine. As with any compound, the efficacy of a particular prostaglandin is dependent upon its inherent potency, formulation, route of administration and metabolic profile. These parameters had a marked influence on the development of fenprostalene, a new $PGF_{2\alpha}$ analogue.

In cattle, the maintenance of pregnancy is dependent upon progesterone derived from the corpus luteum until approximately 163 days of gestation[4]. After this stage of pregnancy, there is a luteo-placental shift in progesterone production and the pregnancy is no longer dependent on progesterone production by the corpus luteum. Thus, cows and heifers pregnant 150 days or less make ideal models for determining the luteolytic activity of a prostaglandin.

INHERENT POTENCY

Laboratory studies indicated that fenprostalene was approximately 750 times more luteolytic than the naturally occurring $PGF_{2\alpha}$ when administered subcutaneously as an aqueous solution to pregnant hamsters.

Studies in cattle revealed that doses of 1.25, 1.75 and 3.0 mg of fenprostalene caused abortion rates of 85, 54 and 69%, respectively (Table 19.1). Such abortion rates would indicate that all of the doses were at the plateau of the dose-response curve and that higher levels of the aqueous solution would not increase luteolysis. However, when the 3.0 mg dose was administered as two 1.5 mg doses of fenprostalene 48 h apart, the abortion rate rose from 69% to 100% in heifers pregnant 100 days or less. In animals pregnant over 150 days, the abortion rate was 50%. In the same study, five heifers, pregnant 120–196 days, received 3.0 mg of aqueous fenprostalene solution by continuous intravenous infusion at a rate of 50 μg/h for 60 h.

Table 19.1 Dose results with aqueous fenprostalene

Group no.	*Dose* (mg)	*No. of animals*	*Abortion rate* (%)	*Mean days pregnant*	*Time to abortion* (h)
1	1.25	13	85	115	11 ± 11
2	1.75	13	54	110	11 ± 8
3	3.0	13	69	107	5 ± 1
4	1.5 (2 ×)	15	100	90	3 ± 1
5	3.0*	5	100	154	5 ± 3

*60 hours infusion

All aborted within 2–8 days after the start of the infusion. These results clearly show that sustaining an effective biological halflife is more important than the total dose of prostaglandin. In addition, fenprostalene may have a mechanism of action other than luteolysis which causes abortion in animals pregnant over 150 days.

FORMULATION

Two studies were conducted to titrate the release rate of fenprostalene over a fixed period of time necessary to result in maximum luteolysis. Luteolysis was determined by measuring both the blood plasma progesterone levels and abortion rates. Osmotic minipumps (Alzet® osmotic minipumps, Alza Corporation, Palo Alto, CA 94304) were filled with various concentrations of aqueous fenprostalene designed to release 7, 21, 42 and 83 μg/h for 72 h amounting to total doses of 0.5, 1.5, 3 and 6 mg, respectively. All pumps were subcutaneously implanted. The release rate of 42 μg/h resulted in 100% luteolysis (Table 19.2). Since it is more difficult to design a formulation that releases drug over 72 h than 24 h, it was important to determine if a 24 h release rate would also result in acceptable luteolysis. In addition, drug delivery rate and duration of release are important to reduce drug dose and

Table 19.2 Summary of results obtained with various release rates of aqueous fenprostalene

Group no.	*No. of animals*	*Release rates* (μg/h)	*Total dose* (mg)	*Mean days pregnant*	*Days to abortion*	*Abortion rate* (%)
1*	13	7	0.5	89	5.5	69
2*	13	21	1.5	100	4.5	85
3*	13	42	3.0	102	3.8	100
4*	13	83	6.0	100	3.7	92
5†	6	21	0.5	92	3	83
6†	9	42	1.0	82	3.5	100
7†	9	83	2.0	81	3	100

*Duration of release in these groups was 72 h.
†Duration of release in these groups was 24 h.

Table 19.3 Average plasma concentrations (ng eq/ml) following single dose of fenprostalene in heifers

Time (h)	*Formulations* *A*	*B*	*C*	*D*	*E*	*F*
2	0.13	0.20	0.13	0.63	0.75	0.90
4	0.20	0.34	0.23	0.54	0.56	0.67
6	0.18	0.29	0.14	0.37	0.35	0.43
8	0.21	0.29	0.16	0.39	0.32	0.35
12	0.13	0.27	0.12	0.24	0.20	0.17
24	0.12	0.13	0.09	0.12	0.14	0.07
36	0.05	0.08	0.06	0.04	0.08	0.04
48	0.05	0.09	0.04	0.03	0.12	0.04
72	0.04	0.08	0.05	0.04	0.10	0.03
96	0.04	0.06	0.03	0.02	0.08	0.02

Formulations: *A* – Propylene glycol, s.c.; *B* – PEG 400, s.c.; *C* – 84.3% Glycerin, s.c.; *D* – Aqueous buffer, s.c.; *E* – PEG 400, i.m.; *F* – Aqueous buffer, i.m.

decrease or eliminate potential side-effects. Therefore, a second study was performed using release rates of 21, 42 and 83 μg/h, which resulted in total doses of 0.5, 1.0 and 2.0 mg, respectively, over a 24 h period of time. Abortion rates and plasma progesterone levels indicated that the dose-response plateau was again reached at 42 μg/h.

Although the minimum duration of the 42 μg/h release rate was not established, it was not practical to pursue this parameter further and formulation studies were begun.

Early formulation studies compared [13,14,-^{3}H]-fenprostalene in buffered saline, polyethylene glycol 400 (USP), 100% glycerin (USP) and propylene glycol (USP). Subcutaneous administration of these formulations to heifers revealed that absorption was slow from all vehicles, except the aqueous buffer (Table 19.3). Based on the urinary excretion rate (Table 19.4), the relative release rates from slowest to most rapid are propylene glycol, polyethylene glycol 400, glycerin, and aqueous buffer. The net result was an increase of the biological halflife to approximately 24 h. Polyethylene glycol 400 was selected for further development because it is well-tolerated upon subcutaneous injection in cattle.

Table 19.4 Urinary recovery of 13,14,^{3}H-fenprostalene in heifers

Formulation	*Route of administration*	*% of 0–72 h total* 0–24	24–48	48–72	*% of dose* 0–72
A	s.c.	83.2	16.0	0.8	62.6
B	s.c.	85.1	13.9	1.0	65.3
C	s.c.	89.0	10.7	0.3	57.2
D	s.c.	96.9	2.8	0.2	72.6
E	i.m.	94.6	5.2	0.1	70.9
F	i.m.	98.7	1.0	0.4	80.8

Formulations: A – Propylene glycol; B – PEG 400; C – 84.3% Glycerin; D – Aqueous buffer; E – PEG 400; F – Aqueous buffer

ROUTE OF ADMINISTRATION

The effect that the route of administration has on the plasma absorption profile and urinary excretion is shown in Tables 19.3 and 19.4. The polyethylene glycol 400 formulation administered intramuscularly is rapidly absorbed by the very vascular muscle tissue and excreted nearly as fast as aqueous formulations, thus decreasing its biological halflife.

METABOLISM

Another factor influencing a drug's efficacy, in addition to inherent activity, formulation and route of administration, is the effect that structural modifications exert on its metabolic disposition. The slower the metabolism of the parent or any active metabolites, the smaller the therapeutic dose that will be required. The modifications that distinguish fenprostalene from naturally-occurring $PGF_{2\alpha}$ are the deletion of carbons 17 through 20, substitution of a phenoxy group on carbon 16, and introduction of a Δ^4 unsaturated bond. The phenoxy substitution blocks metabolic degradation of fenprostalene by the actions of 15-hydroxy dehydrogenase and/or 13,14 reductase, while the introduction of the Δ^4 unsaturated bond, resulting in a $\Delta^{4,5,6}$ allenic system, restricts degradation by conventional β-oxidase enzyme activity[1–3]. The net result of these modifications is apparent in the comparatively long halflife of fenprostalene and small therapeutic dose required.

DOSE RESPONSE STUDIES

Three dose response studies were conducted using the same basic protocol with the exception of varying the dose levels of the final fenprostalene-polyethylene glycol 400, USP, formulation. Following treatment with fenprostalene, the animals were observed once daily for visual signs of abortion and examined rectally on days +1, +4, +8, +12, +21 and +60 for the presence or absence of a fetus and any possible complications. In addition, blood samples were obtained from each heifer and assayed for progesterone levels on days 0, +1, +4, +8 and +12.

Fenprostalene in doses of 0.0625, 0.125, 0.25, 0.50, 1.0 and 2.0 mg per animal resulted in abortion rates of 31, 31, 58, 84, 88 and 100%, respectively. No statistical differences could be detected in the abortion rates obtained in the 0.5, 1.0 or 2.0 mg groups. However, the time to abortion following treatment was 6.9 ± 10.4 days in animals treated with 0.5 mg of fenprostalene compared to 5.7 ± 3.8 and 5.5 ± 2.2 days for animals treated with 1.0 and 2.0 mg, respectively. The greater variability was the primary reason that the 0.5 mg dose was considered unsatisfactory for further development. The actual abortion rate obtained with 1.0 mg of fenprostalene was 88%, with a 95% confidence interval of 68–97%, as compared to an abortion rate of 100% with 2.0 mg of fenprostalene and a 95% confidence interval of 72–100% (Figure 19.1). Quite clearly, the abortion rate plateaued at the 1.0 mg dose without a significant increase in efficacy at the 2.0 mg dose.

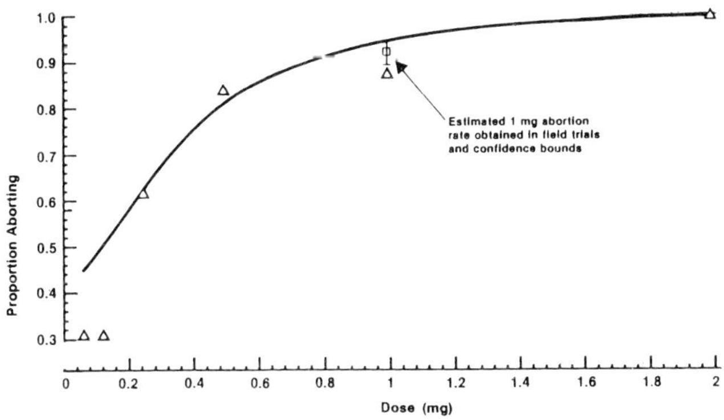

Figure 19.1 Estimated fenprostalene abortion rate dose response curve

Blood plasma assays conducted throughout the course of these studies indicated that, in order to cause abortion in animals pregnant 150 days or less, blood progesterone levels must fall below 2.0 ng/ml by day 4 following treatment (Figure 19.2).

No differences could be detected in the plasma progesterone levels in heifers that aborted, regardless of the dose of fenprostalene administered. Examination of the mean plasma progesterone levels of fenprostalene-treated animals that failed to abort by day 12 shows that the 1.0 mg dose depressed the values to lower levels by day 4 (with an associated smaller standard deviation) than did thc 0.5 mg dose. This also supports the selection of 1.0 mg of fenprostalene as the optimum luteolytic dose in the bovine.

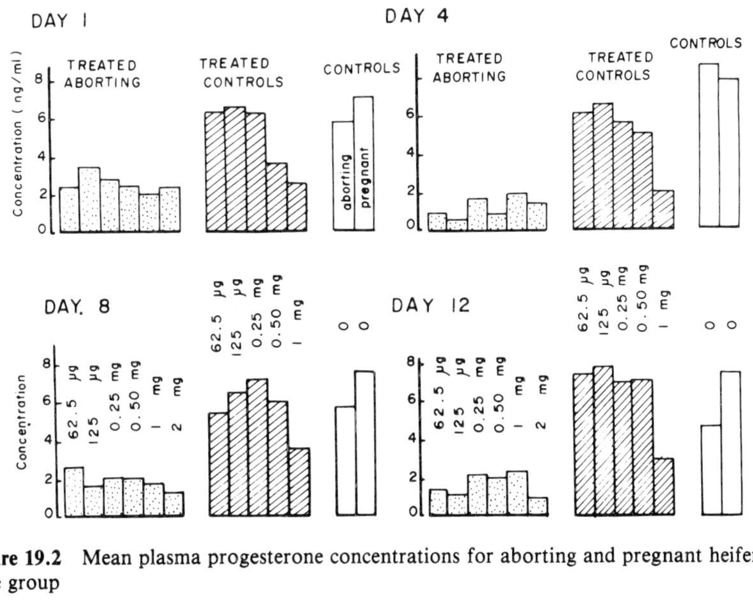

Figure 19.2 Mean plasma progesterone concentrations for aborting and pregnant heifers by dose group

The dose-response studies showed that 1.0 mg of fenprostalene was an effective luteolytic dose causing a high abortion rate, a precipitous and consistent drop in progesterone levels, and a predictable interval from treatment to abortion. Therefore, the 1.0 mg dose was selected for further testing in controlled field trials.

FIELD TRIAL STUDIES

Ten investigators located in different geographical areas of the United States conducted 11 studies to evaluate the efficacy of fenprostalene as an abortifacient. A total of 1835 heifers were each treated with a single subcutaneous injection of 1.0 mg of fenprostalene in the final formulation and were evaluated for efficacy and safety. Of the 1835 treated heifers, 869 were pregnant 150 days or less, 145 were pregnant over 150 days, and 821 were non-pregnant.

Table 19.5 Summary of fenprostalene abortion rates stratified by length of pregnancy

Length of pregnancy (days)	*Treated*		*Controls*	
	Aborted/pregnant	*% aborted*	*Aborted/pregnant*	*% aborted*
1–30	15/15	100.0	2/4	50.0
31–60	195/198	98.5	5/37	13.5
61–90	203/208	97.6	7/36	19.4
91–120	231/244	94.7	8/57	14.0
121–150	155/204	76.0	6/56	10.7
>150	56/145	38.6	5/29	17.2
Cumulative				
≤30	15/15	100.0	2/4	50.0
≤60	210/213	98.6	7/41	17.1
≤90	413/421	98.1	14/77	18.2
≤120	644/665	96.8	22/134	16.4
≤150	799/869	91.9	28/190	14.7
>150	56/145	38.6	5/29	17.2

In those fenprostalene-treated heifers pregnant 150 days or less, the cumulative abortion rate was 91.9% (Table 19.5) while in those pregnant over 150 days, the abortion rate was 38.6%. The decrease in abortion rate in animals pregnant over 150 days was expected since the conceptus in most cattle no longer depends solely on the corpus luteum for survival.

When the stages of pregnancy are stratified into 30 day increments (Table 19.6), it can be seen that between 121 and 150 days of gestation the abortion rate decreases only slightly to 76%.

The short biological halflife of $PGF_{2\alpha}$ in aqueous solution suggests that luteolysis, and hence abortion rate, will plateau at levels similar to those seen with aqueous fenprostalene described earlier. The intramuscular administration of $PGF_{2\alpha}$ to cattle pregnant 100 days or less in doses of 10 mg, 20 mg and 40 mg results in abortion rates of 54%, 75% and 68%, respectively, with a marked decrease in efficacy in animals pregnant over 100 days (Table 19.6)[7].

Table 19.6 Comparison of abortion rates for $PGF_{2\alpha}$ and fenprostalene, 14 days after treatment

Gestation stage (days)	$PGF_{2\alpha}$ 10 mg %	20 mg %	40 mg %	*Fenprostalene* 1 mg %
0–100	54	75	68	97.7
0–150	50	62	63	91.9
101–150	38	49	59	85.2
>150	12	26	57	38.2

The recommended dose of $PGF_{2\alpha}$ for abortion is 25 mg intramuscularly, but data have not been reported regarding efficacy at this dose. A comparative study was therefore conducted between aqueous $PGF_{2\alpha}$ and the new, longer-acting fenprostalene formulation at recommended dose rates (Table 19.7). A total of 573 feedlot heifers pregnant 150 days or less were randomized into two groups. One group received 25 mg of $PGF_{2\alpha}$ intramuscularly, and the other received 1 mg of fenprostalene subcutaneously. The results indicated a statistically significant superiority of the longer-acting fenprostalene preparation in animals pregnant over 100 days.

Table 19.7 Abortion rate summary 14 days after treatment, stratified by gestation length

Pretreatment gestation (days)	*% Abortion rate (no. aborting/no. pregnant)* $PGF_{2\alpha}$	*Fenprostalene**	p value
1–30	—	100.0 (1/1)	—
31–60	66.7 (6/9)	100.0 (10/10)	0.087
61–90	95.0 (38/40)	100.0 (29/29)	0.505
91–120	70.9 (29/55)	87.2 (41/47)	0.055
121–150	67.9 (124/182)	83.4 (166/199)	0.0005
1–150	72.1 (207/287)	86.4 (247/286)	0.0001
1–100	89.8 (44/49)	100.0 (40/40)	0.0618
101–150	68.5 (163/238)	84.2 (207/246)	0.0001

*Dose: $PGF_{2\alpha}$ – 25 mg; Fenprostalene – 1 mg

FUTURE STUDIES

By extending the biological halflife of fenprostalene, it is possible to reap the benefits of other prostaglandin actions, such as contraction of smooth muscle tissues. The contractile effect of prostaglandin $F_{2\alpha}$ on the smooth muscle of the bovine uterus has been well-documented[5,6]. However, this effect lasts only 1–2 min due to the rapid metabolism of $PGF_{2\alpha}$ in the body. Recent studies with the delayed release formulation have proved fenprostalene to be helpful in the treatment of retained placentas in cows. Animals with retained placentas and treated with fenprostalene shed their placentas significantly sooner following calving than conventionally-treated animals ($p<0.001$).

In this study, a retained placenta was defined as any placenta retained for 8 h or more following calving. Animals treated with fenprostalene shed the placenta 59.7 h after calving while animals treated with conventional therapy required 94.1 h ($p < 0.001$). In addition, only 27% of the cows treated with fenprostalene developed metritis while conventional treatment resulted in a 63% infection rate ($p < 0.00002$).

In conclusion, as compounds become available that have profound physiological activity but relatively short biological halflives, new delivery systems must be developed which will maximize their potential use in animals. Particular attention must also be made to the route of administration, subsequent absorption, and plasma halflife to optimize drug effect.

References

1. Bourne, G. R., Mass, S. R., Phillips, P. J. *et al.* (1979). The disposition of the synthetic prostaglandin analogue cloprostenol ('Estrumate') in the rat and marmoset. *Xenobiotica*, **9**, 623
2. Granstrom, E. and Hansson, G. (1976). Effect of chemical modifications on metabolic transformation of prostaglandins. In Samuelsson, B. and Paoletti, R. (eds.) *Advances in Prostaglandin and Tromboxane Research.* Vol. 1, p. 215. (New York: Raven Press)
3. Green, K., Samuelson, B. and Margerlein, B. J. (1976). Decreased rate of metabolism induced by a shift in the double bond in prostaglandin $F_{2\alpha}$ from the Δ^5 to the Δ^4 position. *Eur. J. Biochem.*, **62**, 527
4. McDonald, L. E., McNutt, S. H. and Nichols, R. E. (1953). On the essentiality of the bovine corpus luteum of pregnancy. *Am. J. Vet. Res.*, **14**, 539
5. Singh, L. P., Sadiku, A. and Verma, O. P. (1979). Prostaglandin $F_{2\alpha}$-induced response of the bovine ovary, oviduct (uterine tube), and uterus. *J. Am. Vet. Res.*, **40**, 1789–91
6. Speroff, L. and Ramwell, P. N. (1970). Prostaglandins in reproductive physiology. *Am. J. Obstet. Gynecol.*, **107**, 1110–30
7. Upjohn Veterinary Report n° 12. *Abortion Induction in Feedlot Heifers.* (Kalamazoo, Michigan, USA: The Upjohn Company)

20
Worm diseases: economic aspects of anthelmintic treatment

H. Van den Bossche

Knowledge of some of the common parasitic helminths must go back to prehistoric times. It is unthinkable that our primitive ancestors never encountered *Ascaris* or tapeworms. The ancient Egyptians were certainly familiar with intestinal worms and haematuria, the most common clinical manifestation of *Schistosoma haematobium*, is mentioned in four medical papyri, for example 28 times in *Papyrus Ebers*[6].

Galen (AD 170) recognized three human species of intestinal worms, *Ascaris*, *Enterobius* and *Taenia*. Later on, some idea of their medical importance was gained. But it was not until about the middle of the nineteenth century that attempts were made to assess the size of the problem in terms of the effects of parasitic helminths on the health of man and animals. It was also at that time that the bladderworm (*Echinococcus*) already known by Hippocrates, was recognized as one of the most dangerous and incurable parasitic diseases[12]. This disease is still a very serious problem in sheep-raising parts of the world. Furthermore, goats, camels and pigs, together with dogs, maintain the life cycle in various countries. Despite efforts to control echinococcosis, this disease still constitutes a substantial economic and health problem in most livestock-raising areas of the world.

Although the experimental proof[8] that *Cysticercus cellulosae* changes into *Taenia solium* within the human intestine was published by Küchenmeister in 1855 only, the cystic stage must have been noticed since man killed animals for food or for sacrificial purposes. According to Küchenmeister[5] the Mosaic prohibition of the flesh of the pig, hare and rabbit was probably because of their being known to harbour cysticerci (it should be mentioned that Deuteronomy, Chapter 14, verse 8 has been related to trichinosis too). Aristote speaks of the cysticerci of pigs as having been known for ages[5]. This zoonosis also causes economic losses but it is difficult to obtain estimates of actual figures. A study[10] done in Chile indicates that, over a 15 year period *T. solium* cysticercosis has resulted in a loss of US $2 400 320.

Taeniasis in man due to *Taenia saginata* is not a serious human health problem. However, condemnation of cattle carcasses due to cysticercosis leads to a considerable loss of protein.

The common liver fluke, *Fasciola hepatica*, is another helminth causing considerable loss of protein resulting from condemnation of livers. This parasite has been known as an important parasitic helminth of sheep since mediaeval times. An accurate description of the manner of acquisition of *Fasciola* in sheep and its damage to the liver can be found in *Le Bon Berger*, a book completed in 1379 by Jean de Brie. He wrote: 'The malady of the fluke can remain hidden for a year or more, but finally the sheep dies because the fluke destroys the liver'. Thomas[11], in a classic description of the natural history of the liver fluke and of the prevention of liver-rot, suggested that in view of the complex nature of the parasite's life cycle, farmers should use a combination of control measures including drainage, grazing management and molluscicides to ensure a satisfactory degree of control. He also proposed a system once the sheep were infected: 'Unless sheep are very valuable it may be better to kill them instantly they are known to be infected; for we shall thus prevent the production of more eggs and the propagation of the fluke. The cure of sheep, if cure be possible, will probably cost more than it is worth . . . Above all, livers of fluked sheep should be destroyed, for if every egg succeeded in producing a fluke a single liver might contain sufficient eggs to destroy a flock of 50 000 sheep.'

Generations of cattlemen have also recognized the damage caused by liver flukes and it is commonly accepted that *Fasciola hepatica* and *Fasciola gigantica* cause a considerable economic loss. For example, Armstrong[2] found that, 42 days after infection, calves weighed about 11 kg less than the uninfected controls. This study shows that the liver fluke can cost the cattleman as much as $20 per head. This is one of the few attempts that have been made to assess, in economic terms, the losses due to helminthiasis.

To control worm diseases other possibilities than those suggested by Thomas[11] are currently available. A variety of anthelmintics may play a role in livestock parasitism. Thanks to the strategic use of these anthelmintics, we no longer hear of outbreaks of haemonchiasis in Australia or of acute fascioliasis in the United Kingdom[3].

Crossland *et al.*[4] did field trials to investigate the effects of fascioliasis control on the productivity of lowland sheep. The molluscicide trifenmorph and the fasciolicide, oxyclozanide, were used. After 3 years the ewe flock was slaughtered and at postmortem examinations 33 (means per plot: 1.3–134) liver-flukes were recovered per ewe from untreated plots compared with 0.1 (means per plot: 0–0.6) per ewe from treated plots. Ewes from untreated plots gained significantly less weight and were significantly less productive than ewes from treated plots. There was a negative correlation between the numbers of liver-flukes per ewe and the weight of lambs produced.

The economic value of the treatment with the flucicide closantel of lambs infected naturally with *F. hepatica* was investigated by Kearney[7]. Twelve weeks after treatment a weight gain of 1.86 kg per lamb was found as compared with 0.32 kg per lamb in the untreated control group.

Anderson and colleagues published an interesting study on the economic returns from two schemes for the anthelmintic control of helminthiasis in weaned lambs[1] and in breeding ewes[9]. The results were compared with those from sheep receiving no anthelmintic treatment, and with those from sheep given an anthelmintic every 2 weeks. The first scheme called the 'critical treatment' was based on results reported by the authors who showed that in Australia the late spring and summer period was a critical period in the life cycle of *Ostertagia* and *Trichostrongylus* spp. The first treatment was given when the pasture was noticeably drying off as a result of hot weather and the second treatment was applied during midsummer. The second scheme called the 'traditional treatment scheme' was based on a survey of local control programmes. It was found that when routine treatments were given to breeding ewes, they were restricted to before or before and after lambing. Signs of parasitism may or may not have been present. In this experiment lambs were given anthelmintic treatment in December, at weaning, next April and January. The anthelmintic used was levamisole (320 mg for ewes and 160 mg for lambs).

All schemes of anthelmintic treatment gave better livestock production than the 'no treatment' scheme. The results showed that the 'critical' treatment scheme was the most profitable, yielding a net return of A $70 per 100 sheep (based on 1970–1971 prices). The benefit from this scheme was not adversely affected by economic conditions, e.g. variations in wool or sheep prices. The 'traditional' treatment scheme also yielded positive net returns but the benefits were adversely affected by even a small change in mortality rate.

In breeding ewes the 'critical' treatment scheme also was the most financially rewarding one in all years and under all circumstances evaluated. The net benefit per 100 sheep as compared with the 'no treatment' group was in the first year A $213 and in the second A $255. The benefit was derived from higher fleece weight per ewe, higher prices per kilogram for better quality wool and from higher values of lambs at weaning and of ewes.

Clearly these studies show that a critical utilization of anthelmintics will maximize net return. Obviously, anthelmintics make the modern intensive production of food animals more profitable.

A critical utilization of anthelmintics should be based on a better knowledge of the life cycle of the parasites, of the ecological aspects and above all on a better knowledge of the pharmacology, pharmacokinetics and mode of action of the available anthelmintics. The pharmacological basis of the use of anthelmintics will be discussed in the subsequent papers.

References

1. Anderson, N., Morris, R. S. and McTaggart, I. K. (1976). An economic analysis of two schemes for the anthelmintic control of helminthiasis in weaned lambs. *Aust. Vet. J.*, **52**, 174–80
2. Armstrong, D. A. (1979). Liver fluke: economic effect on feedlot cattle. Paper presented at the *Western States Veterinary Conference, Sheep and Goat Section*, Las Vegas, March 5–8
3. Campbell, W. C. (1977). The control of parasites: the role of drugs. *Proc. Helminthological Soc. Washington*, **44**, 17–28

4. Crossland, N. O., Johnstone, A., Beaumont, G. and Bennett, M. S. (1977). The effect of control of chronic fascioliasis on the productivity of lowland sheep *Br. Vet. J.*, **133,** 518–25
5. Foster, W. D. (1965). *A History of Parasitology*. (Edinburgh: E. & S. Livingstone)
6. Jonckheere, F. (1944). *Une Maladie Egyptienne*. Edition de la Fondation Egyptologique Reine Elisabeth, Brussel
7. Kearney, A. (1978). Comparative activity of closantel against *Fasciola hepatica* in sheep. Janssen Research Products Information Service. Nov. Serial Number: R 12 564 and R 31 520
8. Küchenmeister, F. (1855). Experimenteller nachweis, daß *Cysticercus Cellulosae* innerhalb der menschlichen Darmkanales sich in *Taenia solium* umwandelt. *Wien. Med. Wochenschr.*, **5,** 1–4
9. Morris, R. S., Anderson, N. and McTaggart, I. K. (1977). An economic analaysis of two schemes for the control of helminthiasis in breeding ewes. *Vet. Parasitol.*, **3,** 349–63
10. Smyth, J. D. (1980). Importance of larval cestodiasis to man in developing countries. In Wood, C. and Rue, Y. (eds.) *Health Policies in Developing Countries*. Royal Society of Medicine. International Congress and Symposium Series, No. 24, p. 89
11. Thomas, A. P. W. (1881). Report of experiments on the development of the liver fluke (*Fasciola hepatica*). *J. R. Agric. Soc. Engl.*, 1–28
12. Thudicum, J. L. (1864). Seventh report of the medical officer to the Privy Council, London. p. 465. (Mentioned by Foster loc. cit.)

21
Pharmacological basis of the treatment of helminth in cattle

A. Dakkak and M. Kessabi

Parasitic helminth infections in cattle are widespread and cause severe economic losses throughout the world[13]. The use of anthelmintic agents is therefore extensive.

For many years the introduction of anthelmintic drugs was empirical, but with the discovery of the anthelmintic properties of phenothiazine new concepts and standards of efficacy and safety were developed. This led to the discovery of thiabendazole, with which the era of modern anthelmintics began.

In recent years interest in physiological processes and biochemical pathways of helminths has increased, but the mode of action of anthelmintics is still, in many instances, poorly understood[4,7,20,24,27,28]. Sites of action can often be defined but the precise biochemical changes induced by anthelmintics are not known for many of them. However, it has been possible to identify and exploit differences in neurotransmitters and in energy generating metabolic processes between the host and parasite. These differences have led, through selective toxicity, to the development of less toxic agents[24,28].

Modern anthelmintic research has provided a considerable array of efficient drugs. However, several factors limit the use of anthelmintics. These factors may be connected with the host (route of administration, oesophageal groove reflex, etc.), the worms (hypobiosis of fourth-stage larvae), or related to the drug itself (route of administration, dose volumes, particle size of insoluble anthelmintics, chemical structure, etc.).

TESTS FOR ANTHELMINTIC EFFICACY

Faecal worm egg count

This is a rapid, inexpensive and mostly the only available method of assessing drug efficacy against adult worms, but it does not give any indication of efficacy against immature worms.

Anthelmintic test for 'normal immature' and adult worms

Experimentally infected animals are treated when worms are present as third- or fourth-stage larvae or as adults and slaughtered when the remaining larvae have developed to adults. The major disadvantage of this method is that the third and the fourth moults vary within and between species[23].

Anthelmintic test for inhibited larvae

Since attention was focused on the clinical disease resulting from maturation of larvae of *Ostertagia ostertagi* inhibited in the early fourth stage[1], research has been directed towards developing an anthelmintic against inhibited larvae. Armour and Duncan[2] and Armour and Bairden[3] used the following method. During a season known to be favourable to induce inhibition of nematode larvae, calves are grazed on a field known to be heavily contaminated with infected larvae. Animals are slaughtered 4–7 days after anthelmintic treatment and mucosae from the abomasum and large intestine are digested in HCl/pepsin solution to allow counting of the parasites. The histotropic fourth-stage larvae are divided into early-L_4 (probably hypobiotic larvae) and late-L_4 (considered not to be inhibited).

Anthelmintic test for several species of helminths

The assessment of anthelmintic efficacy against several helminth species is made by comparing the mean worm burden of a group of treated animals with the worm burden of an untreated control group. The results are expressed in terms of percentage reduction.

SOURCES OF VARIATION IN ANTHELMINTIC EFFICACY

Despite the remarkable success of the modern anthelmintics used in cattle, there are still some factors which account for variation in efficacy. These may be broadly classified, as proposed by Kelly *et al.*[17] and Gibson[13], into three categories.

Factors relating to the anthelmintic

The efficacy of some insoluble or sparingly soluble anthelmintics depends upon the particle size of the active component. In general, fine particle suspensions are more active than coarse material against nematode parasites[25]. Particle size of an anthelmintic influences its dissolution rate, absorption characteristics and plasma concentration which in turn influences efficacy[22,25].

Factors relating to the parasite

The resistance of nematodes to anthelmintics is almost unknown in cattle. The major source of variation in anthelmintic efficacy relating to the parasite in cattle is arrested development or hypobiosis of histotropic fourth-stage larvae. This hypobiosis phenomenon has a variety of causes[21]. The best known example is that of *Ostertagia ostertagi*[1]. Hypobiotic larvae are embedded in the gut mucosae and are metabolically inactive. Hence, these larvae exhibit little or no sensitivity to anthelmintics known to be effective against worms developing at the 'normal' rate[1,21]. In recent years, however, a number of broad spectrum anthelmintics (some benzimidazole carbamates and ivermectin) have been shown to be active on hypobiotic larvae[2,3].

Factors relating to the host

In cattle the major host-related variation noted with some orally-administered anthelmintics is associated with the oesophageal groove reflex[14,19]. When the groove is closed, the rumen is by-passed and drenches pass directly into the omasum and abomasum. This may result in a reduction in activity (see below). The use of low dose volumes, deposition of drenches into the posterior oral cavity, and rapid administration reduce the intensity of the stimuli which induce the oesophageal groove reflex[17].

MODE OF ACTION OF ANTHELMINTICS

Anthelmintic reviews by van den Bossche[26–28], Coles[7], Rew[24], Prichard[20], Behm and Brayant[4] and Mansour[18] have concentrated on the biochemical aspect of their actions on helminths. Most investigations have been concerned with identifying systems within the helminths that are different in some way from those used by the host. Present information indicates two primary sites of action: interference with energy-generating metabolism or modification of neuromuscular transmission.

Host–parasite comparative biochemistry and neurophysiology

In contrast to the aerobic metabolism of vertebrate tissues, the major parasitic helminths derive energy largely by anaerobic fermentation of carbohydrate to reduced end-products[4,20]. A number of pathways of carbohydrate metabolism are found in parasites which have no parallel in their vertebrate hosts (Figure 21.1). This is the case with the formation of acetate or ethanol from pyruvate, the fixation of CO_2 into phosphoenolpyruvate and the subsequent conversion of the product oxaloacetate to succinate and propionate via fumarate reductase and the decarboxylation of succinate, and also the process of ATP synthesis which occurs anaerobically in helminth mitochondria[4,24].

The metabolic pathway of the helminth parasites may vary between species[6,7]. Parasitic helminths of cattle may be divided into two broad types. The first includes the essentially homolactic fermenters (*Schistosoma* spp and filarial worms) which depend entirely on glycolysis[6,24]. The second includes parasites in which there are fairly normal glycolytic sequences as far as phosphoenolpyruvate conversion.

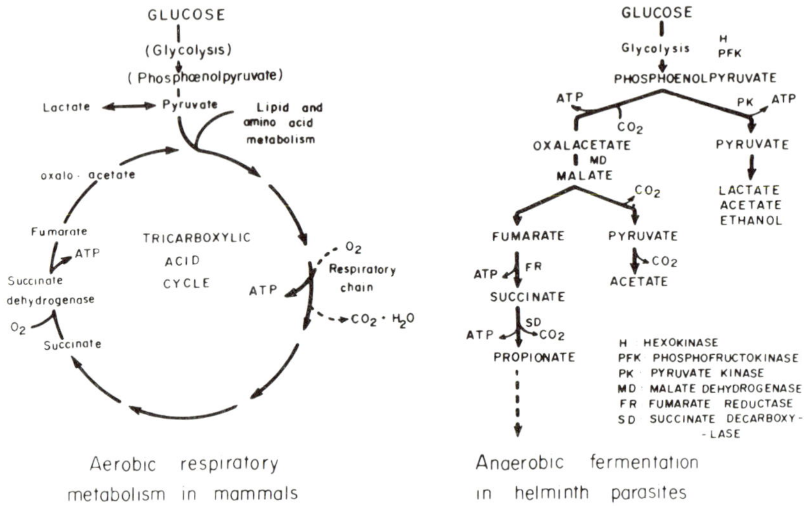

Figure 21.1 Comparative energy-generating metabolism in helminth parasites and in mammals. Helminth parasites, except *Schistosoma* and filarial worms, derive energy from anaerobic fermentation. *Schistosoma* and filarial worms obtain their energy by simple glycolysis

Less information is available on mechanisms of nerve transmission in helminths than in the area of glucose metabolism. Debell *et al*[8] found a resting potential in nematode and trematode muscles of $-30\,mV$ which is very different from the vertebrate muscle resting potential of $-90\,mV$.

Cholinergic receptors have been identified in *Ascaris* spp. and in *Fasciola hepatica*[18]. Since neither atropine nor d-tubocurarine affected the neuromuscular activity of the nematodes, acetylcholine receptors in these parasites may be different from those found in mammalian synapses containing nicotinic receptors[18].

The results of several studies (for review see ref. 18) strongly implicate serotonin as the putative neurotransmitter in the regulation of neuromuscular activity in parasitic flatworms. In parasitic roundworms, the excitatory neurotransmitter is acetylcholine and the inhibitory transmitter is γ-aminobutyric acid[8,10]. Although histamine has been found in roundworms, its function is unknown[24].

Principles of mode of anthelmintic action

Host–parasite comparative biochemistry and neurophysiology show that the parasitic helminths have few life support functions to serve as sites for chemical attack. The life support functions of these worms are based mainly on remaining at advantageous feeding sites where they can transport and metabolize essential substrates. The maintenance of feeding sites requires proper neuromuscular co-ordination, the energy of which is derived to a large extent by anaerobic fermentation of carbohydrate to reduced end-products.

The major forms of pharmacological treatment of helminths generally involve, at the usual dosages, interference with one of these functions vital to the parasite.

Mode of action of common anthelmintics

The anthelmintics that interfere with energy-generating metabolism are:

(1) Inhibitors of glucose transport (e.g. mebendazole) block the uptake of glucose. The worms may then starve when endogenous energy stores have been exhausted[28]. The effects on glucose uptake may originate from a disruption of tegumentary and intestinal cytoplasmic microtubules[26].

(2) Inhibitors of mitochondrial reactions (e.g. thiabendazole, parbendazole, oxibendazole, fenbendazole, oxfendazole, albendazole, febantel and thiophanate-ethyl) inhibit energy production in mitochondria. This target is particularly important since its properties differ significantly from those of the host[11,15,24,28].

(3) Uncouplers of electron transport-associated oxidative phosphorylation (e.g. nitroxynil, salicylanilides and bithionol-sulphoxide) uncouple the mitochondrial reactions involved in electron transport events from ATP generation[20,24,26].

The anthelmintics that modify neuromuscular transmission[24] are:

(1) Acetylcholinesterase inhibitors (organophosphates) inhibit the breakdown of the excitatory neurotransmitter acetylcholine. This results in maintained stimulation of the muscle[26].

(2) Cholinergic agonists (e.g. imidazothiazoles and tetrahydropyrimidines) act by mimicking the action of the excitatory neurotransmitter causing a continual acetylcholine-libre response which results in spastic paralysis[7,24,28].

(3) Muscle hyperpolarizers such as piperazine, acting by mimicking the inhibitory neurotransmitter γ-amino-butyric acid (GABA)[10,24] which results in flacid paralysis, and Ivermectin acting by inducing GABA liberation and its fixation on the postsynaptic receptors[3].

PHARMACOKINETIC BEHAVIOUR AND ITS RELATIONSHIP TO DRUG EFFICACY

Administration and absorption

Anthelmintics used in cattle are frequently water-insoluble, crystalline solids (except levamisole, tetramisole and piperazine). They generally exhibit good physicochemical stability during storage and at the pH of the digestive tract. These characteristics determine the routes of administration and the efficacy of these drugs[17,22]. The gastrointestinal absorption of anthelmintics in cattle depends on their chemical structure. Thus, benzimidazole carbamates which have the 5-position of the benzene blocked are more insoluble than benzimidazole thiazolyls. This slows down their rate of metabolism and excretion. The nature of the group substituted in the 5-position of the benzene and the replacement of the thiazole by methylcarbamate affect the rate of elimination. These modifications confer to benzimidazole carbamates broader activity spectrums than benzimidazole thiazolyls.

Because they are frequently water-insoluble, anthelmintics are most often given orally as a suspension, paste, tablet, capsule or powder. Their gastrointestinal absorption is then influenced by the pharmaceutical formulation (Figure 21.2) and by the oesophageal groove reflex (see above) and it is often prolonged and incomplete. Peak plasma concentrations, which may be an indicator of efficacy[14, 25], are reached a few hours after administration (4–6 h for tetrahydropyrimidines, 12–24 h for salicylanilides and benzimidazoles) or even after a few days (3–4 days for bithionol sulphoxide)[15, 20]. The non-absorbed fraction is generally large (50% for benzimidazoles, 60% for phenothiazine and 50–70% for tetrahydropyrimidines)[15, 20].

In general, anthelmintics given orally are more effective in ruminant animals where the rumen presumably serves to deliver the drugs over an extended period, which increases their absorption and delays their effects[19, 22, 25]. Some benzimidazole carbamates, which are metabolized to sulphoxides (major anthelmintically-active metabolite) and sulphones, seem more effective in sheep than in cattle (Figure 21.3).

The absorption of anthelmintics given parenterally (nitroxynil, trichlorfon, tetramisole and levamisole) is rapid and complete. Peak plasma concentrations are reached 30–60 min after dosing[15, 20]. Some products may be

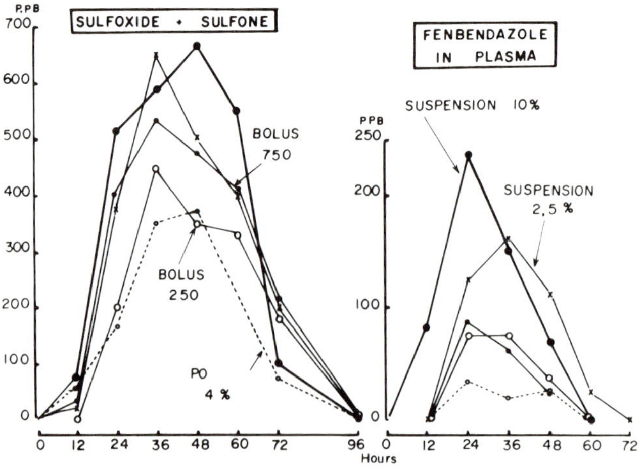

Figure 21.2 Plasma concentrations of fenbendazole and its two metabolites (sulphoxide + sulphone) in cattle after administration of the drug as a suspension, powder (PO) or bolus[9]

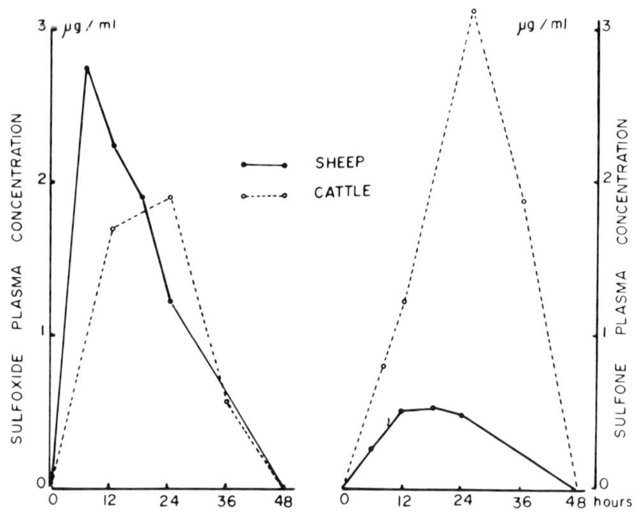

Figure 21.3 Sulphoxide and sulphone albendazole plasma concentrations in sheep and cattle[9]

used either orally or parenterally (tetramisole and levamisole). Recently interest has been shown in 'mass medication' with anthelmintics. Thus, some of these drugs such as the tetrahydropyrimidines are incorporated in the feedstuffs[16,20], while others (phenothiazine and benzimidazoles) are incorporated in the drinking water[12], and others (levamisole) are applied dermally[5]. Other application methods use special carriers allowing slow release into the rumen; the latter practice increases the efficacy of the drug[22].

Metabolism and excretion

Anthelmintics pass to various tissues and organs (digestive tract, liver, lung, etc.). They can be classified into two types: (1) non-absorbable drugs that remain in the digestive tract (niclosamide) and are thus recommended against parasites that develop in the gut, and (2) anthelmintics that cross the intestinal barrier and end up either bound to plasma proteins (salicylanilides) or are present in non-bound form in the plasma. The plasma anthelmintic concentrations may be related to the efficacy of these drugs[14]. The efficacy of some anthelmintics, such as the benzimidazoles, is increased when the duration of exposure of parasites to the drugs increases[12,15,16].

The biochemical breakdown of anthelmintics may start in the digestive tract (nitroxynil), a fact which excludes their oral administration. However, the liver is usually the site of degradation by oxidation, reduction, hydrolysis and conjugation reactions which yield products which are more water soluble[15,16]. Some molecules (e.g. febantel and thiphanate-ethyl) are active only after biotransformation in the treated animal[11,14].

Some anthelmintics are rapidly degraded and inactivated (tetrahydropyrimidines and imidazothiazoles) while others (salicylanilides) are degraded more slowly[20]. The latter property enhances clinical efficacy[12,22].

The elimination of anthelmintics in the faeces is by far the most important process. It is complete for the partially absorbed products or their metabolites which are secreted back into the tract (e.g. benzimidazoles). Frequently, secretion occurs from the liver into the bile. This may be important for anthelmintics which are active against liver parasites. Urinary elimination predominates for the water-soluble forms (conjugated substances mainly); its importance is often secondary. Some products are also partially eliminated in the milk (e.g. benzimidazoles, oxyclosanide, nitroxynil, etc.)[15,16].

The anthelmintics are usually well-tolerated by cattle because of their low absorption rate from the digestive tract and their mode of action on the parasites which generally have no parallel in the host (except organophosphates) at the usual dosages. However, serious and even lethal poisoning may occur with some drugs (e.g. phenothiazine, tetramisole and levamisole)[15]. Side-effects are relatively more frequent. They are due to digestive intolerance (e.g. piperazine) or nervous and muscular disorders related to the mode of action of the drugs (organophosphates).

At the usual dosages, benzimidazoles do not induce embryotoxicity in cattle as some of them do in sheep.

The relatively good tolerance of cattle to anthelmintics should not be taken as a general rule by toxicologists. Toxicity studies of anthelmintics and their metabolites should be pursued in order to gain an in-depth understanding of their effects and to assess the withholding period for animals from slaughter or milk from human consumption until residues have fallen to acceptable levels.

References

1. Armour, J., Jennings, F. W. and Urquhart, G. M. (1969). Inhibition of *Ostertagia ostertagi* at the early 4th larval stage. *Res. Vet. Sci.*, **10**, 232–44
2. Armour, J. and Duncan J. L. (1978). Activity of oxfendazole against inhibited larvae of *Ostertagia ostertagi* and *Cooperia onchophora. Vet. Rec.*, **25**, 263–4
3. Armour, J. and Bairden, C. (1980). Anthelmintic efficacy of Ivermectin against naturally acquired bovine gastrointestinal nematodes. *Vet. Rec.*, **107**, 226–7
4. Behm, C. A. and Brayant, C. (1979). Anthelmintic action: a metabolic approach (a review). *Vet. Pharmacol.*, **5**, 39–49
5. Brooker, P. J. and Goose, J. (1975). Dermal application of levamisole to sheep and cattle. *Vet. Rec.*, **96**, 249–50
6. Coles, G. C. (1975). Flack biochemistry – *Fasciola* and *Schistosoma. Helminthological Abstr.*, **44A**, 147–62
7. Coles, G. C. (1977). The biochemical mode of action of some modern anthelmintics. *Pestic. Sci.*, **8**, 536–43
8. Debell, J. T., Del Castillo, J. and Sanchez, V. (1963). Electrophysiology of somatic muscle cells of *Ascaris lumbricoides. J. Cell. Comp. Physiol.*, **62**, 159–78
9. Delatour, P. (1982). Biodisposibilité comparée de six forms galénique du fenbendazole (PANACUR N.D.) chez les bovins. (Personal communication)
10. Del Castillo, J., De Mellow, W. C. and Morales, T. A. (1964). Mechanism of the paralysing action of piperazine on *Ascaris* muscle. *Br. J. Pharmacol. Chemother.*, **22**, 463–77
11. Douch, P. G. C. (1974). The metabolism of some thioureidobenzen fungicides in mice and sheep. *Xenobiotica*, **4**, 457–63

12. Downey, N. E. and O'Shea, J. (1977). Calf parasites: control by means of low level anthelmintic administrated via the drinking water. *Vet. Rec.*, **100**, 265–6
13. Gibson, T. E. (1980). Factors influencing the application of anthelmintics in practice. *Vet. Parasitol.*, **6**, 241–54
14. Hennessy, D. R. and Prichard, R. K. (1981). The role of absorbed drug in relation to its efficacy. *Proc. Aust. Soc. Parasitol.*, Perth
15. Jaussaud, P., Delatour, P. and Gevrey, G. (1980). *Pharmacie et Toxicologie des Antiprotozoaires et des Anthelminthiques.* (France: Ecole Nationale Vétérinaire de Lyon)
16. Jones, R. M., Pott, J. M. and Cornwell, R. L. (1978). Low level feed administration of Morantel tartrate in the prophylaxis of experimental nematode infections in lambs and calves. *Br. Vet. J.*, **134**, 166–70
17. Kelly, J. D., Gordon, H. Mc L. and Whitlock, H. V. (1976). Anthelmintics for sheep historical, perspectives, classification/usage, problem areas and future prospects. *New South Wales Vet. Proc.*, **12**, 18–31
18. Mansour, T. E. (1979). Chemotherapy of parasitic worms. *New Biochem. Strat. Sci.*, **205**, 462–9
19. Marriner, S. and Bogan, J. A. (1979). Ruminal by-pass with benzimidazole anthelmintics. *Vet. Rec.*, **105**, 161–3
20. Prichard, R. K. (1978). Anthelmintics. In Proceedings of *39th Refresher Course for Veterinarians*, University of Sydney, Vol. 6, pp. 421–63.
21. Prichard, R. K., Donald, A. D. and Hennessy, D. R. (1978). Factors involved in the relative anthelmintic tolerance of arrested 4th stage larvae of *Ostertagia ostertagi. Vet. Rec.*, **102**, 382–3
22. Prichard, R. K., Hennessy, D. R. and Steel, J. W. (1978). Prolonged administration of a new concept for increasing the spectrum and effectiveness of anthelmintics. *Vet. Parasitol.*, **4**, 309–15.
23. Reinecke, R. K. and Anderson, P. J. S. (1967). Modifications to the larval anthelmintic test. *J. S.Afr. Vet. Med. Assoc.*, **38**, 231–8
24. Rew, R. S. (1978). Mode of action of common anthelmintics. *J. Vet. Pharmacol. Ther.*, **1**, 183–98
25. Shastri, S., Mroszak, E., Prichard, R. K. *et al.* (1980). Relationship among particle size, distribution, dissolution, efficacy of oxygendazole. *Am. J. Vet. Res.*, **41**, 2095–101
26. van den Bossche, H. (1976). The molecular basis of anthelmintic action. In van den Bossche, H. (ed.) *Biochemistry of Parasites and Host-Parasite Relationships.* pp. 553–72. (Amsterdam: North Holland)
27. van den Bossche, H. (1978). Chemotherapy of parasitic infections. *Nature (London)*, **273**, 626–30
28. van den Bossche, H. (1980). Peculiar targets in anthelmintic chemotherapy. *Biochem. Pharmacol.*, **29**, 1981–90

22
Pharmacokinetics of albendazole, fenbendazole and oxfendazole

J. A. Bogan and S. E. Marriner

The benzimidazole anthelmintics have broad spectrum activity and are now used in many species of animals against a wide variety of helminth parasites. We believe that a study of the pharmacokinetics of these compounds could assist parasitologists in choosing more appropriate dosages and dose intervals, especially for use against some of the parasites which are more difficult to eradicate.

These studies have been conducted with the three benzimidazole anthelmintics which have the broadest spectrum of activity including activity against lungworm and inhibited larval species and which are used at the lowest dosage rates, namely fenbendazole, oxfendazole and albendazole.

In all species studied, the principal route of metabolism appears to be by oxidation of the sulphide to the sulphoxide and the sulphone metabolites. Activity is associated with both the sulphide and sulphoxide but appears to be minimal or absent in the sulphone. However, it is interesting that the sulphide–sulphoxide metabolism can be shown to be reversible (Figure 22.1). There are few metabolic conversions of xenobiotics by hepatic microsomes which are known to be reversible. These are prednisone–prednisolone, possibly because of their similarity to the endogenous cortisone–cortisol metabolism[4] and the anti-inflammatory drug sulindac which also undergoes a sulphide–sulphoxide conversion[1]. Ruminal fluid causes reduction of sulphoxide to sulphide only. After *in vitro* incubation of sulphide (fenbendazole) or sulphoxide (oxfendazole) with bovine hepatic microsomes, the presence of sulphoxide or sulphide respectively can be readily demonstrated. The rate constants for this conversion are difficult to determine because of the problems of preparing accurate concentrations in aqueous solutions, due to the exceedingly low solubilities of fenbendazole and albendazole ($< 1\ \mu g/ml$ in phosphate buffer, pH 7.4). Nevertheless, when either fenbendazole or oxfendazole is administered to sheep the ratio of sulphoxide to sulphide in plasma samples is about 4:1. It can, therefore, be concluded that the rate constants for the sulphide–sulphoxide conversion are rapid

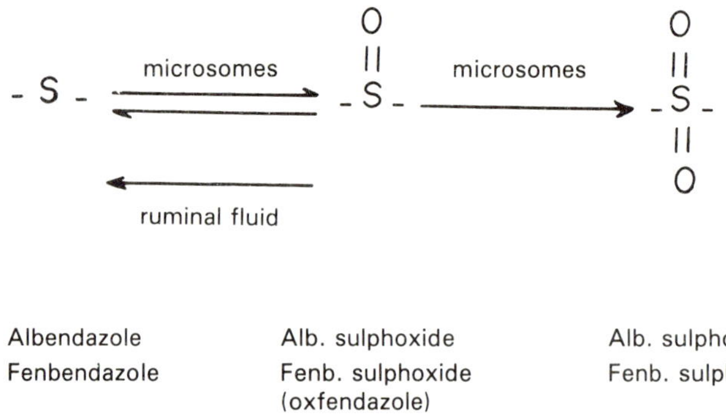

Figure 22.1 Principal route of metabolism of albendazole, fenbendazole and oxfendazole

relative to the rate constants for absorption, excretion or conversion to sulphone[11]. It should be noted that, although the sulphoxide–sulphide ratios in plasma are similar, the *total* bioavailability (AUC sulphide + AUC sulphoxide) is about 40% after fenbendazole of that after oxfendazole at the same dose rate (10 mg/kg) in the same six sheep. After albendazole, although reversible metabolism can also be demonstrated, the conversion is in favour of the sulphoxide, such that only low or negligible concentrations of the sulphide (albendazole) are found in plasma. The mean concentrations of the sulphoxide metabolites in plasma after administration of albendazole, fenbendazole and oxfendazole at dose rates of 10 mg/kg to the same six sheep

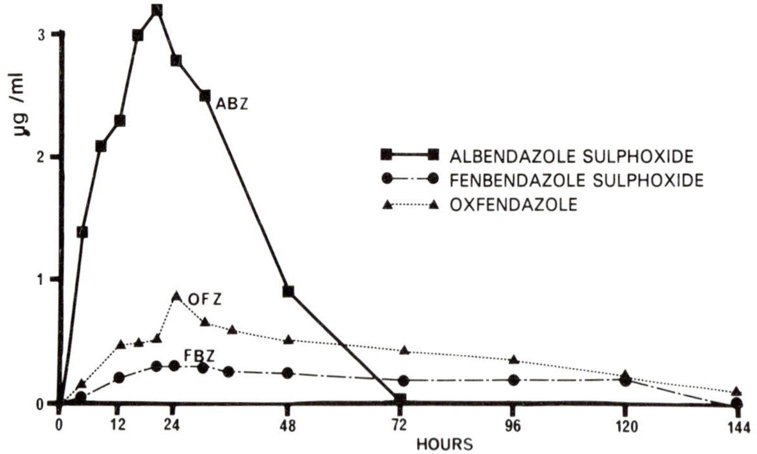

Figure 22.2 The mean concentrations in plasma of oxfendazole, fenbendazole sulphoxide (oxfendazole), and albendazole sulphoxide obtained after administration of oxfendazole, fenbendazole and albendazole respectively at a dose rate of 10 mg/kg as suspension formulations to the same six sheep

on different occasions are shown in Figure 22.2. Concentrations in abomasal fluid of the sulphoxides are greater than those in plasma and parallel those in plasma.

The concentrations of albendazole sulphoxide reached in plasma of species other than ruminant are considerably less and are shown in Figure 22.3. In the ruminant animal, orally administered drug is deposited to large extent in the rumen followed by slow dissolution in ruminal fluid, or possibly to a greater extent, passage of benzimidazole as particulate material to the more acidic abomasal fluid followed by dissolution. Either of these processes supports the concept of the rumen acting as a reservoir for the benzimidazoles giving an extended time period for dissolution to take place and for increased plasma bioavailability. In sheep given fenbendazole (10 mg/kg) via an abomasal cannula, neither fenbendazole nor oxfendazole was detectable in

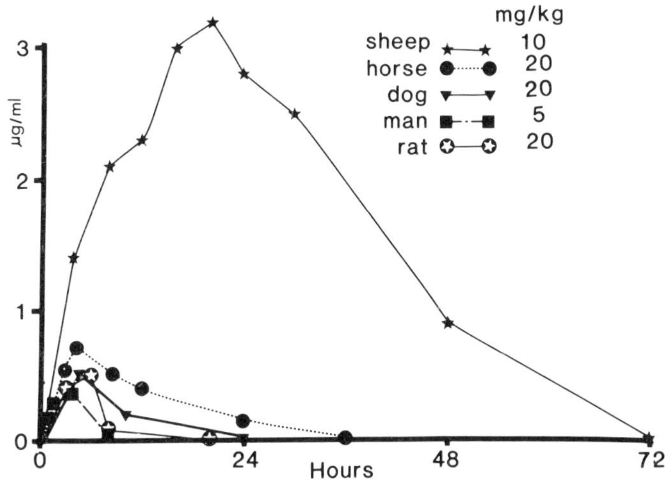

Figure 22.3 The mean concentration in plasma of albendazole suphoxide obtained after administration of albendazole to different species (sheep, $n = 6$; horse, $n = 3$; dog, $n = 3$; man, $n = 4$; rat, $n = 3$)

fluid taken from the rumen. Drug given directly into the abomasum in sheep leads to much reduced concentrations in plasma[5] and has led some authors[2] to suggest that rumen bypass via the oesophageal (reticular) groove reflex is responsible for the occasional anthelmintic failure with these drugs. In our experience, rumen bypass, as assessed by measuring abomasal fluid and plasma concentrations soon after oral administration, occurs frequently in adult sheep but we have not experienced a situation in more than 40 sheep examined where 100% of the orally-administered drug was considered to have totally bypassed the rumen. This conflicts with the observations of McEwan and Oakley[7] in cattle who observed total rumen bypass in 20% of animals. However, we suspect that with the small volumes of suspension being administered in our experiments (< 10 ml) it is probable that much of the particulate material in the administered suspension is deposited in the oesophagus and ruminal and omasal walls. With large volumes of solutions, as in the experiments of McEwan and Oakley[7], bypass may be more significant.

In two separate experiments with albendazole, administration of albendazole (10 mg/kg) to six sheep as a paste and as a suspension did not result in plasma concentrations of albendazole sulphoxide and sulphone which were significantly different at any time (paired Student *t*-test)[6] and similarly, in six other sheep, administration as a suspension and as a pellet formulation also did not result in significant differences in plasma concentrations.

The benzimidazoles produce their anthelmintic action by affecting the uptake of nutrients by helminth parasites[10]. This has been shown with mebendazole to be caused by effects on the gut epithelium in helminths, by destruction of the microtubular structure of the cells lining the epithelium, accumulation of secretory granules in the cells and subsequent autolysis. Other suggested modes of action such as effects on fumarate reductase activity are probably consequent to effects on the helminth gut epithelium and the resultant reduced glycogen content of benzimidazole-treated helminths. As a result, anthelmintic activity is related not only to the concentrations achieved but also to the duration of these concentrations. Thus divided dosage regimes even in ruminant species can lead to increased efficacy[9]. From the concentrations achieved (Figure 22.3) suitable dosage intervals for albendazole in man would be about 12 h and for the horse daily dosage would be appropriate. In man, using a dose rate of 5 mg/kg at 12 h intervals three out of four patients with active hydatid disease showed evidence of regression[8].

Benzimidazole anthelmintics are frequently given to animals suffering from clinical helminthiases and in these animals considerably altered pharmacokinetics may result. We report here on preliminary results investigating the effect of parasitism on the pharmacokinetics of fenbendazole. Fenbendazole (10 mg/kg) was administered to three sheep which had previously been surgically implanted with permanent abomasal cannulae. The concentrations of fenbendazole suphoxide in abomasal fluid were determined. *Ostertagia circumcincta* larvae were administered (7000/day per *os*) over 30 days to these sheep. 15 days after the last larval dose the same dose of fenbendazole was administered and the concentrations again determined. In each sheep there was an increased bioavailability (AUC) of fenbendazole sulphoxide in the abomasal fluid. In the most severely affected animal (clinically ill, abomasal fluid pH increased to 6.1) the increase in sulphoxide bioavailability was most marked (249% of non-parasitized. See Figure 22.4) and was less affected in the other two sheep (132% and 111% of non parasitized). The effects of infection with *O. circumcincta* on the abomasum are twofold: abomasal pH rises and the abomasal epithelial lining is severely disrupted. The pH effect would tend to lower sulphoxide concentrations in the abomasum, while the second effect may lead to increased concentration due to more rapid diffusion through the disrupted epithelium. However, after fenbendazole treatment of the parasitized sheep the abomasal pH had returned to pH 2 within 24 h of treatment, even although the helminths could

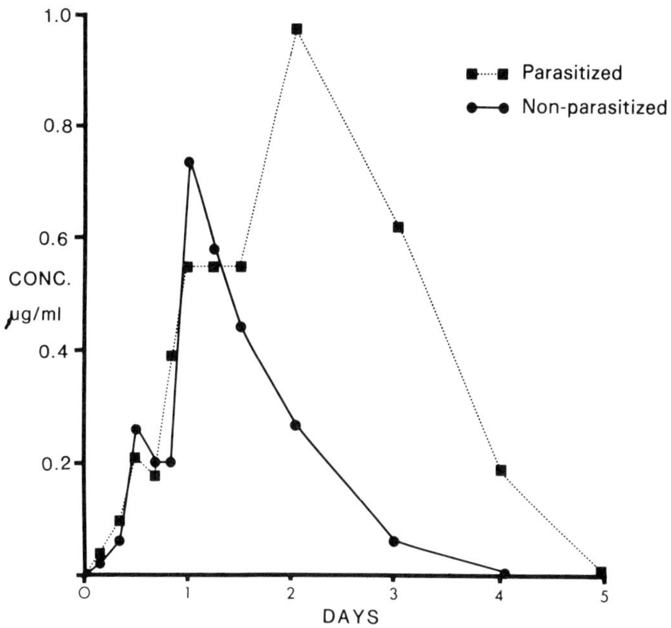

Figure 22.4 Concentrations of fenbendazole sulphoxide (oxfendazole) in the abomasum of the most severely affected sheep of a group of three sheep artifically infected with *Ostertagia circumcincta* larvae, given a dose of fenbendazole (10 mg/kg) before and after infection

be observed to be alive in abomasal samples. This supports the hypothesis that the elevated pH is not a result of the disrupted epithelium[3]. Further, if the elevated pH is a consequence of some secretion by the helminths, the return of pH to normal demonstrates early effects by fenbendazole on the worms although still motile, and probably a much more rapid clinical improvement than might be expected.

References

1. Duggan, D. E., Hooke, K. F. and Hwang, S. S. (1980). Kinetics of the tissue distributions of sulindac and metabolites. *Drug Metab. Disp.*, **8,** 241–6
2. Duncan, J. L., Armour, J., Bairden, K. *et al.* (1977). The activity of fenbendazole against inhibited 4th stage larvae of *Ostertagia ostertagi. Vet. Rec.*, **101,** 249
3. Eiler, H., Baber, W., Lyke, W. A. *et al.* (1981). Inhibition of gastric hydrochloric acid secretions in the rat given *Ostertagia ostertagi* (a gastric parasite of cattle) extract. *Am. J. Vet. Res.*, **42,** 498–502
4. Jenkins, J. S. and Sampson, P. A. (1967). Conversion of cortisone to cortisol and prednisone to prednisolone. *Br. Med. J.*, **2,** 205–7
5. Marriner, S. E. and Bogan, J. A. (1981). Pharmacokinetics of fenbendazole in sheep. *Am. J. Vet. Res.*, **42,** 1146–8
6. Marriner, S. E., Bogan, J. A. and Vandaele, W. (1981). Comparison of the pharmacokinetics of albendazole and its major metabolites after oral administration of albendazole as a suspension and as a paste formulation to sheep. *Zentralbl. Veterinaermed. Reihe B.*, **28,** 19–26

7. McEwan, A. D. and Oakley, G. A. (1978). Anthelmintics and closure of the oesophageal groove in cattle. *Vet. Rec.*, **102,** 314–15
8. Morris, D. L., Dykes, P. W., Dickson, B. *et al.* (1983). Albendazole in hydatid disease. *Br. Med. J.*, **286,** 103–4
9. Prichard, R. K., Hennessy, D. R. and Steel, J. W. (1970). Prolonged administration: a new concept for increasing the spectrum and effectiveness of anthelmintics. *Vet. Parasit.*, **4,** 309–15
10. van der Bossche, H. and de Nollin, S. (1973). Effects of mebendazole on the absorption of low molecular weight nutrients by *Ascaris suum*. *Int. J. Parasit.*, **3,** 401–7
11. Wagner, J. G., Di Santo, A. R., Gillespie, W. R. *et al.* (1981). Reversible metabolism and pharmacokinetics: application to prednisone–prednisolone. *Res. Comm. Chem. Pathol. Pharmacol.*, **32,** 387–405

23
Pharmacokinetics of levamisole in goats and pigs

P. Nielsen and F. Rasmussen

Tetramisole was introduced as an anthelmintic for veterinary use in 1965. It is a racemic mixture of two optical isomers and it has been demonstrated that the anthelmintic activity rests almost solely with the l-isomer, levamisole. In addition to its anthelmintic properties, levamisole also possesses an immunomodulating effect[8], which has led to its widespread use in human as well as in veterinary medicine. This extensive use makes pharmacokinetic studies desirable and the purpose of the present study has therefore been to determine pharmacokinetic parameters for levamisole in goats and pigs and to measure its excretion in urine and faeces.

MATERIALS AND METHODS

The experiments were performed on three goats and six pigs. [^{3}H]levamisole (5 mg/kg b.w., spec. activity 2 μCi/mg) was administered intravenously. Blood samples were collected at the times indicated in Figure 23.1. The animals were kept in metabolic cages for quantitative collection of urine and faeces during the experimental period which lasted as long as ^{3}H was detectable in urine samples. [^{3}H]levamisole in plasma, urine and faeces was measured by liquid scintillation counting.

Unchanged levamisole and its metabolites were separated by TLC (0.25 mm silica gel plates developed in chloroform:methanol-25% aq. ammonia = 150:8:1). The amounts of unchanged drug and its metabolites were determined by liquid scintillation counting.

RESULTS AND DISCUSSION

Figure 23.1 illustrates a semilogarithmic plot of the concentration of levamisole in plasma vs. time after intravenous administration of the drug to a goat. The biexponential curve may be resolved into its two components

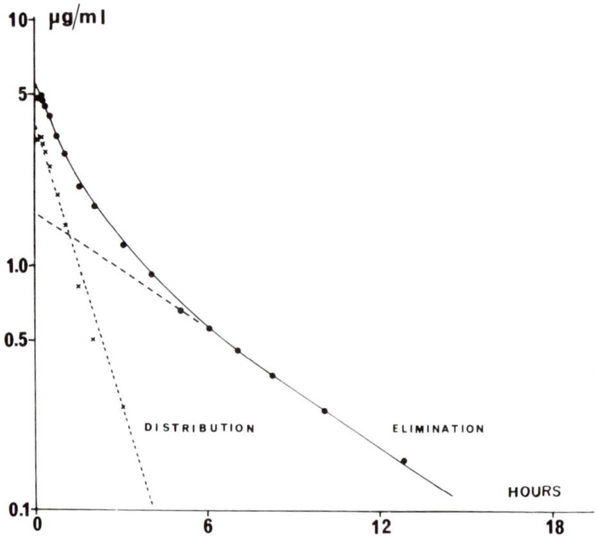

Figure 23.1 Concentration of levamisole in plasma *vs.* time after intravenous administration of the drug to a goat

representing distribution of the drug in the organism and elimination from plasma. The elimination phase is rapid and a level of 0.1 μg/ml is reached approximately 15 h after administration of the drug.

The distribution of levamisole is faster in goats than in pigs. Moreover, the elimination is also faster in goats (Table 23.1).

Table 23.1 Elimination halflife and volume of distribution for levamisole in goats and pigs

	Goats	*Pigs*
Elimination halflife (min)	222 ± 26	310 ± 100
Volume of distribution (l/kg)	3.1 ± 1.4	2.5 ± 0.7

Values are means ± SD

As a weak organic base of high lipid solubility, levamisole has an apparent volume of distribution greater than 1 which indicates that it is accumulated in tissues. The reason for the larger volume of distribution of levamisole in goats than in pigs may be diffusion of the organic base into the rumen of the goat. The accumulation of levamisole in tissues is in agreement with the results of Graziani & DeMartin[1], who investigated the distribution of [^{14}C]levamisole in bulls and pigs. (Subsequent chromatography and autoradiography of extracts of liver, kidney and blood showed that most of the extracted radioactivity was due to the parent drug.) Tissue levels of levamisole were determined 24, 48 and 72 h after the administration of a single 8 mg/kg dose to bulls and a 10 mg/kg dose to pigs. Tissue levels were higher in pigs, even allowing for the somewhat greater dose administered to pigs. Of the tissues studied, the highest levels were observed in liver in both species. However, with the exception of pig liver, tissue levels were less than 1 ppm 24 h after drug administration. Within 48 h in cattle and 96 h in pigs, residual tissue levels of levamisole were negligible (<0.1 parts/10^6). Such studies indicate the importance of analyses of tissue levels of a drug together with pharmacokinetic studies and show clearly that differences in rates of elimination of a drug from plasma and tissues may occur.

Table 23.2 shows the elimination halflife of levamisole in some other species. It is clear that elimination is particularly rapid in the rat and the rabbit. Table 23.3 shows the excretory routes for levamisole and its metabolites in goats and pigs. The goats excreted 55% of the administered dose in urine and 30% in faeces, giving a total recovery of 85% of the administered dose. In milking goats a small amount of the drug was excreted in milk, but this did not exceed 1% of the dose. The pigs excreted the major part of the dose (80–85%) in urine and only 5–10% was recovered from faeces samples. Similar differences in excretion in urine and faeces between goats and pigs have been noted for other drugs. In experiments with trimethoprim in pigs and goats it was reported[5] that goats excreted approximately equal amounts of this drug and its metabolites in urine and faeces whereas the figures for pigs[6] were almost the same as for levamisole. In rats 46% of levamisole is excreted in urine and about 32% in faeces[1].

Table 23.2 Elimination halflife for levamisole in other species

Species	*Elimination halflife*	*Reference*
Rat	30 min	3
Rabbit	45 min	4
Dog	3–4 h	3
Cattle	4–6 h	2
Man	2–6 h	3

Table 23.3 Excretion of [^{3}H]levamisole and its metabolites in urine and faeces from goats and pigs (% of dose)

	Urine	*Faeces*
Goats	55	30
Pigs	85	5

Most of the metabolites of levamisole were highly polar compounds and only about 20% of the labelled compounds excreted in urine was extractable with chloroform. Thin-layer chromatographic investigations revealed that many minor metabolites are formed and that only 5–10% of the labelled compounds excreted in urine was unchanged levamisole.

The pathways involved in the renal excretion of levamisole were not studied in the present experiments. Plante *et al.*[7] investigated the renal excretion of levamisole in dogs and found that about 15% of the drug was excreted by glomerular filtration while 85% was excreted by active tubular secretion at plasma concentrations of 0.9–6.7 μg/ml. In some experiments the clearance of levamisole was almost as high as the clearance of PAH. However, the pathway for the excretion of levamisole and PAH is not the same; PAH is an organic acid while levamisole is a base and as such they are excreted by different transport systems in the proximal convoluted tubule. Active tubular secretion of levamisole was further confirmed by the fact that it was possible to block it by simultaneous loading of the dogs with thiamine, which is a competitive inhibitor for active renal secretion of organic bases.

SUMMARY

Levamisole is an organic base which is distributed widely in the organism and accumulates in tissues such as liver and kidney. It is eliminated relatively quickly from plasma, but elimination from tissues is much slower. Levamisole is metabolized to a very high extent and only a small percentage is excreted unchanged. Pigs excrete levamisole and its metabolites almost entirely in urine, while goats excrete them in both urine and faeces.

References

1. Graziani, G. and DeMartin, G. L. (1977). Pharmacokinetic studies on levamisole. Absorption, distribution, excretion and metabolism of levamisole in animals. *Drugs Exptl. Clin. Res.*, **2**, 221–33
2. Heykants, J., Wynants, J. and Scheijgrond, H. (1975). The absorption, excretion and metabolism of levamisole in man. *Clinical Research Report*, November. Janssen Research Products Information Service
3. Langley, B. W. (1968). Blood level studies with l-tetramisole. *Biological Research Report*, July. (Acc. No. 6179). Janssen Research Products Information Service
4. Michiels, M., Woestenborghs, R. and Heykants, J. (1978). Absorption and plasma levels of oral levamisole in the rabbit. *Preclinical Research Report*, June. Janssen Research Products Information Service
5. Nielsen, P. and Rasmussen, F. (1975). Elimination of trimethoprim in swine. Comparison of results obtained by three analytical methods. *Acta Pharmacol. Toxicol.*, **37**, 307–16
6. Nielsen, P. and Rasmussen, F. (1976). Elimination of trimethoprim, sulphadoxine and their metabolites in goats. *Acta Pharmacol. Toxicol.*, **38**, 104–12
7. Plante, G. E., Erian, R. and Petitclerc, C. (1981). Renal excretion of levamisole. *J. Pharmacol. Exp. Ther.*, **216**, 617–23
8. Symoens, J. and Rosenthal, M. (1977). Levamisole in the modulation of the immune response: the current experimental and clinical state. *J. Reticuloendothelial Soc.*, **21**, 175–221

APPENDIX

Two pharmacokinetic studies of levamisole in ruminants were recently published with the following summaries:

'Quantitation of levamisole in biological fluids of ewes and goats was obtained by the use of HPLC after oral (10 mg/kg), intramuscular (7.5 mg/kg), and subcutaneous (7.5 mg/kg) administrations. Greater efficiency was obtained in both species after intramuscular rather than subcutaneous or oral administrations. After intramuscular injection, levamisole levels in nasal secretion and saliva were five to twenty times higher than in plasma. Because of the high susceptibility of goats to levamisole, the subcutaneous route is preferred in this animal.'

Galtier, P., Escoula, L., Camguilhem, R. and Alvinerie, M. (1981). Comparative bioavailability of levamisole in non-lactating ewes and goats. *Ann. Rech. Vét.*, **12**, 109–15

'Levamisole, at a dose rate of 7.5 mg/kg, produced mean peak plasma concentrations of 3.1, 0.7 and 0.8 μg/ml in four sheep after administration by the subcutaneous, oral and intraruminal routes, respectively. The mean peak concentrations in abomasal fluid were 33, 164 and 21 μg/ml, respectively. The bioavailability of levamisole to the systemic compartment was less after oral and intraruminal administration than after subcutaneous administration. In six sheep there were no significant differences in the plasma concentration in the thoracic, neck or gluteal regions. Dividing the dose between five sites in the gluteal region produced higher peak plasma concentrations than when injected into a single site.'

Bogan, J. A., Marriner, S. E. and Galbraith, E. A. (1982). Pharmacokinetics of levamisole in sheep. *Res. Vet. Sci.*, **32**, 124–6

24

The prophylactic activity of imidocarb against tick-transmitted parasitic infections

N. McHardy

Imidocarb – 3,3′bis-(2-imidazolin-2-yl) carbanilide dipropionate (Carbesia®, Imizol®) is highly active against all species of the protozoan parasite *Babesia*, with the possible exception of *B. gibsoni* of dogs, and *B. felis* in cats. It is very active against *Anaplasma marginale*, a rickettsia-like parasite of ruminants. It is not effective against *Theileria*. Imidocarb exerts a prophylactic effect against some species of *Babesia*[3,5] which may last for several weeks. The duration of prophylaxis seems to depend on the severity and virulence of challenge[4]. Imidocarb has no prophylactic effect on *Anaplasma*. The mode of action of imidocarb is not certain, although two mechanisms have been suggested. The effect of imidocarb on *Trypanosoma brucei* has been antagonized with excess polyamines, which suggests that the drug interfered with the production or utilization of polyamines[1]. Imidocarb blocks the entry of inositol, an essential nutrient, into the erythrocyte containing the *Babesia* parasite, apparently resulting in the 'starvation' of the parasite (Elford, unpublished). This mechanism would readily explain the prophylactic effect of imidocarb since the presence of very small quantities of imidocarb on the surface of the erythrocyte could make it unattractive to the parasite.

The experiments reported here were aimed at clarifying the mechanism of prophylaxis of imidocarb by comparing its activity with that of several other antibabesial compounds. The model used was *B. rodhaini*, Beveridge strain[2] in CD-1 male mice, weighing 16–20 g or in male Wister rats, weighing about 60 g.

METHODS

Three main experimental designs were used with mice:

(1) Therapeutic model. The mice were infected by the intravenous injection of 2×10^7 erythrocytes infected with *B. rodhaini*. After 24 h experimental compounds, appropriately dissolved and diluted, were injected

subcutaneously. The course of the infection was monitored by the examination of stained smears of tail blood, and by recording the time of death of the mice.

(2) Prophylactic model. The design of the experiment was essentially similar to the therapeutic model, except that compounds were injected s.c. up to 14 days before i.v. challenge with 2×10^7 or 2×10^5 infected erythrocytes.

(3) *In vitro/in vivo* model. Blood from mice with approximately 50% parasitaemia was withdrawn and diluted with minimum essential medium to give mixtures of 2×10^8 infected erythrocytes in known concentrations of experimental compounds. The mixture was incubated for 2 h at 37°C, after which the erythrocytes were washed twice and 2×10^7 erythrocytes were injected i.v. into mice. The infection was then monitored as above.

The experiments in rats were essentially similar to the therapeutic and prophylactic models in mice except that implantable mini-pumps (Alzet, model 2002, Scientific Marketing, London) were also used. They released compound at a known rate over 14 days following subcutaneous insertion under anaesthesia.

EXPERIMENTAL

Therapeutic effects

The therapeutic efficacy of four standard antibabesials – imidocarb dipropionate, amicarbalide, quinuronium sulphate and diminazene aceturate,

Table 24.1 Comparison of efficacy of antibabesials in mice treated s.c. 1 day after i.v. challenge with 2×10^7 *B. rodhaini*

		Survival at day 14 (groups of 5 mice)						
	ED_{50}* mg/kg	*Dosage* (mg/kg s.c.)						
Compound	*(+fiducial limits)*	10	5	2.5	1.0	0.5	0.25	0.125
Imidocarb	0.49 (0.43–0.56)	5	5	5	5	5	5	4
Diminazene	8.89 (7.68–10.16)	5	4	3	0			
Amicarbalide	2.41 (2.08–2.82)	5	5	5	1	0	0	
Quinuronium	0.46 (0.41–0.52)	T†	T	5	5	2	2	
Monensin	1.86 (1.76–1.97)	0	0	0	0	0		
Isometamidium	0.84 (0.68–1.01)	1	1	0	0	0		

Untreated mice died in 4.2 days (mean)
*ED_{50} – dose of drug which reduces parasitaemia to 50% of that in untreated controls on day 4
†T – lethally toxic

together with the ionophore antibiotic monensin, and the trypanocidal compound isometamidium, was compared (Table 24.1). The results reflect, approximately, the relative efficacies of the standard antibabesial compounds against *B. bovis* and *B. bigemina* in cattle[7]. Survival was greatest among mice treated with imidocarb even in groups treated with less than the ED_{50}, in which parasitaemia reached relatively high levels. Although monensin and isometamidium were very effective in controlling parasitaemia at day 4, as shown by their relatively low ED_{50}, they failed to cure mice.

Table 24.2 Comparison of activity of antibabesials as determined by the *in vitro/in vivo* system with *B. rodhaini*

Compound	*EC_{50}** mg/l (*+fiducial limits*)	*Concentration of compound* (mg/l) 10	2.5	0.6	0.15	0.04	0.01	0.0025
		% Parasitaemia on day 4 (±SD)						
Imidocarb	0.028 (0.025–0.032)	0	0	0.25	6.2 ±2.34	33.8 ±6.76	83.0 ±4.30	90.2 ±3.96
Diminazene	0.57 (0.47–0.66)	6.4 ±2.51	12.8 ±2.68	45.0 ±4.0	86.2 ±1.92	92.8 ±3.19	91.6 ±1.52	90.2 ±2.59
Amicarbalide	0.17 (0.14–0.21)	1.1 ±0.55	2.0 ±1.00	9.0 ±2.74	51.2 ±17.4	89.8 ±1.48	92.2 ±1.79	93.0 ±2.35
Quinuronium	1.22 (1.17–1.29)	1.4 ±0.55	10.6 ±1.67	81.8 ±4.44	91.2 ±1.92	92.8 ±1.30	93.2 ±2.59	92.8 ±1.30
Monensin	0.043 (0.038–0.047)	0	0.2 ±0.11	3.8 ±1.64	11.2 ±2.59	48.0 ±3.54	53.6 ±8.02	64.0 ±12.51

Untreated mice had parasitaemia 92.4% ±3.91 on day 4
*EC_{50} – concentration of drug which reduces parasitaemia to 50% of that in untreated controls on day 4

Next, the performance of compounds in the *in vitro/in vivo* system was examined (Table 24.2). The activity of the three bisamidines, imidocarb, diminazene and amicarbalide, was shown to be high, and the ratio of ED_{50} (in mg/kg): EC_{50} (in mg/l) was, respectively, 17.5, 15.5 and 12.5 : 1. With the bisquinolyl compound quinuronium sulphate, the ratio was 0.38 : 1, indicating a basically different mode of action, or a different rate of uptake or binding with quinuronium sulphate. The mode of action of none of these compounds is proven, as discussed earlier[1,4]. Monensin gave an $ED_{50}:EC_{50}$ ratio of 43.25 : 1. While its mode of action as an antibabesial is not known, it is believed to act as an ionophore, particularly for K^+ ions, in its action on coccidia. Monensin shows only slight activity against *B. bovis* in cattle (McHardy, unpublished) and is extremely toxic when injected into cattle[6], so is unlikely to be used as an antibabesial in the field.

Prophylactic effects

Of the antibabesial drugs, imidocarb has the greatest prophylactic effect in the field, and is used for this purpose at around 2.5 mg/kg. The prophylactic effect of imidocarb in mice was examined in groups of ten mice injected with

Table 24.3 Prophylactic effect of imidocarb and isometamidium in groups of 10 mice challenged with *B. rodhaini*

	Challenged 2 × 10^7 i.v.				*Challenged* 2 × 10^5 i.v.			
	Imidocarb 10 mg/kg s.c.		*Isometamidium* 10 mg/kg s.c.		*Imidocarb* 10 mg/kg s.c.		*Isometamidium* 10 mg/kg s.c.	
Treatment	*% Parasitaemia Day 4*	*± SD*	*% Parasitaemia Day 4*	*± SD*	*% Parasitaemia Day 7*	*± SD*	*% Parasitaemia Day 7*	*± SD*
Untreated	88.3 ±4.16	(0)*	—	—	88.3 ±4.06	(0)	—	—
Day −14	86.3 ±5.73	(0)	89.7 ±4.83	(0)	84.1 ±8.07	(0)	88.0 ±4.32	(0)
Day −10	41.3 ±19.34	(6)	87.1 ±6.08	(0)	11.5 ±14.5	(5)	89.0 ±5.08	(0)
Day −7	16.3 ±7.70	(9)	90.0 ±5.42	(0)	0.8 ±0.89	(8)	89.2 ±5.33	(0)
Day −4	4.1 ±1.20	(5)	40.7 ±20.31	(3)	0.0 —	(5)	72.0 ±21.34	(1)
Day −2	0.7 ±0.26	(10)	65.1 ±22.19	(0)	0.0	(10)	84.5 ±11.83	(0)
Day −1	1.7 ±0.48	(9)	14.6 ±17.30	(4)	0.0	(10)	29.4 ±32.34	(4)

*Figure in parenthesis is number of mice surviving to day 21

imidocarb at 10 mg/kg s.c. up to 14 days before challenge with either 2 × 10^7 or 2 × 10^5 *B. rodhaini*, injected i.v. (Table 24.3). Isometamidium (Samorin) was also included in this experiment. It shows a prophylactic effect against African trypanosomes in cattle of up to 3 months following a dosage of only 0.5 mg/kg i.m., and its ED_{50} against *B. rodhaini* (Table 24.1) was 0.84 mg/kg.

Imidocarb at 10 mg/kg showed marked prophylactic effects against *B. rodhaini* when injected up to 10 days before challenge with either 2 × 10^7 or 2 × 10^5 organisms, using depression of parasitaemia or survival of mice as parameters. There was no significant protection when imidocarb was injected 14 days before challenge. Isometamidium at 10 mg/kg gave some protection at 4, but not 7 days before challenge. So, while the prophylactic effect of imidocarb in mice infected with *B. rodhaini* was significant, it was not as prolonged as that seen in cattle challenged with *B. bovis* or *B. bigemina*[3]. However, the severity of parasitaemia following challenge was greater with high than with low challenge, as seems to occur in the field. Despite its use at 12 times its ED_{50} against *B. rodhaini* and 20 times the field usage rate against trypanosomes, isometamidium failed to show marked prophylaxis against *B. rodhaini*. This indicates that prophylaxis against *Babesia* may not be simply a manifestation of persistence of drug, and again indicates that the prophylactic effect of imidocarb may be peculiar to this class of compound. To investigate this further, diminazene aceturate – a

Table 24.4 A comparison of the prophylactic effect of diminazene aceturate and imidocarb dipropionate in groups of ten mice challenged with 2×10^5 *B. rodhaini* i.v.

	Imidocarb 2.5 mg/kg s.c.				*Diminazene* 10 mg/kg s.c.			
	% Parasitaemia		*Mean survival*		*% Parasitaemia*		*Mean survival*	
Treatment	*Day 7*	*±SD*	*(Days)**	*±SD*	*Day 7*	*±SD*	*(Days)**	*±SD*
Untreated	90.7 ±3.06		7.7 ±0.67	(0)	—		—	
Day −7	61.7 ±26.05		9.0 ±1.15	(0)	9.0 ±3.65		10.1 ±0.32	(0)
Day −4	1.4 ±2.11		18.1 ±4.7	(7)	2.6 ±1.50		11.2 ±0.42	(0)
Day −2	0		18.5 ±2.13	(9)	0.42 ±0.19		12.0 ±1.04	(0)
Day −1	0		21	(10)	0.1 —		13.5 ±2.72	(1)

*Mice which survived to end of experiment (day 21) scored as 21. Figure in parenthesis is no. alive on day 21

bisamidine like imidocarb, was also tested for prophylactic effect; 10 mg/kg was injected up to 7 days before challenge with 2×10^5 *B. rodhaini*. In this trial imidocarb was used at 2.5 mg/kg (Table 24.4).

Imidocarb at 2.5 mg/kg s.c. demonstrated marked prophylaxis when given up to 4 days before challenge, but only a marginal effect at day 7. Diminazene, 10 mg/kg s.c., was very effective in reducing parasitaemia, even when given 7 days before challenge, but it did not prevent the mice dying, even when given only 1 day before challenge. This suggests that imidocarb has a true prophylactic effect while diminazene may have been released slowly from the injection site for about 4 days, before being rapidly excreted or metabolized, so demonstrating no true prophylactic effect.

Further confirmation of the prophylactic effect of imidocarb was obtained by comparing the effects in rats infected with *B. rodhaini* by daily s.c. injections of low doses of imidocarb and the continuous release of similar quantities of imidocarb from osmotic mini-pumps implanted s.c. on the abdomen. As a control, further groups of rats were injected s.c. with a single dose of imidocarb equivalent to the total dose delivered by these methods.

In the first trial (Table 24.5) the rats were infected by the i.v. injection of 1×10^8 *B. rodhaini* in infected mouse blood. Five rats were left untreated while groups of four rats received 14 daily s.c. injections of 0.1 or 0.3 mg/kg imidocarb or were implanted with pumps continuously delivering 0.1 or 0.3 mg/kg imidocarb per day for 14 days. These treatments began on the day after infection. Two further groups of four rats received a single dose of 1.4 or 4.2 mg/kg s.c. on the day after infection. The untreated controls developed severe babesiosis (maximum parasitaemia 57.6%) but recovered within 12 days, having shown maximum parasitaemia on day 4.4 (mean). The course of infection in all the treated groups was remarkably similar to each other.

Table 24.5 Comparison of the effect of administration of imidocarb by daily s.c. injection or from implantable mini-pump beginning on the day *after* infection in rats* infected with 1×10^8 *B. rodhaini*

Treatment	*Maximum %* *Parasitaemia* $\pm SD$	*Duration of* *Parasitaemia* (Days) $\pm SD$	*Day of maximum* *Parasitaemia* $\pm SD$
Untreated	57.6 ±5.03	12.6 ±2.41	4.4 ±0.55
Imidocarb s.c. injn. 1.4 mg/kg × 1 day +1	6.75 ±4.19	6.25 ±0.96	2.75 ±0.5
Imidocarb s.c. injn. 0.1 mg/kg × 14 days +1 to +14	10.5 ±6.60	6.0 ±0.82	2.75 ±0.5
Imidocarb s.c. pump 0.1 mg/kg/day × 14 days +1 to +14	7.25 ±3.77	6.25 ±0.5	3.0 ±0.0
Imidocarb s.c. injn. 4.2 mg/kg × 1 day +1	0.9 ±0.82	4.75 ±1.71	2.0 ±0.0
Imidocarb s.c. injn. 0.3 mg/kg × 1 days +1 to +14	10.5 ±6.95	6.0 ±0.82	3.0 ±0.0
Imidocarb s.c. pump 0.3 mg/kg/day × 14	9.75 ±8.92	6.5 ±0.58	3.0 ±0.0

*4 rats per group except untreated controls (5). All rats survived

The single dose of 4.2 mg/kg imidocarb limited peak parasitaemia to only 0.9% but in all other groups mean peak parasitaemia was 6.75–10.5%. The peak occurred on day 2.0–3.0, and lasted for 4.75–6.5 days in all the treated groups.

In the second experiment (Table 24.6), which shared the untreated controls with the first, groups of five rats received 0.1 mg/kg imidocarb daily for 14 days by s.c. injection or pump, beginning on the day before infection, or a single s.c. injection of 1.4 mg/kg on the day before infection. They were challenged i.v. with either 1×10^8 or 1×10^6 *B. rodhaini* in infected mouse blood. In the rats challenged with 1×10^6 parasites maximum parasitaemia was 20%, reached its peak on day 9.4 (mean) and persisted for 14.0 days, i.e. the infection was less severe than that in rats challenged with 1×10^8 organisms (above). In the treated rats all three regimens at each challenge dose gave remarkably similar results, and with the 1×10^6 challenge parasitaemia did not attain countable levels in any treated rat.

These two experiments indicate that imidocarb acted in a truly prophylactic manner in controlling *B. rodhaini* infection – a single high dose around the time of infection gave very similar initial effect and persistent effect to daily administration of low doses. In all cases infections were effectively suppressed in comparison with untreated controls.

Table 24.6 Comparison of the effect of administration of imidocarb by daily s.c. injection or from implantable mini-pumps, beginning on the day *before* infection, in rats infected i.v. with 1×10^8 or 1×10^6 *B. rodhaini*

Treatment	*Maximum % parasitaemia ±SD*		*Duration of parasitaemia ±SD*		*Day of maximum parasitaemia ±SD*	
	Challenge 1×10^8	*Challenge* 1×10^6	*Challenge* 1×10^8	*Challenge* 1×10^6	*Challenge* 1×10^8	*Challenge* 1×10^6
Untreated*	57.6 ±5.03	20.0 ±11.33	12.6 ±2.41	14.0 ±1.22	4.4 ±0.55	9.4 ±2.30
Imidocarb s.c. injn. 1.4 mg/kg × 1 day −1	4.4 ±0.55	+ve	6.25 ±3.59	3.6 ±1.34	2.2 ±0.45	3.0 ±0.0
Imidocarb s.c. injn. 0.1 mg/kg × 14 day −1 to +12	4.0 ±1.41	+ve	6.0 ±1.41	3.6 ±2.19	2.0 ±0.0	3.75 ±0.5
Imidocarb s.c. pump 0.1 mg/kg/day × 14 day −1 to +12	3.7 ±2.11	+ve	5.0† ±1.63	2.4 ±1.34	2.2 ±0.45	‡

*5 rats in each group
†1 rat which shed pump on day 3 excluded
‡3 rats +ve, 2 rats −ve

Drug levels in cattle

In order to relate these findings to the situation in cattle following injection of imidocarb, the *in vitro/in vivo* method was used to monitor the level of antibabesial activity in two calves following the i.m. injection of imidocarb at 2.5 mg/kg, an effective prophylactic dose[3]. Samples of venous blood were taken, using heparin as anticoagulant, at timed intervals after dosing. Plasma was separated by centrifugation and samples were stored at −70° C until used. Plasma samples were then assayed in the *in vitro/in vivo* system by incorporation in the incubation mixtures at 5% concentration of plasma. A series of known concentrations of imidocarb was also tested to provide a reference standard curve for inhibition by imidocarb, and from which the equivalent concentration in the plasma samples could be calculated.

It was found (Table 24.7) that inhibition was already maximal at the time that the first plasma sample was taken – 30 min after administration. It was equivalent to about 3.4 mg/l, which is far in excess of the *in vitro* EC_{50} of imidocarb (0.028 mg/l, Table 24.2). The concentration of imidocarb in the plasma had begun to fall significantly 4 h after injection, and was around the EC_{50} at 48 h. It had fallen below detectable levels (0.001 mg/l) at 72 h. This result is in agreement with earlier results (Nimmo-Smith, unpublished) which showed that concentrations in the plasma of nine calves injected i.v. with 0.5 mg/kg imidocarb fell from 2.17 mg/l 5 min after injection to 0.02 mg/l at 24 h, when assayed by a chemical method.

Table 24.7 Concentration of imidocarb in plasma of calves following injection of 2.5 mg/kg imidocarb i.m., monitored by *B. rodhaini in vitro/in vivo* test

Time after treatment (h)	*Concentration of imidocarb in plasma* (mg/l) *Calf* 1469	*Calf* 1473
0	0	0
0.5	2.69	4.03
1	2.12	4.03
2	1.14	2.57
4	0.75	1.52
7	0.40	1.10
24	0.034	0.23
48	0.010	0.086
72	0.008	0.00

CONCLUSIONS

The results reported here indicate that the mouse and rat infected with *B. rodhaini* provide useful models for the prophylactic effect of imidocarb in cattle, and the *in vitro/in vivo* system can be used to monitor drug levels in bovine blood. Concentrations of available imidocarb in the plasma of cattle fell below inhibitory concentrations within 3 days of injection of 2.5 mg/kg s.c. The extended prophylaxis seen in the field therefore could be due either to mobilization from other sites[8] or to imidocarb bound to erythrocytes inhibiting entry or survival of parasites in the erythrocytes. This latter explanation fits well with the mode of action of imidocarb proposed but unpublished by Elford, that the drug acts at the surface of the infected erythrocyte.

References

1. Bacchi, C. J., Nathan, H. C., Hutner, S. H. *et al.* (1981). Prevention by polyamines of the curative effect of amicarbalide and imidocarb for *Trypanosoma brucei* infections in mice. *Biochem. Pharmacol.*, **8**, 883–6
2. Beveridge, E. (1953). *Babesia rodhaini*: a useful organism for the testing of drugs designed for the treatment of piroplasmosis. *Ann. Trop. Med. Parasitol.*, **47**, 134–8
3. Callow, L. L. and McGregor, W. (1970). The effect of imidocarb against *Babesia argentina* and *Babesia bigemina* infections of cattle. *Aust. Vet. J.*, **46**, 195–200
4. Euzeby, J., Moreau, Y., Gauthey, M. *et al.* (1981). Studies on the efficacy of imidocarb against *Babesia divergens* and *B. canis*, agents of bovine and canine piroplasmosis in Europe. *Bull. Soc. Sci. Vét. Méd. Comp. Lyon*, **83**, 129–34
5. Haigh, A. J. B. and Hagan, D. H. (1974). Evaluation of imidocarb dihydrochloride against 'redwater' disease in cattle in Eire. *Vet. Rec.*, **94**, 56–9
6. McHardy, N. and Rae, D. G. (1982). Antitheilerial activity of the coccidiostat monensin. *Trop. Anim. Hlth Prod.*, **14**, 13–14
7. Purnell, R. E. (1981). Tick-borne diseases. *Br. Vet. J.*, **137**, 221–40
8. Wood, J. C. (1971). The activity of imidocarb against *Babesia* infections of cattle. *Irish Vet. J.*, **25**, 254–7

Section III
Non-Ruminant Pharmacology

25
The distribution and function of histamine receptors

P. Eyre and K. B. Mirbahar

From the first description of the biological actions of histamine by Dale and Laidlaw[20] in 1910, histamine has provided a constant stimulus to pharmacologists and immunologists who have attempted to define this amine in various physiological and pathological roles. It was 40 years ago that Bovet and Staub[10] first reported that compound 929F antagonized the actions of histamine on smooth muscle and protected guinea-pigs from anaphylaxis. It soon became clear that although many of the effects of histamine could be specifically blocked by low concentrations of these 'classical' antihistaminics, there were other actions of histamine which were refractory even to toxic doses of the antihistaminics then available. These resistant actions include inhibition of the rat uterus[7], stimulation of the heart[42] and stimulation of gastric secretion[3].

Ash and Schild[2] systematically studied the receptors mediating the actions of histamine and concluded that there were two separate receptor classes, based on the fact that histamine analogues showed two distinctly different activity profiles when assayed on a variety of tissues. Ash and Schild[2] suggested the symbol H_1 to denote histamine receptors which were sensitive to low doses of the classical[10,28] histamine antagonists. Non-H_1 receptors were later classified by Black *et al.*[4] and designated as H_2-receptors.

The H_1-receptor antagonist group of drugs includes mepyramine, diphenhydramine, chlorpheniramine, chlorcyclizine and promethazine, each representing a different chemical class[2,28]. Burimamide, metiamide and cimetidine comprise the H_2-receptor antagonists[4,5,12]. 2-Methylhistamine and 2-pyridylethylamine[2,4,21] are histamine H_1-agonists, whereas 4-methylhistamine and dimaprit are H_2-agonists[4,38] (Figure 25.1).

The judicious use of the above selective H_1- and H_2-receptor agonists and antagonists has now firmly established the concept of two distinct receptors which mediate the numerous biological effects of histamine.

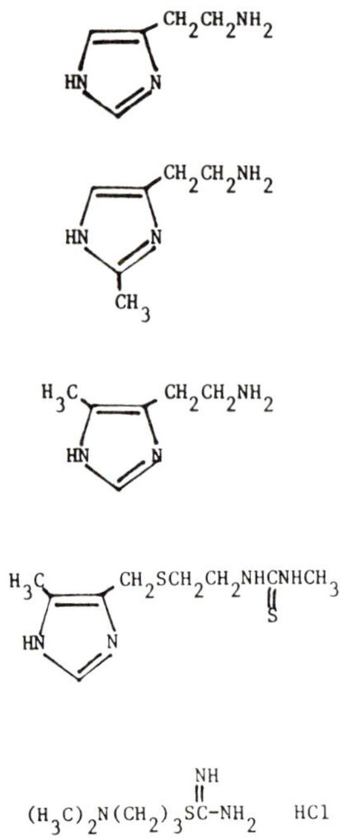

Histamine

2-Methylhistamine (selective H_1-agonist)

4-Methylhistamine (selective H_2-agonist)

Metiamide (selective H_2-antagonist)

Dimaprit (selective H_2-agonist)

Figure 25.1 A selection of histamine analogues

GASTROINTESTINAL SYSTEM

The ability of histamine to contract the guinea-pig ileum is one of the best known H_1-mediated responses[2], and it is generally true to say that histamine-induced motility of the alimentary tract is mediated by H_1-receptors. Histamine has also been shown to inhibit neurogenic, atropine-resistant tetanic spasms of the ileum[1]. This action of histamine was blocked by burimamide, which suggests that the participating receptors are H_2-receptors. In a similar way, histamine-induced relaxation of the rat uterus is presumed to be caused by H_2-receptor stimulation[2], but the evidence is not absolutely conclusive. Histamine stimulates gastric parietal cells to secrete hydrochloric acid[3]. This effect is blocked by H_2 receptor antagonists[4].

THE CARDIOVASCULAR SYSTEM

Blood pressure

Histamine causes a fall in blood pressure which is sometimes followed by a secondary pressor response. The depressor effects of small doses of histamine are antagonized by H_1-antagonists, whereas those of large doses of histamine usually are not[28]. The concept of a second type of cardiovascular histamine receptor was postulated in the 1940s and 1950s. It is now clear that the mepyramine-resistant actions of histamine on systemic blood pressure are mediated by H_2-receptors. Evidence for this statement may be summarized using three examples. The systemic response to histamine in the rabbit is variable, often biphasic with a pressor response predominating. Very large doses of histamine may induce a depressor effect. H_1-antagonists convert the biphasic or pressor effect to depression, whereas H_2-antagonists abolish the depressor effect and convert it to a purely pressor one[4,5]. In cats and dogs both H_1- and H_2-antagonists inhibit the depressor response to histamine[6,39], whereas in calves[23] the depressor effect of histamine is partially blocked by mepyramine and potentiated by burimamide, suggesting that an H_2-receptor mechanism is playing a modulatory pressor role. Further studies revealed that H_2-antagonists potentiated anaphylactic shock in calves[23].

Regional bloodflow and vascular permeability

Local application of histamine causes vasodilatation in most vascular beds including the skin, skeletal muscle and digestive tract, among others. Vasodilatation is usually accompanied by increased vascular permeability and sometimes by alterations in bloodflow. Studies in the cat and dog closely parallel those on systemic blood pressure. Histamine-induced vasodilatation in the hind limb may be antagonized by either or both H_1- and H_2-receptor blockers, suggesting the participation of both H_1- and H_2-receptors[27]. However, there is little or no evidence that H_2-receptors play more than a minor role in histamine-induced vascular permeability changes[17].

Pulmonary vasculature

Histamine may cause vasoconstriction or vasodilatation in the pulmonary vasculature with the former usually dominating. The vasoconstrictor effect of histamine is abolished by H_1-antagonists or converted to a depressor response, which is in turn blocked by H_2-antagonists[29,40]. H_2-blockers themselves enhance the pulmonary vasoconstrictor response of histamine.

The heart

Actions of histamine on the heart are highly complicated because it is difficult to distinguish between the direct effects of histamine and indirect actions caused by reflex vascular and respiratory changes and humoral substances such as catecholamines released by histamine. Histamine causes increased rate and force of contraction in isolated spontaneously-beating heart preparations[25,33]. These effects are usually accompanied by increased cardiac output and increased coronary bloodflow[26]. The positive chronotropic effects of histamine on the heart are mimicked by H_2-agonists and are effectively blocked by H_2-antagonists[33], but are not affected by H_1-blockers. The inotropic action of histamine has been more difficult to define. The action of histamine on electrically driven left atria was blocked by mepyramine, whereas the inotropic effect of histamine on spontaneously beating hearts was blocked by H_2-antagonists. Arrhythmias induced by histamine are also antagonized by H_2-blocking agents[43].

AIRWAY SMOOTH MUSCLE

There is considerable species variation in airway reactivity to histamine[13]. Histamine does not cause contraction of isolated bronchi of rat, cat or sheep[22]; it has variable action in the rabbit and ferret but in all other species produces powerful bronchoconstriction which is regarded as an important component in the aetiology of bronchial asthma. Mepyramine partially antagonizes histamine-induced bronchoconstriction. If the tracheobronchial muscle is partially contracted by carbachol in the presence of mepyramine (H_1-blocked), further addition of histamine causes bronchodilatation. These relaxations of airway smooth muscle are blocked by H_2-antagonists in some species (e.g. man, horse and guinea-pig[15,41]) but in some other species H_2-agonist-induced airway relaxation is not blocked by H_2-antagonists (cat, rat and rabbit[14,16]). This gives rise to a suggestion that there may be *two* sub-types of histamine H_2-receptors in airways[14–16].

THE NERVOUS SYSTEM

The exact role of histaminergic synapses in the central nervous system has not been well defined although it seems probable that H_2-receptor mechanisms are involved. It was shown recently that metiamide may interact pharmacologically with the antihypertensive drug clonidine[30]. It seems that the hypotensive action of clonidine is antagonized by centrally-administered metiamide or cimetidine. This suggests that H_2-receptors are somehow involved in the central mechanism of action of clonidine. It is interesting that clonidine has also been reported to have H_2-agonist activity on the heart[19].

Histamine stimulates autonomic ganglia. In the cat superior cervical ganglion, H_1-receptors mediate facilitation while H_2- receptors mediate inhibitory effects of histamine on ganglionic transmission[11].

TISSUE UPTAKE AND METABOLISM OF HISTAMINE

Histamine H_2-antagonists increase histidine decarboxylase activity[34], thereby enhancing histamine formation. H_2-blockers also inhibit the uptake of histamine by the cardiovascular system[24] and may also interfere with histamine catabolism, especially with the enzyme histamine-*N*-methyltransferase[24].

INFLAMMATION AND HYPERSENSITIVITY

It is well-known that leukocytes and mast cells possess specific receptors for a variety of hormones such as insulin, catecholamines, prostaglandins and histamine. Interactions with these hormones mediate important modulatory mechanisms in a variety of immunological and pharmacological cellular phenomena[8,35]. Histamine inhibits IgE-dependent release of chemical mediators from mast cells and basophils, a process which is accompanied by increased intracellular cyclic AMP concentrations[9]. H_2-antagonists themselves enhance the release of mediators and, predictably, inhibit the histamine-induced inhibition of mediator release[31,32].

It has been suggested that the activity of lymphocytes is governed by the number of histamine receptors carried by the cells. Histamine inhibits T-lymphocyte cytotoxicity and this property increases with time after immunization[36,37]. In a similar way, histamine inhibits the immunological release of leukocyte lysosomal enzymes[35] and enhances eosinophil migration[18]. Thus endogenously-released histamine plays an important part in the regulation inflammation.

ACKNOWLEDGEMENT

Supported in part by the National Research Council of Canada, Agriculture Canada, Ontario Ministry of Agriculture and Ontario Racing Commission.

References

1. Ambache, N., Killick, S. W. and Zar, M. A. (1973). *Br. J. Pharmacol.*, **48**, 362P-3P
2. Ash, A. S. F. and Schild, H. O. (1966). *Br. J. Pharmacol.*, **27**, 427–39
3. Ashford, C. A., Heller, H. and Smart, G. A. (1949). *Br. J. Pharmacol.*, **4**, 153–6, 157–61
4. Black, J. W., Duncan, W. A. M., Durant, G. J. *et al.* (1972). *Nature (London)*, **236**, 385–90
5. Black, J. W., Duncan, W. A. M., Emmett, J. C. *et al.* (1973). *Agents Actions*, **3**, 133–7
6. Black, J. W., Owen, D. A. A. and Parsons, M. E. (1975). *Br. J. Pharmacol*, **54**, 319–24
7. Blyth, D. I. (1972). *Br. J. Pharmacol.*, **45**, 126–8
8. Bourne, H. R., Lichtenstein, L. M., Melmon, K. L. *et al.* (1974). *Science*, **184**, 19–28
9. Bourne, H. R., Melmon, K. L. and Lichtenstein, L. M. (1971). *Science*, **173**, 743–5
10. Bovet, D. and Staub, A. (1937). *C.R. Soc. Biol.* **124**, 547–9
11. Brimble, M. J. and Wallis, D. I. (1973). *Nature (London)*, **246**, 156–9
12. Brimblecombe, R. W., Duncan, W. A. M., Durant, G. J. *et al.* (1975). *J. Int. Med. Res.*, **3**, 86–92
13. Chand, N. and Eyre, P. (1975). *Agents Actions*, **5**, 277–95
14. Chand, N. and Eyre, P. (1977). *Agents Actions*, **7**, 183–90
15. Chand, N. and Eyre, P. (1978). *Agents Actions*, **8**, 191–8
16. Chand, N. and Eyre, P. (1978). *Res. Comm. Chem. Path. Pharmacol.*, **21**, 55–65
17. Church, M. K. and Miller, P. (1975). *Br. J. Pharmacol.*, **55**, 315P
18. Clark, R. A. F., Sandler, J. A., Gallin, J. I. *et al.* (1977). *J. Immunol.*, **118**, 137–45
19. Csongrady, A. and Kobinger, W. (1974). *Arch. Pharmacol.*, **282**, 123
20. Dale, H. H. and Laidlaw, P. P. (1910). *J. Physiol.*, **41**, 318–49
21. Durant, G. J., Ganellin, C. R. and Parsons, M. E. (1975). *J. Med. Chem.*, **18**, 905–9
22. Eyre, P. (1973). *Br. J. Pharmacol.*, **48**, 321–3
23. Eyre, P. and Wells, P. W. (1973). *Br. J. Pharmacol.*, **49**, 364–7
24. Fantozzi, R., Mannaioni, P. F. and Moroni, F. (1973). *Br. J. Pharmacol.*, **49**, 361–3
25. Flacke, W., Atanackovic, D., Gillis, R. A. *et al.* (1967). *J. Pharmacol. Exp. Ther.*, **155**, 271–8
26. Flynn, S. B., Gristwood, R. W. and Owen, D. A. A. (1977). *Br. J. Pharmacol.*, **59**, 530P
27. Flynn, S. B. and Owen, D. A. A. (1975). *Br. J. Pharmacol.*, **55**, 181–8
28. Folkow, B., Haeger, K. and Kahlson, G. (1948). *Acta Physiol. Scand.*, **15**, 264–78

29. Goadby, P. and Phillips, E. A. (1973). *Br. J. Pharmacol.*, **49**, 368–9
30. Karppanen, H., Paakkari, I., Paakkari, P. *et al.* (1976). *Nature (London)*, **259**, 587–8
31. Krell, R. D. and Chakrin, L. W. (1977). *Eur. J. Pharmacol.*, **44**, 35–44
32. Lichtenstein, L. M. and Gillespie, E. (1973). *Nature (London)*, **244**, 287–8
33. McNeill, J. H., Verma, S. C. (1974). *J. Pharmacol. Exp. Ther.*, **188**, 180–8
34. Maudsley, D. V., Kobayashi, Y., Williamson, E. *et al.* (1973). *Fed. Proc.*, **32**, 808
35. Melmon, K. L. and Bourne, H. R. (1974). *Clin. Pharmacol. Ther.*, **16**, 886–91
36. Melmon, K. L., Bourne, H. R., Weinstein, Y. *et al.* (1972). *Science*, **177**, 707–9
37. Melmon, K. L., Weinstein, Y., Shearer, G. M. *et al.* (1972). *Isr. J. Med. Sci.*, **8**, 641
38. Parsons, M. E., Owen, D. A. A., Durant, G. J. *et al.* (1977). *Agents Actions*, **7**, 31–7
39. Powell, J. R. and Brody, M. J. (1974). *Fed. Proc.*, **33**, 585
40. Okpako, D. T. (1973). *Arch. Pharmacol.*, **279**, R35
41. Okpako, D. T., Chand, N. and Eyre, P. (1978). *J. Pharm. Pharmacol.*, **30**, 181–2
42. Trendelenburg, U. (1960). *J. Pharmacol. Exp. Ther.*, **130**, 450–60
43. Zavecz, J. H. and Levi, R. (1976). *Fed. Proc.*, **35**, 645

26
Serotonin and S_2 antagonists in veterinary medicine

L. Ooms, F. Awouters, A. Degryse and T. Jageneau

PHARMACOLOGY

Peripherally-acting serotonin affects mainly the cardiovascular, respiratory and gastrointestinal systems in which smooth muscles are very sensitive to the contractile activity of this biogenic amine[15]. In mammals serotonin (5-HT; 5-hydroxytryptamine) is present in the enterochromaffin cells of the gut (major part), in nervous tissue and in platelets. In rats, it was shown that the lung plays a major role in the total body clearance of circulating serotonin[64]. In rats and also in other animal species, serotonin is also abundant in mast cells, from which it is released in allergic reactions and by polyamines, such as compound 48/80. Very heterogeneous stimuli may cause release of serotonin from these cellular sources and thereby activate pathological pathways.

Table 26.1 Pharmacological activity spectrum of R 41468

System	*Potent*	*Weak*	*Absent*
Receptor preparations	Binding to 5-HT_2	Binding to - histamine - noradrenaline	Binding to 5-HT_1
Isolated tissues organs and cells	5-HT antagonism in - blood vessels - airways - platelets	Antagonism of - histamine - noradrenaline	- 5-HT antagonism in gastric and intestinal smooth muscle - own agonist activity
Whole animal	Antagonism of endogenous or injected serotonin	Antagonism of - histamine - noradrenaline - tryptamine	Generalization with LSD

In our laboratories, antagonism of endogenous serotonin was studied by a new method. An intravenous injection of compound 48/80 in rats is known to induce lethal shock, which can be prevented by the administration of any specific histamine H_1-antagonist[47]. Despite adequate antihistamine treatment, severe gastric ulceration gradually develops after compound 48/80 injection and these ulcers were found to be fully prevented by additional administration of drugs with known serotonin antagonistic activity. This provided a simple way to screen new compounds and the quinazolinedione derivative, R 41468, proved to be a potent serotonin antagonist with an oral ED_{50} of 0.15 mg/kg. Detailed studies of the pharmacological activities of R 41468, summarized in Table 26.1, have revealed marked differences between the known serotonin antagonists and the new class of pure and selective S_2-antagonists, of which R 41468 (ketanserin) is the prototype.

The new compounds did not mimic the action of serotonin in any test and were not generalized with LSD in a drug discrimination procedure (Table 26.2). They showed high affinity binding to S_2 (5-HT_2) receptors of the

Table 26.2 *In vitro* receptor binding profiles (K_i-value in nmol/l) of 5-HT_2 receptor ligands

Compound	*5-HT_2*	*5-HT_1*	*Ratio 5-HT_1/ 5-HT_2*	*H_1*	*α_1*	*α_2*	*DA*	*Ach-M*
LSD	*8.2**	20	2.4	n.a.	160	58	20	n.a.
Methysergide	*12*	99	8.3	n.a.	2300	2600	200	n.a.
Metergolin.	*0.9*	20	22	1100	10	n.a.	220	n.a.
Metitepine	1.9	62	32	4.9	*0.47*	48	4	n.a.
Mianserin	13	1100	85	*2.9*	82	60	620	n.a.
Cyprohept.	6.5	700	108	*2.7*	100	860	31	19
Spiperone	1.2	160	133	n.a.	10	n.a.	*0.16*	n.a.
R 41468	*2.1*	n.a.	>1000	10	10	n.a.	220	n.a.
Pirenperone	*2.0*	n.a.	>1000	14	6.8	3.3	16	n.a.
R 46700	*2.8*	n.a.	>1000	13	12	n.a.	147	n.a.
R 50970	*2.6*	n.a.	>1000	16	2.7	3.3	50	n.a.

*Figures in italic not significant

frontal cortex but none to S_1 (5-HT_1) serotonin receptors of the hippocampus. Serotonin responses of blood vessels, the respiratory tract and platelets were inhibited at low concentrations, but not those of gastrointestinal smooth muscle. To study the involvement of serotonin in peripheral pathology, particularly of cardiovascular origin, R 41468 has the further advantage of being only weakly active against histamine, noradrenaline and central tryptamine. The activity spectrum of other S_2-antagonists, however, may include significant antagonism of biogenic amines other than serotonin, providing combinations that are better adapted to particular applications, e.g. substances combining the high S_2 antagonist activity with a high α_1 adrenergic blockade and histamine$_1$ antagonist activity, a high α_2 agonist activity and a moderate or high dopamine antagonist activity.

VETERINARY APPLICATIONS

Prevention of malignant hyperthermia (MH) and exercise-induced muscle damage in stress-susceptible pigs

The predominant clinical features associated with malignant hyperthermia (MH) in pigs are gross musculature rigidity, hyperthermia, rapid rise in body temperature and blotchy cyanosis. There is also a severe metabolic acidosis with a rise in serum electrolytes. In pigs, MH is a manifestation of a generalized susceptibility to stress. MH is not confined to pigs. Anaesthetic-induced MH has also been described in dogs, cats, horses, birds and also in wild animals during capture[13, 31, 55, 65]. The immediate cause of MH appears to be a sudden rise in myoplasmic calcium concentration. However, the abnormality that could account for the rapid rise in myoplasmic calcium is not yet known. From literature, the possibilities are multiple: defective accumulation of calcium in the sarcoplasmic reticulum, defective accumulation of calcium in the mitochondria and excessively fragile sarcolemma with passive diffusion of calcium into the myoplasm from the extracellular fluid. Stress and the sympathetic nervous system are obviously intimately involved in MH in pigs. Serotonin has been shown to be involved in the stimulation of motor neurons and also in the development of tremor and myoclonus[48]. Also, transmitter release at the mammalian neuromuscular junction is enhanced by serotonin[16]. Since nerve terminals containing 5-HT make intimate contact with motorneurons, a functional role for 5-HT in the regulation of muscle tone seems implicated. Serotonin is also involved in the muscle necrosis in functional ischaemic skeletal muscle and in the development of degenerative changes in skeletal muscle[62]. S_2 antagonists were tried out to prevent halothane-induced MH and exercise-induced muscle damage in stress-susceptible pigs.

(1) Halothane-induced MH. Pietrain pigs (±20 kg body weight) were injected with 5-HT_2 antagonists or isotonic saline before (−30 min) exposure to 12 min halothane anaesthesia (4% halothane during first 5 min followed by 2–3% halothane). Clinical observations (cyanosis and muscle stiffness) were combined with measurement of rectal temperature. Blood samples and muscle biopsies were taken before and 19 min after start of anaesthesia. In a few pigs also the systolic and diastolic blood pressure and the venous distensibility were measured by plethysmography. The central venous pressure, the respiratory rate and the tidal volume were continuously recorded.

(2) Exercise-induced muscle damage. Belgian Landrace pigs and Pietrain pigs (±80 kg) were injected with 5-HT_2 antagonists or with isotonic saline 20 min before running on a treadmill for 10 min (speed: 6 km/h). Each pig was tested with saline and with 5-HT_2 antagonists with at least 1 week of interval. Blood samples (venous blood) were taken before running, immediately after running and 4 h later from a catheter (jugular vein) implanted at least 10 days before the first exposure to exercise stress.

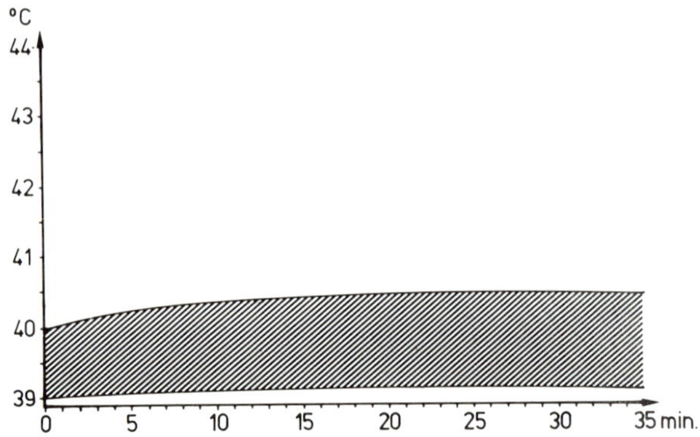

Figure 26.1 Rectal temperature of pigs pretreated with R 41468 (0.25–0.5 mg/kg i.m.) from t = 0 to t = 12 min and after exposure to halothane. All animals survived

Table 26.3 (a) Serum values of control pigs and pigs pretreated with R 41468 or R 50970 before (0 min values) and after exposure (19 min values) to halothane

N	*Parameter*	*0 min values*	*SD*	*19 min values*	*SD*	p-*value*
Control pigs						
8	K (mEq/l)	4.98	0.57	8.98	0.72	0.011*
8	A. phosph. (mg/100 ml)	7.37	1.04	14.82	2.39	0.011*
8	Lactate (mg/100 ml)	23.5	5.23	119.75	22.49	0.011*
7	LDH (U/1)	970.28	113.387	1749.57	203.11	0.017*
8	Cholesterol (mg/100 ml)	84.75	10.36	114	4.14	0.011*
8	CPK (U/1)	980.26	236.46	3446.25	1054.73	0.011*
Pretreated pigs						
16	K (mEq/l)	5.06	0.51	5.15	0.46	0.46
16	A. phosph. (mg/100 ml)	6.76	0.37	6.65	0.39	0.33
16	Lactate (mg/100 ml)	20.56	3.68	20.56	3.99	0.94
15	LDH (U/1)	1052.53	138.45	1150.67	132.25	0.043*
16	Cholesterol (mg/100 ml)	79.87	4.33	83.75	5.54	0.039*
16	CPK (U/1)	951.56	399.41	995.43	421.01	0.014*

*Significant

Table 26.3 (b) Comparison of the increase of the various parameters between not pretreated and pretreated pigs

Parameter	p-*value*
Potassium	0.000089†
Inorganic phosphate	0.000088†
Lactate	0.000086†
LDH	0.00021†
Cholesterol	0.00018†
CPK	0.000089†

†Mann-Whitney U-test

Results

Pigs, which were susceptible to halothane-induced malignant hyperthermia pretreated with 5-HT_2 receptor blocking agents (0.25–0.5 mg/kg), and survived a subsequent exposure to halothane. No muscle stiffness was noted. Rectal temperature increased by 0.2–0.4° C or decreased below the initial rectal temperature (Figure 26.1). Measured plasma values did not change significantly (Table 26.3 (a)). Without pretreatment, all pigs showed the typical clinical syndrome of MH: muscle stiffness 30 sec to 3 min after the application of halothane, hyperthermia (42.5–44° C, Figure 26.2) and blotchy

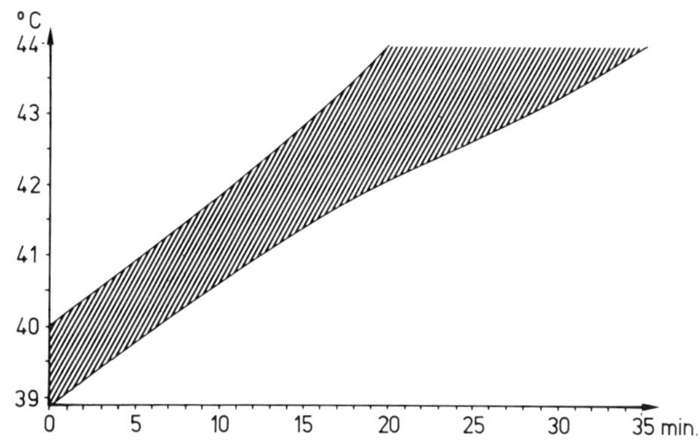

Figure 26.2 Rectal temperature of non-pretreated pigs from t = 0 to t = 12 min and after exposure to halothane. All animals died

cyanosis of the skin. All pigs died after a variable time period (12–40 min). Plasma values of potassium, calcium, inorganic phosphate, lactate and cholesterol were significantly increased (Table 26.3 (b)). Electron microscopy of muscles of not pretreated pigs showed swollen mitochondria with a clear increased calcium content and damage of the cristae (Figure 26.3). In pretreated pigs no morphological damage was seen. The calcium content of the mitochondria was only moderately increased (Figure 26.3). In control pigs, exposed to halothane, a significant decrease in venous distensibility accompanied with a high increase in peripheral resistance and central venous blood pressure was seen (Figure 26.4). This increase in peripheral resistance is accompanied by a significant increase of arterial blood pressure (systolic and diastolic). A few minutes before the animals die, arterial blood pressure (systolic and diastolic pressure) decreased sharply. A decreased cooling of the muscles by a lower bloodflow through the muscles and the skin is most probably involved in the development of hyperthermia. Pigs pretreated with 5-HT_2 antagonist activity showed an increase of the venous distensibility and no significant increase of the peripheral resistance (Figure 26.5) in comparison with untreated pigs (Figure 26.6). Arterial and central venous blood pressure did not change significantly. In the treadmill experiments, pigs pretreated with isotonic saline showed after 10 min a significant increase of

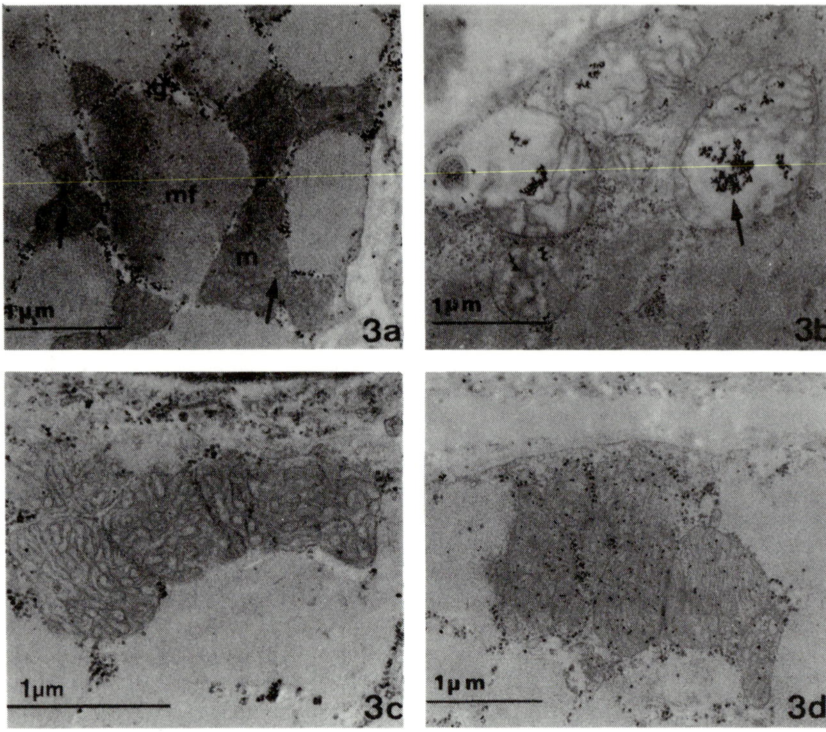

Figure 26.3 Ultrastructural localization of calcium in the mitochondria of skeletal muscle tissue observed in four different samples taken from the same pig. (a) Pre-anaesthesia sample; no pretreatment. The low amount of calcium in the normal mitochondria (m) is visualized by the presence of a few spots of precipitate (arrows) in the matrix. Glycogen (g); myofilaments (mf) (×34 000). (b) Postanaesthesia sample; no pretreatment. The large conglomerates of precipitate (arrows) in the clarified matrix of these swollen mitochondria (m) indicate the presence of large amounts of intramitochondrial calcium (×27 000). The greatly increased amounts of calcium are most probably deleterious to these skeletal muscle mitochondria. (c) Pre-anaesthesia sample; pretreatment with R 41468. A comparably low amount of calcium is seen in these normal mitochondria as shown in (a) (×34 000). (d) Postanaesthesia sample; pretreatment with R 41468. The amount of calcium is increased in the otherwise normal looking mitochondria (×34 000). The moderate increase in myoplasmic calcium which may have occurred after halothane anaesthesia in this pretreated pig can probably be managed by the mitochondria

blood lactate, base excess, potassium and inorganic phosphate. After 4 h, LDH and CPK values were significantly increased. These blood values were only moderately increased after pretreatment with 5-HT_2 antagonists (Table 26.4). The percentage of increase depends on the potency of the substance as a 5-HT_2 antagonist and the other pharmacological properties of the same substance (α_1 antagonism, dopamine antagonism).

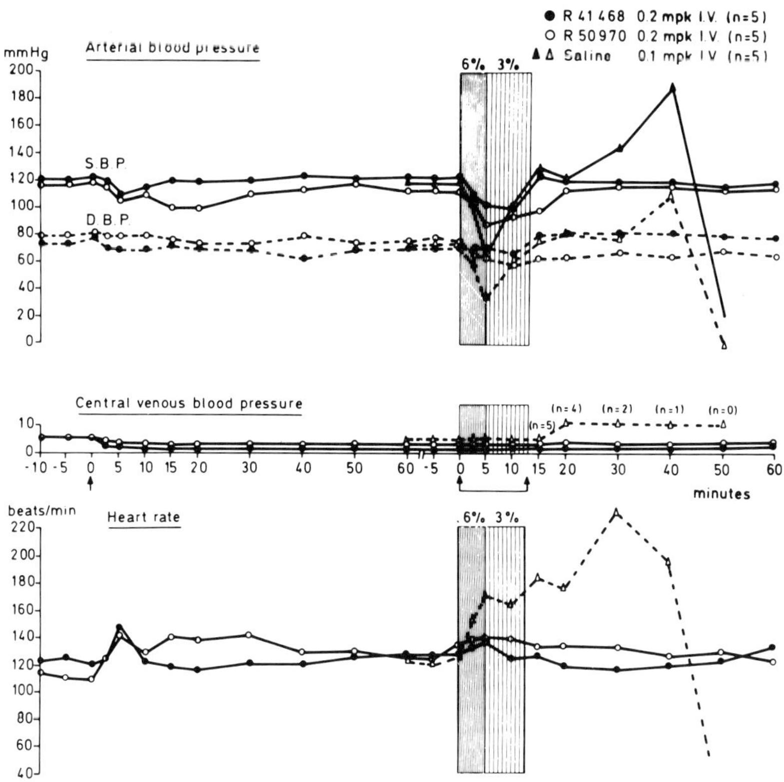

Figure 26.4 Measurement of arterial blood pressure, central venous blood pressure and heart rate of pigs pretreated with R 41468 and R 50970 and control pigs pretreated with saline before, during and after halothane anaesthesia

Table 26.4 Serum values of two pigs (B and G) during control run and running after pretreatment with R 41468 or R 50970 (20 mg i.v.)

Parameter	*Control*	*Pig B* *R 50970*	*R 41468*	*Pig G* *Control*	*R 41468*
Increase or decrease within 10 min					
Potassium	+ 1.5	+ 0.2	+ 0.5	+ 0.7	+ 0.0
Glucose	+ 181	+ 36.0	+ 58.0	+ 51.0	+ 1.0
Inorganic phosphate	+ 2.1	+ 0.4	+ 0.1	+ 1.0	− 0.4
Lactate	+ 136	+ 28.0	+ 26.0	+ 17.0	+ 4.0
pH	− 0.53	− 0.1	− 0.14	− 0.06	+ 0.0
pO_2	+ 17.5	+ 16.0	+ 22.6	+ 3.5	− 1.8
BE	− 28.8	− 10.4	− 12.2	− 6.2	− 1.0
Increase or decrease within 4 h					
CPK	+ 4794	+ 225	+ 526	+ 5929	+ 128
LDH	+ 1312	+ 281	+ 310	+ 1387	− 582

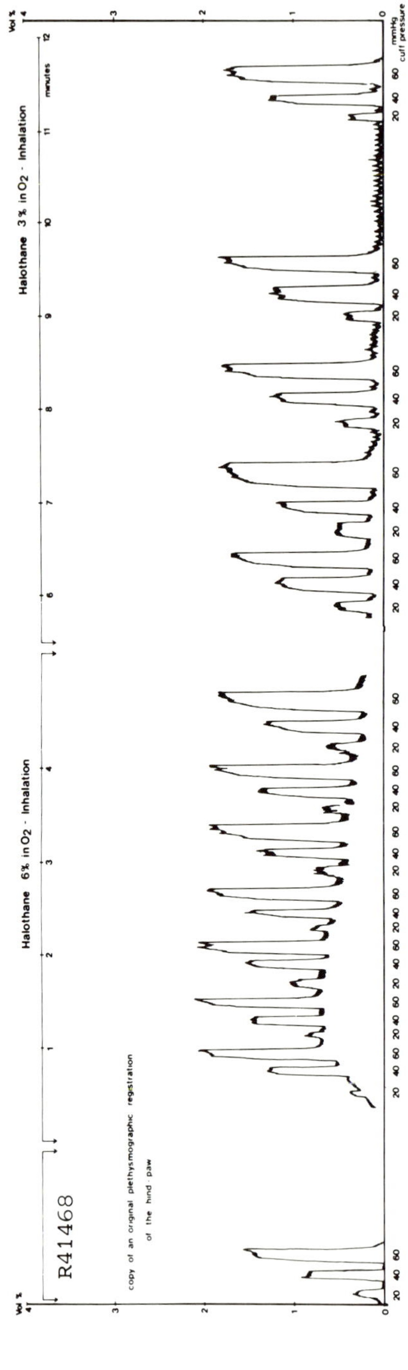

Figure 26.5 Plethysmographic measurements of venous distensibility of the hind-paw before, during and after halothane anaesthesia on a pig pretreated with R 41468

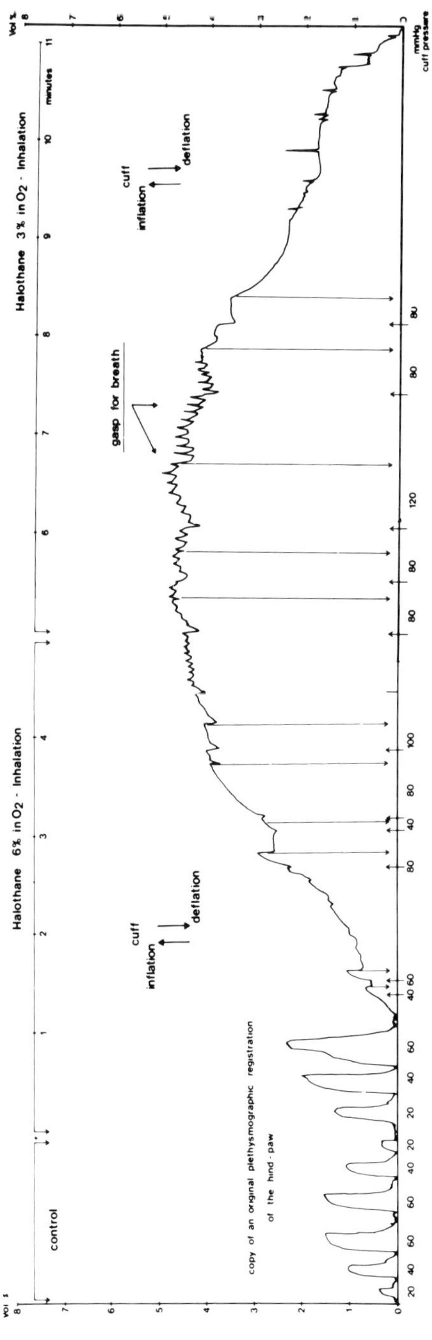

Figure 26.6 Plethysmographic measurement of venous distensibility of the hind-paw before, during and after halothane anaesthesia on a control pig pretreated with isotonic saline

Discussion

5-HT_2 antagonists prevent the development of malignant hyperthermia in susceptible pigs and also muscle damage in pigs submitted to physical stress. *In vitro*, our substances did not show a protective activity on halothane (1%) nor on caffeine (2 mmol/l) induced contractions. So no antagonist activity was stated on isolated muscles *in vitro*. *In vivo*, stress and the sympathetic nervous system are obviously intimately involved in MH and muscle damage in pigs. Pietrain pigs are extremely sensitive to α-adrenergic stimulation and develop a fatal hyperthermia. Serotonin has been shown to reverse blockade induced by the non-depolarizing agents and hemicholinium and to potentiate blockade produced by the depolarizers. What is most important in the development of MH: a primarily abnormal membrane structure as suggested by *in vitro* experiments or an increased release or decreased metabolism of serotonin or both? The action of serotonin seems to be on the circulatory system by increasing the peripheral resistance to flow. Also a direct involvement on the skeletal muscle membrane itself by increasing the membrane permeability for calcium seems possible. The observation that substances combining S_2 antagonist activity with an α_1-adrenergic blockade and dopamine blockade (central sedation) are more potent in the prevention of halothane-induced MH and/or muscle damage due to stress or exercise, indicates that more than one mediator is involved, but finally having an additive effect on the action of serotonin.

Diarrhoea

About 65% of the total body serotonin is present in the gastrointestinal tract. In preparations of longitudinal muscle (with myenteric plexuses attached) from the guinea-pig ileum, 5-HT concentrations of 81 ± 11 ng/g and 110 ± 20 ng/g have been reported[50]. Within the enteric neurons, 5-HT appears to be stored together with a specific binding protein (serotonin binding protein) that is similar in its properties to the serotonin binding protein found in serotonergic neurons in the brain. In the remaining layers of the intestine (including the mucosa) concentrations of 6350 ± 860 to $89\,000 \pm 600$ ng/g were found[36]. High concentrations of serotonin are present especially in the enterochromaffin cells (endocrine cells). 5-HT is taken up by both nerve plexuses and mucosa, with a high affinity mechanism. 5-Hydroxytryptophan (5-HTP) is converted to 5-HT[26,27]. 5-HTP decarboxylase in the gut might be involved in the regulation of 5-HT synthesis and is likely to be involved as a limiting step. Tryptophan hydroxylase was also shown in intrinsic neurons of the intestine (myenteric and submucous plexuses of guinea-pig, mice and rats). So 5-hydroxytryptamine is an endogenous constituent of the enteric nervous system.

Physiological stimulators releasing serotonin from the enterochromaffin cells

Stimulation from the luminal side Luminal stimulation by instillation of hypertonic glucose solutions or by acidification of the duodenum caused a degranulation of the enterochromaffin cells (EC) and a release of 5-HT into the circulation[38]. In rats, glucose load caused a significant decrease in duodenal concentration of serotonin and an increase in pancreatic serotonin.

Stimulation from the circulation Several circulating substances and drugs have been shown to influence the release of 5-HT from EC. Catecholamines, morphine, nicotine, and reserpine have been shown to release 5-HT from the intestine or to decrease the 5-HT content of EC[5–7]. Acetylcholine also decreased the 5-HT content of EC but was much less potent than the adrenergic substances. Dopamine had no effect. *In vitro* incubations with noradrenaline, adrenaline and isoprenaline caused a minor decrease of 5-HT in EC, indicating that a cholinergic control may also contribute to the 5-HT content of EC.

Neural stimulation In both cats and guinea-pigs, stimulation of the vagus decreases the 5-HT content of the EC[1, 58]. Fluorescence histochemical studies have shown that adrenergic nerves run with the vagus[40]. The response was prevented by destroying noradrenergic nerves by the injection of 6-hydroxy-dopamine or by injecting antibodies to nerve growth factor and also by prior removal of the superior cervical ganglia. So it was illustrated that 5-HT can be released through nerve activity, even though the source of 5-HT is not the nerves themselves[49]. Also the splanchnic nerves participate in the regulation of 5-HT release from EC into the portal circulation by an adrenergic mechanism. Splanchnic nerve stimulation in the cat significantly increased the portal 5-HT levels. This effect could be blocked by α and β adrenoreceptor antagonists. Ultrastructurally, nerve terminals of three different kinds were observed in very close relationship to the basal part of the EC cells in the guinea-pig duodenum (cholinergic, purinergic and adrenergic). In addition, sensory nerve endings were demonstrated near the base of the EC.

Involvement of serotonin in secretory diarrhoea induced by cholera toxin

In 1974 Fujita *et al.*[22] showed that crude cholera toxin introduced into the duodenum of the anaesthetized rabbit caused release of the basal granules in the EC. These EC cells are stimulated by cholera toxin at their apical microvilli and release serotonin. In a more recent study it was shown that cholera toxin causes a depletion of the endocrine cells of serotonin (60–70%). Most of the 5-HT was secreted in the intestinal lumen[12].

Serotonin acting from the serosal side *In vitro* and *in vivo*, it was shown that 5-HT increased the electrical activity of the rat jejunum. The increased potential difference and short circuit current resulted from a stimulation of electrogenic chloride secretion and a reduction of NaCl absorption. 5-HT did not alter cyclic AMP level on isolated enterocytes. 5-HT and acetylcholine acted independently in inducing intestinal secretion. Since certain intestinal secretagogues, including the cholinergic agonists and serotonin from the serosal side, do not cause mucosal cAMP to increase and require extracellular calcium to produce a full electric response, these substances may act as calcium ionophores on the epithelial cells. It is likely that the intestinal secretory effect of 5-HT is initiated by an influx of calcium, since the effect of 5-HT was diminished in Ca-free media and mimicked by the Ca ionophore A23187. It was also shown that the 5-HT response was inhibited by the calcium channel blocker verapamil and also that the presence of 5-HT was associated with an increased rate of calcium movement between the intestinal mucosa and its environment[14].

In cat experiments, there was a continuous decrease in the VIP release in control animals, while the VIP release increased steadily from intestines exposed to cholera toxin. The release could be inhibited by tetrodotoxin give i.a. or lidocaine administered into the gut lumen[8]. Nervous reflex arcs are activated via the release of 5-HT from the EC cells. 5-HT stimulates the dendrites located closely adjacent to the EC cells. One of the transmitters released at the efferent end of the reflex arc in the crypts and/or in the villi is VIP. To test this hypothesis, it was shown that rats exhibiting choleraic secretion did not show fluid secretion after being made tachyphylactic against serotonin or after 5-HT blocking agents (methysergide or chorpromazine) given i.v.

Serotonin acting from the luminal side *In vitro*, on the descending colon from Sprague-Dawley rats, electrogenic transport was estimated from the short-circuit current measured *in vitro* with a four-electrode voltage clamp and the tissue mounted in Frizzel–Schultz chambers. Serotonin, harmaline and melatonin (structurally similar to amiloride) inhibited the SCC similar to amiloride with onset of inhibition in seconds, inhibition only from the luminal side, reversible inhibition and inhibition only of the portion of SCC that is amiloride-sensitive. The concentration of half maximal inhibition for serotonin in the rat colon is 12 mmol/l. The maximal inhibition with serotonin and amiloride is similar, suggesting a single site of action[39].

Serotonin and intestinal motility

After an oral ingestion of 5-HTP (30 mg/kg) in dogs, the spiking activity during the recording time rose from 25% (control) to 50% during the first hour. A percentage of 90–95 is reached for the next 5 h[51]. The release of 5-HT after distension or after intraluminal application of hypertonic glucose load also facilitates contraction of the intestine. In the dog small intestine, Burks provided evidence that 5-HT excited intraneural cholinergic nerve elements since the intestinal contracting effect of 5-HT was blocked by tetrodotoxin, nicotonic depolarization and atropine, but not by TEA[4]. 5-HT, applied by microelectrophoresis to neurons of the submucous plexus of the guinea-pig small intestine, depolarized all neurons and, if the amount of depolarization by 5-HT was sufficient, action potentials were initiated[32]. The effect of 5-HT was depressed by d-tubocurarin, but remained unaffected by methysergide.

5-HT$_2$ antagonists and diarrhoea

With the knowledge that serotonin in one way or another is involved in the mechanisms of cholera and *E. coli* enterotoxins-induced diarrhoea, we used serotonin$_2$ antagonist in an *in vivo* model on young pigs.

Ten day old animals were operated under general anaesthesia (metomidate i.v.) after a 24 h period of fasting (only water available). Loops ($n = 5$) were made in the jejunum with thick cotton wires and injected intraluminally with 10 μg of pure cholera toxin. Animals were treated 1 h before and 2 h after introduction of cholera toxin with 1 ml of isotonic saline (control animals) or with a serotonin$_2$ antagonist (R 50970; 0.3 mg/kg i.m.). Postoperatively, only isotonic saline solution was available *ad libitum*. 6 h later, the animals received an overdose of barbiturates i.v. The contents were centrifuged and the fluid volume measured and indicated as ml fluid per cm of intestinal loop (Table 26.5).

From these preliminary results, it seems that serotonin is involved in secretory diarrhoea. However, further experiments on animals showing spontaneous diarrhoea of different origin seem necessary to further evaluate these substances.

Table 26.5 Results of pigs treated with isotonic saline and R 50970 (5-HT$_2$ antagonist)

	Isotonic saline	*R 50970*
Number of pigs	25	27
ml/cm of intestine (mean)	0.971	0.666
SD	0.282	0.362
P-value		0.002
Significancy		*

*Mann-Whitney U-test

Rumen motility

Rumen motility is under control of the central nervous system (medulla oblongata) and depends mainly upon autonomic control systems[29, 54, 59], ensuring a co-ordinate function of the reticulum, rumen and omasum. The motor events happen in cycles lasting about 1 min. A contraction starts by a biphasic contraction of the reticulum followed by the primary contraction of the rumen with secondary rumen contractions occurring in the interval between two primary contractions of the reticulo-rumen for about 40–60% of the motor cycles[52]. Secondary retrograde contractions seem to be necessary for eructation. An increase in their number is associated with a higher rate of eructation[11].

Substances, such as dopamine and apomorphine, caused inhibition of extrinsic ruminal contractions that could be prevented by domperidone pretreatment[41]. Substance P also inhibits extrinsic rumen contractions[61]. Morphine depressed both frequency and amplitude of ruminal contractions, while naltrexone and naloxone significantly increase the frequency of ruminal contractions.

In vitro, on the longitudinal smooth muscle from the rumen and reticulum of the bovine forestomach, 5-HT potentiated the contraction evoked by stimulation of the intramural cholinergic nerves but did not show any effect on the relaxation produced by the non-adrenergic inhibitory nerve excitation. 5-HT alone caused a contraction and relaxation of the ruminal strips while it produced only an excitatory effect on the reticular strips. These effects were blocked by methysergide, LSD-25 and phenoxybenzamine. 5-HT seems to have a direct effect on the smooth muscle, but also to induce presynaptic activation of the local cholinergic nerves[57].

However, serotonin, injected intravenously, inhibits the rumino-reticular motility in sheep[53]. In sheep it was shown that R 41468 (specific serotonin$_2$ antagonist) at a dose level of 0.05 mg/kg significantly increased the volume of eructated gas when the intraruminal pressure was maintained at 2 mmHg and increased the frequency of primary and secondary contractions of the rumen by 41.5 and 24.3% respectively. At an intraruminal pressure of 4 mmHg, R 41468 at a dose level of 0.1 mg/kg significantly increased the volume of eructated gas and also the frequency of both primary (23.6%) and secondary contractions (23.7%). From these results it seems that specific serotonin$_2$ antagonists offer the ability to treat bloating in ruminants (Table 26.6)[21].

Table 26.6 Effects of increased doses of R 41468 on the volume of eructated gas and rumen motility in fasted sheep (Mean ± SD for three experiments performed in four ewes)

Intraruminal pressure (mmHg)	*R 41468* (mg/kg)	*Eructated*† *volume* (1/5 min)	*Frequency of rumen contractions*† *Primary* (/5 min)	*Secondary* (/5 min)
2	control	2.33 ± 0.26	4.01 ± 0.71	3.75 ± 0.46
	0.05	3.33 ± 0.81*	5.66 ± 0.57*	4.66 ± 0.58*
	0.1	2.91 ± 0.54*	5.12 ± 0.15*	3.33 ± 1.53
4	control	3.92 ± 0.35	5.12 ± 0.15	4.31 ± 0.52
	0.05	4.32 ± 0.24	6.03 ± 0.21*	5.05 ± 0.61
	0.1	5.23 ± 0.17*	6.33 ± 0.42*	5.33 ± 0.37*

†Measured during a 15 min period before and after treatment
*Significantly different from control ($P<0.05$) using the paired *t*-test

Laminitis in horses

Laminitis in horses has been associated with the intake of high concentrates and changes in caecal and colonic microbial populations. After carbohydrate overload, increases in lactic acid-producing bacteria and decreases in Gram negative bacteria were stated during the onset of acute laminitis. Progressive decreases in caecal fluid pH were also seen[25]. The damage of the gastro-intestinal mucosa seems to permit absorption of endotoxins into the circulation. Local infections, such as metritis or retention of the placenta, frequently induce laminitis. In laminitis of alimentary and reproductive origin, endotoxins seem to be involved. Also endurance riding (local trauma) may result in the development of laminitis. Anti-inflammatory corticosteroids have been associated with laminitis. Local intra-articular injections may cause laminitis[63]. Even long term treatment with dexamethasone (i.m.), can result in the development of laminitis for no apparent reason[46]. Chronic administration of glucocorticoids or androgens predisposes the animals to a disseminated intravascular coagulation type condition and some types of consumptive coagulopathy[33]. On spirally cut digital arteries and veins *in vitro*, it was shown that addition of hydrocortisone or betamethasone alone did not cause contractions. But added to vessel strips that were partially contracted by epinephrine, norepinephrine or serotonin, each vessel strip invariably underwent an additional contraction[19]. Corticosteroids seem to have an additive effect on some vasoactive substances. Biogenic amines (e.g. serotonin, noradrenaline, histamine and prostaglandins) have been shown to be involved in the development of laminitis. On isolated strips of digital arteries and veins it was shown that all contracted dose-dependently in response to histamine, serotonin, epinephrine and norepinephrine. The threshold potency was greater in the venous than in the arterial strips. Comparing the maximal contractions, the effectiveness of these amines in causing vasoconstriction was greater in the veins than in the corresponding arteries taken from the same individual animal[19]. Serotonin is one of the mediators released by endotoxin, taken up by the reproductive system or produced by bacterial organisms giving sepsis. From the available evidence it seems that the disease is primarily vascular and local. The lesion in the foot is generally characterized by decrease capillary filtration, increased arterio-venous shunting, ischaemic necrosis, pain and finally resulting in rotation of the pedal bone[23,34]. The adrenal-stress phenomenon that develops during the onset of laminitis also seems to be of importance in that glucocorticoids and also serum testosterone values are increased[2]. However, it has also been claimed that the vascular changes, which occur in the foot are only part of a general vascular change in which peripheral resistance to bloodflow is increased by the causative agents. This also results in a significant increase in arterial blood pressure[24,30].

Table 26.7 Treatment of laminitis in horses with serotonin$_2$ antagonists

Body weight (kg)	*Aetiology*	*Time**	*Treatment* mg/kg i.v.	days	*Result†*
±600	Retention	12 day	1×0.16	3	+
190	Endurance riding	0.5 h	1×0.10	3	+ +
450	Endurance riding	1 h	1×0.10	2	+ +
±500	Overfeeding	1 day	1×0.10	2	+ +
±600	Overfeeding	1 day	2×0.10	2	+ +
460	Overfeeding	1 day	2×0.10	1	+ +
±500	Lameness (one leg)	1 day	2×0.15	2	+

*Time period between the first clinical observations and the first treatment
†+: sufficient clinical effect; + +: total clinical disappearance of the syndrome

Thrombocytopenia, eosinopenia and lymphocytopenia coagulopathies usually characterize the onset of acute laminitis[42]. Abnormalities in blood coagulation may be causative or be part of the syndrome. From the findings, hypertension, increased vascular resistance and abnormal platelet aggregation, it seems that serotonin could be involved as one of the final mediators. We used $serotonin_2$ antagonists for the treatment of horses with laminitis of different origin. Preliminary findings of the successful treatment are reported in Table 26.7.

Fever

A large variety of stimuli can induce fever: several types of endotoxins, tissue damage, antigen-antibody reaction, tumours, etc. The fever producing agent (pyrogen) can be of exogenous or endogenous origin.

On a molecular level, fever is associated with endogenous pyrogens and endotoxins, cell-mediated (phagocytosis) and antibody-mediated mechanisms (complement activation, immune reactions). The final mediation is realized by endogenous mediators resulting in metabolic and hormonal responses both by central and peripheral mechanisms. Serotonin seems to be involved as one of those endogenous mediators.

5-HT nerve endings terminate in the thermosensitive zone of the anterior hypothalamus[20]. This zone is reactive to endotoxin and also to leukocyte pyrogen. Following intrahypothalamic injection of serotonin, shivering, vasoconstriction and sharp rise in temperature were seen. 5-HT injected locally into the anterior hypothalamus evokes a hyperthermia in virtually all species. This area is also involved in the cellular mechanism which triggers a fever response to a bacterial challenge. So the serotonergic neurons underlying the rostral hypothalamic temperature controller are responsible not only for the defence of an animal's body temperature during exposure to cold, but also for initiating the shift in the temperature set-point during a febrile episode[45].

The observation on intact thermoregulating animals also provides direct evidence that a subtle perturbation in the release of serotonin by lipopolysaccharides and other pyrogenic molecules are part of the final neurohumoral pathway in inducing fever[44].

Fenfluramine (13 mpk i.p.; serotonin agonist) in rats produced a rapid hyperthermia effect in rats housed in a warm environment (26–28 °C. Drugs with known activity on serotonin-mediated pathways were the most effective antagonists of this hyperthermia[56].

The influence of an S_2 antagonist on endotoxin-induced fever is indicated in Figure 26.7.

Respiratory pathology

In neonatal rabbits, it was shown that pulmonary neuroendocrine cells respond to changes in airway oxygen levels. Decreased oxygen stimulates secretion of serotonin which directly or indirectly increases artery wall constriction[37]. Serotonergic agonists decrease tidal volume and minute

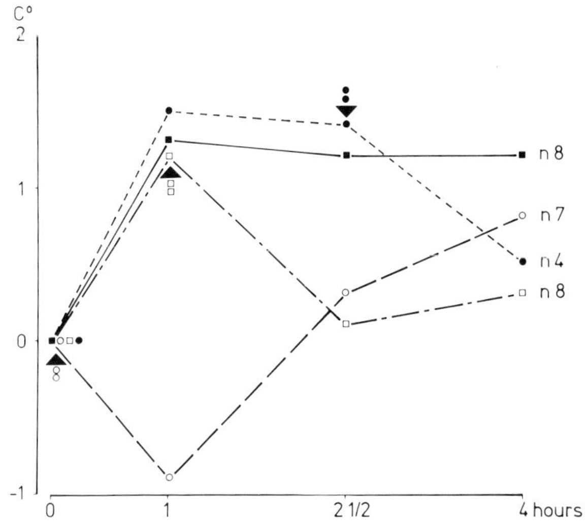

Figure 26.7 Effect of R50970 (0.5 mg/kg) on endotoxin-induced fever. Arrows indicate time of treatment of different groups: ○ treatment before; □ treatment after 1 h; ● treatment after 2.5 h; ■ control pigs; n number of animals

volume in a dose-dependent manner and also produce a respiratory acidosis. So the central nervous system areas involved in respiratory control seem to be modulated by the activity of central serotonergic neurons[43]. Serotonin is also one of the mediators released in type I hypersensitivity in bovine and ovine lung[17]. Serotonin is known to contract both trachea and bronchus in the calf and the sheep[18]. Also dog bronchial tissue[10] contracts to 5-HT. Pulmonary veins seem highly susceptible to the contractile activity of serotonin (horses, dogs and calves)[10, 17, 28]. In the dog it was shown *in vivo* that serotonin not only constricted arterioles, but also raised lung microvascular pressure by constricting postcapillary venules[3]. In the sheep and the goat, serotonin relaxed the pulmonary vein[9, 17]. In dogs it was also shown that serotonin infusion (0.020 mg/kg) caused a pronounced and sustained rise in airway pressure[60]. This effect could be abolished by an intravenous dose of 0.04 mg/kg R 41468 (a specific 5-HT_2 antagonist). In the anaesthetized guinea-pig, serotonin-induced bronchoconstriction was inhibited by R 41468 in a dose-dependent way.

So serotonin seems to contribute in many animal species to the pathophysiology of pulmonary pathology (airways and pulmonary blood vessels) by raising the peripheral resistance, capillary pressure and volume, augment filtration and oedema formation in the pulmonary circulation and also the contraction of the respiratory pathway. Also other substances, such as histamine, slow-reacting substance of anaphylaxis, kinins and prostaglandins are involved in the development of respiratory pathology due to type I hyperimmune reactions.

Pulmonary embolism in dogs, induced by autologous clot injected intravenously, resulted in a fall of platelet count and in an increase of mean pulmonary arterial pressure, pulmonary vascular resistance and physiological dead space. Injection with R 41468 (0.15 mg/kg) reversed pulmonary hypertension and increased the number of perfused arteries in comparison with control animals[35].

Also preliminary observations with 5-HT_2 antagonist in different animal species indicate that these substances, alone or combining this with H_1 antagonism and α_1 antagonism (R 50970), seem to be useful in the symptomatic treatment of respiratory problems of different origin in different animal species.

GENERAL CONCLUSION

With $serotonin_2$ antagonists one can prevent or treat many irregularities in animal pathology. Further research has to elucidate the final involvement and mechanism of action of serotonin in animal physiology and pathology of different origin. Specific $serotonin_2$ antagonists seem very useful potent pharmacological substances and promise to be useful in further research on the involvement of serotonin in animal physiology and pathology.

References

1. Ahlman, H., Lundberg, J., Dahlström, A. *et al.* (1976). *Acta Physiol. Scand.*, **98**, 366
2. Amos, M. S., Hood, D. M., Miller, W. G. *et al.* (1979). *J. Equine Med. Surg.*, **3**, 171–5
3. Bhattacharya, J., Nanjo, S. and Staub, N. C. (1982). *J. Appl. Physiol.*, **52**, 634–7
4. Burks, T. F. (1973). *J. Pharmacol. Exp. Ther.*, **185**, 530–9
5. Burks, T. F. and Long, J. P. (1966). *J. Pharm. Sci.*, **55**, 1383–6
6. Burks, T. F. and Long, J. P. (1967). *J. Pharmacol. Exp. Ther.*, **156**, 267–76
7. Burks, T. F. and Long, J. P. (1967). *Br. J. Pharmacol.*, **30**, 229–39
8. Cassuto, J., Jodal, M., Tuttle, R. *et al.* (1979). *Experientia*, **35**, 1467–8
9. Chand, N. (1981). *Br. J. Pharmacol.*, **72**, 233–7
10. Chand, N. and Eyre, P. (1979). *Agents Actions*, **9**, 4–8
11. Colvin, H. W., Bueno, L. and Ruckebusch, Y. (1981). Paper presented at *16th Conference on Rumen Function*, Chicago
12. Dahlström, A., Ahlman, H., Larsson, I. *et al.* (1981). *Workshop on 5-Hydroxytryptamine in Peripheral Reactions.* (Beerse, Belgium: Janssen Pharmaceutica)
13. de Jong, R. H., Heavner, J. E. and Amory, D. W. (1974). *Anesthesiology*, **41**, 608–9
14. Donowitz, M., Asarkof, N. and Pike, G. (1980). *J. Clin. Invest.*, **66**, 341–52
15. Douglas, W. W. (1980). In Goodman, L. S. and Gilman, A. (eds.) *The Pharmacological Basis of Therapeutics*. pp. 608–9. (New York: MacMillan)
16. Dretchen, K., Ghoneim, M. M. and Long, J. P. (1972). *Eur. J. Pharmacol.*, **18**, 121–7
17. Eyre, P. (1972). *Arch. Int. Pharmacol. Thér.*, **199**, 245–52
18. Eyre, P. (1975). *Am. J. Vet. Res.*, **36**, 1081–4
19. Eyre, P., Elmes, P. J. and Strickland, S. (1979). *Am. J. Vet. Res.*, **40**, 135–8
20. Feldberg, W. and Myers, R. D. (1965). *J. Physiol.*, **177**, 239–45
21. Fioramonti, J., Bueno, L., Ooms, L. *et al.* (1982). *J. Vet. Pharmacol. Ther.*, **5**, 213–15
22. Fujita, T., Osaka, M. and Yanatori, Y. (1974). *Arch. Histol. Jap.*, **36**, 367–78
23. Ganjam, V. K. and Garner, H. E. (1982). *Proc. 1st Equine Endotoxemia-Laminitis Symp., Newsletter*, **2**, 156–9

24. Garner, H. E., Coffman, J. R., Hahn, A. W. *et al.* (1975). *J. Am. Vet. Med. Assoc.*, **166,** 56–8
25. Garner, H. E., Moore, J. N., Johnson, J. H. *et al.* (1978). *Equine Vet. J.*, **10,** 249–52
26. Gershon, M. D. and Ross, L. L. (1966). *J. Physiol.*, **186,** 451
27. Gershon, M. D., Dradontides, A. B. and Ross, L. L. (1965). *Science*, **149,** 197
28. Hanna, C. J. and Eyre, P. (1978). *Can. J. Physiol. Pharmacol.*, **56,** 812–17
29. Harding, R. and Leek, B. F. (1971). *J. Physiol.*, **219,** 587–610
30. Harkema, J. R., Robinson, N. E. and Scott, J. B. (1978). *Am. J. Vet. Res.*, **39,** 741–4
31. Henschel, J. R. and Louw, G. N. (1978). *S. Afr. J. Sci.*, **74,** 305–6
32. Hirst, G. D. S. and Silinsky, E. M. (1975). *J. Physiol.*, **251,** 817–32
33. Hood, D. M., Stephens, K. A. and Amoss, M. S. Jr. (1982). *Proc. 1st Equine Endotoxemia Laminitis Symp., Newsletter*, **2,** 149–51
34. Hood, D. M., Amoss, M. S., Hightower, D. *et al.* (1978). *J. Equine Med. Surg.*, **2,** 439–44
35. Huval, W. V., Stemp, L. I., Mathilson, M. *et al.* (1982). Presented at *43rd Ann. Meet. Cornell Medical Center, New York*
36. Jurio, A. V. and Gabella, G. (1974). *J. Neurochem.*, **22,** 851
37. Keit, I. G., Wiley, L. A. and Will, J. A. (1981). *Cell Tissue Res.*, **214,** 201–5
38. Kellum, J. M. and Jaffe, B. M. (1976). *Ann. Surg.*, **184,** 633–6
39. Legris, G. P., Will, P. C. and Hopfer, U. (1981). *Ann. NY Acad. Sci.*, **372,** 345–6
40. Liedberg, G., Nielsen, K. C., Owman, C. *et al.* (1973). *Scand. J. Gastroenterol.*, **8,** 177
41. Maas, C. L., van Duin, C. T. M., van Miert, A. S. J. P. A. M. (1982). *J. Vet. Pharmacol. Ther.*, **5,** 191–6
42. Moore, J. N., Garner, H. E. and Coffman, J. R. (1981). *Equine Vet. J.*, **13,** 240
43. Mueller, R. A., Lundberg, D. and Breese, G. R. (1980). *Pharmacol. Biochem. Behav.*, **13,** 247–55
44. Myers, R. D. (1977). In Copper, K. E., Lomax, P. and Schönbaum, E. (eds.) *Drugs, Biogenic Amines and Body Temperature.* pp. 51–3. (Basel: Karger)
45. Myers, R. D. (1981). *J. Physiol., Paris*, **77,** 505–13
46. Muylle, E. and Oyaert, W. (1973). *Equine Vet. J.*, **5,** 37–44
47. Niemegeers, C. J. E., Awouters, F., van Nueten, J. M. *et al.* (1978). *Arch. Int. Pharmacodyn. Thér.*, **234,** 164–76
48. Parry, O. and Roberts, M. H. T. (1980). *Neuropharmacology*, **19,** 515–8
49. Petterson, G., Dahlström, A., Larsson, I. *et al.* (1978). *Acta Physiol. Scand.*, **103,** 219–24
50. Robinson, R. G. and Gershon, M. D. (1971). *J. Pharmacol. Exp. Ther.*, **178,** 311
51. Ruckebusch, Y. and Bueno, L. (1981). *Workshop on Stress and Serotonin in Animals and Man.* (Beerse, Belgium: Janssen Pharmaceutica)
52. Ruckebusch, Y. and Tomov, T. (1973). *J. Physiol.*, **235,** 447–58
53. Ruckebusch, Y., Fargeas, J. and Bueno, L. (1969). *Ann. Rech. Vét.*, **3,** 131–48
54. Ruckebusch, Y., Tsiamitas, C. and Bueno, L. (1972). *Life Sci.*, **11,** 55–64
55. Short, C. E. and Paddleford, R. R. (1973). *Anaesthesiology*, **39,** 462–3
56. Sulpizio, A., Fowler, P. J. and Macko, E. (1982). *Life Sci.*, **22,** 1439–46
57. Taneike, T. (1979). *J. Vet. Pharmacol. Ther.*, **2,** 59–68
58. Tansy, M. F., Rothman, G., Barlett, J. *et al.* (1971). *J. Pharm. Sci.*, **60,** 81
59. Titchen, D. A. (1968). In Heidel, W. (ed.) *Handbook of Physiology.* pp. 2705–24. (Baltimore: Williams and Wilkins)
60. van de Water, A., Wouters, L., Xhonneux, R. *et al. (1981). Preclinical Research Report on R 41468.* (Beerse, Belgium: Janssen Pharmaceutica)
61. Veenendaal, G. H., Woutersen-Nijnanten, F. M. A. and van Miert, A. S. J. P. A. M. (1980). *Am. J. Vet. Res.*, **41,** 479–83
62. Verheyen, A., Vlaminckx, E., Remeysen, P. *et al.* (1981). *Virchows Arch. Anim. Pathol. Anat. Histol.*, **393,** 265–72
63. Vernimb, G. D., van Hoose, L. M. and Hennessey, P. W. (1977). *Vet. Med. Small Anim. Clin.*, **72,** 241–4
64. Wiersma, D. A. and Roth, R. A. (1976). *J. Pharmacol. Exp. Ther.*, **212,** 97–102
65. Williams, C. H. (1976). *Persp. Biol. Med.*, **20,** 120–30

27
Dopaminergic control of gastrointestinal motility

L. Bueno and J. Fioramonti

Since a specific dopamine receptor in peripheral vessels has been proposed, many studies have proved that dopamine acts on distinct dopamine receptors on peripheral nerves and smooth muscle[3,14].

This assessment has been recently supported by experiments concerning dopamine action on the lower oesophageal sphincter[8,36,41] and on both gastric and colonic motility[27,39,54]. *In vivo* studies have suggested the presence of inhibitory dopamine receptors in the human stomach[28]. Subsequently, an antagonism of peripheral dopamine-mediated inhibition of gastric motility has been suggested to explain the action of the antiemetic drugs domperidone[39] and metoclopramide[54] in man. However, dopamine has also been shown to inhibit gastric motility via stimulation of adrenergic receptors in guinea-pig[11] and rat stomach[21]. More recently[53], it has been demonstrated that the inhibitory effects of dopamine on contractions of human gastric smooth muscle strips are unaffected by haloperidol but abolished by a combination of phenoxybenzamine and propranolol. In addition, an indirect action of dopamine has been proposed via the release of gastrointestinal hormones affecting both exocrine pancreatic secretion and plasma glucagon levels in man.[42]

Many antidopaminergic substances are used in human therapy as antiemetic substances but also in the treatment of flatulent dyspepsia, diabetic gastroparesis, chronic reflux oesophagitis, gastric stasis, gastritis, peptic ulcer and hiccups. All these applications suggest that these substances are active on gastrointestinal motility. Therefore, the principal aim of this review was to establish their effects on intestinal motility and their ability to antagonize the effects of dopamine in different species with special reference to clinical implications in animal medicine.

OESOPHAGEAL GROOVE CLOSURE

In the milk-fed calf or lamb, reflex closure of the oesophageal groove permits the direct transfer of milk from the oesophagus to the abomasum with bypass of the reticulo-rumen. Oesophageal groove motility is controlled by the vagus, and anticholinergic drugs are known to suppress this closure during sucking in lambs and calves[37]. Cholinergic drugs are known to reinforce this closure whereas adrenergic substances administered prior to sucking are able to reduce the closure of the oesophageal groove[1,37].

Using thermodilution to evaluate the amount of milk passing, respectively, into the abomasum and the reticulo-rumen in 3–5 week old calves, we have shown that the intravenous injection of dopamine (0.2 mg/kg) inhibits the closure of the oesophageal groove, thereby increasing the passage of milk into the reticulo-rumen. Both α- and β-adrenergic blockers are unable to antagonize these effects, whereas this action is suppressed by an infusion of an antidopaminergic substance such as metoclopramide ($6\,\mu g\,kg^{-1}\,min^{-1}$) suggesting that inhibitory dopamine receptors control the motility of the oesophageal groove in preruminants (Figure 27.1).

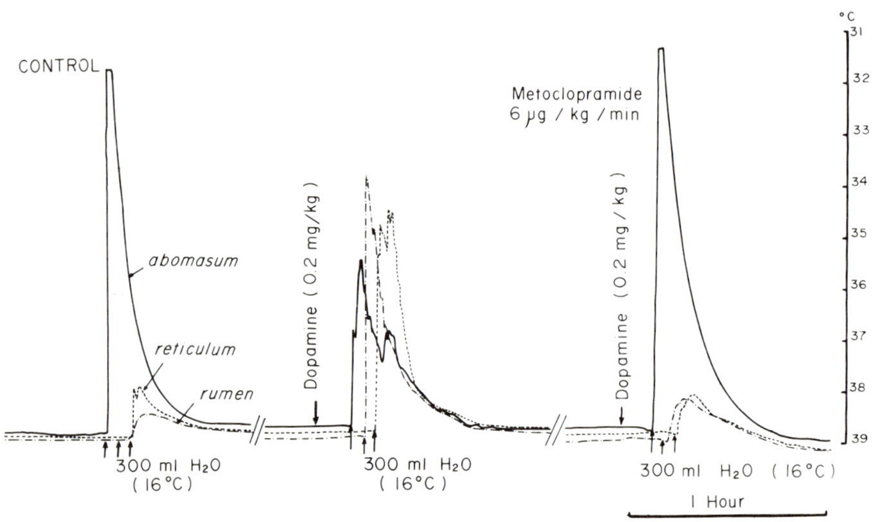

Figure 27.1 Effect of dopamine on abomasal and ruminal temperature changes following cold water suckling in 3 week old calf. Note that dopamine reduced the amount of water passing directly into the abomasum as judged by the reduced fall in abomasal temperature. The inhibiting effect of dopamine on closure of the oesophageal groove was suppressed under metoclopramide infusion

Similar results are obtained with domperidone, which is considered to be a peripheral dopamine antagonist as it does not pass the brain–blood barrier[25]. This is in agreement with the hypothesis of a direct peripheral effect by dopaminergic blocking agents on oesophageal groove motility.

Partial closure of the oesophageal groove is considered as one of the major primary digestive disturbances appearing in milk-fed calves[45]. Since dopamine may be involved, treatment with dopaminergic blocking agents should be tested in clinical trials.

MOTILITY OF THE FORESTOMACH AND LOWER OESOPHAGEAL SPHINCTER

The motility of the ruminant forestomach is under the direct control of the central nervous system (*medulla oblongata*); reticular contractions are abolished when the vagus nerves have been cut[16,48,52]. However, α_2-receptors may be involved in the peripheral adrenergic inhibition of ruminal motility[34].

Site of action of dopamine on rumino-reticular motility

When administered intravenously at a rate of $20\,\mu g\,kg^{-1}\,min^{-1}$, dopamine had a prompt inhibitory effect on forestomach motility. The contractile activity was completely abolished during the first 10–12 min; this effect was accompanied by a slow increase in the basal tone. Then the frequency of contractions was nearly halved during the following 10 min. Administered by intracerebroventricular (i.c.v.) route at $2\,\mu g\,kg^{-1}\,min^{-1}$, dopamine had an inhibitory effect on rumino-reticular motility only after 4-6 min of infusion. However, the period of total motor inhibition was similar to that observed after i.v. infusion (Figure 27.2). These results suggest that dopamine acts peripherally on the tonus of the rumen and centrally on the 'rate circuit' of phasic contractions.

During the i.c.v. infusion of dopamine ($2\,\mu g\,kg^{-1}\,min^{-1}$), the inhibition of forestomach motility was preceded by a period of rumination. When the inhibitory effects of an i.v. infusion of dopamine are blocked by metoclopramide, a period of rumination is also observed. This effect of dopamine on rumination is central and mediated by α_2-adrenergic receptors as indicated by the antagonism produced by preliminary i.c.v. administration of tolazoline ($20\,\mu g/kg$) (Figure 27.3).

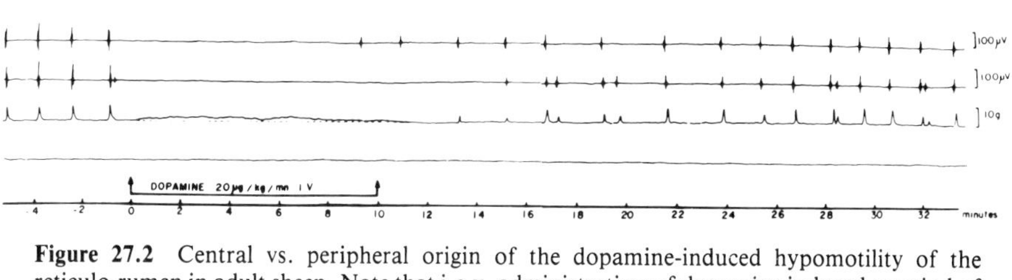

Figure 27.2 Central vs. peripheral origin of the dopamine-induced hypomotility of the reticulo-rumen in adult sheep. Note that i.c.v. administration of dopamine induced a period of rumination which was stopped by the inhibitory effects on rumino-reticular motility

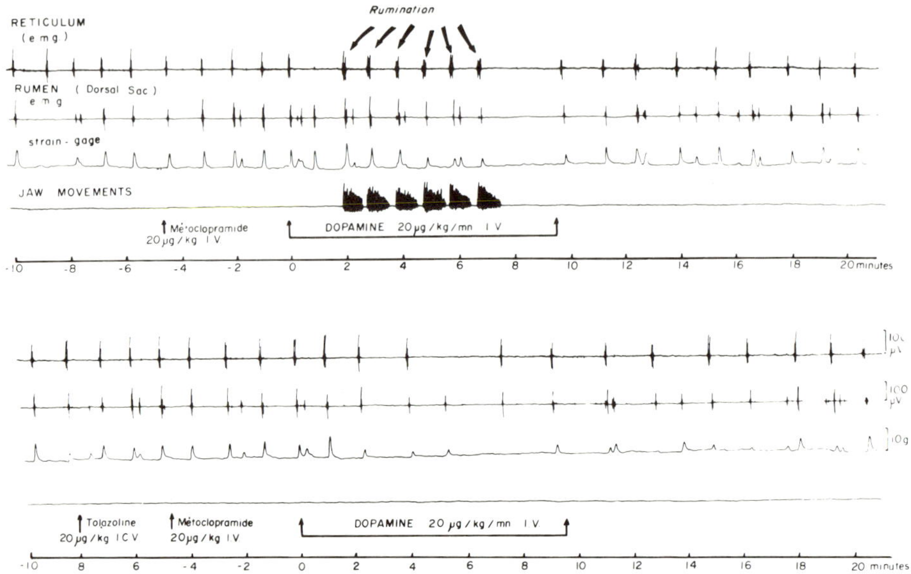

Figure 27.3 Antagonistic effects of tolazoline (i.c.v.) and metoclopramide (i.v.) on respectively rumination and rumino-reticular hypomotility induced by i.v. dopamine infusion in sheep. Note that rumination occurred after blockade of the peripheral effects of dopamine on rumino-reticular motility by metoclopramide (10 μg/kg) and was blocked by central administration of tolazoline (20 μg/kg)

Effect of antidopaminergic substances on rumen motility

The effects of these substances were not equivalent. One major explanation is the antagonism between antidopaminergic and cholinergic drugs according to the well-known 'see-saw' mechanism between the dopamine–acetylcholine (Da-ACh) systems[18], which is only seen with the 'atypical' Da-blocking agents and is not observed with the classical Da antagonist. Also, only some of these agents are able to pass the blood–brain barrier[19,56]. Even then the bulbar centre which controls reticular motility is considered to be peripheral to the blood–brain barrier as with the trigger zone (CTZ)[44], the activity of which is modulated by higher central hypothalamic and cortical structures[47].

In addition, some antidopaminergic substances such as metoclopramide have other pharmacological properties (local anaesthesia activity, cholinergic properties, etc.).

Only metoclopramide is currently used in bovine therapy as an antibloating substance, and in small animals as an antiemetic. Experiments have been developed to analyse its effects on spontaneous reticulo-ruminal motility and its antagonistic effects upon hypermotility induced by emetic substances (acting on dopaminergic receptors of the trigger zone) such as apomorphine. Intravenous infusion of metoclopramide at a rate of 4 μg kg^{-1} min^{-1} for 1 h increased the occurrence of secondary contractions by 24.2%. However, this increase was suppressed by higher rates of infusion and was not observed in fed animals. Intravenous injection of apomorphine (25–100 μg/kg) inhibits the reticular contractions. Under metoclopramide infusion (0.4 mg $kg^{-1} h^{-1}$), the inhibitory effect of apomorphine was reduced in a dose-related manner. A bolus injection of 0.5 mg/kg of metoclopramide reduced the inhibitory effects of apomorphine (0.2 mg/kg) on the amplitude of reticular contractions by 50%.

Lower oesophageal sphincter (LES) and eructation

Eructation in ruminants depends not only upon ruminal motility, but also upon co-ordinated reflexes involved in the opening of the cardiac orifice. Dysfunctions of ruminal motility and of cardiac opening are both involved in bloating phenomenon. Therefore, the pharmacology of ruminal motility alone has limited significance. Simultaneous recording of intraruminal pressure and eructated volume is suitable to study the effect of a drug on eructation and ruminal motility and their relationship. Since specific dopamine receptors are involved in the movements of the LES in monogastric animals, experiments have been performed to test the action of dopamine and antagonists on eructation.

Eructation involves co-ordinated reflexes and aspiration of gases into the lungs; in cattle, the original technique developed for collection of eructated gases from the trachea[6] has been modified several times[9,46]. In our test, in sheep, we have used the original technique[6] in which the animals are prepared with chronic tracheal and ruminal fistulae.

During experiments the anterior trachea was connected to a spirometer to measure the volume of the eructated gases; a strain gauge transducer permitted simultaneous recording of intraruminal pressure.

Two experimental procedures were used.

(1) Intraruminal pressure was elevated to 3 mmHg by insufflation of nitrogen through a T-tube attached to the rumen cannula with the anterior tracheal cannula previously clamped shut to stop eructation. Drugs were administered 30 sec before the opening of the tracheal cannula and the rate of eructation was measured for the following 10 min.

(2) Intraruminal pressure was elevated to between 1 and 4 mmHg by continuous insufflation of nitrogen through the rumen cannula and the flow of nitrogen was adjusted to maintain this pressure throughout the experiment.

The effects of dopamine and antidopaminergic drugs on ruminal motility and eructation were tested using the first experimental procedure. Figure 27.4 shows a normal profile of eructation after ruminal distension (5 min) and the effects on an intravenous injection of dopamine alone or after previous administration of clebopride, an antidopaminergic drug. Both in the control experiment and after dopamine, the volume of the first eructation was so large that gases passed directly into the atmosphere through the mouth, as indicated by the drop in pressure without concomitant gas inhalation. This

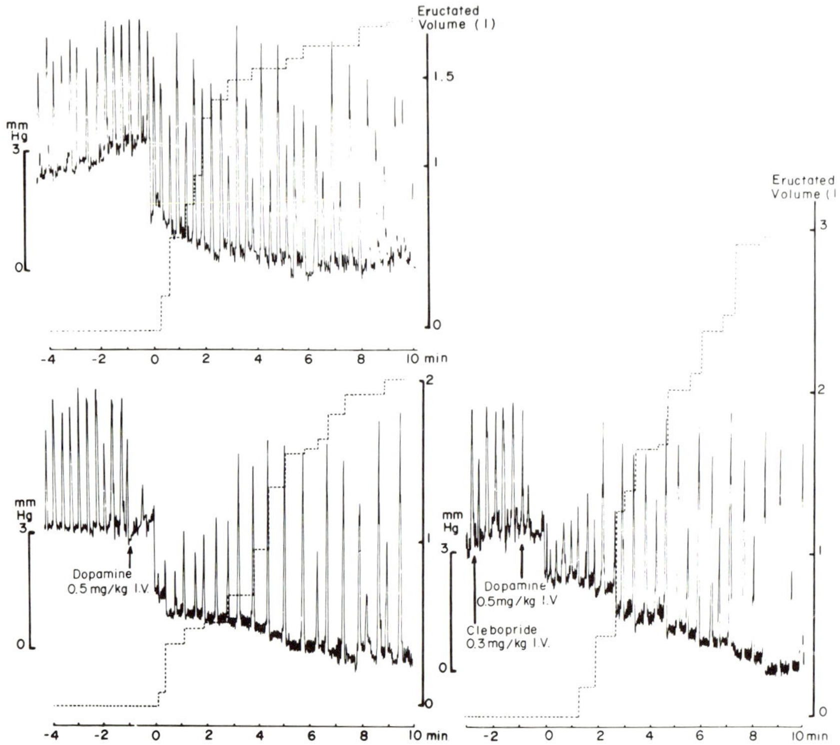

Figure 27.4 Intraruminal pressure (continuous line) and volume of eructated gases (dotted line) after ruminal distension (3 mmHg) with the anterior tracheal cannula clamped shut. At time 0 distension was stopped and the tracheal cannula opened. Note the different slopes of inhaled gases and intraruminal pressures between control and dopamine, with or without clebopride administration

loss of gas was reduced after clebopride, probably because of greater tone of the cardia and because the mean rate of gas inhalation was higher than that observed in the control or dopamine experiments.

In sheep when intraruminal pressure was maintained at 4 mmHg, the volume of eructated gas was 3.92 ± 0.35 l/5 min and was significantly reduced to 2.33 ± 0.26 l/5 min when the pressure was halved. Similarly, the frequency of primary contractions of the rumen decreased from 5.1 to 4.0 per 5 min. When dopamine was infused intravenously at a rate of 62.5 $\mu g\,kg^{-1}\,min^{-1}$ during rumen insufflation, the frequency of secondary contractions of the rumen was maintained. After 2–3 min transient reduction (48%) in the eructated volume, we observed a 110% higher rate of eructation than in the control experiments (Figure 27.4). These results suggest that dopamine in ruminants has an effect on the LES or cardia similar to that observed in monogastrics[41]. The increased rate of eructation observed with dopamine infusion may be the consequence of its relaxant effects on the cardia as well as the increased tonicity of the rumen wall.

Following metoclopramide (1 mg/kg i.v.), dopamine-induced inhibition of primary contractions was abolished and the frequency of secondary contractions was increased by 20 to 50% compared to the control. However, such motor effects did not significantly modify the volume of gases eructated, which was lower than that observed for dopamine alone (Figure 27.5). During rumen insufflation, metoclopramide probably reduced the volume of eructated gases by increasing the tonus of the cardia.

Similar effects were observed only for the other antidopaminergic substances tested (domperidone, clebopride); however, haloperidol, which is also partially able to block the dopamine-induced inhibition of rumen primary contractions, is unable to antagonize the modifications in the volume of eructation produced by dopamine (Figure 27.5).

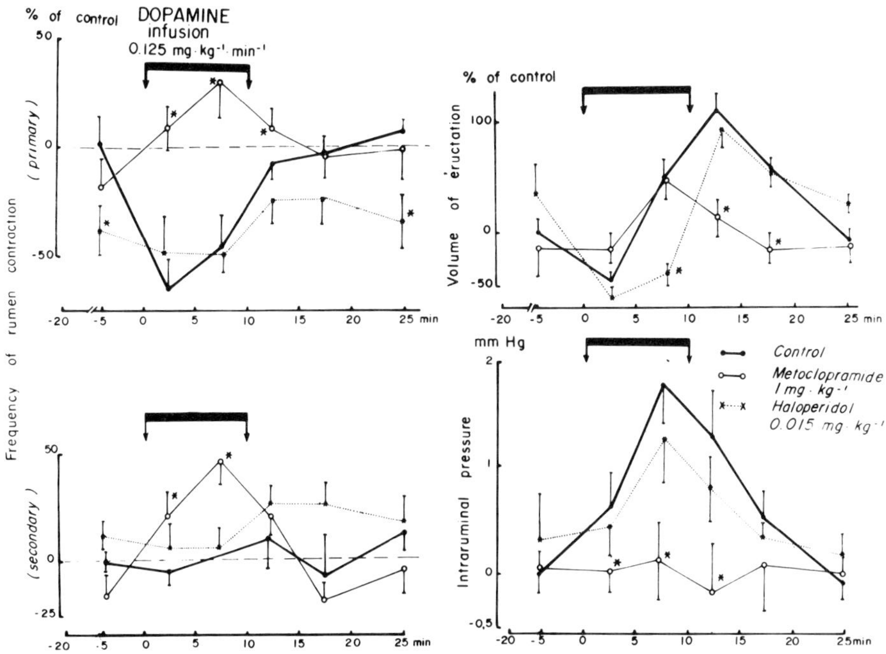

Figure 27.5 Effects of dopamine on ruminal motility and eructation in sheep. Changes induced by dopamine were antagonized by metoclopramide but not by haloperidol which inhibited by itself ruminal motility

MOTILITY OF THE SMALL INTESTINE

Dopamine

In sheep, intravenous administration of dopamine (0.4 mg/kg) was followed by immediate inhibition of both antral and duodeno-jejunal spiking activity. Whereas this inhibition was prolonged on the antrum, after a delay of

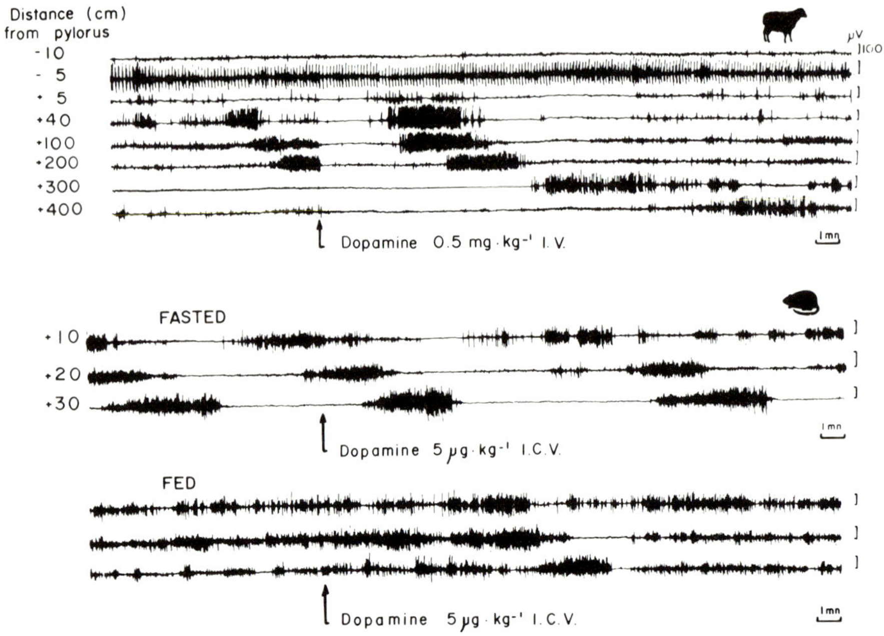

Figure 27.6 Effects of dopamine on small intestine motility in sheep and rat. In sheep dopamine injected intravenously induced a propagated phase of regular spiking activity; a similar effect was obtained only for intracerebroventricular administration in the fed rat

2–3 min the duodenum exhibited a phase of regular spiking activity (RSA) similar to that occurring normally at 90 min intervals, i.e. the migrating myoelectric complex (MMC)[2]. This dopamine-induced activity was propagated over the entire small intestine at a velocity of 15–30 cm/min (Figure 27.6); the effect was suppressed by bilateral vagotomy. No similar effects were observed in dogs and rats. However, in these species the intracerebroventricular administration of dopamine (5 μg/kg) was able to induce the duodenal occurrence of a RSA phase in fed rats (Figure 27.6) and the fasted dog. In the fed dog, the i.c.v. administration of dopamine shortened the disruption of the 'fasted' pattern, i.e. the cyclic occurrence of the MMC (unpublished results). The lack of motor effects on the small intestine by dopamine injected intravenously in rats is in agreement with the absence of changes in gastrointestinal content transit recently observed in rats[15].

Antidopaminergic substances

The effects of dopamine antagonists such as metoclopramide, domperidone, and haloperidol on spontaneous gastrointestinal motility and the antagonism of dopamine-induced relaxation on gastric smooth muscle by these compounds occur at a much lower concentration than those required for the modification of neuronal control[39]. This result is in agreement with the hypothesis that some dopamine receptors are located on smooth muscle. Consequently, metoclopramide and domperidone are used in human therapy to augment gastric and duodenal activity in a number of clinical situations. They can be used as adjuncts to radiological examination of the gastrointestinal tract, in duodenal intubation, functional dyspepsia and in nausea[43]. Studies performed in man have shown that administration of metoclopramide results in prompt evacuation of the stomach, whereas intravenous administration of domperidone apparently results in a smoother but more protracted effect on gastric emptying. For this reason, metoclopramide may be more useful in radiodiagnosis (where prompt evacuation of the stomach is required), whereas domperidone may be more useful in the treatment of diseases which are associated with disordered gastrointestinal motor function.

Studies performed in the dog are only partially in agreement with findings in humans. A 2 h infusion of metoclopramide in conscious fasting dogs enhanced the spike activity during migrating myoelectrical complexes without disruption of the fasted pattern[57]. The effects of metoclopramide were variable, not dose-dependent, and more effective on the proximal than on the distal small bowel (a result similar to that previously reported for human duodenal motor activity)[20, 23]. In addition, there are apparently discrepant data concerning residual drug activity when infusion was terminating. Enhanced irregular spiking activity returned to control levels whereas jejunal hyperactivity remained significantly enhanced.

Such an increase in activity may be responsible for increased gastric emptying. Our results confirm an increase in duodenal peristaltic activity after a bolus injection of metoclopramide (0.1 mg/kg) in the dog; similar stimulation of duodeno-jejunal motility is observed after intravenous and oral administration of other substituted benzamides such as clebopride. In contrast, domperidone did not appear to stimulate duodenal motility in both the dog and sheep when administered intravenously or orally at a dose of 1 mg/kg; sulpiride was able to induce only a very slight and transient (40–60 sec) increase (30%) in the amplitude of duodenal contraction[32], but only with a dose of 12 mg/kg.

These data suggest that the clinical need for an agent such as metoclopramide as a 'regulator' of intestinal motility cannot be objectively assessed until the nature of motility disorders is more clearly defined. It has been suggested that failure to produce MMC may be associated with bacterial overgrowth stasis in man and rats[49, 55].

COLONIC MOTILITY

The role of the adrenergic system in the regulation of colonic motility is not fully elucidated, although catecholamines usually exert an inhibitory motor effect on the gastrointestinal tract[3] and some β-adrenergic drugs are known to have stimulatory effects on the sigmoid colon[26]. Administered intravenously in healthy humans, dopamine exhibits stimulatory effects on the motility of the recto-sigmoid colon which are not opposed by α- and β-antagonists. These data suggest that dopamine does not act as a precursor of noradrenaline and adrenaline, nor does it combine with α- or β-adrenergic receptors. Furthermore, dopamine does not act through cholinergic mediation, because atropine failed to inhibit its motor stimulant effect on the human sigmoid colon; on the contrary, there was a significant increase in this effect after cholinergic blockade[27,28]. All these results suggest that dopamine stimulates the motor function of the human large bowel through specific receptors. However, only the motility of the distal colon has been considered in these experiments and different effects of drugs on the proximal and distal colon have been observed previously in humans which confirms the presence of two distinct neural control areas[13].

In the dog, a species presenting a well-defined cyclic pattern of contraction propagated from the proximal to the distal colon[51], dopamine infusion has

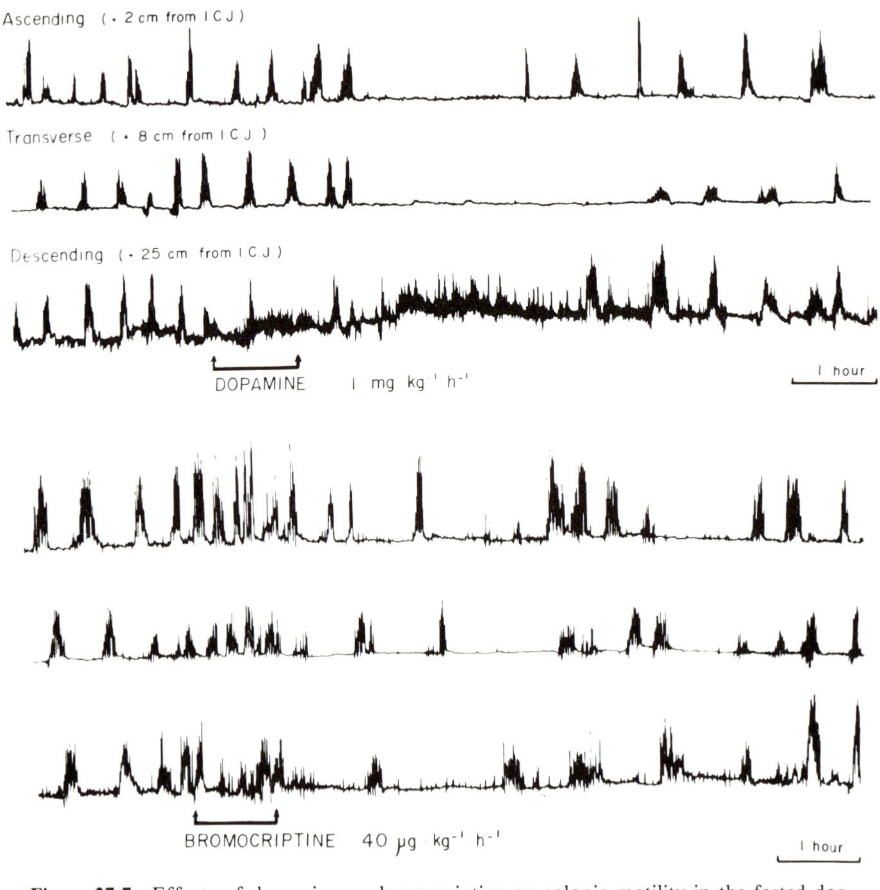

Figure 27.7 Effects of dopamine vs. bromocriptine on colonic motility in the fasted dog. Dopamine, but not bromocriptine, produced inhibition of the contractions of the proximal colon whereas they had a similar stimulatory effect on the distal colon

variable effects depending upon the animal and the site considered. When infused at a rate of 0.5 mg/h (an emetic dose), dopamine has no effect (40%) or inhibits (60%) the motility of the proximal colon, whereas stimulation of the distal part was observed in 30% of the trials in the same dogs (Figure 27.7). In contrast, bromocriptine (0.5 mg/kg) gave more coherent effects, consisting of delayed stimulation of colonic motility at all sites considered (Figure 27.7).

Effect of antidopaminergic substances

If many clinical investigations suggest that the use of dopaminergic blocking agents is efficient in the treatment of 'spastic colon' syndrome, nervous diarrhoea and many psychosomatic disturbances[30], only very few experiments have been performed to analyse the colonic motor effects of these drugs[30]. Similar to the results observed for the small intestine, the results for the colon appeared to be related to the nature of the antidopaminergic drug used, its dosage, and the basal motor activity of the colon. However, haloperidol, sulpiride, pimozide and thioridazine are able to modify the motility of the distal colon. Generally, haloperidol and sulpiride, classical and 'atypical' neuroleptic agents, respectively, induce antagonistic effects[31]. Haloperidol reduces and sulpiride increases sigmoidal motility in patients with high intestinal tone (>30 mmHg). This discrepancy has been related to the fact that haloperidol is preferentially a presynaptic blocking agent[12,29] whereas sulpiride is exclusively a postsynaptic blocking agent[17]. However, both anticholinergic drugs and dihydroergotamine abolished the stimulatory effects of sulpiride on sigmoidal activity and are able to stimulate serotonergic receptors at the central level[7] by producing an increase in serotonin levels[38]. Reversed effects of haloperidol and sulpiride are observed in patients presenting low sigmoidal activity. In this case haloperidol increases and sulpiride does not affect or reduces colonic activity[31], but no clear explanation of these effects has yet been formulated and they may be related to other properties of the dopaminergic blocking agents used. For example, the finding that sulpiride, and not haloperidol, induces cholinergic rebound of motility in the hyperactive colon has been correlated with the fact that antidopaminergic drugs of the butyrophenone family possess antimuscarinic effects[24,35] whereas sulpiride frequently induces cholinergic side-effects in humans[33,38].

In the conscious healthy dog, we have established that each dopaminergic blocking drug studied has unique effects on colonic motility which are identified regardless of the location in the colon. Metoclopramide and clebopride stimulated colonic motility whereas sulpiride produced inhibition (Figure 27.8). Only in dogs, for which dopamine exerts an inhibitory action on colonic motility, were metoclopramide and clebopride, but not sulpiride, able to block the effects of dopamine, suggesting a peripheral site of action of dopamine on the colon. In addition, clebopride, metoclopramide and sulpiride block the effects of 5-hydroxytryptophan (5-HTP) on colonic motility.

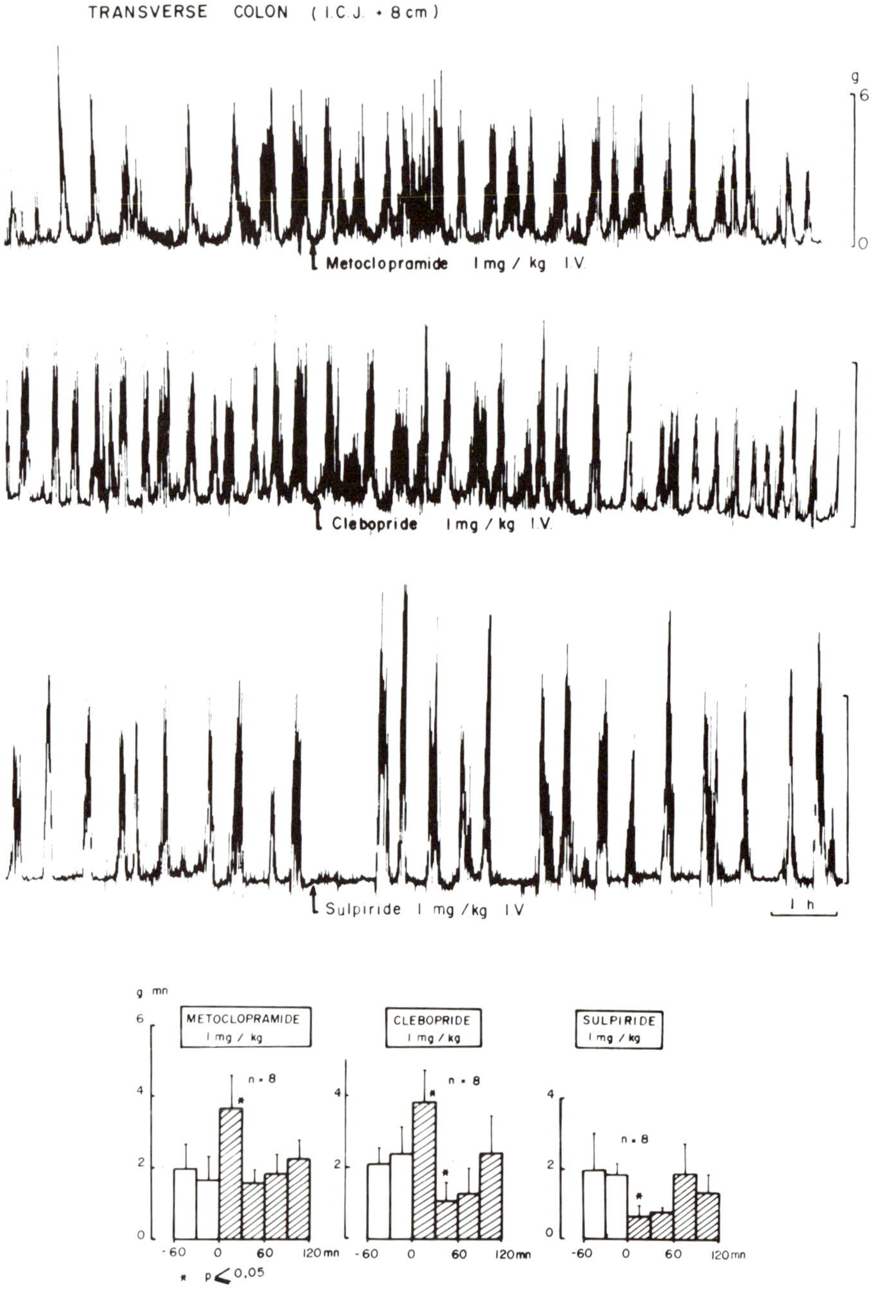

Figure 27.8 Comparative effects of some antidopaminergic drugs on the motility of the transverse colon in the dog. The lower panel corresponds to histograms of the motility indexes over consecutive 30 min periods showing that sulpiride reduced significantly the colonic motility which was enhanced by metoclopramide and clebopride

These results contrast with the observations[27] in humans that haloperidol, but not α- and β-blockers, is able to antagonize dopamine-induced stimulation of recto-sigmoidal motility.

Usually, haloperidol administered intravenously (0.5 mg/kg) blocks both inhibition of the proximal colon and stimulation of the distal colon induced by i.v. infusion of dopamine at a rate of $0.5\,\mathrm{mg\,kg^{-1}\,h^{-1}}$. However, phentolamine (0.2 mg/kg i.v.) seems to block these effects in some dogs with this pattern of activity. These results suggest that, in the dog, dopamine does not act on colonic motility through specific dopaminergic receptors.

CONCLUSIONS

In human therapy, antidopaminergic drugs are used in the treatment of many digestive disturbances such as flatulent dyspepsia, diabetic gastroparesis, chronic reflux oesophagitis, gastritis and peptic ulcer, nausea and vomiting, and emesis in pregnancy. All these clinical uses can be transported to animals. However, all pharmacological studies suggest that there is not a single simple pharmacological explanation of these uses and the mechanism of action remains unknown.

In addition to their dopamine antagonism, many of these butyrophenones or substituted benzamines have other pharmacological properties such as (1) enhancement of cholinergic excitatory processes at postganglionic myoneural junction[5,10,22,40,50], (2) inhibition of non-cholinergic, non-adrenergic motor inhibitory neurons[40], (3) antagonism of serotonin[40], and (4) direct action on smooth muscle[4].

Regardless of the mechanism involved, the present results suggest that antidopaminergic drugs may be useful in specific problems of veterinary medicine, such as closure of the oesophageal groove in milk-fed calves with partial opening due to stress conditions, abomasal stasis, and other digestive disturbances like intestinal infection. By reinforcing the tone of the LES and simultaneously stimulating rumen motility, antidopaminergic substances may be useful in forestomach motor disturbances associated with vagal damage or ruminal hypomotility.

By stimulation of duodenal activity in the sheep and dog, substituted benzamides such as metoclopramide and clebopride may be useful in cases of delayed gastric emptying and intestinal transit. The lack of characteristic and uniform effects on colonic motility does not permit proposal of their use in the treatment of diarrhoea, constipation or defaecation disturbances, or as postoperative treatment to abolish gut hypomotility.

Finally, since an analogue of procainamide, metoclopramide, has been useful in human clinical practice for a number of years in the treatment of gastrointestinal dysfunction, it is appropriate to consider it and other substituted benzamides with antidopaminergic properties for use in veterinary practice. The indications for their use still remain uncertain and have to be carefully examined, particularly for the treatment of digestive disturbances.

References

1. Bueno, L. (1975). Fonctions motrices et digestives du feuillet chez les ruminants. *Thèse Doct. Sci. Nat., Toulouse*
2. Bueno, L. and Fioramonti, J. (1979). Rhythms of abomaso-intestinal motility. In Ruckebusch, Y. and Thivend, P. (eds.) *Digestive Physiology and Metabolism in Ruminants.* pp. 53–80. (Lancaster: MTP Press)
3. Burks, T. F. (1981). Actions of drugs on gastrointestinal motility. In Johnson, L. R. (ed.) *Physiology of the Gastrointestinal Tract.* pp. 495–516.(New York: Raven Press)
4. Cohen, S., Morris, D. W., Schoen, H. J. *et al.* (1976). The effect of oral and intravenous metoclopramide on human lower oesophageal sphincter pressure. *Gastroenterology*, **70,** 484–7
5. Cools, A. R. and van Rossum, J. M. (1976). Excitation-mediating and inhibition-mediating dopamine receptors: a new concept toward a better understanding of electrophysiological, biological, chemical, pharmacological, functional and clinical data. *Psychopharmacologia*, **42,** 243–56
6. Colvin, H. W., Wheat, J. D., Thode, E. A. *et al.* (1957). Techniques for measuring eructated gas in cattle. *J. Dairy Sci.*, **40,** 492–502
7. Costale, B. and Naylor, R. J. (1978). Neuroleptic interaction with the serotonergic-dopaminergic mechanism in the *nucleus accumbens. J. Pharm. Pharmacol.*, **30,** 257
8. de Carle, D. J. and Christensen, J (1976). A dopamine receptor in oesophageal smooth muscle of the opossum. *Gastroenterology*, **70,** 216
9. Dougherty, R. W., Stewart, W. E., Nold, M. M. *et al.* (1962). Pulmonary absorption of eructated gas in ruminants. *Am. J. Vet. Res.*, **23,** 205–12
10. Eisner, M. (1968). Gastrointestinal effects of metoclopramide in man. *In vitro* experiments with human smooth muscle preparations. *Br. Med. J.*, **4,** 679–80
11. Ennis, C., Schnieden, H. and Cox, B. (1978). Effects of the anti-emetic drug domperidone on guinea pig isolated gastrointestinal tissue. *J. Pharm. Pharmacol.*, **30** (Suppl.), 34
12. Farnebo, L. O. and Hamberger, B. (1971). Drug induced changes in the release of ^{3}H monoamines from field stimulated rat brain slices. *Acta Physiol. Scand. (Suppl.)*, **371,** 35–49
13. Fink, S. and Friedman, G. (1960). The differential effect of drugs on proximal and distal colon. *Am. J. Med.*, **28,** 534–40
14. Goldberg, L. I. (1972). Cardiovascular and renal actions of dopamine potential clinical applications. *Pharmacol. Rev.*, **24,** 1–13
15. Gustavsson, S., Johansson, H., Nilsson, F. *et al.* (1979). Gastrointestinal propulsion and mixing in the rat during infusion of dopamine. *Eur. Surg. Res.*, **11,** 277–81
16. Harding, R. and Leek, B. F. (1971). The locations and activities of medullary neurones associated with ruminant forestomach motility. *J. Physiol.*, **219,** 587–610
17. Honda, F., Satom, Y., Shimomura, K. *et al.* (1977). Dopamine receptor blocking activity of sulpiride in the central nervous system. *Jap. J. Pharmacol.*, **27,** 397–404
18. Hornykiewicz, O. (1971). Neurochemical pathology and pharmacology of brain dopamine and acetylcholine; rational basis for the current treatment of parkinsonism. In McDowell, F. H. and Markham, C. H. (eds.) *Recent Advances in Parkinson's Disease.* p. 933. (Philadelphia: Davis)
19. Jenner, P., Elliot, B. N. C., Clow, A. *et al.* (1978). A comparison of *in vitro* and *in vivo* dopamine receptor antagonism produced by substituted benzamide drugs. *J. Pharm. Pharmacol.*, **29,** 46–8
20. Johnson, A. G. (1971). The action of metoclopramide on human gastro-intestinal motility. *Gut*, **12,** 421–6
21. Komissarov, I. V. and Reutskaia, G. I. (1978). Effect of dopamine on smooth muscles of the rat stomach and characteristics of α adrenoreceptors of muscle cells of the gastro-intestinal tract. *Byull. Eksp. Biol. Med.*, **85,** 176–9
22. Kowalewski, K. and Kolodej, A. (1975). Effect of metoclopramide on myoelectrical and mechanical activity of the isolated canine stomach perfused extracorporally. *Pharmacology*, **13,** 549–62
23. Labo, G., Barbara, L. and Lanfranchi, G. A. (1968). Effeti della metoclopramide sulla motilita duodenale. Studio contemporanea dell'activa elettrica electtromanometrica e degli aspetti radiologici. *Riv. Med.*, **82,** 1527–53

24. Laduron, P. M. and Laysen, J. E. (1978). Is the low incidence of extrapyramidal side-effects of antipsychotics associated with antimuscarinic properties? *J. Pharm. Pharmacol.*, **30**, 120–4
25. Laduron, P. M. and Leysen, J. E. (1979). Domperidone, a specific *in vitro* dopamine antagonist, devoid of *in vivo* central dopaminergic activity. *Biochem. Pharmacol.*, **28**, 2161–5
26. Lafranchi, G. A., Marzio, L., Cortini, C. *et al.* (1975). Evidence of β adrenergic receptors with stimulatory motor effect on the sigmoid colon. In Vantrappen, G. (ed.) *5th Symposium on Gastrointestinal Motility*. p. 52. (Leuven: Typoff Press)
27. Lanfranchi, G. A., Marzio, L., Cortini, C. *et al.* (1978). Motor effects of dopamine on human sigmoid colon: evidence for specific receptors *Am. J. Dig. Dis.*, **23**, 257–63
28. Lafranchi, G. A., Marzio, L., Cortina, C. *et al.* (1978). Effect of dopamine on gastric motility in man: evidence for specific receptors. In Duthie, H. L. (ed.) *Gastrointestinal Motility in Health and Disease*. p. 161. (Lancaster: MTP Press)
29. Langer, S. Z. (1977). Presynaptic receptors and their role in the regulation of transmitter release. *Br. J. Pharmacol.*, **60**, 481–97
30. Lechin, F., Van der Dijs, B., Bentolila, A. *et al.* (1977). The 'spastic colon' syndrome: therapeutic and pathophysiologic considerations. *J. Clin. Pharmacol.*, **17**, 431–9
31. Lechin, F. and Van der Dijs, B. (1979). Effects of dopaminergic blocking agents on distal colon motility. *J. Clin. Pharmacol.*, **19**, 617–25
32. Lobello, R., Marzano, L. A., Colantuoni, A. *et al.* (1975). Sulpiride e motilita intestinale. *Bull. Soc. It. Biol. Sper.*, **51**, 1098–103
33. Mielke, D. H., Gallant, D. M. and Kessler, C. (1977). An evaluation of a unique new antipsychotic agent, sulpiride: effects on serum prolactin and growth hormone levels. *Am. J. Psychiatr.*, **134**, 12
34. Miert van, A. S. (1968). Adrenergic receptors in the ruminal wall of sheep. *J. Pharm. Pharmacol.*, **20**, 495–6
35. Miller, R. J. and Hiley, R. C. (1974). Antimuscarinic properties of neuroleptics and drug-induced Parkinsonism. *Nature (London)*, **248**, 596
36. Mukhopadhyay, A. K. and Weisbrodt, N. (1977). Effect of dopamine on oesophageal motor function. *Am. J. Physiol.*, **232**, E19–24
37. Newhook, J. C. and Titchen, D. A. (1974). Effects of vagotomy, atropine, hexamethonium and adrenaline on the destination in the stomach of liquids sucked by milk fed lambs and calves. *J. Physiol.*, **237**, 243–58
38. Nishiura, M. (1976). Clinico-pharmacological studies of sulpiride. *Curr. Ther. Res.*, **20**, 164–6
39. Nueten van, J. M. and Janssen, P. A. (1978). Is dopamine an engogenous inhibitor of gastric emptying? In Duthie, H. L. (ed.) *Gastrointestinal Motility in Health and Disease*. pp. 173–84. (Lancaster: MTP Press)
40. Okwusaba, F. K. and Hamilton, J. T. (1976). The effect of metoclopramide on intestinal muscle responses and the peristaltic reflex *in vitro*. *Can. J. Physiol. Pharmacol.*, **54**, 393–404
41. Rattan, S. and Goyal, R. K. (1976). Effect of dopamine on oesophageal smooth muscle *in vivo*. *Gastroenterology*, **70**, 377–82
42. Rayfield, E. J., George, D. T., Eichver, H. L. *et al.* (1975). L-Dopa stimulation of glucagon secretion in man. *N. Engl. J. Med.*, **293**, 500
43. Reyntjens, A. J., Niemegeers, C. J. E., van Nueten, J. M. *et al.* (1978). Domperidone, a novel and safe gastrokinetic antinauseant for the treatment of dyspepsia and vomiting. *Arzneim. Forsch.*, **28**, 1194–6
44. Royen, van J. M. and Offermeier, J. (1981). Peripheral dopaminergic receptors. *S. Afr. Med. J.*, **25**, 329–32
45. Roy, J. H. B. (1980). *The Calf.* 4th Ed. (London: Butterworth)
46. Ruckebusch, Y. and Ruckebusch, M. (1959). Enregistrement de l'éructation chez les ruminants. *C. R. Soc. Biol.*, **153**, 1049–51
47. Ruckebusch, Y. (1974). Sleep deprivation in cattle. *Brain Res.*, **78**, 495–9
48. Ruckebusch, Y., Tsiamitas, C. and Bueno, L. (1972). The intrinsic electrical activity of the ruminant stomach. *Life Sci.*, **11**, 55–64
49. Scott, L. D. and Cahall, D. L. (1982). Influence of the interdigestive myoelectric complex on enteric flora in the rat. *Gastroenterology*, **82**, 737–45

50. Sell, A. B., Duarte, D. F. and Israel, Jr., G. (1974). Aspectos farmacodinamicos de metoclopramida. *Rev. Bras. Anest.*, **24,** 73–80
51. Templeton, R. D. and Lawson, H. (1931). Studies on the motor activity of the large intestine. Part I: Normal motility in the dog, recorded by tandem balloon method. *Am. J. Physiol.*, **96,** 667–76
52. Titchen, D. A. (1968). Nervous control of motility of the forestomach of ruminants. In *Handbook of Physiology*, Section 6, Alimentary Canal. pp. 2705–24. (Baltimore: Williams & Wilkins)
53. Thompson, B. K. and de Carle, D. J. (1982). The effect of dopamine on human gastric smooth muscle. *Aust. J. Exp. Biol. Med. Sci.*, **60,** 123–7
54. Valenzuela, J. E. (1976). Dopamine as a possible neurotransmitter in gastric relaxation. *Gastroenterology*, **71,** 1019–22
55. Vantrappen, G., Janssens, J., Hellemans, J. *et al.* (1977). The interdigestive motor complex of normal subjects and patients with bacterial overgrowth of the small intestine. *J. Clin. Invest.*, **59,** 1158–66
56. Wauquier, A., Niemegeers, C. J. E. and Janssen, P. A. J. (1981). Neuropharmacological comparison between domperidone and metoclopramide. *Jap. J. Pharmacol.*, **31,** 305–14
57. Wingate, D., Pearce, E., Hutton, M. *et al.* (1980). Effect of metoclopramide on interdigestive myoelectrical activity in the conscious dog. *Dig. Dis. Sci.*, **25,** 15–21

28
Vomiting and antiemetics in small animal practice

G. R. Hewett

Vomiting is a very common clinical sign in dogs and cats. Isolated episodes of vomiting are of little significance and occur more commonly in dogs than in cats. Persistent vomiting, on the other hand, should be considered clinically abnormal and, if left untreated, will cause dehydration, hypokalaemia, hypochloraemia and a variable degree of hyponatraemia.

Vomiting or emesis may be defined as the forceful expulsion of the gastrointestinal contents through the mouth, while retching is the laboured rhythmic activity of the respiratory muscles which usually precedes or accompanies vomiting. However, retching may occur without emesis in dogs and cats. Dogs and cats often show signs of restlessness and salivation prior to vomiting. Yoxall[34] suggests that these signs may indicate that the animal is experiencing nausea, a subjective condition in man which may or may not be associated with vomiting. It has been found[2] that these signs can be stimulated after decerebration, and hence they cannot be considered as indicating that dogs and cats experience nausea.

The ability to vomit is not present in puppies and kittens at birth. Brizee and Vitale[7] studied the functional development of emesis in the cat and found that kittens developed the ability to vomit when weighing between 150 g (about 2 days of age) and 250 g (about 10 days of age). It was also found that the components of the emetic mechanism became functional within a very short period of time. Pi and Peng[27] reported that emesis could not be elicited in puppies aged 2 days by intravenous apomorphine hydrochloride at a dose rate of 1 mg/kg. They did not study the puppies again until 5 days of age when a significant number showed signs of emesis after being given graded doses of 0.1–0.3 mg/kg apomorphine hydrochloride. Smith *et al.*[29] found that vomiting in response to intramuscular apomorphine injection at a dose rate of 1 mg/kg first appeared in puppies at 3 days of age. The fullness of the stomach with milk was found to be an important factor in determining the ability of the puppy to vomit.

There are many possible causes of vomiting, both central and peripheral, which should be considered in making a differential diagnosis[26] but, whatever the aetiology, the physiology of emesis can be considered as a complex motility disorder.

Vomition is preceded by cyclical periods of abnormal peristaltic activity of the small intestine and inhibition of gastric peristalsis. Large antiperistaltic movements of the upper small intestine may occur in the period preceding emesis[28]. Vomition comprises phases of oesophageal dilatation caused by the animal swallowing air, gastric emptying with contraction of the pylorus and relaxation of the body of the stomach, gastric reflux and oesophageal collapse in cyclical repetition. The gastric contents are forcefully expelled by contraction of the abdominal wall musculature against a caudally moving diaphragm. The flattening of the diaphragm serves to open the cardiac sphincter. The glottis is closed and the soft palate presses against the nasopharynx and this prevents vomit entering the nasal cavity.

These complex movements are controlled and co-ordinated through the vomiting centre in the lateral reticular formation of the medulla oblongata. This centre may be activated by several neural pathways (see Figure 28.1) of which the following are examples.

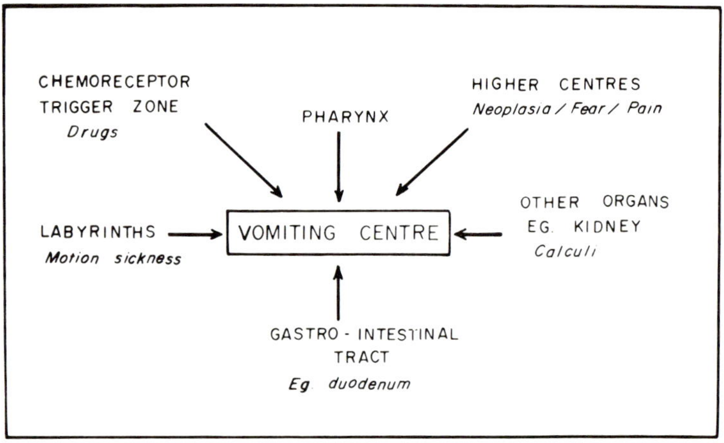

Figure 28.1 Diagram of pathways leading to vomiting centre

Stimulation of the pharynx is transmitted by afferent nerves in the glossopharyngeal nerve, cranial nerve IX. Impulses arising from the stomach, liver, intestines and peritoneum are conveyed to the vomiting centre by visceral afferent fibres in the sympathetic and vagal nerves. Visceral afferent fibres of the sympathetic nerves carry impulses from the kidneys, ureters and urinary bladder. Chemical stimulation and distension are responsible for initiating the vomiting reflex by means of these neural pathways. Caution must be exercised in the use of antiemetic drugs as they may mask clinical signs which may be necessary to establish a diagnosis[12].

Labyrinth stimulation is the primary factor in the aetiology of motion sickness. Labyrinthectomy or section of the auditory nerves, cranial nerve VIII, renders animals immune to the emetic effects of motion.

There are projections from the vomiting centre to the cerebral cortex and the limbic system. Fear and pain may initiate the vomiting reflex through the cortical-vomiting centre pathway. Head injuries, as sustained in a road traffic accident, and increases in intracranial pressure, as a result of neoplasia, may provoke emesis by means of the limbic system.

The chemoreceptor trigger zone (CTZ) is located on the dorsal aspect of the medulla, dorsolateral to the vagal nuclei (area postrema), and is connected to the vomiting centre by neural pathways[32]. The area postrema is in contact with the cerebro-spinal fluid and is devoid of the blood–brain barriers, so that substances can diffuse freely from the capillaries of this region. Borison[1] has shown that cats, in which the area postrema has been destroyed chemically, are indistinguishable from normal cats in their behaviour. However, they consistently present a permanent form of emetic refractoriness to a variety of chemical agents. The chemosensory deficiency is precise, and activation of the vomiting centre through other pathways is not affected.

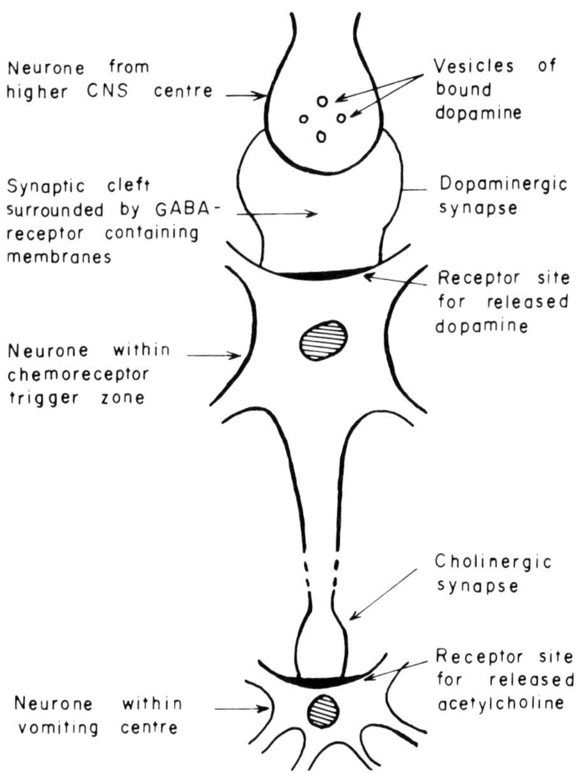

Figure 28.2 Diagrammatic presentation of the transmittter mechanisms associated with chemoreceptor trigger zone. Courtesy of P. A. J. Janssen (1967)[17]

The CTZ is affected by circulating drugs and toxins, and the neurophysiology of the CTZ is relatively well understood. Apomorphine causes depolarization of the small astrocytes containing a reddish fluorescent substance. This electrical activity is transmitted to the dopaminergic neurons which leads to the release of neurotransmitter into the synaptic cleft. The dopamine receptors are activated and a nervous impulse is initiated which is transmitted to the cholinergic synapse of the vomiting centre[17], although other transmitters may also be involved[33] (see Figure 28.2).

ANTIEMETICS

Anticholinergic drugs

Anticholinergic drugs inhibit gastric motility but do not inhibit apomorphine-induced emesis[4,8]. Atropine and l-hycoscine have two main actions in the body: (1) upon the smooth muscle and secretory glands innervated by postganglionic cholinergic nerves, and (2) upon the central nervous system. They owe a large proportion of their antiemetic activity to their central activity. Jaju *et al.*[18] found that anticholinergic drugs are able to suppress activity within the vestibular nuclei of cats, but they may decrease emesis even when the vestibular system is not directly involved in the afferent neural pathways[23]. L-hyoscine may be used to prevent motion sickness in dogs. It has a short duration of action, and the dose rate is 0.03 mg/kg four times daily. It is not suitable for use in cats since it induces hyperexcitability.

Anticholinergics, which reduce motility by inhibiting peristalsis, may increase the time available for gut bacteria to multiply and invade other tissues.

These disadvantages, together with the lack of selectivity of these agents, limit their use in veterinary practice as antiemetics.

Antidopaminergic drugs

GABA-like drugs

The phenothiazine and butyrophenone tranquillizers have similar chemical structures to GABA. Janssen[16] postulated that they have a greater tendency to form a monomolecular film on membranes containing GABA-receptors than on other membranes. Such a film will reduce the excitability of the receptors within the synaptic cleft of the dopaminergic synapse. The phenothiazines block the CTZ at low doses and depress the emetic centre at higher doses[6]. Phenothiazine derivatives are able to produce other effects in the body including α-adrenoceptor block, anticholinergic actions and stimulation of the extrapyramidal system. Chlorpromazine may be used orally to prevent motion sickness at a dose rate of 0.5–1.0 mg/kg, but such doses will induce sedation as well.

Animals showing signs of gastrointestinal disease may be medicated with chlorpromazine at a low dose to prevent emesis[14] but acepromazine should only be used if it is certain that there is no decrease in circulating blood volume[26].

Trifluoperazine, another phenothiazine, is approximately 18 times more potent than chlorpromazine in preventing emesis induced by intravenous injection of 1 mg/kg apomorphine hydrochloride[30]. The peak effect occurred 2 h after administration, and the antiemetic activity lasted more than 12 h. No controlled clinical trials in dogs and cats have been reported but Murdock[25] demonstrated that 0.03 mg/kg twice daily was capable of controlling emesis in small animals. Extrapyramidal side-effects have been reported in man with high doses[11], and it has been found that, after oral and subcutaneous administration of doses of 2 mg/kg, dogs showed miosis, sedation, relaxation of the nictitating membrane, ataxia and lachrymation. These side-effects are very unlikely to be observed in animals medicated using the clinical dose regimen.

Some antihistamines possess antiemetic activity[5]. Promethazine has marked antihistaminic and anticholinergic properties[13], and has been found to be capable of inhibiting apomorphine-induced emesis in dogs[5]. Promethazine, at a dosage rate of 2 mg/kg twice daily, is used in small animal practice for prevention of motion sickness. It has also been found to be effective in increasing tolerance to radiation-induced emesis in dogs[9].

The butyrophenones are more potent antiemetic drugs than the phenothiazines[16], but they are not widely used in veterinary practice as they may induce bizarre behavioural changes[34].

Metoclopramide

Metoclopramide is similar chemically to procainamide and is an antidopaminergic agent with both peripheral and central actions[15,22,24]. The antiemetic activity is equally marked for both apomorphine and copper sulphate induced emesis[24], and it was concluded that metoclopramide acts directly on the emetic centre against copper sulphate and on the CTZ against apomorphine hydrochloride and dihydroergotomine. Metoclopramide does not possess the tranquillizing activity of the phenothiazines, which is an important advantage in the clinical assessment of dogs and cats following therapy.

In the dog, metoclopramide is 35 times more effective in inhibiting apomorphine-induced vomiting than chlorpromazine[20]. Metoclopramide prevented vomiting in the cat encephale isolé preparation induced by electrical stimulation of the nucleus tractus solitari of the brainstem. It was also found to affect the nucleus, suggesting a possible antivertigo action. Kobayashi *et al.*[3] reported that metoclopramide administered intraperitoneally, at a dose of at least 0.5 mg/kg 15–20 min before apomorphine administration, prevented vomiting and the appearance of aggressive behaviour in cats.

Occasional extrapyramidal side-effects of metoclopramide have been reported in man[19], but these have not been reported in dogs.

According to Yoxall[34], metoclopramide would appear to be the antiemetic of choice for most clinical situations unless sedation is required as well. No controlled trials have been reported on its use in small animal practice, but it has been used successfully in small animals for the control of emesis in cases of gastrointestinal disease[34].

It is important to stress that antiemetics should be used in a therapeutic programme designed to treat the underlying disease process, and not simply symptomatically, as they may mask disease processes which need further investigation.

References

1. Borison, H. L. (1974). Area postrema - CTZ for vomiting. Is that all? *Life Sci.*, **14,** 1807–14
2. Borison, H. L. and Wang, S. C. (1953). Physiology and pharmacology of vomiting. *Pharmacol. Rev.*, **5,** 193–230
3. Bowman, W. C. and Rand, M. J. (1982). *Textbook of Pharmacology*. 2nd Ed. (Oxford: Blackwell Sci. Publ.)
4. Boyd, E. M. and Cassell, W. A. (1957). Agents affecting apomorphine induced vomiting. *J. Pharmacol. Exp. Ther.*, **119,** 390–4
5. Boyd, E. M., Cassell, W. A., Boyd, C. A. *et al.* (1955). Inhibition of the apomorphine induced vomiting syndrome by antihistaminic agents. *J. Pharmacol. Exp. Ther.*, **113,** 299–309
6. Brand, E. D., Harris, T. D., Borison, H. L. *et al.* (1954). The anti-emetic activity of 10-(dimethylaminopropyl)-2-chlorophenothiazine (chlorpromazine) in the dog and cat. *J. Pharmacol. Exp. Ther.*, **110,** 86
7. Brizee, F. R. and Vitale, D. (1959). Functional development of the emetic apparatus in the cat. *Am. J. Physiol.*, **196,** 1189–90
8. Cheymol, J. and Quinquaud, A. (1950). Application d'atropine sur le bulbe émétisant. *C. R. Soc. Biol.*, **144,** 662–4
9. Cooper, J. R. and Mattsson, J. L. (1979). Control of radiation induced emesis with promethazine, cimetidine, thiethylperazine or naloxone. *Am. J. Vet. Res.*, **40,** 1057–61
10. Chinn, H. I. and Smith, P.K. (1955). Motion sickness. *Pharmacol. Rev.*, **7,** 33–82
11. Davis, L. E. (1980). Pharmacologic control of vomiting. *Am. J. Vet. Med. Assoc.*, **176,** 241–2
12. Davis, L. E. (1980). In Anderson, N. V. (ed.) *Veterinary Gastroenterology*. (Philadelphia: Lea and Febiger)
13. Douglas, W. W. (1980). In Gilman, A. G., Goodman, L. S. and Gilman, A. (eds.) *The Pharmacological Basis of Therapeutics*. 6th Edn. (New York: MacMillan)
14. Goldston, R. T. and Seybold, I. M. (1982). Management of gastrointestinal problems, V. M./S.A.C., **77,** 171–3
15. Jacobie, H. I. and Brodie, D. A. (1967). Gastrointestinal actions of metoclopramide. *Gastroenterology*, **52,** 676–84
16. Janssen, P. A. J. (1965). The evolution of the butyrophenones, haloperidol and trifluperidol from meperidine-like 4-phenylpiperidines. *Intern. Rev. Neurobiol.*, **4,** 221
17. Janssen, P. A. J. (1967). The pharmacology of haloperidol. *Intern. J. Neuropsych.*, **3,** 10–18
18. Jaju, B. P., Kursten, E. B. and Wang, S. C. (1970). Effects of belladonna alkaloids on vestibular nucleus in the cat. *Am. J. Physiol.*, **219,** 2148
19. Johnson, A. G. (1977). *Metoclopramide Ten Years After, An Independent Review of the Biomedical Literature*. (Amsterdam: Excerpta Medica)
20. Justin-Besancon, L. and Laville, C. (1964). Action antiémétique du métoclopramide vis-à-vis de l'apomorphine et de l'hydergine. *C.R. Soc. Biol.*, **158,** 723–7
21. Kobauashi, T., Murayama, S. and Yoshino, T. (1966). Pharmacology of metoclopramide: its anti-emetic action *Jap. Symp. Ther. New Drugs*, vol. Rapp, 41–4
22. Kowalewski, K. and Kolodej, A. (1975). Effect of metoclopramide on myoelectrical and mechanical activity of the isolated canine stomach perfused extracorporeally. *Pharmacology*, **13,** 549–62
23. Laurence, D. R. (1973). *Clinical Pharmacology*. 4th Ed. (Edinburgh: Churchill Livingstone)

24. Laville, C. (1964). Protection exercée par le métoclopramide contre les effets vomitifs du sulfate de cuivre. *Pathol. Biol.*, **12,** 577–8
25. Murdock, D. Personal communication
26. Murdock, D. (1979). *Canine Medicine and Therapeutics.* (Oxford: Blackwell Sci. Publ.)
27. Pi, W. P. and Peng, M. T. (1971). Functional development of the central emetic mechanism in the puppy dog. *Proc. Soc. Exp. Biol. Med.*, **136,** 802–4.
28. Smith, C. C. and Brizzee, K. R. (1961). Cineradiographic analysis of vomiting in the cat. *Gastroenterology*, **40,** 654–64
29. Smith, D. M., Dirk, G. R. and Shepp, E. (1974). Maturation of the emetic apparatus in the dog. *Am. J. Vet. Res.*, **35,** 1281–3
30. Smith, Kline and French (1958). *Pharmacology of Stelazine.* Science Information Department, Welwyn
31. Takori, S., Nakai, Y. and Shimamoto, K. (1968). The mechanism of antagonism between apomorphine and metoclopramide on unit discharges from nuclear structures in the brain-stem of the cat. *Int. J. Neuropharmacol.*, **7,** 115–26
32. Wang, S. C. and Borison, H. L. (1952). A new concept of organisation of the central emetic mechanism: recent studies on the sites of action of apomorphine, copper sulphate and cardiac glycosides. *Gastroenterology*, **22,** 1–12
33. Wood, C. D. and Graybiel, A. (1970). A theory of motion sickness based on pharmacological reactions. *Clin. Pharm. Ther.*, **11,** 621
34. Yoxall, A. T. (1980). *Physiological Basis of Small Animal Medicine.* (Oxford: Blackwell Sci. Publ.)

29
Diarrhoea and antidiarrhoeal drugs

J. Fioramonti, C. J. E. Niemegeers and F. Awouters

In man, diarrhoea mainly affects children (500 million annually world-wide) and is the leading cause of death in children under 4 years[26]. In animals, diarrhoea also mainly occurs in the neonatal period. One of the main characteristics of diarrhoea in animals as well as in humans is the diversity of aetiologies within the same species.

AETIOLOGY OF DIARRHOEA IN FARM ANIMALS

Acute diarrhoeal disease remains a major limiting factor in cattle production and 5–10% of calves born each year may be lost due to neonatal enteric infection[34]. This occurs despite important advances in knowledge about the intestinal infections which cause diarrhoea, and about the nutrition and management of the neonatal calf.

The aetiology of diarrhoea in calf remains unclear. *Escherichia coli* infection is the most common disease of young calves and occurs mainly during the first 3 weeks of life. Ten years ago, considerable emphasis was given to the involvement of viruses (rotavirus, coronavirus) as a cause of diarrhoea in the neonatal calf[35]. However, the pathogenesis of acute diarrhoea in calf is complex and also involves environmental and dietary factors associated with the intensity of modern production methods.

Swine dysentery is a major disease affecting pigs in large production units, with an acute form of bloody diarrhoea frequently followed by a subacute or chronic form of mucoid diarrhoea without blood.

Investigations over the last 10 years[57] have revealed that *Treponema hyodysenteriae* is the primary pathogen in the aetiology of swine dysentery but the presence of one or more other anaerobes is a prerequisite for expression of its pathogenicity[56]. Adenovirus has been associated also with mild diarrhoea in pig[21]. Environmental and dietary factors may be also important in the development of the disease.

The most important sign of digestive pathology in the young rabbit (5–15 weeks) is diarrhoea. As in other animals the aetiology is complex with non-specific causes. Various kinds of stress are involved (e.g. transport, changes in temperature, noise) and are able to activate the infectious agents. The specific agents mainly include coccidiae but their pathogenic action is very variable since coccidiae are present in the digestive tract of all rabbits[40]. The more pathogenic species are *Eimeria intestinalis* and *Eimeria pellerdyi* while species like *Eimeria perforans* are weakly pathogenic[20].

Chronic diarrhoea is also a disease that affects a wide range of ages and breeds of horse. In this case, it seems that diarrhoea corresponds to an immunologic disorder and not to some chronic infection. The concentration of immunoglobulin A in the serum of horses with diarrhoea was approximately 50% lower than that in the serum of normal horses[49]. Treatment of foals with diarrhoea by intramuscular injection of γ-globulin prepared from serum of normal horses proved successful while antibiotics and anti-diarrhoeal drugs were ineffective[48]. However, the α-adrenergic blocking agent, phenoxybenzamine, has been recently reported to be successful in the treatment of diarrhoea in horses[28] but its mechanism remains unknown; similarities with the efficacy of chlorpromazine in enterotoxic diarrhoea in man and swine[27] can be postulated.

EXPERIMENTAL DIARRHOEA

Many models of experimental diarrhoea have been developed to elucidate aetiology and physiopathological mechanisms and to study potential therapeutic measures.

In calves oral inoculation with enteropathogenic strains of *Escherichia coli* was used to induce diarrhoea and to study the pathogenesis of enteric colibacillosis[39] or the efficacy of some rehydration solutions[16].

A dysentery model in pig was developed using infection with *Treponema hyodysenteriae*[41]. This model was useful for testing the efficacy of various drugs[42], or various dietary supplementations[50] and to study intestinal fluid absorption[2] in swine dysentery. Experimental infections in gnotobiotic pigs also demonstrated the pathogenic synergism between *Treponema hyodysenteriae* and other anaerobes in the aetiology of swine dysentery[56].

Since diarrhoea is the most common sign of coccidiosis in various animal species and since the young rabbit is very sensitive to some coccidiae, experimental coccidiosis was used for determination of hydroelectrolytic[33] or digestive motility disturbances[24]. However, the choice of coccidiae species is difficult because of the high lethality of pathogenic species which does not permit longterm experimental studies; for this reason, *Eimeria magna* has been often chosen.

Beyond these infectious models, other types of experimental diarrhoea have been developed to study the colonic motility during diarrhoea, such as castor oil in cats[18] or Ca-sennosides in dogs[25]. Nutritional diarrhoea was also induced for the analysis of the digestive motility disturbances, e.g. grain overload in sheep[10] and cereal food overfeeding in dogs[22].

DISTURBANCES OF DIGESTIVE MOTILITY IN DIARRHOEA

Disturbances of digestive motility associated with diarrhoeal diseases are very variable. In humans, chronic diarrhoea observed in the irritable bowel syndrome has been found to be associated with chronic hypomotility[19,54]. However, hypermotility or hypomotility are insufficient terms to describe colonic motor disturbances. The colon of all mammalian species investigated is characterized by a duality of contractile activity[23]: tonic contractions of small amplitude, and propulsive phasic contractions. These two kinds of contractions are detected on colonic electromyograms as short and long spike bursts (SSB and LSB) respectively.

Recording of electrical activity of the descending and sigmoid colon in patients with irritable bowel syndrome, manifested by chronic constipation

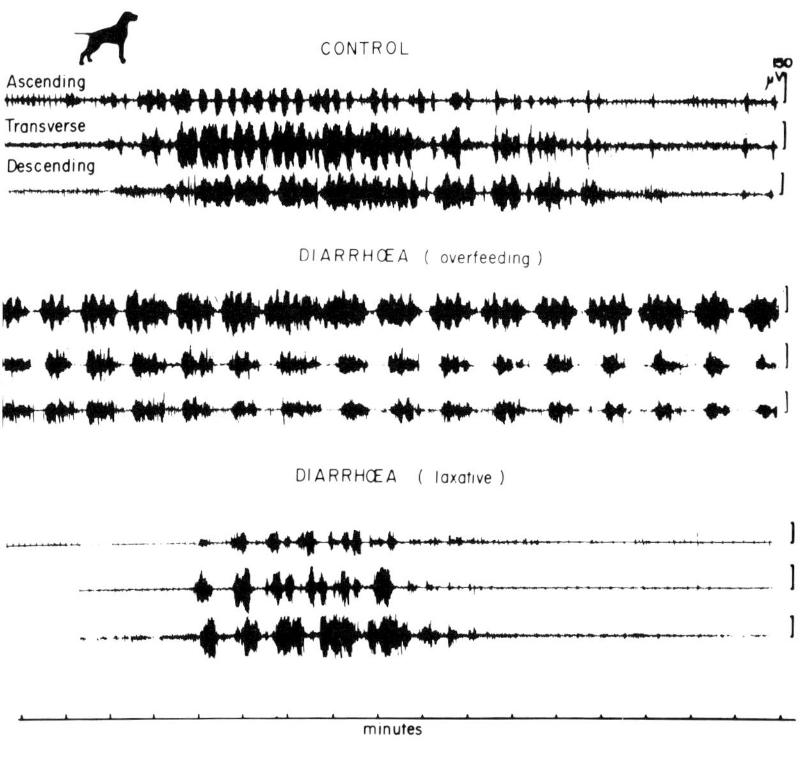

Figure 29.1 Disturbances of colonic motility during diarrhoea in dog. The normal colonic electromyogram consists of bursts of spikes, corresponding to propulsive contractions, grouped in phases lasting about 10 min (upper panel). Feeding large amounts of dry dog food induces production of soft faeces and is associated to propulsive contractions (middle panel). Laxative-induced diarrhoea (senna extracts) corresponds to an hypomotility (lower panel)

or diarrhoea, indicate significant changes in the SSB and LSB activities compared to normal control volunteers[10]. Two major groups of electromyographic changes have been detected. The first, corresponding to an increase in SSB activity was mainly recorded in constipated patients. The second group was characterized by a reduction in both SSB and LSB activity and was often observed in patients with predominantly diarrhoeal symptoms. However, constipation or diarrhoea does not correspond systematically to the afore-mentioned disturbances of colonic motility.

In dogs, the production of abundant and soft faeces induced by feeding a large amount (500 g/day) of dry food is associated with an increase of the propulsive LSB activity and reduction of the SSB tonic activity. In contrast, diarrhoea induced by oral administration of senna extracts corresponds to a strong decrease in both propulsive and tonic contractile activity (Figure 29.1).

In sheep, the spiral colon was characterized by a nearly continuous tonic SSB activity involved in the formation of pellets[46]. In cases of a spontaneous[23]

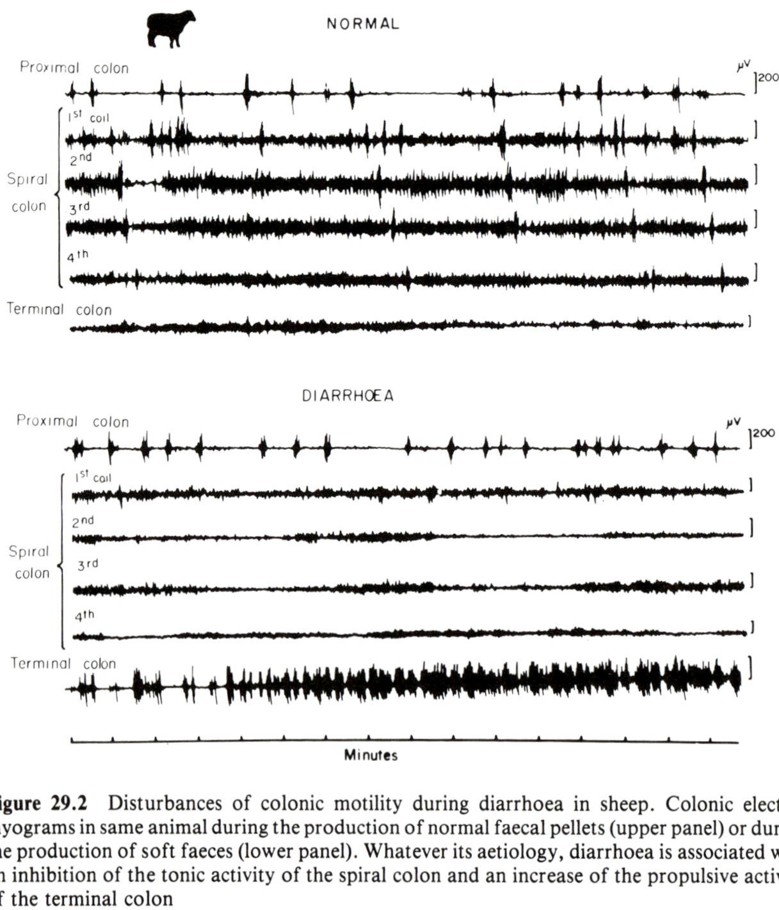

Figure 29.2 Disturbances of colonic motility during diarrhoea in sheep. Colonic electromyograms in same animal during the production of normal faecal pellets (upper panel) or during the production of soft faeces (lower panel). Whatever its aetiology, diarrhoea is associated with an inhibition of the tonic activity of the spiral colon and an increase of the propulsive activity of the terminal colon

or experimental diarrhoea[11] and inhibition of the tonic activity of the spiral colon has always been observed (Figure 29.2).

Thus, inhibition of the tonic activity of the colon is a common finding to the various types of diarrhoea investigated.

Disturbances of the motility of the small intestine have also been described. A general finding is the disorganization of the cyclic motor profile observed in sheep when diarrhoea was induced by intraluminal infusions of hypertonic solutions[45], in rabbits during experimental coccidiosis[24] as well as in a human patient with irritable colon[51].

EFFECTS OF OPIATES AND ANTICHOLINERGIC DRUGS ON DIGESTIVE MOTILITY

The effects of antidiarrhoeal drugs on intestinal motility have been studied largely under *in vitro* conditions. *In vivo* most of the studies concern the digestive transit time but very little information is available on the effects on contractile activity of the digestive tract. Recently, similarities between colonic motor profiles in dogs and humans have been shown[10]. Therefore, colonic motility in the dog was used as a model for studying the effects of some antidiarrhoeal drugs[12,13].

Opiates

The stimulation of colonic motility in dogs by morphine was first demonstrated in 1940 by Adler and Ivy[1]. Studies over long periods[12] show that the typical pattern of colonic motility in the dog is disrupted by intravenous administration of morphine (0.1 mg/kg). A 180–240 min period of significant increase in colonic motility followed the injection. In many cases, this response was biphasic. During the first 25–35 min a sustained increase in the baseline with superimposed phasic contractions was observed. This primary response was followed 2 h later by an additional tonic response accompanied by an increase in the frequency of phasic contractions. These stimulatory effects were abolished by previous administration of naloxone or atropine while methysergide blocked only the second phase of colonic stimulation. Moreover, methysergide blocked the response when injected by the intracerebroventricular route at doses inactive by the intravenous route[13], suggesting that the long-lasting stimulatory effects of morphine on colonic motility are centrally mediated through serotonergic receptors.

Similarly, loperamide (0.5 mg/kg i.v.) significantly increased the colonic motility index in dogs but only during the first 30 min following its administration[32].

However, extrapolation of data obtained on the dog colon would be speculative. For example, morphine also induced a centrally mediated increase in the motility of the small intestine in sheep, but this response was blocked by previous administration of nalorphine[9], while in dogs morphine and nalorphine induced the same stimulatory effects at the colonic level[12].

Moreover, opiates stimulate the motility of the small intestine in dogs[14] and in humans[31] while an inhibition has been found in rats[55]. Similarly, in horses morphine induced a strong inhibition of colonic motility preceding a period of increase in tonic activity (Fioramonti, unpublished results), while in dogs only colonic stimulation has been observed (Figure 29.3).

In summary, the constipating effects of opiates, beyond their action on the movement of water and electrolytes[7], are induced by different modifications of intestinal motility. They are mediated through mechanisms which vary with the animal species and the part of the digestive tract.

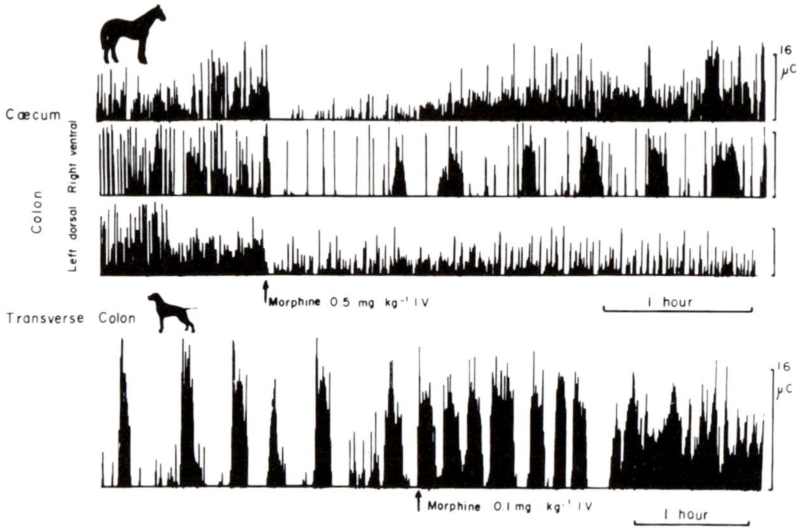

Figure 29.3 Species differences in the response of large bowel motility to morphine. Integrated electromyograms of the caecum, ventral and dorsal colon in horse (upper panel) and of the transverse colon in dog (lower panel). Morphine induces in horse an inhibition of the whole large bowel which shows a localized stimulation of the cyclic activity except for the dorsal colon, while in dog a stimulation of colonic motility is observed

Anticholinergic drugs

Anticholinergic drugs generally have an inhibitory effect on the motility of the digestive tract[6]. These inhibitory effects appear clearly at the colonic level in the dog[32]. A nearly total inhibition was observed during the hour following intravenous administration of atropine sulphate or prifinium bromide (0.5 mg/kg).

However, atropine-resistant contractions of the digestive tract, as evidenced in the taenia of guinea-pig caecum[17], indicate the need for more research on smooth muscle physiology. Recently, an atropine-resistant activity of the descending and sigmoid colon has been found in man[44]. After subcutaneous administration of atropine sulphate (15 μg/kg) tonic contractions and localized phasic contractions were strongly decreased while the occurrence of aborally propagated contractions remained unchanged.

On the small intestine of sheep, the most important effects of anticholinergic drugs consist of a disorganization of the cyclic motor profile associated with an increase in segmental contractions[8]. Compared to the atropine effects, this disorganization was more important for the prifinium bromide while *N*-butyl-hyoscine bromide was less effective.

From these studies it appears that diarrhoea and its treatment depend upon many complex processes: the diversity of the aetiology of diarrhoea, the relationship between digestive motility, transit of chyme and absorption–secretion, the variability of the effects of antidiarrhoeal drugs according to the animal species, the segment of the digestive tract, and the experimental conditions. This would theoretically imply that in the search for new antidiarrhoeals at least several methods and several different animal species should be used.

In practice, great progress may, however, be expected from the use of a single and simple animal model which mimics to a certain extent the basic pathways of the intestinal response to a foreign challenge. Agents effective in such a model and characterized by a safe and sufficiently specific intestinal action may then, later on, be tested for their therapeutic value in the very diverse clinical forms of diarrhoea that are known either in animals or in man and may in a further step help in elucidating the different processes that play a role in diarrhoea.

PHARMACOLOGY OF ANTIDIARRHOEAL AGENTS

The systematic study of the antidiarrhoeal activity of compounds is relatively recent. Up to 20 years ago, relief of diarrhoea and dysentery in man was mainly pursued with opium preparations, which traditional medicine had selected for this purpose from the many drugs that can cause constipation. This selection appeared to be clinically and also pharmacologically acceptable: morphine and codeine show antidiarrhoeal activity at doses below the analgesic dose[37]. At the same time, however, the central effects of opiates, such as drowsiness, analgesia, respiratory depression and addiction, imposed many practical restrictions to their gastrointestinal use.

The pharmacological progress from opiate alkaloids to the synthetic antidiarrhoeal loperamide has been described in detail[3,38]. The development of loperamide resulted from the synthesis of a new chemical series of piperidine derivatives which lacks the pethidine moiety and from the introduction of the castor oil test in rats which measures antidiarrhoeal activity of compounds instead of constipation.

The induction of diarrhoea with castor oil results from the action of ricinoleic acid formed by hydrolysis of the oil (Figure 29.4). Ricinoleic acid produces changes in the transport of water and electrolytes, resulting in a net hypersecretory response. The normal reaction of the intestine to excessive fluid load is increased peristalsis. In addition to hypersecretion, ricinoleic acid sensitizes the intramural neurons of the gut. This effect of ricinoleic acid

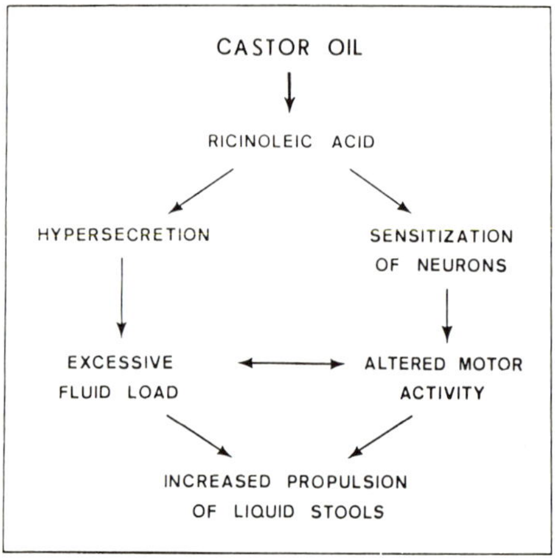

Figure 29.4 Intestinal fate and actions of castor oil

is a general property of hydroxy fatty acids. Ricinoleic acid, therefore, can be considered the prototype of lipids which stimulate the gut, such as the hydroxy fatty acids which are produced by pathogenic bacteria, and the very potent prostaglandins made by the intestine itself. The net result of the neuronal sensitization is to further promote the transport of soft intestinal contents. The described reactions of the gut to ricinoleic acid are the basic mechanisms through which the intestine responds to a wide variety of pathological stimuli. For these reasons castor oil induced diarrhoea was selected for evaluating the effects of antidiarrhoeals.

The standardized castor oil test procedure is as follows. One ml of castor oil applied orally to rats fasted overnight induces profuse diarrhoea within 1 h in all vehicle-treated animals. In rats treated with an antidiarrhoeal, presence or absence of diarrhoea is noted at hourly intervals after the castor oil challenge, and on this basis drug activity is evaluated and expressed in ED_{50}-values which represent doses effective in 50% of the animals.

Castor oil induced diarrhoea in rats has been used for more than 10 years. The test provides reproducible results in control and treated animals, it allows evaluation of the potency of a compound, the onset, and duration of the antidiarrhoeal effect. We further know that the castor oil challenge combines hypersecretion and increased propulsion, and that it gives a reliable prediction of the clinical efficacy of antidiarrhoeal compounds[37].

INTESTINAL ACTION OF LOPERAMIDE: SPECIFICITY AND NATURE

When studied in the castor oil test, loperamide was much more potent than morphine[36]. Protection from diarrhoea up to 2 h was obtained in 50% of the rats with 0.29 mg/kg of orally administered loperamide and with 5.21 mg/kg

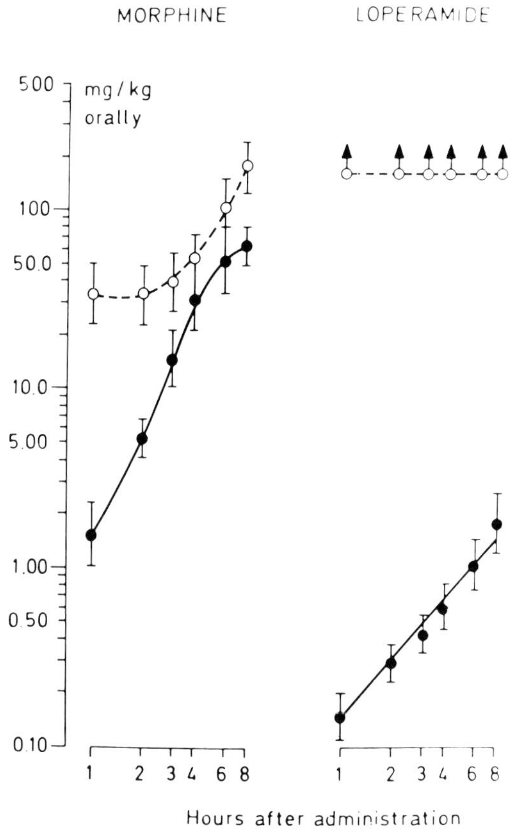

Figure 29.5 Oral ED_{50}-values (with confidence limits) of morphine and loperamide in two tests in rats. Protection from castor oil diarrhoea for 1 up to 8 h (●---●) and inhibition of the tail withdrawal reaction (reaction time >10 s) (○---○) at 1 up to 8 h interval between treatment and test

of morphine (Figure 29.5). This figure also indicates that six times the antidiarrhoeal dose of morphine induced surgical analgesia (tail withdrawal reaction times of more than 10 s), whereas more than 500 times (160 mg/kg) the antidiarrhoeal dose of loperamide did not.

It was found that orally administered loperamide is well absorbed but practically confined to the enterohepatic circulation[15]. Tissues outside the digestive system are therefore, for the most part, excluded from its action. Even when loperamide is deliberately introduced into the general circulation by intravenous injection, central actions were only observed at high, nearly toxic doses[38] and the compound again tended to concentrate in the gastrointestinal tract[58].

Increasing doses of loperamide induce a progressively longer diarrhoea-free period in rats challenged with castor oil. At the same time fluid loss becomes progressively smaller[5]. In contrast to loperamide, aspirin-like drugs

Table 29.1 Some effects of loperamide on intestinal motor function and hypersecretion

Species or preparation	*Process*	*Effect of loperamide*	*Reference*
Guinea-pig ileum (*in vitro*)	Peristaltic reflex	Inhibition	52
Dog colon	Motility	Significant increase during first 30 min	32
Man	Anal sphincter pressure	Significant increase	43
Rat intestine	Cholera toxin or PGE_2-induced fluid accumulation	Antagonism except for increase in cAMP levels	47
Rabbit ileum mucosa (*in vitro*)	Theophylline stimulation of Cl^--secretion	Inhibition	30
Guinea-pig colon	Permeability increase induced by laxative	Dose-dependent reversal	53

produce only a delay in diarrhoea[4]. Although they increase the time available for intestinal absorption, the faecal excretion remains at least as copious as in control animals. Many studies have now established that loperamide changes motor function to a less propulsive pattern, and prevents intestinal fluid accumulation in response to a great variety of secretory agents. Table 29.1 represents a partial list of such studies.

In some of these studies, such as the inhibition of the peristaltic reflex in the guinea-pig ileum[52] loperamide was much more potent than morphine and both drugs could also be qualitatively distinguished.

In the motility studies on the dog[32], loperamide (0.5 mg/kg i.v.) was less active than morphine (0.1 mg/kg i.v.) and had a short duration of action, i.e. there was no second phase of centrally mediated stimulation.

Loperamide and morphine-like drugs have a direct local action on intestinal opiate receptors, which appears to be essential for their antidiarrhoeal activity. However, in binding studies loperamide also shows high affinity binding of large capacity to other receptors. One of these has been identified as the calmodulin binding site, which is considered important in calcium-dependent hypersecretion in the intestine[29] and to which loperamide, in contrast to morphine-like drugs, binds at low concentration[59].

SYMPTOMATIC TREATMENT OF DIARRHOEA AT PRESENT AND IN THE FUTURE

Loperamide acts on the common pathways the intestine follows in response to a variety of diarrhoeal stimuli. Symptomatic treatment of acute and chronic diarrhoea in man with loperamide has found wide acceptance. The medication is, in general, rapidly effective and no side-effects occur, undoubtedly because of the exceptional intestinal specificity of loperamide.

When treatment is considered with other available drugs the pharmacological results of Table 29.2 are of great interest. Eight drugs with known

Table 29.2 Pharmacological results of eight drugs with 'antimotility' and/or 'antisecretory' activity

Compound	ED_{50} *castor oil test* (mg/kg)	ED_{50} *second test* (mg/kg)	*Antidiarrhoeal specificity*
Acetylsalicylic acid	95.3	38.0*	0.40
Atropine	9.3	0.39†	0.042
Clonidine	0.028	0.085‡	3.0
Codeine	10.8	56.6**	5.2
Indomethacin	8.7	6.2*	0.71
Isopropamide	74.6	12.4†	0.29
Lidamidine	1.7	24.9‡	14.9
Loperamide	0.29	>160**	>552

*Nystatin paw oedema test (anti-inflammatory activity)
†Mydriasis (anticholinergic activity)
‡Automatic side-effects (exophthalmos, piloerection and hypotonia)
**Tail withdrawal reaction test (narcotic analgesis activity)

'antimotility' or 'antisecretory' effects were tested in the castor oil test to obtain the dose protecting from diarrhoea for 2 h. The same drugs were studied in another test, which measures the possible primary effect expected from compounds belonging to a particular pharmacological class.

Compounds with very different mechanisms of action, including blockade of intestinal muscarinic receptors, inhibition of prostaglandin synthesis and clonidine-like (adrenergic) action showed antidiarrhoeal activity, but generally at high doses when compared to their primary activity. The first restriction to their clinical use appears to be the lack of intestinal specificity. As in the case of the progress from codeine to loperamide, more specific drugs may be found in the future.

CONCLUSIONS

The incidence and severity of diarrhoea in the neonatal period remains a serious health problem in farm animals as well as in man. A wide range of infectious agents, environmental factors, motility patterns and responses to drugs that act on intestinal smooth muscle have been detected by studying diarrhoea and motility in different species.

As a result a large number of experimental models are now available, which more closely mimic particular types of diarrhoea and which allow a more detailed evaluation of the field of application of the available drugs. The development of a new drug is for practical reasons, such as, for example, a systematic study of structure activity relationships, only possible by using carefully selected animal models. Castor oil diarrhoea in rats is clearly an appropriate model, which has been of great value in the development of synthetic antidiarrhoeal drugs and in the discovery of loperamide. Antagonism of intestinal propulsion as well as of fluid accumulation can be obtained with loperamide in the absence of undesirable systemic effects. The same high degree of intestinal specificity should be pursued in new compounds that have a different mechanism of action. Such new drugs may be excellent tools to further clarify the pathogenesis of the multiple forms of diarrhoea and may perhaps become the treatment of choice for a particular type of diarrhoea.

References

1. Adler, H. F. and Ivy, A. C. (1940). Morphine atropine antagonism on colon motility in dog. *J. Pharmacol. Exp. Ther.*, **70**, 454
2. Argenzio, R. A. (1980). Glucose-stimulated fluid absorption in the pig small intestine during the early stage of swine dysentery. *Am. J. Vet. Res.*, **41**, 2000–6
3. Awouters, F., Niemegeers, C. J. E. and Janssen, P. A. J. (1983). Pharmacology of anti-diarrhoeal drugs. *Am. Rev. Pharmacol. Toxicol.* (In press)
4. Awouters, F., Niemegeers, C. J. E., Lenaerts, F. M. *et al.* (1978). Delay of castor-oil diarrhoea: a new way to evaluate inhibitors of prostaglandin biosynthesis. *J. Pharm. Pharmacol.*, **30**, 41–5
5. Awouters, F., Niemegeers, C. J. E., Kuyps, J. *et al.* (1975). Loperamide antagonism of castor-oil-induced diarrhoea in rats: a quantitative study. *Arch. Int. Pharmacodyn. Ther.*, **217**, 29–37
6. Bachrach, W. H. (1958). Anticholinergic drugs. Survey of literature and some experimental observations. *Am. J. Dig. Dis.*, **3**, 743–99
7. Beubler, E. and Lembeck, F. (1979). Inhibition of stimulated fluid secretion in the rat small and large intestine by opiate agonist. *Arch. Pharmacol.*, **306**, 113
8. Bueno, L. and Ruckebusch, Y. (1978). Effect of anticholinergic drugs on the electrical activity of antrum and duodeno-jejunum in sheep. *J. Vet. Pharmacol. Ther.*, **1**, 225–32
9. Bueno, L. and Ruckebusch, Y. (1978). Origine centrale de l'action excito-motrice de l'intestin de la morphine. *C.R. Soc. Biol.*, **172**, 972–7
10. Bueno, L., Fioramonti, J., Ruckebusch, M. *et al.* (1980). Evaluation of colonic myo-electrical activity and functional disorders. *Gut*, **21**, 480–5
11. Bueno, L., Fioramonti, J. and Ruckebusch, Y. (1980). Digestive disturbances in ruminants: an electromyographic study. *Vet. Sci. Comm.*, **4**, 29–38
12. Bueno, L., Fioramonti, J. and Ruckebusch, Y. (1981). Comparative effects of morphine and nalorphine on colonic motility in the conscious dog. *Eur. J. Pharmacol.*, **75**, 239–45
13. Bueno, L. and Fioramonti, J. (1982). A possible central serotonergic mechanism involved in the effects of morphine on colonic motility in dog. *Eur. J. Pharmacol.*, **82**, 147–53
14. Burks, T. F. (1973). Mediation by 5-hydroxytryptamine of morphine stimulant actions in dog intestine. *J. Pharmacol. Exp. Ther.*, **185**, 530
15. Butterworth, B. S. (1982). The pharmacokinetics of loperamide in animals. (Unpublished review)
16. Bywater, R. J. (1980). Comparison between milk deprivation and oral rehydration with a glucose–glycine–electrolyte formulation in diarrhoeic and transported calves. *Vet. Rec.*, **107**, 549–51
17. Campbell, G. (1966). Nerve mediated excitation of the taenia of the guinea-pig caecum. *J. Physiol.*, **185**, 148–59
18. Christensen, J., Weisbrodt, N. W. and Hauser, R. L. (1972). Electrical slow wave of the proximal colon of the cat in diarrhoea. *Gastroenterology*, **62**, 1167–73
19. Connel, A. M. (1962). The motility of the pelvic colon. II. Paradoxical motility in diarrhoea and constipation. *Gut*, **3**, 342–8
20. Coudert, P., Licois, D. and Provot, F. (1976). Etude comparée de quatre coccidioses intestinales du lapin: pathogénicité, bilan économique, chimioprévention et chimiothérapie. Paper presented at *1er Cong. Int. Cunicole*, Dijon, France
21. Coussement, W., Ducatelle, R., Charlier, G. *et al.* (1981). Adenovirus enteritis in pigs. *Am. J. Vet. Res.*, **42**, 1905–10
22. Fioramonti, J., Garcia-Villar, R., Bueno, L. *et al.* (1980). Colonic myoelectrical activity and propulsion in dog. *Dig. Dis. Sci.*, **25**, 641–6

23. Fioramonti, J. (1981). Etude comparée des fonctions motrices du gros intestin. *Thèse Doct. Sci. Nat.*, Toulouse
24. Fioramonti, J., Sorraing, J. M., Licois, D. *et al.* (1981). Intestinal motor and transit disturbances associated with experimental coccidiosis (*Eimeria magna*) in the rabbit. *Ann. Rech. Vét.*, **12,** 413–20
25. Garcia-Villar, R., Leng-Peschlow, E. and Ruckebusch, Y. (1980). Effect of anthraquinone derivatives on canine and rat intestinal motility. *J. Pharm. Pharmacol.*, **32,** 323–9
26. Hirschhorn, N. (1980). The treatment of actute diarrhoea in children. An historical and physiological perspective. *Am. J. Clin. Nutr.*, **33,** 637–63
27. Holmgren, J. and Greenough, W. B. (1980). Reversal of enterotoxic diarrhoea by chlorpromazine and related drugs. In Field, M., Fordhan, J. S. and Schultz, D. G. (eds.) *Secretory Diarrhoea*. pp. 211–18. (Baltimore: *Am. Physiol. Soc.*)
28. Hood, D. M., Stephens, K. A. and Bowen, M. J. (1982). Phenoxybenzamine for the treatment of severe nonresponsive diarrhoea in the horse. *J. Am. Vet. Assoc.*, **180,** 758–62
29. Ilundain, A. and Naftalin, R. J. (1979). Role of Ca^{2+}-dependent regulator proteins in intestinal secretion. *Nature (London)*, **279,** 446–8
30. Ilundain, A. and Naftalin, R. J. (1981). Opiates increase chloride permeability of the serosal border of rabbit ileum. *J. Physiol.*, **316,** 56–7
31. Ingram, D. M. and Catchpole, B. N. (1981). Effects of opiates on gastroduodenal motility following surgical operation. *Dig. Dis. Sci.*, **26,** 989–92
32. Latour, A. and Bueno, L. (1980). A micro-computerized system to measure the colonic contractile activity. *Int. J. Bio-Med. Compt.*, **11,** 389–96
33. Licois, D., Coudert, P. and Mongin, P. (1978). Changes in hydromineral metabolism in diarrhoeic rabbits. I. A study of the changes in water metabolism. *Ann. Rech. Vét.*, **9,** 1–10
34. Martin, S. W. and Wiggins, A. D. (1973). A model of the economic costs of dairy calf mortality. *Am. J. Vet. Res.*, **34,** 1027–31
35. Mebus, C. A., Stair, E. L., Inderdahl, N. R. *et al.* (1973). Calf diarrhoea of viral etiology. *Ann. Rech. Vét.*, **4,** 71–6
36. Niemegeers, C. J. E., Colpaerts, F. C. and Awouters, F. H. L. (1981). Pharmacology and antidiarrhoeal effect of loperamide. *Drug Dev. Res.*, **1,** 1–20
37. Niemegeers, C. J. E., Lenaerts, F. and Awouters, F. (1976). Preclinical animal studies of modern antidiarrhoeals. *In vivo* pharmacology. In van Bever, W. and Lal, H. (eds.) *Synthetic Antidiarrhoeal Drugs*. pp. 65–114. (New York: Marcel Dekker)
38. Niemegeers, C. J. E., McGuire, J. C., Heykants, J. J. P. *et al.* (1979). Experimental dissociation between opiate-like and antidiarrhoeal drugs. *J. Pharmacol. Exp. Ther.*, **210,** 327–33
39. Pearson, G. R. and Logan, E. F. (1982). Ultrastructural changes in the small intestine on neonatal calves with enteric colibacillosis. *Vet. Pathol.*, **19,** 190–201
40. Peeters, J. E., Geeroms, R., Froyman, R. *et al.* (1981). Coccidiosis in rabbits: a field study. *Res. Vet. Sci.*, **30,** 328–34
41. Raynaud, J. P., Brunault, G. and Patterson, E. B. (1981). A swine dysentery model for evaluation of drug prophylaxis: development of a model involving oral infection plus pen contamination. *Am. J. Vet. Res.*, **42,** 49–50
42. Raynaud, J. P., Brunault, G. and Patterson, E. B. (1981). A swine dysentery model for evaluation of drug prophylaxis: efficacy of various drugs in the control of swine dysentery. *Am. J. Vet. Res.*, **42,** 51–3
43. Read, M. and Read, N. W. (1981). Anal sphincter function in diarrhoea: influence of loperamide. *Clin. Res. Rev.*, **1** (Suppl. I), 73–81
44. Rozental, G., Frexinos, J., Gerardin, A. *et al.* (1982). Modifications de l'activité myoélectrique du côlon humain induites par le sulfate d'atropine. Paper presented at *VIe Journées Francophones d'Hépatologie et de Gastroentérologie*, Paris
45. Ruckebusch, Y. and Bueno, L. (1975). Electrical activity of the ovine jejunum and changes due to disturbances. *Am. J. Dig. Dis.*, **20,** 1027–1934
46. Ruckebusch, Y. and Fioramonti, J. (1980). Motor profile of the ruminant colon: hard vs soft faeces production. *Experientia*, **36,** 1184–5
47. Sandhu, B. K., Tripp, J. H., Candy, D. C. A. *et al.* (1981). Loperamide: studies on its mechanism of action. *Gut*, **22,** 658–62

48. Sitarska, E. and Pytkowski, S. T. (1968). Effects of prophylactical and therapeutical application of gamma-globulin in foal's diarrhoea. *Medycyna Weterynaryjna (Lublin, Poland)*, **24**, 34–6
49. Targowski, S. P. (1976). Treatment of horses with chronic diarrhoea: immunologic status. *Am. J. Vet. Res.*, **37**, 29–33
50. Teige, J., Tollersrud, S., Lund, A. *et al.* (1982). Swine dysentery: the influence of dietary vitamin E and selenium on the clinical and pathological effects of *Treponema hyodysenteriae* infection in pigs. *Res. Vet. Sci.*, **32**, 95–100.
51. Thompson, D. G., Laidlow, J. M. and Wingate, D. L. (1979). Abnormal small-bowel motility demonstrated by radiotelemetry in a patient with irritable colon. *Lancet*, **1**, 1321–4
52. van Nueten, J. M., Janssen, P. A. J. and Fontaine, J. (1974). Loperamide (R 18 553) a novel type of antidiarrhoeal agent. 3. *In vitro* studies on the peristaltic reflex and other experiments on isolated tissues. *Arzneim. Forsch.*, **24**, 1641–5
53. Verhaeren, E. H. C., Dreessen, M. J. and Lemli, V. A. (1981). Influence of 1.8-dihydroxyanthraquenone and loperamide on the paracellular permeability across colonic mucosa. *J. Pharm. Pharmacol.*, **33**, 526–8
54. Wangel, A. G. and Deller, D. J. (1965). Intestinal motility in man. II. Mechanisms of constipation and diarrhoea with particular reference to the irritable bowel syndrome. *Gastroenterology*, **48**, 69–83
55. Weisbrodt, N. W., Sussman, S. E., Stewart, J. J. *et al.* (1980). Effect of morphine sulfate on intestinal transit and myoelectrical activity of small intestine of the rat. *J. Pharmacol. Exp. Ther.*, **214**, 333–8
56. Whipp, S. C., Robinson, I. M., Harris, D. L. *et al.* (1979). Pathogenic synergism between *Treponema hyodysenteriae* and other selected anaerobes in gnotobiotic pigs. *Infect. Immun.*, **26**, 1042–7
57. Windsor, R. S. (1979). Swine dysentery. In Grunsell, C. G. S. and Hill, F. W. G. (eds.) *The Veterinary Annual.* pp. 88–96. (Bristol: John Wright & Sons)
58. Wuester, M. and Herz, A. (1978). Opiate agonist action of antidiarrhoeal agents *in vitro* and *in vivo* findings in support of selective action. *Naunyn-Schmiedeberg's Arch. Pharmacol.*, **301**, 187–94
59. Zavecz, J. H., Jacxson, T. E., Limp, G. L. *et al.* (1982). Relationship between antidiarrhoeal activity and binding to calmodulin. *Eur. J. Pharmacol.*, **78**, 375–7

30
Pharmacology and comparative toxicology of non-steroidal anti-inflammatory agents

G. Mazué, P. Richez and J. Berthe

Non-steroidal anti-inflammatory agents (NSAIA) are widely used drugs in human therapy and to a lesser extent in veterinary practice. They belong to many chemical classes (although most of them are organic acids) and have in common antipyretic, analgesic and anti-inflammatory activity. Their mechanism of action differs from those of the anti-inflammatory steroids and the opioid analgesics. Recent progress in the knowledge of the mode of action makes it possible to understand why such heterogeneous agents have the same basic therapeutic activities and often the same side-effects.

The aim of this report is to present bibliographic and experimental data concerning the principal pharmacological and toxicological properties of NSAIA, mainly in domestic and laboratory animals. These properties can briefly be described as prostaglandin inhibition leading to inflammation relief, but also include gastrointestinal and renal toxicities.

CLASSIFICATION

There are approximately 30 commercially available NSAIA, for which different chemical classifications have been proposed (Figure 30.1).

A classification based on their biological activities does not appear to be possible, owing to the great similarities in the mode of action and the pharmacological activities, despite heterogeneous molecular structures.

PHARMACOLOGICAL PROPERTIES

In 1971, Vane *et al.* demonstrated that low doses of aspirin and indomethacin inhibited the enzymatic synthesis of prostaglandins[11,12]. In subsequent years, the following major points have been established:

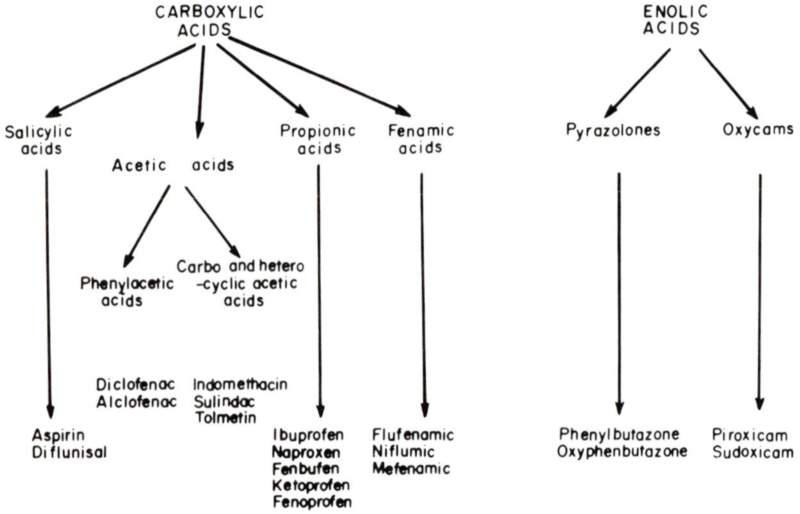

Figure 30.1 Chemical classification of non-steroidal anti-inflammatory agents[28]

(1) All mammalian cell types studied have microsomal enzymes for the synthesis of prostaglandins.

(2) Prostaglandins are always released when cells are damaged and have been detected in increased concentration in inflammatory exudates. Furthermore, prostaglandins are not stored, and their release depends on biosynthesis *de novo*.

(3) All aspirin-like drugs inhibit the biosynthesis and release of prostaglandins in all cells tested.

(4) Other classes of drugs do not, generally speaking, affect the biosynthesis of prostaglandins.

From these observations, it has been admitted that NSAIA exert their pharmacological action mainly by inhibiting prostaglandin synthesis[11] (Figure 30.2). The step in prostaglandin synthesis where NSAIAs are active differs according to the chemical class: (1) cyclo-oxygenase for aspirin, fenamates, indomethacin, phenylpropionates, and (2) endoperoxide isomerase for pyrazolon derivates[13, 27].

These properties allow pharmacological action on: (1) inflammation, mainly by a decrease in PgE_2, PgI_2 or PgE_1 production responsible for erythema and local bloodflow increase, (2) pain, also by a decrease in PgE_1, PgE_2 and $PgF_{2\alpha}$ responsible for hyperalgesia in inflamed tissues (aspirin is not an analgesic in non-inflamed tissues[19]), and (3) fever, caused by most of the prostaglandins (except for PGI_2).

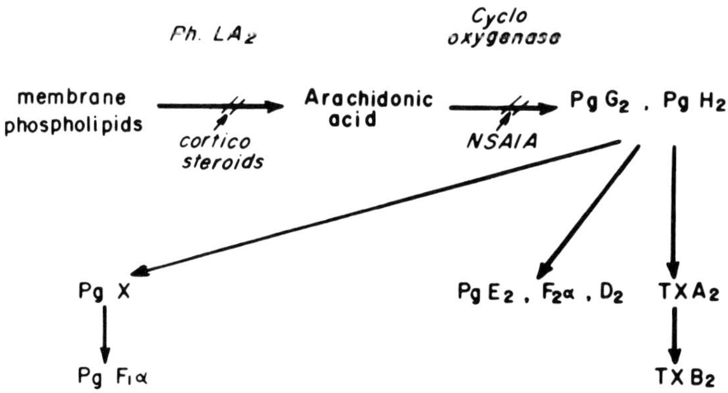

Figure 30.2 Inhibition of the conversion of arachidonic acid to prostaglandins, by inhibition of cyclo-oxygenase for most of the NSAIA, except for pyrazolon derivatives

Pharmacological evaluation

Many *in vivo* and *in vitro* experimental models have been proposed[1] as being able to detect anti-inflammatory effects or action displayed by clinically useful NSAIAs.

The most currently used procedures for *in vivo* assessment of anti-inflammatory activity have been subdivided into two categories: (1) procedures able to detect the drug-induced modification of events occurring during inflammatory processes (erythema, exudation, granulation tissue formation, pain, fever), and (2) experimentally-induced syndromes resembling human rheumatoid diseases.

Among the *in vitro* models proposed, the most satisfactory studies the inhibition of prostaglandin synthesis.

A screening programme can be successfully designed to bring a new compound to clinical trial based upon the following tests:

(1) Action on erythema. Erythema can be experimentally induced by ultraviolet light in albino guinea-pigs or by applying irritant substances directly to the skin (e.g. nicotinic acid).

(2) Action on fever. Hyperpyrexia is obtained after local (plantar tissue) or systemic (subcutaneous or i.p.) administration of an aqueous suspension of brewer's yeast.

(3) Pain. As a result of inflammation, pain is obtained by all types of inflammatory processes, such as local injection of brewer's yeast or carrageenin, or i.p. administration of 2-phenyl-1.4 benzoquinone or acetic acid, both responsible for 'stretching' in rodents (writhing, squirming, abdominal constriction).

(4) Oedema and exudation. Carrageenin-induced paw oedema in rats is classically one of the most used tests but others are also useful, such as determination of leukocyte migration *in vivo* (pleural exudate induced by turpentine, cell collection from artificial skin chambers, etc.).

(5) Cellular phase of inflammatory processes ('repair phase'). This is reproduced by granuloma-induced formation (e.g. cotton pellet subcutaneously introduced in rats, or implantation of pouches containing croton oil or mycobacterial adjuvant in the back of rats, etc.).

(6) Animal models for rheumatic disease. Arthritis is induced by injection in paraffin oil of killed bacteria.

(7) *In vitro* measurement of prostaglandin synthetase degree of inhibition.

These tests allow the classification of the drug from a pharmacological point of view, in comparison with reference drugs, as indicated in Table 30.1.

Table 30.1 Effective doses of NSAIA on pharmacological tests permitting the demonstration of the action on pain, fever, oedema and exudation, experimentally-induced inflammatory disease and prostaglandin synthesis[1]

Drug	*Analgesia Phenyl-B-Benzo Quinone test* ED_{50} mg/kg p.o.	*Antipyresis Yeast fever* mg/kg p.o.	*Carrageenin* ED_{50} mg/kg p.o.	*Adjuvent arthritis* ED_{50} mg kg^{-1} day^{-1} p.o.	*PG synthesis Sheep seminal vesicles* ED_{50} μm
Indomethacin	1.9–3.7	0.9–1.4	2.7–5.2	0.2–1.5	0.4–10
Diclofenac	2.3–4	0.5	2.1–3.5	0.2–1.5	0.3
Naproxen	16–24	75–150	20–29	4–8	4.7–6.1
Flurbiprofen	not reported	not reported	0.8–3.4	1.5–3.5	0.07–1.2
Ibuprofen	38–51	24	23–45	<100	1.5–2.8
Phenylbutazone	75–115	35	28–50	13–50	12.6–58
Sudoxicam	10	120	18–30	0.4–1.8	7

Interspecific and interindividual variations

As for many other drugs[3,5] the main differences encountered for NSAIA are related to pharmacokinetic variations, occurring at any step in the fate of the drug (absorption, distribution, metabolism and elimination).

Table 30.2 Plasma halflife of drugs in four species. Great differences for the same drug among different species need appropriate dosage schedules for inducing adequate therapeutic effect[30]

Drug	*Rat*	*Dog*	*Monkey*	*Man*
Piroxicam	6♂ 16♀	45	5	45
Indomethacin	4	0.3	0.3	2
Naproxen	5	35	1.9	13.9
Ibuprofen	1	2.5	—	3
Phenylbutazone	6	6	7	72
Fenoprofen	8	4	0.3	2.5
Sulindac	4	—	—	8

Interspecific variations

These are numerous and sometimes important, as indicated by the plasma halflife of some selected drugs[30] presented in Table 30.2. The many interspecific differences make it necessary to know the pharmacokinetic parameters of the drug in the animal species used before any initiation of a treatment. This procedure leads to the avoidance of toxicity risks by overdosing or absence of therapeutic effect by inappropriate dose levels or intervals (Table 30.2).

Interindividual variations

These can occur also, according to physiologic or pathologic conditions[20]. Food intake may influence the absorption of drugs, as is demonstrated by a 30% reduced bioavailability of aspirin in dogs when administered during a fat-rich diet[21]. The elimination of the NSAIA, often related to a drug-metabolizing system, can be influenced by hepatic disorders or renal failure.

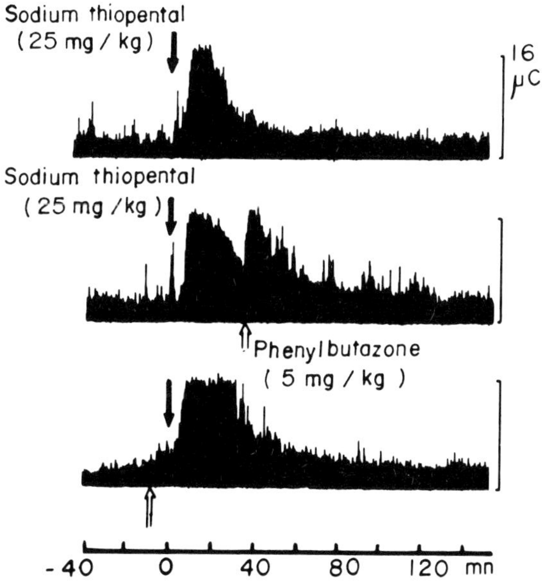

Figure 30.3 Integrated e.c.g. in a sheep anaesthetized with sodium thiopental (25 mg/kg) when phenylbutazone was injected intravenously during recovery or administered before the barbiturate[20].

Another property of some NSAIA is their ability to displace other drugs from their protein-binding sites. For example, phenylbutazone injected intravenously in sheep is able to reinduce sleep in awakened animals previously anaesthetized with sodium thiopental[24]. This action was demonstrated to be related to a liberation of thiopental in blood by protein displacement by phenylbutazone[20] (Figure 30.3).

TOXICOLOGY

Renal and digestive toxicities are the main types encountered. Furthermore, hepatotoxicity and haematotoxicity can be observed but with much lower incidence. Only the two first types will be discussed.

Digestive toxicity

The occurrence of gastrointestinal damage (bleeding, ulceration) is probably among the most prevalent and serious of the side-effects associated with the use of NSAIA. There are no common structural features which can be identified in determining whether or not an NSAIA will be ulcerogenic. Rainsford[18] proposed a classification of relative ulcerogenic activity of NSAIA (Table 30.3), which seems to be in good agreement with clinical reports. From these observations, it is interesting to note that, for example,

(1) Sulindac is markedly less ulcerogenic than the related drug indomethacin.

(2) All the fenamates appear to have comparable (moderate) gastric-ulcerogenic activity.

(3) Of the phenylacetates, only fenclofenac is in the low-ulcerogenic class.

(4) Of the enolic acids, only azopropazone is non-ulcerogenic.

Table 30.3 Classification of NSAIA according to their ulcerogenic activity in the laboratory rat[18]

Low	*Medium*	*High*
Azapropazone	Niflumic acid	Aspirin
Sulindac	Ibuprofen	Diclofenac
Fenclofenac	Salicylic acid	Indomethacin
	Naproxen	Ketoprofen
	Phenylbutazone	
	Flurbiprofen	

As NSAIA are able to exert their effects either on gastric or intestinal (mainly duodenal and colonic) mucosa, indexes such as UD_{50} (ulcerogenic dose 50%), PD_{50} (perforative dose 50% on intestinal mucosa), ED_{50} (pharmacologically effective dose 50%) are useful indexes of the therapeutic safety margin when compared with LD_{50}[6,8,25].

Many hypotheses have been proposed to explain the mode of action of NSAIA on digestive mucosa. NSAIA may lead to the breakdown of small blood vessels before any cytolytic effect. The erosion develops as an ischaemic infarct[22]. Such lesions are associated with a deficiency of gastric mucus macromolecular glycoproteins[2]. Other observations indicating a disruption of the gastric mucosal barrier to hydrogen on ion back-diffusion[14] have now to be considered as a consequence rather than a cause of lesions.

Why vessels in a small area are affected whilst others remain normal is unexplained. However, the erosions produced as an ischaemic infarct could be the underlying cause of many of the isolated observations previously reported as primary but unconnected events: uncoupling of oxidative phosphorylation and reduction in ATP, increase in cAMP, decrease in acid secretion and changes in ionic gradients[22]. The reason for vascular primary action of NSAIA has not been clearly demonstrated until now but could be related to inhibition of the synthesis of vasoactive prostaglandins.

The local action by direct contact with digestive mucosa does not seem to be an important factor in the induction of ulcers[6]. Phenylbutazone is equally toxic by oral or intravenous route, and indomethacin is more toxic for the intestine after intravenous administration than after oral gavage, at least in rats (Table 30.4). But the existence of enterohepatic recirculation may also partly explain why such drugs as indomethacin are more ulcerogenic in species such as the dog or the rat when compared with poorly recycling species such as monkeys or man[9].

Table 30.4 Ulcerogenic dose 50% (UD_{50}) of selected drugs for stomach and intestine after administration in the rat by the intravenous (i.v.) route or orally (p.o.)[6]

	Phenylbutazone		*Indomethacin*		*Ibuprofen*	
	stomach	*intestine*	*stomach*	*intestine*	*stomach*	*intestine*
UD_{50} i.v.	80	120	9	7	210	172
UD_{50} p.o.	75	120	7	11	70	88
Ratio i.v./p.o.	1.1	1	1.3	0.6	3	1.9

From our own experience in toxicology, the most efficient technique for detecting early gastric mucosal injuries is fibroscopy in large species such as pigs, monkeys or dogs. This technique permits the determination of the kinetics of apparition of the lesions, whereas necropsy only gives observations at a given time. In a 1 month oral toxicity study performed in Beagle dogs (Table 30.5). It could be demonstrated that phenylbutazone failed to induce ulcers, even at the dose level of 100 mg/kg/day, whereas others such

Table 30.5 Gastric fibroscopic observations during a 4 week study in Beagle dogs. CB 804 is bucloxic acid

Compound	*Dose level* mg kg^{-1} day^{-1}	*Fibroscopic observations*
CB 804	200	Congestion followed by ulcerations. Gastric ulcers after 20 days
Aspirin	400	Haemorrhages after 1 adm. Gastritis at day 5 leading to ulcers (pyloric) after 1–2 weeks
Phenylbutazone	100	Gastritis after 1 adm. No ulcer produced after 1 month (only some exulcerations)
Indomethacin	25	No effect during some 4 days. Then, gastritis leading to ulcers after 2 weeks

as CB 804 (Bucloxic acid, Clin-Midy, France), aspirin and indomethacin were responsible for a primary gastritis (congestion and haemorrhages in the case of aspirin) followed 1–2 weeks later by gastric ulcers.

This latter technique can be completed by the measurement of faecal blood loss induced by gastrointestinal bleeding (mainly in rats, where fibroscopy is not a suitable method). The injection of labelled compound (^{51}Cr or ^{59}Fe) allows measurement of the exact quantity of blood lost by the digestive tract and shows, for example, micro-bleeding in a dose-dependent manner with aspirin in dogs[17] or a good correlation in rats between EDL_{50} (dose-inducing blood loss 50%) and UD_{50} (ulcerogenic dose 50%)[16].

Owing to great interspecific variations, it is necessary to know the effect of the NSAIAs used in each species concerned with therapeutic effect. For example, indomethacin is not a suitable therapeutic drug in dogs[9], whereas aspirin[21] or phenylbutazone[5] are useful potent drugs presenting a relatively wide margin of safety.

Nephrotoxicity

Tubular nephritis can be observed, mainly at high dose levels, with most of the commercially available NSAIA[26]. The five examinations to be performed on laboratory animals in order to detect potential nephrotoxicity[15] of these drugs are:

(1) Biochemical evaluation in blood and urine, including (a) BUN and creatininaemia, for which the variations observed in tubular nephritis are closely related. (b) Blood lactate dehydrogenase and serum glutamic pyruvic transpeptidase. These examinations have to be performed early in the course of a subacute or chronic treatment, the values increasing during the first days and dropping slowly back to subnormal values after the second week. (c) Urinalysis. In dogs, NSAIA, like aspirin, induce a dose-related decrease in para-aminohippuric acid clearance associated with a slight increase of potassium urinary elimination and a marked decrease in sodium elimination[4]. Nephrotoxicity induced by NSAIA is also accompanied by proteinuria and ketonuria in rats, monkeys and dogs.

(2) Clinical observations of the treated animals. The signs often observed are non-specific: pilo-erection, weakness, or signs of dehydration. Stronger signs (coma, gingival ulcer) are recorded when the uraemic syndrome is detected.

(3) Iterative renal biopsies. Small samples of kidney tissue (about 10 mg) are obtained with biopsy needles (TRU-CUT, Travenol) after surgical heterotropic subcutaneous transposition of the left kidney on anaesthetized animals. More than 20 biopsies can be performed successfully for light or electron microscopy on the same animal at daily or weekly intervals in monkeys, pigs and dogs.

    This procedure shows the kinetics of development of the renal injuries induced by NSAIA when administered at high dose levels. Tubular nephritis is accompanied by tubular cylinder formations, followed by tubular cell necrosis associated with interstitial inflammation. Regeneration of the tubular epithelium occurs within a few days. Fibrosis observed after necrosis may lead in extreme cases to glomerular anoxia and degeneration.

(4) The kidney weight (absolute and relative to the bodyweight). This useful index of nephrotoxicity is easily measurable at necropsy.

(5) Macroscopy and light and electron microscopy of the renal tissue. The main signs observed are tubular degeneration associated with regeneration and interstitial inflammation. In chronic studies, it is not infrequent to observe intense interstitial fibrosis, sometimes leading to irreversible glomerular degeneration.

Macroscopic examination permits the observation of papillary necrosis. This lesion appears more sporadically than chronic interstitial nephritis, often after longterm administrations. The syndrome has been induced mainly in rats and pigs, occasionally in rabbits and in dogs, and rarely in monkeys[28]. NSAIA are rarely implicated in renal papillary necrosis in man[26].

CONCLUSIONS

Non-steroidal anti-inflammatory agents belong to a chemical class of active drugs for which the pharmacological activity has been demonstrated by many authors, by *in vivo* and *in vitro* systems. Their use in veterinary practice appears for most of them to be limited by the occurrence of side-effects, mainly gastrointestinal and renal. This relatively limited use in comparison with human medicine is related to pharmacokinetic differences, possibly leading to limited therapeutic effect or excessive toxicity.

Two long-known NSAIAs (aspirin, phenylbutazone) have been proved during many years of experience to be relatively well tolerated in domestic animals when administered at adequate therapeutic dose levels.

For other NSAIAs which have been proved to be very efficient in pharmacological tests, use in veterinary therapy may be considered possible according to recent studies indicating the lower toxicity of certain drugs when administered together with other NSAIA. For example, the gastric toxicity of indomethacin can be greatly diminished when administered together with aspirin in rats[23]. The same observations are true for such associations as indomethacin and sodium salicylate[10], aspirin and phenylbutazone[18] or indomethacin and diflunisal etc.[7].

The mechanism of inhibition of the gastric toxicity when two NSAIAs are associated remains unclear, although many hypotheses have been advanced[7,10,18,23]. Further studies have therefore to be performed in order to determine the advantages of such associations from a therapeutic and a toxicological point of view.

References

1. Arrigoni, A. and Martelli, E. (1979). Screening and assessment of antiinflammatory drugs. *Meth. Find. Exptl. Clin. Pharmacol.*, **1**, 157–77
2. Azuumi, Y., Ohara, S., Ishiara, K. *et al.* (1980). Correlation of quantitative changes of gastric mucosal glycoproteins with aspirin-induced gastric damage in rats. *Gut*, **21**, 533–6
3. Baggot, J. D. (1977). *Principles of Drug Disposition in Domestic Animals: The Basis of Veterinary Clinical Pharmacology.* (Philadelphia: W. B. Saunders)
4. Berg, K. J. and Bergan, A. (1976). Effects of different doses of acetylsalicylic acid on renal function in dogs. *Scand. J. Clin. Lab. Invest.*, **36**, 1–8
5. Booth, N. H. (1977). Nonnarcotic analgesics, In Meyer Jones, L. *et al.* (eds.) *Veterinary Pharmacology and Therapeutics.* 4th Edn., pp. 351–72. (Ames: Iowa State University Press)
6. Cioli, V., Putzolu, S., Rossi, V. *et al.* (1979). The role of direct tissue contact in the production of gastrointestinal ulcers by anti-inflammatory drugs in rats. *Toxicol. Appl. Pharmacol.*, **50**, 283–9
7. Conti, P. and Continenza, A. (1980). Decreased ulcerogenic effect of indomethacin in the rat when given in association with diflunisal. *J. Pathol.*, **131**, 357–61
8. Dimantis, W., Melton, J., Sofia, R. D. *et al.* (1980). Comparative gastric ulcerogenic effects of meseclazone, 5-chlorosalicylic acid and other nonsteroidal antiinflammatory drugs following acute and repeated oral administration to rats. *Toxicol. Appl. Pharmacol.*, **52**, 454–61
9. Duggan, D. E. *et al.* (1975). Enterohepatic circulation of indomethacin and its role in intestinal irritation. *Biochem. Pharmacol.*, **25**, 1749–54
10. Ezer, E., Palosi, E., Hajos, G. Y. *et al.* (1979). Comparative pharmacology of a 1:10 combination of indomethacin–sodium salicylate. *Agents Actions*, **9**, 117–23
11. Ferreira, S. H. and Vane, J. R. (1974). New aspects of the mode of action of nonsteroid antiinflammatory drugs. *Ann. Rev. Pharmacol.*, **14**, 57–73
12. Flower, R. J., Moncada, S. and Vane, J. R. (1980). Analgesic antipyretics and anti-inflammatory agents. In Goodman, L. S., Gilmann, A. *et al.* (eds.) *The Pharmacological Basis of Therapeutics.* 6th Edn., pp. 682–728. (New York: MacMillan)
13. Flower, R., Gryglewski, R., Herbaczinska-Cedro, K. *et al.* (1972). Effect of antiinflammatory drugs on prostaglandin biosynthesis. *Nature (London)*, **230**, 104–6
14. Guth, P. H. and Paulsen, G. (1979). Effect of parenteral aspirin on the gastric mucosal barrier in the rat. *Digestion*, **19**, 93–8
15. Mazué, G., Vallée, E., Genet, P. *et al.* (1974). Toxicological studies of bucloxic acid (804CB). *Arzneim. Forsch. (Drug Res.)*, **24**, 1298–1413
16. Menasse-Gdynia, R. and Drupp, P. (1974). Quantitative measurement of gastrointestinal bleeding in rats: the effect of nonsteroidal antiinflammatory drugs. *Toxicol. Appl. Pharmacol.*, **29**, 389–96
17. Phillips, B. M. (1973). Aspirin-induced gastrointestinal micro-bleeding in dogs. *Toxicol. Appl. Pharmacol.*, **24**, 182–9
18. Rainsford, K. D. (1977). The comparative gastric ulcerogenic activities of nonsteroid anti-inflammatory drugs. *Agents Actions*, **7**, 573–7
19. Randall, L. O. (1963). Non narcotic analgesics. In Root, W. S. and Hofman, F. G. (eds.) *Physiological Pharmacology.* Vol. 1, pp. 313–416. (New York: Academic Press)
20. Richez, P. (1980). Recherches sur les variations individuelles et interspécifiques en pharmacocinétique. *Thèse Doc. INP*, Toulouse
21. Richez, P., Regnier, A. and Ruckebusch, Y. (1980). Influence of food intake on the absorption of lysine acetylsalicylate in dogs. *J. Vet. Pharmacol. Ther.*, **3**, 121–4
22. Robins, P. G. (1980). Ultrastructural observations on the pathogenesis of aspirin-induced gastric erosions. *Br. J. Exp. Pathol.*, **61**, 497–504
23. Rosenbaum, E. S. and Barbieri, E. J. (1979). Inhibition by aspirin of gastrointestinal toxicity induced by indomethacin in polyarthritic rats. *Toxicol. Appl. Pharmacol.*, **49**, 535–41
24. Ruckebusch, Y. and Richez, P. (1980). L'anesthésiologie vétérinaire, modèle pharmacologique. *Anesth. Analg. Réanim.*, **37**, 573–7
25. Schiantarelli, P. and Cadel, S. (1981). Piroxicam pharmacologic activity and gastrointestinal damage by oral and rectal route. *Arzneim. Forsch. (Drug Res.)*, **31**, 87–97

26. Shelley, S. (1978). Pharmacological mechanisms of analgesic nephropathy. *Kidney Int.*, **13,** 15–26
27. Shen, T. Y. and Winter, C. A. (1977). Chemical and biochemical studies on indomethacin, sulindac and their analogs. *Adv. Drug Res.*, **12,** 89–95
28. Wiseman, E. H. (1982). Pharmacologic studies with a new class of nonsteroidal anti-inflammatory agents – the oxicams – with special reference to piroxicam (Feldene). *Am. J. Med.*, **72,** 2–8
29. Wiseman, E. H. and Reinert, H. (1975). Antiinflammatory drugs and renal papillary necrosis. *Agents Actions*, **5,** 322–25
30. Wiseman, E. H. and Hobbs, D. C. (1982). Review of pharmacokinetic studies with piroxicam. *Am. J. Med.*, **72,** 9–17

31
Clinical pharmacokinetic studies of digoxin and digitoxin in the dog

A. de Rick, F. M. Belpaire, M. G. Bogaert, D. Mattheeuws and S. Chakrabarti

Digitalis glycosides have a narrow therapeutic index. Small changes in the dose, bioavailability, rate of elimination and interactions with other drugs can lead to either subtherapeutic or toxic effects. Some aspects of these clinical pharmacokinetic problems have been reported previously[5–7]. The purpose of this report is to give a summary of the results of studies in our laboratory.

PLASMA CONCENTRATIONS OF DIGOXIN AND DIGITOXIN DURING DIGITALIZATION OF HEALTHY DOGS AND DOGS WITH CARDIAC FAILURE

Loading and maintenance doses for digoxin and digitoxin have often been developed empirically. In this study, an attempt to define a more rational approach to digitalization in the dog was made.

Healthy dogs and dogs with cardiac failure were used. Drug plasma concentrations and physical and e.c.g. signs were followed after administration of digoxin and digitoxin. In some animals, plasma halflives of digoxin and digitoxin were measured as well (see ref. 5).

Digitalization with digoxin, applying the principle of loading until toxicosis occurred, resulted in high plasma concentrations (2.6–7.6 ng/ml) in both healthy dogs and in dogs with cardiac failure. Loading the same dogs with approximately half these doses produced plasma concentrations of 1.5–2.5 ng/ml but toxicosis was avoided (Figure 31.1).

Maintenance doses of digoxin of approximately 0.01 mg/kg every 12 h gave plasma concentrations that exceeded 2 ng/ml in some healthy animals and were lower than 1 ng/ml in others. The mean halflife of digoxin in healthy animals was 31.3 h.

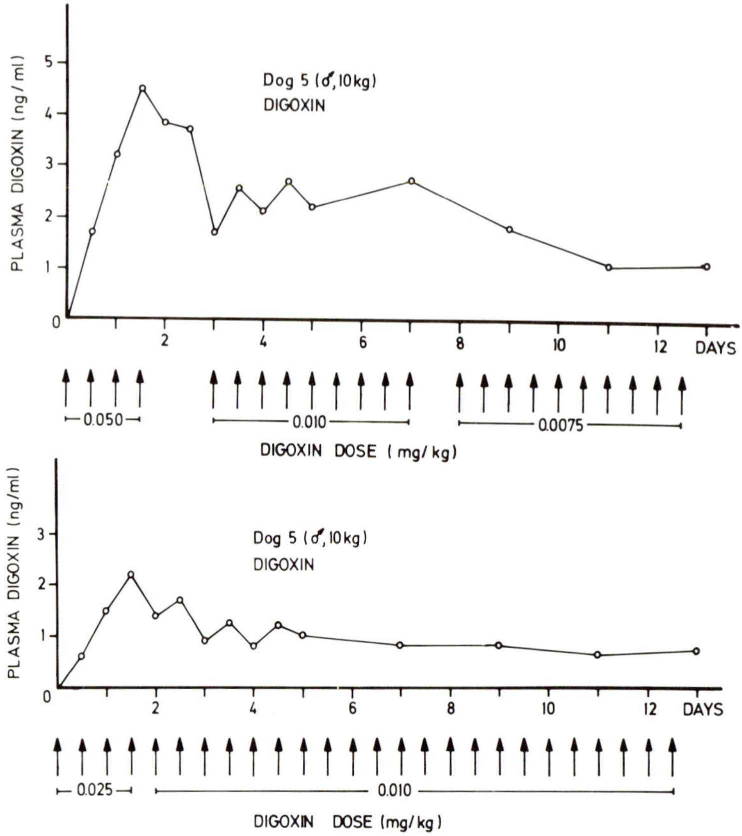

Figure 31.1 Dosage regimen and plasma concentrations of digoxin after oral administration in a healthy dog

The loading dose of digitoxin resulted in maximal plasma concentrations which varied considerably between animals: 26–77 ng/ml (Figure 31.2). Cessation of dosing with digitoxin for 24 h produced almost complete elimination of the drug from plasma in most dogs. This is consistent with the short halflife of digitoxin (mean value 13.1 h) calculated during the first 30 h after administration. Applying therapeutic concentrations accepted in man to dogs, a maintenance dose of 0.03 mg/kg of bodyweight every 12 h of digitoxin elixir resulted in low plasma values (15 ng/ml) in five of eight healthy dogs.

In five of the six dogs with cardiac failure, digoxin maintenance doses of 0.007–0.010 mg/kg every 12 h gave plasma concentrations ranging from 0.8 to 1.9 ng/ml and accompanying clinical improvement. In one dog clinical improvement was not seen although plasma concentrations were as high as 3 ng/ml.

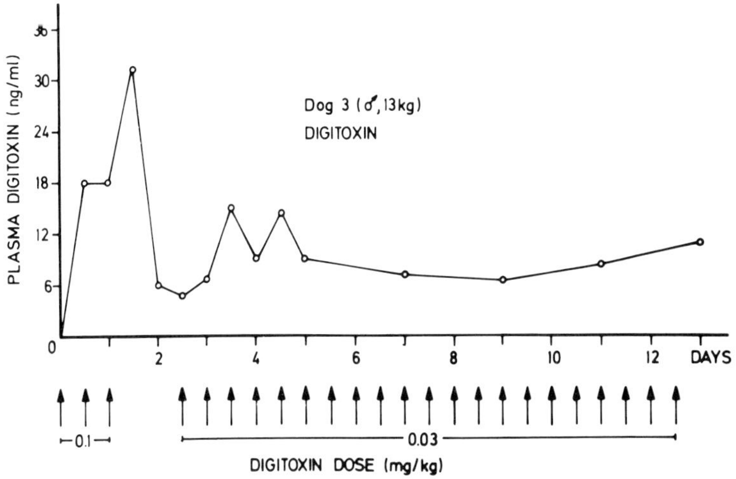

Figure 31.2 Dosage regimen and plasma concentrations of digitoxin after oral administration of digitoxin elixir in a healthy dog

It is concluded that large loading doses of digoxin are not needed to obtain (within 48 h) plasma concentrations in the same range as those obtained during maintenance therapy. On the other hand, the often recommended guideline maintenance dose of 0.02 mg/kg daily for digoxin provided acceptable plasma levels, but the recommended maintenance dose of 0.06 mg/kg daily for digitoxin elixir gave low plasma concentrations.

Rapid elimination of digitoxin during the first 24 h necessitates dividing the daily maintenance doses into several fractional doses. These findings have been confirmed by others[3, 11, 13].

COMPARATIVE BIOAVAILABILITY OF DIGOXIN TABLETS

It is well known that, after oral administration, digoxin is not completely absorbed in both man and dogs. What is more important, however, is variation in bioavailability between different dosage forms. In dogs, for example, digoxin elixir has a higher bioavailability than tablets. Moreover, in man, digoxin tablets of different brands are not bioequivalent[3, 6, 11].

Since information on the comparative bioavailability of digoxin tablets in dogs is scarce, it was decided to compare the bioavailability of three brands of digoxin tablets, commercially available in Belgium, in the dog. In addition, *in vitro* dissolution tests were carried out.

Six healthy dogs, two males and four females, were studied in a cross-over randomized experimental design. On four occasions, with intervals of at least 2 weeks, each dog received 1 mg digoxin, once intravenously and three times orally.

Four tablets, each containing 0.25 mg digoxin, were administered by intragastric intubation. Food was withheld for 10 h before and until 6 h after dosing. Plasma samples were obtained at 0, 0.5, 1, 1.5, 2, 3, 4, 6, 8, 12 and 24 h.

Bioavailability was studied by calculating three parameters: time to peak plasma concentration, peak plasma concentration and area under the curve (AUC). Areas under the time–plasma curve from 0 to 24 h ($AUC_{0-24\,h}$) were calculated by the trapezoidal rule. Plasma digoxin concentrations were measured by radioimmunoassay using tritiated digoxin[1]. Dissolution rate was studied, according to U.S.P. XIX. The amount of digoxin in the samples was determined spectrofluorimetrically[9].

Statistical significance was assessed by the method of Tukey[15].

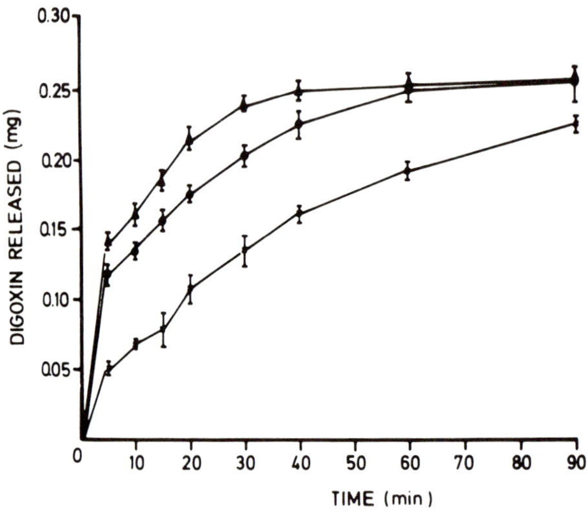

Figure 31.3 Dissolution curves of three commercially available digoxin tablets. Each point represents the mean of three determinations. Vertical bars refer to SEM. Triangles, tablet 1; circles, tablet 2; crosses, tablet 3

For the three oral preparations peak plasma concentrations were always reached within 1 h and often within 30 min of dosing. The mean peak concentrations (±SEM) of preparations 1, 2 and 3 were 11±1.2, 10±0.5 and 8.1±0.6 ng/ml. These values are not significantly different.

The mean areas under the curve relative to the intravenous values were 80, 71 and 65% for preparations 1,2 and 3, respectively. For the same preparation the fraction absorbed varied considerably from dog to dog and the mean AUCs of the different preparations were not significantly different.

Three tablets from each brand were examined for their dissolution characteristics (Figure 31.3). The times for 50% dissolution were 4.5, 7.5 and 25 min for preparations 1, 2 and 3, respectively. Significant differences were found between preparations 1 and 3, and between 2 and 3.

These results indicate that all three preparations had similar rates of absorption as reflected by AUC values and the time to peak serum concentrations. None of the tablets was absorbed completely, although the bioavailability of the tested tablets was higher than the values reported by Krasula *et al.*[12] for encapsulated digoxin (65%), for the elixir (Lanoxin) (58.2%) and for tablets (Lanoxin) (47%).

Although the differences were not significant, for all bioavailability parameters, values were always highest for preparation 1 and lowest for preparation 3 in the present investigation. This ranking order was the same for *in vitro* dissolution of the tablets. Similar findings have been reported in man[2].

These results suggest that it is probably advisable not to change a digitalized dog from one brand or formulation to another, since bioinequivalence could lead to reduced therapeutic effect or increased toxicity.

DIGOXIN-QUINIDINE INTERACTION IN THE DOG

In approximately 85% of human patients taking digoxin, steady state concentrations of digoxin increase when oral quinidine is added to the digoxin treatment, and it has been stated that this could lead to toxicity. The mechanism of this interaction, although studied extensively in man, is yet not fully understood[7,14]. Pharmacokinetic interactions between digoxin and quinidine have also been reported in dogs[8,10,16]. An increase in the plasma digoxin concentration was seen in two studies[8,16], but in another study increases could not be predicted from pharmacokinetic parameters[10].

The experiments reported here were designed to evaluate the clinical significance of the digoxin–quinidine interaction in the dog.

Seven healthy mongrel dogs, weighing 9–12 kg were used. On day 1 the dogs received a loading dose of digoxin (0.05 mg/kg daily) followed by a daily maintenance dose (0.02 mg/kg daily) for the next 14 days. These doses were given orally as tablets. On days 6, 7, 8, 9 and 10 quinidine (200 mg twice daily orally) was added to the dosing regimen.

Three of the seven dogs were trained to lie quietly on a table so that e.c.g. could be taken daily from the fifth day before the start of the experiment until the last day of digoxin administration. PQ-intervals were measured, using at least fifteen P-QRS complexes. Since heart rate, and consequently PQ-intervals, may vary from day to day and even from beat to beat, only PQ-intervals occurring at a heart rate of 90–110 beats/min were used. The e.c.g. was also screened for atrial and ventricular arrhythmias and for other changes that might indicate digitalis toxicity. The same three dogs were also observed for physical signs of digitalis toxicity: anorexia, vomiting and diarrhoea. On a separate occasion the dogs were given quinidine (200 mg twice daily) without digoxin for 8 days.

Blood samples for plasma digoxin and quinidine determinations were taken 10–12 h after the last administration on each day. Plasma digoxin concentrations were measured by radioimmunoassay[1]. Plasma quinidine concentrations were measured fluorimetrically[5].

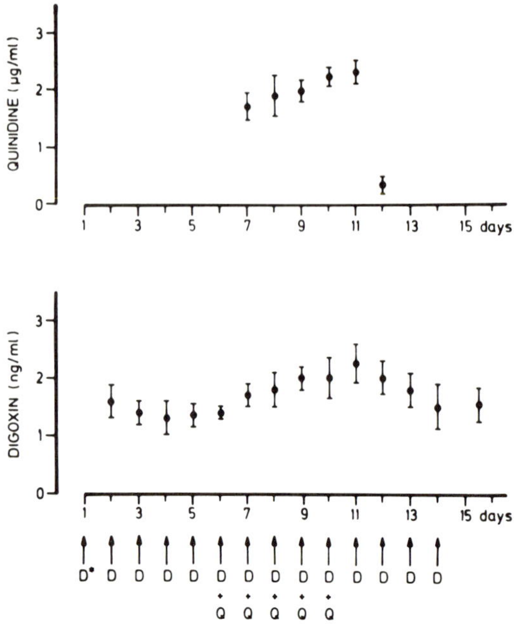

Figure 31.4 Mean plasma concentrations (±SEM) of digoxin and quinidine in seven dogs. An oral loading dose of digoxin (D* = 0.05 mg/kg) was administered, followed by a daily oral maintenance dose (D = 0.02 mg/kg). From day 6 to 10 an oral quinidine dose (200 mg) was added

Statistical evaluation of changes in serum digoxin concentration and PQ-intervals was made using the Student's *t*-test for paired values. Serum concentrations of digoxin and quinidine are given in Figure 31.4. The average steady state digoxin concentration rose during quinidine administration from 1.4 to 2.3 ng/ml ($p<0.01$), while the mean quinidine plasma concentration was about 2 µg/ml. After terminating quinidine administration, the plasma digoxin concentrations again fell to approximately 1.5 ng/ml.

One dog exhibited vomiting and anorexia the day after the loading dose of digoxin was given. None of the three dogs vomited or was anorectic during the following days before quinidine administration was begun. Emesis and anorexia were present in all three dogs during quinidine administration but tended to disappear after quinidine withdrawal. When quinidine was given alone, neither vomiting or anorexia was seen.

Atrial and ventricular arrhythmias were absent in all three dogs. The PQ-interval increased significantly ($p<0.01$) from 0.01 to 0.03 s during the period when digoxin was given without quinidine. No further increase in the PQ-interval occurred during the period of digoxin–quinidine treatment. In one dog, second degree heart block of the Wenckebach type, with ventricular escape, occurred on day 3 and persisted until the end of the experiment.

The finding that the steady state plasma concentrations of digoxin are altered significantly by administration of quinidine is in agreement with the results of others[8, 16], but differs from the findings of Gibson and Nelson[10].

The latter authors found that the halflife and the volume of distribution of digoxin were significantly reduced whereas the total body clearance was not changed in the presence of quinidine. However, the data obtained by Doherty *et al.*[8] and Wilkerson *et al.*[16] were based on multiple dose studies, whereas the data of Gibson and Nelson[11] were derived from single dose.

Cardiac toxicity resulting from the interaction was not seen. It is worth noting that Doherty *et al*[8] found that redistribution of digoxin in the presence of quinidine resulted in a decrease in the concentration of digoxin in the myocardium.

Our results confirm that in dogs treated chronically with digoxin, plasma concentrations of this substance increase when quinidine is added. The increase in plasma concentration was accompanied by pronounced anorexia and vomiting. This finding indicates that the interaction between digoxin and quinidine in the dog is not only of pharmacological interest but also may have clinical implications.

References

1. Belpaire, F. M. and Bogaert, M. G. (1976). Radioimmunoassay of digitalis glycosides. *Acta Clin. Belg.*, **31**, 212–21
2. Bogaert, M. G., Belpaire, F. M., Mussche, M. M. *et al.* (1976). Use of radioimmunoassay of digitalis glycosides in man. *Acta Clin. Belg.*, **31**, 222–7
3. Button, C., Gross, D. R., Johnston, J. T. *et al.* (1980). Pharmacokinetics, bioavailability and dosage regimens of digoxin in dogs. *Am. J. Vet. Res.*, **41**, 1230–7
4. Cramer, G. and Isaksson, B. (1963). Quantitative determination of quinidine in plasma. *Scand. J. Clin. Lab. Invest.*, **15**, 553–7
5. de Rick, A., Belpaire, F. M., Bogaert, M. G. *et al.* (1978). Plasma concentrations of digoxin and digitoxin during digitalization of healthy dogs and dogs with cardiac failure. *Am. J. Vet. Res.*, **39**, 811–5
6. de Rick, A., Chakrabarti, S., Belpaire, F. *et al.* (1979). Bioavailability of three brands of digoxin tablets in dogs. *J. Vet. Pharmacol. Ther.*, **2**, 27–9
7. de Rick, A. and Belpaire, F. (1981). Digoxin–quinidine interaction in the dog. *J. Vet. Pharmacol. Ther.*, **4**, 215–18
8. Doherty, J. E., Straub, K. D., Murphy, M. L. *et al.* (1980). Digoxin–quinidine interaction. Changes in canine tissue concentration from steady state with quinidine. *Am. J. Cardiol.*, **45**, 1196–9
9. Fraser, E. J., Leach, R. H., Poston, J. W. *et al.* (1973). Dissolution and bioavailability of digoxin tablets. *J. Pharm. Pharmacol.*, **25**, 968–73
10. Gibson, T. P. and Nelson, H. A. (1980). Digoxin alters quinidine and quinidine alters digoxin pharmacokinetics in dogs. *J. Lab. Clin. Med.*, **95**, 417–28
11. Hamlin, R. L. (1978). Basis for selection of a cardiac glycoside for dogs. In Proceedings of *First Symposium of Veterinary Pharmacology and Therapeutics*, Baton Rouge, Louisiana
12. Krasula, R. W., Gardella, L. A., Zarolinski, J. F. *et al.* (1976). Comparative bioavailability of four dosage forms of digoxin in dogs. *Fed. Proc. Am. Soc. Exp. Biol.*, **35**, 327
13. Pedersoli, W. M. (1978). Serum digoxin concentrations in healthy dogs treated without a loading dose. *J. Vet. Pharmacol. Ther.*, **1**, 279–84
14. Peters, D. N., Hamlin, R. L. and Powers, J. D. (1981). Absence of pharmacokinetic interaction between digitoxin and quinidine in the dog. *J. Vet. Pharmacol. Ther.*, **4**, 271–5
15. Snedecor, G. W. (1961). In Snedecor, G. W. (ed.) *Statistical Methods.* 5th Edn: (Ames, Iowa: The Iowa State Univ. Press)
16. Wilkerson, D. R., Mockridge, P. B. and Massing, G. K. (1980). Effects of selected drugs on serum digoxin concentration in dogs. *Am. J. Cardiol.*, **45**, 1201–10

32

Influence of anaesthetics and ancillary agents on cardiovascular and respiratory systems in the horse

P. Lees, C. J. Hillidge and L. Serrano

There are several reasons why pharmacologists and anaesthetists devote much of their time to studying changes in cardiovascular and respiratory functions following the administration of anaesthetics and ancillary agents. First, all available agents produce some changes in respiration and the cardiovascular system. These are usually of a depressant nature, involving, for example, decreases in heart rate or blood pressure. There are instances, however, when drug-induced cardiovascular or respiratory stimulation occur. Secondly, there is a clinical requirement for knowledge of changes in physiological variables such as mean arterial pressure (MAP) and arterial oxygen tension (PaO_2) because changes, if too profound or too persistent, may impair a variety of physiological functions. Finally, when mortality is associated with the use of anaesthetics and ancillary agents, it is most commonly due to respiratory failure or cardiovascular depression or both. For example, respiratory depression (reducing PaO_2) and hypotension (potentially reducing tissue perfusion) may occur together with many anaesthetics and related drugs to produce tissue hypoxia.

Similarly, if decreased cardiac output (CO) occurs simultaneously with decreased arterial oxygen content (CaO_2), oxygen supply to tissues will be reduced. Whole body oxygen supply is measured by the variable oxygen flux (FO_2) which is the product of CO and CaO_2. Arterial blood oxygen content and oxygen flux are given by the equations:

$$CaO_2 = \alpha PaO_2 + SaO_2 \times Hb \times 1.39$$

$$FO_2 = CO \times CaO_2$$

where

α = solubility of oxygen in blood (solubility coefficient = 0.003 mlO_2/100 ml blood/mmHg at 37° C),

SaO_2 = arterial oxygen saturation,

Hb = haemoglobin concentration,

1.39 = volume of oxygen (ml) combining with each g of haemoglobin.

From these equations it will be seen that if anaesthetics and ancillary agents reduce CO, PaO_2 and SaO_2 in, say, a clinical case which is anaemic through reduced erythrocyte count (and hence reduced haemoglobin), tissue oxygen supply may be reduced to critical levels. Cardiovascular and respiratory changes occurring during anaesthesia are therefore potentially very important. They may also be of importance following recovery from anaesthesia. For example, hypoxia during anaesthesia may depress the functions of organs such as the liver once recovery has occurred, while severe hypotension in anaesthetized subjects can cause renal failure several days after an apparently normal recovery.

Thus, knowledge of the cardiovascular and respiratory effects of drugs may enable the clinician to use anaesthetics and ancillary agents more safely. However, such knowledge cannot simply be transposed directly from experimental animals to clinical cases because (1) the clinical subject is an individual which cannot be expected to conform to mean values derived from laboratory-based experiments, and (2) clinical cases may be less tolerant of the cardiovascular and respiratory effects of anaesthetics and ancillary agents if they are 'poor risk' anaesthetic subjects.

In addition to studying the nature, magnitude and time-course of the changes in respiration and cardiovascular function produced by anaesthetics and related drugs and considering their clinical significance, pharmacologists are also concerned to establish the mechanisms underlying these changes. This can be difficult, and sometimes impossible, in *in vivo* studies because of the many interacting factors involved. For example, several reports from this and other laboratories indicate that halothane anaesthesia in the horse is associated with hypotension. It has also been shown that this results from decreases in both CO and total peripheral resistance (TPR), MAP being the product of these variables (MAP = CO × TPR). The fall in TPR might result from several known actions of halothane (depression of the vasomotor centre, ganglion blockade, interference with noradrenaline release or action and a direct spasmolytic action) or from some indirect action, such as respiratory acidosis which accompanies halothane anaesthesia and which is known to dilate arterioles. Similarly, the decrease in CO may result from both direct and indirect effects of halothane. The direct negative inotropic action of halothane contributes to the reduced CO, but the respiratory acidosis is an indirect effect which also reduces contractility. In addition, reduced CO may result, in part, from decreased venous return arising from peripheral pooling of blood. The actual contribution of each factor, acting directly or indirectly to lower CO and TPR and hence reduce MAP also, can be difficult to assess in the whole animal.

METHODS

This chapter describes the results of experiments in normal healthy ponies (usually of the Welsh Mountain breed), receiving a variety of anaesthetics, sedative and analgesic drugs alone or in combination. Respiration and cardiovascular function were assessed by measuring several variables in conscious ponies *at rest* (a vital requirement since significant changes are produced by apprehension and stress). Changes from the control levels were then assessed from further measurements taken at predetermined times during the course of action of the drug(s), including the recovery phase. In some instances further experiments were undertaken to elucidate the mechanisms underlying the measured changes.

Cardiac output was measured by dye dilution and arterial pressure was monitored using a strain gauge transducer. These measurements were facilitated by raising 4 cm sections of both common carotid arteries to subcutaneous positions in the neck at prior operation. Arterial blood gas tensions were measured at 37 °C, using standard electrodes, values being corrected subsequently to body temperature. Biochemical and haematological measurements were made using standard laboratory techniques and derived variables, such as TPR and FO_2, were calculated from standard equations.

RESULTS AND DISCUSSION

Tranquillizer-sedatives

The phenothiazine, acepromazine, and the butyrophenone, azaperone, are sedatives used in equine medicine. Neither agent produces significant respiratory depression, as assessed by PaO_2 and $PaCO_2$ measurements, although acepromazine may reduce respiratory rate. Both drugs produce a moderate degree of hypotension and reduce PCV, both effects lasting for several hours[6,9].

The fall in MAP produced by acepromazine was shown to be caused initially (5 min) by a reduction in TPR which probably reflects a decrease in arteriolar tone (Table 32.1). Thereafter, TPR was still reduced, although it

Table 32.1 Acepromazine and cardiovascular function in ponies (mean ± SE for six animals)

Time (min)	*Heart Rate* (beats min^{-1})	CO (ml $min^{-1} kg^{-1}$)	TPR (dyne sec cm^{-5})	MAP (kPa)
Control	42 ± 5	71 ± 9	572 ± 39	15.1 ± 0.8
A + 5	52 ± 7	94 ± 10	365 ± 41	12.1 ± 0.5
A + 15	61 ± 6	64 ± 5	400 ± 27	10.6 ± 0.7
A + 30	51 ± 7	62 ± 6	468 ± 84	10.6 ± 0.9
A + 45	45 ± 6	61 ± 4	499 ± 100	10.9 ± 1.1
A + 60	44 ± 5	56 ± 7	513 ± 73	11.3 ± 0.8
A + 90	44 ± 5	59 ± 7	517 ± 38	11.8 ± 0.5

Acepromazine (100 μg/kg) was administered intravenously to six Welsh Mountain ponies. Cardiovascular measurements were taken before and at pre-determined times after drug administration tended to return towards the control level, and CO was reduced so that both variables contributed to the hypotension. The cause of the decrease in CO is not known, although it cannot be assumed that it is due to myocardial depression; it could simply reflect reduced venomotor tone and a resulting decrease in venous return to the heart. Another consequence of the fall in CO (and also of the reduction in CaO_2 which results from a decrease in haemoglobin concentration) is a decrease in FO_2. However, oxygen supply is still adequate to meet body needs in normal animals at rest.

From experiments in ponies in which acepromazine and azaperone suppressed the rises in MAP and PCV induced by intravenous doses of adrenaline, it was concluded that their hypotensive actions were due, at least in part, to α-adrenoceptor blockade and a consequent decrease in vasomotor tone[6,9]. Thus, blockade of α-receptors in arterioles could reduce arteriolar tone and hence TPR while blockade of α-receptors in venules might decrease venomotor tone and thereby reduce venous return.

Neuroleptanalgesics

The cardiovascular effects of analgesic dose rates of drugs of the morphine type in the horse have been studied by Muir and co-workers[7], who reported mild cardiovascular stimulation (increases in heart rate and MAP). Our studies have involved administration of much larger doses of the related drug, etorphine, which is available for use in combination with acepromazine (Large Animal Immobilon, LAI). In horses it is used to produce the so-called state of neuroleptanalgesia. The drug mixture is supplied with a solution of the competitive antagonist, diprenorphine, which is used to reverse the actions of etorphine. Studies in our laboratory have shown that LAI produces marked increases in heart rate and an initial rise in MAP. This is followed by a return of MAP to near normal levels[5]. A mild to moderate respiratory acidosis (increased $PaCO_2$) and marked hypoxia (decreased PaO_2) also occurred[3]. In spite of the hypoxia FO_2 was not reduced, indeed it was increased, because the fall in PaO_2 was offset by rises in CO and haemoglobin concentration. It will be recalled that $FO_2 = CO \times (\alpha PaO_2 + SaO_2 \times Hb \times 1.39)$.

Mechanisms underlying the recorded cardiovascular and respiratory effects of neuroleptanalgesia in the horse have been studied by comparing the effects of LAI with those produced by etorphine alone (Table 32.2).

Etorphine produced marked and sustained increases in MAP and PCV and a moderate decrease in PaO_2. When the two drugs were given together as LAI, the cardiovascular effects were shown to be intermediate between those produced by etorphine and acepromazine given separately (Tables 32.1 and 2). It is concluded that etorphine causes cardiovascular stimulation by activation of the sympathoadrenal system, probably by acting on the CNS, while acepromazine suppresses those sympathetic responses mediated by α-adrenoceptors. LAI produced a greater rise in $PaCO_2$ and a greater fall in PaO_2 than etorphine alone, the decrease in PaO_2 being particularly profound with LAI. Acepromazine, therefore, seems to potentiate the respiratory

Table 32.2 Effects of Immobilon and etorphine on MAP, PCV and PaO_2 in ponies

Time (min)	*Pony 1* *I*	*E*	*Pony 2* *I*	*E*	*Pony 3* *I*	*E*
Mean Arterial Pressure (kPa)						
Control	17.8	15.2	15.4	14.8	14.6	14.1
E + 5	22.0	39.8	26.6	38.0	17.3	32.5
E + 15	16.1	37.9	21.7	31.9	14.4	30.9
E + 30	14.2	42.2	22.6	31.0	16.0	30.1
PCV (l/l)						
Control	0.32	0.34	0.31	0.30	0.30	0.27
E + 5	0.37	0.47	0.40	0.51	0.33	0.40
E + 15	0.31	0.46	0.37	0.50	0.30	0.44
E + 30	0.30	0.45	0.34	0.51	0.31	0.42
PaO_2 (kPa)						
Control	13.1	14.4	13.0	13.2	13.3	13.7
E + 5	6.3	7.6	6.5	10.0	8.1	9.3
E + 15	6.7	8.9	6.8	9.6	8.7	11.8
E + 30	8.3	10.5	7.5	10.0	8.4	12.8

Immobilon (etorphine 22.5 μg/kg and acepromazine 100 μg/kg) or etorphine (22.5 μg/kg) was administered intravenously to three ponies following which measurements were taken after 5, 15 and 30 min

depressant effects of etorphine. As noted above, however, it is not clear that marked tissue hypoxia occurs in spite of the marked reduction in PaO_2 with LAI since this effect was offset by other recorded changes.

Volatile anaesthetics

Following thiopentone induction (10 mg/kg intravenously), anaesthesia with halothane, ether and chloroform, administered in a closed to-and-fro circuit to produce a deep plane of surgical anaesthesia, was associated with hypotension (maximal after 15–30 min) and respiratory acidosis (greatest after 2 h). The degree of respiratory acidosis was similar with all three volatile agents, indicating that depth of surgical anaesthesia was probably similar also. However, the level of hypotension varied, being greatest with halothane and least with chloroform (Table 32.3). The cause of the partial return of MAP towards control levels after 30 min of anaesthesia with all three agents is not clear. Changes in heart rate were small and, in general, insignificant during halothane and chloroform anaesthesia. Ether, on the other hand, increased heart rate. This tachycardia is almost certainly due to activation of the sympathoadrenal system by ether (see below). As expected, large alveolar-arterial oxygen tension differences existed during anaesthesia, but PaO_2 levels were almost invariably greater than levels for conscious horses because of the high inspired concentration of oxygen. However, it was sometimes difficult to maintain PaO_2 levels in the second hour of chloroform anaesthesia.

Further studies in ponies of thiopentone-induced, halothane-maintained anaesthesia revealed that hypotension during anaesthesia was due to

Table 32.3 Effects of anaesthesia on MAP, heart rate and $PaCO_2$ in ponies

Time (min)	*Ether*	*Halothane*	*Chloroform*
MAP (kPa)			
control	14.5 ± 0.4	14.6 ± 0.5	14.6 ± 0.8
15	10.5 ± 0.5†	6.9 ± 0.5†	12.5 ± 1.1*
30	9.7 ± 0.5†	7.5 ± 0.4†	10.6 ± 1.2†
60	9.8 ± 0.5†	9.4 ± 0.5†	11.8 ± 0.8†
120	11.2 ± 0.5†	9.8 ± 0.4†	13.3 ± 0.7
Heart rate (beats min^{-1})			
control	47 ± 1	47 ± 1	45 ± 2
15	58 ± 2†	51 ± 1*	49 ± 2
30	56 ± 2†	46 ± 1	45 ± 4
60	58 ± 2†	46 ± 1	46 ± 2
120	63 ± 4†	46 ± 2	51 ± 5*
$PaCO_2$ (kPa)			
control	6.0 ± 0.1	6.1 ± 0.1	6.3 ± 0.1
15	7.6 ± 0.1†	8.3 ± 0.4†	8.3 ± 0.4†
30	7.6 ± 0.1†	8.5 ± 0.4†	8.1 ± 0.5†
60	8.8 ± 0.8†	8.9 ± 0.4†	8.4 ± 0.5†
120	9.7 ± 1.0†	9.4 ± 0.5†	9.0 ± 1.0†

Values are means ± SE for 16–18 ponies (halothane and ether) or 6 ponies (chloroform). The significance of differences from control values was examined by *t*-tests and is indicated by: $*p<0.05$, $†p<0.01$. Control values were taken in conscious animals before induction of anaesthesia with thiopentone. Anaesthesia was then maintained for 2 h with a volatile agent administered in a to-and-fro closed circuit.

decreases in CO_2 and TPR (Table 32.4), and a variety of indicators (e.g. left ventricular end-diastolic pressure, maximal rate of rise of left ventricular pressure) demonstrated that myocardial contractility was reduced[4]. It is likely that the well-known direct negative inotropic action of halothane and the acidosis which accompanied anaesthesia both contributed to the reduction in contractility.

Enhancement of activity in the sympathetic nervous system during ether anaesthesia in horses is suggested by the cardiovascular collapse which is

Table 32.4 Effects of thiopentone–halothane anaesthesia on cardiovascular function in ponies

Time (min)	*TPR* (dyne sec cm^{-5})	CO_2 (ml min^{-1} kg^{-1})	*MAP* (kPa)
control	459 ± 43	86.6 ± 6.6	16.1 ± 0.5
15	289 ± 58	51.7 ± 8.7*	6.9 ± 0.6†
30	252 ± 41*	57.6 ± 4.1*	7.4 ± 0.4†
60	314 ± 61	61.0 ± 8.3*	9.4 ± 0.5†
120	299 ± 36*	68.9 ± 6.1	9.9 ± 0.4†

Values are means ± SE for 5 (TPR), 6 (CO) and 15 (MAP) ponies. The significance of differences from control values was assessed by paired *t*-tests and is indicated by: $*p<0.05$, $†p<0.01$. Anaesthesia was induced with thiopentone (10 mg/kg) and maintained for 2 h with halothane-oxygen in a to-and-fro circuit precipitated by administration of the β-adrenoceptor antagonist, propranolol[10]. This also seems likely from a number of indirect indicators, for example from the increases in PCV and blood glucose and lactate concentrations which occur in ponies anaesthetized with ether[2]. It is of interest that these changes not only persist into the recovery phase, they are maximal during recovery. Peak PCV and lactate levels occur at 1 h, while glucose concentration is highest 6 h after the end of anaesthesia (Table 32.5). With the exception of small rises in blood glucose, no such changes were recorded during recovery from halothane anaesthesia. Metabolic changes during recovery from chloroform were similar to those produced by ether but they were generally much less pronounced (Table 32.5).

Table 32.5 Metabolic and haematological changes following anaesthesia in ponies

Time (h)	*Ether*	*Halothane*	*Chloroform*
PCV (l/l)			
control	0.295 ± 0.016	0.335 ± 0.008	0.339 ± 0.018
0.25	0.358 ± 0.025†	0.321 ± 0.016	0.349 ± 0.011
1	0.380 ± 0.023†	0.339 ± 0.015	0.306 ± 0.014*
6	0.300 ± 0.027	0.300 ± 0.007*	0.354 ± 0.029
24	0.306 ± 0.022	0.319 ± 0.013	0.389 ± 0.022*
Glucose (mmol/l)			
control	4.26 ± 0.24	3.68 ± 0.07	3.47 ± 0.11
0.25	7.88 ± 1.29†	3.71 ± 0.03	5.38 ± 0.73*
1	7.49 ± 0.87*	5.06 ± 0.94	5.04 ± 0.47
6	7.93 ± 0.84*	5.88 ± 0.63*	5.68 ± 0.07*
24	5.01 ± 0.64	4.40 ± 0.17*	3.95 ± 0.23
Lactate (mmol/l)			
control	1.16 ± 0.19	0.91 ± 0.28	0.87 ± 0.33
0.25	3.40 ± 0.40†	0.95 ± 0.23	1.51 ± 0.58
1	7.04 ± 1.68†	0.81 ± 0.17	1.20 ± 0.37
6	1.54 ± 0.26	0.62 ± 0.11	0.91 ± 0.07
24	0.89 ± 0.14	0.55 ± 0.08	0.74 ± 0.10

Values are means ± SE for five ponies. The significance of differences from control values was examined by *t*-tests and is indicated by: $*p<0.05$, $\dagger p<0.01$. Control values were taken in conscious animals before induction of anaesthesia with thiopentone and maintenance with a volatile agent for 2 h. Further samples were taken at predetermined times after disconnecting the anaesthetic circuit

There is currently much concern that the large and abrupt decrease in inspired oxygen concentration which occurs on disconnecting horses from an anaesthetic circuit can cause hypoxic hypoxia[1,8]. Several factors are involved, including continuing respiratory depression from the anaesthetic agent and ventilation–perfusion imbalances. We have measured minute-by-minute changes in cardiovascular and respiratory parameters in ponies in the immediate anaesthetic recovery period. After disconnecting the anaesthetic circuit, MAP started to rise immediately (from the depressed level during anaesthesia) (Figure 32.1), and heart rate increased after 5 min (Figure 32.2).

$PaCO_2$ fell rapidly from the elevated levels during anaesthesia (Figure 32.3) and PaO_2 levels were reduced, with considerable variation between ponies (Figure 32.4). For animals in lateral recumbency the lowest recorded value was 6.7 kPa, but in one pony PaO_2 levels were in excess of 13.3 kPa. In

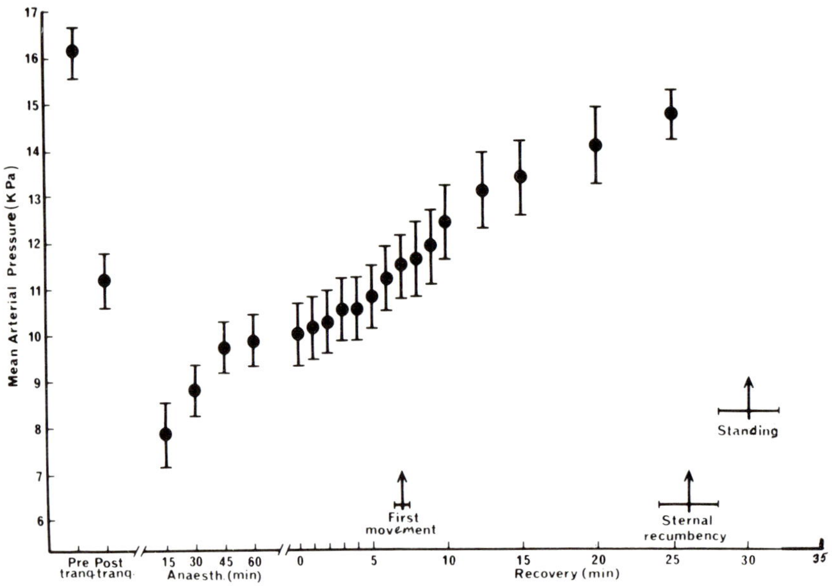

Figure 32.1 Mean arterial blood pressure in ponies: (a) in the standing position at rest (pre-tranq.); (b) standing after azaperone (0.8 mg/kg i.m.) premedication (post-tranq.); (c) in lateral recumbency during halothane/oxygen anaesthesia (after induction with thiopentone, methohexitone or metomidate) at times of 15, 30, 45 and 60 min; (d) in lateral or sternal recumbency after disconnecting the anaesthetic circuit. Arrows indicate the times (and ranges) during recovery of first movement, movement from lateral to sternal recumbency and movement to the standing position. Each point is the mean ± SE for 10 ponies

almost every instance oxygen saturation (SaO_2) was greater than 90%. Moreover, PaO_2 was actually increased slightly in ponies lying in lateral recumbency from conscious control levels because of a small rise in haemoglobin concentration. However, greater decreases in PaO_2 and SaO_2 would be expected in larger breeds of horse.

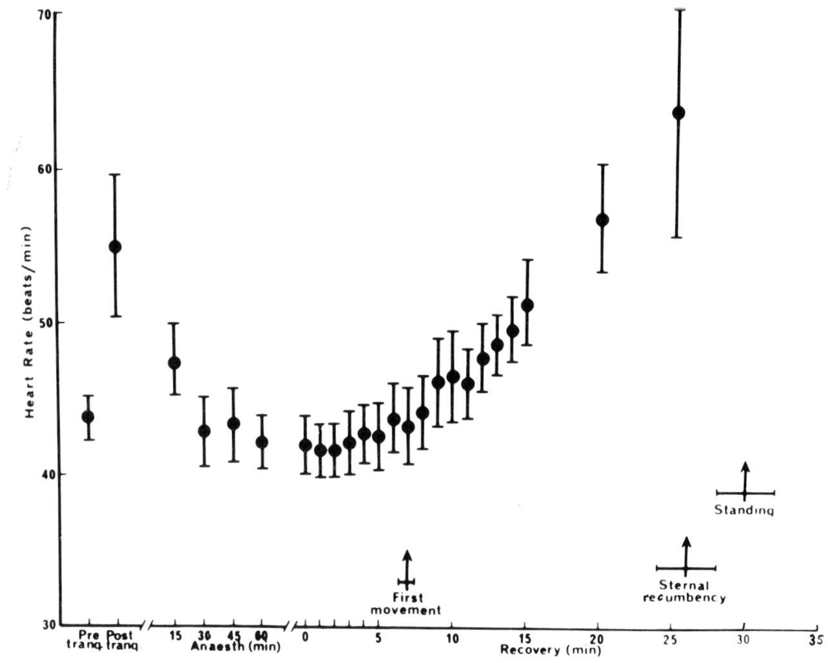

Figure 32.2 Heart rate in ponies in circumstances (a), (b), (c) and (d) as described in Figure 32.1. Each point is the mean ± SE for 10 ponies

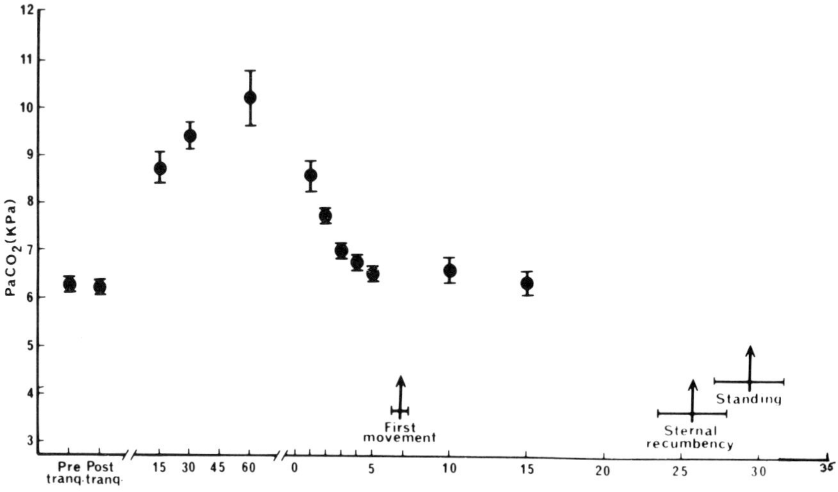

Figure 32.3 Arterial carbon dioxide tension (PaCO_2) in ponies in circumstances (a), (b), (c) and (d) as described in Figure 32.1. Each point is the mean ± SE for 9 ponies

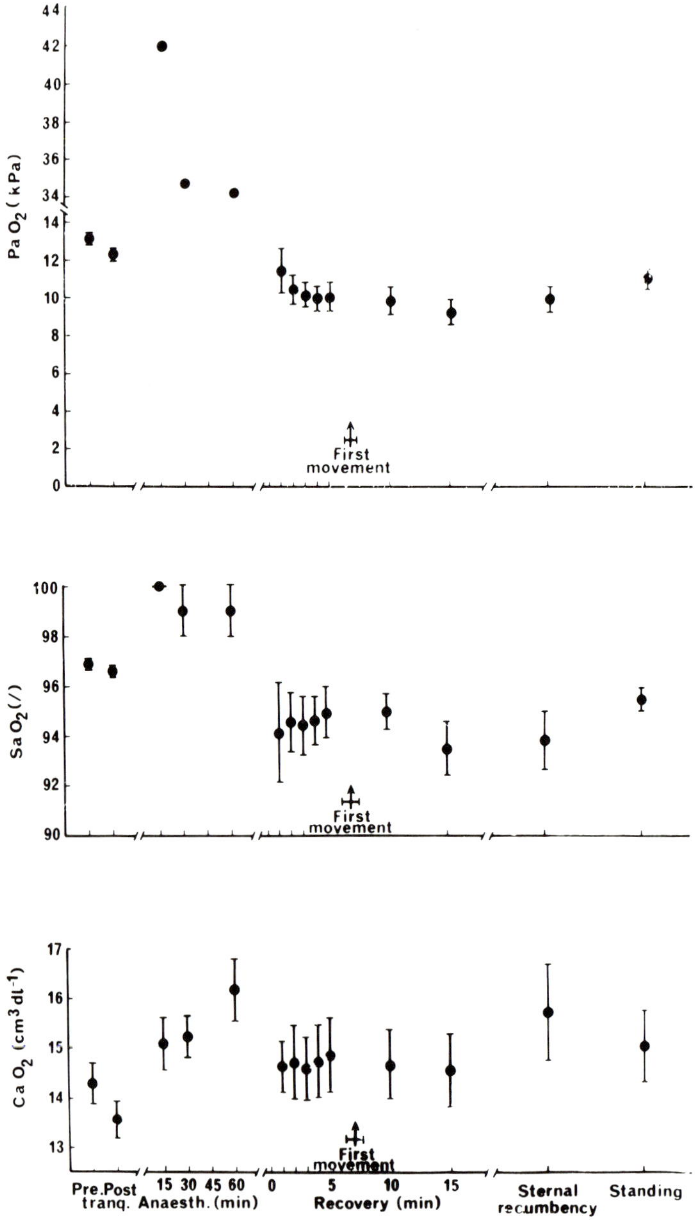

Figure 32.4 Arterial oxygen tension (PaO_2), saturation (SaO_2) and content (PaO_2) in ponies in circumstances (a), (b), (c) and (d) as described in Figure 32.1. Further values in recovery from anaesthesia were recorded in sternal recumbency and when animals had regained the standing position. Each point is the mean ± SE for 9 (PaO_2), 5 (SaO_2) and 5 (PaO_2) ponies. SE levels for PaO_2 during anaesthesia are omitted

References

1. Hall, L. W. (1971). Disturbances of cardiopulmonary function in anaesthetized horses. *Equine Vet. J.*, **3,** 95–8
2. Hillidge, C. J. (1973). Some effects of general anaesthetic agents on cardiovascular function in the horse. *PhD Thesis*, University of London
3. Hillidge, C. J. and Lees, P. (1975). Influence of the neuroleptanalgesic combination of etorphine and acepromazine on the horse: blood gases and acid–base balance. *Equine Vet. J.*, **7,** 148–54
4. Hillidge, C. J. and Lees, P. (1976). The rate of rise of intraventricular pressure as an index of myocardial contractility in conscious and anaesthetised ponies. *Res. Vet. Sci.*, **21,** 176–83
5. Lees, P. and Hillidge, C. J. (1975). Neuroleptanalgesia and cardiovascular function in the horse. *Equine Vet. J.*, **7,** 184–91
6. Lees, P. and Serrano, L. (1976). Effects of azaperone on cardiovascular and respiratory functions in the horse. *Br. J. Pharmacol.*, **56,** 263–70
7. Muir, W. W., Skarda, R. T. and Sheenan, W. C. (1978). Cardiopulmonary effects of narcotic agonists and a partial agonist in the horse. *Am. J. Vet. Res.*, **39,** 1632–5
8. Schatzmann, U., Koehli, M., Dudan, F. *et al.* (1982). Effect of postural changes on certain circulatory and respiratory values in the horse. *Am. J. Vet. Res.*, **43,** 1003–5
9. Serrano, L. and Lees, P. (1976). The applied pharmacology of azaperone in ponies. *Res. Vet. Sci.*, **20,** 316–23
10. Tavernor, W. D. and Lees, P. (1969). The influence of propranolol on cardiovascular function in conscious and anaesthetized horses. *Arch. Int. Pharm. Ther.*, **180,** 89–99

33
Steroidal anti-inflammatory agents in the horse: pharmacokinetics and action on the adrenal gland

P. L. Toutain and R. A. Brandon

Although the non-steroidal anti-inflammatory agents are the most useful anti-inflammatory drugs in equine practice, corticosteroids are also used for a variety of conditions such as endotoxic shock, arthritis, pulmonary diseases, etc. In addition, the psychostimulant effect of corticosteroids has led to their large and uncontrolled misuse in racing horses in order to improve performance. The pharmacological properties and therapeutic indications of synthetic cortiscosteroids are documented for the horse. In contrast, information on the pharmacokinetics and the effects of these agents on the adrenal gland are scant or absent. The objectives of the present report are to review the information available in these two fields and to present unpublished data obtained on dexamethasone and prednisolone in the horse.

RELEVANCE OF PHARMACOKINETIC STUDIES OF CORTICOSTEROIDS

As for other drugs, pharmacokinetic data on corticosteroids are needed to evaluate some basic parameters such as the rate of absorption, bioavailability, extent of metabolism, urinary excretion, etc. Another point of interest is the availability of the corticosteroids from their ester forms. To modify the solubility of steroids, many corticosteroid esters have been introduced. However, only the free alcohol is active and a preliminary hydrolysis in the body is necessary to remove the ester. For example, it was shown in man that dexamethasone-21-sulphate, an ester currently used in certain European and Asian countries, is not hydrolysed and consequently is without therapeutic effects[16]. In this respect, not only the total availability of the steroid from the ester form is important to consider, but also the speed of its availability through hydrolysis, especially in some circumstances (e.g.

in the course of endotoxic shock therapy), when massive corticotherapy is necessary.

One of the main purposes of pharmacokinetic studies is to establish a rational dosage regimen. For corticosteroids, no apparent relationship has been demonstrated between blood levels and therapeutic effects[19]. In addition, steady-state plasma concentrations are not desirable. Consequently, determination of pharmacokinetic parameters will probably not be of help in determining an appropriate dosage regimen which is still largely empirical. In contrast, pharmacokinetics may be able to contribute to the evaluation of the potency and duration of action of corticosteroids. Indeed, it is generally accepted that the halflife in plasma is related to the duration of activity. In addition, relative anti-inflammatory potency of the different corticosteroids in man are approximately correlated with the plasma halflife[15].

ANALYTICAL TECHNIQUES

Pharmacokinetic studies of synthetic corticosteroids and evaluation of their effects on the adrenal gland require sensitive, specific and reproducible analytical techniques; in addition, they must be adaptable to routine use.

In the horse, plasma cortisol has been measured by five methods: fluorometry, thin-layer chromatography, competitive protein-binding (CPB), radioimmunoassay (RIA) and high performance liquid chromatography (HPLC) (Table 33.1). Fluorometric techniques measure the fluorescence developed by the 11-hydroxy group. This technique lacks specificity and

Table 33.1 Basal cortisol values in the horse according to the analytical techniques

Analytical technique	*Cortisol* (ng/ml) *mean* ± *SD*	*Reference*
Fluorometric	58 ± 18.9	11
	110–130	8
Thin-layer chromatography ultraviolet absorption-fluorescence	2190–3950	28
Competitive protein binding	51.2 ± 16.7	9
	13.7 ± 4.0	3
	42 ± 20	14
	85 ± 19	6
Competitive protein binding vs. radioimmunoassay	138.4 ± 30.9 vs. 43.3 ± 9.3	7
Radioimmunoassay	19–31	13
	15–50	21
	about 40	20
	6–23	2
High performance liquid chromatography	73.0 ± 11.19	Toutain (unpublished observation)

detects cortisol, corticosterone and other non-specific fluorescent material. Despite these limitations, fluorometric values reported in the horse[11] are in agreement with other techniques such as CPB and HPLC. Using thin-layer chromatography, ultraviolet absorption and fluorescence, the first plasma cortisol values reported in the literature for the horse (2190–3950 ng/ml) were much too high to be acceptable[28]. Competitive protein binding methods rely on competition between unknown and radiolabelled cortisol for a cortisol binding-protein (i.e. corticosteroid binding-globulin). As for fluorometry, other hydroxycorticosteroids bind to the protein, but their contribution in the horse are probably of little importance because it may be assumed that cortisol is the principal corticosteroid. With this technique, reported normal mean values in the horse vary relatively widely from 13.7 ± 4 to 138.4 ± 30 ng/ml[3,7]. Radioimmunoassay methods are sensitive and give generally lower values than CPB techniques.

The same samples analysed by these two techniques give mean values in the ratio of 1:3. Radioimmunoassay techniques were also used for the analysis of dexamethasone[4,21]. The cross-reactivity of cortisol to the dexamethasone antiserum is only 0.12% (Table 33.2)[21]. Consequently, kinetic studies of dexamethasone, including its effects on the adrenal gland, could be undertaken with the RIA method. In contrast, prednisolone displays a strong cross-reaction against cortisol antibody which prevents a precise pharmacokinetic study with this method. In general, the lack of specificity of the RIA technique developed for dexamethasone analysis is such that it may be used to detect the administration of a wide range of other synthetic corticosteroids and their derivatives[4].

Table 33.2 Cross-reaction of various steroids with dexamethasone and cortisol antisera at 50% binding (from ref. 21)

	% Cross-reaction	
Steroid	*Dexamethasone antiserum*	*Cortisol antiserum*
Dexamethasone	100	0.0113
Cortisol	0.12	100
Betamethasone	15.9	0.03
Triamcinolone	8.1	0.07
Prednisolone	0.6	60.9
Corticosterone	0.08	1.3
Cortisone	0.01	2.2
11-deoxycortisol	0.031	8.2
17β-oestradiol	0	0.003
Progesterone	0.065	0.003
Dihydrotestosterone	0.09	0.015

The characteristics of HPLC techniques when coupled with sensitive UV detectors provide the advantages of simple preliminary treatment of the sample, a very selective separation and a short time analysis[1]. This has been used in our laboratory to evaluate simultaneously both natural and synthetic corticosteroids in the horse. Plasma cortisol values found with this method (73 ± 11.2 ng/ml) are in agreement with those of the CPB technique.

Different synthetic corticosteroids used in the horse (prednisolone, dexamethasone, flumethasone) can be easily and specifically quantified with a level of sensitivity of about 2 ng/ml, which is convenient for kinetic studies.

PHARMACOKINETICS OF DEXAMETHASONE AND ITS ESTERS

Intravenous administration

The plasma concentrations (ng/ml) of dexamethasone (DXM) after intravenous (i.v.) administration of DXM alcohol and DXM-21-isonicotinate (0.05 mg/kg) to six horses are shown in a semilogarithmic plot (Figure 33.1(a)). The plasma concentrations were fitted to the biexponential equation $Cp^t = Ae^{-\alpha t} + Be^{-\beta t}$, where Cp^t is the concentration of drug in plasma at time t, A and B are coefficients and α and β are exponential coefficients. Table 33.3 gives the values of these different parameters. The halftimes of elimination of DXM for these two formulations were, respectively, 53.35 ± 13.91

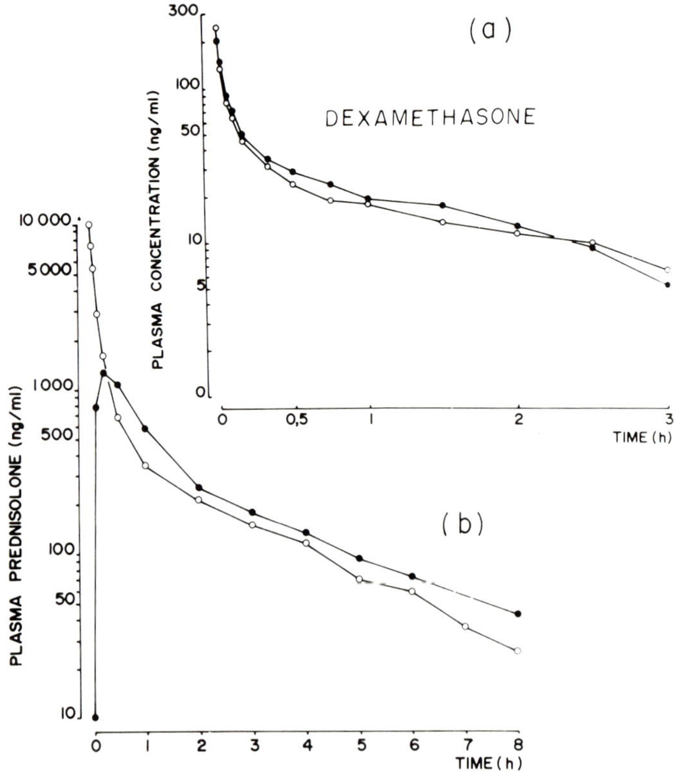

Figure 33.1 The semilogarithmic plot of mean plasma concentration (ng/ml) vs. time (h) of (a) dexamethasone after intravenous administration (0.05 mg/kg) of dexamethasone alcohol (○) and dexamethasone-21-isonicotinate (●) to six horses, and (b) of prednisolone after intravenous (○) and intramuscular (●) administration of prednisolone succinate (0.6 mg/kg) to four horses

Table 33.3 Kinetics of DXM in horse, intravenous route (0.05 mg/kg as DXM alcohol)

Compound	*Parameters*			
	A	*B*	α	β
DXM alcohol	302 (±83.8)	44.6 (±8.79)	0.4473 (±0.1180)	0.01407 (±0.00521)
DXM-21-isonicotinate	251.85 (±123.90)	49.4 (±8.91)	0.4769 (±0.2143)	0.01413 (±0.00370)

and 53.5±16.98 min (mean±SD). In addition, the areas under the curves and the initial concentrations were not statistically different between the two formulations, thus indicating that DXM is totally and immediately available from its isonicotinate ester. Consequently, DXM alcohol and DXM-21-isonicotinate administered by the intravenous route in the horse must be considered as therapeutically equivalent. Similar results have been obtained with DXM-21-sodium phosphate. Following intravenous administration (20 mg *in toto*), the level of DXM in plasma after 15 min was 63 ng/ml and nearly absent after a delay of 12–14 h[21]. In comparison to other species, it appears that the elimination of DXM is more rapid in the horse (see Table 33.4).

Table 33.4 Halflife (min) of DXM in different species

Species	*Horse*	*Cow*	*Dog*	*Man*	*Rat*
Halflife	53	290–335	110–130	140–200	156–324
Authors	Present report	23	24	25	26

Intramuscular administration

In the same six horses used for the i.v. study, the plasma concentrations achieved by intramuscular injection (i.m.) of DXM alcohol and DXM-21-isonicotinate were too low to allow kinetic analysis. However, the suppression of endogenous corticosteroids and the presence of DXM in urine suggest absorption had occurred. After i.m. administration of radiolabelled DXM, DXM was detected in plasma within 15 min; the peak level was obtained approximately after 2 h and between 40 and 50% of administered radioactivity[5] was excreted in urine in the first 24 h thus suggesting a good availability of the DXM solution. Following i.m. administration of a suspension of DXM-21-isonicotinate, it was impossible to detect DXM in plasma and the peak level in urine was achieved 20 h after dosing, indicating relatively slow absorption[21]. Even slower absorption was observed with DXM-21-trimethylacetate since urinary DXM increased to 16 ng/ml within 24 h of the injection and remained slightly elevated[21] for 120 h at least. In summary, DXM alcohol and its soluble esters are rapidly absorbed following i.m. administration. In contrast, water insoluble esters are slowly absorbed which explains the prolonged activity of these formulations.

Table 33.5 The urinary excretion of dexamethasone in the horse—single administration

Compound	*Dose* (μg/kg)	*Route of administration*	*Number of animals*	*Analytical method*	*Time* (h) *to obtain a non-detectable level*	*Authors*
DXM alcohol	50	i.v.	5	HPLC	24–48	Present report
	50	i.m.	6	HPLC	24–72	
21-sodium phosphate	about 50	i.v.	2	RIA	20–30	21
	90	i.m.	1	RIA	24	4
21-sodium metasulphobenzoate	53	i.m.	1	RIA	27	4
	81	i.m.	1	RIA	31	
21-isonicotinate as a solution	50	i.v.	6	HPLC	24–48	Present report
	50	i.m.	5	HPLC	24–72	
21-isonicotinate as a suspension	40	i.m.	1	RIA	88	4
	about 50	i.m.	2	RIA	120	21
21-acetate	53	i.m.	1	RIA	76	4
	80	i.m.	1	RIA	93	
21-trioxaundecanoate	66	i.m.	1	RIA	49	4
	98	i.m.	1	RIA	51	
21-trimethylacetate	about 50	i.m.	1	RIA	120	21

Urinary elimination of dexamethasone and its metabolites

DXM and its metabolites are largely excreted in urine. The total urinary excretion of DXM corresponds to 6–7% of the administered dose[15]. The remaining drug in urine corresponds to different metabolites, the principle of which[22] is 9-fluoro-16α-methyl-6β,11β,16β-trihydroxy-1,4-androstadiene-3,17-dione. Other metabolites[17] are 9α-fluoro-16α-methyl-6,11β-dihydroxyandrost-1,4-diene-3,17-dione,11-dehydroxydexamethasone,20-dihydroxydexamethasone and 6-hydroxydexamethasone.

Kinetics of urinary elimination are important to consider in order to estimate an appropriate clearance time. Table 33.5 gives the values obtained from the literature and from our laboratory. It appears that the clearance times of DXM alcohol and its hydrosoluble esters (phosphate, . . .) are relatively short (from 24 to 48 h). In contrast, after intramuscular administration of a long-acting formulation (acetate, . . .), DXM can persist in urine for more than 4 days.

PHARMACOKINETICS OF PREDNISOLONE

At the present time, no precise pharmacokinetic study has been published on this corticosteroid. It has been suggested[17] that good absorption occurs from the gut and that urinary excretion is complete 3 days after oral administration.

The plasma concentrations (ng/ml) of prednisolone after intravenous and intramuscular administration of prednisolone succinate (0.6 mg/kg) to four horses are shown as a semilogarithmic plot in Figure 33.1(b). A halftime of about 2 h was calculated for both the i.v. and i.m. routes. In addition, rapid and nearly complete absorption (about 85%) were observed. In contrast to other species, the elimination of prednisolone appeared to be slower than DXM. Figure 33.2 shows plasma prednisolone concentrations after the i.m. administration of prednisolone acetate (0.6 mg/kg) to six horses. The rate

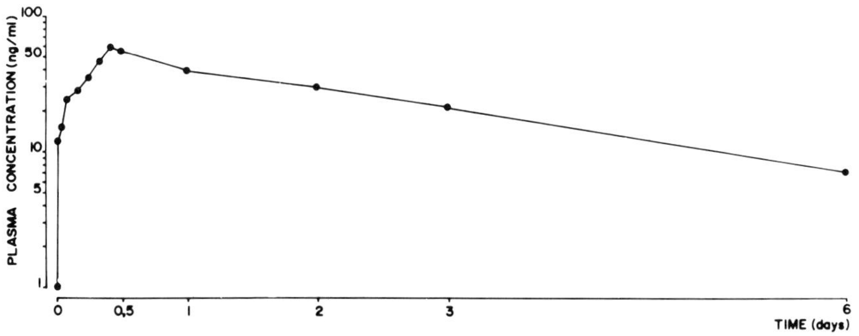

Figure 33.2 The semilogarithmic plot of mean plasma concentration (ng/ml) vs. time (days) of prednisolone after intramuscular administration of prednisolone acetate (0.6 mg/kg) to six horses

of absorption was much slower than that of prednisolone succinate and a halftime of absorption of about 2 days was calculated from the terminal phase of the curve ('flip-flop' model of absorption). This explains the presence of prednisolone in some horses 10 days after its administration as the acetate and the long suppressive effect on the adrenal gland of this formulation (see below).

At the present time, no precise information is available for other corticosteroids in the horse.

SUPPRESSIVE EFFECT OF SYNTHETIC CORTICOSTEROIDS IN THE HORSE

Synthetic corticosteroids inhibit the production of natural corticosteroid by the adrenal gland because insufficient ACTH is released from the pituitary. In addition, repeated administration may result in adrenal atrophy leading to a 'steroid let-down' syndrome when glucocorticoid therapy is stopped. In the horse, as in other species, withdrawal signs consist of myalgia, arthralgia, diarrhoea, electrolyte imbalance, haemoconcentration and severe depression with extreme muscle wastage[12,18]. Thus, medical supervision of adrenal status is required during corticotherapy, especially if it is prolonged. At the present time, measurement of basal cortisol values and responsiveness to an ACTH test are the most useful criteria to evaluate the degree of suppression. Interpretation of basal cortisol level in the horse must include consideration of factors of variation (see Table 33.6). It appears that in the normal horse, age, sex, and breed are of little importance. In addition, the speed of blood sampling and the use of a thin needle cause minimum stress and are probably without effect[11]. Under normal conditions, the most important factor of variability is the sampling time. Wide differences between morning and evening cortisol values have been reported[3,9]. The highest values were reported in the morning (06.00–09.00) and the lowest during the afternoon or the night (16.00–22.00). Such variations must be considered; control blood sampling should be done at the same times and under the same conditions.

Evaluation of the suppressive effect of exogenous corticosteroids, by measuring basal plasma cortisol, is not sufficient. As shown in cattle[23], the basal levels of cortisol may be normal while adrenal responsiveness remains depressed. Consequently, both static (basal cortisol) and dynamic levels (plasma cortisol after ACTH administration) must be evaluated. ACTH tests have been performed in the horse with both natural (corticotropin) and synthetic (tetracosactide) ACTH. Figure 33.3 shows the responses obtained with these two formulations. With natural ACTH administered intramuscularly as a gel, the delay of response appears to be variable[5]. The peak value is obtained after a relatively long delay (i.e. from 4 to 8 h)[6,11,14], and significantly higher values persist until 10–15 h after administration. In addition, rebound depression is observed[11,14]. In contrast, after administration of tetracosactide by the i.v. route, the peak level of cortisol appears earlier (30 min postinjection with 10–50 IU or after 2 h when 100 IU or

Table 33.6 Various factors which influence plasma cortisol concentration in the horse

Factors	*Variations*	*Authors*
Age	no effect	9
Sex	no effect higher values in male than in female: 23.8 ± 4.24 *vs.* 9.06 ± 1.12 ng/ml	8, 9, 11 2
Breed	ponies no different of thoroughbreed: 71.6 ± 20 *vs.* 71.5 ± 16 ng/ml	11
Circadian rhythm	absent present with highest values in the morning 09.00: 75 ± 19.3 ng/ml - 21.00: 51.8 ± 13.7 ng/ml 08.00: 42 ng/ml - 16.00: 17 ng/ml 08.00: about 28 ng/ml - 16.00: about 6 ng/ml 06.00: 65 ng/ml - 18.00: 20 ng/ml	8 11 9 3 14
Exercise	no effect increase of 130%	8 4
Pathologic	increase: shock, colics, etc. no effect: chronic stress (poor performers)	10 2
Venipuncture	no effect on trained horses	11 Present report
Anaesthesia	no effect (acepromazine, thiopentone, halothane)	11
Surgery	large increase similar to that obtained after ACTH administration	11
Adrenaline	no effect	11
Hypoglycaemia	only severe hypoglycaemia induced by insulin (0.8 IU/kg) increase plasma cortisol	11

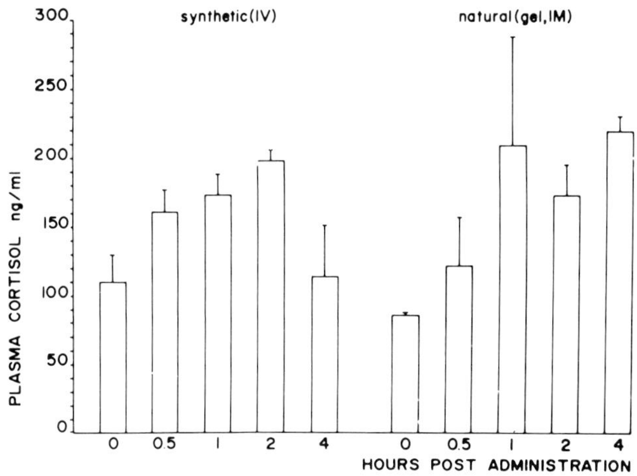

Figure 33.3 ACTH-stimulated plasma cortisol concentration (ng/ml) after intravenous (synthetic) or intramuscular (natural, gel) administration of ACTH (100 IU)[6]

larger doses are given). Return to normal values are seen[6] within 4 h. From these results, it may be concluded that tetracosactide is preferred for testing the adrenal gland in the horse because shorter and more uniform responses are obtained. In addition, a reduced risk of hypersensitive reaction may be expected since the preparation is pure and has a smaller molecular weight.

The degree of adrenal suppression is dependent upon the drug, its formulation and dose and the duration, frequency, time and route of administration. A rational approach to glucocorticoid therapy in the horse requires precise information on these different variables but at the present time only limited data are available.

Short-acting formulations, single administration (i.v., i.m.)

For short-acting preparations (alcoholic solution or hydrosoluble esters such as succinate, hemisuccinate, sulphobenzoate, trihydroundecanoate, isonicotinate, phosphate and phosphate disodium) and for single administration either by the intravenous or intramuscular routes, adrenal suppression is not always total. Return to normal values is observed within 1–5 days according to the drug. Figure 33.4(a) shows the plasma cortisol concentrations after a single administration of prednisolone succinate to four horses (0.6 mg/kg, i.v.). Suppressive effects are significant 15 min after administration; non-detectable values were observed 6–12 h after administration and normal values returned within 24–38 h. Similar results were obtained by the i.m. route. Single administration of DXM-21-isonicotinate as a solution (0.05 mg/kg, i.m.) suppressed cortisol production following a delay of 1–2 h with return to normal values after 4–5 days (Figure 33.4(b)). Similar results were obtained using DXM alcohol by either the intravenous or intramuscular route and for DXM-21-isonicotinate by the intravenous route. Consequently, it appears that the suppressive effect of DXM is of a longer duration than prednisolone in the horse. After injection of DXM-21-sodium phosphate (20 mg, i.v.), plasma cortisol was undetectable within 12 h. After a delay of 18 h, the level increased steadily to normal[21] after about 30 h. Similar observations are reported[7,10,11]

Short-acting formulation, repeated administration[10]

Daily administration of 20 mg of DXM by intramuscular injection for 10 days to one horse resulted in a decrease in cortisol concentration which varied from 11 to 26 ng/ml (value for control horses: 51 ± 16 ng/ml). On the 11th day, this horse was given 500 units of ACTH gel; the plasma cortisol value then increased from 0 to 52 ng/ml. This response was lower than the response of control horses (153 ng/ml) indicating a suppressive effect on both the static and dynamic functions of the adrenal gland.

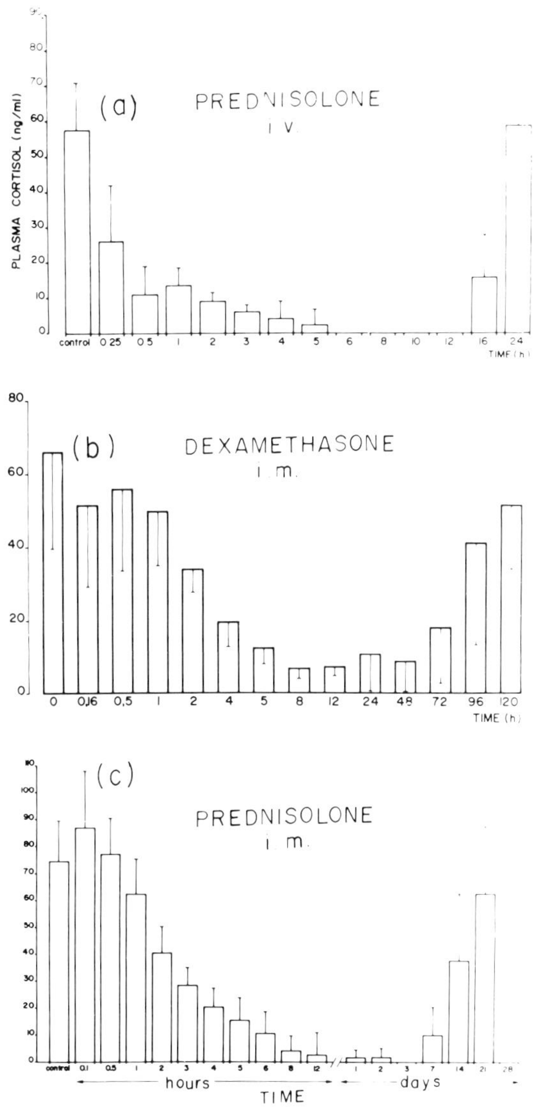

Figure 33.4 Histogram of mean plasma cortisol concentration (ng/ml) vs. time (h) (a) after intravenous administration of prednisolone succinate (0.6 mg/kg) to four horses; (b) after intramuscular administration of dexamethasone-21-isonicotinate (0.05 mg/kg) to six horses; (c) after intramuscular administration of prednisolone acetate (0.6 mg/kg) to six horses. Mean and standard deviation for (a), (b), (c)

Long-acting formulations (i.m.)

After DXM-21-trimethylacetate intramuscular administration (20 mg) no consistent depression of plasma cortisol was observed for 24 h. Thereafter, cortisol levels remained low until the end of the 120 h period of observation[21]. A more precise study of the effect of prednisolone acetate (0.6 mg/kg) was undertaken in our laboratory. Both the cortisol level and ACTH test were used to evaluate the suppressive effects of prednisolone acetate on the adrenal gland. Figure 33.4(c) shows the changes in plasma cortisol after prednisolone acetate injection and Figure 33.5 shows the response to the ACTH test. Plasma cortisol decreased after a delay of 1–2 h and reached a low or undetectable value after 12 h postadministration. Return to normal required about 20 days. Similarly, the ACTH test indicated that the responsiveness of the adrenal gland was depressed equally for 3 weeks (Figure 33.5).

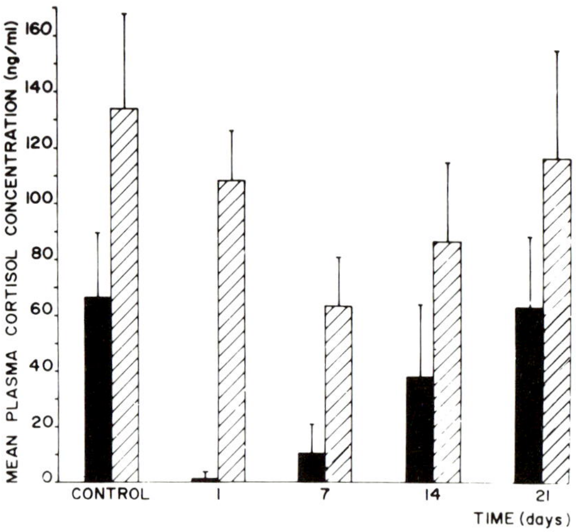

Figure 33.5 Histogram of the mean base-line plasma cortisol concentration and ACTH-stimulated plasma cortisol concentration before and after the intramuscular administration of prednisolone acetate (0.6 mg/kg) to six horses; mean and standard deviation

Local administration

Intra-articular corticosteroid therapy is widely used in the horse in order to avoid systemic side-effects. However, after intra-articular administration, some steroids are absorbed into the systemic circulation. In man, intra-articular injection has been shown to produce adrenal atrophy, but no information is available at the present time in the horse. A probable systemic effect on the adrenal gland of the horse is suggested by evidence that administration of betamethasone dipropionate plus betamethasone sodium phosphate resulted in a decrease in the eosinophil count for 2 weeks[27].

CONCLUSION

Suppression of the hypothalamic-pituitary-adrenal system is the most prevalent and most dangerous side-effect induced by corticosteroids. The main factor appears to be the formulation. Soluble forms (alcohol and phosphate, etc.) depress the adrenal gland for 1–5 days depending upon the drug and route of administration. In contrast, insoluble esters (acetate, etc.) can depress for a much longer time (i.e. several weeks). Such a difference must be related to the speed of absorption from the site of administration as shown by pharmacokinetic studies. For such preparations, repeated administration (i.e. every 2 weeks) can lead to severe adrenal insufficiency. Despite the new results presented here, no precise recommendation can be offered for the conduct of longterm corticotherapy in the horse. Further studies in this field are required to obtain more information, such as the effect of repeated administration of short-acting formulations and the value of the oral route in the horse.

References

1. Alvinerie, M. and Toutain, P. L. (1982). Simultaneous determination of corticosterone, cortisol and dexamethasone in dogs plasma using high performance liquid chromatography. *J. Pharm. Sci.*, **7**, 816–8
2. Baker, H. W. G., Baker, I. D. C., Epstein, V. M. *et al.* (1982). Effect of stress on steroid hormone levels in racehorses. *Aust. Vet. J.*, **58**, 70–1
3. Bottoms, G. D., Roesel, O. F., Rausch, F. D. *et al.* (1972). Circadian variation in plasma cortisol and corticosterone in pigs and mares. *Am. J. Vet. Res.*, **33**, 785–90
4. Chapman, D. I., Moss, M. S. and Whiteside, J. (1977). The urinary excretion of synthetic corticosteroids by the horse. *Vet. Rec.*, **100**, 447–50
5. Dumasia, M. C., Houghton, E., Moss, M. S. *et al.* (1979). Metabolism of dexamethasone in the horse. In Tobin, T., Blake, J. W. and Woods, W. E. (eds.), *Third International Symposium on Equine Medication Control.* pp. 247–52. (Lexington, Kentucky: College of Agriculture)
6. Eiler, H., Goble, D. and Oliver, J. (1979). Adrenal gland function in the horse: effect of cosyntropin (synthetic) and corticotropin (natural) stimulation. *Am. J. Vet. Res.*, **40**, 724–6
7. Eiler, H., Oliver, J. and Goble, D. (1980). Combined dexamethasone-suppression cosyntropin (synthetic ACTH) stimulation test in the horse: a new approach to testing of adrenal gland function. *Am. J. Vet. Res.*, **41**, 430–4
8. Flisinska-Bojanowska, A., Skwarlo, K., Lukaszewska, J. *et al.* (1974). Diurnal variation of serum cortisol and PBI in the thoroughbred horse and effect of physical effort on plasma cortisol concentration. *Bull. Acad. Pol. Sci. (Biol.)*, **22**, 719–24
9. Hoffsis, G. F., Murdick, P. W., Tharp, V. L. *et al.* (1970). Plasma concentrations of cortisol and corticosterone in the normal horse. *Am. J. Vet. Res.*, **31**, 1379–87
10. Hoffsis, G. F. and Murdick, P. W. (1970). The plasma concentration of corticosteroids in normal and diseased horses. *J. Am. Vet. Med. Assoc.*, **11**, 1590–4
11. James, V. H. T., Horner, M. W., Moss, M. S. *et al.* (1970). Adrenocortical function in the horse. *J. Endocrinol.*, **48**, 319–35
12. Kirk, M. D. (1974). Field diagnosis and treatment of secondary adrenocortical insufficiency in the horse. *Vet. Med. Small Anim. Clin.*, **11**, 1383–6
13. Kumar, M. S. A., Liao, T. F. and Chen, C. L. (1976). Diurnal variation in serum cortisol in ponies. *J. Anim. Sci.*, **42**, 1360
14. Larsson, M., Edqvist, L. E., Ekman, L. *et al.* (1979). Plasma cortisol in the horse, diurnal rhythm and effects of exogenous ACTH. *Acta Vet. Scand.*, **20**, 16–24

15. Melby, J. C. (1977). Clinical pharmacology of systemic corticosteroids. *Ann. Rev. Pharmacol. Toxicol.*, **17**, 511–27
16. Miyabo, S., Nakamura, T., Kuwazima, S. *et al.* (1981). A comparison of the bioavailability and potency of dexamethasone phosphate and sulphate in man. *Eur. J. Clin. Pharmacol.*, **20**, 277–82
17. Moss, M. S. and Rylance, H. J. (1967). A thin-layer chromatography study on the metabolism of prednisolone in the horse. *J. Endocrinol.*, **37**, 129–37
18. O'Connor, J. T. (1968). The untoward effects of the corticosteroids in equine practice. *J. Am. Vet. Med. Assoc.*, **153**, 1614–7
19. Pickup, M. E. (1979). Clinical pharmacokinetics of prednisone and prednisolone. *Clin. Pharmacokinetics*, **4**, 111–28
20. Reimers, T. J., Cowan, R. G., Davidson, H. P. *et al.* (1981). Validation of radioimmuno-assay for triiodothyronine, thyroxine and hydrocortisone (cortisol) in canine, feline and equine sera. *Am. J. Vet. Res.*, **42**, 2016–21
21. Seawright, A. A., Ng, J. C., Steele, D. P. *et al.* (1979). The detection of dexamethasone administrations in thoroughbred horses. In Tobin, T., Blake, J. W. and Woods, W. E. (eds.), *Third International Symposium on Equine Medication Control.* pp. 227–46. (Lexington, Kentucky: College of Agriculture)
22. Skrabalak, D. S. and Maylin, G. A. (1982). Dexamethasone metabolism in the horse. *Steroids*, **39**, 233–44
23. Toutain, P. L., Brandon, R. A., Alvinerie, M. *et al.* (1982). Dexamethasone in cattle: pharmacokinetics and action on the adrenal gland. *J. Vet. Pharmacol. Ther.*, **5**, 33–43
24. Toutain, P. L., Alvinerie, M. and Ruckebusch, Y. (1983). The pharmacokinetics of dexamethasone and its effects on adrenal gland function in the dog. *Am. J. Vet. Res.*, **44**, 212–7
25. Tsuei, S. E., Moore, R. G., Ashley, J. J. *et al.* (1979). Disposition of synthetic gluco-corticoid. I. Pharmacokinetics of dexamethasone in healthy adults. *J. Pharmacokin. Biopharm.*, **7**, 249–64
26. Varma, D. R. and Mulay, S. (1980). Antiinflammatory and ulcerogenic effects and pharmacokinetics of dexamethasone in protein deficient rats. *J. Pharmacol. Exp. Ther.*, **214**, 197–202
27. Vernimb, G. D., van Hoose, L. M. and Hennessey, P. W. (1977). Onset and duration of corticosteroid effect after injection of betasone for treating equine arthropathies. *Vet. Med. Small Anim. Clin.*, **72**, 241–4
28. Zolovick, A., Upson, D. W. and Eleftherious, B. E. (1966). Diurnal variation in plasma glucocorticosteroid levels in the horse. *Endocrinology*, **35**, 249–53

34
Spasmolytic analgesic drugs and small intestinal function in the horse

E. L. Gerring and J. V. Davies

Spasmolytic and analgesic drugs are widely used in the treatment of abdominal pain in the horse. Pain in these cases may emanate from a variety of sources and is commonly referred to as colic. Pain in the small intestine may be due to obstruction of the lumen, distension by fluid or gas, or interference with the regional vascular supply. It is frequently not possible, particularly in the early stages of the condition, to make an accurate diagnosis and treatment must be undertaken empirically[2]. Since spasmolytic and narcotic analgesic drugs are frequently administered in such situations, the purpose of this investigation was to measure the effects of such drugs on the function of a small intestinal loop in conscious ponies.

MATERIALS AND METHODS

Three Welsh pony geldings (125–135 kg) aged 12–24 months were studied. Under halothane anaesthesia, 120 cm T-V loops of the jejunum were prepared in each animal, via a left paracostal laparotomy high on the flank. The stomata were placed on the ventrolateral aspect of the abdomen. Two pairs of electrodes and two strain gauge transducers (SGT) were attached to the loop. The electrode and SGT connections were made through perspex cannulae exteriorized through the left flank[1]. The ponies were allowed 3 weeks to recover from surgery and trained to stand in stocks for recording sessions. They were housed individually and fed hay, bran, pony nuts and oats.

During recording the loop was perfused with 0.9% sodium chloride solution at 37 °C. The head of saline was adjusted so that fluid was ejected in distinct jets (deliveries). All fluid collected was measured and returned via a filter to the reservoir. The large volume of the reservoir (20 l) compensated for any small losses of fluid.

Recordings were made over several hours at the same time of day. At least

1 h of steady perfusion was used as the predose control in each experiment. Ponies had access to food prior to recording but were not fed during the experiment. Recordings from the electrodes (electroenterogram) and the SGT (mechanogram) were displayed simultaneously on the polygraph.

All drugs were administered by slow injection into a jugular vein in the following doses: acepromazine 5 mg (2.5 ml), Buscopan: 40 mg hyoscine and 5 g dipyrone (10 ml), pethidine 250 mg (5 ml), methadone 10 mg (1 ml) and in control experiments saline 5 ml.

Mathematical tables were used to randomize the sequence of experiments.

ANALYSIS OF DATA

The traces were analysed together when the experiments had been completed to standardize interpretation. Measurements, made over 5 min units of time, were slow wave frequency (SWF), frequency of superimposition of spiking activity on the slow wave (SA), the rate of delivery of jets of fluid test meal (DR) and the volume of test meal transported (Vtm).

Grand pretreatment control means $\bar{x} \pm 2$ SEM (standard error of the mean) for each parameter were calculated from the pretreatment values of all the experiments. These values were used to construct 96% confidence limits to delineate daily or experimental variation. Pretreatment control means were calculated for each experiment and post-treatment changes from control means were summed every 15 min.

RESULTS

The effects on SWF, SA, DR and Vtm were calculated for each drug. The results for acepromazine gave a 5% ($p \leqslant 0.01$) reduction in slow wave frequency and a 32% peak increase ($p \leqslant 0.01$) in flow rate. Changes in spiking activity and delivery rate were not significant (Figure 34.1).

Drug / $\bar{x} \pm 2$ SEM	SWF 61.3 ± 0.4 c/5 min	SA 21.5 ± 0.4 c/5 min	DR 4.9 ± 0.3 c/5 min	Vtm 850 ± 44 ml/5 min
Acepromazine 5 mg	↓↓	—	—	↑↑↑
Buscopan 40 mg	—	—	↓↓	—
Pethidine 250 mg	↓	↓	↓↓	↑↑
Methadone 10 mg	↓↓	↓↓	—	↑↑

Figure 34.1 Effects of four drugs on the slow wave frequency (SWF), spiking activity (SA), delivery rate (DR) and flow rate (Vtm) in a jejunal loop

Buscopan had less marked effect. There was a tendency for an overall reduction in each of the parameters, but only in the case of DR was this consistently significant ($p<0.05$).

There was a tendency to reduce SWF and DR ($p<0.01$) was consistently decreased with pethidine. The volume of fluid transported was increased overall and significantly so during the 15–45 min period after injection. The pattern was somewhat similar with methadone but the effects were more marked. Both SWF ($p<0.05$) and SA ($p<0.05$) were reduced but no significant change occurred in DR. Flow rate was increased but only after 30 min from the time of injection.

Control injections of saline made no significant difference to any of these measurements of motility.

DISCUSSION

In these experiments the effect of drugs on the motility patterns of a T-V loop were assessed by alterations in the electrical, mechanical and transport profiles. The activity of the phenothiazine group of tranquillizers represented by acepromazine is complex (Lees, 1982, personal communication). Many of their actions may exert an influence on gut motility, particularly parasympatholytic, direct spasmolytic and membrane stabilizing properties. Electrical activity was depressed by a reduction in SWF. Although the delivery rate was unaffected, the flow rate was markedly increased. This increase may be explained by an increase in the force of propulsive contraction or by a decrease in tubular resistance. The atropine-like activity and spasmolytic effects are probably responsible for a decrease in tone, thereby augmenting tubular volume and thus reducing the resistance to flow.

The flow rate (Vtm) is a function of the radius (r) of the intestinal tube and the delivery rate (d) since $\text{Vtm} \propto dr^3$ and thus $r^3 \propto \text{Vtm}$. Any spasmolytic effect will increase r; in the case of acepromazine the marked increase in Vtm with no change in d would lead to the conclusion that there was an increase in the tubal radius due to spasmolysis.

Buscopan contains hyoscine and the anti-inflammatory compound dipyrone. The belladonna alkaloids are reported to produce marked and prolonged inhibitory effects on the motor activity of the gut, characterized by a decrease in tone, amplitude and frequency of peristaltic contractions[3]. In these experiments, however, electrical activity was not significantly altered. The most significant change was a decrease in the frequency of deliveries. Although these productive contractions decreased, the volume of fluid transported remained largely unchanged. Assuming $r^3 \propto (\text{Vtm}/d)$ then a marked decrease in d with no change in Vtm would show a larger value for r and therefore spasmolysis. Buscopan appears therefore to reduce peristalsis by decreasing the number of productive contractions without altering the inherent electrical pattern of the gut, and to reduce tone, thereby allowing fluid to pass through the gut passively.

Both pethidine and methadone decreased the total electrical activity of the T-V loop. Methadone had the more profound and lasting effect. Although these drugs increase intestinal contraction, the net effect of the opiates and their derivatives on the gut is constipating[4].

In a review of the literature surrounding this controversy it was concluded that, although there may be an initial burst of activity, the main effect is to cause a prolonged depression of intestinal propulsion[7]. The internal volume (tone) of a T-V loop in dogs and the work done have been measured in terms of fluid transported[6]. Morphine reduces the amount of propulsive work done, but the immediate effect is to increase the tone of the loop, expelling fluid from both ends. However, raising the perfusion pressure allows fluid to enter the loop which is then vigorously transported. By constantly perfusing the loop in these experiments the effect of pethidine and methadone has been to increase the volume of fluid transported. These drugs therefore reduce the amount of electrical and propulsive activity but greatly increase its force.

Observations incidental to an experimental protocol have demonstrated the initial burst of activity in the jejunum after an injection of morphine, but there was no record of the effects after 10 min. The effect of the drug might also have been modified by the presence of clinical colic[5].

In the clinical treatment of colic each of these preparations is widely used with apparently good results. Both acepromazine and Buscopan are reputed to be spasmolytic but it is likely that the analgesic properties of all four drugs may be the more significant in clinical cases.

References

1. Davies, J. V. and Gerring, E. L. (1983). Small intestinal motility in the horse. *Res. Vet. Sci.* (In press)
2. Gerring, E. L. (1983). Equine colic: causes, diagnosis and treatment. In Bogan, J. A., Lees, P. and Yoxall, A. T. (eds.), *Pharmacological Basis of Large Animal Medicine.* pp. 511–22 (Oxford: Blackwell Scientific Publications) (In press)
3. Goodman, L. S. and Gilman, A. (1970). *The Pharmacological Basis of Therapeutics.* 4th Edn., pp. 531–2. (London: MacMillan)
4. Meyers, F. H., Jawetz, E. and Goldfien, A. (1970). *Review of Medical Pharmacology.* 2nd Edn., p. 241. (Los Altos: Lange Medical Publications)
5. Phaneuf, L. P., Grivel, M. L. and Ruckebusch, Y. (1972). Electromyoenterography during normal gastrointestinal activity, painful, or non-painful colic and morphine analgesia in the horse. *Can. J. Comp. Med.*, **36**, 138–44
6. Vaughan, W. E. M. (1951). The measurement of secretion and absorption by intestinal loops in conscious dogs. *J. Physiol.*, **112**, 32–3
7. Vaughan, W. E. M. (1954). The mode of action of drugs upon intestinal motility. *Pharmacol. Rev.*, **6**, 159–90

35

Physiological, pharmacological and therapeutic aspects of some gastrointestinal disorders in the horse

L. P. Phaneuf and Y. Ruckebusch

A high incidence of acute abdominal diseases is recognized in horses. A retrospective study of causes of death indicates that the alimentary tract was responsible for 33% of the lethal disorders in horses of less than 1 year to more than 15 years of age in UH[3]. An insurance firm has compiled that, in 1981, 20.9% of the claims for euthanasia in USA were caused by colic[4]. In both cases, the highest prevalence of gastrointestinal diseases is in horses of less than 1 year of age.

Abdominal problems are related to difficulties with the rapid progression of abundant digesta in organs of relatively limited volumes: stomach and small intestine. The large intestine, a much larger and more important digestive organ than in other domestic animals, is also vulnerable[2]. To fit into the abdominal cavity, this voluminous intestinal tube is multifolded, its diameter is alternatively dilated and narrowed, whereas the structure of its wall varies considerably from segment to segment. Accordingly, changes in the gastrointestinal transit and motility feedings are more marked than in other species. The morphological characteristics favour impaction, volvulus and intussusception.

Troubles in gastrointestinal motor functions lead to (1) interruption of the internal circulation of fluid and electrolytes, exsorption exceeding insorption, (2) perturbation of the enzymatic and bacterial digestive processes, and (3) intermittent or continuous visceral (sympathetic tracts mediated) or parietal (somatic tracts mediated) abdominal pain.

The first therapeutic intervention is usually to obtund the abdominal pain before a satisfactory examination of the horse can be performed to restore the altered gastrointestinal motility[9]. This review will discuss abdominal pain, normal and abnormal gastrointestinal motor events, mostly during chronic experimental situations, and the effect of drugs on these parameters.

EQUINE ABDOMINAL PAIN

Abdominal pain of the horse is conveniently classified as visceral pain and parietal pain. Visceral pain is associated with the typical signs of colic, where horses exhibit uncontrollable physical activity. External palpation, when possible, is usually not painful unless the troubled viscus is contacted. Parietal pain differs: the horses tend to remain immobile, and palpation of the abdomen causes considerable pain[24].

Specific experimental obstructions have been performed to determine changes in signs of pain and interrelationships with other physical signs. Ponies with ligation of the duodenum survive about 18 h, and most (5/6) show a ruptured stomach. Visceral pain, with body sweat more abundant at the thoracic and abdominal areas, is greatest 2 h before death[8]. Closed loop obstruction of the ileum (simulated volvulus) causes death in about 21 h, visceral pain is continuous, and sweating does not occur. In both duodenal obstruction and ileal volvulus, the sounds of intestinal motility disappear 2 h after onset of the problem[8]. Ponies with obstruction of the small colon display intermittent visceral pain limited to pawing or looking at the flank, mild sweating, and survive more than 36 h[8].

Models to simulate impaction of the large intestine use chronic fistulas at the caecum[10,13] or on the left ventral colon near the pelvic flexure[11]. A balloon inserted in such a fistula and inflated above capillary pressure provokes immediate colic or a visceral pain simulating impaction[10,11,13]. A change from pellets to hay may cause, within 24–48 h, impaction in the pelvic flexure-fistulated ponies[11]. Similarly, intravenous injection of an acaricide, amitraz, incites a progessive obstruction of the large intestine in the area of the pelvic flexure of ponies[15,23].

Some of these objective models for colic pain have been used to evaluate simple analgesic drugs[10,11,13,14] and combination of analgesic drugs[14]. On ponies subjected to induced caecal visceral pain[13], analgesia, obtained with single drugs and with a combination of two drugs have been subjectively ranked[14]. The combination of xylazine hydrochloride and fentanyl citrate has been rated a little better than xylazine alone for the relief of visceral pain (Table 35.1). With the pelvic flexure impaction model, flunixin or xylazine have relieved signs of impaction colic in ponies for 30–60 min[11].

Table 35.1 Performance ranking of drugs in four ponies with visceral pain. The best drug was ranked 4, with values decreasing to the poorest, which was ranked 1[14]

	4 measurements at 2-hour intervals					8 measurements at 4-hour intervals				
	Pony no.					Pony no.				
Treatment	*1*	*2*	*3*	*4*	*Rank values*	*1*	*2*	*3*	*4*	*Rank values*
Xylazine	1	3	4	4	12	2	3	3	4	12
Xylazine + fentanyl	3	4	3	3	13	3	4	4	3	14
Xylazine + meperidine	4	1	1	2	8	4	1	1	2	8
Xylazine + oxymorphone	2	2	2	1	7	1	2	2	1	6

Painful colic, with jejunal spasms detected electromyographically, has been relieved by intravenous administration of 1 mg/kg of morphine, in a pony[12].

GASTROINTESTINAL MOTOR EVENTS

The objective of motility of the stomach and small intestine of the horse is chiefly to mix chyme with secretions, and propel the liquid digesta rapidly into the caecum. The motor events in the caecocolic segments aim to delay the transit time of digesta for bacterial fermentation, and later to propel the residues to be voided as semi-solid faeces.

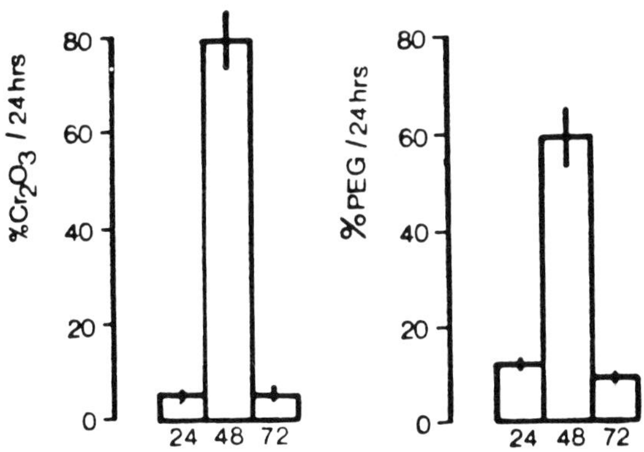

Figure 35.1 The transit time of Cr_2O_3 and of PEG through the gut in the horse. Time in hours after administration[1]

The gastrointestinal transit of particulates of chromic oxide (Cr_2O_3) or liquid polyethylene glycol (PEG) markers administered to ponies[1] takes nearly 72 h (Figure 35.1). In ponies fed chopped or long hay (33% cellulose) coloured with markers, the mean gastrointestinal transit time[26] is from 26 to 37 h. The passage of feeds from mouth to caecum requires about 3–4 h under normal feeding conditions. After a period of fasting of 12 h, this transit is made in less than 1 h because of practically no retention in the stomach[25]. The hyperactivity of feeding results from sensory stimulation during prehension, mastication and insalivation of each bolus of feed[6,25]. This hyperactivity of the intestinal tract has been measured from recordings of intraluminal pressure changes[11,21,23] and from electromyographic modifications[6,7,12,20].

Electromyography, with closely coupled subserosal wire-electrodes chronically implanted in the smooth muscle layers, has helped to gain some insights on the complicated motor activity of the stomach and the intestine of the conscious horse[19]. The concept is based on analysis of the various electrical potentials coinciding with the cellular activity of the longitudinal and circular

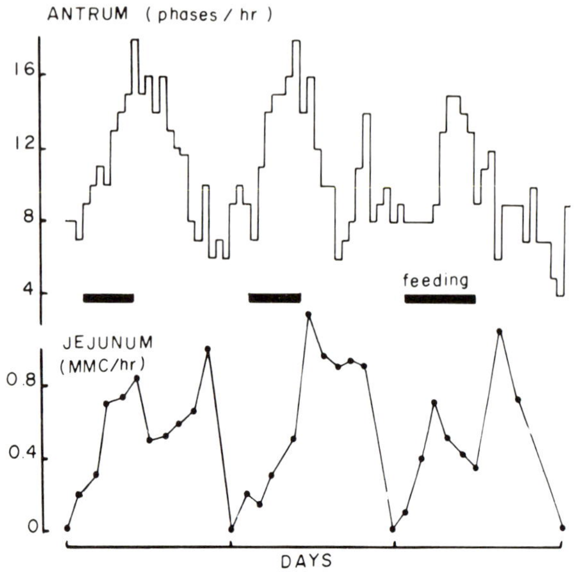

Figure 35.2 Integrated electromyograms of the antrum and jejunum in the horse. Periods of antral activity per hour are doubled during feeding. Migrating myoelectric complexes (MMC) are recorded during feeding but their frequency is enhanced after feeding

muscular layers. In the stomach and small intestine, slow waves originate from the longitudinal smooth muscles. They occur without any mechanical evidence at a rate characteristic for each segment: stomach (5/min), duodenum (15/min), ileum (10/min)[17]. During activity of the circular muscles, bursts of spike potentials are added to the slow waves (Figure 35.2). In the small intestine, this spiking activity can be irregular (ISA), when only some slow waves carry bursts of spike potentials. This type of activity has been identified with peristaltic activity. The regular activity (RSA), where each slow wave is loaded with spike potentials, corresponds to rhythmic segmentation. By electronic integrator analysis these electrical events can be grouped to represent the duration of the sequential phases of a migrating myoelectric complex (MMC)[18]. Ideally a MMC is the succession of a phase of ISA that fuses with a relatively short phase of RSA, itself ending in a phase of slow waves (quiescence or intestinal rest), and it lasts about 50 min in the horse. With normal feeding, the sequence is disorganized as the phases of ISA are extended at the expense of the phases of rest, which disappear or only account for 2–5% of the recording time (See Figure 35.5)[6].

Analysis of caecocolic electromyography is based on the duration of the bursts of spiking activity. Short spike bursts (SSB) last less than 5 s, are usually localized or unpropagated, and occur in series of about 10/min on the haustrations to mix the digesta. Long spike bursts (LSB) last 10–20 s, and show a tendency to be grouped in short periods which recur cyclically at intervals of 10 min during feeding, and at 15 min intervals during

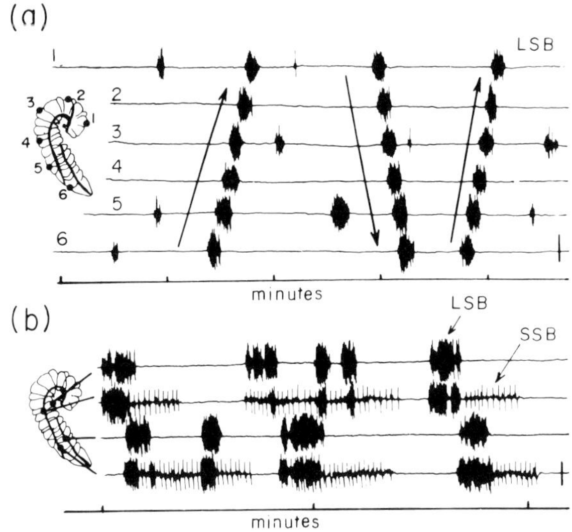

Figure 35.3 Patterns of activity of the caecum in the horse (a) propagated activity along the caecum or long spike bursts (LSB); (b) localized activity or short spike bursts (SSB)

fasting[19,21] (Figure 35.3). They spread orally, aborally, or in both directions from a pacemaker in the pelvic flexure of the large colon[22,23], and contribute to keep the caecum and ventral divisions of the colon (left or LVC, and right or RVC) filled[23]. LSB are associated with caecocolic retropulsion[23] and colic propulsion[18,23,25] while SSB are mainly concerned with storage[19].

The stomach of the horse undergoes almost no receptive relaxation to accommodate and store the ingested feeds. To avoid gastric impaction, immediate emptying is provided by probably a vagal reflex stimulated by buccal receptors. Upon arriving in the duodenum, the chyme activates receptors to cause the MMCs to disappear and be replaced by IRA activity until the end of gastric emptying[19]. As most of the soluble carbohydrates (95%) are absorbed in the duodeno-ileum, the higher insulin level presumably contributes also to augment motor activity in the small intestine. The increase in caecal LSB associated with feeding is due to a gastro-caecal reflex[18]. It regulates the ileal inflow and the colic outflow of digesta and maintains the caecal volume nearly constant[21,25]. Also, during the post-feeding period, metabolites of microbial digestion, first ammonia alone then ammonia volatile fatty acids, exert a chemical stimulation to increase the rate of SSB in the caecum and proximal colon (Figure 35.4(a)). When ammonia concentration predominates, both SSB and LSB hyperactivity occur in the caecum. Feeding elicits a stimulating effect on the colon similar to its action on the caecum: retropulsion–propulsion (LSB), and local activity of the haustrations (SSB)[21,23,25]. The caecocolic segment functions as a unit regulated by a pacemaker area, at the junction of the ventral and dorsal divisions of the colon (pelvic flexure), that keeps this orad part of the large

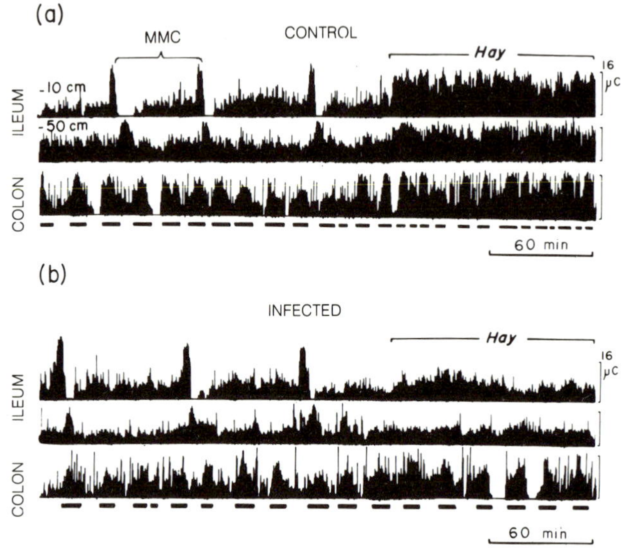

Figure 35.4 Electrical spiking activity summed at 20 s intervals of the ileo-caeco-colic region in the normal (a) and infected (b) pony. Migrating myoelectric complexes (MMC) were recorded at hourly intervals at the ileal level. Phases of increased spiking activity recorded at 20 min intervals on the colon are underlined. Continuous ileal spiking activity and increase in the frequency of the phases of colonic activity were recorded during feeding in the normal but not in the infected pony[6]

intestine filled with digesta[23]. The reservoir activity of that portion of the large intestine is facilitated by retropulsive events (LSB).

These are seen even after resection of the extrinsic nerve supply to the large intestine: vagosympathetic nerve nets surrounding the right colic artery and the colic branch of the ileocolic artery[22]. Lowering of the temperature of digesta from 38 to 20 °C for 2 h has reduced the frequency and amplitude but has increased the duration of the pressure changes in the lumen of the pelvic flexure-left dorsal colon[23]. During feeding, ponies experimentally infected with strongyles have exhibited reduced motor activity at the ileum[6], the caecum[6], the right ventral colon[6], and the left ventral colon[23] (Figure 35.4(b)).

There is a paucity of objective information on the pharmacological basis of intestinal motor disturbances in horses. *In vitro* studies have shown that norepinephrine favours contraction of the longitudinal fibres and inhibits the activity of the circular fibres of horse jejunum[16]. Other drugs, which affect the autonomic nervous system, have performed as expected on strips of duodenum, jejunum and ileum[16]. On tissue from the pelvic flexure, sodium ricinoleate has no effect[22].

In chronic studies with normal ponies, the effect of various drugs on the rate of passage of markers (Cr_2O_3 and PEG) through the digestive tract has been determined[1]. Morphine delays the passage of Cr_2O_3, and with PEG there is haste then a delay in the transit. *Tinct. opii* has the opposite effect to morphine on each marker. Meperidine does not affect the passage of Cr_2O_3, but it speeds then slows the transit of PEG. Atropine and loperamide expedite the passage through the gut of both markers[1]. On the basis of electromyographic evidences, intravenous morphine hydrochloride (1 mg/kg), in a pony, increases the spiking activity at the jejunum and the right ventral colon[12]. Painful (visceral) colic, characterized by long-lasting (15–20 s) spike bursts recurring every 2–3 min in the circular layer of the jejunum, and electromyographic silence at the antrum and right ventral colon, responds also to morphine. The antrum remains silent but the jejunal spasms are replaced by a vigorous regular spiking activity which appears also on the right ventral colon together with irregular activity on the ileum[12]. It is interesting to note that parietal pain due to occlusion of the ileum presents a continuous hyperactivity of the cranial portions of the small intestine with spasms of the jejunum[12]. With the pelvic flexure–impaction model for colic, flunixin corrects the visceral pain without altering the elevated blood flow and lowering the intraluminal pressure changes[11]. In the same colic model, xylazine overcomes the pain but lowers the blood flow of colic by 50%, and relaxes the wall of the large colon near the pelvic flexure for 30–45 min[11].

Intraluminal pressure changes in the large colon are not significantly altered by synthetic gastrin I or by caerulein administered to vagotomized

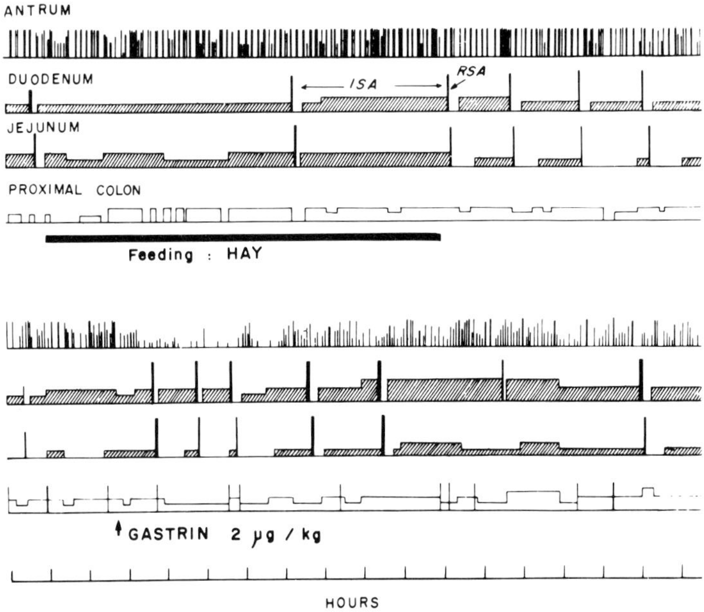

Figure 35.5 Comparative effects of feeding and gastrin on the motor profile of the antrum, the small intestine and proximal colon. Gastric motility was inhibited following the administration of gastrin which in turn increased the number of periods of regular spiking activity (RSA)

ponies[5]. Insulin has little effect on the stomach motility but disorganizes the MMC pattern of the small intestine. Gastrin inhibits the stomach but increases RSA in the small intestine (Figure 35.5).

Mebendazole (10 mg/kg) in control ponies inhibits gastrointestinal activity[6] for 4 h. In strongyle infected ponies, mebendazole produces a greater reduction in electrical motor events that lasts[6] for over 12 h. This anthelmintic affects the colonic feeding hyperactivity: momentarily in normal ponies, and by 50% in strongyle infected ponies (Figure 35.6).

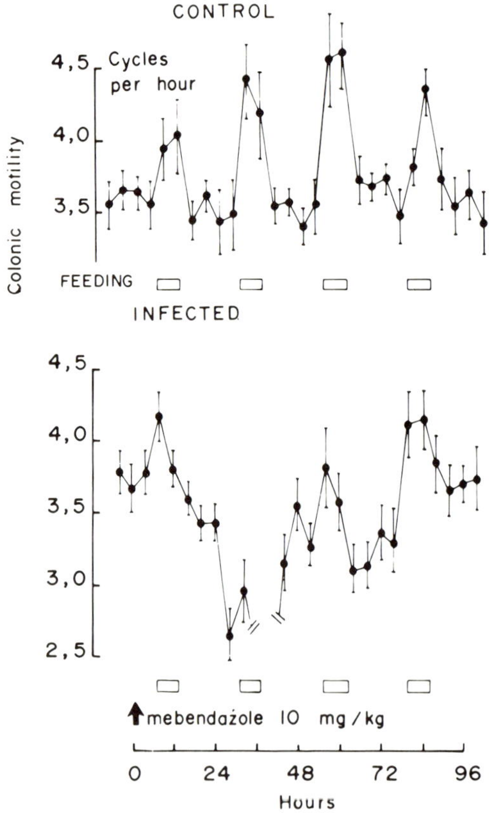

Figure 35.6 Postprandial colonic activity unchanged by mebendazole drenching (control). In the infected pony, mebendazole (10 mg/kg) reduced the number of colonic activity cycles and abolished the increase seen on feeding[6]

An acaricide (amitraz) administered intravenously produces a decrease in the amplitude of intraluminal pressure changes. Dissociation of the pressure-peak activity of the left dorsal colon from that of the left ventral colon perturbes the co-ordination between the segments connected by the pelvic flexure[22].

CONCLUSIONS

From these limited reports, it is evident that equine gastrointestinal pharmacology is in its infancy. Most of the armamentarium recommended is based on anecdotal impressions or interpretations from data obtained in physiologically different species (ponies vs. horses). A conceptual basis for efficient digestive pharmacotherapy in horses is still to be acquired through experimentation with models of the disturbances and objective techniques of measurements.

References

1. Alexander, F. (1978). The effect of some anti-diarrheal drugs on intestinal transit and faecal excretion of water and electrolytes in the horse. *Equine Vet. J.*, **10**, 229–34
2. Argenzio, R. A. (1975). Functions of the equine large intestine and their interrelationship in disease. *Cornell Vet.*, **65**, 303–30
3. Baker, J. R. and Ellis, C. E. (1981). A survey of post mortem findings in 480 horses (1958 to 1980). 1. Causes of death. *Equine Vet. J.*, **13**, 43–6
4. Barkley, J. E. (1982). Euthanasia – two sides of the story. *Equine Vet. Data*, **3**, 119–21
5. Brondum, J. (1978). Effect of synthetic human gastrin I and caerulein on motility of the equine colon. *Physiologist*, **21**, 13
6. Buéno, L., Ruckebusch, Y. and Dorchies, P. (1979). Disturbances of digestive motility in horses associated with strongyle infection. *Vet. Parasitol.*, **5**, 253–60
7. Candau, M. and Vigroux, P. (1974). Sur le mécanisme de l'hypermotilité caecale liée au repas chez le cheval. *C. R. Séances Soc. Biol.*, **168**, 893–7
8. Datt, S. C. and Usenik, E. A. (1975). Intestinal obstruction in the horse. Physical signs and blood chemistry. *Cornell Vet.*, **65**, 152–72
9. Davis, L. E. and Knight, A. P. (1979). Review of the clinical pharmacology of the equine digestive system. *J. Equine Med. Surg.*, **1**, 27–35
10. Lowe, J. E. (1978). Xylazine, pentazocine, meperidine, and dipyrone for relief of balloon induced colic: a double blind comparative evaluation. *J. Equine Med. Surg.*, **2**, 286–91
11. Lowe, J. E., Sellers, A. F. and Brondum, J. (1980). Equine pelvic flexure impaction. A model used to evalute motor events and compare drug response. *Cornell Vet.*, **70**, 401–12
12. Phaneuf, L. P., Grivel, M. L. and Ruckebusch, Y. (1972). Electromyoenterography during normal gastro-intestinal activity, painful or non-painful colic and morphine analgesia in the horse. *Can. J. Comp. Med.*, **36**, 138–44
13. Pippi, N. L. and Lumb, W. V. (1979). Objective tests of analgesic drugs in ponies. *Am. J. Vet. Res.*, **40**, 1082–6
14. Pippi, N. L., Lumb, W. V., Fialho, S. A. G. *et al.* (1979). A model for evaluating pain in ponies. *J. Equine Med. Surg.*, **3**, 430–5
15. Roberts, M. C. and Seawright, A. A. (1979). Amitraz-induced large intestinal impaction in the horse. *Aust. Vet. J.*, **55**, 553
16. Ruckebusch, M., Grivel, M. L. and Fargeas, M. L. (1971). Sur l'action paradoxale de l'adrénaline au niveau de l'intestin grêle chez le cheval. *Arch. Int. Pharmacodyn.*, **194**, 387–402
17. Ruckebusch, Y. (1973). Les particularités motrices du jéjuno-iléon chez le cheval. *Cah. Méd. Vét.*, **42**, 128–43
18. Ruckebusch, Y. (1981). Motor functions of the intestine. *Adv. Vet. Sci. Comp. Med.*, **25**, 345–69
19. Ruckebusch, Y., Buéno, L. and Fioramonti, J. (1981). *La Mécanique Digestive chez les Mammifères.* (Paris: Masson)
20. Ruckebusch, Y., Grivel, M. L. and Hatey, F. (1971). Etude électromyographique du profil moteur de l'intestin grêle chez le cheval *(Equus caballus). C. R. Séances Soc. Biol.*, **169**, 1454–9

21. Ruckebusch, Y. and Vigroux, P. (1974). Etude électromyographique de la motricité du caecum chez le cheval *(Equus caballus). C. R. Séances Soc. Biol.*, **168**, 887-92
22. Sellers, A. F., Lowe, J. E. and Brondum, J. (1979). Motor events in equine large colon. *Am. J. Physiol.*, **237**, E457-64
23. Sellers, A. F., Lowe, J. E., Drost, C. J. *et al.* (1982). Retropulsion-propulsion in equine large colon. *Am. J. Vet. Res.*, **43**, 390-6
24. Stashnak, T. S. (1980). Colic evaluation. *Equine Vet. Data*, **1**, 119-26
25. Vigroux, P., Candau, M. and Ruckebusch, Y. (1975). Motricité caecale et transit caeco-colique chez le cheval. *C. R. Séances Soc. Biol.*, **169**, 1617-22
26. Wolter, R., Durix, A. and Letourneau, J. C. (1974). Influence du mode de présentation du fourrage sur la vitesse du transit digestif chez le poney. *Ann. Zootech.*, **23**, 293-300

36
Pharmacological control of reproductive mechanisms in the equine female

E. Palmer, B. Bour and F. Chevalier

The compounds used to control reproductive phenomena in the equine species are similar to those in other species, except for doses and indications. Time of administration in relation to the oestrous cycle is very important for their efficacy. This chapter reviews first the effects of different chemicals used in experiments in the equine. Secondly, it describes their association in sequences of treatments for control of the time of ovulation. Thirdly, it illustrates how the precise knowledge of the physiological situation is necessary to control the induction of ovulation at the transition from anoestrus to cyclicity.

CHEMICAL COMPOUNDS

Gonadotrophins

Only pregnant mare serum gonadotrophin (PMSG), human chorionic gonadotrophin (hCG) and equine pituitary extracts have been studied extensively.

PMSG has little biological effect[25] at doses up to 100 000 IU. This dose is higher than those used in other domestic species (2000 IU induces superovulation in the cow), but it is much lower than physiological production in the pregnant mare in which total circulating PMSG reaches several millions of units. Low biological activity is easily explained by low affinity for equine FSH and LH receptors[7,33]. Endogenous PMSG in the mare has the biological effect of luteinizing hormone (LH) rather than follicle stimulating hormone (FSH). At the present time no indication of exogenous PMSG administration can be proposed.

Table 36.1 Induction of (multiple) ovulations in seasonally anoestrus pony mares by injection of pituitary extracts during January (from ref. 9)

	Control	*Experimental group* Ethanolic extract	Purified MPC MF3
No. of mares	4	4	4
No. ovulating	0	4	4
No. of ovulations	0	2.3 ± 0.5	1.5 ± 0.3
Days of ovulations	—	(14, 14, 17) (23) (13, 16) (15, 15, 19)	(15) (16, 17) (14, 22) (25)

Treatment consisted in 14 days of treatment of a total of 0.122 and 13.2 mg/100 kg body weight of pituitary extracts MPCMF3 and EE respectively, equivalent to 6.6 NIHFSHSI + 0.6 NIHLHS1

Equine pituitary extracts (Table 36.1) have been used successfully for two purposes: induction of preovulatory size follicle during anovulatory season, and induction of multiple follicles for multiple ovulations during the breeding season[9,19]. Administration during a prolonged period is necessary to obtain both effects.

Calculation of the dose is tedious due to varying degrees of purity of extracts, and difference in the method for their assay (biological or radioreceptor assays using different species as receptors and different standards). Duration of treatment should be approximately 6 days (day 11–16 post-ovulation or day 1–6 of oestrus) for superovulation in cyclic mares and 14–20 days for stimulation of the anoestrous mare. Two commercial preparations, one of equine pituitaries (Pitropin, Biological Specialities, Middleton, WI, USA)[8] and one of porcine pituitaries (FSH P – Armour, Baldwin Labs, Omaha NE, USA)[17] have been used with success to induce superovulation.

A pure LH effect is obtained with hCG preparations. It is widely used for induction of ovulation of a preovulatory follicle. According to different authors[20,34], 1500–3000 IU, subcutaneously, intramuscularly or intravenously, induce ovulation between 36 and 48 h after injection in 75% of the mares (Table 36.2). Induced ovulation is normal for all criteria, including fertility. Two problems related to use of hCG for induction of ovulation in the mare are the choice of right time for injection (i.e. time of occurrence of preovulatory follicle), and the presence of antibodies against hCG in the serum of mares after repeated injections[31].

Table 36.2 Distribution of time of ovulation following intravenous injection of 2500 IU hCG on the day when a follicle reaches 35 mm in diameter (unpublished data)

Days following injection	1	2	3	4	5	6
Percentage of mares ovulating ($n = 145$)	11	73	4	4	1.5	6

Sexual steroids

Oestrogens (17β oestradiol benzoate, 5 mg/day, or diethylstilboestrol, 2 mg) induced oestrus behaviour in the mare provided the circulating level of progesterone is low. The presence of endogenous[22] or exogenous[14] progesterone will suppress this effect. Practical applications are induction of heat in anoestrous mares for semen collection of stallions, and to test for the presence or absence of an active corpus luteum[22]. The latter effect may provide a pregnancy diagnosis if performed on day 17 postovulation, or a diagnosis to separate ovarian inactivity from persistent corpus luteum conditions. Oestrus induced by oestrogens is usually anovulatory and the treatment has no application in mares for mating.

Progesterone may be used for its direct effect on the genital tract, i.e. to maintain pregnancy. For this purpose very high doses and frequent injections are needed to obtain 'physiological' levels[13] (200 mg per day in water solution). Such a treatment allows pregnancy to continue in spite of castration of the mare on the 35th day[35]. It is, however, difficult to give an indication of use to avoid abortion because death of embryo probably precedes abortion and luteolysis.

Progesterone may be used also for its feedback effects on the brain and pituitary. Oestrus can be suppressed in mares with 100 mg of progesterone daily. However, 200 mg are needed to suppress ovulation and inhibition is not effective for preovulatory follicles which may ovulate during the first 2–3 days of treatment[24]. After 18 days of progesterone treatment, onset of oestrus will occur within 3–5 days[16]. More complex treatments for synchronization of oestrus and ovulation will be discussed below. Progesterone can be replaced by synthetic progestins given either by oral or vaginal route[26, 38]. The association of progesterone and oestrogens has been proposed to enhance the inhibitory effect of progesterone, and to obtain a better synchronization of oestrus and ovulation[21].

Testosterone can induce male sexual behaviour in both the gelding and the mare. In the stallion and the mare its negative feedback on the pituitary reversibly reduces the level of gonadotropin and induces atrophy of the gonads[6, 37]. Some anabolic steroids can have the same inhibitory effects[37].

LHRH

LHRH has been shown to induce a transitory release of both FSH and LH in the mare[17]. The amount and ratio of FSH and LH released are effected by the steroid environment[12]. Practical application of LHRH in horse breeding remains questionable: some authors have induced advanced ovulation with single or multiple[18] injections of LHRH, but others have not[15].

During winter anoestrus a sequence of LHRH and progesterone injections have resulted in induction of ovulation without corpus luteum formation in acyclic mares[11].

Prostaglandins (PG)

Prostaglandin $F_{2\alpha}$ is now considered to be the natural luteolytic factor secreted by the uterus around day 14 postovulation. Its injection (5–10 mg

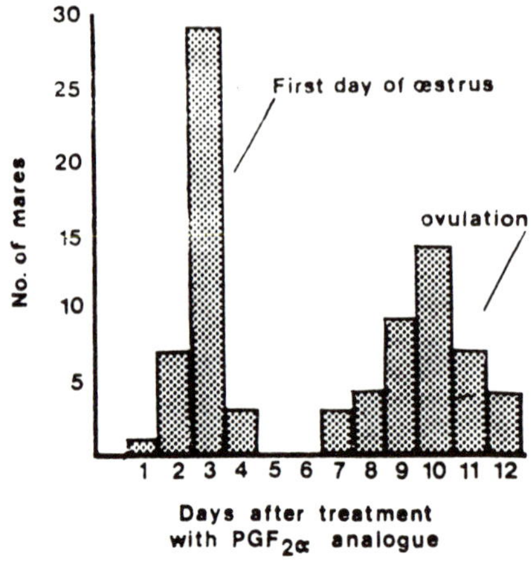

Figure 36.1 Distribution of time of onset of oestrus and ovulation following injection of a $PGF_{2\alpha}$ analogue. Adapted from ref. 1

intramuscularly or subcutaneously) causes lysis of the corpus luteum, provided ovulation has occurred more than 4 days previously. Many analogues[1,23,40] have been used with success to induce oestrus after 3–5 days, and ovulation 5–12 days after treatment (Figure 36.1). Fertility is not affected. The differences between various $PGF_{2\alpha}$ analogues are in the dose needed, and the ratio between luteolytic and side-effects. Practical uses are treatment of persistent corpus luteum, synchronization of oestrus, and early abortion (before 35 days of pregnancy). Induction of foaling at term is possible with a PG analogue[32]. The luteolytic effect is absent, as ovaries are no longer secreting progesterone for 150 days.

Other compounds tested on the mare

Foaling can also be induced[29] by low doses of oxytocin, 2.5–10 IU, or repeated large doses of dexamethasone, 100 mg daily[3]. Dexamethasone was shown recently to suppress oestrus behaviour in ovariectomized mares[5]. Some adrenal steroids are associated probably with oestrus during winter ovarian inactivity as a similarity exists between oestrus of ovariectomized and seasonally inactive mares[4]. Further studies are needed to find some practical consequences.

Anti-oestrogens (clomiphene citrate) have been tested in order to stimulate ovarian activity with conflicting results[14,30].

SEQUENTIAL ASSOCIATION OF TREATMENTS TO OVULATION

The compounds described above affect a very precise step of the ovarian pattern towards ovulation. A clear understanding of the physiological situation of the animal is needed to use the appropriate compound at the right time.

Different approaches to the control of the time of ovulation can serve to illustrate how to combine the diagnosis of ovarian status and the sequence of a hormonal treatment.

(1) In mares, prediction of the time of ovulation, by oestrus signs and rectal palpation, is not too accurate. Induction of ovulation of a follicle at a short and precise interval has been attempted with hCG injection (2500 IU, i.v. or i.m. on a follicle larger than 35 mm diameter. A good prediction of time (Table 36.2) of ovulation has been obtained: 73% of the females ovulating between 24 and 48 h after the injection. Fertility of induced ovulation was not affected in a field trial comparing fertility of ovulations occurring either spontaneously (fertility 48%, $n=50$) or induced by hCG ($f=52\%$, $n=74$). Efficiency of such a system is dependent on the precision of rectal palpation.

(2) When palpation is not possible, another sign is needed to decide when to inject hCG. 70% success is reported with an injection on day 1 or 2 of oestrus (ovulation 24–48 h later) during the breeding season[34]. Very poor results are usual during the transitory season[39] when oestrus is the only criterion of choice.

(3) When oestrus detection is not possible, control of the ovarian events is obtained by synchronization of onset of oestrus, and induction of ovulation.

The synchronization of onset of oestrus is performed by using one of the following combinations:

(a) Two successive PG injections 18 days apart[16],
(b) a PG–hCG–PG sequence[28] on days 0, 6, and 14,
(c) a 18 day regimen of progesterone or progestagen[16],
(d) a 8 day progestagen treatment associated with a prostaglandin injection at the end of the treatment[24].

Although comparison has not shown a significant experimental difference between these systems, for theoretical considerations the last one is preferred. The two PG sequence requires that all females be cycling before treatment and as the mechanism involves control of two ovulations, the risks of failure are increased. Progesterone treatment alone may be more effective when administered earlier in the breeding season; the induced ovulation may be the first of the season. Females with persistent corpus luteum, a very common condition in large mares, will not respond. Best synchronization of onset of oestrus and induction of ovulation results in 50% of mares ovulating within the same 24 h period, and 75% within a 96 h period.

For practical reasons the progestagen is given by vaginal sponges, which, in spite of mild local irritation, have no deleterious effect on fertility[26]. Thus, the synchronization of onset of oestrus is obtained with only two manipulations of the mares one week apart: sponge insertion on day 0, and sponge removal together with prostaglandin administration on day 7.

The mechanism of action of this treatment has been described in details[10] (Figure 36.2): sponge insertion at random time of the cycle causes a sharp decrease of LH, which remains low throughout the treatment. FSH levels are

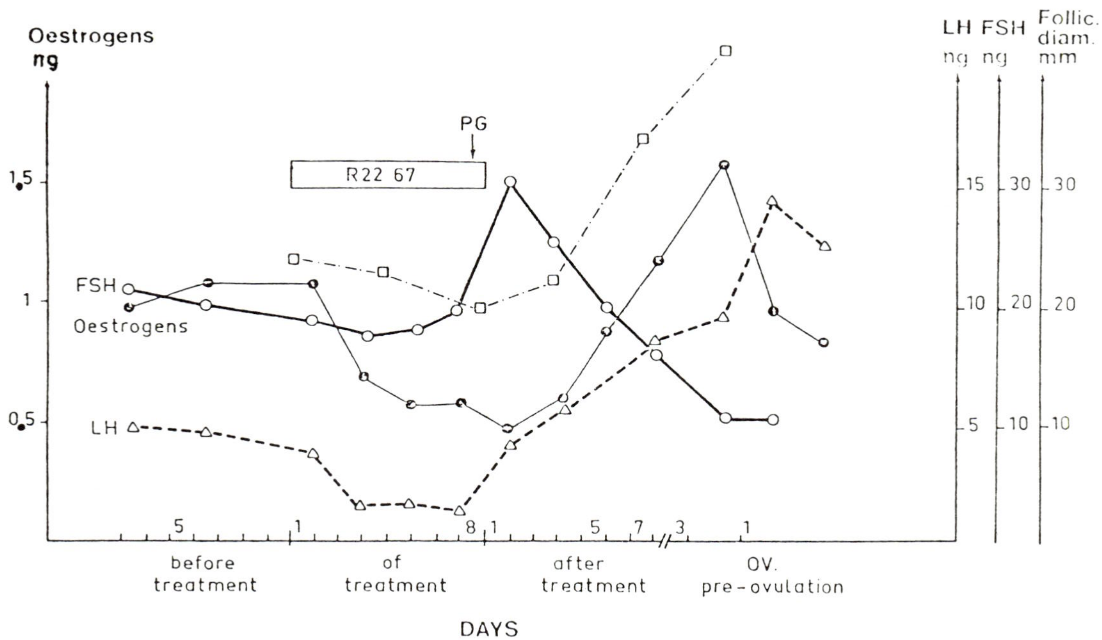

Figure 36.2 Effect of a treatment for synchronization of oestrus on endocrine and ovarian parameters (from ref. 10). Treatment consisted in vaginal sponges impregnated with 0.5 g progestagen (Altrenogest, R2267, Roussel Uclaf, France) and intramuscular injection of a PG analogue (1 ml Estrumate, ICI, UK) at sponge removal. Treatment was started at random time of the oestrous cycle ($n = 32$)

Table 36.3 Field trial of breeding at predetermined time after synchronization of oestrus and ovulation in mares not pregnant at the end of traditional breeding season

Protocol	
Day 0	Echographic selection of mares not pregnant from mating during breeding season
(July 25 ± 7)	Insertion of polyurethane sponges impregnated with 0.5 or 1 g of Altrenogest
Day 7	Withdrawal of sponges, i.m. injection of 1 ml Estrumate ($PGF_{2\alpha}$ analogue)
Day 12	Mating or AI with fresh semen stored for 0–8 h
Day 14	i.m. injection of hCG (2500 or 5000 IU)
Day 15	Mating or AI
Day 35	Echographic pregnancy diagnosis (result)

Result

35 mares pregnant/93 mares treated 38%

Dose of Altrenogest is not significant
1 g 17/45 (38%) 0.5 g 18/48 (38%)

Non-significant effect of dose of hCG
2500 IU 14/47 (30%) 5000 IU 21/45 (46%)

Significant decrease of fertility with AI
Mating 25/44 (57%) AI 10/49 (20%)

unaffected by sponge insertion. The diameter of the largest follicle, and the level of oestrogens progressively decline with the progestagen administration. Within 2 days from sponge removal, and prostaglandin injection, progesterone is low in all animals and FSH and LH show a sudden increase. Later (days 2–8 after removal) a follicle grows, secreting increasing amounts of oestrogens, and progressively inhibiting the FSH secretion. LH continues to increase until synchronized ovulation occurs around day 11 (SD = 2.8 days) post-treatment.

This treatment, associated with injection of hCG 7 days postremoval and breeding at predetermined times, gave satisfactory fertility results when applied in farm practice. In spite of selection of mares which had not conceived during the normal breeding season, and of use of a suboptimal artificial insemination technique in half of the mares (Table 36.3), 38% became pregnant.

When oestrus and ovulation are needed in February, a stimulation of the ovarian activity by 2 months photoperiodic treatment[26] is required prior to hormonal synchronization. This time lag corresponds to the mean interval from onset of photoperiodic stimulation to ovulatory responses without hormonal synchronization (Table 36.4).

INDUCTION OF OVULATION DURING WINTER ANOESTRUS

Many attempts to induce ovulation at different dates of the winter months have shown recently that this problem is a complex one. The mechanism of transition from anoestrus to cyclicity is a progressive phenomenon still poorly understood.

Table 36.4 Effect of combined photoperiodic* and hormonal† treatments on the onset of cyclicity and synchronization of ovulation in Welsh pony mares (from ref. 26)

Group No.	*Treatment*	*No. of mares*	*Day of 1st ovulation of the year*‡	*Proportion of mares with synchronized ovulation*
1	Untreated controls	8	113 ± 7††	
2	Light	11	35 ± 4	
3	Light + synchronization on 10 January**	12	36 ± 5	0/12††
4	Light + synchronization on 1 February**	12	36 ± 3	9/12
5	Light + synchronization on 20 February**	12	45 ± 6	10/12

* Controls = natural variation of daylength; light = 16 h light: 8 h dark from 25 November
† Oral progestagen (20 mg R2267) for 10 days and 2500 IU hCG 10 days after withdrawal of progestagen
‡ Day 1 = 1 January; mean ± SEM, estimated by blood progesterone increase
**Day of hCG injection
††Significantly different from all other values, $p < 0.01$

The hypothesized mechanism involves:

(1) A natural tendency for a 1 year cycle of alternating activity and inactivity, even under constant day length.
(2) Synchronization of this cycle with season via photoperiodic stimulation.
(3) Transformation of a neural signal to an endocrine signal by the pineal gland secreting melatonin.
(4) Successive effect on pituitary secretion of FSH and then of LH.
(5) Responses of the ovary to gonadotrophin secretions by follicular growth, maturation and ovulation.
(6) After first ovulation of the season, continuous cyclicity is helped by feedback mechanisms which lead to surges of gonadotrophins in responses to variations of steroids.

Natural evolution of hormonal levels during transition from inactivity to cyclicity is presented in Figure 36.3. A period of high fluctuating FSH and constant low LH levels is associated with waves of follicular growth occurring at increasing frequency, and reaching progressively larger diameters before atresia then regression of these follicles[14].

Stimulation by photoperiod is now well documented[27]; mares submitted to 14.5–16 h of light per day during winter show recrudescence of cyclicity approximately 2.5 months later. In spite of its efficiency, this method is not sufficient because of the 2.5 months of delay and pharmacological attempts were made to get a more rapid response.

The phenomenon of transition being progressive, the period at which a treatment is started greatly influences its efficiency. This period can be defined in individual mares by clinical examination of the physiological state

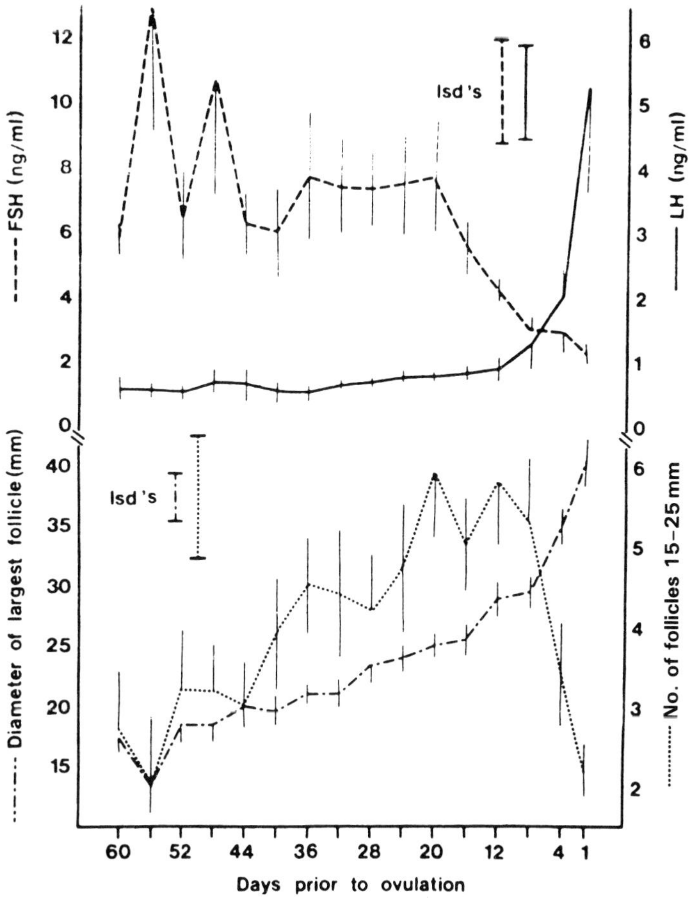

Figure 36.3 Evolution of gonadotropins levels and follicular growth during 2 months before first ovulation of the season. From ref. 14

Table 36.5 Pharmacological stimulation of winter ovarian activity of the mare

Period	*Ovarian status*	*Mechanism*	*Method of treatment*	*Result*	*Reference*
January	anoestrus	FSH & LH deficiency	Equine pituitary extracts	(multiple) ovulation	29
March	early transition	LH deficiency only	LH (hCG) supplementation of basal level	1 ovulation (but anti-hCG)	unpublished
April	late transition	control of rhythmicity by steroid feedback	progestagen treatment	shorter oestrus and more predictable ovulation, but not earlier in the year	2
May	cyclicity				

of reproduction ('deep anoestrus', 'shallow anoestrus'). Experiments with groups of mares selected for homogeneous seasonality have shown the time scale to be equivalent (Table 36.5).

During deep anoestrus, when ovaries are very small and bear no follicle above 10 mm, only pituitary extracts containing both FSH and LH can induce growth of follicles and ovulation[9]. Practical use of this technique is limited by occurrence of multiple ovulations and high cost of horse pituitary extracts which are not easily available to practicians.

Later in the transition period, the hypothesis was that only LH was the limiting factor for follicle maturation and ovulation. As hCG constitutes a potent LH substitute in the mare and does not bind to horse FSH receptors we have tried to mimic an increased basal level of LH by daily injections of hCG to seasonally inactive pony females. Supplementation with low doses of hCG (200 IU/day) during March induced the differentiation of a preovulatory follicle, but this was not successful in February (Table 36.6).

This LH supplementation has the advantage of inducing the growth of only one follicle, and fertility is normal. Unfortunately, when a search for antibodies against hCG was made in the animals of experiment I, all four

Table 36.6 Induction of first ovulation of the breeding season with daily administration of low dose of hCG to anoestrous Welsh pony mares

	Experiment I (not mated)		*Experiment II (mated every 48 h when preovulatory follicle)*					
Treatment started hCG 200 IU/day	*Control*	*Treated March 6th*	*Control*		*Treated Feb. 8th*		*Treated March 8th*	
Additional 2000 IU injection when preovulatory follicle	—	+	—	+	—	+	—	+
No. of ♀	3	4	4	4	4	4	4	4
No. ovulating in February (conceived)	0	0	0	1(1)	2(2)	0	0	0
No. ovulating in March (conceived)	0	4	0	0	0	1(1)	3(3)	4(2)
No. ovulating in April and May (conceived)	3	0	4(3)	3(2)	2(1)	3(3)	1(0)	0
Mean day of first ovulation ± SEM	124 ±8	77 ±3	102 ±6	91 ±14	75 ±15	110 ±15	83 ±8	75 ±2
Proportion of females ovulating before April 1st	0/3	4/4	1/8		3/8		7/8	

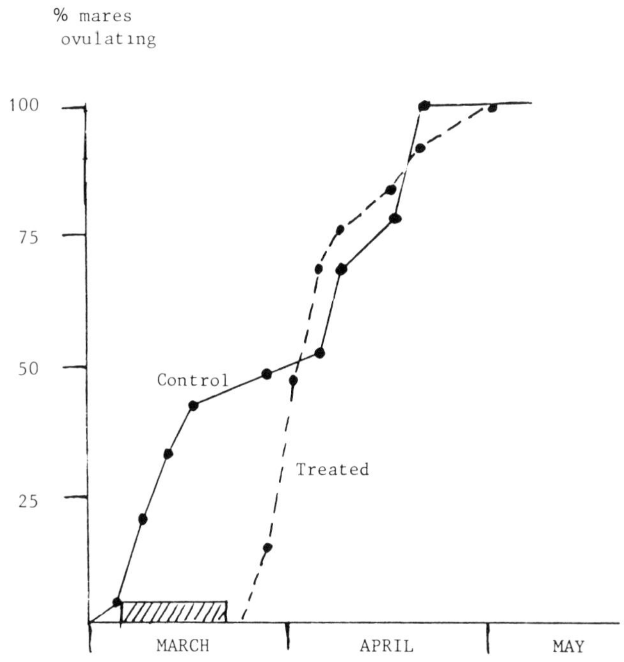

Figure 36.4 Cumulated distribution of first ovulation of the season in 13 Altrenogest treated (----) and 23 control (——) mares. Adapted from ref. 2. The shaded area shows the approximate period of treatment (not exactly the same in all treated mares). First ovulation occurs in a shorter, more predictable period, but not earlier

treated mares were positive. The results of such experiments confirm the theoretical basis of the protocol, but practical use is limited because of the immune response which probably limits its efficiency to 1 year!

In the Southern hemisphere, during September, sequences of LHRH injections and progesterone have induced surges of FSH, some follicular growth, and occasional ovulations without corpus luteum formation, probably because of LH deficiency[11]. Further studies are needed to obtain a simple and efficient treatment based on this mechanism.

In March and April, progestagen treatment of mares during the prolonged oestrous cycle which precedes the first ovulation of the year is followed by an oestrous period of shorter and more predictable duration (Figure 36.4). However, this treatment does not modify the mean date of the first ovulation of the year. Response to progestagen treatment can be predicted from the individual ovarian status of treated mares[36]. In mares with no follicle larger than 15 mm neither control nor treated mares ovulate within 1 month. In mares with 15–25 mm follicles, 4/7 control and 2/7 treated mares ovulate, and 3/6 and 5/6 if a 30 mm follicle is present at initiation of treatment.

CONCLUSION

In spite of numerous studies on reproductive physiology of the mare, few compounds have a precise practical application for the veterinarian. Prostaglandins, hCG, and progestagen are the only compounds available, efficient, and of practical interest. Pituitary extracts are less available, and further studies are needed to give a practical standardized method of use. LHRH remains at the research level.

With this limited number of compounds, control of ovarian activity is possible during the whole breeding season. Treatments for synchronization of oestrus and ovulation are new management tools that do not increase fertility. However, one must keep in mind that they have no potential for increasing fertility compared to natural ovulation.

Control of transition from anoestrus to cyclicity by pharmacological agents remains at the experimental level. Progress has been made in the theoretical approach to this problem but no practical treatment can be proposed to induce, without adverse effects, an ovulation earlier than the spontaneous first ovulation of the year. For the breeder, the solution consists in mating mares during their breeding season or to induce cyclicity with photoperiodic treatments.

References

1. Allen, W. R., Stewart, F., Cooper, M. J. *et al.* (1974). Further studies on the use of synthetic prostaglandin analogues for inducing luteolysis in mares. *Equine Vet. J.*, **6**, 31–5
2. Allen, W. R., Urwin, V., Simpson, D. J., *et al.* (1980). Preliminary studies on the use of an oral progestagen to induce oestrus and ovulation in seasonally anoestrus thoroughbred mares. *Equine Vet. J.*, **12**, 141–5
3. Alm, C., Sullivan, J. and First, N. L. (1972). Dexamethasone induced parturition in the mare. *J. Anim. Sci.*, **35**, 1115
4. Asa, C. S., Goldfoot, D. A., Garcia, M. C. *et al.* (1980). Sexual behavior in ovariectomized and seasonally anovulatory pony mares *(Equus caballus)*. *Horm. Behav.*, **14**, 46–54
5. Asa, C. S., Goldfoot, D. A., Garcia, M. C. *et al.* (1980). Dexamethasone suppression of sexual behaviour in the ovariectomized mare. *Horm. Behav.*, **14**, 55–64
6. Bernstson, W. E., Hoyer, J. H., Squires, E. L. *et al.* (1979). Influence of exogenous testosterone on sperm production seminal quality and libido of stallions. *J. Reprod. Fert., Suppl.*, **27**, 13–17
7. Combarnous, Y. (1981). Hypothèse originale sur la spécificité de liaison des hormones glycoprotéiques à leurs récepteurs. *C. R. Acad. Sci. Paris*, **293**, 229–32
8. Douglas, R. H. (1979). Review of induction of superovulation and embryo transfer in the equine. *Theriogenology*, **2**, 33–46
9. Douglas, R. H., Nuti, L. and Ginther, O. J. (1974). Induction of ovulation and multiple ovulation in seasonally anovulatory mares with equine pituitary fractions. *Theriogenology*, **2**, 133–42
10. Driàncourt, M. A. and Palmer, E. (1982). Seasonal and individual effects on ovarian and endocrine response to synchronization treatment. Third International Symposium on Equine Reproduction. *J. Reprod. Fert. Suppl.*, **32**, (In press)
11. Evans, M. J. and Irvine, C. H. G. (1977). Induction of follicular development, maturation and ovulation by GnRH administration to acyclic mares. *Biol. Reprod.*, **16**, 452–62
12. Foster, J. P., Evans, M. J. and Irvine, C. H. G. (1979). Differential release of LH and FSH in cyclic mares in response to GnRH. *J. Reprod. Fert.*, **56**, 567–72

13. Ganjam, V. K., Kenney, R. M. and Flickinger, G. (1975). Effect of exogenous progesterone on its endogenous levels: biological half life and lack of progesterone binding in mares. *J. Reprod. Fert. Suppl.*, **23**, 183–8
14. Ginther, O. J. (1979). *Reproductive Biology of the Mare.* (Ann Arbor, Michigan: McNaughton & Gunn)
15. Ginther, O. J. and Wentworth, B. C. (1974). Effect of a synthetic gonadotropin-releasing hormone on plasma concentrations of luteinizing hormone in ponies. *Am. J. Vet. Res.*, **35**, 79–81
16. Holtan, D. W., Douglas, R. H. and Ginther, O. J. (1977). Estrus ovulation and conception following synchronization with progesterone, prostaglandin F_2 and human chorionic gonadotropin in pony mares. *J. Anim. Sci.*, **44**, 431–7
17. Irvine, C. H. G. (1981). Endocrinology of the estrous cycle of the mare: applications to embryo transfer. *Theriogenology*, **15**, 85–104
18. Irvine, D. S., Downey, R., Parker, W. G. *et al.* (1975). Duration of oestrus and time of ovulation in mares treated with synthetic Gn-RH (AY-24031). *J. Reprod. Fert. Suppl.*, **23**, 279–83
19. Lapin, D. R. and Ginther, O. J. (1977). Induction of ovulation and multiple ovulations in seasonally anovulatory and ovulatory mares with an equine pituitary extract. *J. Anim. Sci.*, **44**, 834–42
20. Loy, R. G. and Hughes, J. P. (1966). The effects of human chorionic gonadotrophin on ovulation,, length of estrus and fertility in the mare. *Cornell Vet.*, **56**, 41–50
21. Loy, R. G., Pemsteim, R., O'Canna, D. *et al.* (1981). Control of ovulation in cycling mares with ovarian steroids and prostaglandin. *Theriogenology*, **15**, 191–9
22. Nishikawa (1959). *Studies on Reproduction in Horses.* (Tokyo: Japan Racing Assoc.)
23. Oxender, W. D., Noden, P. A., Bolenbaugh, D. L. *et al.* (1975). Control of estrus with prostaglandin $F_{2\alpha}$ in mares: minimal effective dose and stage of estrous cycle. *Am. J. Vet. Res.*, **36**, 1145–7
24. Palmer, E. (1976). Different techniques for synchronization of ovulation in the mare. *Proc. Int. Cong. Anim. Reprod. Artif. Insem.*, **3**, 495–8
25. Palmer, E. (1978). Control of the oestrous cycle of the mare. *J. Reprod. Fert.*, **54**, 495–505
26. Palmer, E. (1979). Reproduction management of mares without oestrous detection. *J. Reprod. Fert., Suppl.*, **27**, 263–70
27. Palmer, E. and Driancourt, M. A. (1981). Photoperiodic stimulation of the winter anoestrous mare: what is a long day? In *Photoperiodism and Reproduction in Vertebrates.* pp. 67–82. (Nouzilly: INRA Colloques)
28. Palmer, E. and Jousset, B. (1975). Synchronization of oestrus and ovulation in the mare with a two PG–HCG sequence treatment. *Ann. Biol. Anim. Biochim. Biophys.*, **15**, 471–80
29. Pashen, R. L. (1980). Low dose of oxytocin can induce foaling at term. *Equine Vet. J.*, **12**, 85–7
30. Robinson, J. R. (1977). Use of clomiphene citrate to induce oestrus in anoestrous mares. *Vet. Med. Small Anim. Clin.*, **72**, 605–7
31. Roser, J. F., Keifer, B. L., Evans, J. W. *et al.* (1979). The development of antibodies to human chorionic gonadotropin following its repeated injection in the cyclic mare. *J. Reprod. Fert., Suppl.*, **27**, 173–9
32. Rossdale, P. D. (1976). Foaling induced by synthetic prostaglandin analogue (fluprostenol). *Vet. Rec.*, **99**, 26–8
33. Stewart, F. and Allen, W. R. (1979). The binding of FSH, LH and PMSG to equine gonadal tissue. *J. Reprod. Fert., Suppl.*, **27**, 431–40
34. Sullivan, J. J., Parker, G. and Larson, L. L. (1973). Duration of estrus and ovulation time in nonlacting mares given HCG during three successive estrous periods. *J. Am. Vet. Med. Assoc.*, **163**, 895–8
35. Terqui, M. and Palmer, E. (1979). Oestrogen pattern during early pregnancy. *J. Reprod. Fert., Suppl.*, **27**, 441–6
36. Turner, D. D., Garcia, M. C., Webel, S. K. *et al.* (1981). Influence of follicular size on the response of mares to allyl trembolone given before the onset of the ovulatory season. *Theriogenology*, **16**, 73–84

37. Turner, J. E. and Irvine, C. H. G. (1982). Effect of prolonged administration of anabolic and androgenic steroids on reproductive function in the mare. Third International Symposium on Equine Reproduction. *J. Reprod. Fert., Suppl.*, **32.** (In press)
38. Webel, S. K. (1975). Estrus control in horses with a progestin. *J. Anim. Sci.*, **41**, 359
39. Webel, S. K., Franklin, V., Harland, B. *et al.* (1977). Fertility, ovulation, and maturation of eggs in mares injected with hCG. *J. Reprod. Fert.*, **51**, 337–40
40. Witherspoon, D. M., Lamond, D. R., Thompson, F. N. *et al.* (1975). Efficacy of a prostaglandin analogue in reproduction in the cycling mare. *Theriogenology*, **3**, 21–30

Section IV Pharmacological Methods

37
Clinical utility and limitations of pharmacokinetics

J. D. Baggot

Techniques provide a practical means for measuring changes in a physical, chemical or biological system by describing activity of the system in quantitative terms. In applying a technique certain procedures have to be followed, while interpretation of the results requires an understanding of the limitations associated with the technique.

Pharmacokinetics may be defined as the mathematical description of drug concentration changes in the body. It is basically a technique which is concerned with the study and characterization of the time course of drug absorption, distribution and elimination, and also with the relationship between these processes and the observed pharmacological effect. The clinical utility of pharmacokinetics largely rests on the premise that the therapeutic range of plasma concentrations for a drug can be at least tentatively defined. While accepting this to be the only practical approach, it should be realized that it is the biophasic concentration rather than the plasma concentration *per se* which directly relates to the intensity of the observed effect. Drug metabolites may also have to be considered when they have pharmacological activity that contributes to the clinical response (Table 37.1). The activity of a drug depends not only on its biophasic concentration but, in addition, on both the affinity of the drug for the receptor sites and its intrinsic activity (efficacy).

Table 37.1 Some drugs and their metabolites, both of which possess pharmacologic activity

Drug	*Metabolite*
Propranolol	4-Hydroxypropranolol
Diazepam	*N*-Desmethyl diazepam
Flunitrazepam	*N*-Desmethyl flunitrazepam
Valproic acid (VPA)	2-en-VPA,3-keto-VPA
Primidone	Phenobarbital, phenylethylmalonamide
Phenylbutazone	Oxyphenbutazone
Acetylsalicylic acid	Salicylic acid

Hence, it follows that species variations in the response produced by a fixed dose (mg/kg) of drug can be attributed to species differences either in disposition processes (mainly the rate of biotransformation) or in the sensitivity of tissue receptor sites.

For drugs which are extensively metabolized by the liver and the elimination process obeys first-order kinetics, interspecies comparisons of their metabolism rates should use intrinsic clearance, and not half-life, as the parameter of choice[10]. Intrinsic clearance is a distinctive characteristic for any particular drug in a given situation and as such it reflects only the inherent ability of the organ (e.g. hepatic metabolic activity) to remove the drug[49].

Clinical pharmacology provides the applied scientific basis for drug therapy. It is a basic aim of clinical pharmacology to understand the dose–effect relationship for drugs. This objective can generally be achieved by linking the pharmacokinetic behaviour of a drug with information on its pharmacodynamic action. The former is concerned mainly with the dose–concentration relationship and the latter with the concentration–effect relationship (Figure 37.1). A parameter that is quantifiable and central to the

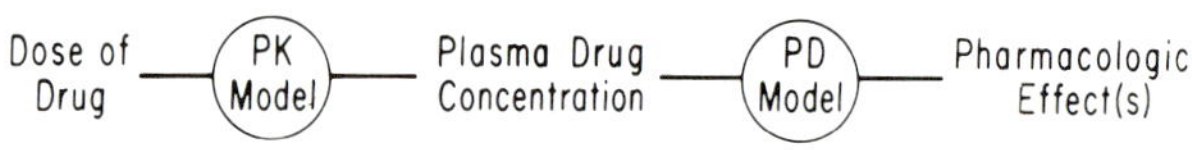

Figure 37.1 Schematic representation of the dose–effect relationship using pharmacokinetic (PK) and pharmacodynamic (PD) models

dose–effect relationship for a drug is the therapeutic (i.e. safe and effective) range of plasma (or serum) concentrations. Definition of therapeutic plasma concentrations requires skilled clinical evaluation of the response produced by the drug in a sufficient number of appropriately selected individuals. A predictable and constant relationship exists for some, but not for all, drugs between the time course of drug effect and the plasma concentration profile. The relationship applies to observable effects between 20 and 80% of maximum and predicts that the pharmacological response will decline linearly while the plasma drug concentrations are declining exponentially[36]. The drugs to which this relationship applies are homogeneously distributed, do not form active metabolites, and are eliminated by first-order kinetics. The usual therapeutic concentration range for an antimicrobial agent defines the serum concentrations that are likely to be effective against the majority of sensitive (or susceptible) micro-organisms and that are non-toxic to the animal. Therapeutic serum concentrations for antimicrobial agents must always be related to the sensitivity of the infecting micro-organisms.

This paper is based on and represents a continuation of that in which the principles of clinical pharmacokinetics are described[1]. The intention here is to point out potential sources of error in calculating pharmacokinetic terms and to discuss aspects of certain concepts that are subject to misinterpretation. In this way, the clinical utility and limitations of the discipline should become more readily apparent.

THE DISPOSITION CURVE

The disposition curve describes graphically the plasma concentration profile of a drug given as a single dose by intravenous injection. The curves for most drugs used in clinical medicine can be fitted to a sum of exponential terms:

$$C_p = \sum_{i=l}^{n} A_i e^{-k_i t}$$

where C_p is the plasma drug concentration at time t after a single intravenous dose, A_i and k_i represent a series (n) of 'hybrid' coefficients and exponents, respectively, that can be related to intrinsic rate constants of appropriate compartmental pharmacokinetic models. It appears that two or, for some drugs, three exponential terms are usually sufficient for a good fit of the data points. This implies that four or six terms will fully characterize the disposition curve (Table 37.2). The hybrid kinetic terms may be obtained from

Table 37.2 Kinetic terms and exponential equations which are associated with compartmental pharmacokinetic models

Pharmacokinetic model	*Experimental constants* *Coefficients* (μg/ml)	*Exponents* (min^{-1})
Two-compartment	A	α
	B	β
Equation:	$C_p = Ae^{-\alpha t} + Be^{-\beta t}$	
Three-compartment	P	π
	A	α
	B	β
Equation:	$C_p = Pe^{-\pi t} + Ae^{-\alpha t} + Be^{-\beta t}$	

the experimental plasma concentration–time data by iterative least-squares regression analysis. The best approach is to fit the disposition curve by means of a digital computer program (NONLIN), which provides a non-linear least-squares regression analysis of the entire plasma concentration–time data.

The completeness of the disposition curve depends not only on the frequency and duration of blood sampling but also on the sensitivity of the analytical method used for quantitative determination of the plasma drug concentrations. The incomplete determination of the disposition curve can lead to error in values of the experimental constants and, inevitably, error in the area under the curve (AUC). This, generally, is due to poor experimental design rather than representing a limitation of pharmacokinetic analysis. The merit of a pilot study, which will provide an outline of the disposition curve and on which sampling times for the subsequent complete study can be based, should be stressed. The most common error is overestimation of the terminal exponent (β) because the duration of sampling was not long enough to allow reliable estimation of this variable[26]. Since the terminal exponent is the major determinant of drug accumulation, the predicted steady state plasma concentration will differ from the observed concentration that multiple-dose therapy will produce[27].

PHARMACOKINETIC MODELS

Pharmacokinetic models conceive the body to consist of distribution compartments and are used to interpret the pharmacokinetic behaviour of drugs. Although such models are often schematically depicted as consisting of two or more interconnected compartments, they represent a set of mathematical equations and do not correspond to anatomical body spaces. The compartments are postulated to account for the experimental observation that drugs distribute to various body fluids and tissues at different rates. This distribution process depends on the bloodflow to the tissues, the mass of various organs and tissues, and certain physicochemical properties (in particular, lipid solubility and degree of ionization) of the drug. Weak organic electrolytes, that have a high degree of lipid solubility, exist predominantly in the non-ionized form in blood plasma and are not extensively bound to plasma proteins, would be expected to undergo rapid and widespread distribution. Lipid solubility may be more important than degree of ionization in determining the rate as well as the pattern of distribution, which are ultimately limited by bloodflow to tissuess. This has been shown for amphetamine (organic base, pK_a 9.9) and thiopental (organic acid, pK_a 7.6). Organs with high perfusion rates, such as heart, brain, liver and kidneys, achieve higher drug concentrations than skeletal muscle and adipose tissue, with equilibrium between these tissues and blood being rapidly attained. Protein binding both in the plasma and in tissues can markedly affect drug distribution, when a high binding affinity exists. It has been calculated that when the drug–albumin association constant exceeds 10^4 l/mol, a change in protein binding can alter drug distribution[38].

Certain assumptions are associated with the use of compartmental pharmacokinetic models. A drug injected intravenously is presumed to equilibrate instantaneously in the fluids and tissues which comprise the volume of the central compartment (V_c). From this compartment, the drug diffuses into one or more peripheral (sometimes called tissue) compartments (Figure 37.2). Pseudodistribution equilibrium can be attained relatively rapidly when only one peripheral compartment exists, but is slowly established when there is, in addition, a deep compartment. It is generally assumed that once pseudodistribution equilibrium has been established, the concentrations of

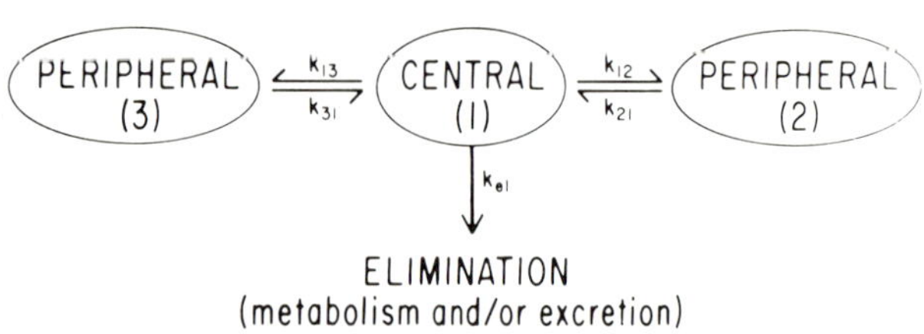

Figure 37.2 Three-compartment pharmacokinetic model. The drug is introduced directly into the central compartment, from which it distributes into the peripheral compartments. The rate constants represent the first-order distribution and elimination processes. Elimination is assumed to take place exclusively from the central compartment

drug in the plasma and in those organs and tissues that contain a 'significant fraction' of the total amount in the body will decline in a parallel fashion. The level of drug that constitutes a significant fraction of the amount in the body may be crucial in determining which compartmental model appropriately describes the pharmacokinetic behaviour of the drug. Elimination, which refers to biotransformation and excretion, is a first-order process for the majority of therapeutic agents and is always assumed to take place exclusively from the central compartment.

The analysis and interpretation of the disposition curve depend on the number of compartments in the pharmacokinetic model selected. The two-compartment open model, which employs a biexponential equation to characterize the disposition curve, may be considered to adequately describe the pharmacokinetic behaviour of the majority of therapeutic agents. According to this model, the body is conceived as consisting of a central compartment and a relatively rapidly equilibrating peripheral compartment. After pseudodistribution equilibrium has been established, the ratio of the diffusible amounts of drug in the central and peripheral compartments is assumed to remain constant; first-order elimination from the central compartment is assumed. First-order disposition processes, which are dose-independent, imply that the rate at which a drug is removed from a compartment is proportional to the concentration of the drug in the compartment.

Values of the actual rate constants associated with the two-compartment pharmacokinetic model (k_{12}, k_{21}, k_{el}) can be calculated from the coefficients (A, B) and exponents (α, β) that characterize the disposition curve:

$$k_{21} = \frac{A\beta + B\alpha}{A+B}$$

$$A + B = C_p^\circ$$

$$k_{el} = \frac{\alpha\beta}{k_{21}}$$

$$k_{12} = \alpha + \beta - k_{21} - k_{el}$$

Determination of the microconstants permits an assessment of the relative contribution of distribution and elimination processes to the disposition of a drug. A knowledge of their values may also assist with interpretation of the changes in the disposition processes that can occur in certain physiological conditions, disease states and, possibly, as a result of drug interactions.

The pharmacokinetic behaviour of drugs which either bind selectively or slowly accumulate in a particular tissue may be more appropriately interpreted in terms of a three-compartment open model. It has been shown that a triexponential equation can best characterize the plasma concentration profiles of pentazocine[47] and diazepam[33] in man, pyrimethamine in the pig[44], oxytetracycline in dogs[6], sulphadoxine in horses[42], and sulphadimethoxine in cattle[11]. Likewise, the pharmacokinetic behaviour of digoxin was interpreted in terms of a three-compartment open model in man[35], the horse[15] and the dog[14].

Interpretation of the pharmacokinetic behaviour of thiopental deserves special consideration as the pharmacological effect is associated with the early phase of its disposition and the clinical use of the drug is dependent on the technique of administration. When given as an intravenous bolus dose the drug very rapidly penetrates the blood–brain and blood–CSF barriers to produce an anaesthetic effect. The duration of clinical anaesthesia is determined mainly by redistribution of the drug from the brain to skeletal muscle and other tissues. The localization of the drug in body fat[13], which takes place slowly due to the limited blood supply of adipose tissue, has little influence. A comparison of the equations using a two- and a three-compartment model to interpret the kinetic behaviour of the drug (Table 37.3) shows that, for clinical purposes, the biexponential equation adequately describes the plasma concentration profile[12]. The half-life of the initial phase of the disposition curve, which is comprised of distribution/redistribution, correlates with the duration of clinical anaesthesia.

Table 37.3 Kinetic behaviour of thiopental, given as an intravenous bolus dose (20 mg/kg), in dogs

Model	*Mathematical presentation of results*
Two-compartment equation	$C_p = 28.0e^{-2.43t} + 25.9e^{-0.0988t}$
Body clearance	$Cl_B = 1.22$ ml/min kg
Three-compartment equation	$C_p = 6.1e^{-20.88t} + 25.8e^{-2.11t} + 25.3e^{-0.0943t}$
Body clearance	$Cl_B = 1.19$ ml/min kg

The pharmacokinetic behaviour of aminoglycoside antibiotics is usually interpreted in terms of a two-compartment open model, since a biexponential equation describes the serum concentration profile that is obtained experimentally[2,4]. Although the aminoglycosides are eliminated entirely by renal excretion and their half-lives are less than 2.5 h, urinary recovery of the dose over a 24 h collection period is incomplete, even when renal function is normal[18]. This situation may be explained by incomplete determination of the disposition curve due to lack of sensitivity of the microbiological assay procedure. The omission of the true terminal (elimination) phase would lead to underestimation of the steady state distribution volume, which is proportional to the average amount of drug in the body following prolonged treatment. This pharmacokinetic parameter may be more relevant to chronic toxicity than serum concentrations[24]. A dosage regimen designed to maintain serum concentrations within the therapeutic range inevitably leads to progressive drug accumulation in the body and especially in renal tissue, where toxicity can occur. It is a logical recommendation to limit the duration of treatment with an aminoglycoside (particularly gentamicin) to the shortest period that will effect a cure.

LIMITATIONS OF THE ONE-COMPARTMENT MODEL

The plasma concentration profile of some drugs (e.g. amphetamine in a variety of species[3], meclofenamic acid in the horse[45], and warfarin in the dog[39]) can be adequately described by a monoexponential equation, which implies that the drugs confer on the body the characteristics of a one-compartment model. According to this model, pseudodistribution equilibrium is so rapidly attained that the drug is considered to be distributed in a single volume. This does not necessarily mean that the drug concentrations in all body tissues at any given time are the same. However, it is assumed that any changes which occur in the plasma quantitatively reflect changes occurring in tissue drug levels. The decline in plasma drug concentration can be described by:

$$\log C_p = \log C_p^\circ - \frac{k_{el}}{2.303} t$$

where C_p° is the plasma drug concentration immediately after intravenous injection of a single dose and k_{el} is the apparent first-order elimination rate constant for the drug. It follows that a plot of the logarithm of tissue drug concentration vs. time should be linear and have exactly the same slope ($-k_{el}/2.303$) as the plasma concentration–time curve.

By converting to natural logarithms this equation becomes:

$$\ln C_p = \ln C_p^\circ - k_{el} t$$

which is

$$C_p = C_p^\circ e^{-k_{el}t}$$

or, in practical terms,

$$C_p = Be^{-\beta t}$$

where B is the extrapolated zero-time intercept and $-\beta$ the slope of the least-squares regression line. The monoexponential equation which is used to describe the plasma concentration profile corresponds to the linear terminal (elimination) phase of the bi-and triexponential equations that relate to two- and three-compartment models, respectively.

When a one-compartment model is employed to describe the disposition of drugs which have a more complex pharmacokinetic behaviour, the following errors may be introduced:

(1) Overestimation of the distribution volume by the extrapolation method, since $V_{d(B)} > V_{d(\text{area})}$ (Table 37.4),
(2) Overestimation of the body clearance, and
(3) Use of the overall elimination rate constant (β), instead of the true elimination rate constant (k_{el}).

The value of β is always smaller than that of k_{el} when a drug confers on the body the characteristics of a two-compartment model since $\beta = k_{el} \times f_c$, where f_c represents the fraction of drug in the central compartment. When the

Table 37.4 Comparison of extrapolation and area methods for estimating apparent volume of distribution (ml/kg) of drugs which show 2-compartment model kinetic behaviour

Drug	*Extrapolation method* $V'_{d(B)} = \text{Dose}/B$	*Area method* $V'_{d(area)} = \text{Dose}/\text{AUC}\,\beta$
Penicillin G	273	156
Kanamycin	278	255
Gentamicin	448	335
Sulphadimethoxine	523	410
Valproate	837	492
Pentylenetetrazol	841	786
Thiopental	851	843
Oxytetracycline*	3100	2096
Xylazine	4575	2517

*3-compartment model

kinetic behaviour of a drug which does not rapidly attain pseudodistribution equilibrium is interpreted in terms of a one-compartment model, it can be predicted that increasing apparent half-lives will be observed on repetitive dosing[26].

The validity of dosage adjustment in patients with impaired renal function is critically dependent on the assumptions that the renal clearances of creatinine and of the drug are proportional, and that non-renal elimination processes are unaffected by the uraemic state[23]. Furthermore, the calculations of dosage are based on the assumption that the disposition kinetics of the drug can be approximated by a one-compartment model.

STEADY STATE PLASMA CONCENTRATIONS

Kinetic parameters derived from single dose studies can be used to predict the steady state plasma concentrations that multiple-dosing schedules will produce. Assuming that a fixed dose is administered repeatedly at a constant dosage interval (τ), the steady state plasma concentration at any time during a dosage interval can be predicted:

$$C_{p(ss)} = \sum_{i=1}^{n} A_i \left(\frac{1}{1 - e^{-k_i \tau}} \right) e^{-k_i t}$$

where A_i and k_i have been previously defined. It is useful to compare the kinetic profile of the drug after administering the last dose with the profile following the single dose on which the predictions were based. This will verify whether the assumption that the disposition processes are dose-independent is valid. Deviation between the observed and predicted steady state concentrations suggests that the wrong model was chosen to explain the drug's kinetic behaviour[27]. The most common error is overestimation of the terminal exponent, which is the principal determinant of drug accumulation.

When a fixed dose is injected intravenously at constant dosage intervals, the 'average' plasma concentration at steady state can be predicted from a single dose study:

$$\bar{C}_{p(ss)} = \frac{\text{AUC}}{\tau}$$

where AUC represents the total area under the plasma concentration–time curve after the administration of a single intravenous dose. This equation is model-independent, assuming that the kinetics are linear and that elimination takes place from the central compartment. The predictive value of the equation relies on the assumption that the body (total plasma) clearance of the drug remains constant over the entire dosing period. It is useful to know that the area under the curve, calculated from arithmetic mean concentration data by the trapezoidal rule from time zero to the last detectable concentration sampling point, is equal to the mean of the individual subject areas under the curve for the same time span[19]. On the other hand, the selection of a compartmental model and estimation of model-dependent pharmacokinetic parameters (such as apparent volume of distribution, rate constants and half-life) from arithmetic mean concentration data can lead to the use of inappropriate models and give biased parameter estimates.

The 'average' plasma concentration of a drug calculated by this last equation gives no idea of the extent of fluctuation in steady state concentrations. It represents neither the arithmetic nor the geometric mean of the maximum and minimum concentrations that are obtained during a dosage interval. Rather, it is the plasma concentration at steady state which, when multiplied by the time between successive doses, equals the area under the plasma concentration-time curve for the dosage interval.

DRUGS SHOWING NON-LINEAR KINETIC BEHAVIOUR

The equations associated with compartmental models which allow calculation of pharmacokinetic parameters and prediction of steady state plasma concentrations are valid only for drugs which show dose-independent or linear pharmacokinetic behaviour. For drugs obeying Michaelis–Menten elimination kinetics, an experimental procedure has been described which allows estimation of their volumes of distribution[37]. Also, a mathematical approach with equations has been developed which allows prediction of steady state concentrations from concentrations 'observed' before steady state is attained[48]. It was suggested that, in the therapeutic monitoring of serum phenytoin concentrations, the blood sample should be collected just before administration of the next dose, in which case C_{ss}^{min} rather than $\bar{C}_{ss}$ is measured. When C_n^{min} values are measured, the fitting of C_{ss}^{min} vs. dose rate (D/τ) data leads to operationally useful parameters, V_m^{app} and K_m^{app}, which are not the true kinetic parameters.

PHYSIOLOGICAL PHARMACOKINETIC MODELS

The purpose of developing pharmacokinetic models is to describe the time course of drug disposition processes in the body. The derived kinetic parameters can be used to calculate safe and effective dosage regimens and to predict steady state plasma concentrations that multiple doses will attain. The choice of compartmental model is based on curve fitting of the plasma concentration profile with a single or multiexponential equation, in which the number of compartments in the model is equal to the number of exponents in the equation. The compartments, which are mathematical entities, give no insight as to the distribution pattern of the drug. This limits the physiological interpretation of species differences in drug disposition, which is the usual source of species variations in response to a fixed dose. To overcome this limitation, attempts have been made to develop physiological pharmacokinetic models[8]. These models would enable the selection of a species from which extrapolation of pharmacokinetic data to other species might validly be made.

A physiological pharmacokinetic model aims at incorporating into the model the bloodflow rate and volume of the various organs and tissues as

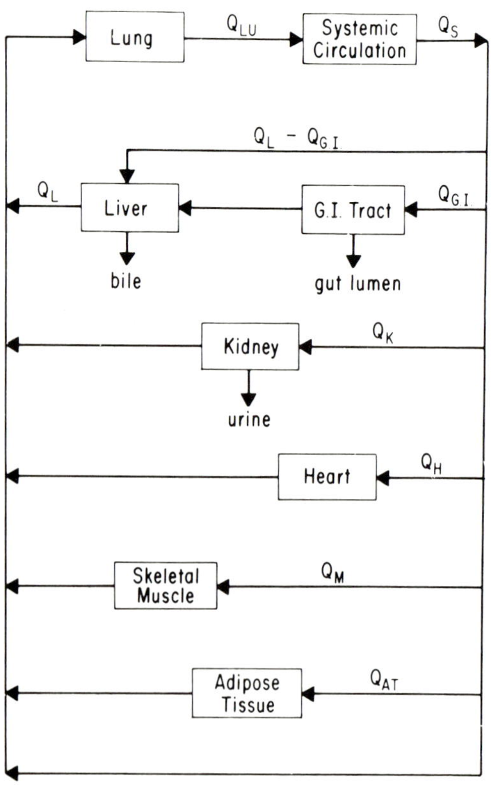

Figure 37.3 Physiological pharmacokinetic model for drug disposition

well as biochemical information on the drug (such as plasma protein binding, lipid solubility and, in particular, tissue/plasma partition coefficients). The model is composed of a series of compartments representing organs or tissue spaces in which drug concentrations are assumed to be uniform (Figure 37.3). Differential mass balance equations are written for each compartment to describe the inflow, outflow, accumulation or disappearance of the drug. An important parameter in the development of physiological pharmacokinetic models is the tissue-to-plasma concentration ratio (partition coefficient) of the drug for each compartment[16]. This type of model has been applied with reasonable success to describe the disposition of thiopental[9] and digoxin[30] in dogs.

The physiological approach to pharmacokinetic modelling may provide the means for predicting drug concentrations in the target tissues and it can be adapted to changing physiological circumstances. A serious drawback, however, is the large amount of data that is required initially to develop the model. The estimation of the tissue-to-plasma partition coefficients is difficult and the values obtained can vary with the mode of drug administration. It has been shown that the tissue-to-plasma concentration ratio at pseudodistribution equilibrium after an intravenous injection is always greater than the ratio at infusion equilibrium[25].

BIOAVAILABILITY

Many drugs are available in a variety of products and dosage forms. When a drug is given orally in solid dosage form, disintegration of the drug product and dissolution of the drug in gastrointestinal fluids precede absorption. Passive non-ionic diffusion is the most important mechanism of drug absorption, while the small intestine is the principle site of absorption in monogastric species. The rate of gastric emptying greatly affects the rate at which drugs are absorbed and, for compounds that are unstable at gastric pH, delayed emptying of the stomach can reduce the extent as well as the rate of their absorption. The plasma concentration vs. time curve reflects the net effect of release of drug from the dosage form administered and the processes of absorption, presystemic metabolism (should it occur), distribution and elimination. A peak concentration is reached when drug absorption no longer exceeds its removal from the systemic circulation by distribution to tissues, metabolism and excretion. It should be emphasized that absorption continues after the peak plasma concentration has been reached.

The term bioavailability is defined as the rate and extent to which the drug administered as a particular dosage form enters the systemic circulation intact (or unchanged). The usual technique for estimating the systemic availability, or extent of absorption, employs the method of corresponding areas. This entails comparison of the total areas under the plasma concentration vs. time curves which are obtained after oral (or other non-intravascular route) and intravenous administration of equal doses of the drug (in appropriate dosage forms) to the same animals:

$$F = \frac{(\text{AUC})_{\text{p.o.}}}{(\text{AUC})_{\text{i.v.}}}$$

The area under the curves (AUC) may be calculated using the trapezoidal rule. The absorption rate can be estimated by deconvolution of the plasma concentration vs. time curve after intravenous drug administration from that obtained after oral administration[7]. The assumption is made that the kinetics of drug distribution and elimination (i.e. body clearance) remain unchanged within and between treatments. This assumption can be avoided when absolute bioavailability and absorption rate are determined by simultaneous administration of an intravenous, stable isotope-labelled drug preparation and the oral drug formulation that is being evaluated[46].

Since intravenous injection delivers the drug directly into the systemic circulation, this route of administration provides complete systemic availability (sometimes called bioavailability). Should an intravenous preparation of the drug not be available, an oral reference standard (usually a well-known aqueous solution or an elixir) may be used as a basis for comparison, in which case the relative, rather than absolute, bioavailability is measured. The relative pharmacodynamic bioavailability of different preparations of the same drug may be estimated by comparing the areas under the pharmacological effect vs. time curves. This technique is particularly appropriate when plasma concentrations of the drug cannot be accurately measured. In the same way that pharmacokinetic bioavailability studies are limited to drugs with concentration-independent or linear kinetic behaviour, pharmacodynamic bioavailability studies should be limited to linear pharmacodynamic models[31].

When estimating the relative bioavailability of chemical analogues, it is incorrect to compare directly their AUC values or the relative amounts of drug excreted unchanged in the urine. Rather, the systemic availability of each analogue must be determined separately and these values can then be compared. It is necessary to adopt this procedure since the plasma concentration–time curve is influenced not only by absorption but also by distribution into tissues and elimination (metabolism and excretion).

ESTIMATION OF AREA UNDER THE CURVE

The integral $\int_0^\infty C_p \, dt$ is the area under the plasma concentration–time curve plotted on rectilinear coordinates from time zero to infinity. Estimation of the area under the curve commonly employs the linear trapezoidal rule. The accuracy of this method depends upon the number of plasma concentration–time points and the interval between successive data points. Following oral administration of a drug both the absorption and postabsorption phases of the curve give rise to error in estimation of the total area. The net effect of the opposing types of error, which are underestimation during absorption and overestimation during the postabsorption phase, will vary with the relative contribution of the areas occupied by these phases to the total area under the curve. Since the intervals between plasma data points are longer during the postabsorption phase and this phase usually occupies the major part of the area, use of the linear trapezoidal rule is likely to overestimate the total area under the curve. This would lead to error in the pharmacokinetic parameters that are based on AUC. They include the extent of absorption, volume of distribution (area method), body clearance and amount of drug absorbed into and eliminated from the body.

To improve the accuracy of estimating total area under the curve, it has been recommended that the linear trapezoidal method be used for calculating area during the absorption phase and the integration or logarithmic trapezoidal method be used during the exponential postabsorption phase[17]. The area under the curve between any two points, $C_{p(1)}$ and $C_{p(2)}$, during exponential postabsorption phase is given by:

$$\mathrm{AUC}_{t1-t2} = \frac{(C_{p(1)} - C_{p(2)})\,(t_2 - t_1)}{\ln C_{p(1)} - \ln C_{p(2)}}$$

When the drug is given as an intravenous bolus dose and confers on the body the characteristics of a two-compartment open model, the total area under the curve can be calculated:

$$\mathrm{AUC} = \frac{A}{\alpha} + \frac{B}{\beta}$$

where A, B, α and β are the experimental pharmacokinetic constants which characterize the biexponential disposition curve.

INCOMPLETE SYSTEMIC AVAILABILITY

The incomplete systemic availability of a drug, whether due to defective absorption or presystemic elimination, will be manifested as a ratio of less than one (or $< 100\%$) for the area under the curves. Presystemic elimination can be attributed to metabolism or degradation in the gut lumen, metabolism in the gut epithelium occurring during absorption, or metabolism in the liver preceding entry of the drug into the systemic circulation (Table 37.5). Isoproterenol[21] and progesterone[40] are extensively metabolized in the gut (intestinal) wall of the dog. The isoproterenol forms mainly a sulphate conjugate whereas conjugation reactions seem to play only a minor role in progesterone metabolism. A distinction must be made between the extent of absorption and the systemic availability of a drug, since these can differ after oral dosage. The extent of absorption refers simply to the proportion of the dose that is absorbed, changed or unchanged, through the gut-mucosa, whereas systemic availability refers to the fraction of the dose that enters the systemic circulation in an unchanged form. Using bioavailability estimates alone, incomplete systemic availability of a drug due to significant presystemic elimination could be misinterpreted as defective absorption.

Table 37.5 Some drugs which undergo presystemic elimination in the dog

Drug (dosage form)	*Dose* (mg/kg)	*Systemic availability* (%)	*Site of elimination*	*Reference*
Lidocaine (solution)	10	15	liver	28
Salicylamide (solution)	30	22	gut wall and liver	28
Acetylsalicylic acid (solution)	250 mg (total)	45	gut wall and liver	29
L-Dopa (solid in gelatin capsule)	25	44	gut lumen and/or gut wall	22
Sulphadimethoxine (aqueous suspension)	55	50	liver	5
Flunitrazepam (micronized drug in gelatin capsule)	2	0	gut wall and liver	32
Propranolol (tablet)	80 mg (total)	2–17	liver	34

In an attempt to differentiate preabsorptive, gut epithelial and hepatic first-pass metabolism, a specialized physiological pharmacokinetic model has been developed[20]. The major portion of the total hepatic blood supply directly perfuses the liver ($Q_S - Q_G$), while the remainder (Q_G) perfuses the gastrointestinal tract prior to the liver (Figure 37.4). Since the gut lumen is not

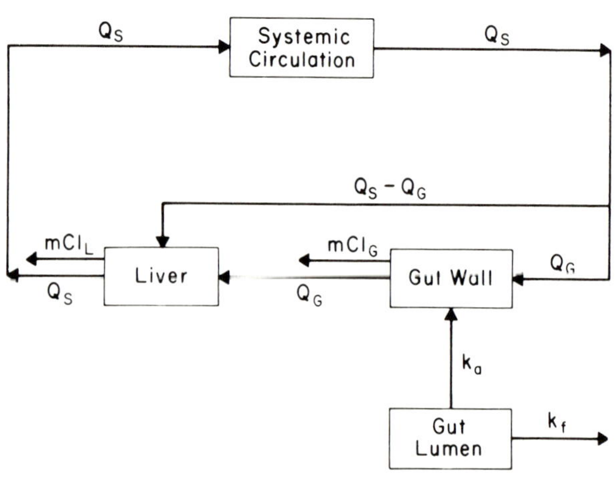

Figure 37.4 Physiological pharmacokinetic model used to describe presystemic drug elimination. Intrinsic metabolic clearance in the gut wall and liver is represented by mCl_G and mCl_L, respectively, while k_a and k_f are the apparent first-order absorption and gut floral metabolic rate constants

a perfused organ, it is incorporated into the model as a classical compartment where the absorption rate constant (k_a) and the gut lumen (flora) metabolic rate constant (k_f) compete for drug present in the gut[41]. Metabolic clearance takes place in the gut (mCl_G) and/or in the liver (mCl_L) and is assumed to be independent of the drug concentration. Another assumption is that the fraction of the dose not metabolized in the gut lumen is completely absorbed. In conjunction with this model, Colburn[20] has derived a set of equations to estimate the fraction of the administered dose which is metabolized at each of the three sites (namely, in the gut lumen, intestinal epithelium and the liver) and to establish the limits of the true absorption rate constant.

An indirect experimental approach to determining the relative contribution of first-pass hepatic metabolism to presystemic elimination is to show the presence (or absence) of quantitative consistency between the magnitude of presystemic elimination ($AUC_{p.o.}/AUC_{i.v.}$, using plasma concentrations) and the value of the hepatic extraction ratio. The latter is estimated from the systemic drug clearance (which must be based on whole blood concentrations) and the liver bloodflow[43]. Hepatic presystemic elimination is most important for highly extracted drugs (such as diazepam, propranolol and lidocaine).

SUMMARY AND CONCLUSIONS

Pharmacokinetics is primarily a technique which allows the absorption, distribution and elimination of drugs to be described in quantitative terms. Various dosage forms of a drug are administered by different routes and the concentrations of the drug (and pharmacologically active metabolites) are precisely determined in plasma (and other biological fluids). Appropriate compartmental (and physiological) pharmacokinetic models with their associated mathematical equations are employed to analyse and interpret the experimental data. It is essential to understand the assumptions and to have an appreciation of the limitations that are associated with pharmacokinetic models.

It is a basic aim of clinical pharmacology to understand the dose–effect relationship for therapeutic agents. This objective can generally be achieved by linking the pharmacokinetic behaviour of a drug with information on its pharmacodynamic action. The therapeutic range of plasma concentrations for a drug is central to the dose–effect relationship. The utility of pharmacokinetics in clinical pharmacology largely rests on the premise that the therapeutic concentration range can be defined.

Kinetic parameters derived from single dose studies may be used to predict the steady state plasma concentrations that multiple-dosing schedules will produce. The accuracy of the predictions depends on certain criteria being fulfilled. These include dose-independent disposition processes and accurate determination of the terminal exponent, in addition to compliance with the recommendation on dose rate. Oral dosage must allow for incomplete systemic availability. When it becomes necessary to extrapolate pharmacokinetic parameters from normal to diseased animals, a knowledge of the elimination mechanisms and margin of safety of the drug are essential for modifying the dosage regimen. Pharmacokinetic predictions aim at optimizing drug therapy, while 'titration by patient response' can achieve this goal. It is well to remember that pharmacokinetics is the servant rather than the master of therapeutics.

Pharmacokinetics is a useful experimental approach for comparing species variations in the extent of distribution and the rate of drug elimination. It provides a basis for the selection of a test species, from which pharmacokinetic information might be extrapolated for application to man. The discipline is well suited for evaluation of test substances which can measure the efficiency of an excretion mechanism or the activity of a metabolic pathway.

The use of pharmacokinetics in the design and evaluation of dosage forms provides an approach to the rational choice and administration of a drug product. While there are definite limitations associated with the technique, inadequate experimental design and misinterpretation of the kinetic parameters detract from its value as a means for predicting optimal dosage under varying circumstances. The study of the correlation between pharmacokinetic behaviour and pharmacodynamic action of a drug serves to greatly enhance the predictive power and thereby clinical utility of pharmacokinetics.

References

1. Baggot, J. D. (1977). *Principles of Drug Disposition in Domestic Animals.* Chap. 6, pp. 144–89. (Philadelphia: Saunders)
2. Baggot, J. D. (1978). Pharmacokinetics of kanamycin in dogs. *J. Vet. Pharmacol. Ther.*, **1**, 163–70
3. Baggot, J. D. and Davis, L. E. (1973). A comparative study of the pharmacokinetics of amphetamine. *Res. Vet. Sci.*, **14**, 207–15
4. Baggot, J. D., Love, D. N., Rose, R. J. *et al.* (1981). The pharmacokinetics of some aminoglycoside antibiotics in the horse. *J. Vet. Pharmacol. Ther.*, **4**, 277–84
5. Baggot, J. D., Ludden, T. M. and Powers, J. D. (1976). The bioavailability, disposition kinetics and dosage of sulphadimethoxine in dogs. *Can. J. Comp. Med.*, **40**, 310–7
6. Baggot, J. D., Powers, T. E., Powers, T. E. *et al.* (1977). Pharmacokinetics and dosage of oxytetracycline in dogs. *Res. Vet. Sci.*, **24**, 77–81
7. Benet, L. Z. and Chiang, C.-W. (1972). The use and application of deconvolution methods in pharmaceutics. *Abstract 13th Natl. Meeting Am. Pharm. Assoc. Acad. Pharm. Sci., Chicago & Washington DC*, **2**, 169–71
8. Bischoff, K. B. and Brown, R. G. (1966). Drug distribution in mammals. *Chem. Eng. Progr. Symp. Ser.*, **62**, 32–45
9. Bischoff, K. B. and Dedrick, R. L. (1968). Thiopental pharmacokinetics. *J. Pharm. Sci.*, **57**, 1346–51
10. Boxenbaum, H. (1980). Interspecies variation in liver weight, hepatic blood flow, and antipyrine intrinsic clearance: extrapolation of data to benzodiazepines and phenytoin. *J. Pharmacokinet. Biopharm.*, **8**, 165–76
11. Boxenbaum, H. G., Fellig, J., Hanson, L. J. *et al.* (1977). Pharmacokinetics of sulphadimethoxine in cattle. *Res. Vet. Sci.*, **23**, 24–8
12. Brandon, R. A. and Baggot, J. D. (1981). The pharmacokinetics of thiopenone. *J. Vet. Pharmacol. Ther.*, **4**, 79–85
13. Brodie, B. B., Bernstein, E. and Mark, L. C. (1952). The role of body fat in limiting the duration of action of thiopental. *J. Pharmacol. Exp. Ther.*, **105**, 421–6

14. Button, C., Gross, D. R., Johnston, J. T. *et al.* (1980). Pharmacokinetics, bioavailability, and dosage regimens of digoxin in dogs. *Am. J. Vet. Res.*, **41**, 1230–7
15. Button, C., Gross, D. R., Johnston, J. T. *et al.* (1980). Digoxin pharmacokinetics, bioavailability, efficacy, and dosage regimens in the horse. *Am. J. Vet. Res.*, **41**, 1388–95
16. Chen, H-S., G. and Gross, J. F. (1979). Estimation of tissue-to-plasma partition coefficients used in physiological pharmacokinetic models. *J. Pharmacokinet. Biopharm.*, **7**, 117–25
17. Chiou, W. L. (1978). Critical evaluation of the potential error in pharmacokinetic studies of using the linear trapezoidal rule method for the calculation of the area under the plasma level-time curve. *J. Pharmacokinet. Biopharm.*, **6**, 539–46
18. Clarke, J. T., Libke, R. D., Regamey, C. *et al.* (1974). Comparative pharmacokinetics of amikacin and kanamycin. *Clin. Pharmacol. Ther.*, **15**, 610–6
19. Cocchetto, D. M., Wargin, W. A. and Crow, J. W. (1980). Pitfalls and valid approaches to pharmacokinetic analysis of mean concentration data following intravenous administration. *J. Pharmacokinet. Biopharm.*, **8**, 539–52
20. Colburn, W. A. (1979). A pharmacokinetic model to differentiate preabsorptive, gut epithelial, and hepatic first-pass metabolism. *J. Pharmacokinet. Biopharm.*, **7**, 407–15
21. Conolly, M. E., Davies, D. S., Dollery, T. *et al.* (1972). Metabolism of isoprenaline in dog and man. *Br. J. Pharmacol.*, **46**, 458–72
22. Cotler, S., Holazo, A., Boxenbaum, H. G. *et al.* (1976). Influence of route of administration on physiological availability of levodopa in dogs. *J. Pharm. Sci.*, **65**, 822–7
23. Dettli, L. (1974). Drug dosage in patients with renal disease. *Clin. Pharmacol. Ther.*, **16**, 274–80
24. Follath, F., Vozch, S. and Wenk, M. (1980). Pharmacokinetic models and dosage regimens. In Gladtke, E. and Heimann, G. (eds.) *Pharmacokinetics.* pp. 109–115. (Stuttgart: Fischer Verlag)
25. Gibaldi, M. (1969). Effect of mode of administration on drug distribution in a two-compartment open system. *J. Pharm. Sci.*, **58**, 327–31
26. Gibaldi, M. and Weintraub, H. (1971). Some considerations as to the determination and significance of biologic half-life. *J. Pharm. Sci.*, **60**, 624–6
27. Greenblatt, D. J. (1979). Predicting steady state serum concentrations of drugs. *Ann. Rev. Pharmacol. Toxicol.*, **19**, 347–56
28. Gugler, R., Lain, P. and Azarnoff, D. L. (1975). Effect of portacaval shunt on the disposition of drugs with and without first-pass effect. *J. Pharmacol. Exp. Ther.*, **195**, 416–23
29. Harris, P. A. and Riegelman, S. (1969). Influence of the route of administration on the area under the plasma concentration-time curve. *J. Pharm. Sci.*, **58**, 71–5
30. Harrison, L. I. and Gibaldi, M. (1977). Physiologically based pharmacokinetic model for digoxin disposition in dogs and its preliminary application to humans. *J. Pharm. Sci.*, **66**, 1679–83
31. Holford, N. H. G. and Sheiner, L. B. (1981). Understanding the dose–effect relationship: clinical application of pharmacokinetic–pharmacodynamic models. *Clin. Pharmacokinet.*, **6**, 429–53
32. Kaplan, S. A., Alexander, K., Jack, M. L. *et al.* (1974). Pharmacokinetic profiles of clonazepam in dog and humans and of flunitrazepam in dog. *J. Pharm. Sci.*, **63**, 527–32
33. Kaplan, S. A., Jack, M. L., Alexander, K. *et al.* (1973). Pharmacokinetic profile of diazepam in man following single intravenous and oral and chronic oral administration. *J. Pharm. Sci.*, **62**, 1789–96
34. Kates, R. E., Keene, B. W. and Hamlin, R. L. (1979). Pharmacokinetics of propranolol in the dog. *J. Vet. Pharmacol. Ther.*, **2**, 21–6
35. Kramer, W. G., Lewis, R. P., Cobb, T. C. *et al.* (1974). Pharmacokinetics of digoxin: comparison of a two- and three-compartment model in man. *J. Pharmacokinet. Biopharm.*, **2**, 299–312
36. Levy, G. (1964). Relationship between elimination rate of drugs and rate of decline of their pharmacologic effects. *J. Pharm. Sci.*, **53**, 342–3
37. Lin, Y-Z., Weidler, D. J., Garg, D. C. *et al.* (1978). Novel method of estimating volume of distribution of a drug obeying Michaelis–Menten elimination kinetics. *J. Pharmacokinet. Biopharm.*, **6**, 197–207

38. Martin, B. K. (1965). Potential effect of the plasma proteins on drug distribution. *Nature (London)*, **207**, 274–6
39. Neff-Davis, C. A., Davis, L. E. and Gillette, E. L. (1981). Warfarin in the dog: pharmacokinetics as related to clinical response. *J. Vet. Pharmacol. Ther.*, **4**, 135–40
40. Nienstedt, W. and Hartiala, K. (1969). Steroid metabolism by the canine intestine. 1. Qualitative experiments with progesterone. *Scand. J. Gastroenterol.*, **4**, 483–8
41. Notari, R. E., DeYoung, J. L. and Reuning, R. H. (1972). Effect of parallel first-order drug loss from site of administration on calculated values for absorption rate constants. *J. Pharm. Sci.*, **61**, 135–8
42. Rasmussen, F., Gelså, H. and Nielsen, P. (1979). Pharmacokinetics of sulphadoxine and trimethoprim in horses. Half-life and volume of distribution of sulphadoxine and trimethoprim and cumulative excretion of [^{14}C]- trimethoprim. *J. Vet. Pharmacol. Ther.*, **2**, 245–55
43. Routledge, P. A. and Shand, D. G. (1979). Presystemic drug elimination. *Ann. Rev. Pharmacol. Toxicol.*, **19**, 447–68
44. Shimoda, M., Kokue, E-I., Kurebayashi, Y. *et al.* (1981). Three compartment model for pyrimethamine disposition in the pig. *J. Vet. Pharmacol. Ther.*, **4**, 165–70
45. Snow, D. H., Baxter, P. and Whiting, B. (1981). The pharmacokinetics of meclofenamic acid in the horse. *J. Vet. Pharmacol. Ther.*, **4**, 147–56
46. Strong, J. M., Dutcher, J. S., Lee, W-K. *et al.* (1975). Absolute bioavailability in man of *N*-acetylprocainamide determined by a novel stable isotope method. *Clin. Pharmacol. Ther.*, **18**, 613–22
47. Vaughan, D. P. and Beckett, A. H. (1974). An analysis of the intersubject variation in the metabolism of pentazocine. *J. Pharm. Pharmacol.*, **26**, 789–98
48. Wagner, J. G. (1978). Time to reach steady state and prediction of steady-state concentrations for drugs obeying Michaelis–Menten elimination kinetics. *J. Pharmacokinet. Biopharm.*, **6**, 209–25
49. Wilkinson, G. R. and Shand, D. G. (1975). A physiological approach to hepatic drug clearance. *Clin. Pharmacol. Ther.*, **18**, 377–90

38
Pharmacological approach of drugs used in coronary insufficiency and cerebrovascular pathology

P. Lacroix and P. Linée

The choice of animal models in vascular diseases is as difficult as that of atherogenic diets (see Appendix). Atherosclerosis may be considered as the main cause of coronary insufficiency due to a progressive reduction of the internal size of the epicardial coronary arteries. Spasm of a coronary artery is also involved in more than one third of coronary insufficiencies. The resulting desequilibrium between oxygen supply and oxygen demand of the myocardium of a hypoperfused area acts as a trigger for haemodynamic, metabolic and electric disturbances.

A prerequisite for the search and selection of drugs which could be used in the treatment of both myocardial and brain vascular diseases is that of suitable animal models.

CORONARY VASODILATOR DRUGS

An increase in the oxygen blood supply might be of interest as far as the ischaemic areas of the myocardium are concerned. Unfortunately, arteriolar coronary dilation may be the cause of a coronary steal to the detriment of ischaemic area. To evaluate the true effect of an increase in the oxygen blood supply, an infarction is provoked by the ligation of the left anterior descending coronary artery in dogs. Five weeks later, animals are set up for the study of coronary haemodynamics. In the normal area, the circumflex coronary flow, termed perfusion coronary flow, is measured by means of an electromagnetic flow probe. Perfusion coronary pressure is recorded in the aorta. Using these parameters, perfusion coronary resistance can also be calculated. The same parameters are recorded in the ischaemic area: retrograde coronary flow by collecting in a test tube the blood emerging from the occluded artery; retrograde coronary pressure and then retrograde coronary resistance. Drugs are administered intravenously (Figure 38.1).

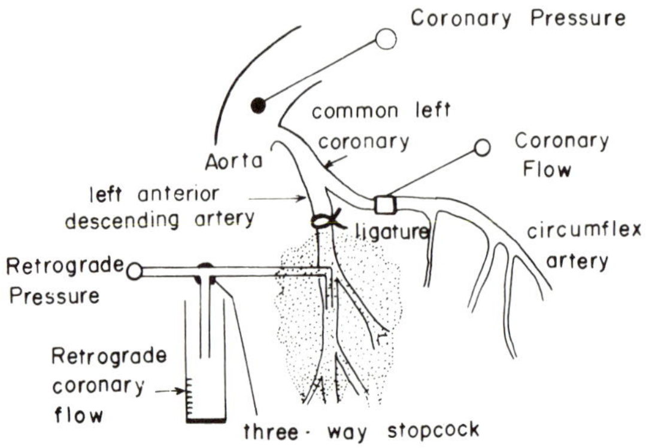

Figure 38.1 Coronary occlusion carried out in dogs 5 weeks before the study of the effects of drugs administered intravenously on the subsequent ischaemic area (shaded zone)

Coronary occlusion was accompanied by 33% mortality including instantaneous (11.5%) and sudden (21.5%) death in an experiment performed on 346 dogs. Five weeks after the coronary occlusion, the average retrograde coronary pressure was 76% of that of the aorta (instead of 24% for experiments carried out 2 or 3 h after the occlusion). This suggested a satisfactory development of collateral circulation on such a model. Nitroglycerin, a nitrate-like compound (molsidomine), calcium entry blockers like diltiazem and bepridil, smooth muscle fibre relaxant agents like papaverine and ethaverine were able to promote an appropriate redistribution, recorded as an increased flow in the ischaemic area. Atenolol, but not propranolol, was active. In contrast, coronary arteriolar vasodilators, like dipyridamole or calcium entry blockers like verapamil and nifedipine, were at the origin of a coronary steal evidenced by a decrease in retrograde coronary flow.

Other trials in animal models resembling human coronary insufficiency are numerous and involve the measurement of the retrograde coronary flow of an ischaemic area in dogs using radiolabelled microspheres.

(1) Epicardial mapping of myocardial ischaemia after coronary ligation in dogs which permits the evaluation of the infarct size and progression.

(2) Biochemical disorders of ischaemia by measurements of enzymatic leakage and calcium entry in both dogs and rats.

(3) Sudden death after left coronary artery ligation in rats or spontaneous death in Japanese quails treated with cholesterol.

(4) *In vitro* measurement of drug induced cardioprotection in the guinea pig.

(5) Coronary vasospasm obtained by agents like vasopressin in both dogs and rats and methylergometrine in anaesthetized rats (Figure 38.2).

Nifedipine, diltiazem, verapamil and molsidomine administered orally were active in the vasopressin rat model but neither dipyridamole nor naftidrofuryl. Nitroglycerine and hexobendine were active intravenously in the vasopressin dog model and both nifedipine and diltiazem were found active orally in the methylergometrine rat model.

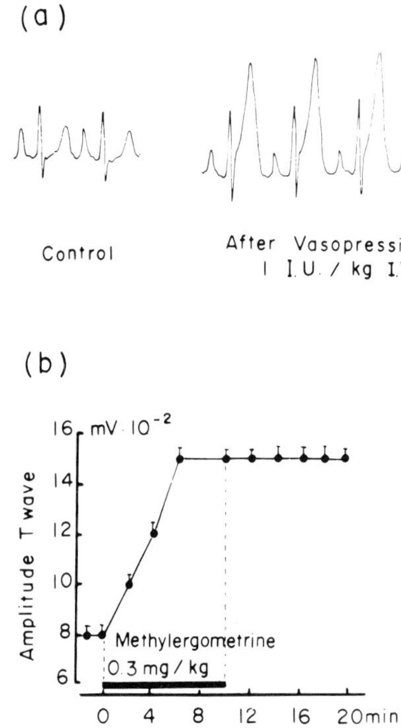

Figure 38.2 Coronary vasospasm. (a) The intravenous injection of vasopressin (1 IU/kg) in the unanaesthetized dog increases the T wave magnitude. (b) A similar long-lasting effect is obtained by the infusion of 0.3 mg/kg of methylergometrine within 10 min

ANTIHYPOXIC DRUGS

An experimental approach to the questions of cerebral ageing and of the prevention or treatment of chronic vascular disorders is very complex for many reasons. The chronic organic brain syndrome is poorly defined, proceeds from both cerebral and extracerebral (cardiovascular, respiratory) disorders and involves many forms of disturbances (memory, self-care). Species differences between animals and man are other factors to be considered. Finally, cerebral ageing in animals has not yet been defined and 'aged' animals could not be used for current research. The commonly induced disturbances include cerebral oxygen insufficiency obtained by hypoxia[1–5]. However, such acute experimental models fail to reproduce any of the progressive changes recorded in chronic therapy. In addition, any drug can be accepted as a standard because of the lack of any controlled clinical trial showing an improvement in the glucose cerebral extraction or consumption and in the cerebral neurotransmitters' turnover.

The four screening tests which have been used to describe the pharmacological profile of the so-called antihypoxic drugs are (1) survival time in mice after an intraperitoneal injection of potassium cyanide[2], (2) mnesic retention of a passive avoidance conditioning following an acute hypobaric hypoxia in rats placed in a two-compartment box[3], (3) partial or total protection against brain oedema obtained in rats by successive oral administration of triethyltin hydrochloride, and (4) in anaesthetized dogs, the cerebral bloodflow including pH, pO_2, pCO_2, glucose, lactate and haemoglobin values in order to calculate changes in cerebral blood supply and metabolism[1].

Table 38.1 Effects of five antihypoxic drugs in the following tests: KCN-induced hypoxia, mnesic retention, brain oedema and cerebral haemodynamics

Compound	*KCN-induced hypoxia* (mice)	*Mnesic retention after hypobaric hypoxia* (rats)	*Triethyltin-induced brain oedema* (rats)	*Cerebral vasodilatation and metabolism* (dogs)	
Dihydroergotoxine	No increase (survival time)	No effect	Yes	No effect	Stimulation (metabolism)
(-) Eburnamonine	Increase	Improvement	Yes	No effect	Stimulation (metabolism)
Papaverine	No increase	No effect	No	Vasodilatation	No effect
Piracetam	No increase	Improvement	No	Not studied	
Vincamine	No increase	No effect	Yes	No effect	No effect

Table 38.1 shows the pharmacological 'profile' of five different drugs. It is worth noting that papaverine is inactive in the tests used, like most of the cerebral vasodilators. In contrast, cerebral metabolism stimulants like dihydroergotoxine and eburnamonine increase survival time or at least prevent the accumulation of water and sodium in white matter of the brain and spinal cord.

The results suggest the possibility of an experimental approach to active drugs in cerebrovascular disorders. However, the experimental data obtained in acute cerebral failure revealed rather a mechanism of action than an efficiency in chronic failures.

References

1. Lacroix, P. *et al.* (1979). Cerebral metabolic and haemodynamic activities of 1-erbunamonine in the anaesthetized dog. A comparison with vincamine. *Arzneim. Forsch.*, **29**, 1094–101
2. Linée, P. and Laville, M. P. (1981). Mesure du temps de survie de la souris en hypoxie histotoxique aiguë provoquée par le cyanure de potassium. *J. Pharmacol., Paris*, **12**, 847–9
3. Linee, P. *et al.* (1977). Action protectrice cérébrale de la 1-éburnamonine étudiée sur 3 modèles d'agression hypoxique aiguë. Comparaison avec la vincamine. *Ann. Pharm.*, **35**, 97–110
4. Meier-Ruge, W. (1977). Experimental pathology and pharmacology in brain research and aging. *Life Sci.*, **17**, 1627–36
5. Rossignol, P. and Ebigwei-Ibru, M. (1980). Drugs against brain hypoxia. *Trends Pharm. Sci.*, **1**, 287–9

APPENDIX
Experimental diet induced atherosclerosis

T. H. Nguyen and O. Guillevic

Among the 219 diet procedures used from 1979 to 1982 to obtain experimental atherosclerosis, 186 referred to mammals in the following order of frequency: rabbit 62, pig 45, monkey 40, dog 18, rat 14, mouse 1, wild rodent 1. Among birds, hens and chicken *(Gallus gallus)* have been used in 25 experiments, the pigeon in six experiments and only one trial in turkey and in quails.

The nature of athcrogcnic diets consisted of cholesterol-enriched diets and high-fat diets, or both of them. The high fat contents were obtained from 19 fats and oils (ground nut oil, butter, cottonseed oil, safflowerseed oil, cocoa fat, coconut oil, crisco oil, rapeseed oil, undetermined fat, hydrogenated oils or margarine, lard, maize oil, olive oil, palm kernel oil, beef tallow, sesame oil, soybean oil, *Stercula foetida* oil and sunflowerseed oil.

Other sterols than cholesterol were cholecalciferol (pig), sistosterol (rabbit), ergocalciferol (rat), cholic acid (rat, rabbit, dog, monkey) and sodium taurocholate (hens).

Egg yolk was used in the rabbit, monkey, pig and *Gallus gallus*. High sugar diets were used in rabbit and monkey. The thyroid inhibitors, propylthiouracyl and iodine-131, were given in dogs. Vitamin E and C deficiencies were induced in rabbit and guinea-pig, respectively. In the pig, atherosclerosis was obtained by injuries of the arterial endothelium and intravenous injection of heterologous serum.

In spite of data collection over many years, no reference was found to the use of the cat as an experimental animal. Are cats really resistant to experimental diet-induced atherosclerosis?

39
Fever, trace metals and disease. The effect of antipyretic agents

A. S. J. P. A. M. Van Miert, D. Zwart, J. H. M. Verheijden and A. J. H. Schotman

---

Many infectious diseases are accompanied by fever associated with a rapid decline in plasma iron concentration and plasma zinc concentration[3,10,14,26]. Similar responses occur in experimental animals when sterile inflammation is produced, such as *E. coli* endotoxin-induced mastitis[22,27] or following intravenous injection of pyrogens[3,4,10,22–24,27]. It is generally believed that fever is mediated by an endogenous pyrogen (EP), a protein which is released from cells of the reticulo-endothelial system and which acts on central nervous system temperature regulating centres[1]. An analogous endogenous substance produced by phagocytic cells has subsequently been found to mediate the changes in plasma trace metals, which occur in conjunction with fever[3,11]. This substance has been termed leukocytic endogenous mediator (LEM). The relationship between EP and LEM has not been determined with certainty[12,17].

One of the beneficial mechanisms of fever in laboratory animals is the decrease in availability of iron to pathogenic micro-organisms[13,28]. Growth inhibition *in vitro* due to iron deprivation has been reported for most pathogenic bacteria[18] whereas injection of iron reduces the survival of experimentally infected animals[5,8]. This effect was also observed[19] following injection of zinc in animals experimentally infected with *E. coli* or *S. typhimurium*. It has been demonstrated that *Pasteurella multocida* was unable to grow at febrile temperatures and low iron concentration[13], whereas rabbits that developed low-grade fever after infection with *P. multocida* were shown to have decreased survival as compared to rabbits that developed high fever[15]. Moreover, effective antipyretic therapy with sodium salicylate eliminated the enhanced survival[25]. It has been shown for *S. typhimurium*[9] and for *E. coli*[16] that the ability of these bacteria to produce bacterial iron transport compounds is diminished at febrile temperatures. These findings suggest that the changes in plasma trace metal concentration and in body temperature act together as a co-ordinated host defence mechanism.

A couple of years ago, we studied the effect of flurbiprofen-induced antipyresis in acute *Trypanosoma vivax* infected goats. It was apparent that the drug had a deleterious effect on these infected goats. Parasitaemia was overwhelming and terminated in early death[21].

The purposes of our recent studies were:

(1) To identify any alteration in parasitaemia during flurbiprofen-induced antipyresis in goats infected with other pathogenic trypanosomes than *T. vivax*. Additional studies were performed to characterize the effects of other antipyretic drugs in this model. Moreover, the influence of flurbiprofen was studied during long-standing trypanosome infections.

(2) To identify any alteration in plasma zinc and iron concentration during fever due to a trypanosome infection or induced by leukocytic and bacterial pyrogens.

(3) To evaluate the effects of flurbiprofen upon the responses to bacterial pyrogens. Flurbiprofen was chosen because, in the goat, this agent is more potent than other antipyretic drugs[20].

RESULTS AND DISCUSSION

Flurbiprofen (1 mg/kg i.v. twice daily) inhibited the febrile reactions during the acute phase of *T. congolense* or *T. brucei* infection. Again, parasitaemia of a progressive type could be observed during drug treatment (Table 39.1). All of the *T. congolense* infected goats treated with flurbiprofen died, in

Table 39.1 The effect of flurbiprofen* (1 mg/kg BW, i.v., twice daily) on the number of parasites per field (8 × 45; less than 1, 10 and from 10 to 20) in the blood from goats experimentally infected with *T. brucei* 1066 or *T. congolense* S 104

Day	T. brucei					T. congolense					
0–3	–	–	–	–	–	–	–	–	–	–	–
4	+	ND	ND	+	–	–	–	–	–	–	–
5	–	+	+	+*	–	–	–	–	+	–	–
6	+	+	+	+*	+*	–	–	–	1	–	–
7	+	+	+	1*	1*	ND	–	ND	+	+	–
8	+	1	ND	10*	10–20*	ND	–	ND	1	+	+
9	+	+	+	10–20*	10–20*	ND	+	+	1	1	+
10	+	+	ND	10–20*	10–20*	+*	+*	+	ND	1	+
11	+	+	+	10–20*	10–20*	1*	+*	+	ND	+	1
12	+	+	1	1*	1*	1*	+*	+	+	+	1
13	+	+	1	1*	1*	10*	10–20*	1	+	1	–
14	1	+	+	1*	1*	1*	10*	+	+	1	1
15	+	+	+	1*	+*	†	10*	ND	–	1	1
16	+	+	–	1*	+*		†	ND	+	1	1
17	+	ND	ND	10*	+*			0	ND	1	1
18	+	+	+	†	1*			+	ND	+	+
19	–	+	+		†			ND	–	+	ND
20	+	+	–					ND	+	+	ND

–, neg.; +, pos. using the haematocrit centrifuge technique; ND, not determined; † died contrast to the infected control animals. However, a number of the *T. brucei* infected goats treated with the drug survived. This was also the case during long-standing trypanosome infections. Nevertheless, flurbiprofen induced a marked increase in the number of circulating parasites in these patients. In the next series of experiments other antipyretic agents were tested in *T. vivax* infected goats. Suprofen, an antipyretic agent which is less potent than flurbiprofen, induced parasitaemia of a progressive type as compared with the intermittent type in the controls. Treatment of *T. vivax* infected goats with sodium salicylate or flunixine meglumine only had a partial inhibitory effect upon the febrile reactions, whereas no significant effects upon the number of circulating trypanosomes could be seen. In conclusion, in goats both flurbiprofen and suprofen induce a progressive increase in the number of circulating trypanosomes, which often terminate in early death. We have measured also the plasma zinc and iron concentration in *T. vivax* and *T. congolense* infected goats (Figure 39.1). During the course of infection

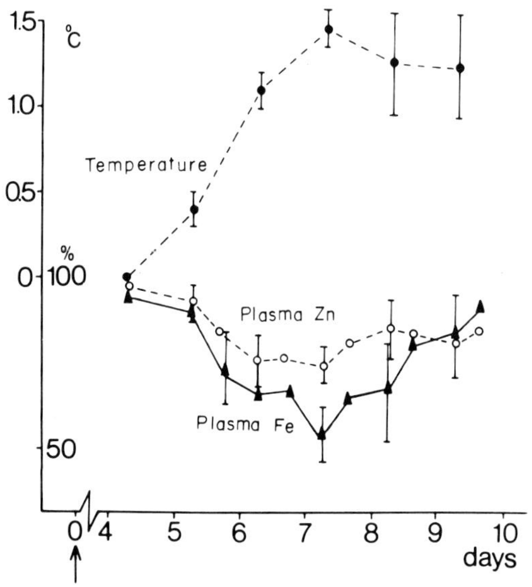

Figure 39.1 Fever and changes in plasma zinc (○) and iron concentrations (▲) in *Trypanosoma vivax* infected goats ($n = 8$). The animals were infected by subcutaneous inoculation using 10^6 parasites (↑)

hardly any significant changes in plasma zinc concentration could be found. Plasma levels of iron, on the other hand, tended to undergo some decline after temperature peaks, although the reduction was much less pronounced as compared with the values found during bacterial pyrogen-induced fever.

When goats were injected i.v. with staphylococcal enterotoxin B (SEB) or *E. coli* endotoxin (LPS), a variety of clinical effects were observed such as febrile responses accompanied by malaise, changes in heart rate and inhibition of rumen motility[22]. The febrile reactions after SEB were less progressive, which demonstrates that in goats the enterotoxin is not a potent pyrogenic agent. Furthermore, *E. coli* LPS caused a short-lasting neutrophylic leukopenia, which was followed by a significant increase in the number of circulating neutrophylic leukocytes; lymphopenia was also seen, causing significant changes in the lymphocyte: neutrophil ratio. SEB induced a long-lasting decrease in the number of white blood cells caused by a decline in circulating lymphocytes and neutrophils, with a marked shift to less mature cells. Within 6 h after *E. coli* LPS or SEB administration, significant decreases were seen in both plasma zinc and plasma iron concentrations. The decline in these trace metal levels was more persistent after SEB than after *E. coli* LPS. Moreover, no clear relationship could be found between the temperature reactions (Fever index) and the alterations in zinc and iron levels[22].

The intramammary infusion of *E. coli* LPS (1 mg) was followed by a certain lag-period before the onset of local signs of inflammation. Approximately 1.5 h after infusion, the gland started swelling markedly, the phenomenon progressing rapidly to its maximum towards the second and third hour. At this time the udder was very firm, hot and painful. Among the systemic signs observed were shivering, rise in body temperature and an increase in heart rate. The absence of marked effects on rumen motility was striking[22, 27].

In the next experiment, SEB was given intramammarily to four lactating goats (1 mg). Typical inflammatory reactions such as swelling and palpate sensitivity developed in the udders within 6 h, but the intensity of this response was less pronounced than after *E. coli* LPS. About 3 h after infusion, rumen contractions gradually diminished and body temperature started to rise. A fall in total white blood cell count was observed after SEB infusion. This was caused by a decline in both lymphocytes and neutrophils, accompanied by an increase in the number of less mature neutrophils[22]. Both toxins induced significant decreases in plasma zinc and plasma iron concentrations. Furthermore, and most remarkable, the drop in plasma iron concentration developed more rapidly after SEB than after *E. coli* LPS, whereas the decline in plasma zinc concentration after SEB was more delayed. When kids were injected i.v. with *E. coli* LPS, biphasic temperature responses coupled with significant decreases in plasma zinc and iron were seen. The i.v. injection of leukocytic pyrogen (EP) induced characteristic monophasic temperature responses in these animals. However, no significant changes in plasma trace metals were observed during and after the febrile episodes[23]. Our findings that (1) leukocytic pyrogen induces fever without changes in plasma zinc and iron concentrations, and (2) that no clear relationship could be found between the temperature responses and the alterations in zinc and iron plasma levels after SEB and *E. coli* LPS administration or in the course of a trypanosome infection, support the theory that febrile reactions and the changes in plasma trace metals are mediated by different proteins (e.g. EP and LEM are not identical proteins). Moreover, in trypanosome infections and after intramammary SEB administration, the pattern of changes in plasma zinc and iron concentrations was different in comparison with the pattern observed after i.v. *E. coli* LPS and SEB administration. These results suggest that plasma zinc and iron do not behave in a similar way.

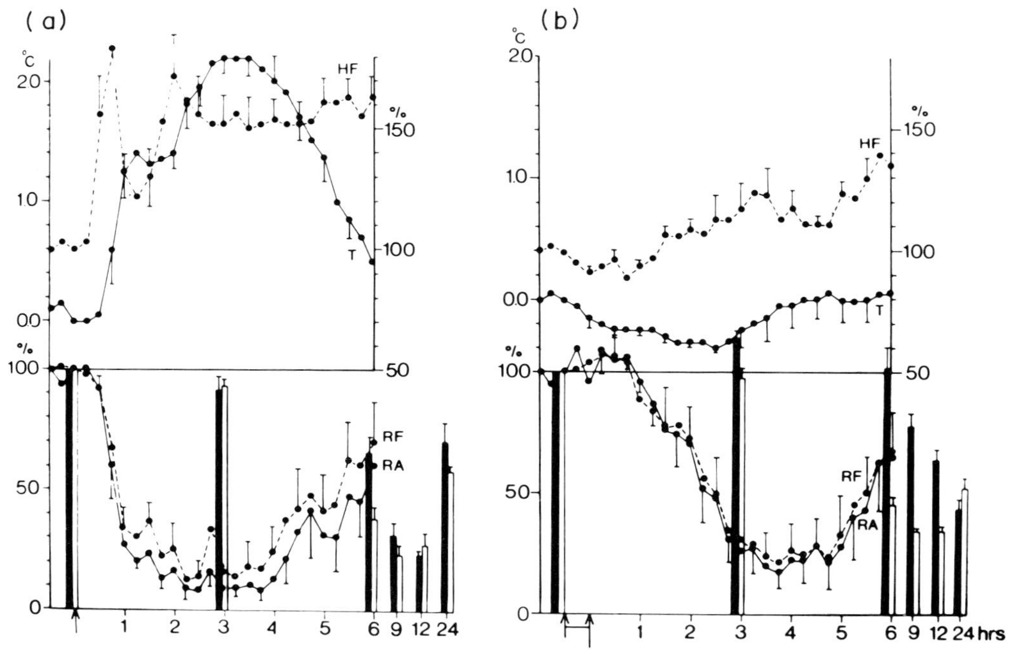

Figure 39.2 (a) Effect of *E. coli* LPS 0.1 μg/kg i.v. (↑) on body temperature, heart rate, rumen contractions and plasma Fe and Zn concentrations in the goat ($n = 6$). (b) Effect of *E. coli* LPS injected immediately after flurbiprofen administration in the same group of animals. The drug was given as an i.v. infusion (↑⎵↑: 2 mg/kg) followed by a bolus injection of 1 mg/kg at the 6th hour. HF = frequency of heart beat per min expressed in percentage of the initial value; T = change in body temperature (°C). Rumen contractions and trace metals are expressed in percentages of the initial values: RF = frequency of contractions per 15 min; RA = summation derived from 15 min intervals of amplitude. Solid vertical bars: plasma Fe values and open vertical bars: plasma Zn values. Values are given as mean ±SEM

Antipyretic agents inhibit both endogenous and bacterial pyrogen-induced fever. However, these agents have no influence upon the synthesis and release of EP[6]. Pretreatment with flurbiprofen completely abolished the febrile reactions to *E. coli* LPS. However, the LPS-induced inhibition of rumen contractions was only delayed (Figure 39.2). The drug blocked the initial tachycardia to LPS, but it did not prevent the secondary biphasic increase in heart rate. Moreover, flurbiprofen failed to modify the LPS-induced decrease in plasma zinc concentration, whereas the decline in plasma iron concentrations was delayed. This again suggests that plasma zinc and iron concentrations are regulated by different mechanisms. After drug pretreatment the changes in circulating white blood cells were more pronounced[24]. These data demonstrate that most of the haematological, blood biochemical and clinical effects to *E. coli* LPS cannot be blocked by flurbiprofen, and that these effects are not due to the increase in body temperature alone. In the control goats, flurbiprofen (2 mg/kg, which is a somewhat high dose) slightly depressed both body temperature and rumen motility, whereas urea nitrogen concentrations gradually increased. Plasma iron concentration and the number of circulating lymphocytes were significantly lower[24]. Many antipyretic agents, given in relatively high doses, induce renal papillary necrosis, acute tubular damage and interstitial nephritis. In men, these pathomorphological effects are often associated with raised blood urea and creatinine levels[7]. Tissue lesions induce non-specific host responses, termed the acute phase reaction[2]. These include infiltration of activated leukocytes, changes in the concentration of certain plasma proteins and trace metals and various associated metabolic adjustments. Previous work in our laboratory has documented renal lesions following the administration of flurbiprofen in goats[21]. Consequently, there might be a relationship between flurbiprofen-induced renal lesions and the drop in plasma iron concentrations. If this is correct, plasma iron concentration might be an interesting criterion for tissue lesions during toxicity studies.

References

1. Atkins, E. and Bodel, P. (1979). Clinical fever: its history, manifestations and pathogenesis. *Fed. Proc.*, **38**, 57–63
2. Beisel, W. R. (1975). Metabolic response to infection. *Ann. Rev. Med.*, **26**, 9–20
3. Beisel, W. R. (1976). Trace elements in infectious processes. *Med. Clin. N. Am.*, **60**, 831–49
4. Blatteis, C. M., Mashburn, T. A. and Ahokas, R. A. (1981). Fever and trace metal changes in endotoxin-challenged neonates. *Pflügers Arch.*, **389**, 177–9
5. Bullen, J. J. and Rogers, H. J. (1969). Bacterial iron metabolism and immunity to *Pasteurella septica* and *Escherichia coli. Nature (London)*, **224**, 380–2
6. Clark, W. G. (1979). Mechanisms of antipyretic action. *Gen. Pharmacol.*, **10**, 71–7
7. del Favero, A. (1981). Anti-inflammatory analgesics and drugs used in rheumatism and gout. In Dukes, M. N. (ed.) *Side Effects of Drugs.* Annual 5, pp. 88–117. (Amsterdam: Excerpta Medica)
8. Elin, R. J. and Wolff, S. M. (1974). The role of iron in nonspecific resistance to infection induced by endotoxin. *J. Immunol.*, **112**, 737–45
9. Garibaldi, J. A. (1972). Influence of temperature on the biosynthesis of iron transport compounds by *Salmonella typhimurium. J. Bacteriol.*, **110**, 262–5

10. Groothuis, D. G., van Miert, A. S. J. P. A. M. and Schotman, A. J. H. (1981). Zinc concentration in plasma during experimental *Salmonella dublin* infection and endotoxin induced fever in calves. *Vet. Rec.*, **109**, 176–7
11. Kampschmidt, R. F. (1978). Leukocytic endogenous mediator. *J. Reticuloendothel. Soc.*, **23**, 287–97
12. Kampschmidt, R. F., Pulliam, L. A. and Merriman, C. R. (1978). Further similarities of endogenous pyrogen and leukocytic endogenous mediator. *Am. J. Physiol.*, **235**, C118–21
13. Kluger, M. J. and Rothenburg, B. A. (1979). Fever and reduced iron: their interaction as a host defence response to bacterial infection. *Science*, **203**, 374–6
14. Kluger, M. J. and Rothenburg, B. A. (1980). Fever, trace metals and disease. In Lipton, J. M. (ed.) *Fever*. pp. 31–8. (New York: Raven Press)
15. Kluger, M. J. and Vaughn, L. K. (1978). Fever and survival in rabbits infected with *Pasteurella multocida*. *J. Physiol. (London)*, **282**, 243–51
16. Kochan, I. (1977). Role of iron in the regulation of nutritional immunity. *Adv. Chem.*, **162**, 55–77
17. Mapes, C. A. and Sobocinski, P. Z. (1977). Differentiation between endogenous pyrogen and leukocytic endogenous mediator. *Am. J. Physiol.*, **232**, C15–22
18. Marcelis, J. H. (1980). Interactions between bacteria and iron binding proteins. *Vet. Res. Commun.*, **4**, 151–64
19. Sobocinski, P. Z., Canterbury, W. J. and Powanda, M. C. (1977). Differential effect of parenteral zinc on the course of various bacterial infections. *Proc. Soc. Exp. Biol. Med.*, **156**, 334–9
20. van Miert, A. S. J. P. A. M., van der Wal-Komproe, L. E. and van Duin, C. Th. M. (1977). Effects of antipyretic agents on fever and ruminal stasis induced by endotoxins in conscious goats. *Arch. Int. Pharmacodyn. Thér.*, **225**, 39–50
21. van Miert, A. S. J. P. A. M., van Duin, C. Th. M., Busser, F. J. M. *et al.* (1978). The effect of flurbiprofen, a potent non-steroidal anti-inflammatory agent, upon *Trypanosoma vivax* infection in goats. *J. Vet. Pharmacol. Ther.*, **1**, 69–76
22. van Miert, A. S. J. P. A. M., van Duin, C. Th. M., Verheijden, J. H. M. *et al.* (1983). Staphylococcal enterotoxin B: fever and associated clinical, haematological and blood biochemical changes in the goat. Comparative observations after intravenous and intramammary administration. *Am J. Vet Res.*, **44**, 955–63
23. van Miert, A. S. J. P. A. M., van Duin, C. Th. M., Verheijden, J. H. M. *et al.* (1983). Fever and changes in plasma zinc and iron concentrations in the goat. The role of leukocytic pyrogen. *J. Physiol. (London)*. (Submitted)
24. van Miert, A. S. J. P. A. M., van Duin, C. Th. M., Verheijden, J. H. M. *et al.* (1983). Endotoxin-induced fever and associated haematological and blood biochemical changes in the goat. The effect of repeated administration and the influence of flurbiprofen. *Res. Vet. Sci.*, **33**, 248–55
25. Vaughn, L. K., Veale, W. L. and Cooper, K. E. (1980). Antipyresis: its effect on mortality rate of bacterially infected rabbits. *Brain Res. Bull.*, **5**, 69–73
26. Verheijden, J. H. M., van Miert, A. S. J. P. A. M., Schotman, A. J. H. *et al.* (1980). Das absinken des zinks im plasma von rindern mit coliformen mastitis und nach intramammären applikation von endotoxinen. *Der Prakt. Tierarzt*, **7**, 596–8
27. Verheijden, J. H. M., van Miert, A. S. J. P. A. M., Schotman, A. J. H. *et al.* (1980). Reduction of plasma zinc and iron concentrations in febrile cows with *E. coli* mastitis. The role of endotoxin. In Szeléryi, Z. and Székely, M. (eds.) *Satellite 28th Congress Physiol. Sci. Pécs*. pp. 157–60. (Budapest: Akadémia Kiado Press)
28. Weinberg, E. D. (1978). Iron and infection. *Microbiol. Rev.*, **42**, 45–66

40
Efficacy of penicillin against *Streptococcus zooepidemicus*. Infection model in the horse

K. J. Varma, T. E. Powers, R. C. Garg,
S. L. Spurlock and J. D. Powers

INTRODUCTION

Experimental infectious models of target animal species are useful for determining *in vivo* pharmacological efficacy and dosage regimens of antimicrobial agents[4]. In antimicrobial therapy, the ultimate aim is to maintain the drug in the biophase surrounding the pathogen at a concentration and for the duration that is optimum for eliminating the pathogen from the body. In clinical practice, the minimum inhibitory concentration (MIC) of the antibiotic for the pathogen may be determined and efforts are made to maintain the drug concentration in blood equal to or higher than the MIC.

In our investigations, we have produced an experimental disease model using β-haemolytic Gram positive *Streptococcus zooepidemicus*. The disease was treated with sodium penicillin G by constant intravenous infusion to maintain concentrations of $4 \times$ MIC, $1 \times$ MIC and $0.25 \times$ MIC in groups of six animals each to observe the effects of different blood levels in curing the experimental *Strep. zooepidemicus* infection.

MATERIALS AND METHODS

The characteristics of the disease model desired were that (1) it be caused preferably by a single pathogen, (2) it should produce clinically observable signs of the disease in an acute and chronic phase, (3) it should run a course of 15–20 days, and (4) it should be treatable by commonly available antibiotics to provide positive controls.

The following parameters were titrated to produce the effective disease model:

(1) Age of the animal,
(2) Route of inoculation,
(3) Inoculum size (number of pathogens and volume of inoculum),
(4) Frequency and interval between inoculations,
(5) Preparation of culture suspension for inoculation.

Streptococcus zooepidemicus model

The organism, quick frozen and stored at −70 °C, was thawed and inoculated in 10 ml Brain Heart Infusion media (BHI) and incubated for 18 h. Of this culture suspension, 0.1 ml was inoculated in 400 ml BHI and incubated for 18 h. This was centrifuged later, the bacterial pellet washed twice with normal saline and reconstituted in 35 ml of normal saline for i.v. inoculation.

All the parameters listed above were titrated in preliminary experiments and the final dose titration was performed based on conclusions from previous experiments as described in Table 40.1.

Table 40.1 Final dose titration

Time of inoculation	*Group I* (40 and 28)†	*Group II* (35 and 48)†	*Group III* (50 and 63)†
Day 1	1×10^{10}*	1×10^{10}*	1×10^{10}*
Day 2	1×10^{10}*	1×10^{8}*	1×10^{6}*

*Size of inoculum (cfu of *Strep. zooepidemicus*); route = intravenous;
† = horse number

In Group I, the animals showed intense signs of the disease and in Group III, one animal did not show the signs at all. The Group II animals showed all the signs of the disease and these could be observed until postinfection day (PID) 15.

After this, we challenged six horses with 10^{10} colony forming units (cfu) as the first i.v. challenge, and 10^{8} cfu, 24 h later, as the second i.v. challenge. This was done to test the reproducibility of the disease model and to determine the effects of the infection upon blood cell counts and blood chemistry parameters. The horses were observed for clinical signs of the disease up to PID 13.

Penicillin study

Sodium penicillin G was infused intravenously at a constant rate starting from PID 3 for 5 days in groups of six horses to maintain 4 × MIC, 1 × MIC and 0.25 × MIC of the drug in the blood. One group of six infected animals received only the diluent (normal saline) and another group of six healthy animals received the drug to maintain 4 × MIC and served as a healthy control. The blood cell counts, blood chemistry parameters and clinical evaluations were done until PID 13, which was 5 days after cessation of therapy. The animals were necropsied on PID 13.

RESULTS AND DISCUSSION

Strep. zooepidemicus model

Blood counts

The blood cell counts of infected animals demonstrated a neutrophilic leukocytosis with both the relative and absolute increase in neutrophils (Tables 40.2 and 40.3). This change was first noticed in all the animals between PID 1 and PID 4.

Table 40.2 Changes in total blood leukocytes (counts/μl) in horses infected with *Strep. zooepidemicus* (mean ± SE, $n = 6$)

Preinfection day	Postinfection day 1	3	5	7	9	11	13
10667	11933	14100	14817	15300	17417	19717	20067
±656	±1063	±1343	±1014	±1880	±2383	±3045	±2905

Table 40.3 Changes in neutrophils (counts/μl) in horses infected with *Strep. zooepidemicus* (mean ± SE, $n = 6$)

Preinfection day	Postinfection day 1	3	5	7	9	11	13
5649	6516	8801	9427	10808	12747	13095	15205
±794	±893	±1779	±1098	±1934	±2242	±2452	±3005

Blood chemistry

The levels of blood chemistry parameters, such as glucose; electrolytes sodium, potassium, chloride; enzymes SGOT, SGPT; minerals, calcium, phosphorus; and total proteins, remained in the normal range until PID 13.

The level of alkaline phosphatase showed a gradual fall up to PID 13, although it stayed in the normal range (Table 40.4). Due to young horses

Table 40.4 Changes in alkaline phosphatase (IU/l) in horses infected with *Strep. zooepidemicus* (mean ± SE, $n = 6$)

Preinfection day	Postinfection day 1	3	5	7	9	11	12
382	402	320	282	269	270	299	277
±6	±12	±22	±32	±30	±30	±29	±33

(3–6 months of age) used in this experiment, the levels at the start of the experiment were almost two times higher than the normal level in adult horses. The gradual fall in alkaline phosphatase may be indictive of the slowing of the growth process in these animals because of infection.

There was a drastic fall in the serum iron level even one day after the challenge, and it remained low until PID 13 (Table 40.5).

Table 40.5 Changes in serum iron (μg/dl) in horses infected with *Strep. zooepidemicus* (mean ± SE, $n = 6$)

Preinfection	*Postinfection day*						
day	1	3	5	7	9	11	12
157	59	52	27	38	48	36	54
±28	±9	±22	±7	±11	±15	±10	±14

The infections lead initially to hypoferraemia and, in chronic processes, result in anaemia[2]. The agents which block the reticulo-endothelial system prevent the development of hypoferraemia and it appears that this is the site of deposition of serum iron[1].

Kluger and Rothenburg[3] grew *Pasteurella multocida in vitro* at various temperatures and different concentrations of iron and found that these bacteria do not grow well at febrile temperatures in iron-poor media, which supports the hypothesis that fever coupled with reduction in serum iron may be part of co-ordinated host defence response.

Clinical signs

The clinical signs observed are give in Table 40.6. All the infected animals were depressed by PID 2. The abnormal lung sounds were heard as early as PID 1. The horses started to show lameness by PID 2.

Table 40.6 Clinical signs observed in horses infected with *Strep. zooepidemicus*

Sign	*Earliest observation*	*Latest observation*
Temperature	Afternoon of 1st challenge	Afternoon of 1st challenge
Depression	PID 2	PID 2
Abnormal lung sounds	PID 1	PID 4
Lameness	PID 2	PID 5
Joint involvement	PID 3	PID 7

Lameness was associated with enlarged joints although it preceded joint swelling. Up to four joints were involved in different animals. The carpal and tarsal joints were most commonly affected. Occasionally, the fetlock, stifle and pastern joints were also involved.

Penicillin in *Strep. zooepidemicus* challenged and unchallenged horses

Blood cell counts

Marked leukocytosis was observed in the horses which only received the diluent. In all the groups receiving penicillin treatment at different dose levels, the white cell counts remained in the normal range, although there was a relative increase in neutrophils. In the healthy control group, the white cell counts remained in the normal range (Table 40.7).

Table 40.7 Changes in total blood leukocytes (counts/μl) in *Strep. zooepidemicus* challenged and unchallenged horses receiving different doses of penicillin G (mean ± SE, $n = 6$)

Group	*Pre-infection day*	*Postinfection day* 1	3	5	7	9	11	13
Diluent	12383 ±791	14116 ±1290	13717 ±3798	14133 ±923	15600 ±1299	16867 ±2023	18200 ±2066	21150 ±2053
025 MIC	12150 ±1334	16750 ±1039	15768 ±737	13268 ±932	15117 ±1521	13600 ±958	16500 ±1273	19717 ±2204
1 MIC	11750 ±2707	13783 ±1519	12467 ±867	12000 ±629	12633 ±897	11850 ±1104	15883 ±1333	16533 ±693
4 MIC	11033 ±1166	13083 ±1087	12733 ±989	10067 ±837	12017 ±448	12283 ±480	17200 ±1482	16417 ±1502
4 MIC*	12150 ±1262	11967 ±1123	11967 ±1444	11917 ±1144	12483 ±1167	12417 ±1459	11900 ±1533	11900 ±1234

*Healthy control

Blood chemistry

The levels of blood chemistry parameters, such as glucose, sodium, potassium, chloride, SGOT, SGPT, calcium, phosphorus and total proteins remained in the normal range throughout the experimental period.

The mean alkaline phosphatase levels are given in Table 40.8. There was a progressive fall in alkaline phosphatase level in all infected animals and this may indicate slowing of growth process in these horses.

The serum iron levels in the healthy control group remained constant throughout. There was a drastic fall in serum iron levels even 1 day after infection (Table 40.9). The levels started to return to normal after PID 7 in all treatment groups, but started to decline again in post-treatment period, i.e. by PID 11. This may be indicative of a flaring up of infection again by organisms seated in deep tissues. A serum iron level as low as $20 \pm 2\,\mu g/dl$ was observed on PID 13 in the horses receiving only normal saline.

Table 40.8 Changes in alkaline phosphatase (IU/l) in *Strep. zooepidemicus* challenged and unchallenged horses receiving different doses of penicillin (mean ± SE, $n = 6$)

Group	*Pre-infection day*	*Postinfection day* 1	3	5	7	9	11	13
Diluent	347 ± 23	365 ± 34	243 ± 24	195 ± 25	197 ± 30	195 ± 27	208 ± 30	203 ± 39
0.25 MIC	369 ± 63	392 ± 43	294 ± 37	236 ± 34	228 ± 37	226 ± 33	218 ± 39	209 ± 28
1 MIC	382 ± 23	374 ± 14	258 ± 14	221 ± 25	252 ± 25	284 ± 25	281 ± 24	268 ± 22
4 MIC	406 ± 49	387 ± 38	249 ± 18	212 ± 15	239 ± 24	272 ± 30	271 ± 36	244 ± 35
4 MIC*	399 ± 28	1408 ± 33	404 ± 33	397 ± 29	404 ± 38	403 ± 41	406 ± 50	408 ± 45

*Healthy control

Table 40.9 Changes in serum iron (μg/dl) in *Strep. zooepidemicus* challenged and unchallenged horses receiving different doses of penicillin (mean ± SE, $n = 6$)

Group	*Pre-infection day*	*Postinfection day* 1	3	5	7	9	11	13
Diluent	206 ± 53	90 ± 36	28 ± 8	35 ± 17	36 ± 16	41 ± 19	36 ± 16	20 ± 2
0.25 MIC	224 ± 28	60 ± 9	28 ± 4	41 ± 9	56 ± 15	67 ± 15	59 ± 18	65 ± 22
1 MIC	220 ± 53	37 ± 6	19 ± 1	30 ± 4	79 ± 27	103 ± 27	77 ± 30	59 ± 19
4 MIC	160 ± 37	52 ± 10	23 ± 5	44 ± 10	103 ± 27	108 ± 20	37 ± 16	42 ± 10
4 MIC*	184 ± 39	179 ± 23	193 ± 26	162 ± 48	189 ± 33	206 ± 43	243 ± 38	219 ± 52

*Healthy control

Necropsy

The animals receiving the diluent and penicillin to maintain 0.25 × MIC showed pulmonary congestion and hyperaemic splenic and mesenteric lymph nodes. No gross abnormality was observed in any organ in horses receiving the drug to maintain 1 × MIC and 4 × MIC.

CONCLUSION

The *Streptococcus* disease model developed in this study has both an acute and chronic phase. Acutely, the disease was characterized by fever, anorexia, bacteraemia, leukocytosis, abnormal lung sounds and lameness. The chronic phase was characterized by lameness, joint swelling, emaciation, loss of weight and anorexia.

This model can be of great value in testing the *in vivo* pharmacological efficacy and pharmacokinetics of newer antimicrobial agents in horses. The animals receiving penicillin to maintain 1 × MIC and 4 × MIC levels in serum showed improvement but relapsed 3–4 days after cessation of therapy. The animals receiving 0.25 × MIC showed no improvement over the control animals.

References

1. Cartwright, G. E., Gubler, C. J. and Wintrobe, M. M. (1950). The anemia of infection. XII. The effect of temperature and coloidal thorium dioxide on the plasma iron and plasma copper in dogs. *J. Biol. Chem.*, **184,** 579–87
2. Cartwright, G. E., Lauritsen, A., Humphries, S. *et al.* (1946). The anemia of infection. II. The experimental production of hypoferremia and anemia in dogs. *J. Clin. Invest.*, **25,** 81–8
3. Kluger, M. J. and Rothenburg, B. A. (1979). Fever and reduced iron: their interaction as a host defense response to bacterial infection. *Science*, **203,** 374–6
4. Powers, T. E., Powers, J. D., Garg, R. C. *et al.* (1980). Trimethoprim and sulfadiazine: experimental infection of Beagles. *Am. J. Vet. Res.*, **41,** 1117–22

41
Receptor binding methods: application to the study of cyclopyrrolones, a new family of minor tranquillizers

J. C. Blanchard and L. Julou

The receptor theory is not a new one. It was first introduced at the beginning of this century between 1905 and 1910 by Ehrlich working on tetanus toxin and trypanocidal dyes and Langley working on the action of nicotine and curare on muscle[16]. At that time, of course, very limited proof supported this notion which was almost purely conceptual[1]. However, many pharmacological studies thereafter, especially those of Clark around 1926, reinforced the interest in this concept which became very fruitful and was finally validated during the 1960s when the existence of receptors was directly established, thanks to the development of binding techniques with radiolabelled ligands[1]. A new and decisive stage was reached with the isolation around 1977 of the nicotinic receptor from the electric organ of electric fishes[11].

We must recall that, in the field of binding techniques, a major impetus came from earlier studies on cytoplasmic hormone receptors (estradiol, around 1960) and peptide hormone receptors (insulin, 1971). The technological background which they provided was especially useful for designing adequate models for the study and characterization of binding (or recognition) sites of opiates (1973) and soon thereafter of neurotransmitters such as dopamine, norepinephrine and serotonin[18].

From about 1973 the use of receptor binding methods became introduced widely in pharmacology and especially neuropharmacology. These techniques are basically similar to classical competitive protein binding assays: after incubation for various times, of an isotopically labelled hormone, neurotransmitter or drug (ligand) with a suitable receptor preparation, the ligand–receptor complex is separated from the free ligand by centrifugation or filtration. The receptor-bound radioactivity is then measured. As stated by

Cuatrecasas *et al.*[8], binding properties of ligands are considered to be specific and to correspond to the existence of specific receptor sites if the following criteria are fulfilled:

(1) High affinity for physiological or pharmacological concentrations of the ligand.

(2) Saturability, which indicates a finite number of binding sites.

(3) Tissue specificity, in accordance with those organs or regions on which the ligand is known to act.

(4) Reversibility, which is consistent with the physiological mechanism involved in the termination of the action of a natural ligand.

(5) Correlation between the binding affinities of the ligand and of its analogues and their biological activities.

It was thus possible to demonstrate the existence of specific brain receptors for many neurotransmitters such as dopamine, serotonin, norepinephrine, etc. and also for drugs such as opiates and, more recently, for the minor tranquillizers of the benzodiazepine family.

Our paper will be mainly devoted to a part of the work which we have performed on benzodiazepine binding sites using new ligands belonging to a quite original chemical family, the cyclopyrrolones. However, we have first to indicate the major contributions that specific binding techniques have brought in the field of pharmacology.

MAJOR CONTRIBUTIONS OF RECEPTOR BINDING METHODS IN PHARMACOLOGY

The usefulness of these techniques as screening methods is well recognized, their major advantages being:

(1) Their rapidity.

(2) The need for only small samples of drugs.

(3) The possibility of analysing the interaction of a drug with a broad spectrum of receptors by using various ligands.

(4) The establishment of direct relationships between chemical structures of drugs and their activities at the receptor level (this can be especially helpful for directing the synthesis of new potentially active compounds).

However, since these are *in vitro* techniques and have inherent limits, a promising compound must be studied *in vivo* as soon as possible to be sure that it can reach its specific receptors. Moreover, one drawback of these *in vitro* techniques must not be forgotten: a compound which is only active *in vivo* after it has been metabolized will not be detected.

The use of receptor binding techniques makes it possible to measure the change in the number of receptor sites in pathological conditions such as Parkinson's disease, myasthenia gravis and insulin-resistant diabetes. In addition, similar measurements following experimental subacute treatments have allowed the explanation of side-effects of some drugs such as tardive dyskinesia induced by neuroleptics.

Moreover, when no sensitive analytical method is available to study blood levels, receptor binding techniques can be used. However, it may be pointed out that the radioreceptor assay not only measures the plasma level of the drug itself but also that of its possible active metabolites. If other drugs which also recognize the same receptor are given simultaneously, the results of the radioreceptor assay cannot be interpreted.

The discovery of specific binding sites for drugs can lead to the discovery of new neurotransmitters: the discovery of opiate sites and the enkephalin–endorphin system is probably the best known example.

Finally, for the study of the mechanism of action of drugs at the molecular level, receptor binding methods are of paramount importance. It is this aspect which we would like to develop now, taking into account the work we have performed with zopiclone (RP 27 267) and suriclone (RP 31 264), two new compounds discovered in our laboratories of the cyclopyrrolone family whose chemical structures are completely different from those of the benzodiazepines (Figure 41.1).

In spite of their original chemical structures, zopiclone and suriclone have the same spectrum of activities by classical psychopharmacological techniques as minor tranquillizers of the benzodiazepine family[2, 10], i.e. anticonvulsant, antiaggressive, myorelaxant, sedative-hypnotic and anxiolytic properties (Table 41.1). Moreover, both compounds have a high margin of safety (ratios of acute LD_{50} to ED_{50} in the pentylenetetrazole test in rats)

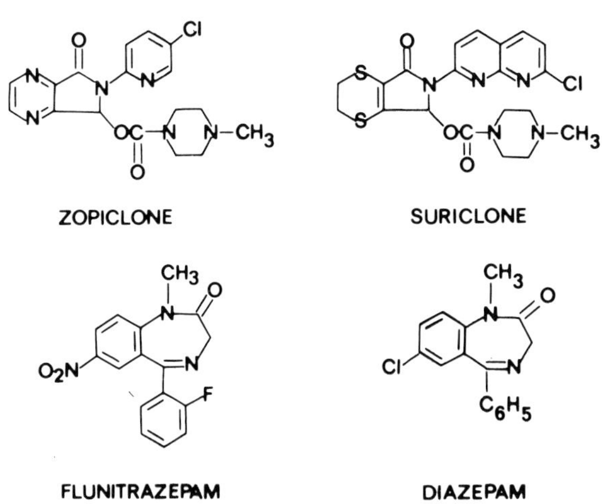

Figure 41.1 Chemical structure of cyclopyrrolones (upper part) and benzodiazepines (lower part)

Table 41.1 Main pharmacological properties of zopiclone and suriclone in comparison with nitrazepam and diazepam

Activity	*Test*	*Species*	*ED_{50} (mg/kg p.o.)* Zopiclone	*Suriclone*	*Nitrazepam*	*Diazepam*
Anticonvulsant	Pentylenetetrazole (150 mg/kg s.c.)	mouse rat	5.4 1.2	2.7 2.4	0.17 0.8	0.4 7.9
Antiaggressive	Fighting behaviour (intermittent electrical foot shocks for 3 min)	mouse	11.9	12.5	0.3	2.3
Myorelaxant	Block of polysynaptic reflex (anterior tibial muscle)	cat	0.3	0.3	0.1	0.1
Sedative-hypnotic	Confinement motor activity (decrease of up and down movements)	rat	5.2	11.6	4.1	13.8
	Righting-reflex in chlorpromazine (5 mg/kg s.c.) treated animals (loss of righting-reflex for 20 s or more)	mouse	32.5	6.0	0.4	2.0
Anxiolytic	Conflict conditioning test (range of active doses)	rat	2.5–20	2.5–20		1.25–40
Safety margin	$\frac{\text{Acute } LD_{50} \text{ (p.o.)}}{ED_{50} \text{ (p.o.) pentylenetetrazole}}$	rat	1925	>2250	2750	300

which is at least as high as those of some well-known benzodiazepines. Both drugs have been found to be useful in therapeutics, zopiclone as a hypnotic (as potent as nitrazepam) and suriclone as an anxiolytic (more potent than diazepam).

APPLICATION OF RECEPTOR BINDING METHODS TO THE STUDY OF THE MECHANISM OF ACTION OF MINOR TRANQUILLIZERS: CYCLOPYRROLONES VS. BENZODIAZEPINES

Studies of the cyclopyrrolones using classical psychopharmacological techniques had been performed in our laboratories for about 10 years when, in 1977, two groups of scientists, Squires and Braestrup from Denmark[19] and Möhler and Okada from Switzerland and Japan[13], demonstrated the presence in the rat brain of high affinity binding sites for diazepam. Moreover, a few months later the same two groups demonstrated the presence of similar specific binding sites in human brain[6, 14]. In their papers, these authors emphasized the specifity of benzodiazepines for their binding sites since no other compounds, even barbiturates or meprobamate, or known neurotransmitters–neuromodulators, had been shown to be able to displace benzodiazepine ligands from their binding sites. In addition, a good correlation was shown between the affinities of the different benzodiazepines for their binding sites and their activities in pharmacological tests such as inhibition of pentylenctctrazole-induced convulsions in mice or reversal of conflict-induced suppression of performance in rats. Thus many criteria were fulfilled leading to the assumption that benzodiazepine binding sites could be considered as receptors. It was, therefore, very interesting to investigate whether cyclopyrrolone derivatives, which had pharmacological properties close to those of benzodiazepines, were also able to recognize the

Table 41.2 Inhibition of [^{3}H]zopiclone, [^{3}H]suriclone and [^{3}H]flunitrazepam binding to rat hippocampus

Compound	[^{3}*H*]*zopiclone**† K_i (nmol/l)	[^{3}*H*]*suriclone**† K_i (nmol/l)	[^{3}*H*]*flunitrazepam**† K_i (nmol/l)
Flunitrazepam	3.4 (2.9–3.9)	4 (4.6–3.4)	2.3 (2.1–2.4)
Nitrazepam	18 (12–24)	14.5 (10–19)	9 (7–11)
Diazepam	19 (13–25)	19.5 (17–22)	14.5 (15–14)
Chlordiazepoxide	428 (303–553)	561‡	397‡
Zopiclone	19 (10–27)	29 (27–31)	36 (35–37)
Suriclone	1.1 (0.9–1.3)	1.0 (1.0–1.0)	0.8 (0.8–0.8)

*The K_i values were calculated using the following equation:

$$K_i = \frac{IC_{50}}{1 + [L]/K_D}$$

where $[L]$ is the concentration of ligand and K_D the dissociation constant of the complex with the ligand

†Results are the mean of two experiments with individual values in brackets

‡For this value only one experiment

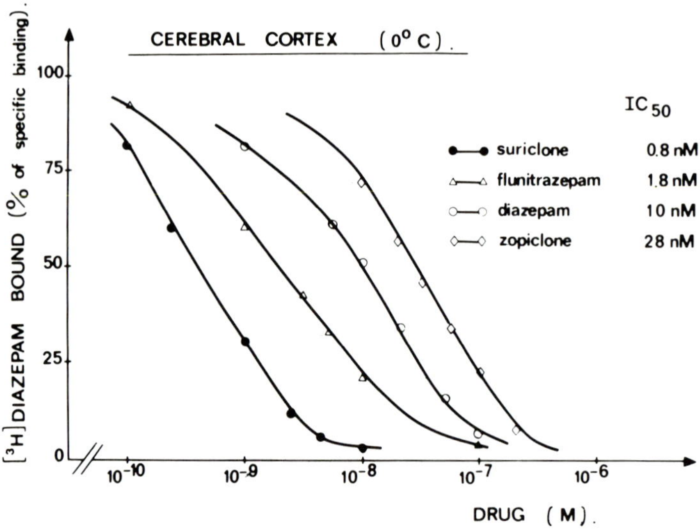

Figure 41.2 Inhibition of specific [^{3}H]diazepam binding by suriclone, zopiclone, flunitrazepam and diazepam. Membranes were incubated with 3nmol/l of [^{3}H]diazepam for 15 min in the presence of unlabelled compounds

benzodiazepine binding sites. Preliminary experiments that we performed with zopiclone seem to confirm this point[3].

Using tritiated diazepam as a ligand, we have found that zopiclone and suriclone also possess high affinity (expressed here by the IC_{50} value) for benzodiazepine binding sites (Figure 41.2). The IC_{50} of the two cyclopyrrolones are, like those of the benzodiazepines, in the nanomolar range, that of suriclone being somewhat lower than that of flunitrazepam and that of zopiclone being very similar to that of diazepam. This demonstration that pharmacologically rather similar, but chemically very dissimilar, compounds compete for common binding sites supports the concept that benzodiazepine sites are not only chemical recognition sites but are, in fact, true biologically relevant receptors.

The availability of [^{3}H]zopiclone and [^{3}H]suriclone has allowed us to study in more depth the nature of the binding sites of the minor tranquillizers of the benzodiazepine and cyclopyrrolone families. As shown in Figures 41.3 and 41.4 equilibrium binding studies with tritiated zopiclone and suriclone have confirmed the existence of high affinity binding sites for the cyclopyrrolones. The Scatchard plots of these equilibrium binding curves were linear, suggesting that zopiclone and suriclone bind to a single or homogeneous population of binding sites without co-operative interaction. With both ligands, the Hill coefficient (n_H) is close to 1 which also supports this contention. The dissociation constant (K_D) calculated from different experiments is 13.24 ± 1.14 nmol/l for zopiclone and 0.5 ± 0.04 nmol/l for suriclone. The total number of binding sites in the hippocampus is 0.70 ± 0.02 pmol/mg protein for zopiclone and 1.5 ± 0.28 pmol/mg protein for suriclone.

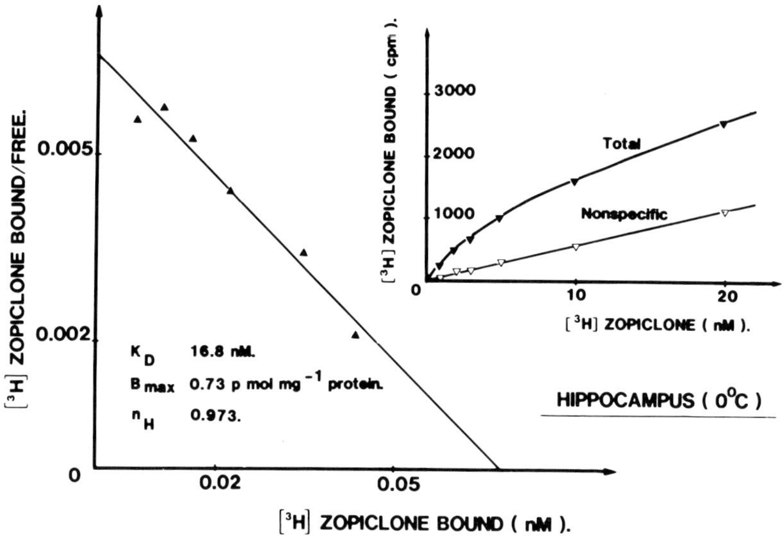

Figure 41.3 Scatchard plot of [^{3}H]zopiclone binding to rat hippocampus membranes. Inset: saturation curve (incubation time 30 min)

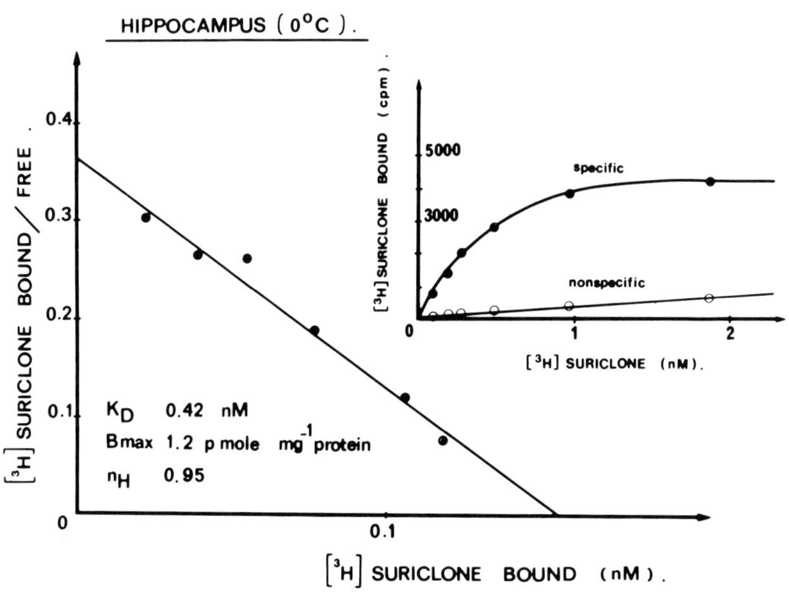

Figure 41.4 Scatchard plot of [^{3}H]suriclone binding to rat hippocampus membranes. Inset: saturation curve (incubation time 2 h) (From *J. Neurochem.* In Press)

As shown in Table 41.2, the binding sites labelled by zopiclone and suriclone are also well recognized by benzodiazepines. Moreover, the potencies of the different benzodiazepines to inhibit cyclopyrrolone binding is very similar to their potencies for inhibiting flunitrazepam binding. We must add that, as in the case of benzodiazepines, neither neurotransmitters nor other compounds (even sedatives such as phenobarbital and meprobamate) are able to recognize the cyclopyrrolone binding sites[4,5].

All these facts suggest the existence of close similarities between cyclopyrrolone and benzodiazepine binding sites. However, by using special experimental conditions, we have been able to compare in more depth the interaction of cyclopyrrolones and benzodiazepines with the 'minor tranquillizer receptors' and this has permitted us to detect some possible differences between the two families.

First of all, it is known that there exist, for at least some benzodiazepines, peripheral sites and especially renal sites in addition to central benzodiazepine binding sites. As shown in Figure 41.5, using equilibrium binding studies, we have confirmed the existence of renal flunitrazepam sites but we have not found such specific renal sites for suriclone. Displacement studies of flunitrazepam have also confirmed that neither suriclone nor zopiclone recognize the renal flunitrazepam binding sites.

Certain factors, such as the inhibitory neurotransmitter γ-aminobutyric acid (GABA), chloride anion and some barbiturates, have been described as able to modify benzodiazepine binding[9,15]. The use of such agents is particularly interesting for more precise study of the nature of benzodiazepine and cyclopyrrolone sites.

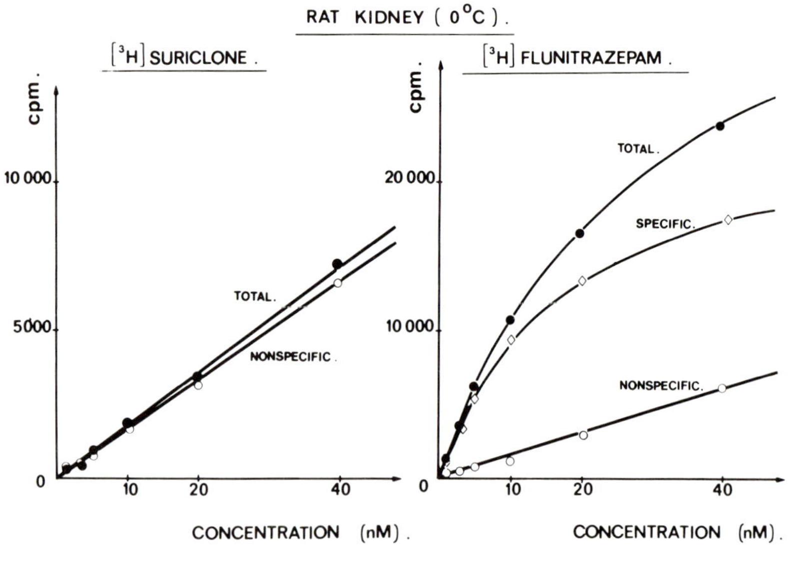

Figure 41.5 Equilibrium binding of [^{3}H]suriclone and [^{3}H]flunitrazepam on rat kidney membranes. Membranes were incubated for 2 h with each ligand

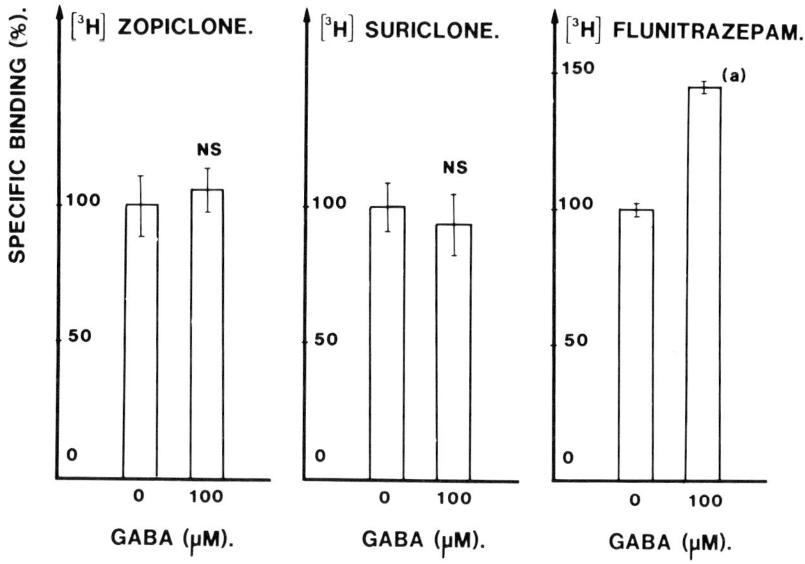

Figure 41.6 Effect of GABA (100 μmol/l) on specific zopiclone (15 nmol/l) suriclone (0.4 nmol/l) and flunitrazepam (1 nmol/l) binding to washed (three times) hippocampus membranes. Results are the mean of six (zopiclone) or three (suriclone and flunitrazepam) determinations. (a) $p<0.001$, NS = not significant

As shown in Figure 41.6, we have confirmed that GABA at the high concentration of 100 μmol/l is able to enhance flunitrazepam binding to washed rat hippocampus membranes*. On the contrary, GABA does not enhance the binding of suriclone or zopiclone at the same concentration†. Moreover, as shown in Figures 41.7 and 41.8, two barbiturates (secobarbital and pentobarbital) and the chloride anion induce a concentration-dependent enhancement of flunitrazepam binding, while zopiclone binding is not modified or only partially enhanced (a slight increase for the highest concentration of NaCl). Similar results have been obtained with suriclone.

Binding properties of ligands can be modified not only by the previous agents which probably induce a conformational change in the receptor, but also by certain agents which interfere with some amino acids entering into the chemical structure of the receptors. With this latter idea in mind we have used diethylpyrocarbonate ($Et_2C_2O_5$) which interacts with the imidazole moiety of histidine to form *N*-carbethoxy histidine[7]. As shown in the upper right hand part of Figure 41.9, this interaction results in a 54% decrease in the number of sites labelled with flunitrazepam (B_{max} control = 1.3 pmol/mg protein; B_{max} $Et_2C_2O_5$ = 0.6 pmol/mg protein) without modification of the affinity of the ligand (K_D control = 1.9 nmol/l; K_D $Et_2C_2O_5$ = 1.7 nmol/l). As shown in

*This effect of GABA is due to an increase in the affinity of the benzodiazepines for their binding sites with no modification of the number of sites.

†It is worth mentioning, however, that zopiclone and suriclone binding sites, like flunitrazepam sites, are protected by GABA (10 μmol/l from thermal inactivation[4,5]).

the upper left hand part of Figure 41.9, suriclone binding sites are less sensitive to $Et_2C_2O_5$ interaction: the decrease in binding sites is only 28% (B_{max} control = 1.8 pmol/mg protein; B_{max} $Et_2C_2O_5$ = 1.3 pmol/mg protein) without modification of affinity. Similarly, acetylation of the phenolic group of tyrosine with *N*-acetylimidazole induces a decrease in flunitrazepam

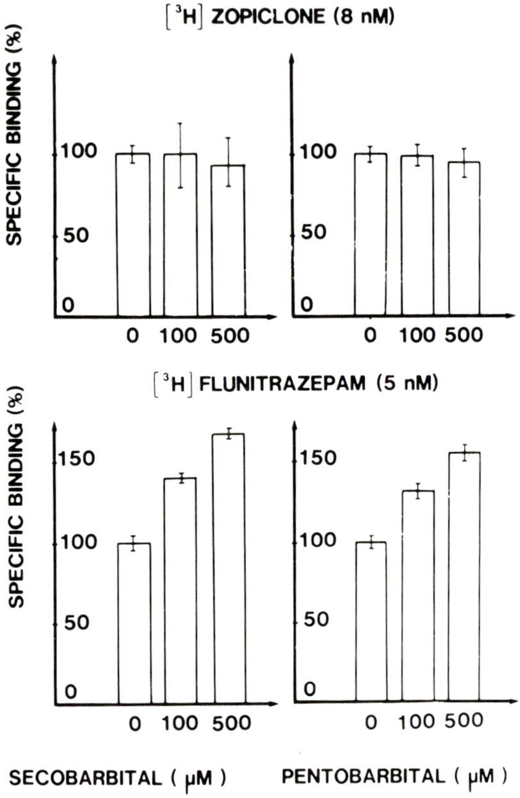

Figure 41.7 Effect of barbiturates (secobarbital and pentobarbital) on zopiclone and flunitrazepam specific binding in rat cerebellum. Results are the mean of six determinations

binding[17] which is *N*-acetylimidazole concentration-dependent [*N*-acetylimidazole (10 mmol/l gives a 47% decrease (Figure 41.9(b))]. At this concentration, *N*-acetylimidazole has no effect on suriclone binding [6% decrease (Figure 41.9(b))]. These differences between the effects of diethylpyrocarbonate or *N*-acetylimidazole on suriclone and flunitrazepam binding indicate that there might be some differences in the amino-acid functional groups involved in the recognition sites for these two minor tranquillizers.

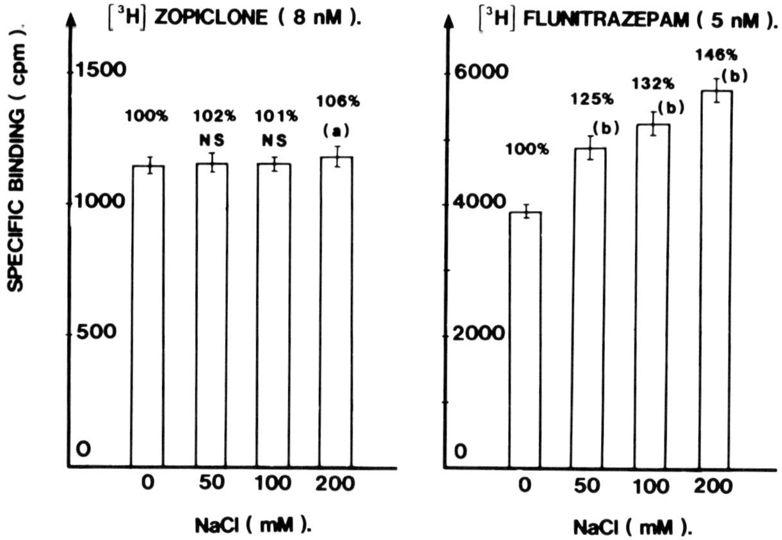

Figure 41.8 Effect of NaCl on zopiclone and flunitrazepam specific binding in rat cerebellum. Results are the mean of six determinations (a) $p<0.05$ (b) $p<0.001$

DISCUSSION

The introduction of receptor binding techniques has been a fundamental step in the validation of the 'receptor concept' put forward at the beginning of this century. In addition to their contributions to basic research (such as in the discovery of the mechanism of disease caused by impaired receptor function), receptor binding techniques have also provided very fruitful new tools for pharmacologists. Their usefulness as screening methods is clear but they have some drawbacks which must be taken into account. It is also worth mentioning the practical importance of radioreceptor assays. However, one of the most exciting applications of receptor binding techniques is probably the study of the mechanism of action of drugs which possess specific binding sites. It must be pointed out that such studies can lead to the discovery of new endogenous ligands (neurotransmitters, hormones, etc.).

We have illustrated this application of binding techniques by presenting the results we have obtained with zopiclone and suriclone, two new hypnotic or anxiolytic compounds of the cyclopyrrolone family which recognize the 'so-called benzodiazepine receptors' described for the first time in 1977.

Displacement studies indicate similarities between cyclopyrrolone and benzodiazepine central binding sites. However, contrarily to some benzodiazepines such as flunitrazepam and diazepam, zopiclone and suriclone do not possess peripheral renal binding sites. Similarly, zopiclone and suriclone binding, in contrast to that of flunitrazepam, is not enhanced by barbiturates and chloride anion. GABA protects zopiclone, suriclone and flunitrazepam binding from thermal inactivation, while it enhances only flunitrazepam

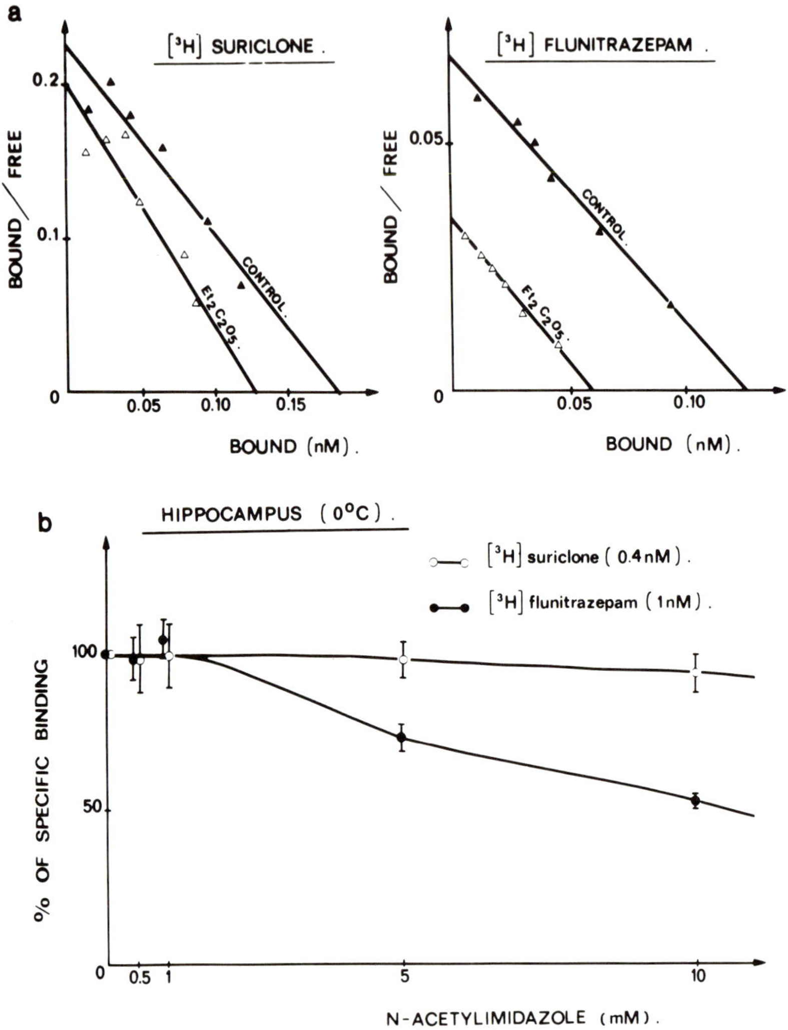

Figure 41.9 (a) Scatchard plot of [^{3}H]suriclone and [^{3}H]flunitrazepam binding for control and diethylpyrocarbonate (1 mmol/l)-treated rat hippocampus membranes. Results are the mean of one experiment in triplicate (b) Effect of increasing concentrations of *N*-acetylimidazole on specific suriclone and flunitrazepam binding to rat hippocampus membranes

binding and not zopiclone and suriclone binding. Moreover, the effects of diethylpyrocarbonate and *N*-acetylimidazole on the sites result in a more pronounced impairment of binding in the case of flunitrazepam than with suriclone. All these facts indicate that, although the receptors recognized by the benzodiazepines and cyclopyrrolones are probably rather similar, the interactions with these receptors and their subsites are probably somewhat different by the two chemical families.

The discovery of specific receptors for benzodiazepines in the brain suggests that there probably exists a natural ligand which might be expected to have anxiolytic or anxiogenous effects. Many research teams are working on this subject[12], but up to now none of the proposed substances seem to correspond to a natural ligand. Finally, the availability of new ligands such as zopiclone and suriclone, belonging to chemical families other than the benzodiazepines, can be of great help in learning more about the exact nature of the 'so-called benzodiazepine receptors', and in this way contribute to the search for the natural ligand. Indeed, the more we know about the 'minor tranquillizer receptors', their natural ligands, and their role, the sooner we can hope to find still more specific anxiolytic drugs.

References

1. Ariens, E. J. (1979). Receptors: from fiction to fact. T.I.P.S., **1**, 11–15
2. Bardone, M. C., Ducrot, R., Garret, C. *et al.* (1978). Benzodiazepine-like central effects of RP 27 267, a dihydro-7-oxo-5 H-pyrrolo [3, 4-b] pyrazine derivative. Presented at *7th International Congress of Pharmacology, Paris.* Abstract 2319
3. Blanchard, J. C., Boireau, A., Garret, C. *et al.* (1979). *In vitro* and *in vivo* inhibition by zopiclone of benzodiazepine binding to rodent brain receptors. *Life Sci.*, **24**, 2417–20
4. Blanchard, J. C. and Julou, L. (1983). Suriclone: a new cyclopyrrolone derivative recognizing receptors labelled by benzodiazepines in rat hippocampus and cerebellum. *J. Neurochem.*, **50**, 601–7
5. Blanchard, J. C., Boireau, A. and Julou, L. (1982). Brain receptors and zopiclone. Presented at *13th C.I.N.P. Congress*, Jerusalem. Abst. p. 799
6. Braestrup, C., Albrechtsen, R. and Squires, R. F. (1977). High densities of benzodiazepine receptors in human cortical areas. *Nature (London)*, **263**, 702–4
7. Burch, T. P. and Ticku, M. K. (1981). Histidine modification with diethylpyrocarbonate shows heterogeneity of benzodiazepine receptors. *Proc. Natl. Acad. Sci.*, **78**, 3945–9
8. Cuatrecasas, P., Hollenberg, M. D., Chang, K.-J. *et al.* (1975). Hormone receptor complexes and their modulation of membrane function. *Rec. Prog. Horm. Res.*, **31**, 37–84
9. Gallager, D. W., Mallorga, P., Thomas, J. W. *et al.* (1980). GABA-benzodiazepine interactions: physiological, pharmacological and developmental aspects. *Fed. Proc.*, **39**, 3043–9
10. Garret, C., Bardone, M. C., Blanchard, J. C. *et al.* (1982). Pharmacological studies of suriclone (RP 31 264) a cyclopyrrolone derivative with anxiolytic properties. Presented at *13th C.I.N.P. Congress*, Jerusalem. Abst. p. 244
11. Heidmann, T. and Changeux, J. P. (1978). Structural and functional properties of the acetylcholine receptor protein in its purified and membrane bound states. *Ann. Rev. Biochem.*, **47**, 317–57
12. Marangos, P. J., Paul, S. M. and Goodwin, F. K. (1979). Putative endogenous ligands for the benzodiazepine receptor. *Life Sci.*, **25**, 1093–102
13. Möhler, H. and Okada, T. (1977). Benzodiazepine receptor: demonstration in the central nervous system. *Science*, **198**, 849–51
14. Möhler, H. and Okada, T. (1978). Biochemical identification site of action of benzodiazepines in human brain by ^{3}H diazepam binding. *Life Sci.*, **22**, 985–96
15. Olsen, R. W. (1981). GABA–benzodiazepine–barbiturate receptor interactions. *J. Neurochem.*, **37**, 1–13
16. Parascandola, J. (1980). Origins of the receptor theory. *T.I.P.S.*, **1**, 189–92
17. Sherman-Gold, R. and Dudai, Y. (1981). Involvement of tyrosyl residues in the binding of benzodiazepines to their brain receptor. *FEBS Letters*, **131**, 313–6
18. Snyder, S. H. (1978). Overview of neurotransmitter receptor binding. In *Neurotransmitter Receptor Binding*. pp. 1–11. (New York: Raven Press)
19. Squires, R. F. and Braestrup, C. (1977). Benzodiazepine receptors in rat brain. *Nature (London)*, **266**, 732–4

42
Multiplicity of kappa opiate sites in the central nervous system

Y. Audigier, B. Attali, C. Gouardères,
H. Mazarguil and J. Cros

The pharmacochemical requirements for morphinomimetic action[21,39] have led to the search for and characterization of an opiate receptor in the central nervous system of mammals[43,46,48]. The existence of this receptor suggested the presence of an endogenous substance for which this binding site would be the physiological target and for which the exogenous opiates would substitute to induce their pharmacological effects. Such a hypothesis was corroborated by the isolation of the enkephalins[26], two related pentapeptides, whose biological actions[7,23,26] and regional distribution[14,27] corresponded to the pharmacological effects of opiates and the localization of the opiate binding sites[32].

These findings suggested, therefore, the existence of a 'single' endogenous ligand interacting with a homogenous population of opiate receptors. However, recent discoveries of a plurality of endogenous opioid peptides and a multiplicity of opiate receptors have challenged this simple idea.

Although all the opioid peptides possess the common feature of containing the amino-acid sequence of either Met-enkephalin[25,35,47] or Leu-enkephalin[17,40], their gene sequences[12,13,29,41,42], their biosynthetic pathways[30,37] and their regional distribution[6,18,40,45,50] favour their distinct physiological functions. Furthermore, this plurality of opioid peptides has been followed by the characterization of multiple opiate receptors in the central and peripheral nervous tissues[36]. According to biochemical[8,9,31,36] and pharmacological[16,28,38,49] experiments, the opiate receptors have been subdivided into three main types:

(1) The μ receptors of which pentacyclic opiates such as morphine are potent agonists.

(2) The δ receptors with which the enkephalins and some opioid peptides such as (D-Ala^2, D-Leu^5)enkephalin[8] or (D-Ser^2, Thr^6)Leu-enkephalin[15] preferentially interact.

(3) The κ receptors which are recognized by tricyclic opiates such as the benzomorphan drugs, ketazocine and ethylketazocine.

All these data raised the question of the physiological relationship between an endogenous ligand and a receptor subtype as well as the pharmacological relationship between an opiate subtype and a definite biological response. The main biological effect of this pharmacological class is the analgesic activity which involves some brain areas (supraspinal sites)[5] and some regions of the spinal cord (spinal sites)[34]. Whereas the antinociceptive action has been shown to preferentially implicate the μ subtype in the supraspinal structures[3], the pharmacological nature of the spinal opiate receptors remain to be elucidated, and especially in the lumbo-sacral part of the spinal cord where the intrathecal administration of opiates induces a long-lasting and naloxone-reversible analgesia[33,51,53].

Preliminary experiments described the absence of [^{3}H]morphine (μ agonist) and [^{3}H](D-Ala^2, D-Leu^5)enkephalin (δ agonist) binding in the lumbo-sacral spinal cord from various mammals[19], suggesting the absence of these two subtypes in this tissue. On the other hand, specific binding sites for [^{3}H]etorphine and [^{3}H]ethylketazocine can be characterized in the spinal cord from the rat[2] and other species[1,19,20]. In the rat spinal cord, the binding characteristics and the binding properties of [^{3}H]etorphine and [^{3}H]ethylketazocine clearly show that these two ligands are interacting with the same class of binding sites[20]. In this context, the absence of μ and δ sites suggested that these binding sites would correspond to the third subtype, the κ subtype.

We report here that these binding sites are not related to the κ sites and binding studies performed on different tissues from various species strongly favour the subdivision of the κ binding sites into two distinct subclasses, κ_1 and κ_2 sites.

MATERIALS AND METHODS

Binding assays

Rats (300–350 g) or guinea-pigs (300–400 g) were killed by decapitation and selected tissues (lumbo-sacral spinl cord or striatum) quickly removed and placed on ice; the spinal or striatal tissue was homogenized with a Teflon-glass homogenizer (V = 1500 rpm; 5 strokes) in 12 volumes 0.05 mol/l Tris-HCl buffer, pH 7.4. After preincubation at 37 °C for 30 min, the homogenate was centrifuged at 49 000 × g for 10 min; the resulting pellet was homogenized as described before. After a second centrifugation, the pellet was resuspended in sufficient Tris buffer to obtain a final concentration of 1 mg protein per ml.

The membranes (0.8 ml) were incubated with [^{3}H]ligand (0.1 ml) either at 37 °C for 30 min for opiate drugs (0.1 ml) or at 0 °C for 150 min for endogenous opioid peptides (0.1 ml). Non-specific binding was determined with 10 μmol/l levorphanol. The incubation mixture was filtered and counted as previously described[3].

Data analysis

In competition experiments, the IC_{50} of drugs were estimated from Hill plots with 5–10 concentrations of unlabelled ligands. Assuming a competitive interaction, the K_I values were calculating according to the formula $K_I = IC_{50}/(1+S/K_D)$ in which S is the concentration and K_D the dissociation constant of the radioligand.

Drugs

Bremazocine (gift from Sandoz, Basle); SKF 10 047 (*N*,allylnorcyclazocine, kindly gift from Dr J. P. Vincent, Nice); ketazocine, ethylketazocine and cyclazocine (Sterling-Winthrop, USA); MR 2034 ((−)5,9-dimethyl-2′hydroxy-2-tetrahydrofurfuryl-6,7-benzomorphan) and MR 2035 ((+) inactive enantiomer of MR 2034) were kindly provided by Dr. H. Merz (Boehringer, Mannheim FRG); morphine (Francopia, Paris); naloxone (Endo, USA); dextrorphan and levorphanol (gift from Hoffman-La Roche, Basle); diprenorphine and etorphine (Reckitt and Colman, England); fentanyl (Janssen Pharmaceutica, Beerse, Belgium); FK33824 [(D-Ala^2, N-Me-Phe^4, Met-(0)^5-ol-enkephalin) gift from Sandoz, Basle)] (D-Ser^2, Thr^6)Leu-enkephalin (gift from Professor B. Roques, Paris); human β endorphin and dynorphin (1→17) (Bachem, Budendorf, Switzerland); Morphiceptin, (D-Ala^2, D-Leu^5)enkephalin, (Arg^6, Phe^7)Met-enkephalin, Met-enkephalin and Leu-enkephalin (synthetized by Dr H. Mazarguil, Toulouse); [^{3}H]etorphine (46 Ci mmol^{-1}) was purchased from the Radiochemical Centre, [^{3}H]ethylketazocine (15 Ci mmol^{-1}) from New England Nuclear.

RESULTS

Binding studies in rat spinal cord

[^{3}H]etorphine binds to a single class of high affinity sites ($K_D = 0.21 \pm 0.04$ nmol/l) whereas [^{3}H]ethylketazocine interacts with a homogenous population of lower affinity sites ($K_D = 2.2 \pm 0.4$ nmol/l) (Figure 42.1). The similar binding capacity and the homogeneity of K_I values (calculated from displacement experiments) and K_D values (extrapolated from saturation curves) for the two radioligands strongly suggest that [^{3}H]etorphine and [^{3}H]ethylketazocine are labelling the same binding sites. This assumption is confirmed by the identical order of potency of opiates and opioid peptides which compete for [^{3}H]etorphine or [^{3}H]ethylketazocine binding (Table 42.1): etorphine and benzomorphan-like drugs are the most potent competitors; naloxone and morphine (μ ligands) display a lower affinity, (D-Ala^2, D-Leu^5)enkephalin has an intermediate K_I value equal to 250 nmol/l whereas (D-Ser^2, Thr^6)Leu^5-enkephalin (δ agonist) interacts poorly with these binding sites. The K_I values of the endogenous opioid peptides against [^{3}H]etorphine binding range from 20 nmol/l to 190 nmol/l (Table

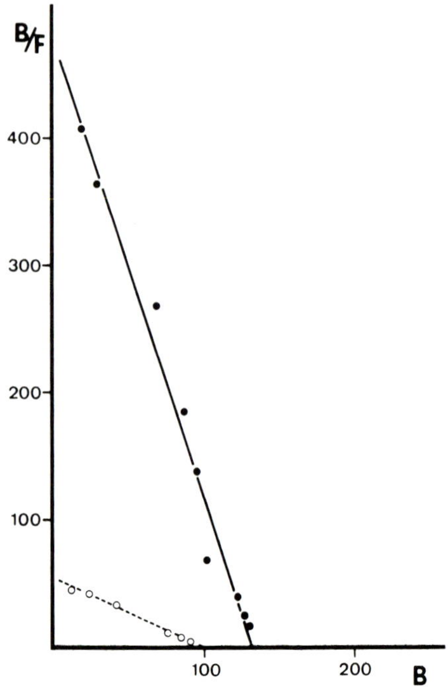

Figure 42.1 Scatchard analysis of [^{3}H]etorphine (●—●) and [^{3}H]ethylketazocine (○---○) binding in rat lumbo-sacral spinal cord

Table 42.1 Affinity of opiates and opioid peptides for [^{3}H]etorphine and [^{3}H]ethylketazocine binding sites in rat lumbo-sacral spinal cord. Opiates and exogenous peptides were assayed at 37 °C for 30 min against [^{3}H]etorphine (0.3 nmol/l) and [^{3}H]ethylketazocine (3 nmol/l) binding. The affinity of endogenous opioid peptides was determined at 0 °C for 150 min against [^{3}H]etorphine (1.5 nmol/l) binding. Results are expressed as mean ± SEM for the number of separate experiments indicated in parentheses

Substance	[^{3}*H*]*ethylketazocine* K_I (nmol/l)	[^{3}*H*]*etorphine* K_I (nmol/l)
Etorphine (3)	0.6 ± 0.1	1.0 ± 0.1
Bremazocine (3)	0.7 ± 0.1	2.1 ± 0.1
Diprenorphine (4)		3.0 ± 0.5
Cyclazocine (3)	1.3 ± 0.4	3.1 ± 0.1
Ethylketazocine (5)	5.7 ± 0.8	9.5 ± 1.2
Naloxone (3)	8.0 ± 0.4	13 ± 1
Ketazocine (6)	9.7 ± 1.6	18 ± 1
Fentanyl (3)		44 ± 2
Morphine (6)	48 ± 3	52 ± 5
(D-Ala^2,D-Leu^5)-enkephalin (3)	269 ± 14	220 ± 55
(D-Ser^2, Thr^6)-Leu-enkephalin (3)	1010 ± 309	853 ± 75
Morphiceptin (3)		1490 ± 164
Endogenous opioid peptides		
β-endorphin (5)		18 ± 2
(Arg^6, Phe^7)Met-enkephalin (7)		32 ± 4
Dynorphin (1–17) (7)		40 ± 4
Met-enkephalin (4)		61 ± 13
Leu-enkephalin (5)		185 ± 11

42.1). β-endorphine and (Arg^6,Phe^7)Met-enkephalin possess the highest affinity, whereas dynorphin (1–17) has a K_I value equal to 40 nmol/l. Met-enkephalin and especially Leu-enkephalin are the less active compounds.

Binding studies in guinea-pig spinal cord

In this species, the binding characteristics of [^{3}H]etorphine and [^{3}H]ethylketazocine are very different since [^{3}H]ethylketazocine binds to two classes of high affinity sites ($K_D = 1.02 \pm 0.06$ nmol/l) and low affinity sites ($K_D = 5.8 \pm 0.5$ nmol/l) and its total binding capacity ($B_{max} = 218 \pm 14$ fmol/mg protein) is larger than that of [^{3}H]etorphine ($B_{max} = 73 \pm 4$ fmol/mg protein) (Figure 42.2 and Table 42.2).

Preliminary displacement experiments revealed that 5 μmol/l of (D-Ala^2,D-Leu^5)enkephalin could only displace 70% of the high affinity binding of [^{3}H]ethylketazocine, suggesting that the high affinity sites represented two different types of interaction, one sensitive to (D-Ala^2,D-Leu^5)enkephalin (DAL sensitive sites) and the other unaffected by (D-Ala^2,D-Leu^5)enkephalin (DAL insensitive sites). In these same conditions, the specific binding of [^{3}H]etorphine is completely abolished and the total number of these sites strictly corresponds to the partial loss of [^{3}H]ethylketazocine binding (Table 42.2).

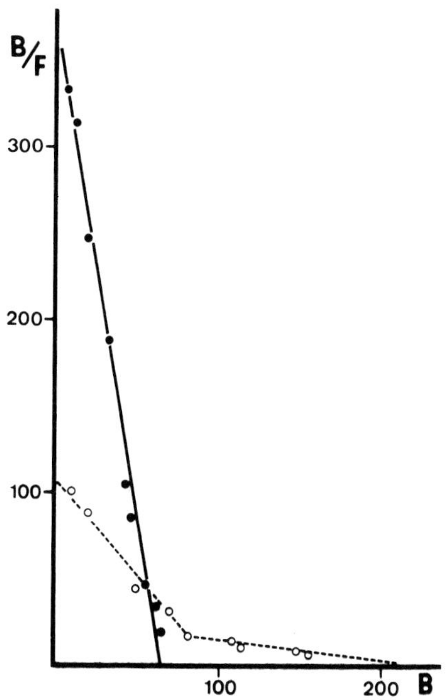

Figure 42.2 Scatchard analysis of [^{3}H]etorphine (●—●) and [^{3}H]ethylketazocine (○---○) binding in guinea-pig lumbo-sacral spinal cord

Table 42.2 Binding characteristics of [^{3}H]etorphine and [^{3}H]ethylketazocine in guinea-pig lumbo-sacral cord. Results are expressed as mean ± SEM for the number of separate experiments indicated in parentheses

Ligands		*Equilibrium dissociation constant* K_D (nmol/l)	*Maximal number of binding sites* B_{max} (fmol/mg protein)
[^{3}H]Etorphine	high affinity sites	0.18 ± 0.03 (15)	73 ± 4 (15)
[^{3}H]Ethylketazocine	high affinity sites	1.02 ± 0.06 (23)	107 ± 5 (23)
	low affinity sites	5.83 ± 0.48 (23)	111 ± 9 (23)
In the presence of 5 μmol/l (D-Ala^2,D-Leu^5)enkephalin			
[^{3}H]Etorphine	loss of specific binding (10)		
[^{3}H]Ethylketazocine	high affinity sites	0.36 ± 0.05 (6)	30 ± 2 (6)
	low affinity sites	6.30 ± 0.90 (6)	121 ± 5 (6)

Table 42.3 Affinity of opiates and opioid peptides for [^{3}H]ethylketazocine binding in the presence of 5 μmol/l (D-Ala^2,D-Leu^5)enkephalin and [^{3}H]etorphine binding in guinea-pig lumbo-sacral spinal cord. Opiates and opioid peptides were assayed at 37 °C for 30 min against [^{3}H]ethylketazocine (0.8 nmol/l) residual binding and [^{3}H]etorphine (0.5 nmol/l) binding. The affinity of endogenous opioid peptides was determined at 0 °C for 150 min against [^{3}H]ethylketazocine (0.8 nmol/l) residual binding and [^{3}H]etorphine (0.6 nmol/l) binding. Results are expressed as mean ± SEM for 3–4 separate experiments

Substance	*[^{3}H]ethylketazocine in the presence of 5 μmol/l DAL* K_I (nmol/l)	*[^{3}H]etorphine* K_I (nmol/l)
Bremazocine	0.4 ± 0.03	0.6 ± 0.15
Ethylketazocine	1.1 ± 0.07	3 ± 0.12
Cyclazocine	1.3 ± 0.11	0.9 ± 0.09
Ketazocine	8.1 ± 1.5	12 ± 1
Naloxone	8.9 ± 0.5	10 ± 2
Etorphine	12.5 ± 2	1.6 ± 0.18
Diprenorphine	14 ± 2	0.3 ± 0.09
Morphine	242 ± 67	35 ± 5
Fentanyl	640 ± 103	28 ± 2
FK33824	1373 ± 28	9.5 ± 1
(D-Ala^2,D-Leu^5)-enkephalin	> 10 000	57 ± 6
(D-Ser^2, Thr^6)-Leu-enkephalin	> 10 000	329 ± 49
Endogenous opioid peptides		
Dynorphin (1–17)	0.36 ± 0.08	10.3 ± 1.8
β-endorphin	111 ± 7	4.9 ± 1.3
[Arg^6, Phe^7]Met-enkephalin	225 ± 4	4.5 ± 1.4
Met-enkephalin	1819 ± 115	11.8 ± 1.09
Leu-enkephalin	4991 ± 140	16.7 ± 1.3

These results demonstrate that [^{3}H]ethylketazocine interacts with two classes of high affinity sites, DAL sensitive and DAL insensitive, whereas [^{3}H]etorphine only binds to DAL sensitive sites. The binding properties of DAL sensitive sites have therefore been investigated with [^{3}H]etorphine and those of DAL insensitive sites with [^{3}H]ethylketazocine in the presence of 5 μmol/l (D-Ala^2,D-Leu^5)enkephalin.

Although benzomorphan-like drugs poorly discriminate between DAL sensitive and DAL insensitive sites, some opiates and many opioid peptides differentially interact with these two binding sites (Table 42.3). In agreement with the selective labelling by [^{3}H]etorphine of DAL sensitive sites, the oripavines display a lower affinity for DAL insensitive sites. Furthermore, the opioid peptides except dynorphin (1–17) interact better with DAL sensitive sites than with DAL insensitive sites. The most active compound at DAL insensitive sites is dynorphin (1–17) whereas (Arg^6, Phe^7)Met-enk has the highest affinity for DAL sensitive sites.

Preliminary displacement experiments performed on the low affinity sites for [^{3}H]ethylketazocine suggest that this binding site cannot be considered as an opiate binding site (B. Attali, personal communication).

Binding studies in guinea-pig striatum

The binding capacity of [^{3}H]etorphine ($B_{max} = 267 \pm 47$ fmol/mg protein) and [^{3}H]ethylketazocine ($B_{max} = 270 \pm 30$ fmol/mg protein) are very similar and each radioligand appears to interact with a homogenous population of binding sites (Figure 42.3). In the presence of 5 μmol/l (D-Alpha^2,D-Leu^5)

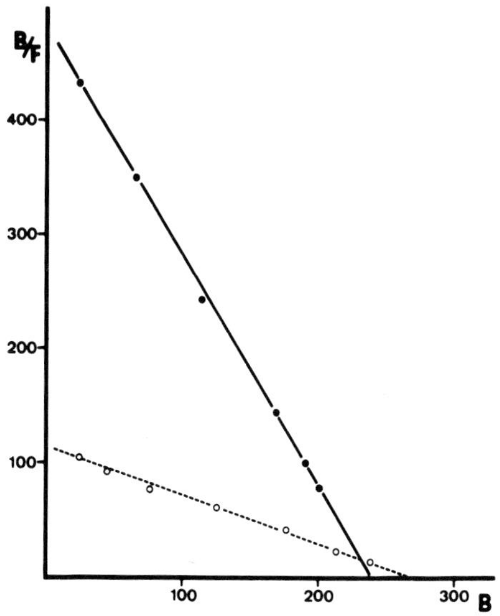

Figure 42.3 Scatchard analysis of [^{3}H]etorphine (●—●) and [^{3}H]ethylketazocine (○---○) in guinea-pig striatum

Table 42.4 Binding characteristics of [^{3}H]etorphine and [^{3}H]ethylketazocine in guinea-pig striatum. Results are expressed as the mean ± SEM for the number of different experiments indicated in parentheses

Ligands	*Equilibrium dissociation constant* K_D (nmol/l)	*Maximal number of binding sites* B_{max} (fmol/mg protein)
[^{3}H]ethylketazocine	1.43 ± 0.43 (4)	270 ± 30 (4)
[^{3}H]etorphine	0.56 ± 0.12 (6)	267 ± 47 (6)
In the presence of 5 μmol/l (D-Ala^2,D-Leu^5)enkephalin		
[^{3}H]ethylketazocine	2.16 ± 0.55 (3)	137 ± 17 (3)
[^{3}H]etorphine	loss of specific binding (3)	
In the presence of 1 μmol/l morphiceptin and 0.1 μmol/l (D-Ser^2,Thr^6)Leu-enkephalin		
[^{3}H]etorphine	0.34 ± 0.12 (3)	165 ± 48 (3)

enkephalin, a concentration which also saturates μ and δ sites present in this tissue, [^{3}H]ethylketazocine still binds to a homogenous population of high affinity sites ($K_D = 2.16 \pm 0.55$ nmol/l) which represent 50% of the specific binding ($B_{max} = 137 \pm 17$ fmol/mg protein). On the other hand, specific binding of [^{3}H]etorphine is completely abolished (Table 42.4).

The binding properties of this residual binding are identical to those of DAL insensitive sites (guinea-pig spinal cord): the oripavines again interact with a lower affinity with these binding sites and among the endogenous opioid peptides, dynorphin 1–17 is the most active substance (Table 42.5).

Table 42.5 Affinity of opiates and opioid peptides for [^{3}H]ethylketazocine binding in the presence of 5 μmol/l (D-Ala^{2}D-Leu^5)enkephalin in guinea-pig striatum. Opiates and all the opioid peptides were assayed at 0 °C for 150 min against [^{3}H]ethylketazocine (5 μmol/l) residual binding. Results are expressed as mean ± SEM for 3–4 separate experiments

Substance	K_I (nmol/l)
Bremazocine	0.76 ± 0.09
Ethylketazocine	5.7 ± 0.7
Ketazocine	7.0 ± 0.8
Naloxone	9.1 ± 1.7
Etorphine	15 ± 2.0
Diprenorphine	8.1 ± 1.2
Morphine	185 ± 19
Fentanyl	819 ± 117
FK33824	1782 ± 624
Morphiceptin	> 20 000
(D-Ser^2,Thr^6)-Leu-enkephalin	> 20 000
(D-Ala^2,D-Leu^5)-enkephalin	> 15 000
Endogenous opioid peptides	
Dynorphin (1–17)	0.90 ± 0.15
β-Endorphin	89 ± 16
(Arg^6, Phe^7)-Met-enkephalin	127 ± 24
Leu-enkephalin	5251 ± 321
Met-enkephalin	2207 ± 242

Table 42.6 Affinity of opiates and opioid peptides for [^{3}H]etorphine binding in the presence of 1 μmol/l morphiceptin and 0.1 μmol/l (D-Ser^2,Thr^6)Leu^5-enkephalin in guinea-pig striatum. Opiates and opioid peptides were assayed at 37 °C for 30 min against [^{3}H]etorphine residual binding (0.6 nmol/l). Results are expressed as the mean ± SEM of 3–4 separate experiments

Substance	K_I
Bremazocine	0.55 ± 0.08
Etorphine	1.93 ± 0.50
Diprenorphine	2.20 ± 0.20
Ethylketazocine	2.97 ± 0.88
Ketazocine	3.81 ± 0.70
Naloxone	10.2 ± 0.3
Morphine	54.9 ± 1.4
Fentanyl	101 ± 11
FK33824	145 ± 9
(D-Ala^2,D-Leu^5)enkephalin	471 ± 67
(D-Ser^2,Thr^6)Leu-enkephalin	4476 ± 655
Morphiceptin	4748 ± 783

After the blockade of μ sites by 1 μmol/l morphiceptin and δ sites by 0.1 μmol/l (D-Ser^2,Thr^6)Leu^5-enkephalin, an important residual binding of [^{3}H]etorphine is still observed which corresponds to 60% of the total specific binding (Table 42.4). The binding properties are similar to those of the same radioligand in rat and guinea-pig spinal cord (Table 42.6): benzomorphan-like drugs and oripavines have a high affinity for these binding sites, whereas naloxone and morphine display a lower affinity. (D-Ala^2,D-Leu^5)enkephalin has an intermediate K_I value equal to 470 nmol/l and (D-Ser^2,Thr^6)Leu^5-enk poorly interacts with these residual binding sites.

DISCUSSION

In the rat spinal cord where the absence of μ and δ sites has been previously reported[19], the similar binding capacity and the identical binding properties of [^{3}H]etorphine and [^{3}H]ethylketazocine indicate the existence of a homogenous population of opiate binding sites. The high K_I values of μ agonists such as morphine[8] or morphiceptin[10] and of δ agonists such (D-Ala^2,D-Leu^5)enkephalin[8] or (D-Ser^2,Thr^6)Leu-enkephalin[15] confirm that these binding sites do not correspond to either the μ nor to the δ subtype. However, the affinity of morphine, (D-Ala^2,D-Leu^5)enkephalin and dynorphin (1–17) is very different from that reported for the third subtype, the κ binding sites in guinea-pig brain[31]. Interestingly, these binding properties are very similar to those of the benzomorphan sites characterized in rat brain[11].

Since the κ sites have not been detected in rat brain[22,24], the question arose concerning a possible phylogenetic variation without any pharmacological consequence. Indeed, the benzomorphan binding sites and the κ binding sites could only represent a phylogenetic modification of the pharmacochemical requirements from the rat to the guinea-pig. Such an assumption is ruled out by the coexistence of κ and benzomorphan binding sites in guinea-pig spinal cord and guinea-pig striatum.

In the guinea-pig spinal cord, the differential affinity of (D-Ala^2,D-Leu^5)enkephalin (DAL) for benzomorphan and $\varkappa$ sites has been useful to characterize their coexistence in terms of DAL sensitive sites (benzomorphan sites) and DAL insensitive sites ($\varkappa$ sites). Furthermore, their distinct binding properties have been extended to the oripavines and many opioid peptides. The DAL insensitive sites have the same binding properties which have been characterized for the $\varkappa$ sites in guinea-pig brain[31], except for oripavines. In fact, our experimental conditions which represent a simple methodology for the *direct* characterization of the $\varkappa$ subtype, clearly demonstrate that the oripavines cannot label at low concentrations the $\varkappa$ sites in agreement with their higher K_I values for $\varkappa$ sites than for benzomorphan sites.

In the guinea-pig spinal cord, the denomination of DAL sensitive sites is strictly referred to benzomorphan sites since the presence of μ and δ sites has not been detected in the lumbo-sacral spinal cord[19]. Although the K_I values of opiates and opioid peptides are lower than those obtained in rat brain[11] and spinal cord[20], the relative order of potency is very similar to that at the benzomorphan site characterized in rat brain and spinal cord.

In the guinea-pig striatum where the presence of μ and δ sites has been reported[8], the characterization of benzomorphan and $\varkappa$ sites required a different methodology. However, since (D-Ala^2,D-Leu^5)enkephalin interacts better with δ and μ sites than with benzomorphan sites[8,9], the DAL insensitive sites always correspond to the $\varkappa$ subtype; the binding properties of the residual [^{3}H]ethylketazocine binding in the presence of 5 μmol/l (D-Ala^2,D-Leu^5)enkephalin are strictly identical to those of the $\varkappa$ sites characterized in guinea-pig brain[31] and spinal cord[1,2]. Consequently, [^{3}H]etorphine does not label $\varkappa$ sites and unlabelled etorphine and diprenorphine display high K_I values for $\varkappa$ sites. After the blockade of μ and δ sites, [^{3}H]etorphine still binds to an important population of opiate binding sites whose binding properties strongly correspond to those of the benzomorphan sites described in rat brain[11] and spinal cord[20] and to those of DAL sensitive sites characterized in guinea-pig spinal cord[2].

Taken together, these results clearly show that benzomorphan and $\varkappa$ sites do not correspond to the same binding entity and that their coexistence in the guinea-pig central nervous system would indicate their distinct physiological relevance. Furthermore, preliminary protection experiments clearly establish the absence of cross-protection for the binding to each binding site (B. Attali, personal communication). Finally, the differential affinity of oripavines and many opioid peptides suggest that the pharmacochemical requirements are different for the binding to these two sites: this conclusion is illustrated by the high affinity of dynorphin (1–17) for $\varkappa$ sites and by the preferential interaction of (Arg^6, Phe^7)Met-enkephalin with benzomorphan sites.

From a pharmacological point of view, the similar affinity of the benzomorphan-like drugs, the similar K_I value of naloxone related to the Ke value for the antagonism of $\varkappa$ agonists in guinea-pig ileum[28] and the differential affinity of opioid peptides are better distinguished as a subdivision into two subclasses rather than to a real dissociation between two classes of opiate binding sites. For these reasons, we propose a different denomination based upon the subdivision of $\varkappa$ binding sites into two subclasses, $\varkappa_1$ sites ($\varkappa$ or DAL insensitive sites) and $\varkappa_2$ sites (benzomorphan or DAL sensitive sites).

The phylogenetic differences between rat and guinea-pig raise some questions concerning the generalization of $\varkappa_1$ and $\varkappa_2$ sites to other species and man. Indeed, the rat brain and spinal cord would contain only $\varkappa_2$ sites whereas $\varkappa_1$ and $\varkappa_2$ sites coexist in guinea-pig brain and spinal cord. Binding studies performed in human brain reveal the presence of two '$\varkappa$' sites, dynorphin-sensitive sites ($\varkappa_1$ sites) and dynorphin-insensitive sites[44]. Although dynorphin has a lower affinity for $\varkappa_2$ sites in guinea-pig[2] and rat spinal cord, the relation between these dynorphin-insensitive sites and $\varkappa_2$ sites remains to be clarified.

The relationship between the affinity of some endogenous opioid peptides and one subclass of $\varkappa$ binding sites is still a question of debate. The high affinity of dynorphin (1–17) for $\varkappa_1$ sites would favour its preferential implication in the endogenous activation of these sites. On the other hand, the high affinity of (Arg^6, Phe^7)Met-enkephalin for $\varkappa_2$ sites characterized in the spinal cord and the presence of high amounts of this peptide in this region[50] could argue for its physiological role in relation to $\varkappa_2$ sites. However, no conclusion can be drawn before the demonstration of a strict correlation between the localization of an endogenous peptide and the distribution of one subclass.

It is noteworthy that this subdivision of $\varkappa$ binding sites is mainly based upon biochemical investigations and therefore the biological effects induced by the stimulation of each subclass are far from known. A recent study provides some evidence for the subdivision of $\varkappa$ 'receptors' in isolated organs[52], but the biological response would represent the same phenomenon, i.e. the modulation of neurotransmitter release.

The characterization of a homogenous population of $\varkappa_2$ sites in *rat* spinal cord is in good agreement with the preferential spinal site of action of the benzomorphan-like drugs[51]. However, the heterogeneity of $\varkappa$ sites in *guinea-pig* spinal cord raises the problem, in this species and others, of the distinct involvement of $\varkappa_1$ and $\varkappa_2$ sites in the modulation of medullary systems.

In conclusion, although a subdivision of $\varkappa$ binding sites has been established in guinea-pig central nervous system, it is tempting to speculate upon its existence in human cerebral tissues where it would lead to many biochemical, pharmacological and clinical applications.

References

1. Attali, B., Gouarderes, C., Audigier, Y. *et al.* (1981). Multiple binding sites for [^{3}H]ethylketocyclazocine on the lumbo-sacral portion of the guinea-pig spinal cord. In *Advances in Endogenous and Exogenous Opioids*. pp. 33–5. (Tokyo: Kodansha Ltd)
2. Attali, B., Gouarderes, C., Mazarguil, H. *et al.* (1982). Differential interaction of opiates to multiple "kappa" binding sites in the guinea-pig lumbo-sacral spinal cord. *Life Sci.*, **31**, 1371–5
3. Audigier, Y., Mazarguil, H., Gout, R. *et al.* (1981). Structure-activity relationships of enkephalin analogs at opiate and enkephalin receptors: correlation with analgesia. *Eur. J. Pharmacol.*, **63**, 35–46
4. Audigier, Y., Attali, B., Mazarguil, H. *et al.* (1982). Characterization of [^{3}H]-etorphine binding in guinea-pig striatum after blockade of mu and delta sites. *Life Sci.*, **31**, 1287–90

5. Besson, J. M., Le Bars, D. and Oliveras, J. L. (1978). L'analgésie morphinique: données neurobiologiques. *Ann. Anesth. Franç.*, **19**, 343–69
6. Boarder, M. R., Lockfield, A. J. and Barchas, J. D. (1982). Met-enkephalin (Arg[6], Phe[7]) immunoreactivity in bovine caudate and bovine adrenal medulla. *J. Neurochem.*, **39**, 149–54
7. Bradley, P. B., Briggs, I., Gayton, R. J. *et al.* (1976). Effects of microiontophoretically applied methionine-enkephalin on single neurons in rat brainstem. *Nature (London)*, **261**, 425–6
8. Chang, K. J., Cooper, B. R., Hazum, E. *et al.* (1979). Multiple opiate receptors: different regional distribution in the brain and differential binding of opiates and opioid peptides. *Mol. Pharmacol.*, **16**, 91–104
9. Chang, K. J. and Cuatrecasas, P. (1979). Multiple opiate receptors: enkephalins and morphine bind to receptors of different specificity. *J. Biol. Chem.*, **254**, 2610–8
10. Chang, K. J., Killian, A., Hazum, E. *et al.* (1981). Morphiceptin (NH_4-Tyr-Pro-Phe-Pro-$CONH_2$): a potent and specific agonist for morphine (μ) receptors. *Science*, **212**, 75–7
11. Chang, K. J., Hazum, E. and Cuatrecasas, P. (1981). Novel opiate binding sites selective for benzomorphan drugs. *Proc. Natl. Acad. Sci. (USA)*, **78**, 4141–5
12. Cochet, M., Chang, A. C. Y. and Cohen, S. N. (1982). Characterization of the structural gene and putative 5′-regulatory sequences for human proopiomelanocortin. *Nature (London)*, **297**, 335–9
13. Comb, M., Seeburg, P. H., Adelman, J. *et al.* (1982). Primary structure of the human Met- and Leu-enkephalin precursor and its mRNA. *Nature (London)*, **295**, 663–6
14. Elde, R., Hökfelt, T., Johansson, O. *et al.* (1976). Immunohistochemical studies using antibodies to leucine-enkephalin: initial observations on the nervous system of the rat. *Neuroscience*, **1**, 349–51
15. Gacel, G., Fournie-Zaluski, M. C. and Roques, B. P. (1980). Tyr-DSer-Gly-Phe-Leu-Thr, a highly preferential ligand for δ-opiate receptors. *FEBS Lett.*, **118**, 245–7
16. Gilbert, P. E. and Martin, W. R. (1976). The effects of morphine- and nalorphine-like drugs in the non-dependent, morphine-dependent and cyclazocine-dependent chronic spinal dog. *J. Pharmacol. Exp. Ther.*, **198**, 66–82
17. Goldstein, A., Tachibana, S., Lowney, L. I. *et al.* (1979). Dynorphin (1–13), an extraordinarily potent opioid peptide. *Proc. Natl. Acad. Sci. (USA)*, **76**, 6666–70
18. Goldstein, A. and Ghazarossian, V. E. (1980). Immunoreactive dynorphin in pituitary and brain. *Proc. Natl. Acad. Sci. (USA)*, **77**, 6207–10
19. Gouarderes, C., Attali, B., Audigier, Y. *et al.* (1981). Opiate binding sites in the lumbo-sacral spinal cord from various species. In *Advances in Endogenous and Exogenous Opioids.* pp. 18–20. (Tokyo: Kodansha Ltd)
20. Gouarderes, C., Audigier, Y. and Cros, J. (1982). Benzomorphan binding sites in rat lumbo-sacral spinal cord. *Eur. J. Pharmacol.*, **78**, 483–6
21. Hardy, R. A. and Howell, M. G. (1965). Synthetic analgesics with morphine-like actions. In *Analgesics.* Vol. 5, pp. 179–279. (New York: Academic Press)
22. Harris, O. W. and Sethy, V. M. (1980). High affinity binding of [^{3}H]ethylketocyclazocine to rat brain homogenate. *Eur. J. Pharmacol.*, **66**, 121–3
23. Hill, R. G., Pepper, C. M. and Mitchell, J. F. (1976). Depression of nociceptive and other neurons in the brain by iontophoretically applied met-enkephalin. *Nature (London)*, **262**, 604–6
24. Hiller, J. M. and Simon, E. J. (1980). Specific, high affinity [^{3}H]ethylketocyclazocine binding in rat central nervous system: lack of evidence for K receptors. *J. Pharmacol. Exp. Ther.*, **214**, 516–9
25. Huang, W. Y., Chang, R. C. C., Kastin, A. J. *et al.* (1979). Isolation and structure of pro-methionine-enkephalin: potential enkephalin precursor from porcine hypothalamus. *Proc. Natl. Acad. Sci. (USA)*, **76**, 6177–80
26. Hughes, J., Smith, T. W., Kosterlitz, H. W. *et al.* (1975). Identification of two related pentapeptides from the brain with potent opiate agonist activity. *Nature (London)*, **258**, 577–9
27. Hughes, J., Kosterlitz, H. W. and Smith, T. W. (1977). The distribution of methionine-enkephalin and leucine-enkephalin in the brain and peripheral tissues. *Br. J. Pharmacol.*, **61**, 639–47

28. Hutchinson, M., Kosterlitz, H. W., Leslie, F. M. *et al.* (1975). Assessment in the guinea-pig ileum and mouse vas deferens of benzomorphans which have strong antinociceptive activity but do not substitute for morphine in the dependent monkey. *Br. J. Pharmacol.*, **55**, 541–6
29. Kakidani, H., Furutani, Y., Takahashi, H. *et al.* (1982). Cloning and sequence analysis of cDNA for porcine β-neo-endorphin/dynorphin precursor. *Nature (London)*, **298**, 245–9
30. Killpatrick, D. L., Jones, B. N., Lewis, R. W. *et al.* (1982). An 18 200 dalton adrenal protein that contains four (Met)enkephalin sequences. *Proc. Natl. Acad. Sci. (USA)*, **79**, 3057–61
31. Kosterlitz, H. W., Paterson, S. J. and Robson, L. E. (1981). Characterization of the K-subtype of the opiate receptor in the guinea-pig brain. *Br. J. Pharmacol.*, **73**, 939–49
32. Kuhar, M. J., Pert, C. B. and Snyder, S. H. (1973). Regional distribution of opiate receptor binding in monkey and human brain. *Nature (London)*, **245**, 447–50
33. Lazorthes, Y., Gouarderes, C., Verdie, J. C. *et al.* (1980). Analgésie par injection intrathécale de morphine. Etude pharmacocinétique et application aux douleurs irréductibles. *Neurochimie*, **26**, 159–64
34. Le Bars, D., Menetrey, D., Conseiller, D. *et al.* (1975). Depressive effects of morphine upon lamina V cell activities in the dorsal horn of the spinal cat. *Brain Res.*, **98**, 261–77
35. Li, C. H. and Chung, D. Isolation and structure of an untriakontapeptide with opiate activity from camel pituitary glands. *Proc. Natl. Acad. Sci. (USA)*, **73**, 1145–8
36. Lord, J. A. H., Waterfield, A. A., Hughes, J. H. *et al.* (1977). Endogenous opioid peptides: multiple agonists and receptors. *Nature (London)*, **267**, 495–9
37. Mains, R. E., Eipper, B. A. and Ling, N. (1977). Common precursor to corticotropins and endorphins. *Proc. Natl. Acad. Sci. (USA)*, **74**, 3014–8
38. Martin, W. R., Eades, C. G., Thompson, J. A. *et al.* (1976). The effects of morphine- and nalorphine-like drugs in the non-dependent and the morphine-dependent chronic spinal dog. *J. Pharmacol. Exp. Ther.*, **197**, 517–32
39. May, E. L. and Sargent, L. J. (1965). Morphine and its modifications. In *Analgesics*. Vol. 5, pp. 123–77. (New York: Academic Press)
40. Minamino, N., Kiturama, K., Hayashi, Y. *et al.* (1981). Regional distribution of α-neo-endorphin in rat brain and pituitary. *Biochem. Biophys. Res. Comm.*, **102**, 226–34
41. Nakanishi, S., Inoue, A., Kita, T. *et al.* (1979). Nucleotide sequence of cloned cDNA for bovine corticotropin-β-lipotropin precursor. *Nature (London)*, **278**, 423–7
42. Noda, M., Furutani, Y., Takahashi, H. *et al.* (1982). Cloning and sequence analysis of cDNA for bovine adrenal preproenkephalin. *Nature (London)*, **295**, 202–8
43. Pert, C. B. and Snyder, S. H. (1973). Opiate receptor: demonstration in nervous tissue. *Science*, **179**, 1011–4
44. Pfeiffer, A., Pasi, A., Mehraein, P. *et al.* (1981). A subclassification of K-sites in human brain by use of dynorphin (1–17). *Neuropeptides*, **2**, 89–97
45. Rossier, J., Vargo, T., Minick, K. *et al.* (1977). Regional distribution of β-endorphin and enkephalin contents in rat brain and pituitary. *Proc. Natl. Acad. Sci. (USA)*, **74**, 5162–5
46. Simon, E. J., Hiller, J. M. and Edelman, I. (1973). Stereospecific binding of the potent narcotic analgesic [^{3}H]etorphine to rat brain homogenates. *Proc. Natl. Acad. Sci. (USA)*, **70**, 1947–9
47. Stern, A. S., Lewis, R. V., Kimura, S. *et al.* (1979). Isolation of the opioid heptapeptide Met-enkephalin (Arg^6, Phe^7) from bovine medullary granules and striatum. *Proc. Natl. Acad. Sci. (USA)*, **76**, 6680–3
48. Terenius, L. (1973). Stereospecific interaction between narcotic analgesics and a synaptic membrane fraction of rat cerebral cortex. *Acta Pharmacol. Toxicol.*, **32**, 317–20
49. Waterfield, A. A., Smockum, R. W. J., Hughes, J. *et al.* (1977). *In vitro* pharmacology of the opioid peptides, enkephalins and endorphins. *Eur. J. Pharmacol.*, **43**, 107–16
50. Weber, E., Evans, C. J., Samuelsson, S. J. *et al.* (1981). Novel peptide neuronal system in rat brain and pituitary. *Science*, **214**, 1248–51
51. Wood, P. L., Rackham, A. and Richard, J. (1981). Spinal analgesia: comparison of the mu agonist morphine and the kappa agonist ethylketazocine. *Life Sci.*, **28**, 2119–25
52. Wuster, M., Schultz, R. and Herz, A. (1981). Multiple opiate receptors in peripheral tissue preparations. *Biochem. Pharmacol.*, **30**, 1883–7
53. Yaksh, T. L. (1978). Analgesic actions of intrathecal opiates in cat and primate. *Brain Res.*, **153**, 205–10

43

Hepatocyte cultures as a research tool in pharmacology and toxicology

F. R. Althaus

Because of the central role of the liver in homeostasis this organ is the site as well as the target of complex regulatory processes, which keep its functions in tune with the metabolic requirements of the whole body system[39]. In studies of liver-specific functions in whole animals, almost invariably various endogenous and exogenous factors influence the specific function under study. Because of complex interactions of the liver with other organs and physiological processes, a large number of investigators have turned to simpler model systems. This is to distinguish primary effects of a particular experimental manipulation from those inflicted secondarily. Hepatocyte cultures are a widely used model system to study the regulation of gene expression[62]. This has led to the accumulation of a large number of research data on the physiology, pathophysiology, biochemistry and pathobiochemistry of the liver[51]. A particular advantage of the model system of hepatocyte cultures is that new research findings can be weighed against this broad background of information.

This paper summarizes recent developments in the use of hepatocyte cultures in pharmacology and toxicology research. Various aspects of this topic have been comprehensively reviewed in the recent past and for a general overview I refer to those publications[24,30,55,60,64]. Because of the limited space the emphasis will be first on the use of hepatocyte cultures in the study of the regulation of drug metabolism. The second part will focus on the role of hepatocyte cultures in toxicology research, particularly in the area of chemical carcinogenesis.

METHODOLOGICAL ASPECTS OF THE ISOLATION OF HEPATOCYTES AND THEIR MAINTENANCE IN CULTURE

First attempts to isolate hepatocytes from rat liver were reported almost 40 years ago[54]. It was not until the development of non-destructive enzymatic techniques[10,34,35] that experimental work with isolated viable hepatocytes became feasible. Today, most laboratories use various modifications of these principle techniques[49]. This technique involves preperfusion of the liver to flush the organ free of blood, and to obtain relatively low Ca concentrations. Then enzymatic digestion of intercellular matrix is achieved by perfusing the liver with crude collagenase at 37 °C. The third step is a gentle mechanical dissociation of the collagenase-digested liver followed by differential pelleting of the isolated hepatocytes, in order to separate intact cells from cell debris and non-parenchymal liver cells. This technique allows for the isolation of viable hepatocytes with high yields. The collagenase–perfusion technique has been successfully used to isolate hepatocytes from different species such as eel[33], frog[63], fetal chicken[8], guinea-pig[21], mouse[36] and rat[10].

Hepatocytes have also been isolated from the livers of other species by techniques without perfusion of the organ[24, 25]. These techniques require less manual skills but yield lower recoveries of cells. However, they can be easily adapted to other species, and even to biopsy material[24].

The high recovery of viable hepatocytes obtained with the collagenase–perfusion technique has also opened the way for biochemical studies in hepatocytes maintained in primary culture.

Conditions to maintain liver specific functions of isolated hepatocytes for several days in culture have been described[2] and used to culture hepatocytes at high initial density onto plastic dishes (Figure 43.1). Subsequent efforts were directed to increase the survival of hepatocytes in culture. A major improvement of viability was achieved by using collagen gels reconstituted from an acid extract of rat tail fibre collagen as a substratum for the culture of hepatocytes[43]. Hepatocytes cultured on the collagen gel substratum were viable for over 3 weeks. This technique was modified by including a piece of nylon mesh in the collagen gels which allowed for easier handling of these cultures[61]. Moreover, hepatocytes have been removed from the collagen gel–nylon meshes in a viable state by short collagenase treatment. A considerably longer survival time (5 months and more) has been reported

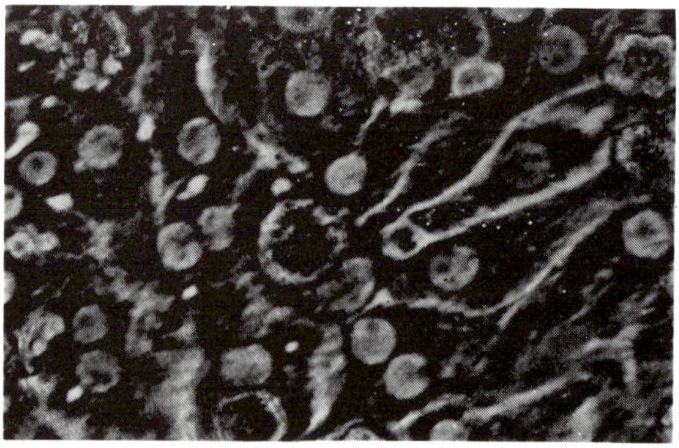

Figure 43.1 Hepatocytes derived from an adult rat liver (male 230 g Holtzman rat) after 44 h in monolayer culture. The amorphous material on the monolayer surface represents non-viable cells. Phase contrast, approx. ×700

recently for hepatocytes that were cultured on a novel substratum, called biomatrix[53]. This material, an extract from the fibrous extracellular liver matrix, has a composition which is not yet fully defined. Although this method offers some promise, it requires comparatively low seeding densities for high attachment efficiency[51]. This may be inconvenient for the maintenance of large numbers of cells over a long period of time.

HEPATOCYTE FUNCTIONS EXPRESSED IN CULTURE

Convincing evidence from a number of laboratories shows that the phenotypic expression of hepatocellular function undergoes fairly dramatic changes during culture[58]. For example, some functions typical of adult liver are rapidly lost when adult rat hepatocytes are established in primary monolayer culture. Meanwhile, other functions that are specific for fetal liver start to be expressed. On the other hand, fetal hepatocytes express various adult genes during monolayer culture. A well-studied example for this is the synthesis of adult types of plasma proteins by cultured chick embryo hepatocytes[29]. However, some functions remain unaltered throughout prolonged culture and therefore the battery of functions expressed *in vitro* is a combination of gene products which would never be expressed simultaneously during the normal ontogeny of the liver *in vivo*[16,58]. Thus a 'hybrid' phenotype is expressed by cultured hepatocytes in response to the new environment represented by the culture conditions. In view of these dynamic changes, it is not surprising that the microsomal drug-metabolizing system also undergoes some adaptive changes in response to the artificial environment of tissue culture (*vide infra*).

THE MICROSOMAL BIOTRANSFORMATION SYSTEM OF CULTURED HEPATOCYTES

Metabolism of drugs by enzymes ('biotransformation') is the principle mechanism affecting intensity and duration of the action of most drugs. A large number of endogenous and exogenous factors affect biotransformation and there is increasing evidence that these factors act on the function of microsomal drug-metabolizing enzymes[17]. A large number of studies have focussed on the microsomal enzymes that are involved in the metabolism of xenobiotics[17]. The uptake of drugs by hepatocytes or their intracellular transport to the site of enzymatic modification play a negligible role in the overall fate of xenobiotics that undergo metabolic modification[31].

Among the enzymes involved in the metabolism of xenobiotics, the cytochrome P-450 system located in the endoplasmic reticulum of the liver has a key role[65]. Essential parts of this system are a group of haemoproteins collectively called cytochrome P-450, a NADPH-requiring flavoprotein (NADPH-cytochrome P-450 reductase) and a lipid part of the membrane. Cytochrome P-450 enzymes play an important role in determining the substrate specificity of microsomal biotransformation. They have the ability to adaptively increase their concentration in response to various substrates ('enzyme induction'); any influence on these enzymes may differentially alter the metabolic capacity of the whole enzyme system[22]. Any factor altering the actual concentration of the eight or more postulated cytochrome P-450 species[38] present in microsomal membranes may change the rate of formation and pattern of metabolites formed from a specific substrate. A number of laboratories have investigated the function of cytochrome P-450 enzymes in hepatocytes during culture. Unfortunately, the maintenance of these hepatocytes is associated with a rapid and selective decrease in cytochrome P-450 concentration and in the activity of NADPH-cytochrome P-450 reductase. This leads to a differential loss of biotransformation capacity[60]. In addition, drug-mediated induction of cytochromes P-450 could not be demonstrated in the first 48 h in these primary cultures[60] and this was paralleled by the lack of an induction response of the rate-limiting enzyme of haem biosynthesis, δ-aminolevulinic acid synthetase (ALA-S), to these same drugs[41]. However, addition of the product of ALA-S reaction, δ-aminolevulinic acid, to these cultures does not restore the inducibility of cytochrome P-450 by drugs, although the rapid loss of cytochromes P-450 is somewhat diminished when hepatocytes are cultured in the presence of this acid[32, 33]. This demonstrates the complex nature of the interactions between haem biosynthesis and the formation of cytochromes P-450[42].

Various manipulations of culture conditions have succeeded in maintaining cytochromes P-450 near *in vivo* levels, at least for a short period of time. These manipulations included supplementation of the culture medium with hormone cocktails[18], vitamins[11], and pyridines[47] as well as modification of the substratum for attachment of cells. In regard to the latter, the cytochrome P-450 maintenance was improved by culturing hepatocytes on a collagen gel substratum[45]. In addition, an increase in spectral cytochrome P-450 was observed in response to phenobarbital. A more elaborate study of this phenomenon, however, indicated that this response of cytochrome P-450 in phenobarbital-treated hepatocyte cultures markedly differs from the differential induction of cytochromes P-450 by barbiturates *in vivo*[23].

Thus, despite attempts by a number of laboratories, a satisfactory maintenance of cytochrome P-450 concentrations over longer culture periods and a preservation of the differential induction response of these enzymes by drugs, similar to the liver *in vivo*, have not yet been achieved in hepatocyte cultures derived from adult rodents. The key factors involved in the regulation of adult drug-metabolizing function in these hepatocytes remain to be elucidated. In view of the fetal changes discussed in the preceding section, it is interesting to note that the cytochrome P-450 system of these hepatocytes also undergoes alterations during culture that lead to a fetal-like phenotypical state.

In contrast to hepatocytes derived from adult mammalian liver, chick embryo hepatocytes maintain inducible haem biosynthesis in culture[28]. Some pioneering work in this area was based largely on the use of this culture system[15]. These studies prompted the use of chick embryo hepatocyte cultures to investigate the regulation of haemoproteins involved in microsomal mono-oxygenase function. Further investigations have demonstrated that

Table 43.1 Effect of drugs and chemicals on microsomal cytochrome P-450 concentrations and on the activities of aminopyrine-*N*-demethylase and aryl hydrocarbon hydroxylase of chick embryo hepatocytes in culture

Drug	*Dose* (μg/ml)	*Exposure time* (h)	*Peak CO-binding spectrum* (nm)	*Cytochrome P-450 % of control*	*AP-N-DME % of control*	*AHH % of control*
Control (DMSO)	—	19	450.6	100*	100†	100‡
Phenobarbital	400	19	451.1	290, 310	240, 270	990, 1060
Aprobarbital	25	19	450.4	220, 160	260, 240	220, 220
Allylisopropylacetamide	50	15	451.0	130, 140	150, 160	100, 100
Propylisopropylacetamide	10	15	451.1	190, 180	270, 250	210, 200
Mephenytoin	4	20	450.6	220, 240	280, 280	320, 340
3-Methylcholanthrene	1	16	448.7	290, 340	200, 230	1010, 1100
β-Naphthoflavone	6	16	449.0	210, 220	200, 210	1820, 1950
Aroclor 1254	2	16	449.4	220, 180	150, 140	310, 250
Pregnenolone-16α-carbonitrile	3	19	449.8	170, 170	130, 140	790, 890

Each drug was tested in two groups of four plates. Control values: *Cytochrome P-450: 78 and 90 pmol/mg micros. protein. †AP-N-DME: 29.4 and 31.6 nmol HCOH/mg protein/h. ‡AHH: 0.64 and 0.96 nmol/mg protein/min[9]

chick embryo hepatocytes maintain high levels of cytochromes P-450 and drug-metabolizing enzymes in culture[9,50]. In addition, these studies showed that a number of inducing agents, most notably phenobarbital, increased the concentration of several forms of cytochromes P-450[9] (Table 43.1). This differential induction of drug-metabolizing enzymes could be achieved under chemically defined culture conditions and this opened the way to the investigation of the regulation of cytochrome P-450 enzymes in this culture system.

Hormones have a differential influence on the induction of cytochrome

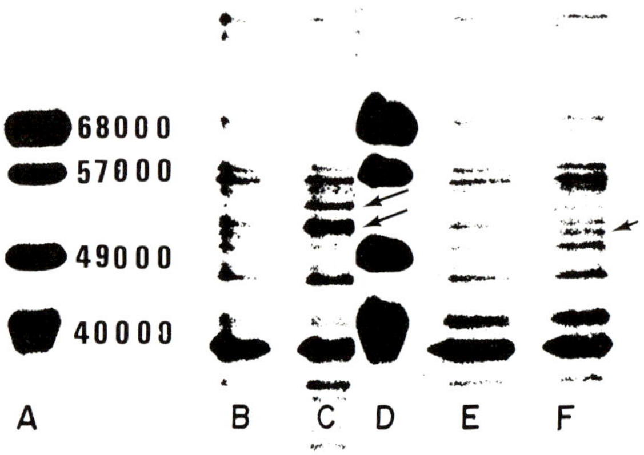

Inducer	*M_r of induced protein*	$t_{1/2}$[a]	*No. of experiments*
		h	
β-Naphthoflavone	56,000	9.60 ± 2.67	4
	54,000	7.87 ± 2.02	4
Phenobarbital	52,000	9.01 ± 2.15[b]	2
Control (solvent)	56,000	11.31 ± 2.13	4
	54,000	9.59 ± 1.35	4
	52,000	10.44 ± 2.39	4

[a]Mean ± S.D. [b]Averaged values

Figure 43.2 Halflives ($t_{1/2}$) of drug-inducible microsomal proteins from cultures chick embryo hepatocytes. Top, SDS-polyacrylamide gel electrophoresis of microsomal proteins from cultured chick embryo hepatocytes. Cultures were treated with solvent (0.02 ml of dimethylsulphoxide, B and E), β-naphthoflavone (22 μmol/l, C), or phenobarbital (1.57 mmol/l, F) for 9 h prior to preparation of microsomes for gel electrophoresis. The molecular weight positions of induced bands (see arrows) were extrapolated from the positions of marker proteins A and D (from ref. 8). Below, estimated half-lives of three drug-inducible microsomal proteins, which on the basis of their molecular weights, spectral and catalytic properties have been identified as cytochrome P-450 haemoproteins (from 8, 9)

P-450 and δ-aminolevulinic acid synthetase, the rate-limiting enzyme of the pathway that provides haem for the association with newly formed cytochrome P-450 apoprotein[56]. This effect of hormones was permissive in its nature, i.e. the hormones by themselves apparently did not induce any of these functions.

A double isotope technique in this culture system was used to demonstrate that drug-mediated induction of three cytochrome P-450 species, characterized by electrophoretic, spectral and catalytic properties, is almost exclusively the result of *de novo* enzyme synthesis and not due to inhibited enzyme degradation[8,9]. The halflives of three different inducible forms of cytochrome P-450 apoproteins in these hepatocyte cultures were also calculated[8] (Figure 43.2). These studies allowed for the characterization of modulatory influences on drug-mediated cytochrome P-450 induction. For example, treatment of these hepatocytes with chemicals that affect their proliferative rate was shown to enhance drug-induced *de novo* synthesis of a number of microsomal proteins including cytochromes P-450. These findings clearly illustrate that drug-mediated induction of cytochrome P-450 enzymes is only part of a pleiotropic response of these hepatocytes.

The use of the cultured chick embryo hepatocyte system has also allowed for the demonstration of nutritional effects on the induction of microsomal mixed-function oxidases and this has shed some light on the interdependence of hepatic haem biosynthesis and microsomal drug oxidation during hepatic porphyria. Recently a phenomenon in these cultures was described which closely resembled what has been termed the 'glycose effect' on δ-aminolevulinic acid synthetase in rodents *in vivo*[14,27]. Also observed was a dose-dependent inhibition by glucose of the induction of δ-aminolevulinic acid synthetase by phenobarbital. Secondarily, the induction of cytochromes P-450 was also diminished in these hepatocyte cultures. These effects could be obtained in the complete absence of extrahepatic factors such as serum or hormones and, therefore, allowed for the identification of glucose, glucose-6-phosphate and non-glycolytic metabolites as the agents responsible for this action[14]. With cultured chick embryo hepatocytes[26], it was found that the induction of cytochrome P-450 by phenobarbital proceeds independently from haem biosynthesis. These data support the concept that the supply of haem for the association with apocytochrome P-450 does not play a rate-limiting role in the synthesis of cytochrome P-450 in these hepatocytes[42]. These findings clearly illustrate the usefulness of chemically defined hepatocyte culture systems in the study of a regulatory mechanism which would not lend itself to experimental investigation in the complex environment of the liver *in vivo*.

The identification of ethanol as an inducer of cytochrome P-450 in chemically defined chick embryo hepatocyte culture[57] is another example where the use of this culture system provided a solution to a problem that is difficult to approach in animals *in vivo*. The *in vitro* approach led to the conclusion that ethanol-induced cytochromes P-450 can be a major factor in the altered pharmacological response of humans chronically exposed to ethanol. It is again important to realize that the contributions of complex extrahepatic influences could be excluded in these studies[57].

HEPATOCYTE CULTURES IN TOXICOLOGY RESEARCH

By virtue of its blood supply, the liver *in vivo* tends to receive higher concentrations of xenobiotics than do most other organs. A large number of these xenobiotics undergo enzymatic conversion that leads to less toxic and/or more readily excretable metabolites. However, this same process may lead to more toxic metabolites that impair hepatocellular or other organ functions. Because of this central role of the liver in the prevention and enhancement of toxicity, hepatocyte cultures have become a very important research tool in biochemical toxicology. The important role of hepatocyte cultures in biochemical toxicology research has been comprehensively reviewed[24, 30].

In the spectrum of toxic actions by xenobiotics, carcinogenic effects often pass unrecognized. The initial perturbation of cellular function by carcinogens is often very discrete and only recognizable by means of biochemical analysis[48]. In contrast to conventional acute cytotoxicity, carcinogen-mediated alterations in cellular physiology are not only compatible with, but advantageous for, the survival of the target cells. Another aspect of carcinogenic action is the long latency period between the 'first hit' and the development of morphologically manifest neoplasia[48]. These characteristics of chemical carcinogenesis have prompted a great deal of research into the development of short-term *in vitro* test systems which allow for the early detection of potential carcinogens[19]. In the hierarchy of test systems available, cultured hepatocytes have become increasingly important because of their differentiated procarcinogen metabolizing capacity[44]. This capacity makes liver cells also a probable site for the early interaction with carcinogens.

The widely accepted concept is that the carcinogenic properties of a large number of chemicals arise from the metabolic activation of their precursors, procarcinogens[46]. This metabolic activation leads to the 'ultimate' metabolite(s) that actually interact(s) with cellular constituents to cause neoplastic transformation. A common property of these ultimate metabolites is that they contain relatively electron-deficient atoms that seek to react with nucleophilic sites, particularly in nuclear DNA[44]. This interaction with nuclear DNA causes structural modification of DNA ('DNA damage') which can be reversed by mechanisms of DNA repair[40]. The occurrence of DNA repair, particularly DNA repair synthesis, is more amenable to rapid analysis than the direct identification of DNA damage by carcinogens. Therefore, for practical purposes, analysis of DNA repair synthesis is a suitable method for large scale screening of potentially carcinogenic agents. DNA repair synthesis in cultured hepatocytes can be determined by autoradiographic analysis of [^{3}H]thymidine incorporation into nuclear DNA[60]. Due to the large differences in [^{3}H]thymidine incorporation into DNA during replicative synthesis and repair synthesis of DNA, these two processes can be readily distinguished by nuclear grain counting. However, the autoradiographic procedure for determination of DNA repair synthesis in hepatocyte cultures has some technical shortcomings, the most notable one being that this technique is fairly time consuming. This is a serious handicap in regard to its application for testing large numbers of chemicals.

Table 43.2 Utility of hepatocyte cultures for screening potential carcinogens in the hepatocyte-DNA repair test. The agent under study and [methyl-^{3}H]thymidine were simultaneously added to the culture medium containing 10 mmol/l hydroxyurea and the amount of [methyl-^{3}H]thymidine incorporated into DNA during an 18 h treatment period was quantified (see refs. 3–6)

Test compound	*Dose range tested* (mol/l)	*DNA repair of ED_{max} (% of control)*	*Interpretation*†
Direct acting carcinogens			
N-acetoxy-2-acetylaminofluorene	10^{-4}–10^{-5}	1174 ± 290 (4)*	Positive
Methyl methanesulphonate	10^{-3}–10^{-5}	521 ± 54 (19)	Positive
N-nitrosomethylurea	1.8×10^{-3}–8.9×10^{-9}	827 ± 77 (2)	Positive
Proflavine	10^{-3}–10^{-6}	193 ± 8 (3)	Positive
Procarcinogens			
Aflatoxin B_1	10^{-5}–10^{-9}	432 ± 81 (2)	Positive
Benzidine	10^{-3}–10^{-6}	142 ± 5 (2)	Positive
Benzo(a)pyrene	1.6×10^{-3}–4.0×10^{-9}	271 ± 40 (2)	Positive
Diethylnitrosamine	10^{-2}–10^{-6}	149 ± 8 (2)	Positive
Safrole	10^{-2}–10^{-6}	135 ± 12 (4)	Positive
Tumour promoters			
α-Hexachlorocyclohexane	10^{-4}–10^{-6}	115 ± 6 (3)	Negative
Phenobarbital	2.0×10^{-3}–2.0×10^{-4}	103 ± 7 (4)	Negative
2,3,7,8-tetrachlorodibenzo-p-dioxin	2.0×10^{-7}–10^{-8}	101 ± 4 (2)	Negative
Non-tumourigenic chemicals			
L-ascorbic acid, Na-salt	5.7×10^{-3}–5.7×10^{-7}	109 ± 10 (3)	Negative
Methionine	6.7×10^{-3}–1.3×10^{-7}	104 ± 18 (2)	Negative
Retinylacetate	3.0×10^{-3}–3.0×10^{-7}	112 ± 11 (2)	Negative

*Number of tests in separate cell preparations, at least two measurements in each cell preparation

†The interpretations were based on a paired *t*-test analysis of a minimum of two measurements per cell batch, in at least two different cell preparations per compound

Our laboratory has been involved in the development of alternative procedures for the rapid and sensitive determination of DNA repair synthesis in cultured hepatocytes[3,4,44,59]. By using chemical analysis of DNA repair synthesis, we were able to get quantitative results within a few hours after exposing hepatocyte cultures to carcinogens[6,7] (Table 43.2). The usefulness of this *in vitro* screening system was documented in a test series involving more than 40 chemicals, including procarcinogens, direct-acting carcinogens, tumour promoters, and non-carcinogenic compounds[6,7]. It was interesting to see that the antihistaminic drug, methapyrilene hydrochloride, which had passed unrecognized in several *in vitro* carcinogenesis tests, scored positive in our test system[4]. Methapyrilene hydrochloride has been shown to be a potent liver carcinogen in the rat[37].

Beyond the practical aspects of the use of hepatocyte cultures in toxicological screening batteries, this culture system has recently been used in our laboratory for the investigation of a novel mechanism by which the vitamin nicotinamide or the widely used drug theophylline can modify the biological response of hepatocytes to chemical carcinogens[1,3]. The recent observation, that nicotinamide enhances DNA repair synthesis in carcinogen treated

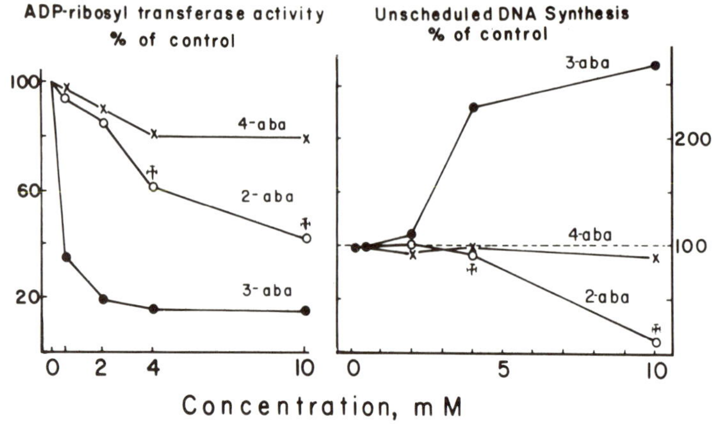

Figure 43.3 Structure–activity relationship of the action of 3-, 2- and 4-aminobenzamides (aba) on the nuclear enzyme ADP-ribosyltransferase and on DNA repair synthesis in cultured rat hepatocytes following exposure during 16 h to the carcinogen methyl methanesulphonate (5×10^{-4} mol/l)

hepatocytes, prompted us to hypothesize that the nuclear enzyme ADP-ribosyltransferase might act to modify the process of DNA repair[3]. ADP-ribosyltransferase catalyses the cleavage and transfer of ADP ribose from NAD to various acceptor sites, particularly chromatin proteins that become ADP-ribosylated. Among the inhibitors of ADP-ribosyltransferase activity are nicotinamide and other pyridines, theophylline, benzamides, and

Table 43.3 Effect of the ADP-ribosyl transferase inhibitor, isonicotinamide (10 mmol/l), on DNA repair synthesis of cultured hepatocytes treated with various carcinogens. The following carcinogens stimulated different levels of repair synthesis which was either enhanced or unaffected by isonicotinamide treatment. Accordingly, carcinogens which induced repair synthesis that is sensitive to isonicotinamide treatment can be classified 'isonicotinamide-positive' in order to contrast them with carcinogens which stimulate isonicotinamide-insensitive repair ('isonicotinamide-negative')

Isonicotinamide-positive	*Isonicotinamide-negative*
2-acetylaminofluorene	4-acetylaminofluorene
N-acetoxy-2-acetylaminofluorene	3,4 benzpyrene
aflatoxin B_1	methapyrilene hydrochloride*
4-aminobiphenyl	2-methyl-4-dimethylaminoazobenzene
benzidine	α-naphthylamine
1,2 benzpyrene	β-naphthylamine*
cyclophosphamide	4-nitroquinoline-*N*-oxide*
diethylnitrosamine	proflavine*
9,10-dimethyl-1,2-benzanthracene	
3-methylcholanthrene	
methyl methanesulphonate	

*Repair synthesis elicited by these compounds was also tested in 3-aminobenzamide (5 mmol/l) treated hepatocytes and found equally unresponsive to this treatment[5]

others[52]. All these enzyme inhibitors enhanced DNA repair synthesis of cultured hepatocytes following carcinogen treatment and, for three isomers of benzamide, there was a structure–activity relationship for the action on ADP-ribosylation as well as on DNA repair synthesis (Figure 43.3). These data and others indicated that ADP-ribosylation interacts with the process of DNA repair at the level of repair synthesis and removal of DNA strand breaks[5, 13, 20]. Another interesting aspect of these observations was that this interaction depended on the chemical nature of the DNA damaging agent[5] (Table 43.3).

These findings have some relevance for an understanding of the complex series of events that ultimately lead to the initiation of tumour formation. In view of recent evidence for an involvement of ADP-ribosylation in differentiation processes, the further investigation of this enzyme function might help clarify the mechanisms leading from DNA damage by carcinogens to altered gene expression in early stages of neoplasia.

Results from our laboratory indicate that ADP-ribosylation might also play a regulatory role in the fetal-genic expression of hepatic functions in cultured hepatocytes[2]. Further investigations are required along these lines.

The examples of ongoing research from our laboratory presented above are intended to demonstrate the versatility of the hepatocyte culture system as a research tool in biochemical toxicology. Complex regulatory mechanisms can be dissociated from extrahepatic influences and can be subjected to experimental manipulation. This approach has not yet been fully explored in biochemical toxicology.

OUTLOOK

The model system of hepatocytes in primary monolayer culture has offered many insights into a large number of cellular functions and mechanisms. The last decade of research work with this system has brought about some major improvements regarding the preservation of hepatocellular functions over extended time periods under chemically defined *in vitro* conditions. However, the preservation of some other liver functions, that are invariably lost during culture of these cells, poses a challenge for future research. In rat hepatocyte cultures, conditions will have to be defined that prevent the loss of cytochrome P-450 species typical of the differentiated drug-metabolism of the adult liver *in vivo*. In addition, for the study of basic regulatory mechanisms in drug metabolism, it will be important that all cytochrome P-450 species retain their differential inducibility under culture conditions. The preservation of this adaptive response to inducing substrates eventually will be closely related to the maintenance of inducible δ-aminolevulinic acid synthetase activity in these cells. Further knowledge of these conditions would offer substantial advantages for research directed towards an understanding of the interactions between the haem biosynthesis pathway and haemoproteins involved in drug metabolism.

Another line of future research will have to be directed towards the study of conditions that can trigger hepatocellular proliferation *in vitro* similar to the response observed in the liver *in vivo* following partial hepatectomy. This manipulation could eventually become the basis of experiments where tumour initiation and promotion can be studied in hepatocytes under completely defined *in vitro* conditions.

References

1. Althaus, F. R. (1981). Evidence for the participation of poly (ADP ribose) polymerase in unscheduled DNA synthesis of cultured hepatocytes. *Proc. Am. Assoc. Canc. Res.*, **22**, 89
2. Althaus, F. R., Lawrence, S. D., He, Y. Z. *et al.* (1982). Effects of altered [ADP-ribose]$_n$-metabolism on expression of fetal functions by adult hepatocytes. *Nature*, **300**, 366–8
3. Althaus, F. R., Lawrence, S. D., Sattler, G. L. *et al.* (1980). The effect of nicotinamide on unscheduled DNA synthesis in cultured hepatocytes. *Biochem. Biophys. Res. Commun.*, **95**, 1063–70
4. Althaus, F. R., Lawrence, S. D., Sattler, G. L. *et al.* (1982). DNA damage induced by the antihistaminic drug methapyrilene hydrochloride. *Mutat. Res.*, **103**, 213–18
5. Althaus, F. R., Lawrence, S. D., Sattler, G. L. *et. al.* (1982). ADP-ribosyl transferase activity in cultured hepatocytes: interactions with DNA repair. *J. Biol. Chem.*, **257**, 5528–35
6. Althaus, F. R., Lawrence, S. D., Sattler, G. L. *et al.* (1982). Chemical quantitation of unscheduled DNA synthesis in cultured hepatocytes as an assay for the rapid screening of potential chemical carcinogens. *Cancer Res.*, **42**, 3010–15
7. Althaus, F. R. and Meyer, U. A. (1979). Drug-mediated induction of cytochrome P-450 in hepatocyte culture: modulation by dexamethasone. *Experientia*, **35**, 946
8. Althaus, F. R. and Meyer, U. A. (1981). Effects of phenobarbital, β-naphthoflavone, dexamethasone and formamidoxime on the turnover of inducible microsomal proteins in cultured hepatocytes. *J. Biol. Chem.*, **256**, 13079–84
9. Althaus, F. R., Sinclair, J. F., Sinclair, P. *et al.* (1979). Drug-mediated induction of cytochrome(s) P-450 and drug metabolism in cultured hepatocytes maintained in chemically defined medium. *J. Biol. Chem.*, **254**, 2148–53
10. Berry, M. N. and Friend, D. S. (1969). High-yield preparation of isolated rat liver parenchymal cells. *J. Cell Biol.*, **43**, 506–20
11. Bissell, D. M. and Guzelian, P. S. (1979). Ascorbic acid deficiency and cytochrome P-450 in adult rat hepatocytes in primary monolayer culture. *Arch. Biochem. Biophys.*, **192**, 569–76
12. Bissell, D. M., Hammaker, L. E. and Meyer, U. A. (1973). Parenchymal cells from adult rat liver in nonproliferating monolayer culture. *J. Cell Biol.*, **59**, 722–34
13. Bohr, V. and Klenow, H. (1981). 3-Aminobenzamide stimulates unscheduled DNA synthesis and rejoining of strand breaks in human lymphocytes. *Biochem. Biophys. Res. Commun.*, **102**, 1254–61
14. Bonkowsky, A. L., Collins, A., Doherty, J. M. *et al.* (1973). The glucose effect in rat liver: studies of delta-aminolevulinate synthetase and tyrosine aminotransferase. *Biochim. Biophys. Acta*, **320**, 561–76
15. Bonkowsky, H. L., Sinclair, P. R. and Sinclair, J. F. (1979). Hepatic heme metabolism and its control. *Yale J. Biol. Med.*, **52**, 13–37
16. Borek, C. and Williams, G. M. (eds.) (1980). Differentiation and carcinogenesis in liver cell culture. *Ann. N.Y. Acad. Sci.*, 349
17. Coon, M. J., Conney, A. H., Estabrook, R. W. *et al.* (eds.) (1980). *Microsomes, Drug Oxidations and Chemical Carcinogenesis.* (New York: Academic Press)
18. Decad, G. M., Hsieh, D. P. H. and Byard, J. L. (1977). Maintenance of cytochrome P-450 and metabolism of aflatoxin B_1 in primary hepatocyte cultures. *Biochem. Biophys. Res. Commun.*, **78**, 279–87
19. de la Iglesia, F. A., Lake, R. S. and Fitzgerald, J. E. (1980). Short-term tests for mutagenesis and carcinogenesis in drug toxicology: how to test and when to test is the question. *Drug Metab. Rev.*, **11**, 103–46
20. Durkacz, B. W., Omidiji, O., Gray, D. A. *et al.* (1980). (ADP-ribose)$_n$ participates in DNA excision repair. *Nature (London)*, **283**, 593–6

21. Elliot, K. R. F. and Pogson, C. I. (1977). Preparation and characterization of isolated parenchymal cells from guinea pig liver. *Mol. Cell. Biochem.*, **16**, 23–9
22. Estabrook, R. W. and Lindenlaub, E. (eds.) (1979). *The Induction of Drug Metabolism.* (Stuttgart: F. K. Schattauer)
23. Fahl, W. E., Michaelopoulos, G., Sattler, G. L. *et al.* (1979). Characteristics of microsomal enzyme controls in primary cultures of rat hepatocytes. *Arch. Biochem. Biophys.*, **192,** 61–72
24. Fry, J. R. and Bridges, J. W. (1979). Use of primary hepatocyte cultures in biochemical toxicology. *Rev. Biochem. Toxicol.*, **1**, 201–47
25. Fry, J. R. (1981). Preparation of mammalian hepatocytes. *Methods Enzymol.*, **77**, 130–7
26. Giger, U. and Meyer, U. A. (1981). Role of haem in the induction of cytochrome P-450 by phenobarbitone. *Biochem. J.*, **198**, 321–9
27. Giger, U. and Meyer, U. A. (1981). Induction of delta-aminolevulinate synthetase and cytochrome P-450 hemoproteins in hepatocyte culture. *J. Biol. Chem.*, **256**, 11182–90
28. Granick, S. (1966). The induction *in vitro* of the synthesis of delta-aminolevulinic acid synthetase in chemical porphyria: a response to certain drugs, sex hormones and foreign chemicals. *J. Biol. Chem.*, **241**, 1359–75
29. Grieninger, G. and Granick, S. (1978). Synthesis and secretion of plasma proteins by embryonic chick hepatocytes. *J. Exp. Med.*, **147**, 1806–23
30. Grisham, J. W. (1979). Use of hepatic cell cultures to detect and evaluate the mechanisms of action of toxic chemicals. *Int. Rev. Exp. Pathol.*, **20**, 123–210
31. Grundin, R., Moldeus, P., Vadi, H. *et al.* (1975). Drug metabolism in isolated rat liver cells. *Adv. Exp. Med. Biol.*, **58**, 251–69
32. Guzelian, P. S. and Bissell, D. M. (1976). Effect of cobalt on synthesis of heme and cytochrome P-450 in the liver. Studies of adult rat hepatocytes in primary monolayer culture and *in vivo. J. Biol. Chem.*, **251**, 4421–7
33. Hayashi, S. and Ooshiro, Z. (1978). Preparation of isolated cells of eel liver. *Bull. Jap. Soc. Sci. Fish.*, **44**, 499–503
34. Howard, R. B., Christensen, A. K., Gibbs, F. A. *et al.* (1967). The enzymatic preparation of isolated intact parenchymal cells from rat liver. *J. Cell Biol.*, **35**, 675–84
35. Howard, R. B., Lee, J. C. and Pesch, L. A. (1973). The fine structure, potassium content, and respiratory activity of isolated rat liver parenchymal cells prepared by improved enzymatic techniques. *J. Cell Biol.*, **57**, 642–58
36. Klauvnig, J. E., Goldblatt, P. J., Hinton, D. E. *et al.* (1981). Mouse liver cell culture. *In Vitro*, **17**, 913–25
37. Lijinsky, W., Reuber, M. D. and Blackwell, B. N. (1980). Liver tumors induced in rats by oral administration of the antihistaminic drug methapyrilene hydrochloride. *Science*, **209,** 817–19
38. Lu, A. Y. H. and West, S. B. (1980). Multiplicity of mammalian microsomal cytochromes P-450. *Pharmacol. Rev.*, **31**, 277–95
39. Lunquist, F. and Tygstrup, N. (eds.) (1974). *Regulation of Hepatic Metabolism.* (Copenhagen: Munksgaard)
40. Maher, V. M. and McCormick, J. J. (1979). DNA repair and carcinogenesis. In Grover, P. L. (ed.) *Chemical Carcinogens and DNA*. Vol. 2, pp. 133–58. (Boca Raton, Florida: CRC Press)
41. Meyer, U. A. Personal communication
42. Meyer, U. A., Meier, P. J., Hirsiger, H. *et al.* (1980). Induction of drug-metabolizing enzymes by phenobarbitone: structural and biochemical aspects. *Exerpta Medica*, **76,** 101–10
43. Michalopoulos, G. and Pitot, H. C. (1975). Primary culture of parenchymal liver cells on collagen membranes. *Exp. Cell Res.*, **94**, 70–8
44. Michalopoulos, G., Sattler, G. L., O'Connor, L. *et al.* (1978). Unscheduled DNA synthesis induced by procarcinogens in suspensions and primary cultures of hepatocytes on collagen membranes. *Cancer Res.*, **38**, 1866–71
45. Michalopoulos, G., Sattler, G. L. and Pitot, H. C. (1976). Maintenance of microsomal cytochrome b_5 and P-450 in primary cultures of parenchymal liver cells on collagen membranes. *Life Sci.*, **18**, 1139–44

46. Miller, E. C. (1978). Some current perspectives on chemical carcinogenesis in humans and experimental animals: presidential address. *Cancer Res.*, **38**, 1479–96
47. Paine, A. J., Hockin, L. J. and Legg, R. F. (1979). Relationship between the ability of nicotinamide to maintain nicotinamide-adenine-dinucleotide in rat liver cell culture and its effect on cytochrome P-450. *Biochem. J.*, **184**, 461–3
48. Pitot, H. C. (1979). Biological and enzymatic events in chemical carcinogenesis. *Ann. Rev. Med.*, **30**, 25–39
49. Pitot, H. C. and Sirica, A. E. (1980). Methodology and utility of primary cultures of hepatocytes from experimental animals. *Methods Cell Biol.*, **21B**, 441–56
50. Poland, A. and Kappas, A. (1973). Chlorcyclizine N-demethylase activity in chick embryo hepatic cell culture. *Biochem. Pharmacol.*, **22**, 749–58
51. Popper, H. and Schaffner, F. (eds.) (1979). *Progress in Liver Diseases*. Vol. 6. (New York: Grune & Stratton)
52. Purnell, M. R., Stone, P. and Whish, W. J. D. (1980). ADP-ribosylation of nuclear proteins. *Biochem. Soc. Trans.*, **8**, 215–27
53. Rojkind, M., Gatmaitan, Z., Mackensen, S. *et al.* (1980). Connective tissue biomatrix: its isolation and utilization for long-term cultures of normal rat hepatocytes. *J. Cell Biol.*, **87**, 255–63
54. Schneider, W. C. and Potter, V. R. (1943). The assay of animal tissues for respiratory enzymes. *J. Biol. Chem.*, **149**, 217–27
55. Seglen, P. O. (1979). Hepatocyte suspensions and cultures as tools in experimental carcinogenesis. *J. Toxicol. Env. Health*, **5**, 551–60
56. Sinclair, J. F., Sinclair, P. R. and Bonkowsky, H. L. (1979). Hormonal requirements for the induction of cytochrome P-450 in hepatocyte cultures in a serum-free medium. *Biochem. Biophys. Res. Commun.*, **86**, 710–17
57. Sinclair, J. F., Sinclair, P. J., Smith, E. L. *et al.* (1981). Ethanol-mediated increase in cytochrome P-450 in cultured hepatocytes. *Biochem. Pharmacol.*, **30**, 2805–9
58. Sirica, A. E., Althaus, F. R. and Hayao, G. (1981). Characteristics of adult rat hepatocytes in primary culture on collagen gel-nylon mesh. In Reid, E., Cook, G. M. W. and Morré, D. J. (eds.) *Cancer-Cell Organelles: Isolation and Characterization of Cells and Cell Components*. pp. 111–21. (England: Chester, Ellis Horwood)
59. Sirica, A. E., Hwang, C. G., Sattler, G. L. *et al.* (1980). Use of primary cultures of adult rat hepatocytes on collagen gel–nylon mesh to evaluate carcinogen-induced unscheduled DNA synthesis. *Cancer Res.*, **40**, 3259–67
60. Sirica, A. E. and Pitot, H. C. (1980). Drug metabolism and effects of carcinogens in cultured hepatic cells. *Pharmacol. Rev.*, **31**, 205–28
61. Sirica, A. E., Richards, W., Tsukada, Y. *et al.* (1979). Fetal phenotypic expression by adult rat hepatocytes on collagen gel/nylon meshes. *Proc. Natl. Acad. Sci.*, **76**, 283–7
62. Spence, J. T., Haars, L., Edwards, A. *et al.* (1980). Regulation of gene expression in primary cultures of adult rat hepatocytes on collagen gel. *Ann. N.Y. Acad. Sci.*, **349**, 99–110
63. Stanchfield, J. E. and Yager, J. D. (1978). Estrogen responsive primary amphibian liver cell culture system. *Exp. Cell Res.*, **116**, 239–52
64. Thurman, R. G. and Kauffman, F. C. (1980). Factors regulating drug metabolism in intact hepatocytes. *Pharmacol. Rev.*, **31**, 229–51
65. Ullrich, V. (1977). The role of cytochrome P-450 in the activation of drugs. *Drug Res.*, **27**, 1821–35

44
Metabolic radical formation from halothane and enflurane and its modification by enzyme induction and inhibition

W. Beuter and A. Schmid

Of the side-effects of halogenated inhalation anaesthetics, damage to the liver and kidneys is the most prominent[21].

The incidence of the so-called 'halothane hepatitis' in humans is given to be 1 in 10 000 cases[12, 13] with extensive cell necroses, especially after repeated halothane anaesthesias and/or anaesthesias with oxygen-deficiencies. The rate of lethality supposedly amounts up to 50%[13].

Damage of the liver caused by halothane has been detected in animals as well, so obviously no species can be excluded with certainty[10, 11, 14, 18, 22, 23, 25]. Particularly revealing tests are reported by Chang and Katz[4], who exposed rats to halothane concentrations from 10 to 500 parts per million for 4–8 weeks and examined their brain, liver and kidneys under an electron microscope. Their result was that in all three organs very subtle pathomorphological changes of the plasma membrane, the endoplasmic reticulum, the mitochondria, the Golgi apparatus and the nuclear membrane had taken place. The authors therefore conclude that the primary cell damage caused by halothane and/or its metabolites obviously happens on cellular and subcellular membranes; at the same time they point out that 'the pathogenic mechanism of halothane or its metabolites still needs to be investigated and cannot be determined at the present time'.

Could the mentioned generalized damage of the membrane caused by halothane and to a lesser extent by enflurane, whose rate of metabolism amounts to only about one sixth of that of halothane[9], result from its metabolic transformation into radicals, as radicals are pronounced membrane poisons, due to their reactivity and their oxidative effect[8]?

EXPERIMENTS

Male mice, weighing about 40 g were tested without prior food reduction. They received halothane (Halothan®, Hoechst, Frankfurt) in six doses from 250 to 1250 mg/kg, or enflurane (Ethrane®, Abbott, Delkenheim) in seven doses from 234 to 1285 mg/kg; some of the animals were injected additionally with 3-methylcholanthren puriss. (Fluka, Basel) at a dose of 20 mg/kg daily for 3 days before the test, or with piperonylbutoxide p.a. (Serva, Heidelberg) at a dose of 400 mg/kg 1 day before the test, on induction or inhibition of mixed-function mono-oxygenases (MFO) respectively. For that purpose, substances were dissolved in paraffinum liquidum (Merck, Darmstadt) – 3-methylcholanthrene in propanediol(1,2) (Merck, Darmstadt) – and applied in a total volume of 5 ml/kg.

As indicators of radical formation *in vivo*, ethane was determined gas chromatographically[17] in the expired air of the animals, and malone dialdehyde production in the liver was determined spectrophotometrically[24].

For each experiment four mice were put into a glass desiccator with a total volume of 860 ml after the application of halothane or enflurane, which contained synthetic air (Linde, Unterschleißheim) and 100 g soda lime (Dräger Sorb® 650 CH 508, Drägerwerk, Lübeck) for the absorption of CO_2 and was provided pressure-free with oxygen (99.995% by volume; Linde, Unterschleißheim). After 3 h, the animals were anaesthetized with nitrogen and decapitated to be bled.

With each dose of halothane or enflurane a double test was performed, i.e. for the six resulting dose–effect curves 312 mice had been used as well as 48 animals for the corresponding controls.

RESULTS

Figure 44.1 shows a typical polyculminating dose–effect curve of the expiration of ethane following halothane injection. The same result was found following enflurane injection.

To obtain a quantitative comparability of various dose–effect curves, the control areas (control value multiplied by maximum dose) were subtracted from the dose–effect areas (below the dose–effect curves) and have been summed up in Table 44.1 as 'effect areas' in the form of the arithmetic mean ($\bar{x}$) including ranges (R).

Table 44.1 shows that:

(1) The application of halothane or enflurane to unpretreated animals results in a distinct increase of ethane expiration ($p \leqslant 0.01$) and a slight increase of malone dialdehyde production in the liver.

(2) With an enzyme induction by 3-methylcholanthren(20), the expiration of ethane is raised even further after halothane ($p \leqslant 0.01$) or enflurane ($p \leqslant 0.05$), respectively, whereas the production of malone dialdehyde in the liver is slightly inhibited.

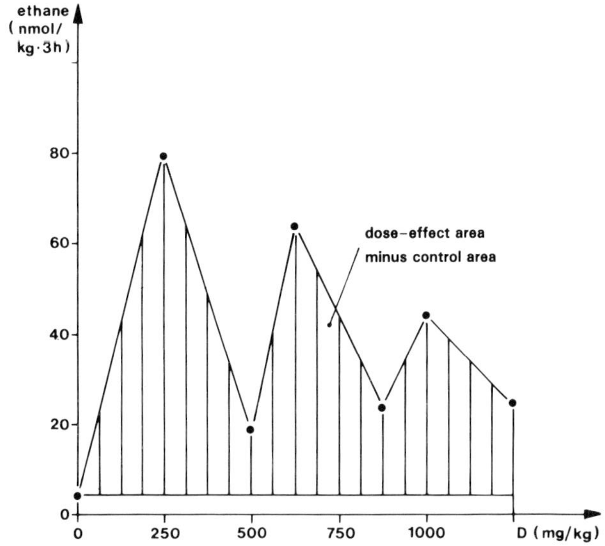

Figure 44.1 Ethane expiration of male mice as function of the halothane dose

Table 44.1 Effect areas of ethane expiration and of malone dialdehyde production in the liver of male mice

Treatment	*Ethane* (nmol mg/kg² 3h)	*Malone dialdehyde* (nmol mg/g kg 3h)
Halothane		
Halothane	46311†	10011
	45566↔47055	6498↔13523
Halothane + 3-CH_3 cholanthren(20)	53607†	−3618
	53316↔53898	−8134↔898
Halothane + Piperonylbutoxide	34234†	2171
	32181↔36287	−258↔4600
Enflurane		
Enflurane	29488†	14015
	27806↔31170	9658↔18372
Enflurane + 3-CH_3 cholanthren(20)	35752†	1290
	35459↔36044	−3467↔6046
Enflurane + Piperonylbutoxide	18868*	−4845
	16841↔20894	−3766↔ −5923

*resp. †mean dose–effect area greater/smaller than mean control area at $p \leqslant 0.05$ resp. $p \leqslant 0.01$

(3) Following an enzyme inhibition with piperonylbutoxide the expiration of ethane is inhibited after halothane ($p \leqslant 0.01$) or enflurane ($p \leqslant 0.05$), respectively; there are corresponding results for the production of

malone dialdehyde in the liver, the inhibiting effect of enflurane ($p \leqslant 0.01$), however, being stronger than that of halothane.

(4) In the tests with halothane, the expiration of ethane and the production of malone dialdehyde in the liver are influenced qualitatively in the same way as in the tests with enflurane. Concerning the quantity, expiration of ethane in the tests with halothane is more evident than in the tests with enflurane, while the production of malone dialdehyde remains comparable.

DISCUSSION

The results can be interpreted as evidence that halothane and enflurane caused a lipid peroxidation (of cellular and subcellular membranes) in unpretreated male mice due to biotransformation into radicals, because ethane expiration of the observed kind is interpreted in this way by numerous authors[1,5,6,17,19,20].

It is striking, however, that radical formation from halothane is obviously higher than that from enflurane, which can be explained by the more intensive biotransformation of halothane[9].

This interpretation of ethane expiration only seems to be a contradiction to the inhibition of malone dialdehyde production in the liver after an enzyme stimulation with 3-methylcholanthren(20), which was observed simultaneously. Although malone dialdehyde production – like ethane expiration – is taken as an indicator for lipid peroxidation[3,7,24], the malone dialdehyde production, or radical production respectively, in the liver comes to a standstill after a high initial rate of radical formation, because mixed-function mono-oxygenases are increasingly damaged, as is known from the metabolic radical formation from carbon tetrachloride[15]. The same is true for the ethane formation in the liver. As the expired and measured ethane, however, originates from the whole organism and not only from the liver, and as halothane, or enflurane respectively, exist in the different distribution volumes in different concentrations, and as they are further transformed into radicals to a different degree (due to different enzyme activities), the expiration of ethane after an enzyme stimulation is not correlated to the production of malone dialdehyde in the liver.

A different inactivation of radical-inducing mono-oxygenases in the distribution volumes of halothane and enflurane, which depend on the dose given, could be the most probable explanation of the fact that the dose–effect curve of the expiration of ethane is unorthodoxically polyculminating[20].

More understandable is the explanation of the effects of piperonylbutoxide. These are thought to originate from an inhibition of halothane and enflurane metabolizing MFO, i.e. reduced production of radicals from both inhalation anaesthetics. Potentially, there exists now a possibility of avoiding prophylactically the supposedly most damaging side-effects of both anaesthetics. As mentioned in the introduction, the morphological halothane damage in the rat described by Chang and Katz[4] can be explained without difficulty with a metabolic radical formation in all tissues or organs with mono-oxygenase activity. This mechanism of damage is underlined also by the clinical experience that 'halothane hepatitis' occurs especially after repeated halothane anaesthesias (enzyme induction) and/or anaesthesias with oxygen deficiencies (since a reductive dehalogenation is discussed as the mechanism of metabolic radical formation[2,16].

If this is true, then the parenchyme damaging side-effect of halothane and enflurane is correlated to the mono-oxygenase activity, which means that it differs between different species and maybe depends on an existing enzyme induction. Moreover, the parenchyme toxicity will be dependent on the metabolizability of the halogenated inhalation anaesthetic, i.e. it will decline in the following order: methoxyflurane > halothane > enflurane > isoflurane[9].

The results lead to the conclusion that halothane and enflurane are biotransformed *in vivo* into radicals whose production is stopped after an induction of MFO due to radical damage to the enzymes and is reduced in animals with inhibited mono-oxygenases.

References

1. Abramson, H. (1949). The oxidation of unsaturated fatty acids in normal and scorbutic guinea pigs. *J. Biol. Chem.*, **178**, 179–83
2. Ahr, H. J., King, L. J., Nastainczyk, W. and Ullrich, V. (1982). The mechanism of reductive dehalogenation of halothane by liver cytochrome P 450. *Biochem. Pharmacol.*, **31**, 383–90
3. Bernheim, F., Bernheim, M. L. C. and Wilbur, K. M. (1945). The reaction between thiobarbituric acid and the oxidation products of certain lipids. *J. Biol. Chem.*, **174**, 257–64
4. Chang, L. W. and Katz, J. (1976). Pathologic effects of chronic halothane inhalation: an overview. *Anesthesiology*, **45**, 640–53
5. Cohen, G. (1979). Lipid peroxidation: detection *in vivo* and *in vitro* through the formation of saturated hydrocarbon gases. In *Oxygen Free Radicals and Tissue Damage*. (Amsterdam, Oxford, New York: Excerpta Medica)
6. Cohen, G., Riely, C. and Lieberman, M. (1968). Ethane formation from lipid peroxides in mammalian cells. *Fed. Proc.*, **27**, 648 (abstract 2436)
7. Dahle, I. K., Hill, E. G. and Holman, R. T. (1962). The thiobarbituric acid reaction and the auto-oxidation of polyunsaturated fatty acid methyl esters. *Arch. Biochem. Biophys.*, **98**, 253–61
8. Demopoulos, H. B. (1973). The basis of free radical pathology. *Fed. Proc.*, **32**, 1859–61
9. Fiserova-Bergerova, V. and Holaday, D. A. (1979). Uptake and clearance of inhalation anesthetics in man. *Drug Metab. Rev.*, **9**, 43–60
10. Hughes, H. C. and Lang, C. M. (1972). Hepatic necrosis produced by repeated administration of halothane to guinea pigs. *Anesthesiology*, **36**, 466–71
11. Hull, M. W. and Reilly, M. G. (1968). Effect of repeated halothane anesthesia on sheep. *Am. J. Vet. Res.*, **29**, 1161–5
12. Liehr, H. and Kasper, H. (1975). *Leberkrankheiten*. p. 161. (Munich: Aesopus Verlag)
13. Marshall, B. E. and Wollmann, H. (1980). General anesthetics. In Goodman Gilman, A., Goodman, L. S. and Gilman, A. (eds.) *The Pharmacological Basis of Therapeutics*. 6th Edn. (New York: MacMillan)
14. Norby, M. A. and Link, R. P. (1970). Effect of halothane anesthesia on liver function in the horse. *Vet. Med. Small Anim. Clin.*, **65**, 946–9

15. Recknagel, R. O. and Glende, Jr., E. A. (1973). Carbon tetrachloride hepatotoxicity: an example of lethal cleavage. *CRC Crit. Rev. Toxicol.*, **2**, 263–97
16. Reynolds, E. S. and Moslen, M. T. (1980). Free-radical damage in liver. In *Free Radicals in Biology*. Vol. IV. (New York: Academic Press)
17. Riely, C., Cohen, G. and Lieberman, M. (1974). Ethane evolution: a new index of lipid peroxidation. *Science*, **183**, 208–10
18. Ross, W. T. and Cardell, R. R. (1972). Effects of halothane on the ultrastructure of rat liver cells. *Am. J. Anat.*, **135**, 5–21
19. Schmid, A. and Christoph, M. (1980). Untersuchungen zur Genese der parenteralen Eisenvergiftung. *Der Prakt. Tierarzt*, **61**, 589–96
20. Schmid, A. and Beuter, W. (1982). Metabolische Radikalbildung aus Tetrachloräthylen und ihre Beeinflussung durch Enzyminduktion und -hemmung. *Zbl. Vet. Med. A.*, **29**. 481–8
21. Stee, E. W. van (1976). Toxicology of inhalation anesthetics and metabolites. *Ann. Rev. Pharmacol.*, **16**, 67–79
22. Stevens, W. C., Eger, E. I. and White, A. (1975). Comparative toxicities of halothane, isoflurane and diethyl ether at subanesthetic concentrations in laboratory animals. *Anesthesiology*, **42**, 408–19
23. Swerczek, T. W. and Prickett, M. E. (1971). Post-surgical liver damage following halothane anesthesia in the horse. *Proc. Am. Assoc. Equine Pract.*, p. 137
24. Terao, J. and Matsushita, S. (1981). Thiobarbituric acid reaction of methyl arachidonate monohydroperoxide isomers. *Lipids*, **16**, 98–101
25. Wolff, W. A., Lumb, W. V. and Ramsay, M. K. (1967). Effects of halothane and chloroform anesthesia on the equine liver. *Am. J. Vet. Res.*, **28**, 1363–72

45
Anaesthesia in pharmacological research

R. Boivin

General anaesthetic drugs are substances which produce a reversible state of unconsciousness and insensibility. In addition to these principal effects, anaesthetic drugs nearly always modify the major functions of the organism. As Claude Bernard[9] remarked more than a century ago, 'An anaesthetic is not merely a special poison for the nervous system. It anaesthetizes all the cells, it invades all the tissues.' Despite these drawbacks, anaesthetic drugs are widely used today for *in vivo* experiments. However, it must be borne in mind that their use may considerably modify the outcome of a physiological or pharmacological experiment. While a great amount of data has been accumulated with respect to the physiological effect of general anaesthesia, little information is available on pharmacological effects.

The aim of this report is to provide information on the possible interactions between general anaesthetic drugs and other pharmacological agents. This review is limited to drugs currently used only in experimental work.

METHODOLOGY

A specific, defined methodology is necessary to observe the effects of anaesthetic drugs. While the procedure itself is fairly straightforward and amounts to the compilation of two comparative series of data (one with and the other without anaesthetic drug use), it cannot always be followed. All too often, physiological determinants demand surgery with difficult to control situations such as haemorrhage, vasomotor disturbances, stimulation or destruction of sensitive nerve fibres, and, finally, endocrinological changes. Under such conditions, the comparisons between anaesthetic and non-anaesthetic conditions lose their significance. It is difficult to distinguish the physiological effects due to anaesthesia from those effects derived from the surgical procedure itself (or any combination of the two). Thus, irregardless of the intervention required, and whether it be simple (catheterization under general anaesthesia) or complicated (laparotomy, thoracotomy), it should be carried out well in advance of the proposed study (several days to 2 weeks). Complete recuperation of the subject must occur before beginning experimentation. Furthermore, it is advisable not to consider results obtained without separation of effects due to anaesthesia and those linked to surgical procedures.

Another difficulty is to maintain a constant level of anaesthesia during the experiment. Cardiac output, blood pressure, and systemic resistances, depend upon the degree of anaesthesia (Figure 45.1 (a)). Moreover, for a given constant level of anaesthesia, the possibility of physiological adaptation has been shown, e.g. during anaesthesia with halothane, a number of

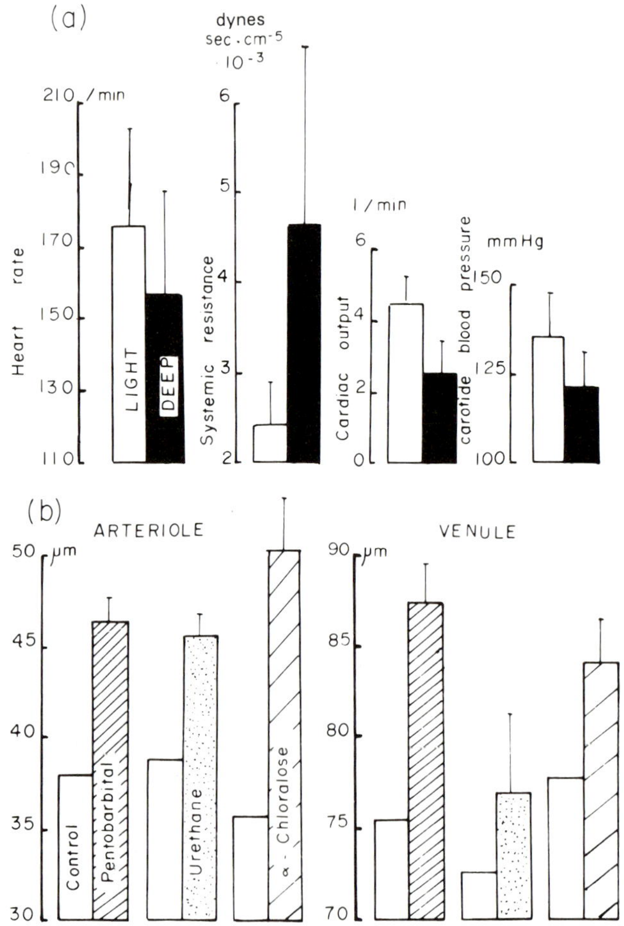

Figure 45.1 (a) Influence of anaesthesia level on some cardiovascular parameters in dogs. Light anaesthesia: chloralose 53 mg/kg, urethane 535 mg/kg, and deep anaesthesia: chloralose 98 mg/kg, urethane 980 mg/kg (from ref. 34). (b) Effect of pentobarbital, urethane and chloralose on diameter (μm) of second order vessels in the bat wing (from ref. 33)

physiological parameters regain their original values; adaptation seen when ether is employed is even more rapid. On the other hand, some physiological parameters might deteriorate, e.g. during more severe drop in cardiac output in the third than in the second hour after administration of chloralose-urethane. Accordingly, a close monitoring of the chronological evolution of all parameters is necessary during an experiment. Variations in the results from different authors often seem to be linked to inadequate monitoring.

ANAESTHESIA AND PHARMACOKINETICS

The concentration of a pharmacological agent at its receptor sites and target organs will depend on its absorption, distribution, metabolism, and its elimination. Very often anaesthesia alters factors considerably.

Absorption

The quantity of drug at the site of absorption, its solubility, and local circulation are involved. During digestive or pulmonary absorption, anaesthesia may have an influence on the quantity of substance actually absorbed. Respiratory depression, which almost always accompanies general anaesthesia, retards the alveolar penetration of an inhalated drug. Motor inhibition of various portions of the digestive tract by anaesthetics would account for irregularities seen in oral drug absorption[28]. This is illustrated by the variations incurred in the dog's gastric emptying time depending on the anaesthetic used. Indeed, an increase of 15% in gastric emptying time can be observed with nitrous oxide as compared to 40% with ether, and 64% with chloroform.

In addition, regardless of the route of drug administration, local circulation at the site of absorption may be affected by the changes of the cardiovascular function under anaesthesia. Changes in blood supply to the canine digestive tract under pentobarbital anaesthesia have been studied with two types of marked microspheres[17]. In the unanaesthetized animal, the amount of blood received by the jejunum was greater than that of the ileum and colon. During the first 15 min of anaesthesia, however, the amount of blood received by the digestive system increased in equal proportion in all regions of the digestive tract, and returned to original levels only 1 hour later. These results confirm those obtained in the rat anaesthetized with chloral, which consisted of a reduction of 68% in the blood supply of the femoral muscles, and an increase in that of the duodenum (96%), colon (74%) and kidney (25%) without any modification in the blood supply to heart, lung, skin and liver[13].

These considerations favour, as a corollary, the intravenous administration of pharmacological agents in anaesthetized animals.

Distribution

The distribution of a drug will depend largely on circulatory parameters, especially the partition of the cardiac output to various tissues, which is profoundly modified under anaesthesia[13,21]. Cardiac output, local circulation and vascular resistances of several organs have been measured in the anaesthetized (pentobarbital 30 mg/kg) and non-anaesthetized monkey[24]. The fraction of the total cardiac output delivered to the kidney, skin, lungs and bone increased at the expense of that of the brain, skeletal muscles, adrenals and thoracic wall without significant changes for the liver. Regardless of the mechanisms involved in these circulatory modifications, the tissue distribution of the drug is altered and consequently the induced pharmacological changes. Not only must one take into consideration the repartition of cardiac output but also the absolute value of blood supply to the tissues themselves. An increase in the retention time of sulphobromophtalein (SBP) in the dog under methoxyflurane anaesthesia has been attributed to a decrease in hepatic circulation. In the rat under ether anaesthesia the shortening of the halflife of an ethylcarbamate derivative was linked to the reduction in the enterohepatic cycle.

The distribution of a drug depends also on the extent of its binding to plasma proteins. Sodium acetrizoate is more highly bound in an animal anaesthetized with pentobarbital, and sodium acetrizoate increases the free fraction of plasma pentobarbital, which may then diffuse with greater ease into the nervous system and thus contribute to a prolongation of the anaesthesia[15]. Competition between certain anaesthetics and other drugs exists for pharmacological receptor sites as well. An antagonism exists between dehydromorphine and xylazine or ketamine[31]. Further studies will, however, be necessary to elucidate differences in analgesic activity between various anaesthetics.

Metabolism

A recent review considered the long discussed interferences of anaesthetics with biotransformations[43]. The mechanisms involved are oxidations mediated by hepatic microsomes. Microsomal induction is especially clear for cytochrome P-450, the key-enzyme of oxidative metabolism, the concentration of which considerably increases following the administration of barbiturates. Microsomal induction has important pharmacological consequences for many agents such as coumarine, prednisone, and the barbiturates, as their length of activity is greatly reduced. However, the hypnotic effects of barbiturates are increased and prolonged with ether and this is most likely due to the inhibition of microsomal enzymes.

When rats inhale various anaesthetics such as chloroform, ether, enflurane, halothane, isoflurane or methoxyflurane the length of sleep produced by hexobarbital is decreased. This is believed to be due to enzymatic induction by volatile anaesthetics[32]. Other workers[22] have demonstrated that longterm exposure to volatile anaesthetics causes a smoothening of the rough endoplasmic reticulum and an increase in cytochrome P-450 concentration, as well as in other enzymes involved in drug metabolism. In the rat, diphenylhydantoine metabolism is particularly inhibited, likely due to effects on hydroxylation. In the same species, a delay in antipyrine and paracetamol elimination is caused by ether, whereas the same agent slightly stimulates the acetylation of sulphanilamide[4]. A recent study[30] of an ether–antipyrine–paracetamol interaction indicates that this lag may be attributed to a lower hepatic catabolism of those substances. The effects of ether are seen even if the substances studied are administered after awakening. In this case, however, paracetamol elimination shows a greater time lag than that of antipyrine in comparison to the conscious rate. This difference is linked to the halflife of these drugs (15 and 75 min for paracetamol and antipyrine, respectively). In the apparently conscious rat, the ether concentration in the liver inhibits paracetamol catabolism for several halflives[30]. On the other hand, one could assume that a greater amount of the ether remaining in the liver would be eliminated during the first halflife of antipyrine. While the use of ether is prohibitive for the study of those substances with short halflives, it may be used in the study of substances with long halflives. *In vitro*, ether inhibits the normal function of mitochondria and protein synthesis in isolated hepatocytes from the rat. In homogenized hepatic tissue, certain oxidative as well as conjugative reactions are inhibited by powerful volatile anaesthetics such as halothane. A decrease in the catabolism of hypnotics, barbiturates and local anaesthetics has also been demonstrated[43] as well as the *in vitro* dose-dependent oxidation of antipyrine and the conjugation of paracetamol due to ether.

Elimination

Any disturbance in tissues or organs necessary for the elimination of a drug or its metabolites affects the clearance rate of this drug. A decrease in the speed of elimination is most frequently noted for volatile agents because of their depressive action on pulmonary ventilation. Any change in the blood supply to the liver, with consequent effects on the enterohepatic cycle, affects the rate of elimination of drugs by the liver. The effects of anaesthesia on hepatic circulation have been widely studied[13,21,24,30,50]. The blood supply to the liver is diminished in the dog anaesthetized with halothane, due to a decreased cardiac output[50]. The amount of drug captured by hepatocytes depends not only on the blood supply but also on the efficiency of extraction. Elimination of agents whose extraction is low (antipyrine, oxyphenbutazone) is slightly and less affected by changes in hepatic circulation. However, changes in hepatic circulation affect substances whose extraction is high (propranolol).

While a great number of studies have dealt with the influence of anaesthesia on urinary output[10], little work exists on the relationship between renal blood supply and the renal clearance of drugs eliminated in the urine. It is clear that the renal clearance of drugs eliminated by filtration alone depends on the level of glomerular filtration. Since glomerular filtration rate remains fairly constant, it may be assumed that general anaesthetics have little effect on the elimination of such drugs. Renal elimination of drugs by active secretion is influenced by circulatory conditions which vary according to the anaesthetic employed. High, moderate and low vasoconstriction is seen with cyclopropane, ether and barbiturates, respectively[45].

ANAESTHESIA AND PHARMACOLOGICAL ACTIVITY

Besides affecting the pharmacokinetics of drugs, general anaesthetics can even inverse the organism's responses to drugs. Such modifications may result from anaesthetic effects on the function of organs or their endocrine and nervous regulation. Most of the research on the effects of anaesthesia on major body functions concern cardiovascular physiology and its regulation.

Circulation

The previous section illustrated the great imporances of the cardiovascular system in pharmacokinetics. Anaesthesia demonstrates the earliest and most far-reaching effects on the cardiovascular system, and while relatively good descriptions for the changes in cardiovascular response during anaesthesia exist, the actual mechanisms involved remain somewhat unclear. Thus, the conclusions reached by various authors are from time to time at odds with one another.

Table 45.1 Effects of parenteral administrations of different non-volatile anaesthetics on arterial pressure of rat, rabbit, dog, pig, sheep, and monkey

Anaesthetic	*Dose* (mg/kg)	*Route of administration*	*Species*	*Change in arterial pressure from awake state* (mmHg)	(%)	*Reference*
Chloralose	60	i.v.	dog	+20	+18	3
	60	i.v.	dog	0	0	27
	80	i.v.	dog	−4	−4	19
	100	i.v.	dog	+9	+9	18
	80	i.p.	rat	−29	−21	14
Ketamine	100–150	i.p.	rat	−29	−21	14
	4	i.v.	dog	+30	+30	23
Ketamine + Xylazine	55 +5	i.m.	rabbit	−29	−30	46
Pentobarbital	30	i.v.	dog	0	0	25
	25–30	i.v.	dog	−10	−8	40
	27	i.v.	dog	−42	−35	36
	25	i.v.	dog	−10	−8	19
	30	i.v.	dog	+6	+5	12
	30	i.v.	dog	−2	−2	44
	40	i.p.	rat	−15	−12	14
	30	i.v.	monkey	−35	−43	24
	38 +16*	i.v.	pig	+10	+8	47
Thiamylal	26 +16†	i.v.	pig	+40	+34	47
Urethane	1300	i.p.	rat	−15	−12	14
Vinbarbital	40	i.v.	sheep	+15	+16	11

*Additional hourly dose
†Additional dose when required

The measurement of *blood pressure* allows for the most straightforward evaluation of the activity of the circulatory system. The effects of anaesthesia on blood pressure are summarized in Tables 45.1 and 45.2. Pentobarbital – depending upon experimental conditions and the authors – produces a rise, drop, or no change in blood pressure. With chloralose, frequently either a slight rise or no change occur in blood pressure, whereas the volatile anaesthetics always show a marked hypotension. Blood pressure is the resultant of two main factors: the cardiac output which itself depends on the rate and force of contraction of the heart, and the peripheral vascular resistance.

Table 45.2 Effects of different volatile anaesthetic agents on arterial pressure in rat, rabbit, dog, and pig

Anaesthetic	*Administration*	*Species*	*Change in arterial pressure from awake state* (mmHg)	(%)	*Reference*
Cyclopropane		dog	+ 15	+ 13	38
Ether		rat	− 10	− 8	14
Ethrane	3% in O_2	rabbit	− 25		35
Halothane	1–3%	dog	− 24	− 22	19
	—	dog	− 47	− 40	38
	1.5%	pig	− 40	− 41	47
Methoxyflurane	1.5%	pig	− 30	− 29	47

Modifications in the *cardiac output* vary with: barbiturate used, species, time of measurement, and authors themselves. Cardiac output increases with thiopental[29], which may first decrease blood pressure before raising it. This phenomenon has also been observed in the dog with pentobarbital and would appear to be due to a decrease in the systolic ejection volume (− 40%) which was partially compensated by an increase in the heart rate (+ 65%)[40]. After 1 h, cardiac output was slightly superior to that of the control (+ 7%), the decrease in systolic ejection volume (− 35%) being compensated by a strong increase in heart rate (+ 71%)[17,37,40]. A prolonged reduction in cardiac output in the pig is linked to a decrease in the systolic ejection volume, which is attributed to an increase in peripheral resistance along with a decrease in venous return and thus ventricular filling[47]. The increase in cardiac rate is generally related to the vagolytic effects of pentobarbital[26,28], although it may be that barosensitive reflexes contribute as well. Finally, pentobarbital has been shown to depress the contractibility of heart muscle fibre. Barbiturates have the ability to influence the action of those substances which normally affect calcium metabolism. Hence, the interactions between anaesthetics and aminoside antibiotics which are known to have effects on the mechanism of calcium[1].

Generally speaking, cardiac output is not modified by chloralose, but decreases with halothane from 25 to 60% in the dog. This reduction, also seen in the heart–lung preparation, is proportional to the plasma concentration of halothane and to the decrease in the volume of systolic ejection. The myocardial depression is linked to the depth of the narcosis itself[16]. As the tachycardia observed with halothane is eliminated by the use of atropine, the depressive action of this anaesthetic may be due, partially, to its parasympathomimetic action. Methoxyflurane also shows a dose-dependent decrease in cardiac output which varies from 27 to 65% depending on the concentration inhaled. The decreased cardiac output is a consequence of a simultaneous reduction in cardiac rate and the volume of systolic ejection.

Vascular resistance is often diminished by general anaesthesia. Chloralose is responsible for a moderate and transitory vasodilatation, which would account for the hypotension frequently observed during induction. Despite the peripheral vasodilatation and an increase in cardiac output incurred in the onset of anaesthesia, pentobarbital causes an increase in peripheral resistance with a drop in cardiac output[40, 44]. In the dog, resistance increases by 7% for the first 5 min after induction, and 26% 1 h later. Variations and even contradictions in some of the results obtained may be explained by differences in procedure, especially in cases where premidication is used. Many barbiturates, acting on the contractibility of isolated vascular muscle, will often inhibit spontaneous contractions of arteries and veins, and will also increase the response to adrenaline, calcium and serotonin[2]. Both halothane and methoxyflurane inhibit smooth muscle in main vasular fields according to a mechanism already described. A direct action may be involved[41] or these drugs may inhibit the action of norepinephrine[16]. With isoflurane, progressive vasodilatation is seen which increases as the anaesthesia deepens.

Control of blood pressure

Modification of control mechanisms is another source of blood pressure variation seen in general anaesthesia. The sinocarotid reflex is often examined in physiology and cardiovascular pharmacology as an excellent indicator of the function of the autonomic nervous system. Variations of blood pressure in the carotid sinus are a function of the anaesthetic employed. The respective influences of the three most widely used anaesthetics in the dog (chloralose, halothane, pentobarbital) have been compared recently [19]. It is concluded that baroreceptor functions are less affected by chloralose or halothane than with pentobarbital. The effect of occlusion of the carotids has been compared in both anaesthetized and non-anaesthetized dogs. The hypertension thus created was more marked when the dog was under chloralose anaesthesia. Yet, as with urethane, a fall in blood pressure may be observed with pentobarbital. With identical studies no variation occurred when cyclopropane was administered, but less marked hypertension was seen under halothane[38].

Bradycardia, following hypertension induced by an i.v. injection of norepinephrine (0.5 or 1 μg/kg), has been reported in the rat. This reflex is reduced by 25–80% in the rat under pentobarbital, totally suppressed under ketamine, and increased by 20% with chloralose[14]. Both ether and urethane caused fluctuations in reflex bradycardia, attributed to great fluctuations in cardiac rate, before norepinephrine was administered. This would explain the interest still seen today in the use of chloralose as an anaesthetic in cardiovascular experimentation. It is clear that only chloralose can allow a cardiovascular response to norepinephrine which is similar to that of the non-anaesthetized animal.

Local circulation and microcirculation are affected by general anaesthesia[33]. Calibre changes are related to both the anaesthetic used and the vessels involved (Figure 45.1 (b)). A possible explanation for anaesthetic influence in the toxicity of cardiac drugs may be found here. Indeed, the toxicity of ouabaine is less in cats anaesthetized with pentobarbital than those under chloralose-urethane[49]. It is suggested that this difference is due to the disparity of anaesthetic effects on cardioregulator innervation. Pentobarbital, for example, reduces vagal tone during induction, and shows minimal effects on sympathetic tone with but a slight inhibition in the secretion of medullar catecholamines by the adrenal glands. This is contrary to chloralose which strengthens sympathetic tone, and urethane which stimulates epinephrine secretion in the adrenal medulla. The differences in the toxicity of ouabaine can be linked to differences seen in sympathetic tone.

Respiration

Respiratory depression is likely to result from any general anaesthetic, provided that the dose administered is of sufficient magnitude[36,39]. The mechanisms involved are related to the diminished responsiveness of respiratory centres, changes in vagal afferences, and curariform effects on the respiratory muscles themselves. Thus, general anaesthesia cannot be recommended for the study of drugs with respiratory effects. This has been illustrated by a decrease in the response of subjects to CO_2 inhalation while under anaesthesia. Prudence is advised in the study of antitussive drugs, as anaesthesia depresses the cough reflex in the organism. It is necessary to work with chronic preparations or with animals under light narcosis.

Digestive tract

The effects of anaesthesia on the motility of the digestive tract has aroused much interest. Recently, the influence of thiopental was studied on the gastrointestinal motility of the dog[28]. As soon as this drug was administered, a brief but powerful stimulation of motility occurred in both the duodenum and jejunum, although the ileum and the pyloric area of the stomach remained unaffected. Ketamine had no effect. Halothane not only inhibited motor responses to vagal stimulation by a ganglioplegic action, but responses to β-methylcholine and barium chloride are inhibited as well, this suggesting a musculo-depressive action.

It is known that secretory responses of the stomach to both physiological and pharmacological agents may be modified considerably by an anaesthetic. For a given dose of gastrin or synthetic peptide (ICI 50 123), a rise in gastric secretion of acid is noted when urethane was administered to the rat (i.m.). Gastric secretion is decreased with barbital (i.m.) and is reduced with halothane. It is believed that a reduction in vagal tonus due to barbital and halothane was responsible for the diminished gastric secretion. In addition, it is claimed - although without providing a satisfactory explanation - that the gastric secretion curves (gastric secretion/gastrine dose or gastric secretion/ICI 50 123) are quite different, depending upon the route of administration (i.m. vs. i.v.). In the second case, the response decreases with increasing doses of secretagogues.

Urinary secretion

Anaesthetics are responsible for considerable disturbances in renal function, and are invariably responsible for a reduction in diuresis. These modifications are the results of: circulatory effects (augmentation or diminution of blood pressure), variations in renal vasoconstrictor tone, or effects on endocrine regulatory systems (ADH, catecholamine, renin-aniotensing, aldosterone). Besides their influence on the elimination of drugs by the kidney, anaesthetics are liable to modify renal responses to various pharmacological agents. Thus, in non-anaesthetized sheep, papaverine or acetylcholine, when administered in the renal artery, produce considerable vasodilatation with an increase in glomerular filtration, but without increasing the amount of Na^+ excreted[11]. In sheep, anaesthetized with pentobarbital, the same agents produced not only vasodilatation and increased glomerular filtration, but also a considerable increase in the excretion of Na^+. It appears that the differences noted in anaesthetized sheep were due to concurrent increases in arterial blood pressure. An increase in peritubular capillary blood pressure would appear to be the cause of decreased reabsorption of Na^+. It is also possible that the above changes may vary with species or age. Modifications in the renal function of the neonate pig were not observed after anaesthesia with ether, halothane or N_2O/ketamine despite a general reduction in blood pressure and cardiac output[5]. On the other hand, in the adult a decrease in urinary secretion was observed. The differences are linked to incomplete sympathetic innervation of the kidneys in the neonate along with high and fixed renal vascular resistances.

Neurovegetative system

Most general anaesthetics modify the activity of the autonomic nervous system. Certain anaesthetics such as pentobarbital have marked parasympatholytic action and tachycardia is noted. This effect is not seen in a dog having previously received atropine. In the same fashion, the absence of atropinic action in a dog under pentobarbital is an additional argument for powerful vagolytic action. Absence of atropinic effect on cardiac rate was noted in the rat anaesthetized with pentobarbital, while atropine produced tachycardia in the rat under urethane (Figure 45.2 (c))[7].

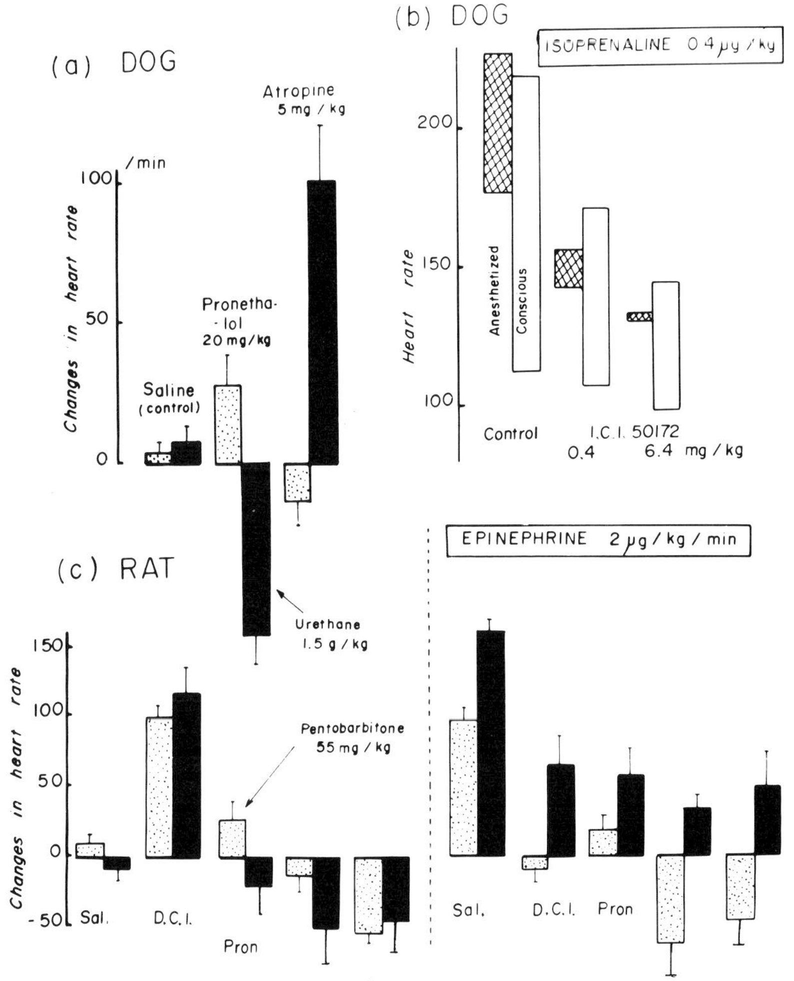

Figure 45.2 (a) Effect of anaesthesia on heart rate response in dogs to atropine and pronethalol (from ref. 7). (b) Increase in heart rate produced by isoprenaline (0.4 μg/kg) in conscious or anaesthetized dogs, after administration of ICI 50 172 (from ref. 20). (c) Effect of pentobarbitone and urethane on heart response of rats to β-adrenergic blockade by pronethalol (PRON), propranolol (PRO) and sotalol (SOT) at 5 mg/kg i.v., and to an adrenaline infusion of 2 μg/kg per min (from ref. 7)

Many general anaesthetics have sympathomimetic effects demonstrated by an increase in plasma catecholamine levels with nitrous oxide, or preganglionic activity with ether, cyclopropane or halothane in the rabbit. This may explain, in part, the influence of anaesthetics on drugs which are mediators or which modify the autonomic nervous system[42].

Several acetylcholine effects may be modified by pentobarbital. An injection of acetylcholine decreases the volume of systolic ejection in the non-anaesthetized dog but the inverse is true for the dog under anaesthesia. The effects of epinephrine and norepinephrine with respect to the anaesthetic used have been the object of several studies[14] including cardiovascular response to norepinephrine in the rat under ether, urethane, pentobarbital, chloralose and ketamine (Figure 45.3). The hypertensive effects of norepinephrine are very diminished by ether and urethane, little changed by pentobarbital, but augmented in the case of chloralose or ketamine[6]. The increase in cardiac period (and thus a decrease in frequency) due to norepinephrine is less in the dog under chloralose than in the non-anaesthetized animal[18].

The arrhythmogenic effects of catecholamines are considerably increased under halothane as well as halothane-like anaesthetics. Even small quantities of epinephrine induce a bigeminal rhythm in the anaesthetized dog, and under such conditions either tachycardia or ventricular fibrillation can happen

In the rabbit, the hypertensive reaction to dopamine is inversed during urethane anaesthesia. Chloralose does not modify the responses to isoproterenol except for a higher cardiac acceleration in response to hypotension.

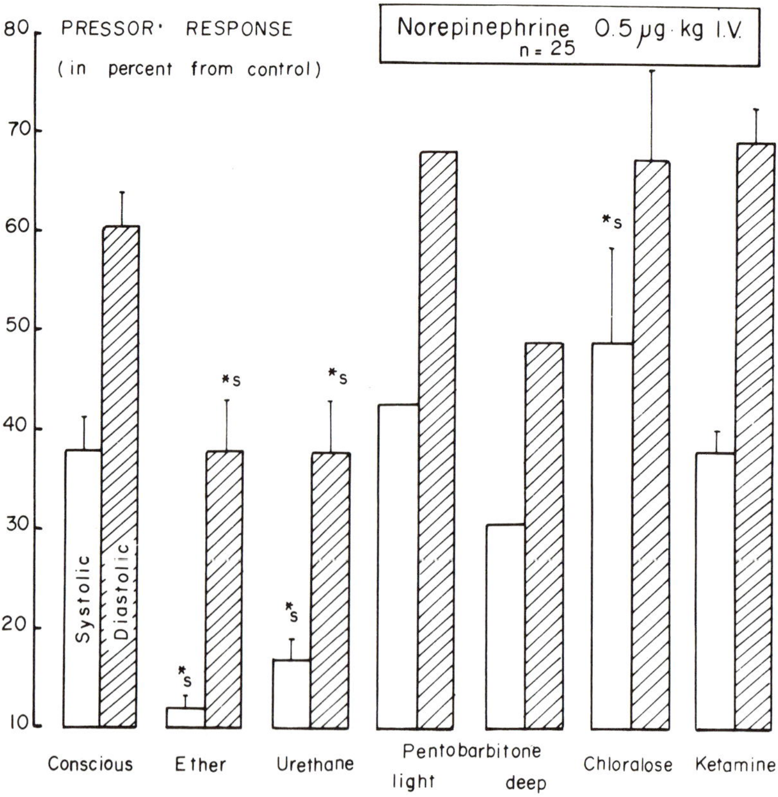

Figure 45.3 Effect of anaesthetics on the pressor response to noradrenaline in rat. Changes are expressed in percentage from pressor response in conscious rat (from ref. 14)

This would suggest an increase in baroreceptor activity seen in this type of anaesthesia. The tachycardia seen after isoproterenol administration is higher for the dog under pentobarbital as compared to the non-anaesthetized animal (Figure 45.2 (b)), but due to the high cardiac rate in the non-anaesthetized dog, the relative increase in cardiac rate is less than in the non-anaesthetized animal.

The decrease in peripheral vascular resistance provoked by isoproterenol is reduced by administration of pentobarbital[17]. The importance in the choice of an anaesthetic in the study of the responses to isoprenaline is illustrated by the fact that, in order to increase the cardiac rate in the pentobarbital-anaesthetized rat by 100, 0.1 μg/kg of isoprenaline is needed, compared to 2 μg/kg for urethane-anaesthetized rat[7]. In order to reduce the resultant tachycardia by 50%, 0.82 mg/kg of propranolol is needed in the case of pentobarbital, while 16.5 mg/kg are required for urethane.

Response to β-sympatholytics will also depend upon the anaesthetic used. An intravenous injection of propranolol modifies neither cardiac rate nor output in the non-anaesthetized animal, but greatly decreases both parameters in the animal under chloralose[8,27]. In a similar fashion, ICI 50 172, a β-sympatholytic, is able to suppress the increase in cardiac rate and contractibility provoked by injections of epinephrine, norepinephrine or isoprenaline, provided the animal has been anaesthetized with pentobarbital. ICI 50 172 in the non-anaesthetized subjects shows no such effects (Figure 45.2 (b)).

Indeed, isprenaline, as all β-sympathomimetics has a double action mechanism:

(1) Direct action on the sino-atrial node which can be blocked by ICI 50 172.

(2) Reflex action as a consequence of hypotension induced by vasodilatation. This latter effect is not blocked by ICI 50 172 but can be blocked by anaesthetics such as chloralose or barbiturates.

The effects of pronethalol were compared in two groups of rats anaesthetized either with pentobarbital or with urethane[7]. While tachycardia was seen in the group under pentobarbital, bradycardia was seen in the group under urethane (Figure 45.2 (c)). Propranolol had no effect on the heart rate of the non-anaesthetized rat but bradycardia was seen in the rat under urethane. The results depend on the pre-existing sympathetic tone of the individuals. When the tone is reduced (e.g. pentobarbital) no effect is observed with antagonists; inversely, when the tone is high (e.g. urethane) β-blockers have marked effects. Thus, propranolol provokes hypertension in the rat under urethane as a consequence of the inhibition of peripheral vasodilatation by catecholamine, vasodilatation being reinforced by the anaesthetic. Certain β-sympatholytics such as oxprenolol, alprenolol or practolol do not show negative inotropic properties in the non-anaesthetized subject. On the other hand, such properties can be clearly seen under halothane anaesthesia[48]. Indeed, in the non-anaesthetized individuals, the reduction in cardiac output due to bradycardia is compensated by an increase in sympathetic tone. However, individuals under halothane may show both myocardial depression as well as peripheral vasodilatation. The adjunction of β-blockers decreases cardiac rate to a still greater degree, and the resultant reduction in cardiac output is therefore more marked. It has also been demonstrated that propranolol decreases coronary supply only when the dog is under anaesthesia; this is explained by the reinforcement of sympathetic tone as compensation for the depressive action of the anaesthetic. Other sympatholytics produce more complex effects as many of these agents show simultaneous agonistic as well as antagonistic effects (Figure 45.2 (c)).

Neuromuscular junction

The inhibition of neuromuscular transmission by ether or enflurane is due to a specific mechanism. In addition, these agents potentiate the effects of curares. A number of years ago, the variations in the interactions of anaesthetics and antibiotics were demonstrated on the cardiovascular system and neuromuscular junction. The way in which aminoglycoside antibiotics inhibit neuromuscular transmission is well known. These antibiotics not only decrease Ca^{2+} availablity at the synapse, and thus inhibit the liberation of acetylcholine, but are also in themselves competitors with acetylcholine, at the cholinergic receptor sites of the motor end plate[1]. These effects are then added to the general depressive effects of such anaesthetic drugs as ether, pentobarbital, halothane and methoxyflurane on the neuromuscular synapse. A case of permanent respiratory failure during pentobarbital administration is reported in the dog undergoing treatment with streptomycin[1].

CONCLUSION

Bearing in mind the complex interactions possible between anaesthetics and drugs, one quickly arrives at the conclusion that pharmacological studies should first be carried out on non-anaesthetized individuals. Indeed, with few exceptions, the great majority of drugs are destined for use in the conscious individual. Despite advances in investigated techniques with the unanaesthetized animal, general anaesthetics are still largely employed, not only for technical reasons, but because of ethical considerations as well. For this reason, systematic observation should be made for possible physiological and pharmacological modifications due to anaesthesia, and interspecies differences. Such observations would allow for the best possible choice of anaesthetic technique. The interpretation of data should take into account not only changes in the responses of effector organs, but also the influences of the anaesthesia on the bioavailability and pharmacokinetics of the drug under investigation.

While some mechanisms such as barbiturate enzymatic induction are clearly understood, others are hypothetical. For this reason caution must be the rule for any extrapolation between anaesthetics and conscious animals.

References

1. Adams, H.R., Tesk, R. H. and Mercer, H. D. (1976). Anesthetic–antibiotic interrelationships. *J. Am. Vet. Med. Assoc.*, **168,** 409–12
2. Altura, B. M., Altura, B. T., Carella, A. *et al.* (1980). Vascular smooth muscle and general anesthetics. *Fed. Proc.*, **39,** 1584–91
3. Arfors, K. E., Arturson, G. and Malmberg, P. (1971). Effect of prolonged chloralose anesthesia on acid–base balance and cardiovascular functions in dogs. *Acta Physiol. Scand.*, **81,** 47–53
4. Aune, H., Olsen, H. and Morland, J. (1981). Diethyl ether influence on the metabolism of antipyrin, paracetamol, and sulphanilamide in isolated rat hepatocytes. *Br. J. Anaesth.*, **53,** 621–6
5. Bailie, M. D., Alward, C. T., Sawyer, D. C. *et al.* (1979). Effect of anesthesia on cardiovascular and renal function in the newborn piglet. *J. Pharmacol. Exp. Ther.*, **208,** 298–302
6. Balis, G. U. and Monroe, R. R. (1964), The pharmacology of chloralose. *Psychopharmacologia*, **6,** 1–30
7. Barret, A. M. (1971). The effect of some autonomic blocking agents on the heart rates of anesthetized and pithed rats. *Eur. J. Pharmacol.*, **15,** 267–73
8. Bergamaschi, M., Shanks, R. G., Caravaggi, A. M. *et al.* (1971). A comparison of the cardiovascular actions of four adrenergic β-receptors blocking agents in resting conscious dogs. *Am. Heart. J.*, **82,** 338–51
9. Bernard, C. (1875). *Leçons sur les Anesthésiques et sur l'Asphyxie.* (Paris: Baillière)
10. Bie, P. (1980). Osmoreceptors, vasopressin, and control of renal water excretion. *Physiol. Rev.*, **60,** 961–1048
11. Blaine, E. H. and Dunlay, M. C. (1981). Renal function during consciousness and anesthesia in sheep: effects of renal vasodilatation by papaverine and acetylcholine.
12. Bond, J. H., Prentiss, R. A. and Levitt, M. D. (1980). The effect of anesthesia and laparotomy on blood flow to the stomach, small bowel, and colon of the dog. *Surgery*, **87,** 313–18
13. Bralet, A. M., Wepierre, J. and Bralet, J. (1973). Influence de l'anesthésie sur la distribution du débit cardiaque chez le rat. *J. Physiol., Paris*, **66,** 101–5
14. Brezenoff, H. E. (1973). Cardiovascular responses to noradrenaline in the rat before and after administration of various anesthetics. *Br. J. Pharmacol.*, **49,** 565–72
15. Chenoweth, M. B. and Vandyke, R. A. (1969). Anesthesia in biomedical research. *Fed. Proc.*, **28,** 1383–5
16. Corbett, T. H. (1979). Pharmacology and toxicology of halogenated anesthetics, *Adv. Pharmacol. Chemother.*, **16,** 195–212
17. Cox, R. H. (1972). Influence of pentobarbital anesthesia on cardiovascular function in trained dogs. *Am. J. Physiol.*, **223,** 651–9
18. Cox, R. H. (1972). Influence of chloralose anesthesia on cardiovascular function in trained dogs. *Am. J. Physiol.*, **223,** 660–7
19. Cox, R. H. and Bagshaw, R. J. (1979). Influence of anesthesia on the response to carotid hypotension in dogs. *Am. J. Physiol.*, **237,** H424–32
20. Dunlop, D. and Shanks, R. G. (1968). Selective blockade of adrenoceptive β-receptors in the heart. *Br. J. Pharmacol.*, **32,** 201–8
21. Dupont, C. and Wepierre, J. (1977). Modification de la réactivité cardiovasculaire à l'égard de l'isoprénaline sous l'influence de l'anesthésique chez le rat. *C.R. Soc. Biol.*, **171,** 1003–7
22. Duvaldestin, Ph., Maze, R. I., Nivoche, Y. *et al.* (1981). Occupational exposure to halothane results in enzyme induction in anesthetics. *Anesthesiology*, **54,** 57–60
23. Folts, J. D., Afonso, S. and Rowe, G. G. (1975). Systemic and coronary haemodynamic effects of ketamine in intact anesthetized and unanesthetized dogs. *Br. J. Anaesth.*, **47,** 686–94
24. Forsyth, R. P. and Hoffbrand, B. I. (1970). Redistribution of cardiac output after sodium pentobarbital anesthesia in the monkey. *Am. J. Physiol.*, **217,** 214–17
25. Gilmore, J. P. (1965). Pentobarbital sodium anesthesia in the dog. *Am. J. Physiol.*, **209,** 404–8

26. Halinen, M. O., Hakumäki, M. O. K. and Sarajas H. S. S. (1978). Suppression of autonomic postganglionic discharges by pentobarbital in dogs. *Acta Physiol. Scand.*, **104,** 167–74
27. Halkola, L., Koivikko, A. and Lansimies, E. (1974). Hemodynamic effects of chloralose and propranolol in dogs. *Acta Physiol. Scand.*, **90,** 505–8
28. Healy, T. E. J., Foster, G. E., Evans, D. F. *et al.* (1981). Effects of some I.V. anesthetic agents on canine gastrointestinal motility. *Br. J. Anaesth.*, **53,** 229–33
29. Horwitz, L. D. (1977). Effects of intravenous anesthetic agents on left ventricular function in dogs. *Am. J. Physiol.*, **232,** H44–8
30. Johannessen, W., Gadeholt, G. and Aarbakke, J. (1981). Effects of diethyl ether anesthesia on the pharmacokinetics of antipyrine and paracetamol in the rat. *J. Pharm. Pharmacol.*, **33,** 365–8
31. Lawrence, D. and Livingstone, A. (1981). Opiate like analgesic activity in general anaesthetics. *Br. J. Pharmacol.*, **73,** 435–42
32. Linde, H. W. and Berman, M. L. (1971). Nonspecific stimulation of drug-metabolizing enzymes by inhalation anesthetic agents. *Anesth. Analg.*, **50,** 656–65
33. Longnecker, D. E. and Harris, P. D. (1980). Microcirculatory actions of general anesthetics. *Fed. Proc.*, **39,** 1580–3
34. Mauck, H. P. Jr., Freund, J. and Porter, R. R. (1961). Variability of cardiac output in dogs under chloralose and urethane anesthesia. *Toxicol. Appl. Pharmacol.*, **3,** 380–5
35. Mohareb, A., El Koussi, A., Osman, F. *et al.* (1979). Evaluation of cardiovascular and respiratory effects of different concentrations of ethrane in rabbits. *Pharmacol. Res. Comm.*, **11,** 747–57
36. Morrison, J. L., Walker, H. A. and Richardson, A. P. (1960). The effect of pentobarbital on the response of cardiovascular system of dogs to epinephrine, acetylcholine and tilting. *Arch. Int. Pharmacodyn.*, **82,** 53–62
37. Nash, C. B., Davis, F. and Woodbury, R. A. (1956). Cardiovascular effects of anesthetic doses of pentobarbital sodium. *Am. J. Physiol.*, **185,** 107–12
38. Ngai, S. H. and Bolme, P. (1966). Effects of anesthetics on circulatory regulatory mechanisms in the dog. *J. Pharmacol. Exp. Ther.*, **153,** 495–504
39. Ngai, S. H., Katz, R. L. and Farhie, S. E. (1965). Respiratory effects of trichlorethylene, halothane and methoxyflurane in the cat. *J. Pharmacol. Exp. Ther.*, **148,** 123–30
40. Olmsted, F. and Page, I. H. (1966). Hemodynamic changes in dogs caused by sodium pentobarbital anesthesia. *Am. J. Physiol.*, **210,** 817–20
41. Parker, J. L. and Adams, R. H. (1978). The influence of chemical restraining agents on cardiovascular function: a review. *Lab. Anim. Sci.*, **28,** 575–83
42. Pitt, B., Green, L. and Sughisit, Y. (1970). Effect of β-adrenergic receptor blockade on coronary haemodynamics in resting unanesthetized dog. *Cardiovasc. Res.*, **4,** 89–92
43. Poppers, P. J. (1980). Hepatic drug metabolism and anesthesia. *Anaesthetist*, **29,** 55–8
44. Priano, L. L., Traver, O. L. and Wilson, R. D. (1969). Barbiturate anesthesia: an abnormal physiological situation. *J. Pharmacol. Exp. Ther.*, **165,** 126–35
45. Price, H. L. (1975). General anesthetics. In Goodman, A. and Gilman, A. (eds.) *The Pharmacological Basis of Therapeutics.* 5th Ed., pp. 89–96. (New York: MacMillan)
46. Sanford, T. D. and Colby, E. D. (1980). Effect of xylazine and ketamine on blood pressure, heart rate and respiratory rate in rabbits. *Lab. Anim. Sci.*, **30,** 519–23
47. Sawyer, D. C., Lumb, W. V. and Stone, H. L. (1971). Cardiovascular effects of halothane, methoxyflurane, pentobarbital and thiamylal. *J. Appl. Physiol.*, **30,** 36–43
48. Stephen, G. W., Dawie, I. T. and Scott, D. B. (1971). Haemodynamic effects of β-receptor blocking drugs during nitrous oxide halothane anesthesia. *Br. J. Anaesth.*, **43,** 320–5
49. Stickney, J. L. (1974). The effect of different types of anesthesia on digitalis toxicity. *Am. Heart J.*, **87,** 734–9
50. Su, J. Y., Amory, D. W., Sands, M. P. *et al.* (1979). Effects of ether anesthesia and surface-induced hypothermia on regional blood flow. *Am. Heart J.*, **97,** 53–60

46
Evaluation of analgesic drug combinations

A. J. M. Seegers, L. P. Jager and J. van Noordwijk

The experimental pharmacological assessment of the therapeutic value of a single drug for a well-defined indication often requires more than one animal model. The evaluation of drug combinations is even more complicated, because it necessitates a quantification of effects, which implies the assessment of dose–response relationships of the individual components of the combination and the efficacy of the combination itself for a specified effect.

ANALYSIS OF EFFICACY

The simplest relationship between dose and effect is given by Clark's classical theory[13]. According to this theory, as extended by Ariëns[2], the analysis of drug–receptor interactions *in vitro* is based on the following postulates: (1) applicability of the law of mass action, (2) proportionality between response and fraction of receptors occupied, and (3) quantitative insignificance of the fraction of drug bound to receptors. A direct relationship between activation of receptors and the response measured is assumed, thus neglecting characteristics of intermediate steps. An S-shaped log dose–response curve of a drug observed *in vivo* can be analysed under the assumption that the response is mediated via one type of receptor, irrespective of its actual existence. In order to evaluate results obtained with drug mixtures a common receptor has to be postulated for the component drugs. This contention derives some support from the fact that different drugs, producing the same qualitative response, generally have at least one step in common.

Consequently, if drugs are administered simultaneously, their actions on different receptors can be projected as interactions at the common step. On the basis of the kinetics of drug–receptor interaction the relationship between the effect observed, v, and the dose of the drug given, A, is presented by:

$$v = \frac{V_{max} \cdot A}{k + A} \qquad (I)$$

The parameters which characterize this equation, and which can be estimated from the observations, are V_{max}, the maximum effect which is theoretically attained when all receptors are occupied by an infinite dose of the drug, and k, the dissociation constant of the drug–receptor complex. Since the relationship between the independent variable, A, and the dependent variable, v, is curvilinear, it has been customary to facilitate estimation of the two parameters by employing linear transformations of Equation I. The suitability of the various transformations in different types of experiments has been evaluated by Dowd and Riggs[28].

Under the hypothesis of additive interactions between component drugs on the same receptor population the *in vitro* efficacy of a drug mixture ($v_{ab\ldots z}$) can be calculated by the following general equation, using estimates of V_{max} and k of the component drugs:

$$v_{ab\ldots z} = \frac{(A/k_a)\cdot V_{max\,a} + (B/k_b)\cdot V_{max\,b} + \cdots + (Z/k_z)\cdot V_{max\,z}}{1 + (A/k_a) + (B/k_b) + \cdots + (Z/k_z)} \qquad \text{(II)}$$

in which for drugs a, b, ..., z, respectively:

$k_a, k_b, \ldots, k_z$ = the dissociation constant of the drug–receptor complex, $V_{max\,a}, V_{max\,b}, \ldots, V_{max\,z}$ = the maximum effect attainable with the drug indicated, and A, B, ..., Z = the dose used in the drug mixture.

In the case of competitive antagonism V_{max} of the antagonist (b) equals zero, yielding the well-known equation:

$$v_{ab} = \frac{A\cdot V_{max\,a}}{k_a + A + B\cdot k_a/k_b} \qquad \text{(III)}$$

Furthermore, Equation II predicts that mixtures of drugs with largely different V_{max}-values, used in concentrations within the range of their k-values, will exhibit dose–response relationships typical for partial antagonism. Thus, the effect of a drug mixture is to be classified as additive when the mean response observed does not differ significantly from the expected value calculated using Equation II. In an optimal experimental design the dosages used in admixture should be equivalent to about half of the individual k-values of the drugs; potentiation or inhibition is hard to discern if the expected efficacy of a drug mixture is close to 100% or to 0%, respectively.

In our experience, using agonists, Equation II proved to be a powerful tool to analyse *in vivo* data providing that the dose–response relationships of the individual drugs can be represented by Equation I and that the component drugs do not exhibit pharmacokinetic interactions[95]. Of course, other methods are used in assessments of the efficacy of drug combinations than that represented by Equation II which involves the law of mass action. Generally, these methods are based on either a comparison of the dose–response curve of one component drug given alone with that of the mixture, or on a comparison of the ED_{50}-values of a component drug in the absence and in the presence of subliminal doses of additives. By now it will be clear that combinations of drugs, with widely different V_{max}-values and/or in dosages outside the range of the dose–response curves, can yield results due to additive interactions but which are interpreted as non-additive. In mice, Grotto *et al.*[46] observed that with the mixture of aspirin + paracetamol (50 + 66 mg/kg) the pain reaction time was longer than that after administration of twice as much aspirin (100 mg/kg) or paracetamol (132 mg/kg) alone. The interaction between these compounds was classified as an augmentative synergism. This classification seems questionable because the dosages of the drugs used in the mixture were half the amounts needed to induce a just detectable increase in pain reaction time when given alone. Apart from the fact that measurement of threshold responses yields relatively large errors, summation of the effects of equipotent amounts of drugs is only justified when their intrinsic activities are similar. Addition of a drug with low intrinsic activity to another drug or drug mixture does not necessarily increase the response. This is illustrated by the observation[46] that addition of caffeine to the combination of aspirin + paracetamol reduced the analgesic effect, as predicted by Equation II[95].

A comparison of a drug combination with one of the component drugs at a dosage unlike that used in the combination cannot yield meaningful information concerning the interactions between the component drugs of the mixture[54].

Furthermore, divergent interpretations of the concepts of inhibition, addition and potentiation contribute largely to the rather confusing results regarding evaluation of drug mixtures. Within the analytical framework outlined above, effects of drug mixtures not significantly different from that predicted using Equation II are classified as due to additive interactions between component drugs. Especially in *in vivo* experiments this class consists of different subtypes of additive interactions, ranging from interactions between full or partial agonists on the same receptor and competitive antagonists to physiological interactions between drugs of which a common intermediate step governs the intensity of the measured response.

In case of non-additive interactions the main advantage of Equation II becomes clear. Subsequent experiments determining whether the drug mixture yields responses significantly smaller or greater than expected in case of addition (one-tailed tests), unambiguously signify a non-competitive inhibition or a potentiation (augmentative synergism), respectively, between component drugs.

MECHANISMS OF ACTION

Since the observation of Vane[100] our understanding of the mechanisms of action of this group of drugs, preferentially referred to as NSAID (non-steroidal anti-inflammatory drugs; aspirin-like drugs; non-narcotic analgesics), is growing rapidly. The involvement of NSAID in the biosynthesis/release of prostaglandins (PGs) is now well-established. Generally, these drugs alter the metabolic pathways of arachidonic acid and structurally related fatty acid precursors (Figure 46.1). This influence can proceed, e.g. via an irreversible or a reversible inhibition of a specific enzyme (cyclo-oxygenase) as with aspirin or indomethacin, respectively. Many defensive

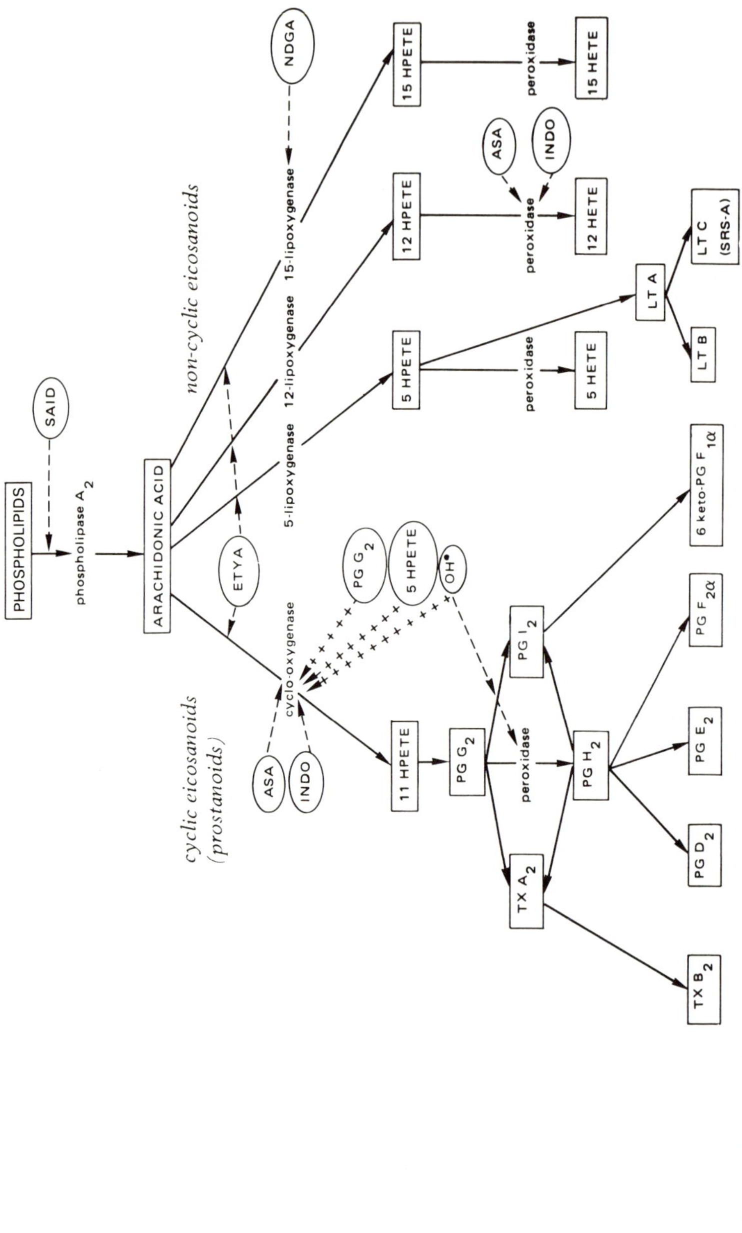

Figure 46.1 Cyclo-oxygenase and lipoxygenase pathways of arachidonic acid. HPETE indicates hydroperoxy eicosatetraenoic acid; HETE, hydroxy eicosatetraenoic acid; PG, prostaglandin; TX, thromboxane; LT, leukotriene; SRS-A, slow-reacting substance-A; SAID, steroidal anti-inflammatory drugs; ETYA, eicosatetraynoic acid; ASA, acetylsalicylic acid; INDO, indomethacin; NDGA, nordihydro guaiaretic acid; OH•, hydroxyl radical; ------▶, inhibitory effect; + + + + ▶, stimulatory effect

responses of the body are triggered by the release of fatty acids from the afflicted locus or loci. The anti-inflammatory action of corticosteroids (SAID) resides mainly in a stabilizing effect on the cell membranes, of which the phospholipids are the main source of the unsaturated fatty acids[48].

The enzyme systems functioning in the metabolic pathways of the unsaturated fatty acids are present throughout the whole body, their presence becoming apparent only when their substrate is liberated. Two main pathways starting from arachidonic acid can be distinguished (1) one starting with the cyclo-oxygenase system yielding the various prostaglandins and thromboxanes, and (2) the other one starting with the lipoxygenases yielding the various eicosatetraenoic acids and leukotrienes (Figure 46.1).

In this overview, emphasis is given to arachidonate, the dominant eicosapolyenoic acid occurring in man, with the Greenland Eskimo still living on a fish diet as the well-known exception. Besides the dienoic PGs derived from arachidonic acid, similar pathways can yield the monoenoic and trienoic PGs from homo-γ-linolenic acid and from eicosapentaenoic acids, respectively. However, although all three precursors yield endoperoxides PGG_1, PGG_2 and PGG_3 as well as PGs of the D, E and F series, PGG_1 does not yield a thromboxane A_1 (TXA_1) or PGI_1. Also, the biological properties of a metabolite depend on its degree of unsaturation. For example, PGE_1 inhibits and PGE_2 facilitates human platelet aggregation. Quantitatively, there is a difference between TXA_2 and TXA_3 on aggregation[82].

The various peroxidases all yield free oxygen-centred radicals (possibly hydroxyl radicals) besides the products indicated[29,30,47,60,61] (Figure 46.1). As these free radicals can modulate the activity of several cellular enzyme systems – including those involved in the metabolism of the eicosanoids – a pivotal role of these short-living reactive intermediates is postulated in the pathophysiology of inflammation. Recently, Lands[62] reviewed the modulating functions of the free radicals on the activity of the cyclo-oxygenase pathway. Besides limiting availability and mutual inhibition of the different polyunsaturated fatty acids, the biosynthesis of prostanoids is, to a large extent, regulated via the level of free radicals. The biosynthesis of prostanoids by the cyclo-oxygenase is regarded as taking place by a lipid peroxide-induced free radical chain reaction mechanism[50]. The instability of a chain reaction might contribute to the self-continuing nature of rheumatic disorders, e.g. polyarthritis in pigs following infection with *Erysipelothrix insidiosa*.

ANALGESIA

Mechanisms of analgesic action

Pain relief afforded by NSAID may result from both a peripheral and a central nervous system (CNS) effect.

If the site of its origin is a locus of inflammation, these drugs modify the pain by protecting the pain receptor from the nociceptive effects of bradykinin, serotonin and other mediators involved in pain[56,63] and by an enhancement of fluid reabsorption from swollen, inflamed tissues[64]. In these processes the inhibitory action of the aspirin-like drugs on the biosynthesis of PGs plays an important role[39, 101]. PGs, at concentrations found in inflammatory exudates, are capable of causing hyperalgesia due to a long-lasting sensitization of pain receptors to mechanical or chemical stimuli[35]. Moreover, they cause erythema and exacerbate oedema induced by other mediators[38]. In addition, the analgesic activity of most classical acidic NSAID correlates with their pK_a-value (around 4). It was demonstrated that weak acidic compounds concentrate in inflamed tissues (as well as in gastric mucosa and kidneys) where they could then exert their PG-synthetase inhibitory action[9, 10].

Besides an involvement in the peripheral component of hyperalgesic processes, PGs may also be involved in the central component and may participate in CNS pain circuits. When injected into the cerebral ventricles of rats they have been shown to enhance hyperalgesia which was induced peripherally by PGs themselves or other inflammatory stimuli[37].

In therapeutic doses, paracetamol and phenacetin, in particular, are thought to act centrally. These drugs probably inhibit the PG-synthetase system in the CNS more strongly than in peripheral tissues; a differential sensitivity of the synthetases from different tissues has been found[40, 41]. This might explain why, for example, paracetamol is an effective analgesic–antipyretic, whereas it only exerts an anti-inflammatory effect at doses considerably in excess of those required for analgesia. Drugs like aspirin, which display a general antisynthetase action, act by blocking both the local and the central release of PGs[36]. Whether the inhibition of PG-biosynthesis and/or -release in the CNS accounts for the suggested interference of the aspirin-like drugs with the transmission of pain impulses at subcortical brain sites is not clear.

Models for evaluation of analgesics

With regard to the models used to evaluate the analgesic activity of drugs different classifications are applicable.

(1) Different types of pain-producing stimuli can be filed into four broad groups: heat, pressure, electricity and chemicals[27]. The chemical production of pain usually results in an inflammatory response in the biological system; therefore, compounds which are evaluated in the presence of chemical algesic stimuli usually exhibit anti-inflammatory activity. Pain produced by all the four groups can be alleviated by NSAID, local anaesthetics, central stimulants, hypnotics, narcotics and anaesthetics. The evaluation of the analgesic activity of NSAID in animal models is thus based on a comparison of dose–response relations observed using chemical stimuli with those observed using stimuli of physical origin.

If the analgesic potency in tests involving chemical stimuli is much larger than that observed using only physical stimuli, the analgesic activity resides mainly or totally in the periphery. On the other hand, an apparently equal or more pronounced pain-reducing activity following physical stimuli indicates a more centrally located mechanism of action. Thus, tests involving hot plates[111], radiant heat[22], microwaves[74], electrical stimulation via electrodes in dental pulp or skin[75, 105], vibrators[45] or artery clips as in Haffner's tailflick test[49] generally produce identical potency profiles for an analgesic relative to others tested simultaneously[2].

However, a far less homogenous picture is obtained when tests are used involving only chemical pain stimuli. Basically, these tests employ the abdominal constriction response in mice[15] and are similar despite the use of a wide variety of chemicals. The stimuli range from injection of non-specific irritating, hypo- or hypertonic salt solutions or acidic solutions to more specific agents like autacoids. Thus, it is not surprising to find a difference of opinion with regard to the usefulness of these tests, particularly when the characterization of the analgesic activity of anti-inflammatory compounds is concerned. Especially for this purpose the use of chemical stimuli producing inflammation (brewer's yeast, carrageenan, etc.) in conjunction with physical pain stimuli is to be preferred[83].

(2) Different types of response towards painful stimuli can be labelled in accordance with the established or supposed extent of participation of the CNS. Although in most experiments different types of responses can be distinguished, ranging from spinal reflexes to struggle and after-vocalization, mostly a single reaction is used to measure the response. A differentiation between the responses following a single pain stimulus, permitting discrimination between different pain projection levels within the CNS, yields more information about the sites of action of the drug in study[75].

(3) A dichotomous classification of tests based on the kind of results obtained, namely population characteristics like ED_{50} using qualitative measurements or dose–response metameters using quantitative measurements, are of importance in order to determine whether a test is suitable for further comparative evaluation; this particularly applies to the evaluation of drug mixtures. As outlined in the preceding paragraph, the assessment of analgesic drug combinations makes sense only if the dose–response metameters of the individual drugs are measured. Results from semi-quantitative tests, e.g. dose–threshold measurements, can readily be converted into dose–response data via the differences between the control value and the experimental values.

In our opinion qualitative analgesic tests employing physical pain stimuli alone and in combination with inflammation give usable indications of analgesic activity in a first screening. However, the appraisal of analgesic activity of single or of compound drugs requires quantitative tests, specified by the presumed or the intended sites of action.

Consequently, the evaluation of analgesic activity of NSAID involves quantitative tests in which physical pain stimuli are employed in conjunction with induced inflammation. As a corollary, the assessment of the therapeutic value of combinations of NSAID with other types of drugs (e.g. narcotics) has to exploit the same NSAID-specific tests.

ANTI-INFLAMMATORY EFFECTS

Mechanisms of anti-inflammatory action

NSAID may affect inflammation and the immune system in several ways.

Inflammation sometimes involves an antigen–antibody reaction activating the complement system. In this way and also as a result of the direct tissue damaging effect of the inflammatory stimulus, substances such as chemotactic factors, histamine, serotonin, bradykinin, slow reacting substance of anaphylaxis (SRS-A) and other metabolites of arachidonic acid (e.g. PGG_2, PGI_2 and PGE_2) are locally liberated[4]. Chemotactic factors, mainly non-cyclic eicosanoids, especially 12-HETE (Figure 46.1), attract leukocytes which migrate into the inflamed tissue, phagocytize inflammatory material and release lysosomal enzymes. These enzymes then cause injury to cartilage and other tissues and enhance inflammation. Histamine, serotonin and bradykinin cause pain and fever and, by causing vasodilation and by increasing vascular permeability, mediate oedema formation. Bradykinin, in addition, activates the release of PGs[55, 102]. In contrast to these mediators, PGs play a modulatory rather than a direct role in acute inflammatory conditions (see ref. 72). By themselves, PGs evoke only some of the local and systemic manifestations of inflammation produced by histamine, serotonin and bradykinin.

However, they intensify the effects of these mediators by enhancing the increased vascular permeability induced by these agents; this may be due to their vasodilatory activity[107]. Furthermore, PGEs appear to enhance migration of leukocytes[104]. In contrast to these inflammatory effects, the actions of PGEs on the proliferative (tissue) component of chronic inflammation appear to be mostly inhibitory (see ref. 5). This may indicate, as proposed by Bonta and Parnham (see ref. 6) that PGEs have a dual function in chronic inflammation, i.e. reinforcement of the vascular processes and inhibition of tissue events. The short-lived, but potentially more active products of PG-synthetase such as the PG endoperoxides (PGG_2 and PGH_2), PGI_2 and TXA_2, may also be involved in the development of inflammation and may even be more important than the PGEs, at least in acute inflammation[72].

Low, therapeutic doses of NSAID, as employed in acute inflammation, exert their anti-inflammatory action mainly via an inhibition of the cyclo-oxygenase enzyme system, and, in this way, suppress the many signs and symptoms of the exudative component of inflammation, enhanced or mediated by the prostanoids. However, by blocking the cyclo-oxygenase pathway in these doses, the drugs cause an increase in the production of non-cyclic eicosanoids, namely 12-HETE (Figure 46.1). In turn, the 5-lipoxygenase enzyme system of the activated leukocytes may produce non-cyclic eicosanoids with much higher chemotactic potency. Thus, the migration of polymorphonuclear leukocytes into inflamed tissue is enhanced by the administration of NSAID in this way (see ref. 51). On the other hand, high therapeutic doses of NSAID, as generally used in chronic inflammatory diseases, also inhibit the several lipoxygenase pathways and thus reduce leukocyte migration. However, the ongoing inhibition of the production of the prostanoids precludes regenerative or beneficial effects of endogenous PGE_2 during the proliferative phase of chronic inflammation[6].

Actions of NSAID which may be related to their anti-inflammatory activity, but probably not related to alterations in arachidonate metabolism, include suppression of antigen–antibody reactions, inhibition of cyclic nucleotide phosphodiesterase, stabilization of lysosomal membranes and uncoupling of oxidative phosphorylation (see ref. 33). However, a number of these actions generally require drug concentrations in excess of those achieved with therapeutic doses.

As the anti-inflammatory action of NSAID is closely related to their peripheral analgesic activity, and models to evaluate the latter include an induced inflammatory response, the anti-inflammatory assessment of these drugs is discussed rather extensively.

Models for evaluation of anti-inflammatory compounds

The animal models used in the evaluation of the anti-inflammatory activity of drugs are usually classified according to the pathological condition induced.

(1) In most reports the acute inflammatory situation is mimicked by the response elicited by one of the following three types of treatment:

  (a) A subplantar injection with chemical stimulants (brewer's yeast, carrageenan, dextran, etc.) into the rat hind paw invariably causes oedema the severity of which can be diminished by both SAID and NSAID[110]. Depending on its pharmacokinetics, the drug studied is given before or simultaneously with the oedema-inducing agent. As cyclic eicosanoids exert their action mainly during the second exudative phase of inflammation, dose-dependent, oedema-reducing effects of NSAID become apparent only 3 h after induction of oedema.

  (b) Injection of a sodium urate crystal suspension into the dog knee joint cavity induces an acute inflammatory response comparable to that above-mentioned and equally susceptible to the actions of SAID and NSAID. This technique, however, has the advantage that other inflammatory parameters as well as oedema size can be monitored[65].

  (c) The experimentally-induced erythema with radiant heat[109] or with UV-illumination[73] resembles the first exudative phase of acute inflammation and is modulated by antagonists of the main mediators active during that phase. Thus, it can only reflect the small augmentative or enhancing role of the cyclic eicosanoids during that phase when used to estimate the activity of NSAID. It is to be expected that the SAID are also hardly effective in these tests. Using a prolonged and/or a more intensive stimulus, these tests are used also to assess the analgesic activity of narcotic analgesics.

(2) The chronic inflammatory condition is usually established 25 days after injection of Freund's adjuvant. The addition of killed, dried *Mycobacterium butyricum* (complete adjuvant) to the oil phase of the water in oil emulsion (incomplete adjuvant) elicits cell-mediated immunity (delayed hypersensitivity) as well as humoral antibody formation[44]. With this technique, a pathological autoimmune condition is evoked which strongly resembles the clinical symptoms of rheumatoid arthritis. The immunomodulatory role of PGs is reflected in the efficacy of NSAID[8]. In this test the anti-inflammatory action of SAID, which restrains all pathways of arachidonate metabolism, is generally more pronounced than that of the NSAID which in high doses interferes only with some of these pathways.

The symptomatic relief obtainable with pharmacotherapy in rheumatoid arthritis seems to correlate well with the results obtained with this test.

(3) The intermediate, subacute or subchronic inflammatory model can be obtained by one of the following procedures:

(a) Induction of a granuloma by implantation, e.g. of cotton pellets impregnated with carrageenan[7]. Fukuhara and Tsurufuji[42] reported that NSAID were mostly effective in reduction of only the developing granuloma, whereas SAID also reduced already developed granulomas.

(b) Induction of an abscess, evolving after injection of carrageenan or turpentine (see acute inflammatory tests) of which the development in time is followed, e.g. by monitoring the migration of radioactive labelled leukocytes into the inflamed locus.

(c) The subplantar injection of Freund's adjuvant in the hind paw of rats, for example, is regularly employed to study the successive inflammatory stages, ranging from acute inflammation to polyarthritis. As is to be expected, the consecutive phases exhibit differential sensitivities towards anti-inflammatory agents.

Most of the inflammatory models yield quantitative data, which are readily converted into dose–response relationships (increasing responses with increasing dosages) suitable for further analysis.

ANTIPYRESIS

Mechanisms of antipyretic action

Body temperature is maintained by a delicate balance between heat production and heat loss, processes which are regulated mainly by the CNS, in particular the hypothalamic nuclei. In fever, endogenous pyrogen, released following infection and/or inflammation, directly interfere with the neurochemical pathways involved in the thermoregulatory function of these nuclei. Ultimately, the set-point temperature is increased, resulting in a decrease in heat loss and an increase in heat gain (see ref. 90).

NSAID inhibit the temperature-elevating effect of both endogenous and bacterial pyrogens, predominantly through a central site of action and not via their anti-inflammatory effect, although this does contribute. Their antipyretic effect, however, is not due to a direct interference with neurochemical pathways, nor to competition between the antipyretic and pyrogen for a receptor site, but probably to modulation of eicosanoid-biosynthesis in the CNS[14]. When injected directly into the thermoregulatory area of the anterior hypothalamus in various species, PGEs stimulate heat gain and inhibit heat loss mechanisms in a manner very similar to that produced by bacterial or endogenous pyrogens[26,103]. Moreover, the level of PGE found in the cerebrospinal fluid is enhanced during fever induced by all kinds of pyrogens. When antipyretic NSAID are administered during fever they inhibit this rise in PGE-levels at the same time as they produce antipyresis[34]. Though the body of data indicating a causal relationship between fever and central PGE-release is impressive, evidence against it has also been put forward[19,20] and the direct relation between PGE and fever still remains in question. Moreover, other metabolites of arachidonic acid, such as the cyclic endoperoxide intermediates (PGG_2 and PGH_2) may be important in central fever production[18].

The fall in body temperature produced by the NSAID 'families' like phenacetin-paracetamol, when given in the absence of fever, is probably not the result of inhibition of PG-biosynthesis in the CNS. This effect seems to be due to an action of the drug on the heat loss mechanisms[70] and is regarded as additional evidence that PGs are not involved in normal thermoregulation.

Apart from inhibition of PG-biosynthesis NSAID-like salicylates may also cause antipyresis by shifting the distribution of body water from intracellular to extracellular compartments, causing haemodilution and sweating. This mechanism may be related to the protein binding affinity of these NSAID, which can alter the affinity of intracellular protein for available water[64].

Although the sites of action of the NSAID in the CNS are far from elucidated, it is remarkable that the NSAID with a clear central analgesic activity are also the NSAID with a pronounced antipyretic or hypothermic potency. It remains to be seen whether this kind of correlation is meaningless or indicates that these NSAID act via similar sites of action or employ similar mechanisms of action in the CNS.

Models for evaluation of antipyretics

A model currently used in the screening of NSAID is hyperthermia induced with brewer's yeast. Two or three hours after an injection of a yeast suspension in the flanks of the animal (generally rats), a fever develops which reaches a peak at about 5 h while the body temperature is back to normal level within 24 h. NSAID are administered according to their pharmacokinetic characteristics and their efficacy in reducing the peak temperature. On the NSAID-induced reduction of this peak temperature quantitative dose–response relations can be based for use in the assessment of drug combinations.

PLATELET AGGREGATION

Although the influence of NSAID on platelet aggregability is of minor interest for the evaluation of analgesic potency, it is mentioned here briefly because of its pertinence for the evaluation of their therapeutic value.

Effects of NSAID on platelet adherence, aggregation and plasticity directly depend on the inhibitory action of these drugs on the cyclo-oxygenase pathway of arachidonate metabolism, possibly leading to a disturbance of the delicate balance between production by platelets of TXA_2 (platelet aggregation and vasoconstriction) and the production by the vessel wall of PGI_2 (inhibition of platelet aggregation and vasodilatation)[71]. As the cyclo-oxygenase in platelets seems to be more sensitive to aspirin than the enzyme in vessel wall, the therapeutic value of aspirin as an antithrombotic is currently under investigation[89]. With a few notable exceptions, e.g. paracetamol, all NSAID prolong bleeding time and thus aggravate their main and common side effect namely gastrointestinal bleeding and ulceration.

GASTROINTESTINAL EROSION

Mechanisms of NSAID-induced gastrointestinal damage

The erosive activity of NSAID on the gastrointestinal mucosa is amply documented[76] and, with regard to the mechanisms underlying this toxicity, the following picture appears to emerge from the literature. By inhibiting the endogenous production of PGs in the gastrointestinal wall NSAID weaken the defensive capacity of the mucosa indirectly[108]. Several types of prostanoids are reported to stimulate production of mucus[3] or to inhibit acid secretion[88] and all PGs tested seem to exert a cytoprotective action in the gastrointestinal tract[86]. Furthermore, back diffusion of hydrogen ions from the stomach lumen into the gastric wall through the broken mucosal barrier seems to be essential for the development of gastric damage (see ref. 104).

Models for evaluation of ulcerogenic compounds

The models currently employed in the evaluation of the mucosal damage of ulcerogenic compounds fall into three main classes: gastrointestinal irritation, gastrointestinal fluid retention and/or secretion, and estimation of faecal blood loss. Ulcerogenic effects of NSAID have been studied mainly in the upper part of the gastrointestinal tract, this because the gastric models of ulceration appear to be most useful for studying the pathomorphology of ulceration and the process of ulcer healing, and for assessing the activity of antiulcer agents[23,52,98,112]. Of all the side effects of the NSAID, the gastric ulcerogenic activity is the one the most frequently compared to their pharmacodynamic potencies[77,78] and involved in studies on structure activity relationships[79].

(1) Gastric ulceration techniques are usually applied in rats, dogs and mice. After administration of the compounds – most orally – the incidence of the mucosal lesions is determined macroscopically several hours later at autopsy. In monitoring the mucosal damage, a large variety of scoring systems is employed ranging from the determination of only the number of animals with haemorrhagic lesions to the more accurate screening of both the number and magnitude of the erosions. With this latter method not only the incidence but also the severity of the mucosal damage is taken into account. Furthermore, it enables the elucidation of dose–response relationships on ulcerogenic activity of NSAID.

Using this method in rats we found the severity of gastric glandular erosions observed 17 h after a single oral dose of aspirin to be closely correlated with the logarithm of the dose administered. This relationship between erosion score and aspirin dose was not affected when phenacetin was added in equal amounts. Addition of caffeine to the aspirin (dose ratio 1:5) increased the erosion scores. Paracetamol in admixture with equal amounts of aspirin appeared not to induce gastric damage at all[91]. Further investigation of the interactions between aspirin and caffeine or paracetamol revealed that both drugs increased or decreased the erosions induced by aspirin, in a log-dose dependent way[92] (Figure 46.2).

In the study of gastric ulcerogenic activity several sensitive techniques have been developed. The animals used can be sensitized by deprivation of food or by exposure to cold[80] or temporary immobilization[12]. Furthermore, for the full expression of gastric ulcerogenic activity mechanical (e.g. distension of the stomach[97]) or chemical (instillation of additional acid[98]) stimuli can be combined with the administration of the compound under investigation. Other factors influencing gastric erosive activity of NSAID include the lodging, species, strain and age of the animals[99,106].

For example our observation that paracetamol, administered orally with aspirin, inhibited aspirin induced erosions in the rat stomach[91,92], was corroborated by van Kolfschoten *et al.* using the same animal species[58], whereas Kawano *et al.*, using comparable doses of aspirin and paracetamol in mice, could not find such a protective effect[57]. In addition, results obtained with the simultaneous administration of paracetamol and indomethacin to rats were contradictory in so far that Rainsford[81] could not demonstrate a protective action of a small dose of paracetamol while data of van Kolfschoten *et al.*[58] show that higher doses of paracetamol do inhibit the gastric erosive activity of indomethacin. Sodium salicylate, on the other hand has been demonstrated unambiguously to reduce gastric ulceration by indomethacin[17,31,32].

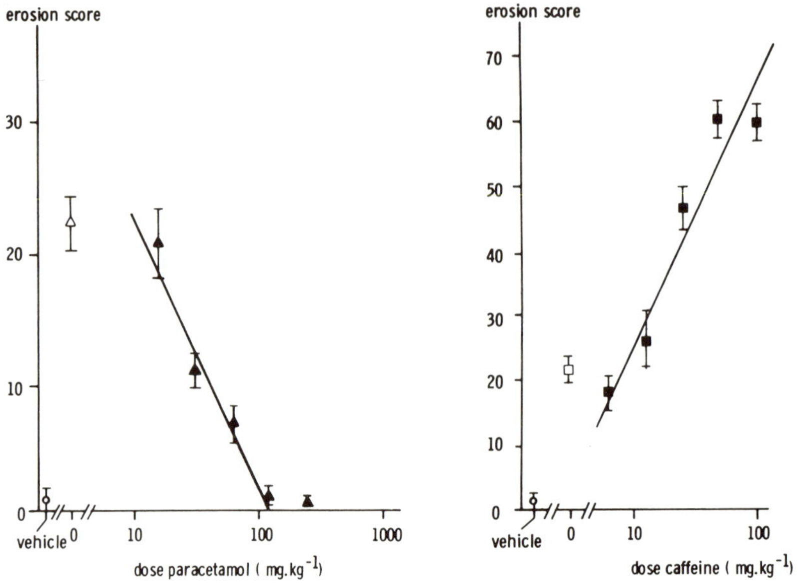

Figure 46.2 Interactions between aspirin and caffeine or paracetamol on gastric erosions observed 17 h after oral administration. □, △: aspirin (250 mg/kg); ■: aspirin (250 mg/kg) and caffeine; ▲: aspirin (250 mg/kg) and paracetamol; ○: vehicle, 5 ml/kg 4% Tween-80 solution; $n = 10$

In experiments on gastric ulcerogenic activity, great importance should be attached also to the development of the erosions in course of time. In our studies to elucidate the interaction between aspirin and paracetamol, surprisingly we found that the gastric damage induced by the mixture of aspirin and paracetamol during the first 2 h hardly differed from that induced by aspirin administered alone. Analysis of the erosion score data indicated that during the first 4 h the number of erosion foculi induced by the mixture of paracetamol and aspirin was not significantly different from that induced by aspirin alone. Thus, paracetamol did not inhibit the induction of erosion foculi by aspirin, but apparently prevented the growth of foculi into erosions. Moreover, after 2 h the foculi started to disappear and 8 h after administration of the mixture the stomachs seemed not to be damaged at all[53, 92, 93]. A study of the absorption of the drugs from the stomach gave no indications that the inhibitory action of paracetamol on the erosive activity of aspirin is accompanied by any effects of paracetamol on the absorption and accumulation of salicylate in the glandular part of the gastric tissue. On the contrary, the absorption of paracetamol into the gastric tissue increased in the presence of aspirin[94].

Since paracetamol has been reported to stimulate PG-synthesis *in vitro*[66, 84] and since co-administration of PGs protects the gastric mucosa against irritation by aspirin, this observation led to the proposition that paracetamol might protect against the erosive activity of aspirin by counteracting the aspirin-induced inhibition of PG-biosynthesis in the glandular part of the stomach[53, 93].

However, van Kolfschoten *et al.*[59] recently found that *in vivo* paracetamol, in the presence of aspirin, did not alter the inhibitory activity of the latter drug on the PG-biosynthesis system of the glandular mucosa of the rat stomach. As an alternative explanation for the protective activity of paracetamol against aspirin-induced gastric damage, they suggested that the drug acts as a scavenger of noxious free radicals. The generation of these radicals, together with lipid peroxides out of alternative pathways of lipoxygenation of arachidonic acid, may be increased during the inhibition of cyclo-oxygenase by the aspirin. Whether a reduction of these peroxides and scavenging of free radicals by paracetamol explain the antagonistic interaction between paracetamol and aspirin on gastric damage in rats or not, needs further investigation. With regard to the interaction between caffeine and aspirin on gastric ulcerogenic acitivity, studies on gastric acid output revealed that both in the absence and in the presence of aspirin, caffeine increased acid secretion[53, 92]. As gastric acid is an important factor in the development of erosions induced by aspirin[16] it seems reasonable to ascribe the potentiating effect of caffeine on the erosive activity of aspirin to this stimulation of acid secretion.

Finally, as another factor influencing the gastric ulcerogenic activity of NSAID, the route of administration should be mentioned. The erosive activities of indomethacin after oral and after subcutaneous administration to rats are similar whereas those of aspirin differ considerably in that subcutaneous aspirin causes far less gastric damage than oral aspirin[59]. In addition, subcutaneously administered paracetamol inhibits indomethacin-induced erosions but is inefficient in reducing aspirin-induced erosions, but orally administered paracetamol is effective in inhibiting both[58, 92]. According to van Kolfschoten *et al.* these observations point to a more important role of direct tissue contact in the erosive mechanism of aspirin that in that of indomethacin[59].

Various other techniques can be employed for the evaluation of gastric mucosal ulceration. These methods include the detection of gastric lesions in pylorus-occluded rats[23, 96], measurement of ionic fluxes and potential difference across the gastric mucosa in dogs with Heidenhain pouches[24, 25], the autoradiographic approach as proposed by Brune[11] and the determination of cellular exfoliation, where the number of gastric cells sloughed off is measured quantitatively[21]. To complete investigations on gastric irritating effects a very precise evaluation of the mucosal damage can be made by microscopical examination and/or by using special photographic techniques[69].

The gastrointestinal fluid retention and/or secretion methods are employed in studies on (gastro-) intestinal dysfunction rather than in evaluations of ulcerogenic activity. In several types of these dysfunctions changes in intestinal PG-biosynthesis may be involved. Using an enteropooling assay as a test for diarrhoea produced by PGs, Robert *et al.*

demonstrated that PGEs give rise to an increase in enteral secretion whereas PGI_2 decreased this phenomenon[85,87].

(3) Faecal blood loss methods take the leakage of labelled blood constituents into the gastrointestinal contents as a measure of the drug-induced mucosal damage. For the determination of the gastrointestinal blood loss ^{51}Cr radioactive labelled erythrocytes are applied most often. Results of animal experiments in which this tracer was used demonstrate that it is suitable and permits reliable quantitative comparisons of the gastrointestinal side-effects of drugs in animals[67,68]. However, this sensitive technique has also considerable disadvantages. The method does not provide any information about the localization, the extent and the depth of the mucosal injury. The pathological changes are only determined *in toto*. Furthermore, drugs which lead to a pronounced increase of bile production may be overestimated in causing gastrointestinal damage as a result of excretion of ^{51}Cr-labelled material with the bile.

To arrive at a meaningful evaluation of the side-effects of combinations of drugs on the gastrointestinal tract it is not only essential that the experimental technique should be sensitive; the selection of a method which yields quantitative data convertible into dose–response relations is just as important.

INTERACTIONS

As can be inferred from the discussion above the experimental assessment of the efficacy of a single drug is far from easy; with drug combinations the same problems are encountered, often in an aggravated form. Furthermore, specific difficulties are to be expected due to interactions between the component drugs. Three types of interaction are possible; they will be discussed with regard to NSAID combinations:

(1) Physicochemical interactions. In animal experiments, drugs can be combined using vehicles which are not suitable for therapeutic use. Mixtures of aspirin and paracetamol suspended in Tween-80 can be administered to laboratory animals, but for therapeutic purpose special formulations have to be developed, e.g. benorylate, an ester of aspirin with paracetamol.

(2) Pharmacokinetic interactions.
   (a) The *absorption* of the component drugs given in admixture can be radically different due to changes in gastrointestinal motility and in other gastrointestinal functions, influenced by prostaglandins.
   (b) The *distribution* of the component drugs may be affected by the albumin binding of many NSAID.
   The component drugs may compete for the same *inactivation* or *excretion* mechanism.

(3) Pharmacodynamic interactions.
   (a) The efficacy of the component drugs may change due to addition or to non-competitive interactions (potentiation and antagonism), as discussed above.
   (b) The *time course* of a given reaction to one of the component drugs can change dramatically.

CLOSING REMARKS

To make use of addition of effects and in the absence of other interactions (especially pharmacokinetic ones) rational dosages of the individual drugs in mixture are those producing about 25% of the maximal response when given alone.

It should be borne in mind that pharmacodynamic interactions may apply to the desired therapeutic effect but also to unwanted effects, such as intestinal dysfunction.

Furthermore, combination with drugs which presumably do not interfere with arachidonic acid metabolism can enhance both the efficacy and/or the side-effects of NSAID in admixture. Thus, addition of caffeine enhances the gastrotoxicity of aspirin but also adds to the analgesic potency.

The precise role of eicosanoids in toxicopharmacology is far from simple and straightforward and inhibition of PG-biosynthesis/release *per se* does not explain entirely the pharmacological effects of NSAID[43].

The data reviewed suggest that although a plethora of NSAID combinations are used in abundance, the experimental pharmacological assessment of their therapeutic value generally still has to be made. Techniques and analyses aimed at evaluation of drug combinations have started to emerge only recently.

Acknowledgments

The authors are indebted to Mrs W. van Kruiningen who supplied the bibliographic data. The assistance of Mr F. J. Propsma and Mrs M. Iedema, in the presentation of this manuscript is gratefully mentioned.

References

1. Ariëns, E. J. (1954). Affinity and intrinsic activity in the theory of competitive inhibition. *Arch. Int. Pharmacodyn. Ther.*, **99**, 32–49
2. Bluth, R. (1981). Zur Prüfung analgetisch wirksamer Substanzen. *Pharmazie*, **36**, 566–72
3. Bolton, J. P., Palmer, D. and Cohen, M. M. (1976). Effects of the E_2 prostaglandins on gastric mucus production in rats. *Surg. Forum*, **27**, 402–3
4. Bonta, I. L. and Parnham, M. J. (1978). Prostaglandins and chronic inflammation. *Biochem. Pharmacol.*, **27**, 1611–23
5. Bonta, I. L. and Parnham, M. J. (1979). Time-dependent stimulatory and inhibitory effects of prostaglandin E_1 on exudative and tissue components of granulomatous inflammation in rats. *Br. J. Pharmacol.*, **65**, 465–72

6. Bonta, I. L. and Parnham, M. J. (1980). Essential fatty acids or prostaglandins: therapeutic modulators of chronic inflammation? *T.I.P.S.*, **1**, 347–9
7. Bonta, I. L., Parnham, M. J. and Bragt, P. C. (1979). Involvement and effects of prostaglandin E in experimental granulomatous inflammation. *Int. J. Tiss. Reac.*, **1**, 51–5
8. Bray, M. A. and Morley, J. (1981). Prostaglandins and immunity. In Berti, F. and Velo, G. P. (eds.) *The Prostaglandin System*. pp. 193–202. (New York: Plenum)
9. Brune, K., Glatt, M. and Graf, P. (1976). Mechanism of action of anti-inflammatory drugs. *Gen. Pharmacol.*, **7**, 27–33
10. Brune, K., Graf, P. and Rainsford, K. D. (1977). A pharmaco-kinetic approach to the understanding of therapeutic effects and side effects of salicylates. *Agents Actions, Suppl.*, **1**, 9–26
11. Brune, K., Schweitzer, A. and Eckert, H. (1977). Parietal cells of the stomach trap salicylates during absorption. *Biochem. Pharmacol.*, **26**, 1735–40
12. Cioli, V., Silvestrin, B. and Dordoni, F. (1967). Evaluation of the potential of gastric ulceration after administration of certain drugs. *Exp. Molecul. Pathol.*, **6**, 68–83
13. Clark, A. J. (1933). *The Mode of Action of Drugs on Cells.* (Baltimore: Williams and Wilkins)
14. Clark, W. G. (1979). Mechanisms of antipyretic action. *Gen. Pharmacol.*, **10**, 71–7
15. Collier, H. O. J., Dinneen, L. C., Johnson, C. A. *et al.* (1968). The abdominal constriction response and its suppression by analgesic drugs in the mouse. *Br. J. Pharmacol.*, **32**, 295–310
16. Cooke, A. R. (1973). The role of acid in the pathogenesis of aspirin-induced gastrointestinal erosions and hemorrhage. *Am. J. Dig. Dis.*, **18**, 225–37
17. Corell, T. and Jensen, K. M. (1979). Interaction of salicylates and other non-steroidal anti-inflammatory agents in rats as shown by gastro-ulcerogenic and anti-inflammatory activities, and plasma concentrations. *Acta Pharmacol. Toxicol.*, **45**, 225–31
18. Cranston, W. I. (1979). Prostaglandins as mediators of pyrexia. *Agents Actions, Suppl.*, **8**, 79–82
19. Cranston, W. I., Duff, G. W., Hellon, R. F. *et al.* (1976). Evidence that brain prostaglandin synthesis is not essential in fever. *J. Physiol.*, **259**, 239–51
20. Cranston, W. I., Hellon, R. F. and Mitchell, D. (1975). A dissociation between fever and prostaglandin concentration in cerebrospinal fluid. *J. Physiol.*, **253**, 583–93
21. Croft, D. N. (1966). The action of analgesic substances on the gastric mucosa. *J. Pharm. Pharmacol.*, **18**, 354–61
22. D'Amour, F. E. and Smith, D. L. (1941). A method for determining loss of pain reaction. *J. Pharmacol. Exp. Ther.*, **72**, 74–9
23. Dai, S. and Ogle, C. W. (1974). Gastric ulcers induced by acid accumulation and by stress in pylorus-occluded rats. *Eur. J. Pharmacol.*, **26**, 15–21
24. Dajani, E. A., Collison, D. A. and Bertermann, R. E. (1978). Effects of E-prostaglandins on canine gastric potential difference. *Am. J. Dig. Dis.*, **23**, 436–42
25. Davenport, H. W., Warren, H. A. and Code, C. F. (1964). Functional significance of gastric mucosal barrier to sodium. *Gastroenterology*, **47**, 142–52
26. Dey, P. K., Feldberg, W., Gupta, K. P. *et al.* (1974). Further studies on the role of prostaglandin in fever. *J. Physiol.*, **241**, 629–46
27. Domer, F. R. (1971). Techniques for evaluation of analgetics. In *Animal Experiments in Pharmacological Analysis*. pp. 275–318. (Springfield: C. C. Thomas)
28. Dowd, J. E. and Riggs, D. S. (1965). A comparison of estimates of Michaelis-Menten kinetic constants from various linear transformations. *J. Biol. Chem.*, **240**, 863–9
29. Egan, R. W., Paxton, J. and Kuehl, F. A., Jr. (1976). Mechanism for irreversible self-deactivation of prostaglandin synthetase. *J. Biol. Chem.*, **251**, 7329–35
30. Egan, R. W., Yale, P. H. and Kuehl, F. A., Jr. (1979). Reduction of hydroperoxides in the prostaglandin biosynthetic pathway by a microsomal peroxidase. *J. Biol. Chem.*, **254**, 3295
31. Ezer, E., Pálosi, E., Hajós, G. *et al.* (1976). Antagonism of the gastrointestinal ulcerogenic effect of some non-steroidal anti-inflammatory agents by sodium salicylate. *J. Pharm. Pharmacol.*, **28**, 655–6
32. Ezer, E., Pálosi, E., Hajós, G. *et al.* (1979). Comparative pharmacology of a 1:10 combination of indomethacin–sodium salicylate. *Agents Actions, Suppl.*, **1**, 117–23

33. Famaey, J. P. (1978). Recent developments about non-steroidal anti-inflammatory drugs and their mode of action. *Gen. Pharmacol.*, **9**, 155–62
34. Feldberg, W. and Gupta, K. P. (1973). Pyrogen fever and prostaglandin-like activity in cerebrospinal fluid. *J. Physiol.*, **228**, 41–53
35. Ferreira, S. H. (1972). Prostaglandins, aspirin-like drugs and analgesia. *Nature New Biol.*, **240**, 200–3
36. Ferreira, S. H. (1981). Prostaglandins and inflammatory hyperalgesia. In Berti, F. and Velo, G. P. (eds.) *The Prostaglandin System*. pp. 127–38. (New York: Plenum)
37. Ferreira, S. H., Lorenzetti, B. B. and Correa, F. M. A. (1978). Blockade of central and peripheral generation of prostaglandins explains the antialgic effect of aspirin like drugs. *Pol. J. Pharmacol. Pharm.*, **30**, 133–40
38. Flower, R. J. (1974). Drugs which inhibit prostaglandin biosynthesis. *Pharmacol. Rev.*, **26**, 33–64
39. Flower, R. J. (1977). The role of prostaglandins in inflammatory reactions. *Naunyn-Schmiedeberg's Arch. Pharmacol.*, **297**, S77–9
40. Flower, R. J. and Vane, J. R. (1972). Inhibition of prostaglandin synthetase in brain explains the antipyretic activity of paracetamol (4-acetamido-phenol). *Nature New Biol.*, **240**, 410–11
41. Flower, R. J. and Vane, J. R. (1974). Inhibition of prostaglandin biosynthesis. *Biochem. Pharmacol.*, **23**, 1439–50
42. Fukuhara, M. and Tsurufuji, S. (1969). The effect of locally injected anti-inflammatory drugs on the carrageenin granuloma in rats. *Biochem. Pharmacol.*, **18**, 475–84
43. Glenn, E. M., Bowman, B. J. and Rohloff, N. H. (1979). Anomalous biological effects of salicylates and prostaglandins. *Agents Actions*, **9**, 257–64
44. Glenn, E. M. and Gray, J. (1965). Adjuvant-induced polyarthritis in rats. I. Biologic and histologic background. *Am. J. Vet. Res.*, **26**, 1180–5
45. Gregg, E. C., Jr. (1952). Effects of non-opiate analgesics and other drugs on the vibratory threshold. *J. Pharmacol. Exp. Ther.*, **106**, 1–13
46. Grotto, M., Dikstein, S. and Sulman, F. G. (1965). Additive and augmentative synergism between analgesic drugs. *Arch. Int. Pharmacodyn. Ther.*, **155**, 365–72
47. Gryglewski, R. J. (1981). Pharmacological interference in arachidonic acid cascade. In Berti, F. and Velo, G. P. (eds.) *The Prostaglandin System*. pp. 85–96. (New York: Plenum)
48. Gryglewski, R. J., Panczenko, B., Korbut, R. *et al.* (1975). Corticosteroids inhibit prostaglandin release from perfused mesenteric blood vessels of rabbit and from perfused lungs of sensitized guinea-pigs. *Prostaglandins*, **10**, 343–55
49. Haffner, F. (1929). Experimentelle Prüfung schmertzstillender Mittel. *Deutsch. Med. Wschr.*, **55**, 731–3
50. Hemler, M. E. and Lands, W. E. M. (1980). Evidence for a peroxide-initiated free radical mechanism of prostaglandin biosynthesis *J. Biol. Chem.*, **255**, 6253–61
51. Higgs, G. A. and Flower, R. J. (1981). Anti-inflammatory drugs and the inhibition of arachidonate lipoxygenase. In Piper, P. J. (ed.) *SRS-A and Leukotrienes*. pp. 197–207. (New York: Wiley)
52. Inatomi, N., Ishihara, Y. and Okabe, S. (1979). Effects of anti-ulcer agents on thermal-cortisone-induced ulcers in rats. *Japan J. Pharmacol.*, **29**, 486–8
53. Jager, L. P., Seegers, A. J. M. and van Noordwijk, J. (1981). Interactions between aspirin and other compounds in analgesic medicines on gastric mucosal damage in rats. In *The Prostaglandin System*. pp. 401–15. (New York: Plenum)
54. Jain, A. K., McMahon, F. G., Ryan, J. R. *et al.* (1978). Aspirin and aspirin–caffeine in postpartum pain relief. *Clin. Pharmacol. Ther.*, **24**, 69–75
55. Juan, H. (1977). Mechanism of action of bradykinin-induced release of prostaglandin E. *Naunyn-Schmiedeberg's Arch. Pharmacol.*, **300**, 77–85
56. Juan, H. and Lembeck, F. (1976). Release of prostaglandins from the isolated perfused rabbit ear by bradykinin and acetylcholine. *Agents Actions*, **6**, 642–5
57. Kawano, O., Sawabe, T., Misaki, N. *et al.* (1978). Studies on combination dosing. III. Aspirin and ethenzamide. *Japan. J. Pharmacol.*, **28**, 829–35
58. van Kolfschoten, A. A., Zandberg, P., Jager, L. P. *et al.* (1982). The influence of paracetamol on the erosive activity of indomethacin in the rat stomach. *Agents Actions*, **12**, 247–53

59. van Kolfschoten, A. A., Dembinska-Kiec, A. and Basista, M. (1981). Interaction between aspirin and paracetamol on the production of prostaglandins in the rat gastric mucosa. *J. Pharm. Pharmacol.*, **33**, 462–3
60. Kuehl, F. A., Humes, J. L., Egan, R. W. *et al.* (1977). Role of prostaglandin endoperoxide PG G_2 in inflammatory processes. *Nature New Biol.*, **265**, 170–2
61. Kuehl, F. A., Humes, J. L., Beveridge, G. C. *et al.* (1977). Biologically active derivatives of fatty acids: prostaglandins, thromboxanes and endoperoxides. *Inflammation*, **2**, 285–94
62. Lands, W. E. M. (1981). Actions of anti-inflammatory drugs. *T.I.P.S.*, **2**, 78–80
63. Lim, R. K. S., Miller, D. G., Guzman, F. *et al.* (1967). Pain and analgesic evaluated by the intraperitoneal bradykinin evoked pain method in man. *Clin. Pharmacol. Ther.*, **8**, 521–42
64. Malseed, R. T. and Malseed, Z. K. (1978). Aspirin: a pharmacologic profile. *Am. J. Pharm.*, **150**, 99–106
65. McCarty, D. J., Jr., Phelps, P. and Pyenson, J. (1966). Crystal-induced inflammation in canine joints. I. An experimental model with quantification of the host response. *J. Exp. Med.*, **124**, 99–114
66. McDonald-Gibson, W. J. and Collier, H. O. J. (1979). Paracetamol potentiates acetylsalicylate in inhibiting prostaglandin synthesis. *Eur. J. Pharmacol.*, **58**, 497–500
67. Menassé-Gdynia, R. and Krupp, P. (1974). Quantitative measurement of gastrointestinal bleeding in rats: the effect of nonsteroidal anti-inflammatory drugs. *Toxicol. Appl. Pharmacol.*, **29**, 389–96
68. Menassé. R. (1979). Evaluation of ulcerogenic effects. *Pharmacol. Ther.*, **5**, 191–7
69. Mikhail, A. A. and Holland, H. C. (1966). Evaluating and photographing experimentally induced stomach ulcers. *J. Psychosomat. Res.*, **9**, 349–53
70. Milton, A. S. (1976). Modern views on the pathogenesis of fever and the mode of action of antipyretic drugs. *J. Pharm. Pharmacol.*, **28**, 393–9
71. Moncada, S., Flower, R. J. and Vane, J. R. (1980). Prostaglandins, prostacyclin, and thromboxane A_2. In Goodman Gilman, A., Goodman, L. S. and Gilman, A. (eds.) *The Pharmacological Basis of Therapeutics*. pp. 668–81. (New York: Macmillan)
72. Moncada, S. and Vane, J. R. (1979). Pharmacology and endogenous roles of prostaglandin-endoperoxides, thromboxane A_2 and prostacyclin. *Pharmacol. Rev.*, **30**, 293–331
73. Mulé, S. J., Clements, T. H., Layson, R. C. *et al.* (1968). Analgesia in guinea-pigs: a measure of tolerance development. *Arch. Int. Pharmacodyn. Ther.*, **173**, 201–12
74. Nicák, A. (1965). New methods of evaluation of analgesics based on ultrasound pain stimulation. *Arch. Int. Pharmacodyn. Ther.*, **153**, 214–17
75. Paalzow, G. and Paalzow, L. (1973). The effects of caffeine and theophylline on nociceptive stimulation in the rat. *Acta Pharmacol. Toxicol.*, **32**, 22–32
76. Prescott, L. F. (1976). Antipyretic analgesics. In Dukes, M. N. G. (ed.) *Meyler's Side Effects of Drugs*. Vol. 8, pp. 154–206. (Amsterdam: Excerpta Medica) (and subsequent annuals)
77. Rainsford, K. D. and Whitehouse, M. W. (1977). Non-steroid anti-inflammatory drugs: combined assay for anti-edemic potency and gastric ulcerogenesis in the same animal. *Life Sci.*, **21**, 371–7
78. Rainsford, K. D. and Whitehouse, M. W. (1980). Are all aspirins really alike? A comparison of gastric ulcerogenicity with bio-efficacy in rats. *Pharmacol. Res. Commun.*, **12**, 85–95
79. Rainsford, K. D. (1978). Structure–activity relationships of non-steroid anti-inflammatory drugs. 1. Gastric ulcerogenic activity. *Agents Actions, Suppl.*, **6**, 587–605
80. Rainsford, K. D. (1978). The role of aspirin in gastric ulceration: some factors involved in the development of gastric mucosal damage induced by aspirin in rats exposed to various stress conditions. *Am. J. Dig. Dis.*, **23**, 521–30
81. Rainsford, K. D. (1979). Prostaglandins and the development of gastric mucosal damage by anti-inflammatory drugs. *Agents Actions, Suppl.*, **6**, 193–200
82. Ramwell, P. W. (1981). Biologic importance of arachidonic acid. *Arch. Int. Intern. Med.*, **141**, 275–8
83. Randall, L. O. and Selitto, J. J. (1957). A method for measurement of analgesic activity on inflamed tissue. *Arch. Int. Pharmacodyn. Ther.*, **111**, 409–19

84. Robak, J., Wieckowski, A. and Gryglewski, R. J. (1978). The effect of 4-acetaminofenol on prostaglandin synthetase activity in bovine and ram seminal vesicle microsomes. *Biochem. Pharmacol.*, **27**, 391–6
85. Robert, A. (1981). Cytoprotection and enteral pooling by prostaglandins. In Berti, F. and Velo, G. P. (eds.) *The Prostaglandin System*. pp. 393–400. (New York: Plenum)
86. Robert, A., Nezamis, J. E., Lancaster, C. *et al.* (1979). Cytoprotection by prostaglandins in rats. *Gastroenterology*, **77**, 433–43
87. Robert, A., Nezamis, J. E., Lancaster, C. *et al.* (1976). Enteropooling assay: a test for diarrhea produced by prostaglandins. *Prostaglandins*, **11**, 809–28
88. Robert, A., Nezamis, J. E. and Phillips, J. P. (1976). Inhibition of gastric secretion by prostaglandins. *Am. J. Dig. Dis.*, **12**, 1073–6
89. Rothschild, B. M. (1979). Hematologic perturbations associated with salicylate. *Clin. Pharmacol. Ther.*, **26**, 145–52
90. de Roij, T. A. J. M. (1978). Neurotransmitters in het centrale thermo-regulatie systeem. In *Dopamine in Central Thermoregulation*, pp. 13–46. State University Utrecht, Thesis
91. Seegers, A. J. M., Jager, L. P. and van Noordwijk, J. (1978). Gastric erosions induced by analgesic drug mixtures in the rat. *J. Pharm. Pharmacol.*, **30**, 84–7
92. Seegers, A. J. M., Jager, L. P. and van Noordwijk, J. (1979). Effects of phenacetin, paracetamol and caffeine on the erosive activity of acetylsalicylic acid in the rat stomach: dose–response relationships, time course of erosion development and effects on acid secretion. *J. Pharm. Pharmacol.*, **31**, 840–8
93. Seegers, A. J. M., Jager, L. P. and van Noordwijk, J. (1980). An hypothesis concerning the protective action of paracetamol against the erosive activity of acetylsalicylic acid in the rat stomach. In Samuelsson, B. *et al.* (eds.) *Advances in Prostaglandin and Thromboxane Research.* Vol. 8, pp. 1547–51. (New York: Raven Press)
94. Seegers, A. J. M., Olling, M., Jager, L. P. *et al.* (1980). Interactions of aspirin with acetaminophen and caffeine in rat stomach: pharmacokinetics of absorption and accumulation in gastric mucosa. *J. Pharm. Sci.*, **69**, 900–6
95. Seegers, A. J. M., Jager, L. P., Zandberg, P. *et al.* (1981). The anti-inflammatory, analgesic and antipyretic activities of non-narcotic analgesic drug mixtures in rats. *Arch. Int. Pharmacodyn. Ther.*, **252**, 237–54
96. Shay, H., Komarov, S. A., Fels, S. S. *et al.* (1945). A simple method for the uniform production of gastric ulceration in the rat. *Gastroenterology*, **5**, 43–61
97. Szelenyi, I. and Thiemer, K. (1978). Distension ulcer as a model for testing of drugs for ulcerogenic side effects. *Arch. Toxicol.*, **41**, 99–105
98. Takeuchi, K., Okabe, S., Takagi, K. *et al.* (1977). Influence of aspirin on healing of chronic gastric ulcers in dogs. *Digestion*, **16**, 51–6
99. Urushidani, T., Okabe, S., Takeuchi, K. *et al.* (1978). Strain differences in aspirin-induced gastric ulceration in rats. *Japan, J. Pharmacol.*, **28**, 569–78
100. Vane. J. R. (1971). Inhibition of prostaglandin synthesis as a mechanism of action for aspirin-like drugs. *Nature New Biol.*, **232**, 232–5
101. Vane, J. R. (1978). The mode of action of aspirin-like drugs. *Agents Actions*, **8**, 430–1
102. Vane, J. R. (1976). Prostaglandins as mediators of inflammation. In Samuelsson, B. and Paoletti, R. (eds.) *Advances in Prostaglandin and Thromboxane Research.* Vol. 2, pp. 791–802. (New York: Raven Press)
103. Veale, W. L. and Cooper, K. E. (1975). Comparison of sites of action of prostaglandin E and leucocyte pyrogen in brain. In Lomax, P. *et al.* (eds.) *Temperature Regulation and Drug Action.* pp. 218–26. (Basle: Karger)
104. Walker, J. R., Smith, M. J. H. and Ford-Hutchinson, A. W. (1976). Anti-inflammatory drugs, prostaglandins and leukocyte migration. *Agents Actions*, **6**, 602–6
105. Weitzman, E. D. and Ross, G. S. (1962). A behavioural method for the study of pain perception in the monkey. The effects of some pharmacological agents. *Neurology (Minneap.)*, **12**, 264–72
106. Wilhelmi, G. and Menassé-Gdynia, R. (1972). Gastric mucosal damage induced by non-steroid anti-inflammatory agents in rats of different ages. *Pharmacology*, **8**, 321–8
107. Williams, T. J. and Peck, M. J. (1977). Role of prostaglandin-mediated vasodilatation in inflammation. *Nature New Biol.*, **270**, 530–2

108. Wilson, D. E. and Kaymakcalan, H. (1981). Prostaglandins: gastrointestinal effects and peptic ulcer disease. *Med. Clin. N. Am.*, **65**, 773–87
109. Winder, C. V., Pfeiffer, C. C. and Maison, G. L. (1946). The nociceptive contraction of the cutaneous muscle of the guinea-pig as elicited by radiant heat. *Arch. Int. Pharmacodyn. Ther.*, **72**, 329–59
110. Winter, C. A., Risley, E. A. and Nuss, G. W. (1962). Carrageenin-induced edema in the hind paw of the rat as an assay for anti-inflammatory drugs. *Proc. Soc. Exp. Biol. Med.*, **111**, 544–7
111. Woolfe, G. and MacDonald, A. D. (1944). The evaluation of the analgesic action of pethidine hydrochloride (Demerol). *J. Pharmacol. Exp. Ther.*, **80**, 300–7
112. Yeomans, N. D. (1976). Electron microscopic study of the repair of aspirin-induced gastric erosions. *Dig. Dis.*, **21**, 533–41

47
Enzyme induction and inhibition

A. Anadón

The pharmacological effect of a drug is partly dependent upon its concentration at its site of action, which in turn is partly dependent upon its rate of elimination. The rate of elimination of many drugs is governed largely by the rate of metabolism, and, therefore, any change in the activity of the drug-metabolizing enzymes may result in a modification of drug action.

Most drugs are taken orally because of the convenience offered by this route of administration. However, the amount of drug which eventually reaches the target tissue in an active form depends not only upon its physico-chemical characteristics but also upon the extent of metabolism occurring in tissues. Metabolism and excretion before a drug can reach the systemic arterial circulation is referred to as presystemic drug elimination.

Extensive presystemic (first pass) metabolism is of considerable clinical, pharmacological and toxicological importance and can limit the usefulness of certain drugs. Thus, many drugs are normally given by injection because when given orally most are destroyed by presystemic metabolism. The major site of drug metabolism is the liver (endoplasmic reticulum), but other tissues such as the lung, kidney, placenta, skin, white blood cells and the gut especially may play an important role in metabolizing drugs or xenobiotic substances. The rough endoplasmic reticulum of the liver is the main site of protein synthesis, whereas the smooth endoplasmic reticulum is probably the most important site of drug metabolism.

Many drugs and foreign compounds are metabolized by an NADPH-dependent microsomal enzyme system. The terminal oxygenase for this enzyme system is thought to be a carbon monoxide-binding cytochrome P-450. The essential physiological action of the drug-metabolizing enzymes is to convert lipophilic drugs into water-soluble metabolites which are more readily excreted. The rate of elimination of many lipophilic drugs is governed by the activity of the hepatic microsomal P-450 mixed-function oxidases. Any alteration in the activity of these enzymes may result in a modification of drug action. A wide range of biologically and chemically unrelated agents are able to alter the activity of the drug-metabolizing enzymes.

The aim of this paper is to discuss the action of these drug-metabolizing enzymes that can be enhanced by enzyme *induction* (increase in the concentration of a particular enzyme), or reduced by enzyme *inhibition* (direct action on the enzyme).

ENZYME INDUCTION

Enzyme induction involves an adaptive increase in the number of molecules of a specific enzyme in response to an enzyme-inducing agent. Inducers of drug oxidation have several features in common, such as lipophilicity, the ability to bind to cytochrome P-450 enzymes, and relatively long biological halflives. Many drugs share these properties without inducing enzyme synthesis.

Animal studies have shown that inducing agents may be divided into groups according to their activity[11]. The first group, represented by phenobarbitone, is characterized by its ability to stimulate the metabolism of a large number of substrates by various pathways. The second group, typified by 3-methylcholanthrene and 3,4-benzopyrene, stimulates a more limited group of reactions. These inducing agents differ, in their time course, in their intensity of induction, and in the production of either cytochrome P-450 or P-448 within the hepatic endoplasmic reticulum. Steroid compounds constitute a third group. This classification is an oversimplification both in terms of enzyme-inducing agents and the oxygenases, the activity of which they alter. The time for onset and offset of induction depends on the halflife of the enzyme, but significant induction generally occurs over a few days and it passes off over 2 or 3 weeks following withdrawal of the inducer. A pharmacokinetic model has been developed to describe the time course of drug concentrations during induction and after removal of the inducing agent[24].

The inducers, when administered over a few days or more, induce an increase in endoplasmic drug-metabolizing enzyme activity (chiefly *hepatic*, but also extrahepatic) which is accompanied by an increase in amino-acid uptake and in total cell protein. That this induction of enzymes (which are proteins) is due to increased synthesis is suggested by the fact that inhibitors of protein synthesis, e.g. actinomycin D, prevent enzyme induction. A great number of reports suggest the presence of several forms of drug-metabolizing enzymes (cytochrome P-450) in liver microsomes of experimental animals[15,23,25,37]. Marked differences exist in the activities of drug-metabolizing enzymes between species and strains of experimental animals. It has been established that drug-metabolizing activities are changed by pathological and non-physiological states, in experimental animals[21]. The pharmacokinetic studies have indicated significant changes in drug-metabolizing activites caused by endogenous and exogenous factors, such as disease states and drug intake. Thus, the next challenge must be to determine relative changes in the amounts of multiple forms of cytochrome P-450 by these numerous factors, and to determine implications of the presence of multiple forms of cytochrome P-450 in veterinary and human therapy.

The phenomenon of enzyme induction is important also in the lungs, gastrointestinal tract and skin. The *lung* can metabolize chemicals of extrapulmonary origin. These include endogenous substances which may originate in the organism (but outside the lungs) and exogenous chemicals which originate outside the organism. Endogenous compounds generally reach the lungs via the circulation, whereas exogenous ones enter via the inhaled air and/or the circulation. Several classes of exogenous compounds are metabolized by the lungs (polycyclic hydrocarbons: benzo(a)pyrene, benzanthracene; aromatic compounds: benzene, aniline, biphenyl; drugs: aminopyrine, acetophenetidin, ethylmorphine; pesticides: parathion, carbaryl). Many simple aromatic hydrocarbons are liquids with high vapour pressures which may enter the body by inhalation, whilst polycyclic hydrocarbons usually enter the lungs adsorbed to inhaled particles. Insecticides such as parathion are often sprayed and may be inhaled in large amounts by animals and farm workers. The lungs appear to be highly active and versatile in their ability to transform oxidatively both endogenous and exogenous substrates. The oxidative metabolism of exogenous compounds by the lungs has been the subject of several reviews[6, 14, 43]. The major pathway is via the cytochrome P-450-dependent mono-oxygenase system, which basically is similar to that present in the liver[33], and accounts for the enormous metabolic versatility of the lungs. The ratio of the concentrations of cytochrome P-450 in liver and lung microsomes varies from about 3:1 in the rabbit[17, 33], to 10:1 in small rodents[28, 33]. Many xenobiotics are metabolized by the pulmonary cytochrome P-450 system and these reactions are, in general, similar to those found for the hepatic system although, when related to the cytochrome, reaction rates are higher within the pulmonary system. Therefore, xenobiotics may act on pulmonary metabolism as enzyme inducers, repressors, activators or inhibitors.

When drugs metabolizing in the *gastrointestinal tract* enter the gut they are exposed to a number of systems with the potential to modify chemically or to chelate the drug molecules that are not found within the tissues of the host. These include extremes of pH, unabsorbed nutrients and xenobiotics, digestive enzymes and the intestinal microflora.

The intestinal micro-organisms represent a potent, diverse and adaptable metabolizing force that has a large potential for the metabolism of drugs and environmental anutrients. The gut flora consists of a complex, dynamic mixture of aerobic organisms that may show large variations (enterobacteria, lactobacilli, enterococci, bacteroides, clostridia and bifidobacteria). This gut flora may be altered by changes in the diet, by diseases and by the administration of foreign compounds. The gut micro-organisms thus represent an adaptable changing source of metabolic activity that may show large inter- and intra-individual variations in the numbers and types of organisms present. In addition, intestinal transit time and defaecation frequency may affect the duration of exposure of a drug to the gut flora *in vivo* and produce pronounced temporal variations in levels of metabolites. The bacteria of intestinal flora have been shown to be capable of performing a large number of different metabolic reactions, most of which are degradative in some way, i.e. hydrolysis, reduction or removal of functional groups. On the other hand, the use of the various tissue preparations has permitted the recognition of a wide variety of drug metabolism reactions in the gut such as *C*-oxidation, hydroxylation, dealkylation, N- and S-oxidation, desulphuration reduction and hydrolysis, and conjugation reactions.

The enzyme activity in the small intestine is less than that detected in the liver but the ratio of hepatic to small intestinal activity is highly variable.

Such differences in enzyme activity suggest that the metabolic pathways of substrates of these enzymes would be different in the two tissues. The small intestine is exposed to a wide range of anutrients present in the diet and it is well established that 'standard animal diets' contain a number of anutrients known to be inducers of hepatic drug metabolism. This raises the possibility that such compounds maintain a constant state of induction of intestinal drug metabolism. Indeed, starvation or the feeding of an artifical diet depresses intestinal drug oxidation considerably[45]. It is possible therefore that, unlike the liver where drug oxidation is always present, the intestinal drug mono-oxygenases are dependent upon exogenous inducers present in foodstuffs.

It is of interest to note that the degree of induction obtained with 3-methylcholanthrene and other so-called cytochrome P-448-type inducers is generally much higher than can be obtained by the administration of phenobarbitone, a potent inducer of the cytochrome P-450-type. This may reflect a difference between the liver and the gastrointestinal tract in terms of the enzymes normally present and in the genetic control of their synthesis in the presence of inducing agents.

Foodstuffs contain a variety of compounds able to induce microsomal drug oxidation in the gut mucosa. These include naturally occurring anutrient chemicals, such as the various indoles present in plants of the genus brassica and xenobiotics produced from food constituents by cooking procedures. Among the latter are the polycyclic aromatic hydrocarbons produced from steroids in meat when cooked over charcoal[27], which, when taken in the diet, exert a selective inductive effect on the intestinal mucosa. Furthermore, inducers such as cigarette smoke and polycyclic hydrocarbons present in industrial and automobile exhausts may be found in the atmosphere but, due to their particular nature, they are usually taken into the body via the gut rather than the airways[12].

The interspecies differences in intestinal drug metabolism are mostly due to genetic factors, but may also result from chemicals ingested with the food.

The *skin* may play an important role in the metabolism of drugs. Many tissues other than liver possess mixed-function oxygenases necessary for drug oxidation. The induction of enzyme activity in skin has been demonstrated in both human and animal models. Cytochrome P-450-dependent mono-oxygenases catalyse the oxidation of many substances, in particular xenobiotics. This system includes several distinct enzymes, each possessing a characteristic spectrum of substrate specificities. The only member of this group which has been extensively studied in skin is aryl hydrocarbon hydroxylase (AHH)[36]; this latter enzyme has recently attracted attention because of the report of a systemic defect in psoriatic patients[9]. Another mono-oxygenase which is of importance in the degradation of xenobiotics is *O*-dealkylase (ODA) and ODA activity has been investigated in mammalian skin[13]. Induction of cutaneous ODA in mice was achieved by subcutaneous injection of phenobarbitone (PB), hexachlorobenzene (HCB) and 20-methylcholanthrene (MC)[13]. Intraperitoneal administration resulted in a similar induction of hepatic ODA but had no effect on the skin, presumably because of rapid clearance of the agent from the circulation by the liver.

Enzyme inducers may modify *toxicological effects*, both short-term and longterm, produced by foreign compounds. Certain types of drug metabolites, so-called chemically reactive metabolites, may produce a range of toxic drug effects by reacting covalently with essential cellular components.

The enzymes responsible for the bioactivation of drugs to these chemically reactive metabolites are microsomal P-450 mixed-function enzymes, and inhibition or induction of these enzymes by drugs or environmental chemicals could therefore play a key role in determining drug toxicity. A pertinent example of increased drug toxicity is the hepatitis observed as a rare complication of halothane anaesthesia, a risk that is greater with repeated exposure within 28 days[19]. Minor highly reactive metabolites of the drug are probably responsible for the liver damage and hepatotoxicity in animals occurs only after induction of the microsomal enzymes[7].

On the other hand, many enzyme-inducing agents can enhance their own metabolism as well as that of other drugs. When prolonged treatment with a drug results in a decrease of its action, a phenomenon known as *tolerance*, enzyme induction may be suspected, but is not always the cause.

Some therapeutic agents are known enzyme inducers: phenobarbital, halogenated anaesthetics, phenylbutazone, phenytoin, griseofulvin, meprobamate, chlorinated hydrocarbons, chloral hydrate, etc. Phenobarbital increases the rate of biotransformation of barbiturates, warfarin, phenylbutazone, testosterone and progesterone.

Chronic administration of low doses of phenobarbital to dairy cows given DDT for 2 months resulted in a significant decrease in the content of DDT-related substances in the milk[2]. Phenylbutazone increases the rate of biotransformation of corticosteroids; griseofulvin increases the rate of biotransformation of warfarin, etc.

Drug *interactions* are the sequelae attending the simultaneous use of two or more drugs. The consequences of enzyme induction for the animal depend upon the relative activity of a drug and its metabolites. The induction of microsomal enzymes by the concomitant use of another drug may lead to increased pharmacological effects, or even toxicity caused by the active metabolites.

Although some substances, such as polycyclic hydrocarbons, which cause enzyme induction, are carcinogens, there is no evidence that the two properties are related. Nonetheless, the possible relationship between enzyme induction and *carcinogenesis* is intriguing. It has long been known that, in experimental animals, administration of polycyclic hydrocarbons, such as 3-methylcholanthrene, can reduce the carcinogenic effect of such compounds as 3-methyl-4-dimethylaminoazobenzene or 2-acetylaminofluorene. Also, substances such as carbon tetrachloride, dimethylnitrosamine and the polycyclic hydrocarbons, are metabolized by microsomes to substances that are probably active carcinogens. Tumours may also appear long after exposure to the carcinogenic agent has ceased. Up to the present, there has been little study of enzyme induction by drugs in relation to carcinogenesis. However, recent work has indicated that enzyme-inducing agents may influence both the initiation and promotion of experimentally-induced carcinogenesis[35]. In mice, certain enzyme-inducing compounds, including dieldrin and DDT, griseofulvin and phenobarbitone, have been found to increase the incidence of hepatic neoplasias. Such an effect has not been found in other species including dogs, rats and monkeys.

With respect to skin metabolism as a determinant of local toxicity, it is known that microsomal mono-oxygenases are capable of metabolizing a wide variety of compounds to reactive, electrophilic intermediates which bind themselves to macromolecules within cells. This process may be important in determining antigenicity, cytotoxicity and carcinogenicity. Skin lesions are one of the most common adverse reactions to drugs and some probably have an immunological basis. In both animals and man the topical application of a variety of polycyclic hydrocarbons produces skin cancers. The carcinogenicity of this diverse group of chemical substances appears to be determined by activation yielding electrophilic metabolites[41]. The carcinogenicity of benzo(a)pyrene appears to be mediated by benzo(a)pyrene-7,8-diol-9,10 epoxide[42]. Recently, the molecular properties and biological functions of microsomal epoxide hydrase have been reviewed[29]. The epoxide hydrase plays a central role in both the activation of mutagenic and carcinogenic metabolites of polycyclic aromatic hydrocarbons as well as in the activation of these metabolites to more toxic compounds. Studies in animals indicate that polycyclic hydrocarbons act as co-carcinogens with ultraviolet light, and it is therefore possible that aryl hydrocarbon hydroxylase and epoxide hydratase play a much wider role than supposed in the pathogenesis of skin cancer. Such an hypothesis would be supported in psoriasis[40].

ENZYME INHIBITION

Variously termed *Kcat inhibitors*, *suicide enzyme inactivators*, and *enzyme-activated irreversible inhibitors*, and *suicide enzyme inhibitors* represent a relatively new approach to specific irreversible inactivation of enzymes. Simply stated, this approach requires that the inhibitor contains a latent reactive grouping and be accepted as a substrate by the target enzyme, following which the normal catalytic activity of the enzyme results in its own irreversible inactivation or 'suicide'.

In vitro, an inhibitor is identified as acting by a suicide mechanism when (1) loss of enzyme activity on incubation with inhibitors which is a time-dependent first-order process, (2) protection by substrate against inactivation is induced by the inhibitor, and (3) irreversible enzyme inhibition shown by techniques such as dialysis and gel filtration. *In vivo*, the desirable consequences of suicide enzyme inhibition in animals are: specificity and a generally long duration of effect. Even when the inhibitor is no longer present, synthesis of new enzyme is required for reversal of the effect. Two points of view are seen about the clinical value of enzyme inhibitors: enzyme inhibitors as potential drugs, and as causing side-effects or drug interactions.

Among enzyme inhibitors currently used in therapy, are monoamine oxidase inhibitors containing an acetylenic moiety. For example, pargyline hydrochloride and the xantine oxidase inhibitor allopurinol, act on their target enzymes by an 'activation' or 'suicide' mechanism. Thus, they may also be considered as pro-drugs. It is a surprising fact that many current drugs exert their therapeutic actions by inhibition of specific enzymes. These range from non-steroidal anti-inflammatory drugs acting on prostaglandin synthetase, to β-lactam antibiotics that inhibit bacterial cell wall transpeptidases, although most of these drugs were discovered on a basis other than biochemical mechanism of action.

The enzyme inhibitor approach to discovery of new drugs may appear rational and predictable; it is not necessarily so in practice. The area of GABA-transaminase (GABA-T) inhibition is very interesting because of the presumed importance of GABA in several functional brain disorders. In the area of ornithine decarboxylase (ODC) inhibition, there are too many types of biological activity resulting from this ODC inhibition. Researchers are in the process of sorting out which of these, if any, is useful. Ornithine decarboxylase (ODC) is a key enzyme in the biosynthesis of the polyamines that exist in all living cells, and play important roles in processes for enhanced cellular growth and replication[8].

One of the more potent of these synthetic inhibitors, DL-α-difluoromethylornithine (DFMO) has inhibitory effects: on experimental tumours, on growth of the prostate gland, on embryogenesis, and on rapidly proliferating non-mammalian cells (parasitic protozoa). Polyamine metabolism had been suggested as a target in the chemotherapy of parasitic disease[10] and specifically against trypanosomes[4]. *Trypanosoma brucei brucei* causes trypanosomiasis in cattle. It seems reasonable to conclude that the ODC inhibition may be a potential therapy for selected protozoal infections. In this field of suicide enzyme inhibitors as potential drugs, it may still be impossible to conceptualize and synthetize a potent specific inhibitor. The chances seem better with enzymes whose mechanisms of action are well defined.

With respect to suicide enzyme inhibitors as causing side-effects or drug interactions: isoniazid impairs microsomal drug-metabolizing capacity and can lead to reduced clearance and elevated plasma levels of other drugs[46]. Phenytoin toxicity is described as a consequence of the use of phenytoin with isoniazid. Rifampicin, on the other hand, stimulates microsomal enzyme activity and may increase clearance of other drugs[34]. The kinetic effect of isoniazid, ethambutol and rifampicin has been assessed on metabolic disposition of diazepam[32]. Short-term administration of the antibiotic rifampicin, a potent enzyme inducer, produces a consistent fall in plasma 25-hydroxy-cholecalciferol (25-OHD), accompanied by increased oxidation of antipyrine and 6β-hydroxycortisol, indicative of hepatic enzyme induction. Since isoniazid is often given with rifampicin for periods up to 1 year the effects of isoniazid on vitamin D metabolism and hepatic monooxygenase activity have been studied[5]. Isoniazid reduced serum calcium and phosphate levels, and also 1α-25 hydroxyvitamin D, the most active metabolite of vitamin D. Isoniazid inhibited hepatic mixed-function oxidase activity, as evidenced by a reduction in antipyrine and cortisol oxidation, and a similar inhibition of the hepatic 25-hydroxylase and renal 1α-hydroxylase would explain the reduction in the corresponding vitamin D metabolites. Thus, both isoniazid and rifampicin interfere with vitamin D metabolism in different ways and the combination may well be synergistic and have important clinical consequences.

The therapeutic problems associated with enzyme inhibition have received much less attention than those associated with enzyme induction. Interactions with the oral hypoglycaemic agent tolbutamide have resulted in hypoglycaemic crises from the administration of chloramphenicol, sulphaphenazole, dicoumarol, phenylbutazone and phenyramidol to patients stabilized on tolbutamide[16]. In each case there was clear evidence for reduced tolbutamide elimination.

Despite the general lack of specificity associated with the drug-metabolizing systems, drug interactions can be subtle and complex. Co-administration of phenylbutazone produced an augmented anticoagulant effect without altering the apparent plasma concentrations of warfarin. Since the *S* isomer is five times more potent an anticoagulant than *R* warfarin, it was concluded that inhibition of the metabolism of *S* warfarin provides one mechanism for the augmented anticoagulation which follows phenylbutazone treatment[26]. Administration of the H_2-antagonist cimetidine may enhance the anticoagulant action of warfarin[39] by inhibition of the microsomal drug-metabolizing enzymes[38]. Imidazole derivates, such as cimetidine, are thought to be potent inhibitors of P-450 enzymes because they can bind to both the oxygen and the substrate binding sites of the enzymes[47].

Drugs may alter the pharmacological action of the other drugs by inhibiting non-microsomal pathways of metabolism.

Disulphuram, used to treat chronic alcoholism, acts by inhibiting the enzyme aldehyde dehydrogenase which is involved in the conversion of ethanol into acetic acid. Allopurinol has been shown to increase both the toxic and therapeutic actions of 6-mercaptopurine *in vivo*.

Furazolidone is widely used in the prevention and treatment of bacterial and protozoal diseases in poultry. At slightly above the therapeutic level the drug inhibits growth, produces anaemia and arrests spermatogenesis in the chicken and may also produce cardiac dilatation and ascites.

The addition of furazolidone to the feed at the therapeutic level inhibits monoamine oxidase activity in chicken duodenal mucosa, heart, and brain, but in the liver the enzyme activity is unaffected by the treatment[3].

At present it is difficult to assess the prevalence of drug toxicity caused by drug accumulation from enzyme inhibition. Drugs that inhibit microsomal enzyme activity in animals include organophosphorous insecticides, pesticide synergics of the methylenedioxyphenyl type (e.g. piperonyl butoxide), quinidine, carbon tetrachloride and chloramphenicol. Intravenous chloramphenicol increases duration of immediately subsequent pentobarbitone anaesthesia by 120% in dogs and 260% in cats[1]. The effect has been shown after administration by oral, intramuscular or intravenous routes and was detectable for up to 24 days after the last dose[44]. Potentiation has also been identified between anaesthetics and aminoglycoside antibiotics. Compounds that inhibit drug-metabolizing enzymes in liver microsomes impair the metabolism of endogenous steroids. Propranolol and metoprolol can inhibit drug metabolism in animals, and the effect of propranolol, the more lipid-soluble agents, is greater than that of metoprolol.

One of the problems in assessing whether or not a drug is an inhibitor of metabolism is that chronic administration of some competitive inhibitors, such as SKF 525-A and piperonyl butoxide produce enzyme induction in animals. Such behaviour may explain why conflicting data are sometimes obtained concerning whether a drug is an inhibitor or an inducer.

FACTORS AFFECTING DRUG METABOLISM

Many factors such as genetic, environmental differences, age, sex, disease, nutritional status, etc. influence drug metabolism and can alter rates of drug elimination (Figure 47.1).

While most clinical pharmacologists recognize the crucial role played by a few factors such as age, certain disease states, and concomitant administration of various drugs, other factors such as genetic constitution, diet, and environmental exposures to chemicals are much less appreciated and insufficiently described.

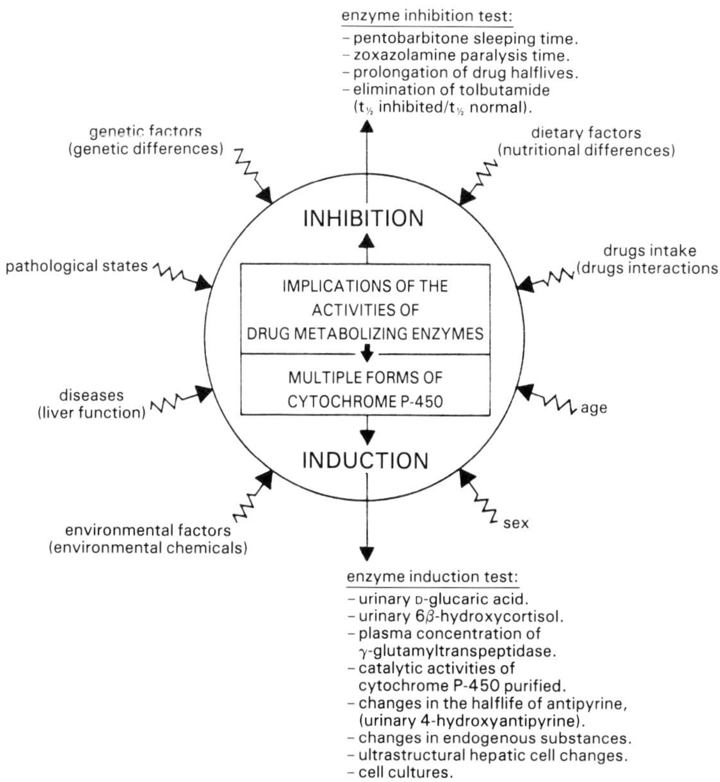

Figure 47.1 Factors affecting drug metabolism

Genetic factors play a prominent role in the determination of an animal's capacity to metabolize certain drugs, but numerous host factors can alter this capacity. They are primarily responsible for controlling the extent to which hepatic drug-metabolizing enzymes are induced in different subjects[7]. A given dose of inducer may induce one enzyme more than another. This type of phenomenon has been seen, comparing the induction of aflatoxin B_1 and B_2 metabolism.

Dietary factors may modify pharmacological and toxicological actions. These modifications concern mostly the nutritional influences on the hepatic drug-metabolizing enzyme system. The main factors important in this sense are simply starvation or deficiencies in macronutrients (carbohydrates, lipids, etc.) or micronutrients (vitamins, minerals) as well as the possible effects of food additives, or certain procedures of preparing food. These factors tend to influence the hepatic microsomal cytochrome P-450 and its catalytic action. Starvation produces rather complex effects on the oxidative drug-metabolizing system which are complicated by a certain sex and species dependency.

Much better known are the effects of artificially unbalanced diets on the drug-metabolizing enzymes. It has been shown that unsaturated fatty acids possess a 'permissive' effect on the endoplasmic reticulum allowing a maximal induction by phenobarbitone only if they are present in the diet. Protein content and quality of the diet seem to be important factors in assessing the influence of macronutrients on toxic manifestations. Protein deficiency has been shown to reduce cytochrome P-450 and microsomal reaction rates for a number of substrates, mostly drugs whose metabolism depends on hydroxylation reactions. Lack of dietary vitamins in general depresses the mono-oxygenase activity and, thus, tends to increase the action of toxicants that are normally detoxified in the liver. Only riboflavin seems to be an obvious requirement for optimal activity since it is an essential component of the cytochrome P-450 reductase. Mineral trace elements are difficult to assess with regard to their influences on the microsomal mixed-function oxidase. Selenium deficiency would lead to a decrease in removal of harmful peroxidases such as those formed in lung tissues, after the ingestion of the dipyridilium herbicide paraquat.

It is conceivable that food additives such as preservatives, antioxidants, flavours, etc., might induce changes that result in altered response to drugs, toxic agents or carcinogens. Antioxidants, within a certain concentration range, are capable of altering the hepatic mono-oxygenase activity by enzyme induction. Butylated hydroxytoluene (BHT) and ethoxyquin increase cytochrome P-450 and the metabolic reactions it catalyses.

The antioxidants can also increase activation of carcinogens (benzopyrene) or accelerate also the detoxification of primary toxicants. However, the inducing doses are several orders of magnitude greater than those ordinarily incorporated.

Many substances are not toxic *per se*, but require metabolic activation by the cytochrome P-450 oxidase enzyme system in the liver microsomes to exert a toxic effect. An increase in the activity of this enzyme system is caused by a variety of chemicals. As more sophisticated techniques for separating forms

Table 47.1 Xenobiotics that stimulate their own metabolism and/or induce unique forms of P-450

Benzo(a)pyrene	Ellipticine
3-Methylcholanthrene	Ethanol
Benzo(a)anthracine	Isosafrole
7,12-Demethylbenzo(a)anthracene	Piperonyl butoxide
Phenobarbital	Ethinyloestradiol
Phenylbutazone	2-Acetylaminofluorene
Aminopyrine	Polybrominated biphenyls
Citrus red dye No. 2	Styrene
Chlorpromazine	trans-Stilbene oxide
Meprobamate	Chlorinated antibacterials
Tolbutamide	TCDD
Hexobarbital	Rifampicin
Pentobarbital	Terpenes and sesquiterpenes
Glutethimide	Lindane
Chlorcyclizine	Isoniazid
Probenecide	α-Pinene
p,p′-DDT	Polychlorinated biphenyls
Chlordiazepoxide	Theophylline
Benzene	Halogenated naphthalenes and terphenyls
Methoxyflurane	Synthetic pyrethroids
Phenytoin	Acetone
Caffeine	Cholestyramine
Pregnenolone-16α-carbonitrile	Carbamazepine 10,11-oxide
Alkanes	Camphor
Volatile deodorants	Cyclohexane
Kepone	Dibromochloropropane
Mirex	Clofibrate
Methadone	Toluene
Griseofulvin	Medroxyprogesterone
Methylated benzenes and naphtalenes	Propanol-2
Ethoxyquin	Pyrazole

of P-450 and for assaying an increased number of mono-oxygenase activities have become available, an increasing number of inducing compounds appear to be neither precisely 3-methylcholanthrene-like nor precisely phenobarbitone-like. Of these xenobiotic inducers have been reported (Table 47.1)[30].

Halogenated aromatic compounds, such as 2,3,7,8-tetrachlorodibenzo-*p*-dioxin (TCDD), polychlorinated biphenyls (PCB) and polybrominated biphenyls (PBB) have become major environmental contaminants. Residues from the use of PCB are now widely distributed in animals associated with polluted waters. Dietary exposure to PBB results in a variety of toxic manifestations in animals: cows exhibited toxic signs including anorexia, decreased milk production, and increased frequency of urination[20]. Interstitial nephritis and gross pathological changes including renal and hepatic degeneration, and haematomas and abcesses in the peritoneal and thoracic cavities were also observed in these animals[20].

Polychlorinated paraffins (CPs) and polychlorinated terphenyls (PTCs) are commonly used as PCB substitutes because of their suitable chemical and physical properties. A widespread distribution can be assumed because of the extensive use of CPs in lubricant and cutting oils, paint, rubber and plastics[18].

The resistance of PCTs and CPs towards degradation, their tendency to accumulate in fish and mammals, the suspected carcinogenicity of PCT and possible synergistic effects with other environmental contaminants, make an uncontrolled industrial use of these substances questionable, although it has been indicated that they are less potent than the PCBs with respect to several effects on the liver[22, 31]. However, it has been shown that PCT is a mixed type of rat liver microsomal cytochrome P-450 inducer[31].

The demonstrated effects of the wide-spread industrial chemicals on the multiple forms of cytochrome P-450 make it highly relevant to perform a further investigation of environmental substances, both with respect to their potential toxicity and their effects on liver microsomal cytochrome P-450.

METHODS OF ASSESSING ENZYME INDUCTION AND INHIBITION

The assessments are based on the effects of inducing agents on the enzymes of the endoplasmic reticulum, the increased turnover of some endogenous substances, and foreign compounds. The induction is usually deduced from an increased rate in the production of drug metabolites in association with the administration of a drug which has been shown to be an inducing agent in animals. The absence of change in the apparent volume of distribution of either the parent drug or its metabolites is essential for assessment.

Theoretically, direct measurement of enzyme activity in liver biopsy samples from domestic animals, before and after administration of the putative inducer, would be the ideal method. Less direct indexes of enzyme induction have been used, such as changes in the pharmacokinetics of a marker drug like antipyrine (antipyrine halflife). Hexobarbitone is often used in animal studies for assessing enzyme induction and is therefore useful for comparative studies. The activity of the drug-metabolizing systems can also be monitored *in vivo* by determination of pentobarbitone sleeping time and zoxazolamine paralysis time. Hexobarbitone and tolbutamide have also been used as drugs, because both are metabolized completely in the liver by microsomal enzymes[48].

As has been shown, following administration of enzyme-inducing agents, there are some considerable physiological changes. Some of these changes afford an increased rate of drug metabolism, others stem from the effect of increased microsomal enzyme activity on endogenous compounds. These physiological changes are liver weight, bile flow, bilirubin, corticosteroid, sex-hormone, vitamin-D and folate metabolisms, etc. Normally standard biochemical liver function tests (bilirubin, aspartate transaminase, alkaline phosphatase and albumin), serum calcium and phosphate, 25-hydroxy-cholecalciferol (25-OHD), 1α-25 hydroxyvitamin D (1,25$(OH)_2$D) levels are estimated as indexes involving enzyme induction.

For studies of assessing gut metabolism *in vivo*, isolated *in situ* intestinal loop preparations have been used. Usually, these preparations are undertaken in anaesthetized animals, and in most studies a loop of jejunum is used because of its good blood supply and high enzyme activity. Drug is introduced into the lumen and venous blood from the loops is collected via a catheter. Parent drug and metabolites in the effluent can then be quantified by specific methods of assay. This method gives not only qualitative information on metabolite patterns, but also some indication of the effect of either physiological or pharmacological interference with *in vivo* metabolism in the gut wall.

References

1. Adams, H. R. and Dixit, B. N. (1970). Prolongation of pentobarbital anaesthesia by chloramphenicol in dogs and cats. *J. Am. Vet. Assoc.*, **156**, 902–5
2. Alary, J. G., Guay, P. and Brodeur, J. (1971). Effect of phenobarbital pretreatment on the metabolism of DDT in the rat and the bovine. *Toxicol. Appl. Pharmacol.*, **18**, 457–68
3. Ali, B. H. and Bartlet, A. L. (1980). Inhibition of monoamine oxidase by furazolidone in the chicken and the influence of the alimentary flora thereon. *Br. J. Pharmacol.*, **71**, 219–24
4. Bacchi, C. J., Hutner, S. H., Lambros, C. *et al.* (1978). Polyamine function in trypanosomatids: activation of cytoplasmic-glycerophosphate dehydrogenase by cationic trypanocides. In Campbell, R. A. *et al.* (eds.) *Advances in Polyamine Research*. Vol. 2, pp. 129–38. (New York: Raven Press)
5. Brodie, M. J., Boobis, A. R., Hillyard, C. J. *et al.* (1981). Effect of isoniazid on vitamin D metabolism and hepatic monooxygenase activity. *Clin. Pharmacol. Ther.*, **30**, 363–7
6. Brown, E. A. B. (1974). The localization, metabolism and effects of drugs and toxicants in lungs. *Drug Metab. Rev.*, **3**, 33–87
7. Brown, B. R. and Sipes, I. G. (1977). Biotransformation and hepatotoxicity of halothane. *Biochem. Pharmacol.*, **26**, 2091–4
8. Campbell, R. A., Morris, D. R., Bartos, D. *et al.* (1978). *Advances in Polyamine Research*. Vol. 1 & 2. (New York: Raven Press)
9. Chapman, P. H., Kersey, P. J., Keys, B. *et al.* (1980). Generalised tissue abnormality of aryl hydrocarbon hydroxylase in psoriasis. *Br. Med. J.*, **281**, 1315–16
10. Cohen, S. S. (1979). Comparative biochemistry and drug design for infectious disease. *Science*, **205**, 964–71
11. Conney, A. H. (1967). Pharmacological implications of microsomal enzyme induction. *Pharmacol. Rev.*, **19**, 317–56
12. Conney, A. H., Pantuck, E. J., Pantuck, C. B. *et al.* (1978). Role of environment and diet in the regulation of human drug metabolism. In Estabrook, R. F. and Lindenlamb, E. (eds.) *The Induction of Drug Metabolism (Symposia Medica Hoechst 14)*. pp. 583–605. (Stuttgart and New York: F. K. Schattaner Verlag)
13. Damen, F. J. M. and Mier, P. D. (1982). Cytochrome P-450 dependent O-dealkylase activity in mammalian skin. *Br. J. Pharmacol.*, **75**, 123–7
14. Gram, T. E. (1980). The metabolism of xenobiotics by mammalian lung. In Gram, T. E. (ed.) *Extrahepatic Metabolism of Drugs and Other Foreign Compounds*. pp. 159–93. (New York: Spectrum Publ.)
15. Guengerich, F. P. (1979). Isolation and purification of cytochrome P-450, and the existence of multiple forms. *Pharmacol. Ther.*, **6**, 99–121
16. Hansen, J. M. and Christensen, L. K. (1977). Drug interactions with oral sulpharylurea hypoglycaemic drugs. *Drugs*, **13**, 24–34
17. Hook, G. E. R., Bend, J. R., Hoel, D. *et al.* (1972). Preparation of lung microsomes and a comparison of the distribution of enzymes between subcellular fractions of rabbit lung and liver. *J. Pharmacol. Exp. Ther.*, **182**, 474–90
18. Howard, P. M., Santodonato, J. and Saxena, J. (1975). *Investigation of Selected Potential Environmental Contaminants:* chlorinated paraffins. EPA-560/2-75-007, p. 122. (Washington: Office of Toxic Substances USA Environmental Protection Agency)
19. Inman, W. H. W. and Mushin, W. W. (1978). Jaundice after repeated exposures to halothane: a further analysis of reports to the committee on safety of medicines. *Br. Med. J.*, **2**, 1455–6

20. Jackson, T. F. and Halbert, M. S. (1974). A toxic syndrome associated with the feeding of polybrominated biphenyls contaminated protein concentrate to dairy cattle. *J. Am. Vet. Med. Assoc.*, **65**, 437–9
21. Kato, R. (1977). Drug metabolism under pathological and abnormal physiological states in animals and man. *Xenobiotics*, **7**, 25–92
22. Kimbrough, R. D. (1974). The toxicity of polychlorinated polycyclic compounds and related chemicals. *Crit. Rev. Toxicol.*, **2**, 445–98
23. Kuntzman, R., Lu, A. Y. H., West, S. *et al.* (1971). The importance of cytochrome P-450 and P-448 in determining the specificity of the reconstituted liver microsomal hydroxylation. *Chem. Biol. Interactions*, **3**, 287–8
24. Lai, A. A., Levy, R. H. and Cutler, R. E. (1978). Time-course of interaction between carbamazepine and clonazepam in normal man. *Clin. Pharmacol. Ther.*, **24**, 316–23
25. Lewin, W. (1977). Purification of liver microsomal cytochrome P-450: hopes and promises. In Ullrich, V. *et al.* (eds.) *Microsomes and Drug Oxidations*. pp. 735–47. (New York: Pergamon Press)
26. Lewis, R. J., Trager, W. F., Chan, K. K. *et al.* (1974). Warfarin, stereochemical aspects of its metabolism and the interaction with phenylbutazone. *J. Clin. Invest.*, **53**, 1607–17
27. Lijinsky, W. and Greenblatt, M. (1972). Carcinogen dimethylnitrosamine production *in vivo* from nitrite and aminopyrine. *Nature (New Biol.)*, **236**, 177–8
28. Litterst, C. L., Mimnaugh, E. G., Reagan, R. L. *et al.* (1975). Comparison of *in vitro* drug metabolism by lung, liver, kidney of several common laboratory species. *Drug Metab. Disposition*, **3**, 259–65
29. Lu, A. Y. H. and Miwa, G. T. (1980). Molecular properties and biological functions of microsomal epoxide hydrase. *Ann. Rev. Pharmacol. Toxicol.*, **20**, 513–31
30. Nebert, D. W., Eisen, H. J., Negishi, M. *et al.* (1981). Genetic mechanisms controlling the induction of polysubstrate monooxygenase (P-450) activities. *Ann. Rev. Pharmacol. Toxicol.*, **21**, 431–62
31. Nilsen, O. G. and Toftgard, R. (1981). Effects of polychlorinated terphenyls and paraffins on rat liver microsomal cytochrome P-450 and *in vitro* metabolic activities. *Arch. Toxicol.*, **47**, 1–11
32. Ochs, R. H., Greenblatt, D. J., Roberts, G. M. *et al.* (1981). Diazepam interaction with antituberculosis drug. *Clin. Pharmacol. Ther.*, **29**, 671–8
33. Oppelt, W. W., Zange, M., Ross, W. E. *et al.* (1970). Comparison of microsomal drug hydroxylation in lung and liver of various species. *Res. Commun. Chem. Pathol. Pharmacol.*, **1**, 43–56
34. Pessayre, D. and Mazel, P. (1976). Induction and inhibition of hepatic drug metabolizing enzymes by rifampicin. *Biochem. Pharmacol.*, **25**, 943–9
35. Pitot, H. C. (1979). In Estabrook, R. F. and Lindenlamb, E. (eds.) *The Induction of Drug Metabolism (Symposia Medica Hoechst 14)*, pp. 472–83. (Stuttgart and New York: F. K. Schattaner Verlag)
36. Pohl, R. J., Philpot, R. M. and Fouts, J. R. (1976). Cytochrome P-450 content and mixed function oxidase activity in microsomes isolated from mouse skin. *Drug Metab. Dis.*, **4**, 442–50
37. Ryan, D., Lu, A. Y. H., Kawalek, J. *et al.* (1975). Highly purified cytochrome P-448 and P-450 from rat liver microsomes. *Biochem. Biophys. Res. Commun.*, **64**, 1134–41
38. Serlin, M. J., Challiner, M., Park, B. K. *et al.* (1980). Cimetidine potentiates the anticoagulant effect of warfarin by inhibition of drug metabolism. *Biochem. Pharmacol.*, **29**, 1971–2
39. Serlin, M. J., Sibeon, R. G., Mossman, S. *et al.* (1979). Cimetidine: interaction with oral anticoagulants. *Lancet*, **2**, 317–19
40. Shuster, S., Chapman, P. H. and Rawlins, M. D. (1979). Psoriasis and skin cancer. *Br. Med. J.*, **2**, 941–2
41. Sims, P. and Grover, P. L. (1974). Epoxides in polycyclic aromatic hydrocarbon metabolism and carcinogenesis. *Adv. Cancer Res.*, **20**, 164–74
42. Sims, P., Grover, P. L., Swaisland, A. *et al.* (1974). Metabolic activation of benzo(a)pyrene proceeds by a diol-epoxide. *Nature (London)*, **252**, 326–8
43. Smith, B. R. and Bend, J. R. (1981). Metabolic interactions of hydrocarbons with mammalian lung. *Rev. Biochem. Toxicol.*, **3**, 77–122

44. Teske, R. H. and Carter, G. G. (1971). Effect of chloramphenicol on pentobarbital induced anaesthesia in dogs. *J. Am. Vet. Med. Assoc.*, **159**, 777–80
45. Watterberg, L. W. (1972). Dietary modification of intestinal and pulmonary aryl hydrocarbon hydroxylase activity. *Toxicol. Appl. Pharmacol.*, **23**, 741–8
46. Weber, W. W. and Hein, O. W. (1979). Clinical pharmacokinetics of isoniazid. *Clin. Pharmacokinet.*, **4**, 401–22
47. Wilkinson, C. F., Hetnarski, K. and Hicks, L. J. (1974). Substituted imidazoles as inhibitors of microsomal oxidation and insecticide synergists. *Pesticide Biochem. Physiol.*, **4**, 299–312
48. Zilly, W., Breimer, D. D. and Reichter, E. (1975). Induction of drug metabolism in man after rifampicin treatment measured by increased hexobarbital and tolbutamide clearance. *Eur. J. Clin. Pharmacol.*, **9**, 219–27

48
Rapid induction of cirrhosis in the liver. A model of hepatic disease

A. A. Seawright, J. S. Lee and J. Hrdlicka

In man the most important cirrhogenic agents are infectious organisms (hepatitis virus) and dietary abnormalities (regular high alcohol intake); hepatotoxins are occasionally responsible for the condition[6]. In domestic animals the hepatotoxins are certainly the main cause of the disorder. The general characteristics of cirrhosis, i.e. loss of hepatic parenchyma, development of fibrosis and bizarre distortions of normal architecture, can readily be produced in experimental animals with a variety of chemical compounds and the resultant hepatic lesions closely resemble naturally occurring forms of cirrhosis in man and domestic animals[6, 23]. Accordingly, such laboratory animal hepatotoxicity models continue to have extensive use in experimental investigations of this condition.

One of the main problems associated with the production of a cirrhosis model by the use of hepatotoxic agents is that many weeks or months of dosing are usually required to achieve the desired effects, and the yield of cirrhotic livers is often unacceptably low[2, 10]. In addition, a high proportion of the test animals may die from intercurrent disease during such a prolonged dosing period.

Most of these difficulties in producing a reliable disease model in the rat were overcome[15] by the use of simultaneous dosing with phenobarbitone and carbon tetrachloride (CCl_4). With this procedure, cirrhosis develops in 4 weeks and the yield of cirrhotic livers can be high. CCl_4 has its necrogenic action preferentially on the centrolobular hepatic parenchyma, subsequently giving rise to annular patterns of fibrosis linking up the central veins, and eventually cirrhosis. Ngaione (Figure 48.1), a furanosesquiterpenoid essential oil isolated from Australasian myoporaceous plants, has its injurious action rather on the periportal hepatocytes (Figure 48.2) after pretreatment of the animal with phenobarbitone[9, 18]. It could well be that experimental conditions are desired that require the initiation of hepatic fibrogenesis leading eventually to cirrhosis, other than around the central veins. Accordingly, the present cirrhosis model, which can be produced equally rapidly[15], is proposed as a similarly satisfactory or even more desirable alternative procedure where appropriate.

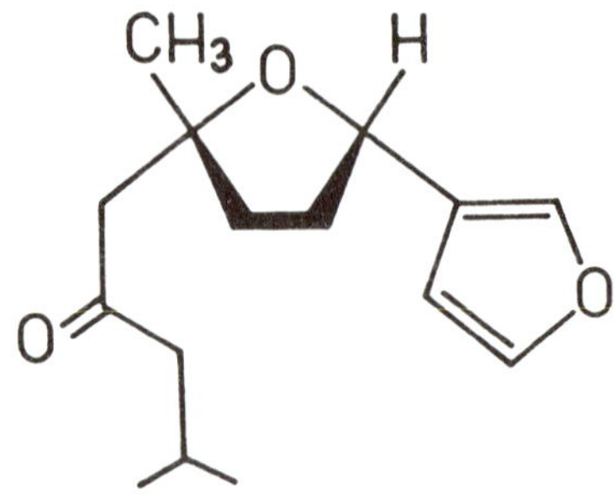

(–)-Ngaione

Figure 48.1 The furanosesquiterpenoid essential oil (–)-ngaione found in Australasian myoporaceous plants

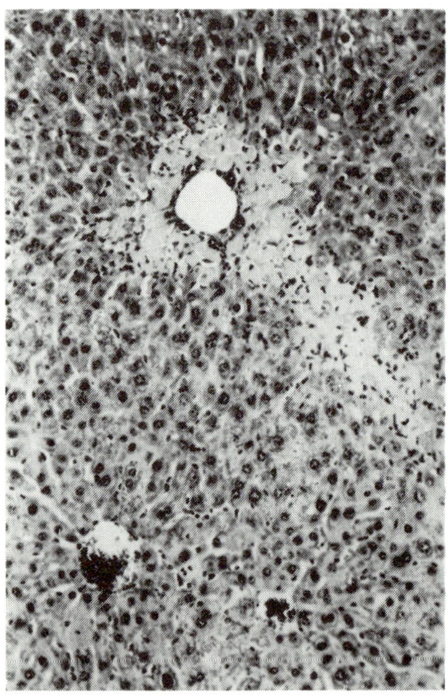

Figure 48.2 Periportal parenchymal injury in the liver due to a single i.p. necrogenic dose (200 mg/kg) of ngaione after pretreatment of the animal with phenobarbitone. H & E ×77

EXPERIMENTAL PROCEDURE

Ngaione was prepared from the fresh leaves of *Myoporum deserti* by steam distillation followed by fractionation[7]. Young male Wistar rats weighing from 100 to 115 g were used. These were kept together in meshed wire cages, fed a proprietary cubed rodent diet, and given tap water *ad libitum*.

The rats were given drinking water containing sodium phenobarbitone at 1 g/l beginning 1 week before daily dosing with ngaione dissolved in arachid oil by the intraperitoneal route beginning at 50 mg/kg, and increasing weekly by 50% until in the fifth week of ngaione dosing, the dose rate of the oil was 255 mg/kg.

At least two of the experimental rats were killed by exsanguination from the carotid artery and jugular vein under light ether anaesthesia before phenobarbitone pretreatment, after a week of phenobarbitone drinking water, and before the start of ngaione dosing, and after each of the successive weeks of ngaione dosing, in order to study the changes taking place in the liver.

PROGRESSIVE CHANGES IN THE LIVER

The rats were apparently normal and grew as well as undosed animals of this strain for the first 3 weeks of the trial. During the fourth week rate of body weight gain was reduced and during the fifth week the animals actually lost weight.

The livers were observed to be pale and swollen after each of the first 3 weeks of dosing. After 4 weeks there were copious amounts of clear yellow serous fluid in the peritoneal cavity and the livers were pale, swollen, of firm

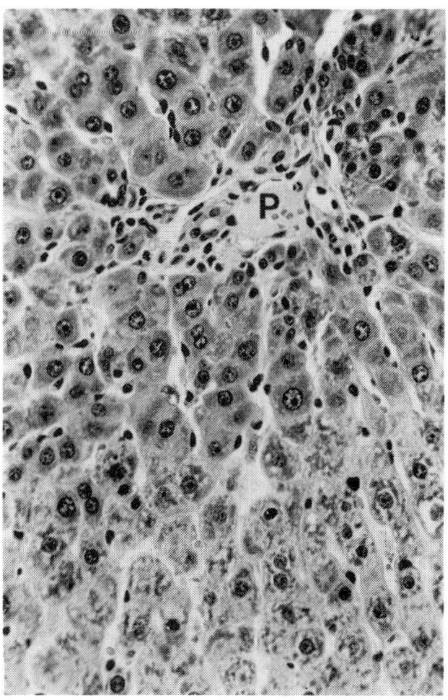

Figure 48.3 The liver of a phenobarbitone-pretreated rat dosed i.p. with 50 mg/kg ngaione for 1 week showing a slight increase in portal connective tissue and mononuclear inflammatory cell infiltration. P = portal vein. H & E ×220

consistency with the surface having a finely granulated appearance suggestive of the early stage of cirrhosis.

Histologically, the livers of the rats before phenobarbitone pretreatment were normal. After a week on phenobarbitone drinking water, there was an enhancement of the size of the hepatocytes of the centrolobular zone due to increased amounts of homogeneously pink-staining cytoplasm. The cells surrounding the portal tracts were slightly smaller than normal and their cytoplasm stained more basically than that of the centrolobular parenchymal cells. The cytoplasm of the centrolobular hepatocytes also contained sporadic vacuoles due to mild fatty infiltration.

After 1 week of ngaione dosing at 50 mg/kg there was no significant alteration to the parenchymal cells except for sporadic nuclear enlargement and occasional mitotic figures. There was however, at this stage, a slight increase in the amount of connective tissue and in the numbers of mononuclear inflammatory cells in the smallest portal tracts (Figure 48.3).

After 2 weeks of ngaione there was sporadic shrinkage necrosis of many of the darkly staining hepatocytes in the periportal zone with mild proliferation of fibroblasts in the smallest portal tracts, spreading out to enclose small groups of hepatocytes to give the appearance of early pseudolobulation. Centrolobular hepatocytes appeared unaffected (Figure 48.4).

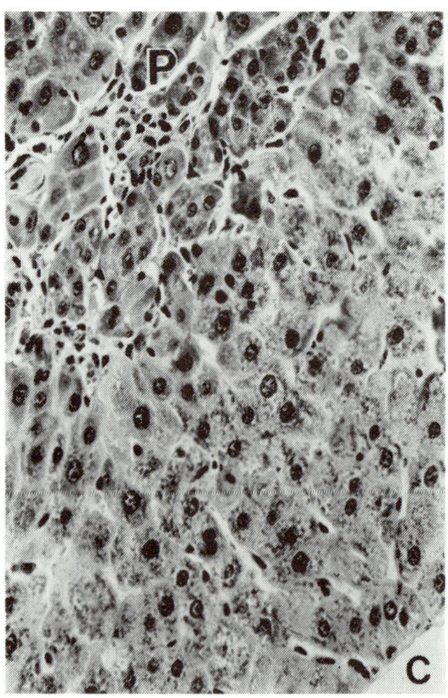

Figure 48.4 The liver of a phenobarbitone-pretreated rat dosed with ngaione at 50 mg/kg daily for the first week followed by 75 mg/kg daily for the second week, showing sporadic necrosis of periportal hepatocytes and mild fibrogenesis with the beginning of separation of periportal from centrolobular parenchyma. P = portal area, C = central vein. H & E × 220

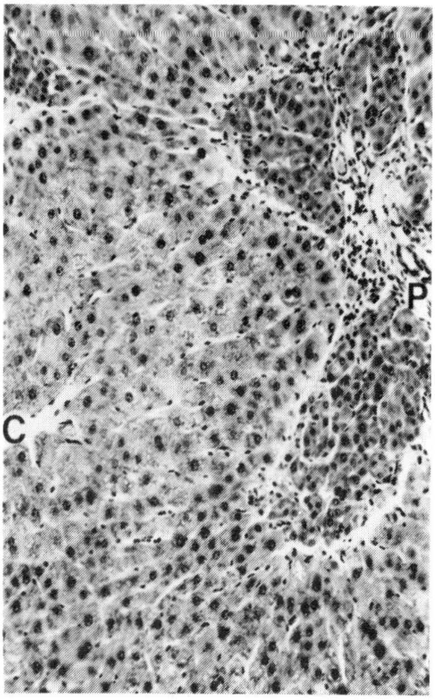

Figure 48.5 The liver of a phenobarbitone-pretreated rat dosed daily with ngaione at 50 mg/kg for the first week, 75 mg/kg for the second week and 113 mg/kg for the third week, showing distinct separation of the periportal and centrolobular parenchyma. P = portal tract, C = central vein. H & E ×110

After 3 weeks there was a distinct separation of the periportal parenchyma from the centrolobular region by a thin band of connective tissue (Figure 48.5). Within the periportal region the hepatocytes were pleomorphic and their arrangement somewhat irregular. Mitotic figures were present, the cytoplasm stained more basically than in the centrolobular zone, and there was mild biliary ductular proliferation which often extended into the encapsulating zone of new connective tissue. These intermediate fibrous tissue zones also contained rudimentary blood vessels and occasional inflammatory cells, and often linked up the separated zones of periportal parenchyma. The hepatocytes of the centrolobular zones were still similar to those seen in livers after 1–2 weeks of dosing except at the margin of the midzonal fibrous tissue where the cytoplasm of most cells became less granular and more homogenous with occasional vacuoles, many nuclei stained darkly and were sometimes pyknotic and occasional apoptotic bodies derived from necrotic hepatocytes could be observed (Figure 48.6).

After 4 weeks the intermediate zone of loose connective tissue separating the centrolobular from the periportal parenchyma was much wider (Figure 48.7) and contained numerous blood vessels together with biliary ductules. The masses of periportal parenchymal cells assumed the form of typical regenerative nodules as the connective tissue appeared to contract around them, and small groups of hepatocytes were split off by connective tissue bands into typical pseudolobules (Figure 48.8).

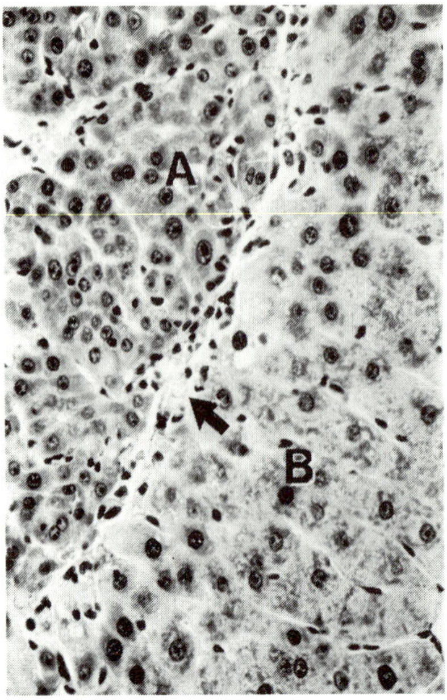

Figure 48.6 The same liver as in Figure 48.5 showing the area of separation of the periportal (A) and centrolobular parenchyma (B). A thin band of connective tissue (arrow) separates these two populations of hepatocytes. Mild degenerative changes are present in the centrolobular hepatocytes adjacent to the fibrous tissue band, while the remaining centrolobular hepatocytes appear normal. H & E ×220

Within the fifth week of dosing there was an acceleration in the necrosis of the residual centrolobular hepatocytes, beginning at the margin of the new midzonal fibrous tissue (Figure 48.9). This allowed a distinct widening of the connective tissue bands which now contained both central veins (Figure 48.10) and other blood vessels appearing to be associated with portal tracts. Bile ductules were plentiful in the new fibrous tissue and appeared to be well separated from parenchymal cells. Histocytes and lymphocytes were present in increased numbers in the new connective tissue. During this week, complete destruction of the remaining centrolobular parenchymal cells occurred in some rats and the widened zone became filled with blood and cellular debris, often obscuring the midzonal loose connective tissue bands. This was followed by collapse of newly nodular periportal parenchyma into the space formerly occupied by the centrolobular parenchyma with the residual veins now caught up in the widened connective tissue bands (Figure 48.11). The liver at the end of the fifth week was then a mass of regeneration nodules and new connective tissue contained biliary ductules, residual portal and central veins with various mononuclear inflammatory cells, the picture in fact, of cirrhosis (Figure 48.12). Despite the high intake of the hepatotoxic essential oil in the final week, the parenchyma constituting the regeneration nodules remained tolerant to its injurious effects through the period of dosing.

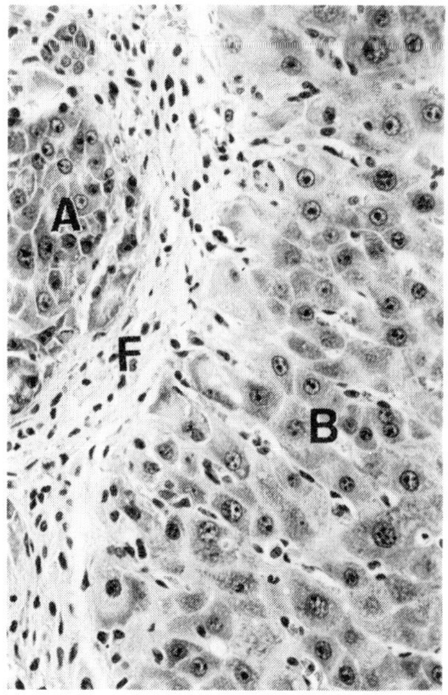

Figure 48.7 The liver of a phenobarbitone-pretreated rat dosed daily with ngaione at 50 mg/kg for 1 week, 75 mg/kg for the second week, 113 mg/kg for the third week and 170 mg/kg for the fourth week. The fibrous band (F) separating the periportal (A) and centrolobular (B) parenchyma is thicker than in Figure 48.6 and there is sporadic necrosis and vacuolation of adjacent centrolobular hepatocytes. H & E ×220

DISCUSSION

Experimental cirrhosis caused by prolonged dosing with hepatotoxic chemicals normally follows persistent and continuous injury to the hepatic parenchyma. In general, such agents preferentially damage the hepatocytes of either the centrolobular zone or the periportal zone. The final picture of cirrhosis, however, is identical in each case[6]. With some of the earliest models to be described, the dose of the respective chemical had to be carefully selected and administered for several weeks or months before cirrhosis could be expected to occur. Examples of such models were chronic phosphorus intoxication in the rabbit and guinea-pig for cirrhosis of periportal origin[12] and carbon tetrachloride intoxication in the rat for cirrhosis of centrolobular origin[2]. With the former, phosphorus is administered by the oral route daily at 1 mg/kg for several months to a year and in the latter, CCl_4 is dosed at the rate of 1 ml/kg every 3 or 4 days for several weeks or months. The procedures have the disadvantages that the yield of cirrhotic livers is unpredictable, and that, due to the severity of liver injury which is likely to occur from time to time throughout the dosage period, intercurrent diseases resulting in death are likely to occur before cirrhosis is established[15].

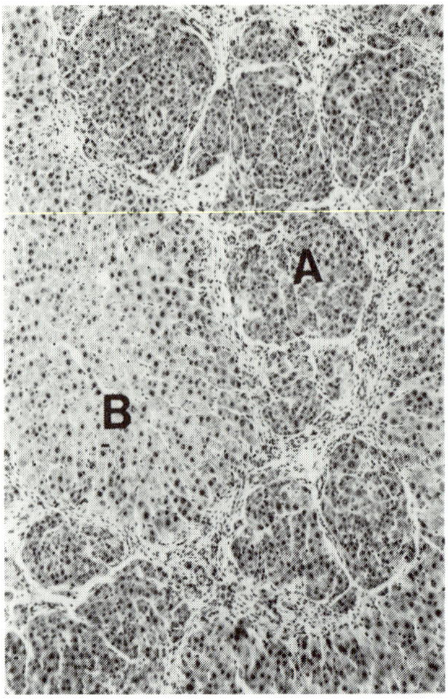

Figure 48.8 The same liver as in Figure 48.7 photographed at lower magnification to show the conversion of the periportal parenchyma (A) to typical regeneration nodules, some of which show early subdivision into pseudolobules. Most of the centrolobular parenchyma (B) still appears normal. H & E ×56

In recent times, however, it has been shown that CCl_4 needs metabolism by the hepatic microsomal mixed-function oxygenases (HMFO) for hepatic injury and overall toxicity for the animal[14]. For any particular set of conditions, the susceptibility of the liver to a given dose of CCl_4 is directly related to the level of hepatic metabolism of the compound, and, accordingly, the activity of the HMFO at the time of dosing[5, 17]. The activity of the latter enzymes may be influenced markedly by numerous factors including the age and sex of the animal, nutrition, previous drug therapy or exposure to environmental chemicals, physiological state and so on[3]. Without prior knowledge of the level of activity of the HMFO, the degree of injury caused by a dose of CCl_4 in any particular animal cannot, therefore, be reliably anticipated and this would have accounted for much of the unpredictability attending early attempts at the induction of cirrhosis in experimental animals following CCl_4 dosing.

This particular difficulty was largely overcome in the model for CCl_4-induced cirrhosis in the rat[15]. In the latter procedure rats were made maximally susceptible to CCl_4 by raising their HMFO by medication of the drinking water with sodium phenobarbitone for 1 week before the start of CCl_4 exposure[5]. This ensured that the degree of hepatocellular injury caused by a selected dose of the CCl_4 would be largely predictable. Following initial exposure to CCl_4, hepatocytes tend to become resistant to subsequently

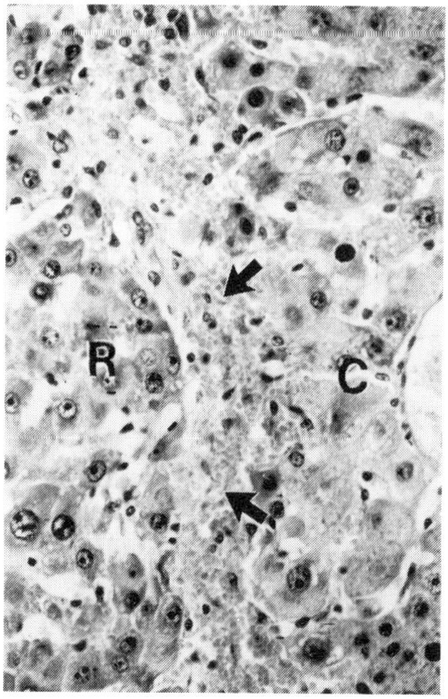

Figure 48.9 The liver of a phenobarbitone-pretreated rat dosed daily with ngaione at 50 mg/kg for 1 week, 75 mg/kg for the second week, 113 mg/kg for the third week, 170 mg/kg for the fourth week and 255 mg/kg during the fifth week. There is accelerated necrosis of the residual centrolobular parenchyma (C) with haemorrhage into the necrotic area and associated midzonal connective tissue (arrows). R = regeneration nodule. H & E ×220

administered doses of the compound[16, 19], mainly because of loss of the microsomal activating enzyme, cytochrome P-450[1, 4]. This latter effect was to some extent prevented by maintaining the rats continuously on the phenobarbitone drinking water to stimulate microsomal enzyme induction throughout the period of CCl_4 dosing. The result was that many centrolobular hepatocytes remained susceptible to the necrogenic effects of subsequently administered doses of CCl_4 and that cirrhosis developed in the animals in only just over 4 weeks of dosing or after only eight exposures to the drug. An important point made by the authors was that, in order for a satisfactory yield of cirrhotic livers to be obtained, particular care had to be exercised in the selection of the first six doses of the hepatotoxin[15]. After this time, surviving parenchyma tends to become more tolerant to further CCl_4 dosing[22], and the dose rate is no longer critical. In the experimental induction of cirrhosis a possible disadvantage arises in using a compound such as CCl_4 which preferentially damages the centrolobular zone. The hepatic microsomal mixed-function oxygenases are concentrated in the centrolobular parenchyma[13, 21]. These enzymes are responsible for the metabolism and detoxification of a wide range of xenobiotic substances as well as various endogenous molecules such as adrenal and sex steroids[3]. The effect of periodic CCl_4 dosing, notwithstanding the continuous ingestion of phenobarbitone,

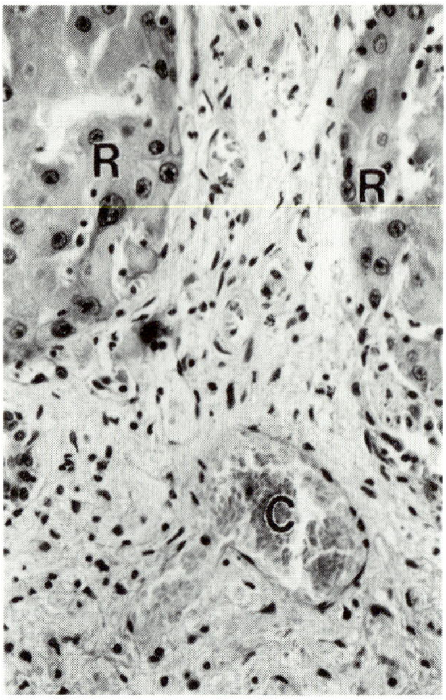

Figure 48.10 Similar liver to that in Figure 48.9 in which loss of centrolobular parenchyma is complete, with replacement of original centrolobular area by haemorrhage and loose new connective tissue. C = central vein, R = regeneration nodules. H & E ×220

would result in the intermittent suppression of these detoxificating enzymes and, accordingly, give rise to significant periods of enhanced susceptibility to possibly noxious chemicals absorbed from the gut or atmosphere, which are normally dealt with by the HMFO and other enzyme systems without harm to the animal. Transient loss of other vital hepatic metabolic functions, due to the periodic episodes of parenchymal cell necrosis, could also be expected to occur after each CCl_4 exposure.

The procedure described here, in which daily ngaione dosing replaced the CCl_4, overcomes such possible disadvantages of the latter compound. For example, only small numbers of periportal parenchyma cells become necrotic following the initial period of ngaione dosing, the centrolobular hepatocytes remaining entirely intact. In addition, the periportal parenchyma very quickly forms regeneration nodules which remain resistant to prolonged dosing with the toxic oil, while connective tissue is gradually built up on their margins, producing unique midzonal annular fibrotic patterns. After 4 weeks, necrosis of the residual centrolobular parenchyma can be accelerated by increasing the dose of ngaione, leaving in the liver only the periportal regeneration nodules and the structures of the portal triads and the central veins caught up in the fibrous tissue band – the final picture in fact, of cirrhosis, within 4–5 weeks.

The histogenesis of the cirrhosis due to simultaneous dosing with phenobarbitone and ngaione is different from that reported for phosphorus[6, 12]

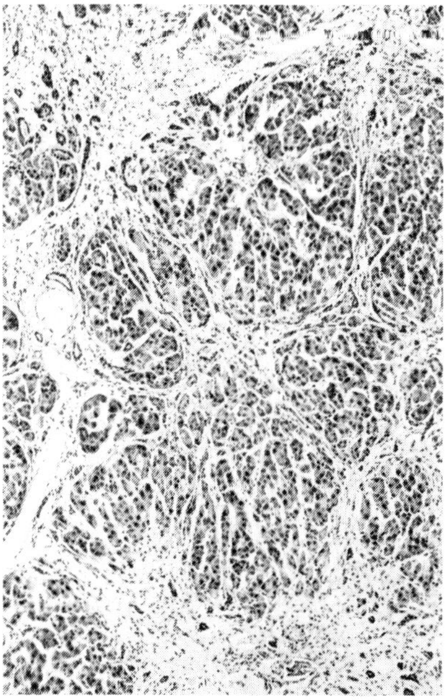

Figure 48.11 Liver of phenobarbitone and ngaione dosed rat at end of 5 week treatment period showing conversion of liver to regeneration nodules dissected by fibrous bands with remainder of liver consisting of fibrous tissue containing portal and central blood vessels and proliferating biliary ductules. H. & E ×56

and other periportal necrosis-producing agents[11]. With the latter there occurs, with prolonged dosing, the development of annular patterns of fibrosis linking up portal tracts and extension of connective tissue into the parenchyma in the direction of the bloodflow until the central veins are involved, permitting porto-central shunting of blood. Regeneration nodules appear to develop rather later in the periportal regions. With the present model, subsequent to the development of the midzonal annular fibrotic patterns within 2–3 weeks, the hepatocytes of the centrolobular zone, most remote from the central veins and lying alongside the midzonal fibrous tissue, appear very susceptible to the ngaione, more so than the immediately perivenular parenchymal cells. Continuous, sporadic parenchymal degeneration and necrosis proceeds in this area, enhancing gradually the regional deposition of connective tissue until all the centrolobular parenchymal region is replaced by it. By 5 weeks the liver may then consist only of regeneration nodules, and new connective tissue containing the hepatic vascular structures, biliary ducts and ductules.

A further advantage of the procedure is that very few, if any, animals are lost during the course of the cirrhosis induction, and that a day or two after cessation of treatment the animals would be suitable for use in experiments in which cirrhotic livers were required.

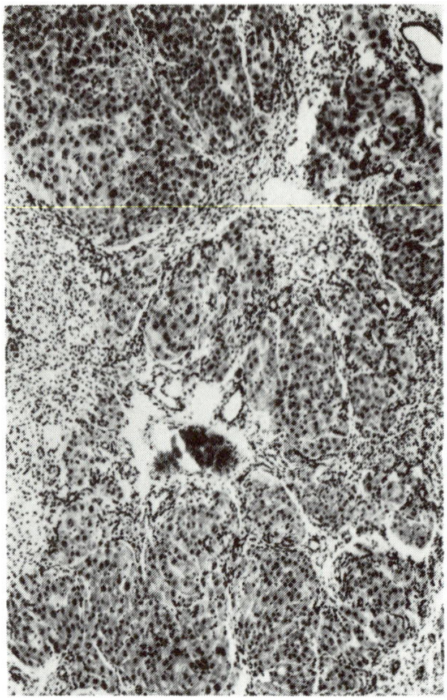

Figure 48.12 Similar liver to that shown in Figure 48.11 after 5 weeks of treatment, showing conversion of parenchyma to regeneration nodules and proliferating connective tissue with more extensive inflammatory cell infiltration. The pseudolobulation of the nodular parenchyma is less marked in this liver. H & E ×56

A problem to be encountered in the exploitation of this model in experimental hepatology might well be considered to be the restricted availability of ngaione since it is found only in Australasian plants. However, the optical enantiomorph of ngaione, ipomeamarone, can be readily formed in sweet potato (*Ipomoea batatas*) tuber tissues treated with 1% mercuric chloride and left to stand for several days at room temperature. Steam distillation of this material yields a fusel oil rich in the compound which can then be further fractionated and purified[20]. Studies in the authors' laboratory with ipomeamarone indicate that its biological action is identical to that of ngaione[8] and that it could serve as a substitute for ngaione in this model should the latter oil be unprocurable.

SUMMARY

Simultaneous administration of phenobarbitone and ngaione results in the induction of cirrhosis in young male rats within 4–5 weeks. Ngaione specifically causes injury to the peripheral parenchymal cells under these conditions and the initial fibrogenic reaction takes place in this zone. This is followed by rapid development of regeneration nodules in the periportal zone which becomes separated from the apparently normal centrolobular zone by a continuous midzonal band of connective tissue. With time and increase in the ngaione dose, the cells of the centrolobular zone remote from the central vein gradually undergo degeneration and necrosis at the midzonal margin, allowing the zone of fibrous tissue to increase in width. Finally, the centrolobular parenchyma is completely lost and entirely replaced by new connective tissue. The liver then consists of regeneration nodules which are resistant to the toxic ngaione, and connective tissue containing the hepatic vasculature and bile ducts and ductules – namely, the complete picture of cirrhosis.

Apart from the short time needed to produce the model, few, if any, animals die in the course of development of the lesion and, for a substantial part of the induction period, the metabolically important centrolobular parenchymal zone remains undamaged. This is in contrast to what occurs with CCl_4 and other well-known hepatotoxic agents which specifically damage the centrolobular zone.

References

1. Barker, E.A., Arcasoy, M. and Smuckler, E. A. (1969). A comparison of the effects of partial surgical and partial chemical (CCl_4) hepatectomy on microsomal cytochrome b_5 and P_{450} and oxidative *N*-demethylation. *Agents Actions*, **1**, 27–34
2. Cameron, G. R. and Karunaratne, W. A. E. (1936). Carbon tetrachloride cirrhosis in relation to liver degeneration. *J. Pathol. Bacteriol.*, **42**, 1–21
3. Conney, A. H. (1967). Pharmacological implications of microsomal enzyme induction. *Pharmacol. Rev.*, **19**, 317–66
4. Dingell, J. V. and Heimberg, M. (1968). Effects of aliphatic halogenated hydrocarbons on hepatic drug metabolism. *Biochem. Pharmacol.*, **17**, 1269–78
5. Garner, R. C. and McLean, A. E. M. (1969). Increased susceptibility to carbon tetrachloride in the rat after pretreatment with oral phenobarbitone. *Biochem. Pharmacol.*, **18**, 645–50
6. Hartroft, W. S. (1964). Experimental cirrhosis. In Rouiller, C. H. (ed.) *The Liver*. Vol. 2, pp. 477–514. (New York: Academic Press)
7. Hegarty, B. F., Kelly, J. R., Park, R. J. *et al.* (1970). Terpenoid chemistry. XVII. (–)-Ngaione, a toxic constituent of *Myoporum deserti*. The absolute configuration of (–)-ngaione. *Aust. J. Chem.*, **23**, 107–17
8. Lee, J. S. (1979). Studies of the toxicity of essential oils in *Myoporum deserti*. pp. 115-30. A. Cunn, PhD *Thesis*, University of Queensland
9. Lee, J. S., Hrdlicka, J. and Seawright, A. A. (1979). The effect of size and timing of a pretreatment dose of phenobarbitone on the liver lesion caused by ngaione in the mouse. *J. Pathol.*, **127**, 121–7
10. Lee, J. S., Hrdlicka, J. and Seawright, A. A. (1981). The effect of daily oral dosing with ngaione for 7 weeks on the liver of the rat. *J. Appl. Toxicol.*, **1**, 165–73
11. Madhavan, T. V., Tulpule, P. G. and Gopalan, C. (1965). Aflatoxin-induced hepatic fibrosis in rhesus monkeys, pathological features. *Arch. Pathol.*, **79**, 466–9
12. Mallory, F. B. (1933). Phosphorus and alcoholic cirrhosis. *Am. J. Pathol.*, **9**, 557–67
13. Massey, E. D. and Butler, W. H. (1979). Zonal changes in the rat liver after chronic administration of phenobarbitone: an ultrastructural, morphometric and biochemical correlation. *Chem-Biol. Interactions*, **24**, 329–44
14. McLean, A. E. M. and McLean, E. K. (1966). The effect of diet and 1,1,1-trichloro-2,2-bis-(p-chlorophenyl)ethane(DDT) on microsomal hydroxylating enzymes and on sensitivity of rats to carbon tetrachloride poisoning. *Biochem. J.*, **100**, 564–71
15. McLean, E. K., McLean, A. E. M. and Sutton, P. M. (1969). Instant cirrhosis, an improved method for producing cirrhosis of the liver in rats by simultaneous administration of carbon tetrachloride and phenobarbitone. *Br. J. Exp. Pathol.*, **50**, 502–6
16. Pound, A. W. and Lawson, T. A. (1975). Reduction of carbon tetrachloride toxicity by prior administration of a single small dose in mice and rats. *Br. J. Exp. Pathol.*, **56**, 172–9

17. Seawright, A. A. and McLean, A. E. M. (1967). The effect of diet on carbon tetrachloride metabolism. *Biochem. J.*, **105**, 1055–60
18. Seawright, A. A., Lee, J. S., Allen, J. G. *et al.* (1978). Toxicity of *Myoporum spp.* and their furanosesquiterpenoid essential oils. In Keeler, R. F., Van Kampen, K. R. and James, L. F. (eds.) *Effects of Poisonous Plants on Livestock*. pp. 241–50. (New York: Academic Press)
19. Ugazio, B., Koch, R. R. and Recknagel, R. O. (1972). Mechanism of protection against carbon tetrachloride by prior carbon tetrachloride administration. *Exp. Mol. Pathol.*, **16,** 281–5
20. Uritani, I., Uritani, M. and Yamada, H. (1960). Similar metabolic alterations induced in sweet potato by poisonous chemicals and by *Ceratostomella fimbriata. Phytopathology*, **50,** 30–4
21. Wattenberg, L. W. and Leong, J. L. (1962). Histochemical demonstration of reduced pyridine nucleotide dependent polycyclic hydrocarbon metabolizing systems. *J. Histochem. Cytochem.*, **10,** 412–20
22. Wong, J. and Finckh, E. S. (1965). Tolerance to carbon tetrachloride in carbon tetrachloride-induced cirrhosis. *J. Pathol. Bacteriol.*, **89,** 611–17
23. Zimmerman, H. J. (1976). Experimental hepatotoxicity. In Eichler, O. (ed.) *Handbook of Experimental Pharmacology*. Vol. XVI. Experimental Production of Diseases. Part 5, Liver. pp. 1–120. (Berlin: Springer-Verlag)

49
Behavioural analysis of drug action

R. Dantzer

In order to understand what are the aims and means of behavioural analysis of drug action, a practical example may be useful.

Mixing unacquainted pigs after weaning usually results in fighting. Such behaviour may last several hours with, in some cases, injury and even death of some of the protagonists. In addition, negative effects on growth have been reported. Let us assume that a drug company has made all the necessary steps to develop a chemical compound with antiaggressive properties and that this compound, referred to as drug A, is a centrally-acting drug. The question with which pharmacologists are confronted is to understand how the antiaggressive effects of drug A are produced. What are the behavioural processes affected by the drug treatment and leading to a reduction of aggression? What are the molecular mechanisms responsible for the behavioural effects of the drug, i.e. how is function at the neuronal level affected by the drug and how does this result in altered behaviour?

If drug A is a neuroleptic agent, acting as an antagonist of dopaminergic postsynaptic receptors, the first question deals with the specificity of the antiaggressive effects, e.g. is the decrease in aggression due to non-specific factors such as impairment of locomotor activity, sensory-motor incoordination or sedation, or to a specific blockade of the aggressive motivation? The second question concerns the role of dopamine in aggressive behaviour and can be answered by looking for correlations between brain dopaminergic activity and fighting, and/or by assessing the behavioural consequences of specific alterations in brain dopaminergic functions.

Both questions are of relevance for any subsequent development of new compounds. If drug A results in suppression of aggression but, at the same time, has profound depressive effects on cardiovascular activity and respiratory function, some animals may die from an overdosage. It would, therefore, be useful to search for more specific compounds, which are devoid of undesirable side-effects. In addition, the pharmacologist may be asked for drugs promoting aggressive behaviour, e.g. in the case of game cocks or fighting bulls. As far as dopamine is a good candidate for the control of aggression, dopaminergic agonists will be useful for their aggression-enhancing effects.

Behavioural analysis of drug action is, therefore, concerned with the study of how drugs affect behaviour. The subject of *behavioural pharmacology* is not limited to the study of psychotropic drugs; it also takes into account a variety of adventitious substances such as solvents and pesticides which may have behavioural side-effects. The contribution of studies using species different from laboratory animals (mainly rodents and primates) is rather limited for two main reasons: (1) the infrequent resort to psychotropic drugs in veterinary medicine, and (2) the limited knowledge available on the behavioural characteristics of many domestic animal species. In spite of these limitations, examples of behavioural studies of drug action in veterinary medicine can be found in the different fields of application of behavioural pharmacology and toxicology.

USE OF BEHAVIOURALLY ACTIVE DRUGS AS A RESEARCH TOOL

If one is interested in emotional behaviour a way of feeling a little more confident about the methods used to assess emotions in animals is to be sure that the behavioural variables selected are sensitive to the effects of antifear agents. In this case, psychotropic drugs are used as a research tool, allowing researchers to categorize the observed behaviour within well-defined classes.

For example, domestic fowls, exposed to a situation where they can see food but are unable to obtain it, develop stereotyped movements. These reactions have been suggested to be motivated by fear or distress elicited by this frustrating experience. In order to test this hypothesis, Duncan and Wood-Gush injected birds having already experienced this frustrating situation once or birds submitted to it for the first time, with a reserpine derivative, metoserpate hydrochloride, claimed to be a specific antifear agent[11]. Metoserpate reduced the severity of already developed stereotyped movements but was unable to prevent them unless it was given to naive hens. These results were interpreted as evidence for involvement of fear in the genesis of stereotyped movements occurring under frustration. However, this interpretation holds true only for metoserpate specifically relieving fear. This is an unlikely event, since neuroleptics have proven to be unable to directly affect motivations: alternative interpretations (e.g. a reduction of arousal or a decreased capacity to switch attention to non-pertinent exteroceptive stimuli) are available to account for their behavioural effects[18].

The limitations of this approach become very clear when considering a recent study in which pigs were treated with a benzodiazepine derivative, diazepam, before being submitted to frustration[1]. Pigs had learnt to push a panel with their snout in order to get food in a modified Skinner box. They were then exposed to this situation but without the availability of more food under two different conditions, with or without access to the response panel and the feeding area. In the first case, when access to the response panel and feeding area was permitted, diazepam enhanced resistance to extinction, i.e. the pigs spent more time pushing the panel and trying to get access to the feeding area, but the treatment did not modify aggression. In the second case, when access to the response panel and the feeding area was not permitted, diazepam increased the severity of aggression observed between the animals

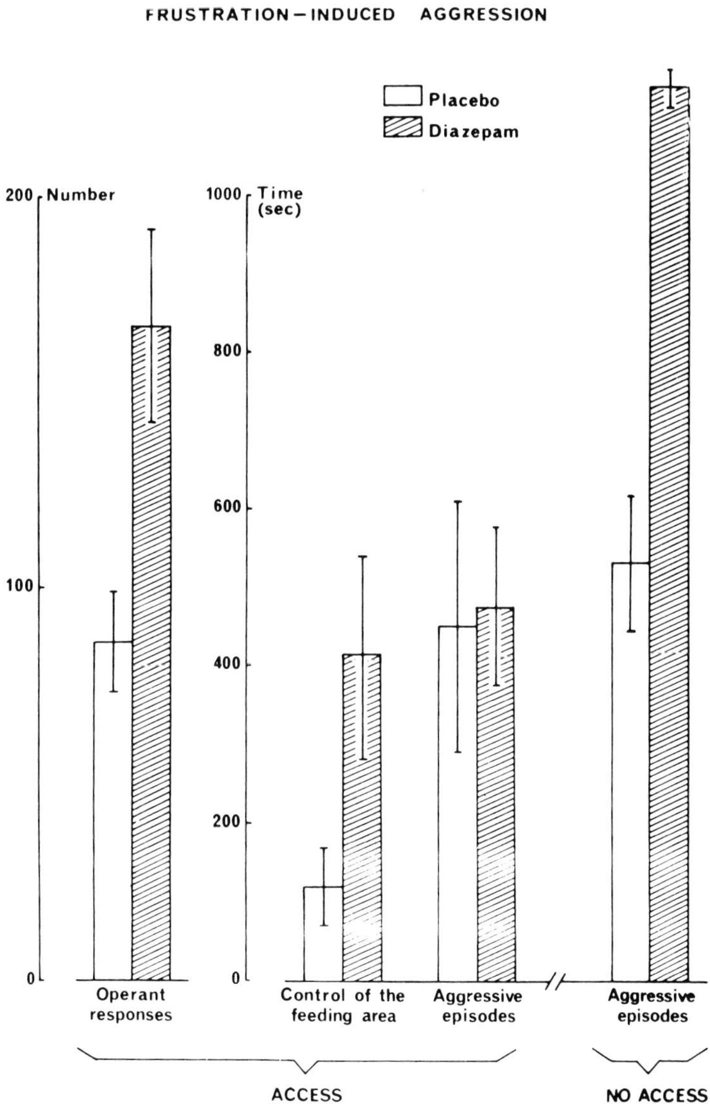

Figure 49.1 Effects of diazepam on extinction-induced aggression in the pig. Pigs were trained to press a panel with their snout to get food in a modified Skinner box. They were then exposed in pairs to this situation but without more food being available (extinction), and under two different conditions, i.e. with, or without, access to the response panel and the feeding area. When access was permitted, pretreatment with diazepam (1–2 mg/kg) increased resistance to extinction but did not modify aggression. When access was prevented, diazepam (2 mg/kg) increased the number of aggressive episodes observed between the animals

(Figure 49.1). These results demonstrate that diazepam does not act on frustration or aggressiveness *per se*, but exerts more complex effects which are critically dependent on the ongoing behaviour and its rate of occurrence. This is true for other psychotropic agents as well and leads to the idea that interpretations of the effects of drugs on behaviour in terms of motivational changes (e.g. changes in fear or anxiety level) have little explanatory value.

As a matter of fact, behavioural pharmacologists have demonstrated for many years that the important concept is not the nature of the event that follows the behaviour (e.g. a food reward or the avoidance of an electric shock) but rather the way the event is occurring in relation to behaviour. In other words, to know how the behaviour is produced, i.e. its ongoing rate and pattern, is more important for the prediction of drug responses than to know why it is produced.

ANALYSIS OF BEHAVIOURAL MECHANISMS OF DRUG ACTION

To arrive at an understanding of the behavioural effects of drugs experimental psychologists describe the behaviour under study in clearly defined elementary steps by which possible alterations under the effect of a drug may be measured.

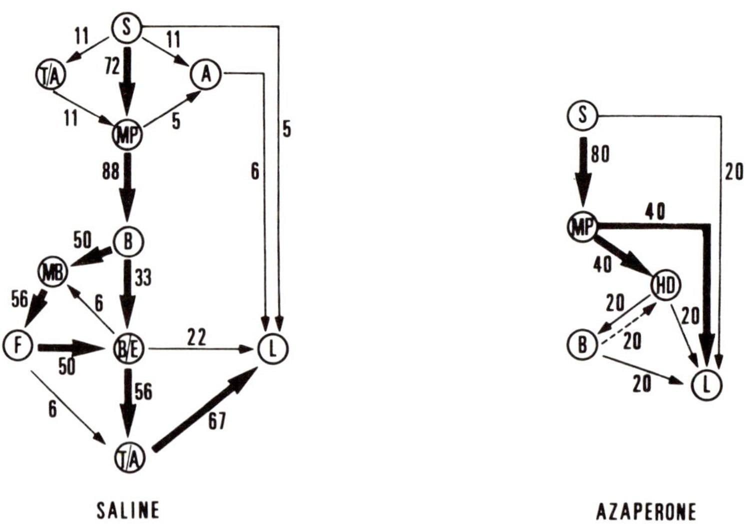

Figure 49.2 Effects of azaperone on the sequence of agonistic interactions occurring when two piglets from different social origins are mixed together. The thickness of the lines and the number besides them indicate the frequency with which one activity is followed by the one to which the line leads. The abbreviations are as follows: *S*, smelling; *T/A*, threat by one animal, avoidance by the other; *A*, avoidance; *P*, pushing; *B*, biting; *MB*, mutual biting; *F*, fighting (shoulder to shoulder posture); *B/E*, biting by one animal, escaping or presenting its back by the other; *HD*, head down, snout to snout (the same attitude in the two opponents); *L*, lying down. Saline or azaperone (2 mg/kg) was injected 10 min before the beginning of the test which lasted 30 min

For example, azaperone, a butyrophenone derivative which is effective in the prevention and cure of aggressiveness in pigs[24] gives a strong sedation within 10–15 min, which lasts for about 2 h. Azaperone-treated pigs lie down during this period instead of fighting like their untreated congeners. However, it can be questioned whether azaperone inhibits fighting by specific antiaggressive effects or if it prevents behavioural expression, because of the sedation. It was stressed that aggression was not simply delayed but that it was inhibited more or less permanently between the members of the newly constituted groups[24]. This has been the subject of some dispute since Blackshaw showed that the agonistic interactions were delayed but did not disappear in azaperone-treated animals[3]. In addition, a sequential analysis of the behavioural patterns observed in pairs of unacquainted pigs mixed together after an injection of azaperone, revealed that the sequence leading to fighting did not disappear but was blocked at an early stage. Treated animals still showed mutual smelling, threats and avoidances and minor agonistic interactions (mainly mutual pushing), but due to sedation they were unable to engage in more elaborate fighting (Figure 49.2).

Similar studies attempting to determine the behavioural processes affected by drugs have been carried out on the effects of neuroleptics on emotional behaviour of sheep[17,20], on the effect of lithium on aggressive behaviour in pigs[10,21] and on the effect of benzodiazepines on emotional behaviour in pigs.[8]

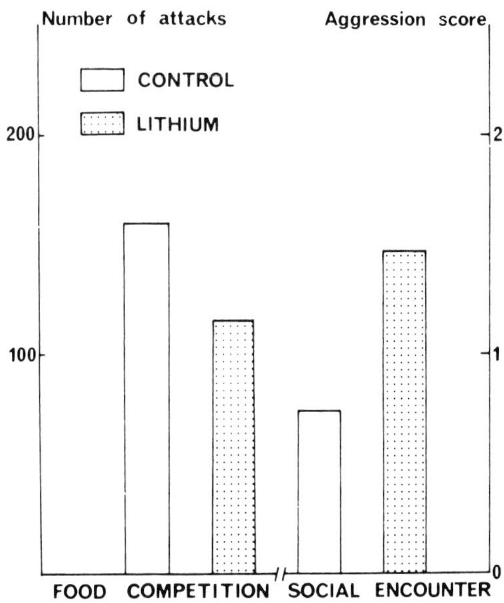

Figure 49.3 Effects of lithium on aggressive behaviour of pigs. Left: mean number of attacks observed in groups of four pigs during a 10 min food competition test run after 10 days of chronic lithium treatment (mean level of plasma lithium: 0.53–0.74 mEq/l). Right: mean score of aggression observed between four pigs from two different pens when brought together in a neutral pen. The test was initiated after 11 days of chronic lithium treatment. Aggression was scored on a 3-point scale, according to intensity (ref. 10)

An interesting issue, raised by the study of the effects of lithium salts on aggressive behaviour, concerns the unitary vs. multiple nature of aggression. Aggression is often seen as a single class, in spite of its different origins and different ways of expression. It was found that non-toxic doses of lithium carbonate decreased aggression occurring among pigs of the same social groups when access to food was restricted, but did not prevent aggression and fighting observed after mixing pigs from different social groups (Figure 49.3). This suggests that aggression elicited by food competition belongs to a functional class different from aggression occurring when unacquainted animals are brought together. Later, we will see other examples of drug-induced dissociations in aggressive behaviour with progestins.

Altogether, these studies have a more pronounced bearing on theoretical issues concerning the mechanisms of action of psychotropic drugs in psychopharmacology than on therapeutic applications in veterinary medicine. However, their contribution to the expansion of knowledge in the field of animal behaviour should not be underestimated. For example, sensitive methods have been developed both in pigs and in sheep for quantitatively assessing emotionality traits using either techniques of observation or operant conditioning methods.

ANALYSIS OF NEUROCHEMICAL MECHANISMS UNDERLYING BEHAVIOUR

In the last two decades, progress in the understanding of neurochemistry led to the concept that psychotropic drugs alter neuronal function by acting at one or a few critical steps in the synaptic transmission. It then became fashionable to use drugs to interfere specifically with a given neurochemical system in order to determine its role by the behavioural alterations such intervention produced. A great deal of interest has focussed on the study of neurochemical mechanisms of feeding, in the hope of finding ways to increase food intake and/or feed efficiency in farm animals.

For example, Simpson *et al.* investigated the role of catecholamines in the chemical control of feeding, by injecting norepinephrine in the lateral ventricles of the brain[23]. In sheep, this injection induced an increased intake of feed (290–390% of control values) which was blocked by, phenoxybenzamine. This α-antagonist alone decreased intake. In contrast, the β-adrenergic antagonist, propranolol, did not modify the effects of norepinephrine. In steer, injection of norepinephrine caused hypophagia, reducing intakes by 50–60%; phenoxybenzamine blocked the norepinephrine-induced hypophagia in steer and, when injected alone, it increased feed intakes to 180% of the control values. These experiments demonstrate, therefore, that the neurochemical coding for feeding is different between sheep and steer. The possibility of eliciting and suppressing feeding behaviour with substances interfering with the neurochemical transmission led the Pennsylvania research group to engage in an intensive search for chemicals capable of increasing the motivation level for feeding. From this work came a new compound, elfazepam, a benzodiazepine derivative, which may hold great promise as a chemical feed intake stimulant[2].

MISCELLANEOUS

Effects of hormones on behaviour

Hormones exert behavioural effects of which the most well known are those of androgens and oestrogens in sexual behaviour and the relationship between androgens and intermale aggression.

Attempts to modify sexually-related behavioural problems in veterinary medicine have mainly focussed on the use of antiandrogens. Progestins have been reported to suppress urine marking, mounting and roaming in dogs and urine spraying and roaming in cats[13]. The same drugs were found to be effective in markedly reducing or eliminating fighting of male dogs with other males but were not able to significantly alter aggression directed towards the owner[15].

Hormones other than sexual steroids are also able to affect behaviour. For example, it has been shown that treatments interfering with the pituitary-adrenal axis (i.e. ACTH or dexamethasone injections) alter reactions of pigs to a fear signal[22] (Figure 49.4). In addition, during the last decade, it has become more and more apparent that hormonal peptides are involved in the control of nervous activity as well as the more classical hormonal roles. This is true for peptides released at the periphery (e.g. ACTH, MSH, vasopressin) and peptides found in the gut (e.g. cholecystokinin) but also for more recently identified peptides with no known hormonal effect. Endorphins, which are endogenous opiate-like peptides able to specifically bind to opiate receptors, belong to this last class. Besides their role in analgesia, they are certainly involved in emotional behaviour[9]. An injection of naloxone decreased the distress reactions observed in piglets separated from their social group and introduced alone into a new environment, but agonists of the opiate receptors had the opposite effect (Figure 49.5). This field of the behavioural effects of peptides is of growing interest since neuropeptides are believed to modulate chemical transmission or to act as transmitters in the brain and, therefore, offer promise for controlling behaviour.

Drug-induced conditioned taste aversion

Drugs can be used for their direct effects on behaviour, but also for their indirect effects, based on their aversive or appetitive consequences. Behaviour which leads to unfavourable consequences, in this case drug-induced toxic effects, tends to be suppressed while behaviour which is followed by pleasant consequences (e.g. euphoria) tends to be repeated. An example of the first case can be demonstrated by attempts to control coyote predation by aversive conditioning as an alternative to killing the predators. Such an

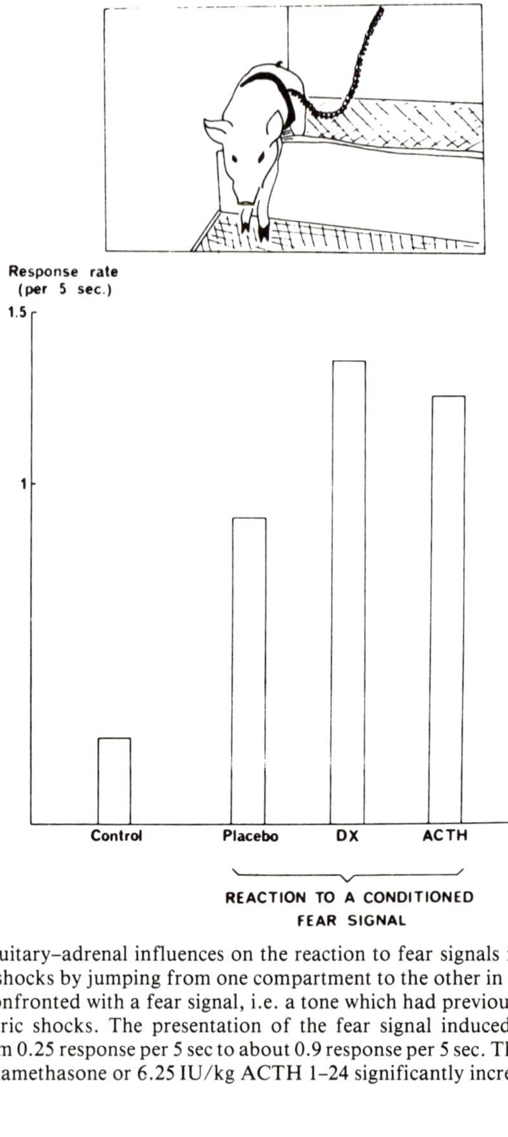

Figure 49.4 Pituitary–adrenal influences on the reaction to fear signals in pigs. Pigs trained to avoid electric shocks by jumping from one compartment to the other in a shuttle-box (upper diagram) were confronted with a fear signal, i.e. a tone which had previously been paired with inescapable electric shocks. The presentation of the fear signal induced an increase of the response rate from 0.25 response per 5 sec to about 0.9 response per 5 sec. The previous injection of 0.2 mg/kg dexamethasone or 6.25 IU/kg ACTH 1–24 significantly increased the reaction to the fear signal

approach makes use of the gustatory avoidance paradigm: when an animal eats a poisoned meal and survives, it will develop an aversion for the flavour of that meal[12]. When ingestion of lamb meat by coyotes is accompanied by illness produced with toxic doses of chloride lithium, a conditioned aversion to that specific food will develop and attack upon lambs will also be suppressed, while attack and eating of other preys will be unaffected[14]. Although the practical effectiveness of this method has been questioned[7], it represents an interesting approach to the problem of controlling undesirable behavioural

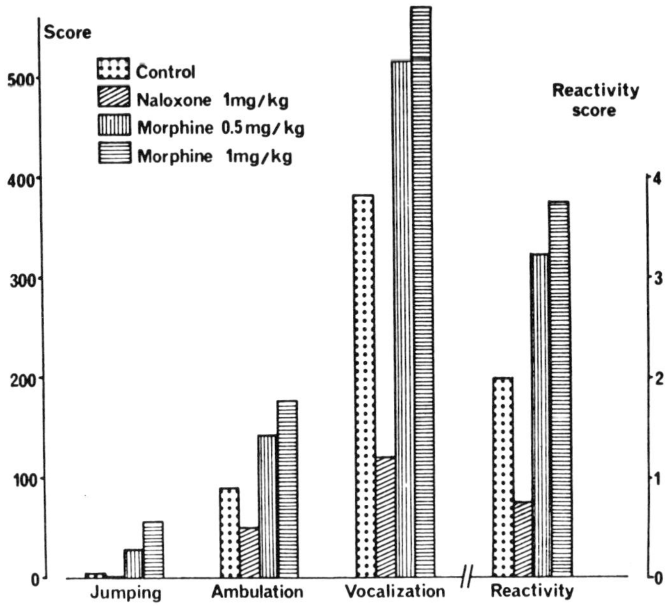

Figure 49.5 Effects of naloxone and morphine on behavioural reactions to social separation in piglets. Piglets were acutely separated from their social group and put alone in a new environment, whilst their behavioural reactions were monitored for 15 min. Under these conditions, control animals showed distress reactions, as evidenced by escape attempts and high levels of locomotion and vocalization. Naloxone decreased these reactions as well as the reactivity score (on a 4-point subjective scale) while morphine increased them

traits and it could certainly be extended to other applications (e.g. acute episodes of tail biting in pigs).

Neurotoxicology and behavioural toxicology

Neurotoxicity is an undesirable side-effect observed with various classes of drugs such as antimicrobial agents (e.g. sulphones, furazolidone) and anthelmintics. It may include not only various neurological disturbances which occur mostly after prolonged administration of drugs but also strong depression or excitation of the central nervous system after a single dose of a drug.

Information on the potential adverse reactions to new drugs is usually obtained in preclinical studies, when the drugs are given to healthy animals, at excessive dosages. However, many untoward side-effects show only in practice, which poses the problem of observing them and their attribution. Such a situation may be due to the fact that toxic reactions of the nervous system occur only with repeated drug administration or as the result of adverse drug interactions. But it can also come partly from the lack of suitable observation methods to quantify behaviour.

Much effort has been invested in this field by combining the resources of toxicology and experimental psychology in order to assess the subtle effects of chronic exposure to low levels of environmental toxicants. Although such studies are usually carried out using laboratory animals, they can be applied as well to farm animals or companion animals. For example, lambs, prenatally exposed to lead and then submitted to discrimination tests, exhibited a reduced learning ability at lead blood levels below the accepted levels[6, 25].

This approach has led to the development of a new discipline known as behavioural toxicology which is of great value for predicting toxic effects of drugs and environmental toxicants.

CONCLUSIONS

From the preceding list of research subjects (which are examples of those generating the most concern in veterinary pharmacology and toxicology at present), it would appear that behaviourally active drugs (among which hormonal treatments should not be forgotten) are used more frequently by fundamental pharmacologists than by clinicians. In fact, chapters dealing with psychotropic drugs in standard veterinary pharmacology textbooks usually only contain rather vague descriptions of the clinical manifestations of psychotropic drugs, besides preanaesthetic purposes and sedation[4]. This is unfortunate in view of the impressive list of psychopathological disorders observed in companion animals, farm animals and zoo animals[19]. It means that the prospects for behavioural analysis of drug action are still extensive in veterinary pharmacology, perhaps indicating the inclusion of more adequate training in basic behavioural science and psychopharmacology in a veterinarians' curriculum.

To give just one example, behavioural therapies involving direct manipulations of organism–environment interactions have been used for curing behavioural abnormalities in animals, especially companion animals. There are well-documented reports on the treatment of excessive fears of specific stimuli ('phobic reactions') in dogs or cats by counterconditioning or desensitization procedures[16], despite the fact that such treatments are usually laborious and give limited results. However, the advantages of psychoactive drugs as an adjunct to behaviour therapy or as a treatment on its own to control abnormal behaviour remains largely unexplored. There is, therefore, a need for systematic, well-controlled clinical trials in this field.

Up to now, one of the main sources of progress has come, not from veterinarians, but from psychopathologists attempting to model human psychopathologies. The use of psychostimulants (mainly methylphenidate) to control hyperkinesis in dogs or the treatment of distress reactions following social separation with tricyclic antidepressants (e.g. imipramine) are examples of by-products from research work on animal models in psychiatry. However, their contribution cannot be expected to continue in the future, due to the fact that, for practical reasons, most of the work in this field is done on laboratory animals rather than on companion or farm animals.

References

1. Arnone, M. and Dantzer, R. (1980). Effects of diazepam on extinction induced aggression in pigs. *Pharmacol. Biochem. Behav.*, **13**, 27–30
2. Baile, C. A. and McLaughlin, C. L. (1979). A review of the behavioral and physiological responses to elfazepam, a chemical feed intake stimulant. *J. Anim. Sci.*, **49**, 1371–95
3. Blackshaw, J. K. (1981). The effect of pen design and the tranquilising drug, azaperone, on the growth and behaviour of weaned pigs. *Aust. Vet. J.*, **57**, 272–6
4. Booth, N. H. (1978). Psychotropic drugs in veterinary medicine. In Clark, W. G. and del Giudice, J. (eds.) *Principles of Psychopharmacology*. pp. 655–87. (New York: Academic Press)
5. Brady, J. P. (1981). Behavioural medicine: scope and promising of an emerging field. *Biol. Psychiatr.*, **16**, 319–32
6. Carson, T. L., van Gelder, G. A., Karas, G. G. *et al.* (1974). Development of behavioral tests for the assessment of neurologic effects of lead in sheep. *Environm. Health Perspect.*, **24**, 233–7
7. Conover, M. R., Francik, J. G. and Miller, D. E. (1977). An experimental evaluation of aversive conditioning for controlling coyote predation. *J. Wildl. Manag.*, **41**, 775–9
8. Dantzer, R. (1978). Dissociation between suppressive and facilitating effects of aversive stimuli on behavior by benzodiazepines. A review and a reinterpretation. *Progr. Neuro-psychopharmacol.*, **2**, 33–40
9. Dantzer, R. (1979). Intervention des endorphines dans le comportement émotionnel du Porc. *C.R. Acad. Sci., Paris*, **289**, 1299–302
10. Dantzer, R. and Mormède, P. (1979). Effects of lithium on aggressive behaviour in domestic pigs. *J. Vet. Pharmacol. Ther.*, **2**, 299–303
11. Duncan, I. J. H. and Wood-Gush, D. G. M. (1974). The effect of a rauwolfia tranquillizer on stereotyped movements in frustrated domestic fowl. *Appl. Anim. Ethol.*, **1**, 67–76
12. Garcia, J., McGowan, B. K., Ervin, F. R. *et al.* (1968). Cues: their relative effectiveness as a function of the reinforcer. *Science*, **160**, 794–5
13. Gerber, H. A., Jochle, W. and Sulman, F. G. (1973). Control of reproduction and of undesirable social and sexual behavior in dogs and cats. *J. Small Anim. Pract.*, **14**, 151–8
14. Gustavsen, C. R., Garcia, J., Hankins, W. G. *et al.* (1974). Coyote predation control by aversive conditioning. *Science*, **184**, 581–3
15. Hart, B. L. (1981). Progestin therapy for aggressive behavior in male dogs. *J. Am. Vet. Med. Assoc.*, **178**, 1070–1
16. Hothersall, D. and Tuber, D. S. (1979). Fear in companion dogs: characteristics and treatment. In Keehn, J. D. (ed.) *Psychopathology in animals*. pp. 239–55. (New York: Academic Press)
17. Hughes, R. N., Syme, L. A. and Syme, G. J. (1977). Open-field behaviour in sheep following treatment with the neuroleptics azaperone and acetylpromazine. *Psychopharmacology*, **52**, 107–9
18. Iversen, S. D. and Iversen, L. L. (1981). *Behavioral Pharmacology*. (New York: Oxford University Press)
19. Keehn, J. D. (ed.) (1979). *Psychopathology in Animals. Research and Clinical Implications*. (New York: Academic Press)
20. Madsen, B. W., Syme, G. J. and Syme, L. A. (1980). Effects of azaperone and acetylpromazine on social and environmental behaviour in sheep. *Br. J. Pharmacol.*, **69**, 179–83
21. McGlone, J. J., Kelley, K. W. and Gaskins, C. T. (1980). Lithium and porcine aggression. *J. Anim. Sci.*, **51**, 447–55
22. Mormède, P. and Dantzer, R. (1978). Pituitary-adrenal effects on avoidance behavior in pigs. *Horm. Behav.*, **10**, 285–97
23. Simpson, C. W., Baile, C. A. and Krabill, L. F. (1975). Neurochemical coding for feeding in sheep and steers. *J. Comp. Physiol. Psychol.*, **88**, 176–85
24. Symoens, J. and van den Brande, M. (1969). Prevention and cure of aggressiveness in pigs using the sedative azaperone. *Vet. Rec.*, **85**, 64–7
25. van Gelder, G. A., Smith, R. M. and Buck, W. B. (1972). Behavioural toxicology: do toxicants alter behavior? *Iowa State University Vet.*, **34**, 17–22

50
Experimental models for respiratory diseases of ruminants and of swine

J. Espinasse, J. P. Raynaud, L. Renault and F. Osdoit

The respiratory diseases dominate the pathology of the ruminants and swine. A study recently carried out by Church and Radostits[25] in Canadian feedlots shows that out of about 250 000 heads, respiratory diseases were responsible for about 60% of the disease conditions, i.e. a cost of about 40 FF per animal. In France, respiratory diseases also produce two thirds of the disease conditions and in some groups and at some seasons affect virtually the whole herd. Enzootic infectious bronchopneumonias sometimes seriously damage fattening units for lambs fed on milk rèplacers, including the exportation from flocks contaminated with the visna-maedi virus. In addition, respiratory disease is one of the major causes of economic loss in swine breeding: mortality at all stages of breeding, delayed growth and an increase of the food efficiency index in fattening pigs.

Knowledge is essentially based on epidemiological research but is also advanced by the use of experimental models. Furthermore, use of such models makes it possible to develop and evaluate many of the methods of control of respiratory disease. This report deals with various experimental models for respiratory diseases of ruminants (and of swine) on the basis of the part of the respiratory system involved, of the major aetiological factors and of clinical development. Practical use of these experimental models in the understanding and therapy of respiratory diseases will be discussed.

EXPERIMENTAL MODELS FOR DISEASES OF THE UPPER RESPIRATORY TRACT

Infectious bovine rhinotracheitis (IBR) and atrophic rhinitis of swine (AR) can be produced using the corresponding aetiological agents: bovine *Herpes virus* 1 in cattle, rabbit and ferret, *Bordetella bronchiseptica* in pig and rabbit.

Infectious bovine rhinotracheitis

Whatever species is used, the test strain of IBR virus is usually cultured on cells: embryonic calf kidney cells or fetal calf cells. Brown and Cabasso[20] used embryo calf cells cultivated in an Earle medium enriched with 20% normal calf serum and lactalbumin hydrolysate. The doses of the virus inoculated via the nasal route by means of a syringe or as an aerosol produced by various types of devices[7, 102] vary between 10^4 and 10^8 T.C.I.D. 50/ml.

The young cattle used for the experimental reproduction of IBR are calves between 2 and 9 months old of any breed and they are raised in the conventional manner. They have routinely been fed with colostrum but do not have any IBR virus neutralizing antibodies. After a short incubation phase (2–5 days) the disease becomes apparent, sometimes by a brief attack of diarrhoea and always by a considerable rise in temperature. The symptoms and the usual lesions of the natural disease then follow: lacrymation, mucopurulent discharge, ptyalism and sometimes involvement of the inner lungs.

In the rabbit[69, 70] and depending on the route of inoculation, the problems may go well beyond the respiratory system.

In the ferret[106] infected by means of a virulent aerosol, the clinical and pathological picture is that of exudative rhinotracheitis.

Atrophic rhinitis of swine

Bordetella bronchiseptica is often associated with respiratory disease of swine and particularly with AR in which it is thought to play a determining role, even though genetic or feed practice may play a role and increase the atrophy of the nasal turbinates.

AR may be produced either using material scraped or washed from the nasal cavities of diseased animals[48] or, with greater accuracy of results, using a pure culture of some strains of *Bordetella bronchiseptica*. The phase 1 strains (encapsulated), which can be recognized because of the smooth round shape of their colonies and which are obtained by culture on Bordet Gengou medium, appear to be the most pathogenic[64]. The bacteria (10^6–10^8) are simply instilled into the nasal cavities or inhaled in aerosol form.

In piglets without colostrum and only a few days old, raised under strictly isolated conditions, born from specific pathogen free (SPF) herds or else SPF themselves and initially free from any respiratory problems and not carrying *Bordetella bronchiseptica* in their nasal cavities, all the signs of AR are produced: cough, nasal discharge, slower growth, distortion of the snout. Two weeks after infection, the atrophy of the ventral nasal concha is seen; 4 weeks later the entire lower and upper nasal turbinate is atrophied or has disappeared. The epithelium of the pituitary mucosa presents the lesions of acute catarrhal rhinitis with epithelium metaplasia. The skeleton shows a diminution and then an atrophy of the bone with a tendency for it to be replaced by cartilaginous tissue which later on tends to disappear.

Other piglets (3–7 weeks old) can be used for the experimental reproduction of AR but the clinical results are less good. Using apparently healthy newborn rabbits without antibodies against *Bordetella bronchiseptica* and raised with their mother until the age of 3 weeks, inoculated via the nasal route with the same dose of inoculum, the lesions are especially marked in the lungs[74,75].

EXPERIMENTAL MODELS FOR DISEASES OF THE LUNG

Viral pneumonia

Pneumoenteritis of lambs due to adenovirus

The pneumoenteritis of lambs due to adenovirus is obtained as follows: colostrum-deprived lambs aged between 1 and 3 weeks or colostrum-free calves a few days old are inoculated with the Belak and Palfi type 4 adenovirus strain[8] or the MacFerran *et al.* type 1 strain[71] cultivated on secondary explant lamb kidney cells. Simultaneous injection via the nasal and intratracheal routes (1.5 ml and 1 ml respectively of a suspension titrating at 10^3 T.C.I.D. 50/ml) quickly produces gastrointestinal and pulmonary symptoms. The intestinal lesions are the same as those of catarrhal enteritis and the respiratory lesions are those of bronchiolitis with exsudative alveolitis.

Visna-maedi of the small ruminants

Visna-maedi is a slowly developing pneumonia of the small ruminants which is produced by a retrovirus related to the visna virus, another slowly developing viral disease which affects the central nervous system.

The maedi virus can be obtained from small ruminants (sheep or goat) aged between 6 and 12 months, raised in isolation after virulent inoculation and which have been obtained from flocks free from this type of pneumonia for the past 10–15 years at least. However, all the animals inoculated do not show the disease and do not always present lesions when sacrificed. It is, therefore, necessary to use groups of about ten animals in order to ensure some experimental cases.

The virulent material is provided either by a 5 or 10% suspension of infected lungs[99] or by a culture of the virus on sheep plexus choroid cells[100] and containing 10^6–10^8 T.C.I.D. 50/ml. The inoculation is usually carried out via various routes: intranasal, intratracheal and intrapulmonary.

Symptoms due to this form of pneumonia are rarely detected without an incubation period of several months, according to De Boer[27] 26–30 months. However, macroscopic and microscopic lesions are often found in animals sacrificed at various intervals during the experimental period and examined for such lesions. These lesions are the same as those found in cases of the spontaneous disease.

Pulmonary adenomatosis of small ruminants

Pulmonary adenomatosis of small ruminants is a carcinoma of the bronchioalveolar cells (the Clara cells and the type 2 pneumocytes) and seems to be produced by the combination of two viruses: a herpes virus (playing an auxiliary role) and a retrovirus different from that of visna-maedi.

The slow development of pulmonary adenomatosis produces the same problems for experimental reproduction of the disease as those described above.

The animals used are lambs from adenomatosis-free flocks usually aged between 3 and 12 months but sometimes much younger (about 12 days). The inoculum is made up of virulent material which differs widely from experimenter to experimenter:

(1) The filtered supernatant of homogenized pulmonary lesions[117].

(2) A culture of tumoural cells removed from an affected lung taken from a recently sacrificed diseased animal[114].

(3) Herpes virus and type C particles bearing a reverse transcriptase[77].

The inoculation may be performed via very varied routes: aerosol, intratracheal, intrabronchial, intrapulmonary and intravenous routes with the addition of gelose to provoke embolisms.

The onset of symptons (discharge, cough, dyspnoea) is always delayed, almost 4 months after infection[116], but macroscopic and microscopic lesions can be used to confirm the disease.

Pleuropneumonia due to mycoplasma or haemophilus

Contagious bovine pleuropneumonia

Contagious bovine pleuropneumonia occurs in zebu cattle or the offspring of a cross of such animals with European breeds of cattle and aged between 1 and 3 years, clinically healthy and free from antibodies against *Mycoplasma mycoides*, after the inoculation of virulent products via the nasal, or more often the endobronchic route. These virulent products are usually an homogenate of lungs from experimentally infected animals[19] or a culture of the Gladysdale strain of the *Mycoplasma mycoides* variety mycoides[97]. Symptoms develop within 2–10 days and are the same as those of the natural disease.

Contagious caprine pleuropneumonia

The experimental model for contagious caprine pleuropneumonia is produced in the female goat aged between 6 months and 3 years, or in the White Swiss mouse weighing between 20 and 25 g and is based on the pathogenicity of the *capri* strain of *Mycoplasma mycoides*, cultivated on media which vary from author to author and inoculated alone or associated with the virus of small ruminant pest[19] by aerosol[1], by the intratracheal, the endobronchial[83], subcutaneous[36] or intraperitoneal[105] routes. Here too, the clinical picture observed after an incubation period of 2–6 days is very similar to that of the spontaneous disease.

Porcine haemophilus pleuropneumonia

Porcine *Haemophilus* pleuropneumonia due to *Haemophilus pleuropneumoniae* or *H. parahaemolyticus* presents various types of development which can be reproduced experimentally by a suitable modification of the doses of a pathogenic strain inoculated into sensitive animals. The piglets used for these trials are usually aged between 9 and 10 weeks, free from respiratory disease and raised either in a conventional environment or SPF and then infected via the nasal route[98] with doses of *H. parahaemolyticus* of between 10^2 and 10^{10}. Under these conditions the disease may develop the three clinical aspects found in practice: hyperacute, acute, subacute–chronic.

Respiratory disease complex

Acute bronchopneumonia

Cattle Acute enzootic infectious bronchopneumonia (EIBP) of young cattle usually involves a complex flora of micro-organisms in which other elements (stress) combine with the pathological effect of various viruses, bacteria, mycoplasma and parasites[33].

Experimental production of EIBP uses calves aged between 2 and 10 months, usually of a dairy breed which may or may not have received colostrum and have been raised in a conventional environment but which are free from serum antibodies against the inoculated micro-organisms.

These organisms include the viruses *Parainfluenza* III (PI3) or IBR and the bacteria *Pasteurella haemolytica* or *Pasteurella multocida*. The experimental models often associate a virus and a bacteria.

Contamination with PI3 virus (10^6–5×10^8 T.C.I.D. 50/ml) is produced using an aerosol by a combination of nasal and intratracheal inoculations[55]. The IBR virus is administered by all the authors in the form of an aerosol using Henderson's apparatus. The Pasteurellas which are inoculated only a few hours after the PI3 virus or 3–5 days after the IBR virus (10^4–10^{10} bacteria) are carried by an aerosol, injected into the trachea or simultaneously introduced into the nasal cavities and into the trachea[6, 78].

Sheep The EIBP of young sheep has many similarities with bovine EIBP and so the experimental protocols for their production are fairly similar.

The experimental animals are lambs of various breeds, aged between 4 and 6 weeks, bred in a conventional or a SPF environment, but in all cases free from circulating antibodies of PI3 virus and not carriers of *Pasteurella haemolytica* in their nasal cavities.

Many authors use the G2 strain of the PI3 virus isolated by Hore[57] and cultivated on fetal lamb kidney cells and at various stages of passage. This strain (10^6–10^8 T.C.I.D. 50/ml) is usually inoculated both by the nasal route and by the intratracheal or intrabronchial route by means of a tracheobronchial catheter and using Smith's technique[104].

Table 50.1 Model of acute bronchopneumonia in the piglet due to oral administration of *Ascaris suum* eggs and intratracheal injection of *Pasteurella multocida*: intratracheal low dose (i.t. low dose): 5.6×10^9 bacteria/animal, intratracheal high dose (i.t. high dose): 2.3×10^{10} bacteria/animal, intravenous (i.v.): 4.5×10^7 bacteria/animal

	Pasteurella: i.t. low dose		*Pasteurella: i.t. high dose*	
	+ i.v.	0 i.v.	+ i.v.	0 i.v.
Ascaris 0	824: no death No clinical effects Hyperthermia Weight loss 269 g		820: dead at P + 3 Septicaemia Weight loss 833 g Pulmonary lesions: 45 826: no death Weight stable Hyperthermia No respiratory symptoms	
Ascaris 10^5	699: dead at P + 2 700: dead at P + 4 689: dead at P + 1 Weight loss 200 g Hyperthermia + + Resp. symp. + + + Pulmonary lesions (26.17.25) = 23 Lesions > Ascaris < Pasteurella		692: dead at P + 2 693: dead at P + 8 Weight loss 350 g Hyperthermia + + + + Resp. symp. + + + + Pulmonary lesions (30.7) = 19 Lesions < Ascaris > Pasteurella	694: dead at P + 2 695: dead at P + 2 Weight loss 200 g Hyperthermia + + Resp. symp. + + + Pulmonary lesions (28.45) = 37 Lesions < Ascaris > Pasteurella
Ascaris 16×10^4	698: dead at P + 2 Weight loss 111 g Hyperthermia + Resp. symp. + + + + Pulmonary lesions: 35 Lesions > Ascaris < Pasteurella	701: dead at P + 2 703: dead at P + 1 Weight loss 121 g Hyperthermia + Resp. symp. + + + + Pulmonary lesions (23.45) = 34 Lesions > Ascaris < Pasteurella		704: dead at P + 1 705: dead at P + 1 Weight loss 188 g Hyperthermia + + + Resp. symp. + + + + Pulmonary lesions (26.45) = 36 Lesions > Ascaris < Pasteurella

The bacteria associated with the PI3 virus is biotype A *Pasteurella haemolytica*. The inoculation takes place 3–9 days after that of the virus by various routes:

(1) Aerosols[118] (10^6–$10^{7.7}$ bacteria),
(2) Intratracheal[12] 5 ml of a suspension containing $5.3–9.7 \times 10^8$ bacteria/ml),
(3) Intranasal 0.5 ml in each nostril and intratracheal, 5 ml of a suspension containing $1–2.5 \times 10^5$ bacteria/ml[26].

As in cattle, the clinical signs and the lesions are similar to those of the naturally occurring disease, sometimes with diarrhoea in the terminal stage.

Swine The first EIBP model in swine was developed in France by Raynaud *et al.*[89]. The initial lesions of the pulmonary parenchyma are produced after oral administration of *Ascaris suum* eggs, and then the infection with *Pasteurella multocida* is done (Table 50.1).

Young piglets (7–8 weeks), free from haemagglutinating antibodies against *Pasteurella multocida*, receive 10^5 embryonated *Ascaris suum* eggs by the oral route. Eight days later they are inoculated by means of an aerosol via the intratracheal route with an highly pathogenic strain of *Pasteurella multocida*.

Under these conditions the authors obtained a typical respiratory disease. However, this was complicated by articular signs (lameness, paralysis, arthritis) and hepatic lesions (jaundice). One of the authors has since suggested another model for Pasteurellosis derived from that of Bentley and Farrington[9] and using a strain of *Pasteurella multocida* type A isolated in

Table 50.2 (a) Clinical development of the subacute form. (b) Pathological, bacteriological and zootechnical assessment after the 10 day observation period

(a)	*Time after inoculation* (h/days)					
	+24 h	+48 h	+72 h	+96 h	+5 days	+10 days
% dyspnoeic animals						
Controls	40	60	80	20	40	20
Treated:						
oxytetracycline (20 mg/kg i.m.)	60	60	40	20	0	0
% animals with T $\geqslant$ 41 °C						
Controls	40	20	60	60	20	0
Treated:						
oxytetracycline (20 mg/kg i.m.)	0	0	0	0	0	0

(b)	*Controls*	*Treated*
Extent of lesions (maximum index[16]: 45) mean values	8/45	1/45
Pasteurella multocida A per gram		
in the lesions	2×10^9	0
in normal lung	1×10^2	1×10^2
Mean weight change during the observation period (10 days)	−3 kg	+1 kg

France, and inoculated via the intratracheal route. Depending on the number of organisms injected (10^{11} or 10^9) in piglets aged 8–10 weeks, weighing on average 20 kg and obtained from a healthy herd, the symptoms recorded were acute or subacute. This model has been used particularly in order to check the clinical activity of an oxytetracycline product for injection (20 mg/kg via intramuscular route) administered at the time of inoculation (Table 50.2 (a) and (b)).

Chronic bronchopneumonia

In both series (sheep and swine) these conditions produce mild respiratory symptoms but, however, have considerable effects on growth. They are essentially interstitial pneumonias with peribronchic, peribronchiolar and perivascular lymphoid proliferation, and alveolar atelectasia following cellular infiltration, expecially by histiocytes, into the alveolar septa with a proliferation of the bronchial epithelium.

Sheep In sheep, the chronic bronchopneumonia models use a mycoplasma or a chlamydia. Ovine mycoplasmosis can be produced in lambs of 5–7 months old raised in a conventional environment and with no *Pasteurella* or *Mycoplasma* infection of the nasal cavities. The inoculum is either a suspension prepared from the lungs of diseased animals containing, for example[4], *Mycoplasma ovipneumoniae* (1.2×10^4/ml), *Pasteurella haemolytica* (10^4/ml), *Neisseria* (10^4/ml), an haemolytic *Streptococcus* (10^4/ml), *Escherichia coli* (10^3/ml) or else a mixed culture of *Mycoplasma ovipneumoniae* and of *Pasteurella haemolytica* isolated from lungs collected from the slaughterhouse[62]. These virulent materials are used in an aerosol (10–15 ml) as a spray administered in each nostril or else via the endobronchial route into both lungs via the main bronchial tube (1 ml) using the technique of Foggie *et al.*[41].

Ovine chlamydiosis is reproduced in the SPF mouse[38] or in normally raised lambs which may or may not have received colostrum and which may be between a few days and a few weeks old. The strain of *Chlamydia psittaci* is cultivated on eggs and inoculated by the intratracheal route by an aerosol[24].

Swine The experimental production of respiratory mycoplasmosis of swine requires piglets between 1 and 15 weeks old reared in a conventional environment but obtained from disease-free herds or removed from the uterus of SPF sows and raised in gnotoxenic conditions.

After the initial studies of Gulrajani and Beveridge[47] the animals were first inoculated with homogenates of lungs from diseased pigs. Since then, cultures of *Mycoplasma hyorhinis* and especially of *Mycoplasma suipneumoniae* have been used more commonly via the intranasal route[76] (simple depots of the culture) or aerosol[88], intratracheal[66] or intrapulmonary[84] routes. It should be noted that the lesions may be aggravated by the simultaneous effect of *Ascaris suum* larvae[113] or of *Metastrongylus sp.* larvae[72].

Parasitic bronchopneumonia

Small laboratory animals (guinea-pig, rabbit and mouse) are suitable for the development of respiratory parasites of ruminants but the target species is preferable for the usual experimental models.

Cattle

The symptoms of dictyocaulosis due to *Dictyocaulus viviparus* can easily be produced within about 3 weeks in calves 2–3 months old following the oral administration via a stomach tube or more simply using a drenching syringe, of 3000–4000 infecting L3 larvae prepared by the Jarret and Urquhart technique[61].

Sheep and goats

This is true also for dictyocaulosis of small ruminants due to *Dictyocaulus filaria* in lambs or in kids of about 2 months old, infected under similar conditions[43].

In the case of bronchoalveolitis due to *Muellerius capillaris*, lambs aged about 4 months are also infected via the oral route with about 60–70 infesting larvae taken from the foot of the molluscs which serve as the intermediate hosts. The lambs are infected 5 days per week for several weeks[90].

Swine

Lungworm infection of the pig due to *Metastrongylus elongatus* and *pudendotectus* also requires an intermediate host, the earthworm *Eisenia foetida*. Piglets aged 6–8 weeks in good health, born either by caesarian or normally and having received colostrum or not, must ingest 2500–5000 larvae before the first respiratory problems appear with 13–14 days[39].

Allergic pneumonia

Type I hypersensitivity

Infecting larvae of *Ascaris suum* produce complex respiratory problems in the ruminants which have ingested them and these problems probably associate with both traumatic lesions and type I hypersensitivity phenomena[13].

An experimental model of atypical interstitial pneumonia of this type was suggested by Fitzgerald in lambs[40] and by Greenway and MacCraw in the calf aged less than 8 days[46].

The latter used eggs produced from *Ascaris* females obtained from the small intestine of adult pigs which then underwent an incubation at 30 °C for at least 3 weeks. The infecting capacity was checked by means of oral administration to rabbits fasted for 24 h (3000–5000 eggs). In our trials piglets were used as well as rabbits.

The infecting doses administered per os, sometimes by means of a stomach tube were variable: 8×10^5–3×10^6 eggs in the lamb, 10^4–10^7 in the calf, depending on whether this was a first dose or subsequent doses given at 3 week intervals.

Symptoms set in 2–3 days after inoculation. First hyperthermia and loss of appetite, then coughing, a rise in heart and respiratory rates, fairly severe dyspnoea accompanied by an expiratory grunt are detected. Auscultation detects bronchial rale and an increase in the tonality of normal sounds. These sounds result from serohaemorrhagic alveolitis complicated with a few weeks

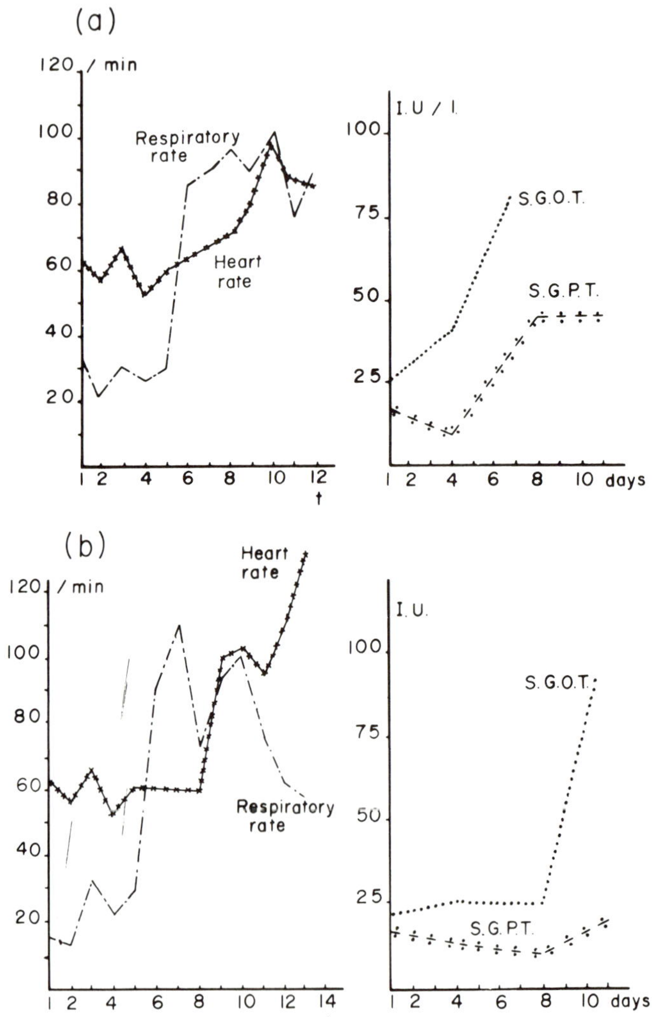

Figure 50.1 (a) Functional symptoms and biochemical lesions in calf 686, produced by *Ascaris suum* larvae (3×10^6 eggs per os at D1). (b) Functional symptoms and biochemical lesions produced in calf 687 by *Ascaris suum* larvae (3×10^6 eggs per os at D1)

to become interstitial pneumonia. After the administration of a second dose, the clinical symptoms become more severe. They may be complicated by urticaria.

During our experiments (Figure 50.1 (a) and (b)) the death of five out of six animals was produced by a single dose of 3×10^6 eggs in less than a fortnight, unlike Eyre *et al.*[37] who used the same amount of larvae both for sensitization and for the challenge dose.

Type III hypersensitivity

In the 'farmer's lung' syndrome particular to cattle from mountain areas eating mouldy hay during the period of winter stabulation, type I hypersensitivity phenomena seem to be associated with type III phenomena, which in fact seem to be predominant.

In cattle, 'farmer's lung' disease can be produced in healthy calves of various breeds and between 4 and 10 weeks old[119]. In most of the protocols, the animals were first sensitized by a subcutaneous injection of 30 mg of soluble *Micropolyspora faeni* antigen in Freund's complete adjuvant and by the intravenous injection of the same amount of this antigen. The clinical onset is usually produced by a 15 min exposure, 5–6 weeks later, to an aerosol of *Micropolyspora faeni* in a 1% aqueous solution prepared with sonic radiated, lyophylized antigen. Administration of the aerosol directly to non-sensitized calves does not produce a clear response even after repeated exposures.

The rabbit[21] and the guinea-pig[120] can also be used as models for 'farmer's lung' using a similar approach.

In all these species, the main symptoms are seen within 3 h of exposure of the sensitized animal to the aerosol: increase of the respiration rate for 3–10 h often complicated by dyspnoea. The animals remain still and refuse to move. Auscultation reveals an increase in the tonality of normal sounds, rales and dry emphysema crepitations.

Toxic pneumonia

Fog fever

Fog fever is no longer considered to be the clinical manifestation of a hypersensitivity reaction but rather an intoxication by various molecules including an L-tryptophan derivative, 3-methyl-indole (3 MI). Symptoms very similar to those of the natural disease appear within 24 h of the oral administration of 3 MI and 6–9 h after i.v. administration of 3 MI.

The administration via the oral route of tryptophan in ruminants produces symptoms of that of fog fever. Adult cattle of various breeds, usually fed with hay and in any case all receiving the same diet for several weeks prior to experimentation, can be used. Various authors administer the DL-tryptophan per os as a suspension in water at doses of between 350 and 700 mg/kg. The D-isomer of tryptophan is inactive at 400 mg/kg whereas the L-tryptophan isomer is active at 350 mg/kg[23]

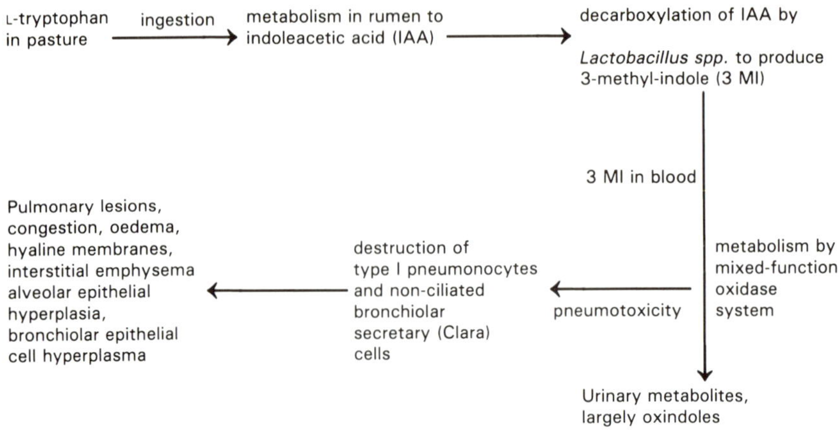

Figure 50.2 Pathogenesis of the pulmonary lesions in cattle caused by ingestion of L-tryptophan

In cattle, 3-methyl-indole (Figure 50.2), given orally or by the intraruminal route, produces fog fever symptoms at a dose varying between 100 and 300 mg/kg according to the authors. The symptoms are produced in sheep with a dose of 200–600 mg/kg[15] and in goat[22]. Our trials in cattle are in agreement with the literature data[34].

Slow intravenous perfusion (for about 12 h) with a solution containing 110 mg/ml 3 MI in propylene glycol at a dose of 60–70 mg/kg body weight produces the symptoms and lesions of fog fever. Similar results are obtained in rabbits with a 1.5–2 h perfusion of 20–40 mg/kg body weight[14].

Since cattle which had eaten mouldy sweet potatoes contaminated by *Fusarium solani* had shown similar symptoms and lesions to those of fog fever, this same material was used by Peckham *et al.*[87] to reproduce the spontaneous disease. This was also possible using *Fusarium solani* mycotoxin, 4-ipomeanol, dissolved in propylene glycol within equal parts with water and given via the oral route[30].

Hydrocarbon intoxications

Oils of varying quality and kerosene introduced via a stomach tube into the rumen of young calves or directly by means of a fistula at a dose of 8 mg/kg body weight per day produce digestive problems (ruminal tympany) and respiratory symptoms[92].

Mechanical pneumonia

Aspiration pneumonia is produced in the calves aged 4–5 months by the administration on two consecutive days of 250 ml of milk[103].

Chronic arterial pulmonary hypertension develops in the pig following pneumectomy or lobectomy[63] and in the calf following ligature of the left pulmonary artery[115]. Chronic arterial and venous pulmonary hypertension occur in the calf following partial obstruction of the pulmonary veins[101].

PRACTICAL USE OF EXPERIMENTAL MODELS

The experimental models of respiratory diseases in ruminants and in swine are of value in comparative pathology due to the lack of spontaneous models (thrombosis of the posterior vena cava of cattle and the Hughes-Stovin syndrome in man as well as heaves of the piglet and hyaline membrane disease in children). They are of special interest in agricultural production with respect to epidemiology, physiopathology, therapeutics and prophylaxis.

Contribution of experimental models to the epidemiology of respiratory diseases

Experimental models for respiratory diseases are an index of the population at risk:

(1) Dhar and Sharma[29] observed that goats are far more sensitive to *Dictyocaulus filaria* infestation than sheep. Wilson[121] shares their opinion.

(2) Montlux *et al.*[80] studied the sensitivity of various breeds of cattle to tryptophan given at an oral dose of 600 mg/kg body weight and confirmed the greater sensitivity of Herefords. Jerseys are slightly less sensitive, Holsteins, Friesians, Angus and Shorthorns are fairly sensitive.

(3) Logomarsino *et al.*[67], having investigated a possible influence of the phosphocalcium content of the diet on the incidence of atrophic rhinitis of swine, noted that a calcium deficiency resulted in osteopenia but not in the lesions characteristic of atrophic rhinitis, and that it had no effect on the development of the experimental condition. On the other hand, in chlamydiosis of sheep, Stevens *et al.*[108] demonstrated the protective role played by vitamin E in animals inoculated 15 days previously with 1000 IU/day per os of α-tocopherol.

(4) Drummond *et al.*[31] defined the role of the levels of atmospheric ammonia in the housing of piglets on the development of experimental atrophic rhinitis. The severity of the rhinitis and the extent of atrophy of the turbinate bone were related to the atmospheric level of ammonia (50 vs. 100 parts/10^6).

Experimental models of respiratory diseases also give information concerning the conditions for infection:

(1) After several trials carried out in parallel, Kobisch *et al.*[64] concluded that lesions of the nasal cavities of atrophic rhinitis in swine were more easily obtained using phase I *Bordetella bronchiseptica*. The amount of bacteria inoculated also plays a determining part: too high a dose results in pneumonia and not in rhinitis.

(2) Dungworth and Cordy[32], and Charton *et al.*[24] found that chlamydia isolated from enzootic abortions, from the faeces of healthy animals or of pneumonia cases had the same pathogenic effect when inoculated via the intratracheal route.

(3) According to Brown and Cabasso[20] the respiratory form of IBR may be produced by conjunctival, intranasal or intratracheal inoculation, but the highest and most consistent rises in temperature were produced by intranasal inoculation.

(4) Shope *et al.*[98] studied the pathogenic power of *Haemophilus pleuropneumoniae* in function of the dose and of the route of inoculation and found that via the subcutaneous route, not only did the symptoms fail to appear but that the piglets resisted to intranasal inoculation with 3.4×10^7 organisms.

(5) MacOwan and Minette[73] demonstrated the possibility of contagion with Contagious Caprine Pleuropneumonia by placing control animals in contact with infected animals. The controls developed the hyperthermia and then the symptoms of pleuropneumonia 10–30 days after the inoculation of the infected animals.

Contribution to the physiopathology of respiratory diseases

Latency, reactivation and re-excretion of the IBR virus

The phenomena of latency, reactivation and re-excretion of the IBR virus were considered only following the use of the experimental model and of immunodepressors.

After six consecutive days of treatment with dexamethasone (0.1 mg/kg body weight via the intravenous route) cattle, which had been inoculated 2 months previously with a pathogenic strain of IBR virus, re-excreted this virus in the nasal discharge. Physical particles appeared well before infectious particles, probably because of neutralization of the infectious particles at the onset of excretion. This re-excretion could occur 24 h after the first injection of dexamethasone; the rapidity of this response seems to suggest a mechanism of action of dexamethasone involving direct cellular activation, rather than an immunodepressive phenomenon[85].

In cattle prepared in the same way as above, the injection of a massive dose of cyclophosphamide via the intravenous route (35–40 mg/kg body weight) produced no such re-excretion, whereas they proved to be still sensitive to dexamethasone. The immunodepression produced by the injection of cyclophosphamide seemed to be unable to produce reactivation and re-excretion of IBR virus in this species[86].

In cattle contaminated with the IBR virus by the method of Pastoret *et al.*[85] and in the latency phase, the oral administration of 3 MI at doses of 50 and 75 mg/kg body weight produced minor clinical signs, a local and systemic immunological response and re-excretion of the IBR virus. At doses of 100 and 200 mg/kg body weight, 3 MI produced severe clinical signs which resulted in death at 200 mg/kg. Local and systemic immunological responses were present but no re-excretion of the IBR virus was detected (Figures 50.3, 50.4, 50.5 (a) and (b)). These results suggest that there may be some connection between disturbances of fermentation in the reticulo-rumen zone and the respiratory problems extending well beyond the clinical syndrome of fog fever[35].

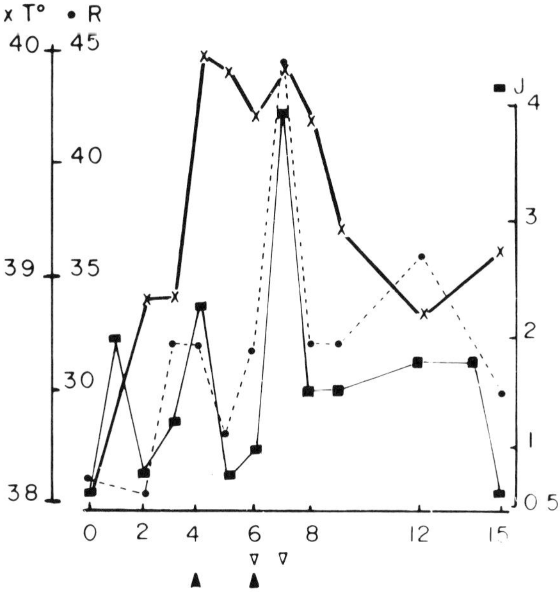

Figure 50.3 Infection by IBR virus. Clinical and laboratory parameters (calf no. 4). The symbols used are rectal temperature (×), respiratory rate (•), volume of nasal secretions (ml) (■), excretion of virus in nasal mucus (▲), presence of antibody neutralizations in the nasal mucus (▽)

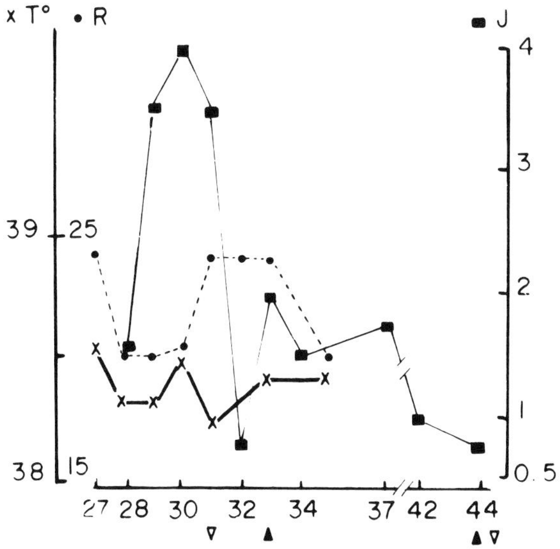

Figure 50.4 Effects of 3 MI (50 mg/kg) on the clinical and laboratory parameters (calf no. 309). Same symbols as in Figure 50.3

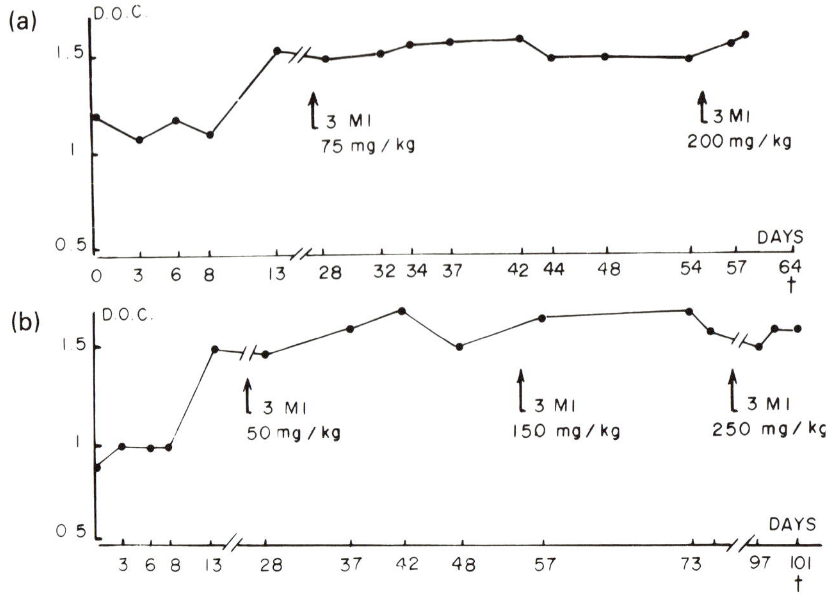

Figure 50.5 Changes in the anti-IBR antibody levels in the serum (Elisa method). (a) Calf No. 4, (b) Calf No. 309

Effects of stress in respiratory diseases

The role of stress in determining the severity of EIBP in cattle has been suggested by several authors, who reach somewhat different conclusions, all of which, however, point to a multifactorial aspect of these disease conditions.

Saunders and Berman[94] applied three types of stress: intramuscular injection of cortisone and of ACTH, transport stress and the i.v. injection of mucosal disease virus. They did not detect any difference between the groups conditioned in this way and the control groups. However, Hamdy *et al.*[50] detected an aggravation of the disease in calves undergoing thermal stress (40 °C during the daytime and 1.1 °C at night), Handy and Pounden[49] reached similar findings in lambs receiving an injection of cortisone acetate.

Stockdale *et al.*[109], comparing the effects of thermal stress (daytime temperature of 25 °C and night-time temperature of 15 °C) with those of transport stress, found that the latter was more active.

In pigs, Fontaine *et al.*[42] investigated the effects of hygiene and of parasitic factors on the extent of the lesions in virus pneumonia. They reported that a fall in the surrounding temperature, a sudden change in the living conditions or in diet produced an aggravation of the lesions.

Synergism of pathogenic agents in respiratory diseases

The EIBP produced by means of the combined effect of a virus and of a bacteria led authors to investigate the possible synergism between these two factors. Baldwin *et al.*[6] in cattle and Sharp *et al.*[96] in sheep investigated the period during which the bacteria were most active following inoculation with the virus. In the mouse, Jakab and Dick[60] showed that the number of live bacteria (*Pasteurella pneumotropica*) taken up by the lung was highest when the virus (*Sendai virus*) developed peak pathogenic effect. Subsequently, Jakab[59] confirmed this by showing that pneumonia was most easily produced by administering the virus 6 days before the *Pasteurella*. In cattle, Lopez *et al.*[68] reached the same conclusions: the number of live bacteria colonizing the lung (83% on average) peaked 7 days after inoculation with PI3 virus.

The part played by *Ascaris suum* larvae in the experimental production of EIBP in swine has already been pointed out. These larvae may also be a factor in the development of chronic bronchopneumonia lesions as indeed may be those of *Metastrongylus sp.*

Immunological, humoral and cellular responses

Diagnostic methods are based on the study of the immunological, humoral and cellular reactions during infectious respiratory diseases of ruminants and swine. Experimental models facilitate the study of these reactions and the development of up to date techniques.

In acute bovine EIBP the level of antibodies neutralizing against PI3 virus peaks 14–21 days after experimental infection[6] whereas that of the haemagglutinating antibodies begins to rise towards day 16 or 17[55].

In chronic bronchopneumonia of the pig due to *Mycoplasma suipneumoniae* the haemagglutination inhibiting antibodies are present within 2–4 weeks of infection and reach peak levels from the 8th or 9th week[56]. Complement-binding antibodies appear at about the same time and the level of these antibodies is a fairly accurate reflection of the progression of these lesions[110].

During trials against swine pleuropneumonia due to *Haemophilus pleuropneumoniae*, Bachman[5] compared various serological tests. He concluded that complement-fixing was a better index (specificity, sensitivity) than agglutination or than precipitation in agar or immunoelectrophoresis.

With the aim of detecting and eliminating from the market recently purchased animals with latent infection of IBR virus in the reactivation/re-excretion phase following the stress caused by transport and modified environmental conditions, the authors are at present attempting to develop an ELISA method for the assay of specific IgM. This study is based on the use of the experimental model of the reactivation/re-excretion of the IBR virus by means of dexamethasone in subjects previously contaminated in the laboratory.

The use of sensitive cattle made it possible for Aguilar-Setien *et al.*[2] to detect a delayed cellular hypersensitivity reaction in experimental IBR infection using a purified virus injected via the intradermal route to detect latent infected animals. The same authors[3], using the same experimental model for the same purposes, have also presented an inhibition test of the migration of plasma leukocytes in the presence of IBR antigen.

Contribution to the treatment of respiratory diseases

Most experimental models of respiratory diseases of ruminants and swine facilitate the carrying out of the controlled therapeutic trials essential to the development of effective drugs and of protocols to check adequate treatments.

Mohanty *et al.*[79] attempted to develop a treatment for IBR by means of 2-desoxy-D-glucose to inhibit the maturation of the virus on the eye surface. The drug was administered for 1 week, either at a dose of 20 mg/kg via the intravenous route or by twice daily instillation on the eye of 20 mg/ml solution from the day of inoculation or for 8 days following the appearance of the first symptoms. 2-desoxy-D-glucose is not active by the systemic route, but via the local route it has a beneficial effect on the ocular symptoms in all cases.

Breeze *et al.*[17] have compared a daily 3-day treatment with oxytetracycline and a single-dose treatment with a long acting oxytetracycline in calves inoculated with *Pasteurella multocida* via the intratracheal route and prepared by thermic stress and the tracheal injection of an 8% solution of acetic acid. The results suggest that the second protocol is much less difficult to apply and equally effective clinically (Table 50.3).

Table 50.3 Effects of experimental *Pasteurella multocida* challenge in control (T1) and treatment groups (T2, T3). Treatment description: T1, *Pasteurella* infected, non-medicated; T2, *Pasteurella* infected and given conventional oxytetracycline (50 mg/ml) intramuscularly in three daily injections of 3 mg/lb body weight (T2X) or two daily injections of 5 mg/lb body weight (T2Y); T3, *Pasteurella* infected and given long-acting oxytetracycline (200 mg/ml) in a single intramuscular injection of 9 mg/lb body weight

Location	Treatment	No. cattle	Depression index* at day Onset	3	Final	Lung lesion score†	Mortality %	Average daily gain, lb
Oregon	T1	5	3.2	1.6	1.9	2.2	0	0.88
	T2X	5	4.3	1.0	1.0	0.8	0	1.44
	T3	5	4.4	1.1	1.0	1.2	0	1.66
Colorado	T1	5	4.0	4.6	2.4	2.0	20	0.20
	T2X	5	4.0	2.2	1.4	1.2	0	0.20
	T3	5	4.6	1.6	0.0	0.8	0	0.31
Indiana	T1	5	4.8	5.6	5.4	3.8	80	−1.57
	T2Y	5	3.8	1.0	0.6	1.8	0	1.03
	T3	5	4.0	0.6	0.2	1.2	0	2.57
Washington	T1	4	6.5	4.8	3.5	3.4	50	0.05
	T2Y	5	6.6	0.0	0.0	1.0	0	1.34
	T3	5	7.0	1.6	0.0	0.5	0	1.61
Summary of four experiments	T1	19	4.6[a]	4.2[a]	3.3[a]	2.9[a]	37[a]	−0.21[a]
	T2X & Y	20	4.7[a]	1.1[b]	0.8[b]	1.2[b]	0[b]	1.00
	T3	20	5.0[a]	1.0[b]	0.3[b]	0.9[b]	0[b]	1.54[b]

*Depression based upon index 0 through 7 (0 = normal; 7 = moribund). Where mortality occurred, index means were derived using last recorded value

†Lung lesions based upon score at necropsy of 0 through 4 (0 = no lesions; 4 = extensive consolidation)

[a, b]Means which do not share a common superscipt are significantly different ($p < 0.05$)

Many anti-infectious agents have been tried in the experimental control of chronic bronchopneumonias in swine:

(1) Penicillin has no effect[11,111].

(2) Streptomycin has little therapeutic effect, but is of prophylactic interest[11,110].

(3) Chloramphenicol has no effect[11].

(4) Chlortetracycline prevents lesions at a dose of 400 parts/10^6 in the feed[76].

(5) Tetracycline has the same properties when administered in the feed at the onset of clinical signs and allows the growth curve to become normal[45].

(6) Oxytetracycline has the same effects as tetracycline[11].

(7) Tylosine at a dose of 10 mg/kg body weight via the intramuscular route for 4 consecutive days, beginning the day before the infectious contact reduces the extent of the lesions[44].

(8) Tiamuline, 200 parts/10^6 in the feed for 10 days, has a similar effect[95].

(9) Lincomycin 200 parts/10^6 in the feed for 3 weeks produces similar results[28].

(10) Sulphamonomethoxine and sulphamethazine are inactive[11,110].

Table 50.4 Clinical signs and treatment* of goats infected with contagious caprine pleuropneumoniae

Group designation and antibiotic employed	*Days to onset of fever*	*Duration of fever after first dose of antibiotic* (days)	*Maximum febrile response within group (days p.f.i.)*†	*No. dose of antibiotic given*
Tylan	3–4	1–3	41.1 °C (3)	1–3
Terramycin	3–4	1–3	42.0 °C (3)	1–3
Leukomycin	3	4–7	41.3 °C (3)	2–7
Penicillin/streptomycin	3–4	5	41.8 °C (4)	4–6
Untreated control	3	20	41.7 °C (3)	0

*Treatment commenced and continued daily as long as individual temperatures exceeded 39.4 °C
†p.f.i.: postnasal first instillation of the organism

The experimental reproduction of caprine pleuropneumonia has confirmed the effects of some antibiotics[82] (Table 50.4).

(1) The association of penicillin–streptomycin and chloramphenicol have poor efficacity.

(2) Oxytetracycline at a dose of 15 mg/kg body weight reduces the symptoms but does not prevent the development of the lesions.

(3) Tylosine is active at a dose of 11 mg/kg body weight.

Many anthelmintics have also been tested on the experimental models of respiratory diseases such as tetramisole[91] and levamisole[18]; fenbendazole[93] and albendazole[10].

With a view to the treatment of atypical interstitial pneumonia Eyre *et al.*[37], using the Greenway MacCraw model[46] and introducing *Ascaris suum* larvae, attempted to determine the efficacy in young calves of various antihistaminic drugs (tripelennamin), anti-5-hydroxytryptamine drugs (methysergide) and anti-inflammatory drugs (aspirin). Only acetyl salicylic acid per os 100 and 250 mg/kg b.i.d. was particularly effective.

Contribution to the prophylaxis of respiratory diseases

Sanitary prophylaxis

The sanitary prophylaxis of infectious respiratory syndromes depends to a large extent on the measures taken to detect infected, latent and carrier animals. The knowledge, by means of experimental models, of the humoral and/or cellular reactions to the respiratory disease agents and the development of techniques making it possible to identify them, also represent important contributions to the methods of sanitary prophylaxis.

Medical prophylaxis

Experimental models of respiratory diseases of ruminants and of swine are also valuable in drawing up protocols for therapy.

Amongst the non-contagious respiratory diseases, the fog fever model using 3 MI has led to attempts of prevention. Hammond *et al.*[54] obtained no protection against the experimental disease with various molecules (acetyl salicylic acid, mepyramine maleate, sodium meclofenamate, dimethylcarbamazine citrate, betamethasone). Better results were obtained with chlortetracycline[51] and especially with monensin at doses of 100–200 mg/kg administered 1 day before and 4 days after the beginning of the trial[52, 53].

The challenge *inoculation of vaccinated and control subjects* with the protection of the former and the onset of the disease in the latter, is a criterion frequently used in the assessment of the usefulness of a vaccine.

Live vaccines Kucera *et al.*[65] have investigated the protection conferred by a thermosensitive strain of the IBR strain following intratracheal vaccination. 4 weeks after vaccination, the 20 vaccinated calves were protected except for one of them, which showed no seroconversion after the vaccination.

Tewari *et al.*[112] investigated the vaccine against dictyocaulosis of small ruminants prepared with irradiated *Dictyocaulus filaria* larvae. The vaccinated lambs were aged between 4 and 6 months and received an initial dose of 1000 irradiated larvae, and then, 28 days later, a second dose of a further 2000 irradiated larvae. The challenge infestation then involved 5000 larvae. A high degree of immunity resulted from this double vaccination.

Inactivated vaccines The authors have studied[107] the protection conferred by an inactivated vaccine in an oily adjuvant against IBR, using an experimental model involving young calves inoculated via the intranasal route by means of a nasal brush. The protection obtained as assessed from the re-excretion of the virus in the nasal discharge, following the challenge inoculation, was better in the animals which had received two injections, at a fortnight's interval (group 1), than in the group which had only received one (group 2) (Figure 50.6). This challenge dose had the effect of a booster on the neutralizing serum antibodies in both groups (Figure 50.7).

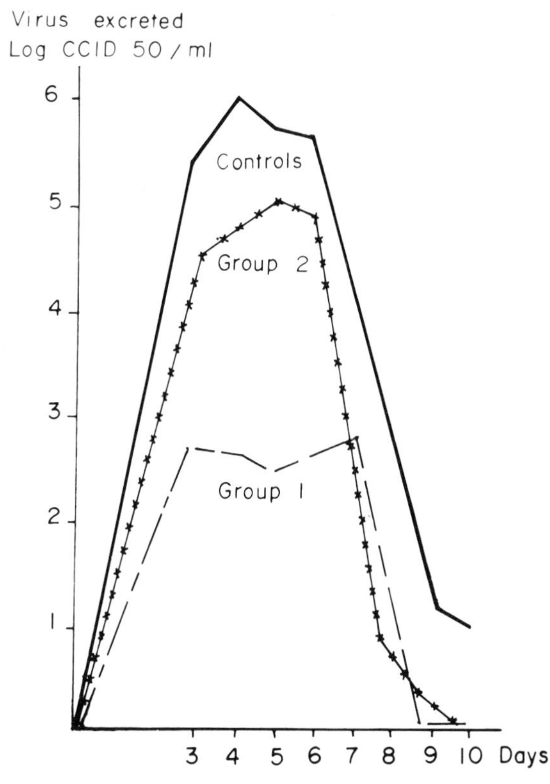

Figure 50.6 Nasal virus excretion post challenge

Mohanty and Lillie[78] administered a vaccine prepared by using the SF4 strain of the PI3 virus, inactivated by formol, and emulsified in a mineral oil with an adjuvant, to vaccinate, via the intramuscular route, calves aged 3–4 months. After 7 weeks, the animals underwent transport stress and then a climatic stress lasting 2 days and were then inoculated via the intranasal route with the virulent SF4 strain. The intratracheal inoculation with *Pasteurella multocida* was carried out 48 h later. All of the non-vaccinated

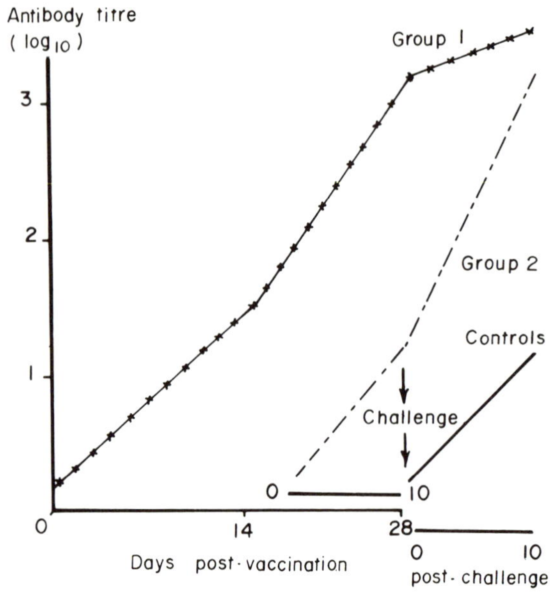

Figure 50.7 Changes in the serum levels of neutralizing antibodies after testing and/or vaccination

calves became ill, the vaccinated animals showed no signs of illness and did not excrete the virus. However, *Pasteurella* could be isolated from some of them.

Nielsen[81] experimented with two formulations of inactivated vaccine against haemophilosis in piglets due to *Haemophilus parahaemolyticus* based on two different adjuvants and 6 and 24 h cultures. 2 weeks after the booster vaccination, he carried out a virulent test and showed that the better protection was given by the 6 h bacterial culture with Freund's complete adjuvant.

Hudson and Turner[58], comparing the efficacy of two vaccines against contagious bovine pleuropneumonia by exposing the vaccinated animals to an inoculation with *Mycoplasma mycoides* variety *mycoides*, reported that the protection afforded by the vaccine prepared on egg was both more rapidly effective and more powerful. However, 1 or 2 months after vaccination, the difference between the two vaccines was very slight.

CONCLUSIONS

Respiratory diseases are difficult to distinguish in practice, and only some of them result from a single aetiological cause. Despite this complexity, experimental models can be devised for most of these syndromes and can lead to a better understanding of the conditions under which respiratory disease appears and develops, hence a more realistic approach to new therapeutic and prophylactic methods. From this point of view, given the multiple difficulties of trials in the field, they not only provide a useful tool for the pharmacologist and the toxicologist, but also an excellent observation base for the clinician.

References

1. Abdulla, A. E. D. and Lindley, E. P. (1967). A study of contagious caprine pneumonia. *Bull. Epizoot. Dis. Afr.*, **15,** 313–17
2. Aguilar-Setien, A., Pastoret, P. P., Burtonboy, G. *et al.* (1978). Test d'hypersensibilité retardée au virus de la rhinotrachéite infectieuse bovine (*Bovine Herpes virus* 1) avec du virus purifié. *Ann. Méd. Vét.*, **122,** 193–9
3. Aguilar-Setien, A., Pastoret, P. P., Michaux, C. *et al.* (1979). Inhibition en présence de l'antigène homologue de la migration des leucocytes circulants provenant de bovins inoculés expérimentalement avec le virus de la rhinotrachéite infectieuse bovine (*Bovid Herpes virus* 1, BHV1). *Ann. Méd. Vét.*, **123,** 249–55
4. Alley, M. R. and Clarke, J. K. (1979). The experimental transmission of ovine chronic non progressive pneumonia. *N.Z. Vet. J.*, **27,** 217–20
5. Bachmann, P. (1972). Beitrag zur Epidemiologie der kontagiösen Pleuropneumonie beim Schwein. *Schw. Arch. Tierh.*, **114,** 362–82
6. Baldwin, D. E., Marshall, R. G. and Wessman, G. E. (1967). Experimental infection of calves with *Myxovirus Parainfluenza* 3 and *Pasteurella haemolytica. Am. J. Vet. Res.*, **28,** 1773–82
7. Beard, C. W. and Easterday, B. C. (1965). An aerosol apparatus for the exposure of large and small animals: description and operating characteristics. *Am. J. Vet. Res.*, **26,** 174–82
8. Belak, S. and Palfi, V. (1974). An adenovirus isolated from sheep and its relationship to type 2 bovine Adenovirus. *Arch. Ges. Virusforsch.*, **46,** 366–9
9. Bentley, O. E. and Farrington, D. O. (1980). Efficacy of a long-acting oxytetracycline formulation in an induced *Pasteurella multocida pneumoniae* model. In *Proceedings of Int. Pig Vet. Soc. Congress*, Copenhagen
10. Benz, G. W. and Ernst, J. V. (1978). Anthelmintic efficacy of albendazole against adult *Dictyocaulus viviparus* in experimentally infected calves. *Am. J. Vet. Res.*, **39,** 1107–8
11. Betts, A. O. and Campbell, R. C. (1956). The action of antibiotics and sulphamethazine on the causal agent of virus pneumonia of pigs. *J. Comp. Pathol.*, **66,** 89–101
12. Biberstein, E. L., Shreeve, B. J., Angus, K. W. *et al.* (1971). Experimental pneumonia of sheep. Clinical, microbiological, and pathological responses to infection with *Myxovirus parainfluenza* 3 and *Pasteurella haemolytica. J. Comp. Pathol.*, **81,** 339–51
13. Black, L. (1979). Hypersensitivity in cattle. II. Clinical reaction. *Vet. Bull.*, **2,** 77–88
14. Bradley, B. J. and Carlson, J. R. (1976). 3 MI effects on goat lungs: electron microscopy. *J. Anim. Sci.*, **42,** 1575
15. Bradley, B. J., Carlson, J. R. and Dickinson, E. O. (1978). 3-methylindole-induced pulmonary edema and emphysema in sheep. *Am. J. Vet. Res.*, **39,** 1355–8
16. Brassine, M., Dewaele, A. and Brouwers, J. (1971). Influence de l'étendue des lésions pulmonaires sur la croissance et l'homogénéité des porcs à l'engrais. *Ann. Méd. Vét.*, **115,** 157–74
17. Breeze, R. G., Lauerman, L. H., Schmitz, J. A. *et al.* (1980). Evaluation of a long-acting oxytetracycline for treatment of *Pasteurella* pneumonia in calves. *Bov. Pract.*, **15,** 96–8
18. Broome, A. W. J. and Lewis, J. A. (1974). Activity of levamisole against developmental stages of *Dictyocaulus viviparus* in experimentally infected calves. *Vet. Rec.*, **94,** 563–6
19. Brown, R. D. (1968). Endobronchial inoculation of cattle with various strains of *Mycoplasma mycoides* and the effect of stress. *J. Comp. Pathol.*, **78,** 383
20. Brown, R. G. and Cabasso, V. J. (1957). Studies on infectious bovine rhinotracheitis (I.B.R.). 2. Experimental transmission to cattle. *Vet. Med.*, **52,** 321–6
21. Burrel, R. and MacCullough, M. J. (1977). Production of thermophilic actinomyces hay aerosols for use in experimental hypersensitivity pneumonitis. *Appl. Environ. Microbiol.*, **34,** 715–19

22. Carlson, J. R. and Dickinson, E. O. (1975). Induction of pulmonary edema and emphysema in goats. *J. Anim. Sci.*, **41**, 404
23. Carlson, J. R., Dyer, I. A. and Johnson, R. J. (1968). Tryptophan induced interstitial pulmonary emphysema in cattle. *Am. J. Vet. Res.*, **29**, 1983–9
24. Charton, A., Faye, P., Parodi, A. *et al.* (1964). Etude d'une pneumopathie expérimentale provoquée chez l'agneau par une souche de virus de l'avortement de la brebis. *Bull. Acad. Vét.*, **37**, 269–76
25. Church, T. L. and Radostits, O. M. (1981). A retrospective survey of diseases of feedlot cattle in Alberta. *Can. Vet. J.*, **22**, 27–30
26. Davies, D. H., Dungworth, D. L., Humphreys, S. *et al.* (1977). Concurrent infection of lambs with *Parainfluenza* type 3 and *Pasteurella haemolytica. N.Z. Vet. J.*, **25**, 263–5
27. De Boer, G. F. (1975). Zwoegerziekte virus, the causative agent for progressive interstitial pneumonia (maedi) and meningo-leucoencephalitis (visna) in sheep. *Res. Vet. Sci.*, **18**, 15–25
28. Degeeter, M. J., Kakuk, T. J., Armstrong, C. H. *et al.* (1979). Liucomycine for the treatment of mycoplasmal pneumoniae. *Proc. 71st Ann. Meet. Am. Soc. Anim. Sci., Abstr.*, **49**, 239
29. Dhar. D. N. and Sharma, R. L. (1978). Studies of the comparative susceptibility of sheep and goats to infection with *Dictyocaulus filaria. Ind. J. Anim. Sci.*, **48**, 29–31
30. Doster, A. R., Mitchell, F. E., Farrel, R. L. *et al.* (1978). Effects of 4-ipomeanol, a product from mold damaged sweet potatoes on the bovine lung. *Vet. Pathol.*, **15**, 367–75
31. Drummond, J. G., Curtis, S. E., Meyer, R. C. *et al.* (1981). Effects of atmospheric ammonia on young pigs experimentally infected with *Bordetella bronchiseptica. Am. J. Vet. Res.*, **42**, 863–8
32. Dungworth, D. L. and Cordy, D. R. (1962). The pathogenesis of ovine pneumonia. 2. Isolation of a virus from faeces. Comparison of pneumonia caused by faecal, enzootic abortion and pneumonitis viruses. *J. Comp. Pathol.*, **72**, 71–9
33. Espinasse, J., Faye, P. and Asso, J. (1977). Infections respiratoires enzootiques. In Mornet, P., *et al.* (eds.) *Le Veau*. pp. 335–58. (Paris: Maloine S.A. Ed.)
34. Espinasse, J. and Savey, M. (1979). Fog fever in France: past, present and future. *Vet. Rec.*, **28**, 397
35. Espinasse, J., Viso, M., Laval, A. *et al.* (1982). Réactivation de l'infection par le virus de la rhinotrachéite infectieuse bovine à l'aide du 3-méthyl-indole. Presented at *XII World Congress on Diseases of Cattle*, Amsterdam
36. El Nasri, M. (1964). The effect of tylosin against experimental and natural infection with *Mycoplasma* in goats. *Vet. Rec.*, **76**, 876–7
37. Eyre, P., Nymeyer, D. H., MacCraw, B. M. *et al.* (1976). Protection by acetyl-salicylic acid and other agents in experimental acute interstitial pneumonia of calves. *Vet. Rec.*, **98**, 64–6
38. Faye, P., Espinasse, J., Le Layec, C. *et al.* (1978). Chlamydiose des ruminants: études expérimentales. 3. Pathogénéicité et antigénicité de *Chlamydia psittaci* (var. *ovis*) par voie aérienne (nébulisation) chez la souris. Rôle adjuvant du phosphate acide de calcium dans la réponse immunitaire. *Bull. Acad. Vét.*, **54**, 81–6
39. Fergusson, D. L. (1971). Anthelmintic activity of L-tetramisole against experimental *Metastrongylus sp.* infection in swine. *Cornell Vet.*, **61**, 681–3
40. Fitzgerald, P. R. (1962). The pathogenesis of *Ascaris lumbricoides* var. *suum* in lambs. *Am. J. Vet. Res.*, **23**, 95
41. Foggie, A., Jones, G. E. and Buxton, D. (1976). The experimental infection of specific pathogen free lambs with *Mycoplasma ovipneumoniae. Res. Vet. Sci.*, **21**, 28–35
42. Fontaine, M., Goret, P., Brion, A. *et al.* (1959). Nouvelles recherches expérimentales sur la pneumonie à virus du porc. *Bull Acad. Vét.*, **32**, 675–94
43. Goldberg, A. (1952). Experimental infection of sheep and goats with the nematode lungworm, *Dictyocaulus filaria. Am. J. Vet. Res.*, **13**, 531–6
44. Goodwin, R. F. W. (1972). Isolation of *Mycoplasma suipneumoniae* from the nasal cavities and lungs of pigs affected with enzootic pneumonia or exposed to this infection. *Res. Vet. Sci.*, **13**, 262–7
45. Goret, P., Fontaine, M., Brion, A. *et al.* (1960). Recherches expérimentales sur la prévention et le traitement de la pneumonie à virus du porc par le chlorhydrate de tétracycline. *Rec. Méd. Vét.*, **136**, 711–30

46. Greenway, J. A. and MacCraw, B. M. (1970). *Ascaris suum* infection in calves. 1. Clinical signs. 2. Circulating and marrow eosinophil responses. 3. Pathology. *Can. J. Comp. Med.*, **34,** 227–55
47. Gulrajani, T. S. and Beveridge, W. I. B. (1951). Studies on respiratory diseases of pigs. 4. Transmission of infectious pneumonia and its differentiation from swine influenza. *J. Comp. Pathol.*, **61,** 118–39
48. Gwatkin, R. and Dzenis, L. (1952). Rhinitis of swine. 6. Topical application of streptomycine in artificially infected pigs. *Can. J. Comp. Med.*, **16,** 330–2
49. Hamdy, A. H. and Pounden, W. D. (1959). Experimental production of pneumonia in lambs. *Am. J. Vet. Res.*, **20,** 78–83
50. Hamdy, A. H., Trapp, A. L., Gale, C. *et al.* (1963). Experimental transmission of shipping fever in calves. *Am. J. Vet. Res.*, **24,** 287–94
51. Hammond, A. C., Bray, T. M., Cummin, K. A. *et al.* (1978). Reduction of ruminal 3-methylindole production and the prevention of tryptophan induced acute bovine pulmonary edema and emphysema. *Am. J. Vet. Res.*, **39,** 1404–6
52. Hammond, A. C., Carlson, J. R. and Breeze, R. G. (1978). Monensin and the prevention of tryptophan induced acute bovine pulmonary edema and emphysema. *Science*, **201,** 153–4
53. Hammond, A. C., Carlson, J. R. and Breeze, R. G. (1980). Prevention of tryptophan induced acute pulmonary edema and emphysema (fog fever). *Vet. Rec.*, **107,** 322–5
54. Hammond, A. C., Carlson, J. R., Breeze, R. G. *et al.* (1980). Progress in prevention of acute bovine pulmonary emphysema. *Bov. Pract.*, **14,** 9–14
55. Heddleston, K. L., Reisinger, R. C. and Watko, L. P. (1962). Studies on the transmission and etiology of bovine shipping fever. *Am. J. Vet. Res.*, **23,** 548–53
56. Holmgren, N. (1974). On the immune response in porcine serum and tracheobronchial secretions following experimental infection with *Mycoplasma hyopneumoniae. Zbl. Vet. Med.*, **21B,** 188–201
57. Hore, D. E. (1966). Isolation of ovine strains of parainfluenza virus serologically related to type 3. *Vet. Rec.*, **79,** 466–7
58. Hudson, J. R. and Turner, A. W. (1963). Contagious bovine pleuropneumonia, a comparison of the efficacy of two types of vaccine. *Aust. Vet. J.*, **39,** 373–85
59. Jakab, G. J. (1974). Effect of sequential inoculation of *Sendai virus* and *Pasteurella pneumotropica* in mice. *J. Am. Vet. Med. Assoc.*, **164,** 723–8
60. Jakab, G. J. and Dick, E. C. (1973). Synergistic effect in viral bacterial combined infection of the murine respiratory tract with *Sendai virus* and *Pasteurella pneumotropica. Infect. Immunol.*, **8,** 762–8
61. Jarret, W. F. H. and Urquhart, G. M. (1954). Husk in cattle. *Vet. Rec.*, **66,** 665–76
62. Jones, G. E., Gilmour, J. S. and Rae, A. G. (1978). Endobronchial inoculation of sheep with pneumonic lung tissue suspensions and with the bacteria and mycoplasma isolated from them. *J. Comp. Pathol.*, **88,** 85–96
63. Kato, H., Kidd, L. and Olley, P. M. (1971). Effects of hypoxia on pulmonary vascular reactivity in pneumonectomized puppies and minipigs. *Circ. Res.*, **28,** 397–402
64. Kobisch, M., Tillon, J. P. and Perrin, G. (1979). Pathologie respiratoire du porc. Détermination du pouvoir pathogène expérimental d'une souche de *Bordetella bronchiseptica. Rec. Méd. Vét.*, **155,** 225–32
65. Kucera, C. J., White, R. G. and Beckenhauer, W. H. (1978). Evaluation of the safety and efficacy of an intranasal vaccine containing a temperature sensitive strain of infectious bovine rhinovirus. *Am. J. Vet. Res.*, **39,** 607–10
66. L'Ecuyer, C. (1969). Enzootic pneumonia in pigs: propagation of a causative *Mycoplasma* in cell cultures and in artificial medium. *Can. J. Comp. Med.*, **33,** 10–19
67. Logomarsino, J. V., Pond, W. G., Krook, L. *et al.* (1974). Effect of dietary calcium phosphorus and nasal irritation on turbinate morphology and performance in pigs. *J. Anim. Sci.*, **39,** 544–9
68. Lopez, A., Thompson, R. G. and Savan, M. (1976). The pulmonary clearance of *Pasteurella hemolytica* in calves infected with bovine parainfluenza 3 virus. *Can. J. Comp. Med.*, **40,** 385–91
69. Lupton, H. W., Barnes, H. S. and Reed, D. E. (1980). Evaluation of the rabbit as a laboratory model of infectious bovine rhinotracheitis virus infection. *Cornell Vet.*, **70,** 77–95

70. Lupton, H. W. and Reed, D. E. (1979). Experimental infection of Eastern Cottontail rabbits (*Sylvilagus floridamus*) with infectious rhinotracheitis virus. *Am. J. Vet. Res.*, **40**, 1329–31
71. MacFerran, J. B., Nelson, R. and Knox, E. R. (1971). Isolation and characterization of sheep *Adenovirus*. *Arch. Ges. Virusforsch.*, **35**, 232–41
72. Mackenzie, A. (1958). Studies on lungworm infection of pigs. 2. Lesions in experimental infections. *Vet. Rec.*, **70**, 903–6
73. MacOwan, K. J. and Minette, J. E. (1977). Contact transmission of experimental contagious caprine pleuropneumonia (CCPP). *Trop. Anim. Hlth Prod.*, **9**, 185–8
74. Maeda, M. (1973). Nasal turbinate atrophy in newborn rabbit infected with *Alcaligenes bronchisepticus* of pig origin. *Nat. Inst. Anim. Hlth Q.*, **13**, 229–39
75. Maeda, M. and Shimizu, T. (1975). Nasal infection of *Alcaligenes bronchisepticus* (*Bordetella bronchiseptica*) and lesions in newborn rabbits. *Nat. Inst. Anim. Hlth Q.*, **15**, 29–37
76. Mare, C. J. and Switzer, W. P. (1966). Virus pneumonia of pigs: drug and ether sensititivy of a causative agent. *Am. J. Vet. Res.*, **27**, 1671–86
77. Martin, W. B., Scott, J. M. and Angus, K. W. (1976). Experimental production of sheep pulmonary adenomatosis (Jaagsiekte). *Nature (London)*, **264**, 183–5
78. Mohanty, S. B. and Lillie, M. G. (1964). Evaluation of a bovine *Myxovirus parainfluenza* 3 (SF4) in calves. *Am. J. Vet. Res.*, **25**, 1653–7
79. Mohanty, S. B., Rockemann, D. D. and Tripathy, R. N. (1980). Chemotherapeutic value of 2 deoxy-D-glucose in infectious bovine rhinotracheitis viral infection in calves. *Am. J. Vet. Res.*, **41**, 1049–51
80. Montlux, W. S., Cutlip, R. C. and Estes, P. C. (1970). Breed susceptibility of tryptophan induced pulmonary adenomatosis in cattle. *Cornell Vet.*, **60**, 547–51
81. Nielsen, R. (1974). Serological and immunological studies of pleuropneumonia of swine caused by *Haemophilus parahemolyticus*. *Acta Vet. Scand.*, **15**, 80–9
82. Onoviran, O. (1974). The comparative efficacy of some antibiotics used to treat experimental induced mycoplasma infection in goats. *Vet. Rec.*, **94**, 418–20
83. Ojo, M. O. (1976). Caprine pneumonia. 4. Pathogenicity of *Mycoplasma mycoides* subspecies *Capri* and caprine strains of *Mycoplasma mycoides* subspecies *mycoides* for goats. *J. Comp. Pathol.*, **86**, 519–29
84. Papageorgiu, C. (1970). Les infections mycoplasmiques du porc. *Bull. Soc. Sci. Vét. Méd. Comp. Lyon*, **72**, 633–49
85. Pastoret, P. P., Aguilar-Setien, A., Burtonboy, G. *et al.* (1978). Mesure de la réexcrétion du virus de la rhinotrachéite infectieuse bovine après injection de dexaméthasone. *Ann. Méd. Vét.*, **122**, 449–56
86. Pastoret, P. P., Aguilar-Setien, A., Burtonboy, G. *et al.* (1980). Effets de la cyclophosphamide sur la latence du virus de la rhinotrachéite infectieuse bovine (*Bovid herpesvirus* 1). *Ann. Méd. Vét.*, **124**, 55–67
87. Peckham, J. C., Mitchell, F. E., Jone, O. H. *et al.* (1972). Atypical interstitial pneumonia in cattle fed moldy sweet potatoes. *J. Am. Vet. Med. Assoc.*, **160**, 169–72
88. Poland, J., Edington, N., Gois, M. *et al.* (1971). The production of pneumonia with or without pleurisy in gnotobiotic piglets with cultures of strain TR 32 of *Mycoplasma hyorhinis*. *J. Hyg. Camb.*, **69**, 145–54
89. Raynaud, J. P., Brunault, G., Maire, C. *et al.* (1977). Pouvoir pathogène de *Pasteurella multocida* pour le jeune porc. Essai de réalisation d'un modèle de pneumonie aiguë expérimentale. *J. Rech. Porc.* en France, INRA-ITP Edit., Paris, pp. 165–9
90. Rose, J. (1958). Site development of the lungworm *Muellerius capillaris* in experimentally infected lambs. *J. Comp. Pathol.*, **68**, 359–62
91. Ross, D. B. (1968). Oral tetramisole. Effect on *Dictyocaulus viviparus, Ostertagia ostertagi* and *Cooperia oncophora* in experimentally infected calves. *Vet. Rec.*, **83**, 69–71
92. Roure, L. D., Dollahite, J. W. and Camp, B. J. (1973). Toxicity of two crude oils and of kerosene to cattle. *J. Am. Vet. Med. Assoc.*, **162**, 61–6
93. Saad, M. B. E. and Rubin, R. (1977). Efficacy of fenbendazole against adult *Dictyocaulus viviparus* in experimentally infected calves. *Am. J. Vet. Res.*, **38**, 1427–8
94. Saunders, J. R. and Berman, D. T. (1969). Epizootiologic studies of shipping fever. 2. Exposure of calves to *Pasteurella* and *Parainfluenza* 3 virus. *Can. J. Comp. Med.*, **28**, 57–62

95. Schuller, W., Laber, G. and Walzl, H. (1977). Chemotherapeutische Untersuchungen mit 81723 hfu (Tiamuline), ein neuen Pleuronutilin Derivat und der experimentellen Myko plasma Pneumonie des Schweines. *Dtsch. Tierärztl. Wosch.*, **84,** 333–72
96. Sharp, J. M., Gilmour, N. J. L., Thompson, D. A. *et al.* (1978). Experimental infection of specific pathogen free lambs with *Parainfluenza virus* type 3 and *Pasteurella haemolytica. J. Comp. Pathol.*, **88,** 237–43
97. Shifrine, M. and Moulton, J. E. (1968). Infection of cattle with *Mycoplasma mycoides* by nasal instillation. *J. Comp. Pathol.*, **78,** 383
98. Shope, R. E., White, D. C. and Leidy, G. (1964). Porcine contagious pleuropneumonia. 2. Studies of pathogenicity of the etiological agent *Haemophilus pleuropneumonia. J. Exp. Med.*, **119,** 369–75
99. Sigurdsson, B., Palsson, P. A. and Tryggvadottir, A. (1953). Transmission experiments with *Maedi. J. Infect. Dis.*, **93,** 166–75
100. Sihvonen, L., Estola, T. and Tuomi, J. (1980). Experimental *Maedi* infection in sheep. 1. Detection of virus, clinical course, histopathology. *Acta Vet. Scand.*, **21,** 113–23
101. Silvoe, E. D., Tavernon, W. D. and Berry, C. L. (1972). Reactive pulmonary arterial hypertension after pulmonary venous constriction in the calf. *Cardiovasc. Res.*, **6,** 36–44
102. Sinclair, I. J. and Tamoglia, T. W. (1972). Intranasal administration of a virulent virus to cattle with a gas-powered atomizer. *Am. J. Vet. Res.*, **33,** 2084–6
103. Singh, S. P. and Singh, N. P. (1980). Milk aspiration pneumonia in calves. *Ind. J. Anim. Sci.*, **50,** 830–3
104. Smith, G. R. (1964). Production of pneumonia in adult sheep with cultures of *Pasteurella haemolytica* type A. *J. Comp. Pathol.*, **74,** 241–9
105. Smith, G. R. (1973). Test in mice on the activity of ronidazole against the causal mycoplasmata of contagious bovine and caprine pleuropneumonia. *Vet. Rec.*, **93,** 440–4
106. Smith, P. C. (1978). Experimental infectious bovine rhinotracheitis virus infections of English ferrets (*mustela putorius furo* L.). *Am. J. Vet. Res.*, **39,** 1369–72
107. Soulebot, J. P., Guillemin, F., Brun, A. *et al.* (1981). Infectious bovine rhinotracheitis. Study on the experimentally induced disease and its prevention using an inactivated adjuvanted vaccine. Presented at *27th International Congress Association Biological Standardization*, Lyon
108. Stephens, L. C., MacChesney, A. E. and Nockels, C. F. (1979). Improved recovery of vitamin E treated lambs that have been experimentally infected with intratracheal chlamydia. *Br. Vet. J.*, **135,** 291
109. Stockdale, P. H. G., Langford, E. U. and Darcel, C. Le Q. (1979). Experimental pneumonic pasteurellosis. 1. Prevention of the disease. 2. Genesis and prevention. *Can. J. Comp. Pathol.*, **436,** 262–71 and 272–9
110. Takatori, I., Huhn, R. G. and Switzer, W. P. (1968). Demonstration of complement fixation antibody against *Mycoplasma hyopneumoniae* in the sera of pigs infected with swine enzootic pneumonia. *Nat. Inst. Anim. Hlth Q.*, **8,** 195–203
111. Takatori, I., Omori, T., Fujiwara, H. *et al.* (1967). The *in vivo* drug sensitivity of a causal agent of swine enzootic pneumonia (SEP). *Nat. Inst. Anim. Hlth Q.*, **7,** 179–86
112. Tewari, H. C., Gangadhara Rao, Y. V. B. and Dhar, D. N. (1972). Studies on radiation attenuated helminth vaccines: laboratory studies on the production and evaluation of gamma irradiated vaccine against the sheep lung-worm *Dictyocaulus filaria. Ind. J. Anim. Sci.*, **42,** 32–7
113. Underdahl, N. R. and Kelley, G. W. (1957). The enhancement of virus pneumonia of pigs by the migration of *Ascaris suum* larvae. *J. Am. Vet. Med. Assoc.*, **130,** 173–6
114. Verwoerd, D. W., Villiers, E. M. de and Tustin, R. C. (1980). Aetiology of Jaagsiekte experimental transmission to lambs by means of cultured cells and cells homogenates. *Onderstepoort J. Vet. Res.*, **47,** 13–18
115. Vogel, J. H. M., Averill, K. H., Pool, P. E. *et al.* (1963). Experimental pulmonary arterial hypertension in the newborn calf. *Circ. Res.*, **13,** 557–71
116. Wandera, J. G. (1968). Experimental transmission of sheep pulmonary adenomatosis (Jaagsiekte). *Vet. Rec.*, **83,** 478–82
117. Wandera, J. G. (1970). Clinical pulmonary adenomatosis of sheep produced experimentally. *Br. Vet. J.*, **126,** 185–93

118. Wells, P. W., Sharp, J. M., Gilmone, N. J. L. *et al.* (1978). The effect of vaccination with *Parainfluenza* type 3 virus on pneumonia resulting from infection with *Parainfluenza* type 3 and *Pasteurella haemolytica*. *J. Comp. Pathol.*, **88**, 253–9
119. Wilkie, B. N. (1976). Hypersensitivity pneumonitis: experimental production in calves with antigens of *Micropolyspora foeni*. *Can. J. Comp. Med.*, **40**, 221–7
120. Wilkie, B. N., Pauli, B. and Gygax, M. (1973). Hypersensitivity pneumonitis: experimental production in guinea pigs with antigens of *Micropolyspora foeni*. *Pathol. Microbiol.*, **39**, 393–411
121. Wilson, G. I. (1970). The strength and duration of immunity to *Dictyocaulus filaria* infection in sheep and goats. *Res. Vet. Sci.*, **11**, 7–17

Section V
Toxicology

51
Environmental pollution: the animal as source, indicator and transmitter

M. Debackere

Environmental sciences are constantly in flux, because new pollutants are identified, new effects are discovered, and old ones are better understood. A precise definition of environmental pollution is difficult, subjective, reflecting the opinion of the contributor. An often cited definition is: 'Environmental pollution is the unfavourable alteration of our surroundings through direct or indirect effects of changes in energy patterns, radiation levels, chemical and physical constitution and abundances of organisms. These changes may affect humans directly or through their supplies of water and of agricultural and other biological products, their physical objects or possessions or their opportunities for recreation and appreciation of nature'[26]. However, this definition is incomplete as it is restricted to human aspects of pollution. Environmental pollution is not limited to the quality of the human environment, but has many harmful consequences and adverse effects on animal health and animal production.

Indeed, it can be suggested that animals occupy an even more complex position in environmental pollution. Although pollution results largely from human activities, animals can be also *sources* of pollution, e.g. by their wastes. Wastes contribute to agricultural pollution by their content in growth promotors, antibiotics, anthelmintics or hormones and infectious agents (bacteria, virus). Clinical signs and toxicological analytical data of poisoned animals are helpful *indicators* for the detection of emissions and immissions of toxic pollutants in the environment. Certain species are reared and used for human consumption, and these edible animal products may be contaminated with pollutants. These animals can be considered as *transmitters* of pollution by way of the food chain.

The purpose of this paper is to discuss the aspects related to this triple function of the animal: source, indicator and transmitter of pollution.

THE FARM ANIMAL AS A SOURCE OF ENVIRONMENTAL POLLUTION

The explosive evolution of animal breeding in the last decades has brought not only a growth of the production capacity, but also certain regional concentrations. The increasing investment of capital and the decreasing dependence on soil has given an industrial character to animal breeding. This is especially so for pig, poultry, and to some extent for cattle breeding. A serious environmental problem with mass production of livestock in 'factory farms' is the large volume of animal waste.

Three cycles can be distinguished in the animal environment relationship[22]:

(1) Primary, which covers metabolic waste products like heat, water vapour, carbon dioxide, methane, faeces and urine.
(2) Secondary, which comprises metabolic waste products broken down and transformed from faeces and urine.
(3) Tertiary, which covers the agents that have been eliminated from the indoor to the outdoor environment, e.g. chemicals from liquid manure (Na, K, nitrate), and pathogenic micro-organisms.

The magnitude of the potential animal waste problem dwarfs that of the human waste problem. For Belgium, it was calculated that the total dry matter production coming from animal manure evolved from 2.45 million metric tonnes in 1959 to 3.5 million metric tonnes in 1978[56]. Daily wet manure production per animal is estimated to average 30 kg for cattle, 3.5 kg for sheep, 3–8 kg for pigs and 0.2 kg for poultry[40,41].

Formerly, farm animal wastes were regarded as important soil fertilizer. The increasing number of farm animals, however, has caused a discrepancy between the manure production and the area of arable land available for manure disposal. This has provoked a waste-supersaturation and waste-overdosage of the available ground with potential harmful consequences. The problem is further aggravated by the liquid wastes from intensive units.

Risks for plants and animals

The nature of the wastes produced depends on the type of animal and the diet. Normal wastes consist of undigested foods, largely cellulose, and fibres. However, the increased use of growth promotors, antibiotics, and other therapeutic substances in farm animal production during the last decade has aggravated the environmental risks already existing from normal components.

Environmental risks from normal animal wastes

Although nitrogen, phosphorus and potassium are essential fertilizers for grass and crops, excess amounts, especially nitrogen, have detrimental effects. The forms of nitrogen returned to the soil from animal wastes are converted into soluble and absorbable nitrates by soil micro-organisms. The absorption from a well-balanced soil is regulated to satisfy the growth demands of the crops. If the soil has an excess of available nitrate, the plant accumulates more than normally required and the plant tissues contain an excess of inorganic nitrates. This accumulation is influenced by many factors[43], and can affect the health of livestock. Inorganic nitrate is not especially toxic, but, reduced to nitrite, it is potentially more toxic as it can oxidize haemoglobin to methaemoglobin and reduce its oxygen-carrying capacity. Nitrate–nitrite poisoning is very well known in cattle. The theorical formation of carcinogenic nitrosamine from these nitrites is possible as for other nitrite-containing foodstuffs[59]. Excessive nitrogen levels in arable land can also lead to negative effects on crops[33]. Dunging of grassland with excessive potassium, especially in the presence of high nitrogen levels in the manure, can adversely influence the magnesium and manganese content of grass. Magnesium deficiency in grass can provoke hypomagnesaemia in cattle, and manganese deficiency can lead to infertility in cattle[56].

Other endogenous compounds excreted by animals and recycled are oestrogens and androgens. Oestrogenic activity can be detected in fresh excreta from almost all livestock and poultry. The quantities are quite variable and the levels are highest in excreta from pregnant dairy cows and high-producing laying hens. The effect of these oestrogenic residues in excreta recycled for feed or fertilizer has not yet been evaluated. Androgenic activity has been found in excreta of livestock and poultry. Microbial conversion of progesterone to androgens seems possible in cattle faeces. Fresh dried poultry excreta show no androgenic activity. It must be incubated in order to become androgenically active. This process is accelerated by fly larvae[7].

The dispersal of pathogenic bacteria.and other micro-organisms, which populate the alimentary tract of domestic animals, by spreading animal wastes and manure on pastures is a real problem. In particular *Enterobacteria*, such as certain strains of *Salmonellae*, can cause sickness in man and animals. These micro-organisms persist for periods up to 12 weeks in animal waste slurries, but the soil is fairly effective in removing these bacteria from liquid slurry, probably by absorption onto mineral components of clay. Nevertheless, bacteria in the top layers of pasture may be a source of infection for grazing animals.

Environmental risks from feed-additives and growth-promotors pollutants

The practice of adding *copper* in concentrations varying from 125 to 250 parts/10^6 in pig feeds is very common in western Europe. This has led to an enhancement of the copper levels in the slurries coming from intensive pig rearing units. Levels even higher than 1000 parts/10^6 copper in dry matter have been reported[2]. Single application of over 50 000 l/ha of copper-rich slurry would increase the copper content of grass for a short period to levels of 10–14 parts/10^6 on dry matter basis. This may be considered as a potential hazard to sheep, which are particularly sensitive to enhanced dietary levels of copper[46]. It was concluded that copper in pig slurry is almost as available to sheep as copper presented as copper sulphate[45, 51]. The main risk from high-copper slurries on pasture comes from the ingestion of copper as a foliar contaminant.

In most countries some *antibiotics* are allowed in animal nutrition as growth stimulating agents. Much attention has been paid to the use of these antibiotics and the risks of their possible residues in foods of animal origin for human consumption[47]. Their use has environmental consequences as they are excreted unchanged or as metabolites in animal wastes that ultimately reach arable grounds and surface waters. Theoretically, these residues of antibiotics may harm the environment by several ways[5]. They disturb the microbiological equilibrium and the cycling processes in water and soil. They accumulate in the environment, are absorbed by plant roots and retain their activity in these plants for a longer time (e.g. streptomycin, tetracyclines). They provoke a selection and propagation of resistance. This is demonstrated for avoparcine, lincomycin, nitrovine and tylosine, used as feed additives in chickens, that increased and prolonged the excretion of resistant *Salmonellae*[49]. Manure from natural dunging not only contains antibiotic residues, but also faecal micro-organisms which disturb the homeostasis of the soil. These effects depend on the persistence of the antibiotic residues in the soil. Therefore biodegradation in the aquatic and solid phases of the soil is of great importance. This biodegradation has been studied for tylosine, oleandomycine, spiramycine and zinc-bacitracin, as has their probable influence on soil homeostasis. For tylosine and oleandomycine, their aerobic and anaerobic catabolism in aquatic systems are limited. Soil degradation for tylosine is very slow, and for oleandomycine is related to the concentration. Lower concentrations of spiramycine show a very quick breakdown, as well in aerobic aquatic systems as in the solid soil phase. At higher concentrations, the breakdown is only completed after 6 months. Under anaerobic conditions there should not be any breakdown at all. Zinc-bacitracin is completely degraded after 3–4 months in aerobic circumstances. In an anaerobic medium the degradation is very slow and only partial.

In some countries *anabolic agents* are legally used in cattle in order to increase growth rate and improve feed efficiency. These compounds and their metabolites, usually excreted in faeces and urine, may have consequences for the environment if recycled in feed and fertilizer. A significant increase of abortions is reported in pregnant cows fed litter from poultry receiving feed containing 35 mg of dienesterol diacetate per kg of feed[20]. More research is needed to determine the levels of anabolic hormone residues in excreta of treated animals, and the effects of these residues on animal performance when recycled in feed. The uptake of diethylstilboestrol (DES) or its metabolites by plants seems to be dependent on soil characteristics and crop variety[7]. Also DES seems to have an inhibitory effect on several species of soil bacteria. There is some discussion about the levels that provoke this effect in relation to the levels found under practical livestock production procedures. Environmental hazards following the use of synthetic grit containing mestranol for pigeon control are reported[50]. The degradation of mestranol in animals and plants is very rapid, and the presence of soil microorganisms seems very important.

Risks for surface waters

Animal wastes are a major problem once they are permitted to enter water supplies. Any *organic matter* oxidized by micro-organisms provokes an increased demand for dissolved oxygen and leads to the depletion of the oxygen content of the water with a detrimental influence on animal life. These wastes are relatively *nitrogen* and *phosphorus* rich so that explosive growths of algae and plankton occur. Their subsequent decay and oxidation leads to a supplemental increase in oxygen demand with even greater destruction of normal animal life in the aquatic environment. Explosive growth of algae, known as eutrophication, may create further serious ecological disturbances like extraordinary growth of dinoflagellates, which occur occasionally in the early summer months on the North Sea coasts of the Netherlands and Belgium. These organisms produce a highly toxic substance absorbed by mussels, and create dangers for human consumption and health.

Liquid waste products from animals may reach the water supplies as run-off into lakes and streams, and by percolation through the soil to underground water sources. This leads to a contamination of drinking water, especially with nitrate and bacteria. Harmful levels of several pathogens from pig and cattle wastes, such as coliform bacteria and faecal streptococci, had been found in drinking water. In the USA, a survey of dairy cattle wastes found in rivers indicates that 90% of the samples exceeded state-accepted bacterial counts[30].

THE ANIMAL AS AN INDICATOR OF ENVIRONMENTAL POLLUTION

It has been estimated that men use about four million different chemical substances. Only 30 000 are commercially produced, the remaining ones being intermediates or waste products. Substances can enter the environment through different and sometimes complex and interrelated paths. A first group, fertilizers, pesticides, and herbicides, enters the environment by direct application. A second group, sulphur oxides, nitrogen oxides, and polycyclic aromatic hydrocarbons, results from combustion processes. A third source is the waste effluents from industry or manufacturing units. Many manufacturing processes generate air- and water-borne wastes which are sometimes more toxic than the raw parent materials. Some chemical substances, once in the environment, undergo physical and chemical changes, and become toxic by-products[53].

Pesticides

Chemical pesticides are used on a great scale and they contribute to an increase in agricultural production, but they have also caused serious ecological damages. Their effects on non-target organisms have been a source of worldwide contention for more than a decade.

Of the three classes of the most-used pesticides, insecticides offer the greatest potential for detrimental non-target effects, fungicides the least, and herbicides are intermediate[62].

The most readily identified insecticide effects on non-targets result from the persistent *organochlorine insecticides* and their metabolites or conversion products. Several of their characteristics, slow rate of biodegradability, persistence, ubiquitous nature, and tendency to concentrate in organisms, make them very appropriate for food chain accumulation and for indirect toxicity on non-target animals of various sensitivities. Besides the adverse effects on non-target organisms, having physiological functions common with those of the target organisms, a second, and usually unpredictable response, is the effect of the pesticide on dissimilar physiological systems in non-targets[62]. One of these effects is biomagnification or bioconcentration which is the accumulation of a pesticide in a living organism[3]. In biomagnification, the key factor is aquatic invertebrates. The role of domestic animals as indicators for environmental pollution through pesticides is negligible. The only role played by livestock is the transfer of pesticides residues in meat and milk when they are exposed to therapeutical doses of persistent insecticides. Bats seem to be the most suceptible mammal to poisoning[42]. The most susceptible non-target animal species seem to be fish and birds. The chlorinated insecticides are outstandingly toxic for fish, especially trout and salmon. Based on this sensitivity, a detection method for pesticides pollutants in drinking water has been devised[29]. This ichtyotest is based on the physiological modification of the electrical activity in the olfactory bulbs of the trout for micro-quantities of pesticides and similar compounds. Concentrations of $10\,\text{parts}/10^{12}$ can be detected in a reproducible way within 0.5 s, which lies in the neighbourhood of the classical analytical methods. A review of the use of biological indicator organisms, such as teleosts or marine mammals, and their major advantages has been produced.

Birds seem to be affected in two ways. Mortality is due to the accumulation of organochlorine residues in their foods, resulting in lethal brain levels of the insecticide. This was noted for the first time in the Californian Lake Clear following routine applications of DDD[27], and a second and similar example was noted some years later in Lake Michigan[23]. Many similar accidents with the death of birds at the top of food chains have been described as a result of biomagnification. In general, predatory birds contain higher residues of these compounds than herbivorous ones, insectivorous species occupy an intermediate position[55].

In the Zoological Park of London after many deaths in owls, livers and brains were found to contain toxic concentrations of dieldrin. This dieldrin residue was traced back to the mice on which they were fed and in turn to the sawdust used as bedding for the mice. This sawdust had been obtained from a builder who was using a timber preservation containing dieldrin to protect against woodworm[32]. A second effect in birds is death of the embryos due primarily to premature cracking of thin egg shells and secondarily to lethal pesticide levels in the embryos[24]. The phenonomenon of thin egg shell has been attributed to induction of hepatic microsomal enzymes that metabolize steroid hormones and hence decrease the blood-calcium levels[62]. Both effects make birds very good indicators for environmental pollution through accumulation of pesticides in concentrations that have no perceptible damaging influences on animals and mankind.

Honey bees also have proven to be very good indicators as they are very sensitive to many insecticides belonging to the carbamate and organophosphate classes. Wettable powders and dusts are particularly hazardous while microencapsulated materials are more toxic than all other formulations because the vinyl spheres are about the size of pollen grains and are treated as such, leading to brood kills[1].

Other organic pollutants

Polychlorinated biphenyls (PCBs) are substances with identical chemical and physical properties to the organochlorine insecticides. Although their toxicity was already known in the 1940s, their persistence in the environment and their accumulation in the food chain were demonstrated only in 1966[31]. Many environmental pollutions with these compounds have been detected and identified thanks to the presence of poultry[36,44], birds[10] and even cattle[60,63]. Later on, it was demonstrated that the toxicity of PCBs was similar to the toxic effects of the chick oedema factor which produces hydropericardium and death. Some toxic properties attributed to PCBs may be due to contamination by the very toxic chlorinated dibenzofurans and dibenzodioxins. The latter were the cause of a large and severe pollution near Seweso (Italy) resulting from an explosion in a chemical plant. On this occasion it was shown that rabbits and rodents were much more sensitive than other animal species. In another study the rabbit populations living on polluted soil had accumulated dioxins in the body up to the concentration of the soil itself, probably through pelt contamination and ingestion of soil particles with the grass[16]. Hence, rabbits are used as indicators for the decontamination of these areas.

It has been known for a long time that cattle feeding on spoiled sweet clover hay develop haemorrhagic disease. Castration of such cattle provoked a staunchless haemorrhage. The active substance was isolated from spoiled clover and found to be bishydroxycoumarine[39].

Outbreaks of an apparently new disease in turkey poults occurred in England in 1960 causing an estimated loss of about 100 000 birds. A short time later similar outbreaks were diagnosed in ducklings and young pheasants. The common factor was the presence of Brasilian groundnutmeal in the food. Simultaneous with the outbreak of Turkey 'X' disease in England, there was a widespread occurrence of hepatomas in trout in the United States. Subsequent research revealed that in all these cases the common toxic factor was a mixture of toxins produced by *Aspergillus flavus* and therefore called 'aflatoxins'. This was the start of an intensive search as it was shown that the most active of these aflatoxins, aflatoxin B_1, which caused trout hepatomas, is one of the most potent carcinogens to date. Therefore ducklings and rainbow trout are used as biological indicators for the presence of aflatoxin-producing fungi in foods and feeds[19].

Trace metals

Trace metals are widely distributed in the environment. Many trace metals are essential to plant and animal life, but in excessive amounts they disturb the environment for animal health. This is especially the case for industrial pollutants and emissions. As metals have no perceptible properties but a very strong cumulative character, the presence of domestic animals on pastures in the vicinity of the immission sources can be of an unexpected value. By eating the contaminated vegetation daily, a progressive accumulation occurs till clinical signs appear at a stage when the presence of the environmental trace metal pollution is still unperceptable[12].

Fluorine injures vegetation and grazing animals as a result of industrial air pollution. For fluoride emissions, cattle, specifically milk-cows, are very good indicators because they are herbivores, and they have a very active calcium metabolism. In Belgium, two severe environmental fluoride pollutions existed, one by a brickworks and one by an enamel factory[13]. Thanks to the presence of cattle, the fluoride pollution was detected before damage happened to humans. From the dental lesions observed and the calculated data of eruption and crown formation of the incisor teeth, it was possible to estimate the start of the fluoride pollution.

As already mentioned, sheep are extremely susceptible to excess *copper*. Forage copper levels of 15–20 parts/10^6 (on a dry matter basis) are critical for sheep and levels of 30–40 parts/10^6 are definitely toxic. Small increases above the normal grass copper levels of 8–15 parts/10^6 will be toxic. Sheep are accepted as very good indicators for environmental pollutions by copper industries and copper smelting works[12].

Lead is one of the most ubiquitous heavy metals in the environment as its use is diverse and widespread. In urban pollution through motor vehicle emissions and contamination of the street dust, dogs and cats can give a very good idea of the lead pollution, as their liver and kidney lead levels increase significantly[15]. The feral pigeon *Clumbia livea* is suggested to monitor lead contamination, and to serve as a model for chronic lead toxicity[28]. The ability of the pigeon to accumulate elevated lead concentrations is due to feeding at ground levels and ingestion of food contaminated with roadside dust. In the case of industrial pollutions or of motor vehicle emissions in the neighbourhood of speedways, where high concentrations of lead are deposited on the vegetation, cattle[4,12], sheep[61] and horses[18] are good indicators of these pollutions. Sheep and even rabbits have been used for the differentiation of oral and inhalatory lead uptake under combined exposure in a polluted area[21]. Terrestrial small mammals have been used for the study of the impact of abandoned metalliferous mines on terrestrial ecosystems[48]. The determination of lead levels in bats and terrestrial small mammals is mentioned for the study of lead emissions near highways[9]. Geese and ducks can easily show lead intoxication by excessive ingestion of lead pellets in the mud of ponds surrounding fields with shooting pits[52].

Industrial poisoning due to *arsenic*-bearing emissions is one of the most commonly occurring poisonings in bees, because bees are very susceptible to arsenic. Death usually occurs within the first few hours after intake or contact and can continue up to 5–6 days afterwards[14].

For *radioactive* pollution and fall-out, special attention is paid to ^{90}Sr and ^{137}Cs, mainly in view of their physical characteristics. Both have a long half-life which determines their persistence, and they are produced in a high yield by nuclear fission. All authorities agree that animal products and especially fresh milk and milk products are important sources of these long-lived radionuclides. Their concentrations in milk and its products have been followed as indicators for environmental pollution through radioactive materials, and have provided the major part of any regular monitoring programme in most countries.

Mercury, especially organic mercury, is another metal that has attracted attention as an extremely hazardous environmental pollutant. The best known case occurred at Minamata Bay in Japan. Before the human cases were recognized, it was noticed that cats in the area became ill, screamed incessantly and jumped of cliffs into the ocean. It was finally established that the link between the feline and the human diseases was the consumption of fish contaminated with Hg, rather than an infectious agent[26].

THE ANIMAL AS A TRANSMITTER OF ENVIRONMENTAL POLLUTANTS

Animals can act as transmitters of pollutants by way of the food chain. For most pollutants there are two possible food chains: (1) sea-water and fish, and (2) soil, plants and herbivores or seed-eating animals.

Pollution of the food chain can be provoked by pollutants: (1) which enter accidentally, e.g. waste products from industrial or traffic sources, or from final products that are used in agriculture or the manufacture of feedstuffs; and (2) which enter the food chain from intentional use in animal production (growth promotors), or in food-processing.

Accidental pollutants

Many *heavy metals* can accumulate in the tissues of fish and food-producing animals. Products of animal origin represent 45% of the total daily diet, fruits and vegetables account for 55%. The daily dietary consumption of *lead* with the latter is three times higher than with the former. From kinetic studies it seems that in cattle and poultry there is a discrimination against lead and, just as with strontium, the observed ratio diet/milk and meat is smaller than one. This means that even for poisoned animals meat concentrations do not differ much from normal animals. Only liver and kidneys can offer exaggerated lead charge that can exceed the tolerable weekly intake of 3 mg[38].

Cadmium is a very controversial pollutant. Its concentration factor, from soil into plants, is about ten. In kidney and liver of cows, pigs and poultry it accumulates with a concentration factor of about ten, in comparison to the level in the dry matter of the rations. Accumulation does not occur in milk, muscle, bones or eggs[54, 58]. In cattle there seems to be a highly significant relationship between the age of the animals and the cadmium content of the kidneys. The kidneys of older cattle often contain many times the quantity of cadmium found in younger animals[37]. Notwithstanding this accumulation of cadmium, obvious toxicological influences on domestic animals have not yet been observed or described. Although the food-producing animals may act as an effective filter of cadmium, consumption of kidney and liver from such animals would supply cadmium above the tolerable level and may pose a hazard. A statistical evaluation shows that about 36% of cadmium ingested by men in West Germany is related to residues in food-producing animals[6].

In the transmission of *mercury*, and especially organic mercury, fish is the only serious source in the human diet. Only in exceptional cases, such as some years ago in the Netherlands with calves, may domestic animals be a potential source of mercury transmission.

For *fluorine*, even in poisoned cattle, milk, meat and visceral organs do not offer hazards for the consumer as there is no accumulation at all in soft tissues.

Pesticides are the most widespread substances that come in contact with animal foods and contaminate edible products from food-producing animals. They can be divided into two groups, the non-persistent compounds, e.g. organophosphate-esters and carbamate-esters, and the more persistent compounds, e.g. organochlorines. Organophosphate- and carbamate-esters are estimated to leave no residues at all or only in such small quantities that they are excreted from the animal body within a short time. There are some species differences, which make residue transmission less problematic. This is the case in ruminants, where rumen metabolization can detoxify a lot of esters by hydrolysis and by anaerobic reduction. This means, that when properly used, meat and edible products from ruminants are not a source of transmission of these pesticides[34].

Organochlorine pesticides and polyhalogenated biphenyls are a problem for the food chain as they are very persistent and cumulative in the ecosystem. Since the ban of DDT in most countries, organochlorine pesticide residue in edible domestic animals is mainly lindane. Some studies have been carried out after oral administration in poultry[35]. It seems that there is an accumulation in eggs and tissues and that this accumulation is dose-related, and proportional with the fat concentration of the tissues. In pigs and cattle the accumulation factor seems to be much higher than in poultry. The quantity of residues found in meat and meat products after oral intake of contaminated food seems to be much lower than the permissible levels fixed in most countries. Only the use of lindane as an ectoparasitical on lactating cows can provoke a sudden contamination of milk with high levels that persist for at least 3 weeks[57]. In the case of accidents with organochlorine pesticides and related compounds, hazards for the consumer can be much more pronounced. This has been proven by the Michigan accident in 1973 with polybrominated biphenyls[8]. Concentrations in bodyfat and milk seem higher. It has been calculated that some farmers, consuming milk from their own cows, could have obtained as much as 10 g of PBB during the period between contamination and identification of the pollutant, which took 250 days[17].

Pollutants after intentional use

Apart from the use of medicines for therapeutic objectives, many of the same substances are used for growth purposes in mass-production units. According to their pharmacotherapeutical properties they are divided into three groups: antibiotics, chemotherapeutics other than antibiotics, and compounds with an hormonal activity.

The literature on the problem of *antibiotic* residues in animals products is very confusing, and agrees that growth stimulating concentrations of 20 and even 50 parts/10^6 result in no measurable residual amounts in the meat, and only parts/10^9 concentrations in the visceral organs. Prophylactic doses up to 100 parts/10^6 give rise to levels of some tenths of parts/10^6 in the meat, and some parts/10^6 in the organs[11]. From acute and chronic toxicity studies there are no indications that these quantities of residues offer hazards for the consumer. Risks of allergic reactions from the most allergenic antibiotics are not fully excluded. The problem of development of microbial resistance seems to be most serious. It is agreed that the practice of using antibiotics as growth-promoting factors has contributed not only to the selection of resistant organisms in animals, but also to the spread of R factors, and such strains may have been transferred to the consumer. Recent publications support the importance of this transfer of resistant micro-organisms from animals to humans.

Among the other *chemotherapeutics*, organic arsenic derivatives are widely used. Levels above 1 part/10^6 (accepted as the permissible level) are found in tissues and muscles of treated swine up to 6 days after the last treatment. Chronic effects only begin to appear above 3 parts/10^6. Different coccidiostatics at their usual doses give detectable amounts of residues in muscles and liver. Their toxicological significance is, however, still unknown.

The use, residues and toxicology of *hormones* as growth promotors are for the moment the subject of a very controversial debate in the Western European countries. Their use for animal fattening is still allowed in some countries. The main health hazard associated with their use is based on residues present at slaughter. The nature, quantity and risks of these residues depend on the type of anabolic agent used[25]. A distinction must be made between endogenous steroids and exogenous anabolic agents.

Endogenous steroids, also called natural hormones, would not present any harmful effects to the health of the consumer when used under the appropriate conditions. They are rapidly metabolized, predominantly in the liver, to compounds with little if any biological activity. These metabolites are eliminated very quickly and only a small percentage can reach the systemic circulation and accumulate in the tissues, particularly in the kidney and the liver. Under appropriate conditions, the treatment of animals with natural steroids results in edible tissues with residues lower than those occurring naturally in mature males, females and pregnant females.

The most dangerous application lies in the use of the synthetic exogenous hormones: diethylstilboestrol (DES), and methyltestosterone, particularly their illegal use, with totally uncontrolled formulations, dosages and treatment-intervals, and without any regard to withdrawal periods. These hazards are not imaginary as has been proven by the detection of high residue levels in canned babyfood of animal origin. Moreover, DES is a proven carcinogen. The risks of two other exogenous anabolic agents, trenbolone, a synthetic steroid with a physiological activity similar to testosterone but with a greater anabolic activity, and zeranol, a non-steroidal oestrogen with anabolic activity, are still under discussion. They are claimed to be the safest products used as hormonal growth promotors[63]. Some data in the hormonal non-effect level and the toxicology of these compounds and their metabolites are still needed to settle the discussion.

CONCLUSIONS

Although incomplete, this study proves that the animal takes a special position in the interrelationship between animal and environment and vice versa. It can be the cause and the victim of environmental pollution. However, as a source it is on a more restricted scale and in complicity with human beings. As victim it can readily be affected and even lethally poisoned before human beings are aware of any change in their environment. This can be a protection for the human population in some chronic and insidious pollutions. Despite the disastrous consequences for the animals themselves and the ecosystem, it is a blessing that animals act as very sensitive indicators. In some cases the animal can be a danger for human beings as it can act as a transmitter for several persistent pollutants by way of the food chain, even to consumers that are far away from the pollution site and the polluted environment. The three functions of the animal as source, indicator and transmitter of pollution indicate an important role for the veterinary profession in the protection of the environment and the ecosystem. As clinician, epidemiologist and food-hygienist, the veterinarian, in cooperation with environmental toxicologists, plays an important role in safe-guarding our environment.

References

1. Atkins, E. L., Anderson, L. D., Kellum, D. *et al.* (1977). Leaflet 2883. (Riverside: Div. Agr. Sci. Univ. Calif.)
2. Batry, T., Berryman, C. and Line, C. (1972). *J. Br. Grassland Soc.*, **27**, 139–43
3. Bevenue, A. (1976). *Residue Rev.*, **61**, 37–59
4. Bhat, R. V. and Krishnamachari, K. A. V. R. (1980). *Bull. Environm. Contam. Toxicol.*, **25**, 142–5
5. Blommaert, M. (1977). Biodegradatie van enkele antibiotica gebruikt als additief in de veevoeding. *Thesis Fac. Landbouwwet. Gent: R.U.G.*
6. Boehncke, F. (1977). *Landwirtsch. Forsch.*, **34**, 44–61
7. Calvert, C. C. and Smith, L. W. (1976). Recycling and degradation of anabolic agents in animal excreta. In Lu, F. C. and Rendel, J. (eds.) *Anabolic Agents in Animal Production, FAO/WHO Symp.* pp. 203–11. (Rome, Stuttgart: G. Thieme)
8. Carter, L. J. (1976). *Science*, **192**, 240–3
9. Clark, D. R. (1979). *Environm. Sci. Technol.*, **13**, 338–41
10. Combs, G. F. and Scott, M. L. (1977). *W. Poult. Sci. A. J.*, **33**, 31–46
11. Craenen, M. (1976). Antibiotica residuen in eetwaren van dierlijke oorsprong. *Lic. Verhandeling Fac. Diergeneeskunde, Gent: R.U.G.*

12. Debackere, M. (1980). Poisoning of domestic animals as an indication of environmental pollution. In van Miert, A. S. J., Frens, J. and van der Kreek, F. W. (eds.) *Trends in Veterinary Pharmacology and Toxicology*. pp. 314–20. (Amsterdam: Elsevier Sci.)
13. Debackere, M. and Delbeke, F. T. (1978). *Intern. J. Environm. Studies*, **11**, 249–52; Ibid., 1979, **13**, 229–31; Ibid., 1981, **17**, 201–7
14. Debackere, M. (1972). *Vlaams Imkersblad*, **2**, 149–55
15. De Corte-Baeten, K. (1972). Lood- an bloodvergiftigingen bij huisdieren. *Med. Fac. Diergeneesk., R.U.G.*, **16**, 3–4
16. Fanelli, R., Castelli, M. G., Martelli, G. P. *et al.* (1980). *Bull. Environm. Contam. Toxicol.*, **24**, 460–2
17. Fries, G. F. (1978). *J. Am. Vet. Med. Assoc.*, **173**, 1479–84
18. Ghergariv, S., Kadar, L. and Bohm, B. (1978). *Rec. Méd. Vét.*, **154**, 633–7
19. Goldblatt, L. A. (1969). *Aflatoxin, Scientific Background, Control and Implications.* (New York: Academic Press)
20. Griel, L. C. Jr., Kredel, D. C. and Wickersham, F. W. (1963). *Cornell Vet.*, **59**, 227
21. Hapke, H. S. and Abel, J. (1978). *Toxicology*, **11**, 83–94
22. Hays, F. C. and Bianca, W. (1975). *Agric. Environm.*, **2**, 311–31
23. Hickey, J. J., Keith, J. A. and Goon, F. B. (1966). *J. Appl. Ecol.*, **3** (Suppl.), 141
24. Hickey, J. J. and Anderson, D. W. (1968). *Science*, **162**, 271
25. Hoffman, B. and Karg, H. V. (1976). Metabolic fate of anabolic agents in treated animals and residue levels in their meat. In Lu, F. C. and Rendel, J. (eds.) *Anabolic Agents in Animal Production, FAO/WHO Symp.* pp. 181–91. (Rome, Stuttgart: G. Thieme)
26. Hodges, L. (1976). *Environmental Pollution.* 2nd Edn. pp. 230–6. (New York: Holt, Rinehart and Winsker)
27. Hunt, E. Q. and Bishoff, H. I. (1960). *Calif. Fish Game*, **46**, 10
28. Hutton, M. and Goodman, G. T. (1980). *Environm. Pollution, Ser. A Biol. Ecol.*, **22**, 207–27
29. Huve, J. J. (1982). *La Recherche*, **13**, 108–10
30. Janzen, J. J., Bodine, A. B. and Luazer, L. J. (1974). *J. Dairy Sci.*, **57**, 260–3
31. Jensen, S. (1966). *N. Scientist*, **32**, 612
32. Jones, D. M., Bennett, D. and Elgar, K. E. (1978). *Nature (London)*, **271**, 52
33. Jorritsma, J. (1975). *Boerderij*, **59**, 46–7
34. Kaemmerer, K. and Buntenkötter, S. (1973). *Residue Rev.*, **46**, 30
35. Kan, A. C. and Jonker-den-Royen, J. C. (1978). *J. Agr. Food Chem.*, **26**, 935–40
36. Kohanawa, W., Shova, S., Ogura, Y. *et al.* (1969). *Nat. Inst. Anim. Hlth Q.*, **9**, 220
37. Kreuzer, W., Kracke, W., Samsowi, B. *et al.* (1978). *Fleischwirtsch.*, **6**, 1022–30
38. Laurier, L. (1978). Lood in het milieu en in de voeding met betrekking tot de dierlijke produktie. *Lic. Verhandeling, Fac. Diergeneeskunde, Gent: R.U.G.*
39. Link, A. (1941). *J. Biol. Chem.*, **138**, 529
40. Loehr, R. C. (1968). Pollution implications of animal wastes, a forward oriented review. (Ada, Okla.: RS Kerr Water Res. Center, US Dept. of the Interior)
41. Loehr, R. C. and Hart, S. A. (1970). *Crit. Rev. Environm. Control.*, **69**, 10
42. Luckens, M. M. and Davis, W. M. (1964). *Science*, **146**, 948
43. O'Hara, P. S. and Frazer, A. J. (1975). *N.Z. Vet. J.*, **23**, 45–53
44. Picharallo, J. (1971). *Science*, **173**, 873
45. Price, J. and Suttle, N. F. (1975). *Proc. Nutr. Soc.*, **31**, 9A–10A
46. Purves, D. (1977). *Trace Element Contamination of the Environment.* p. 174. (Amsterdam: Elsevier)
47. Report of the *Joint Committee on the Use of Antibiotics in Animal Husbandry and Veterinary Medicine (Swann Report)* (1969). Cmnd, 4190. (London: HMSO)
48. Roberts, R. D. and Johnson, M. S. (1978). *Environm. Poll.*, **15**, 61–9
49. Smith, H. W. and Tucker, J. F. (1975). *J. Hyg. Camb.*, **75**, 293–301
50. Sturtevant, J. (1971). *Toxicol. Appl. Pharm.*, **19**, 619–59
51. Suttle, N. F. (1974). *Br. J. Nutr.*, **32**, 395
52. Szymczak, M. R. and Adrian, W. J. (1978). *J. Wildlife Manag.*, **42**, 299–306
53. Tolba, M. J. (1978). *Environm. Intern.*, **1**, 129–40
54. Tomika, T., Sato, T., Saito, K. *et al.* (1979). *Toxicol. Litt.*, **3–5**, 291–7
55. Turner, G. T. (1982). *Vet. Hum. Toxicol.*, **24**, 31–3

56. van Acker, L. (1980). Dierlijke mest: afval of grondstof. *Lic. Verhandeling, Fac. Landbouwwet., Gent: R.U.G.*
57. van Renterghem, R. (1976). *Landbouwtijdschrift*, **29**, 355–76
58. Vemmer, K. and Petersen, U. (1977). *Landwirtsch. Forsch.*, **34**, 66–71
59. Veys, P. (1980). Nitrosaminen in eetwaren van dierlijke oorsprong. Hun toxiciteit, meer speciaal met betrekking tot de carcinogeniteit. *Lic. Verhandeling, Fac. Diergeneeskunde, Gent: R.U.G.*
60. Vos, J. G., Reinders, J. S., Kroneman, S. *et al.* (1971). *Tijdschr. Diergeneesk.*, **96**, 1577
61. Wara, N. I., Brooks, R. R. and Roberts, E. (1978). *Bull. Environm. Contam. Toxicol.*, **20**, 44–51
62. Ware, G. W. (1975). *Residue Rev.*, **59**, 119; Ibid., 1980, **76**, 173–201
63. Williet, L. B. and Hess, J. F. (1975). *Residue Rev.*, **55**, 135–47

52
Residues of drugs and pesticides in milk

W. Heeschen and A. Blüthgen

The occurrence of chemical residues in milk reflects both the increasing number of chemicals in agriculture as well as a more or less polluted environment of the dairy animal or the processing sites.

The first mentioned aspect includes the wide abundance of plant-protecting agents, fertilizers, veterinary drugs, cleaning and disinfecting agents which are more and more essential for economic and sufficient production of agricultural commodities including milk.

On the other hand, chemicals, which are in some cases highly undesirable, may get access into the direct or indirect environment of the cows. This process is, in some cases, additional to the normal site-borne contamination, e.g. with heavy metals.

Table 52.1 Criteria for the hygienic-qualitative property of milk

1.	Pathogens (*Salmonellae, Staph. aureus, Clostridiae et al.*)
2.	Microbial toxins (mycotoxins, enterotoxins *et al.*)
3.	Biocides and environmental chemicals Pesticides (insecticides, fungicides, herbicides) Veterinary drugs (fasciolicides, antibiotics, ectoparasiticides *et al.*) Toxic heavy metals (lead, cadmium, mercury, arsenic) Environmental organics (PCB *et al.*) Cleaning and disinfecting agents (iodine, QAC *et al.*)
4.	Somatic cells (cell count)
5.	Saprophytes (spoilage germs)
6.	Sensory properties (smell, taste)

Despite the different origin of chemical residues in milk, all efforts should be undertaken to protect the consumer as well as possible from any undue impact with food-borne chemicals. As milk is also used as a food for infants, children, sick and elderly people, these efforts have high priority.

From the scientific point of view, the occurrence of chemical residues in milk is part of a larger field of hygienic activities, which is outlined in brief in Table 52.1.

This paper will deal with the more chemical and pharmaceutical aspects of the featured criteria, excluding the microbial and sensory criteria of the problem.

SOURCES AND PATHWAYS OF CONTAMINATION[5]

The chemical contamination of milk is mainly the result of three partially overlapping sources, which are more or less directly associated with the dairy cow or milk production. Figure 52.1 shows the rather complex connection, with selected typical examples. The sources, such as lactating animals, agriculture and environment, production and processing sites, bear the risk of a secretory or postsecretory contamination with one or more chemicals cited in the outlined section. It is evident that contamination in some cases is not restricted to the exclusive source given.

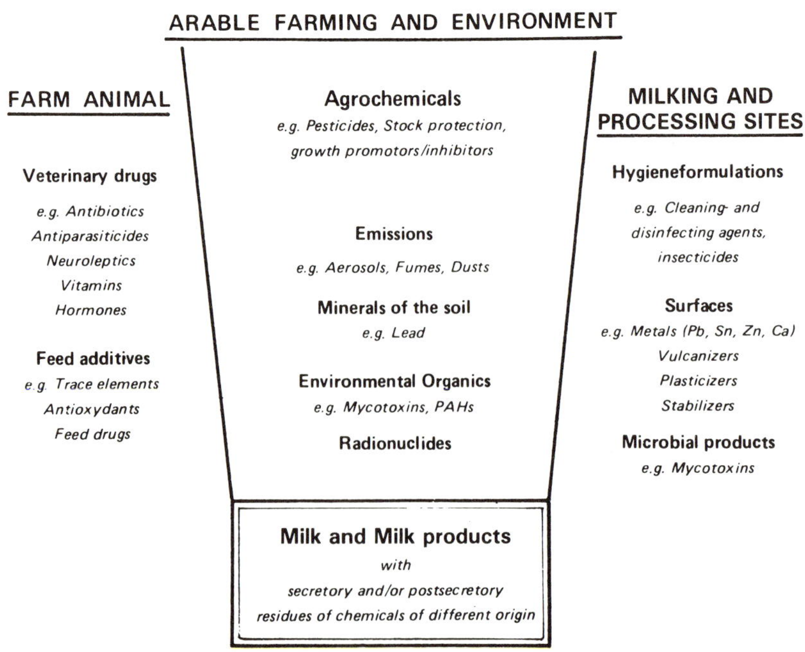

Figure 52.1 Chemical contamination of milk

A well-known phenomenon in the possibility of chemical residues in milk is the kinetics of the included food chain, which begins in the environment with soil and plants, then affects the cow and ends with the human consumer of milk and meat. For substances, which are so stable that they withstand any impact and diminution in the environment including physiology of plants and animals, the food chain will be a pathway of considerable magnification of residues from link to link. The lipophilic chlorinated hydrocarbons are an excellent example of this possibility. On the other hand, less stable or ionic residues will be kept at low levels from link to link, so that these substances will not build up concentrations exceeding the originally low concentration. Figure 52.2 shows the terrestrial food chain including milk and man with the organochlorines as a representative for magnifying residues up to several powers of ten.

The role of the food chain will be briefly mentioned for some residues in the following, if it is of importance in the formation of the specific residue.

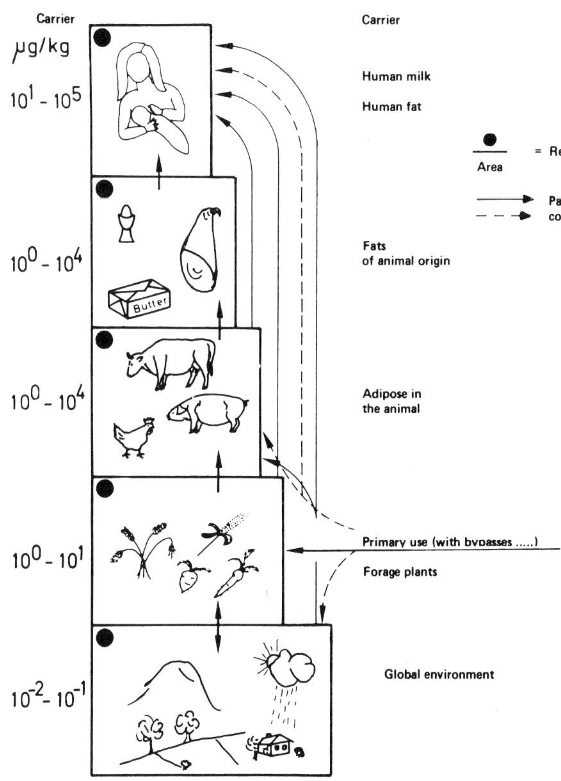

Figure 52.2 Pathways of contamination and accumulation of organochlorine insecticides from the environment in the food chain – air, soil, water – plant – fat – man

SPECIFIC RESIDUES IN MILK[6,8]

As already mentioned, quite a large number of environmental chemicals and drugs can get access into the milk. The following can, of course, only deal with a restricted number of different residues which share special public and scientific attention.

Drugs[1]

The most direct cause of residues in milk is the application of drugs to the farm animal. These substances may be used for the treatment of microbial infections of the mammary gland, the prevention of such infections and for campaigning against any kind of parasites in or on the animals.

Antibiotics[2]

The frequency of so-called inhibitory substances in bulk milk is, after the introduction of suitable test methods, now in the order of 1% or less. The cause is mainly the treatment of the udder with antibiotics against mastitis.

In 1968, our Institute developed the so-called brilliant black reduction test for quick and reliable detection of antibiotic residues in milk, with special attention to fermentation processes in the dairy plant. Table 52.2 features the limits of detection for some inhibitory substances, which may occur in milk. In some cases the borderline limits are still above the limit of technological disturbances, so that there still remains a risk for the dairy industry. This can be overcome by additional specific methods of analysis. Normally, antibiotic residues will not be present in milk when the legal withholding periods are carefully kept or the necessary treatment is carried out, when possible, in the dry-cow phase.

Table 52.2 Limits of detection for so-called 'inhibitory substances' with the brilliant black reduction test (*Bac. stearothermophilus*)

Penicillin G	8 IU/kg
Ampicillin	0.06 mg/kg
Streptomycin	8 mg/kg
Tetracycline	0.8 mg/kg
Chloramphenicol	20 mg/kg
Sulphonamides	1000 mg/kg
Nitrofurazone	20 mg/kg

Teat disinfectants[4,7,14]

An important approach in mastitis prophylaxis is teat dipping with iodophors, containing 3000–5000 mg of active iodine/kg of formulation. This, of course, leads to an increase in the normal milk iodine level, which should be kept below 150 μg/l. As there is a rather narrow span between the maximum daily iodine intake of the adult of 600–700 μg of iodine/day and

Table 52.3 Iodine (μg/kg) in milk in northern Germany (March/May 1980)

Milk	*Number of samples*	*Min.*	*Max.*	*Mean*	*±sd*	*Teat disinfection with iodine yes*	*no*
Herds bulk	130	54	373	118	89	×	×
Herds bulk	63	61	373	155	88	×	
Herds bulk	77	54	226	83	24		×
Road tanker	55	66	128	87	13		×
Market milk	19	66	458	105	86		×
UHT milk	8	111	246	179	54		×

the observed extra in the milk after treatment, the indication should be handled stringently and be limited to so-called problem herds. From our investigations, a risk of undue high iodine intake as the result of mastitis prophylaxis is not apparent (Table 52.3).

Anthelmintics[3, 11]

Though lactating cows are rather resistant to helminths of the juvenile bovine, in some areas the liver fluke *Fasciola hepatica* and its smaller form, the lancet fluke *Dicrocoelium lanceolatum*, lead to massive invasions of the animal, which require specific therapy. These drugs are halogenated and/or phosphorylated phenols, which are, to a small extent (maximum 2% of the dose administered), excreted with the milk. One of the compounds (niclofolane) shows a relatively high mammalian toxicity. Therefore, the treatment should be done in the dry-cow phase or the specific cut-off time carefully observed. From our investigations the following figures are derived. They show the concentration of fasciolicide residues in milk 5 days after treatment, which is the general legal withholding period (Table 52.4). The most favourable compound seems to be oxyclozanide, not only from its excretion in traces, but also from a toxicological point of view. Other anthelmintics, especially fenbendazole, are almost exclusively excreted in urine and faeces, so that milk is not affected by residues of any relevance.

Table 52.4 Excretion of fasciolicides with milk 120 h after treatment

Compound	*Dosage* (mg/kg body wt.)	*Application*	*Residues* (mg/kg)
Niclofolane	3	orally	0.02
Oxyclozanide	10	orally	0.01
Nitroxinil	10	subcutaneous	0.2
Bromphenophos	12	orally	0.01

Ectoparasiticides[6]

Efficient control of ectoparasites including larvae of warbles on the bovine is still a problem of high residuological importance. As the animal is directly in contact with high doses, it is obvious that non-persistent compounds should be used to avoid longterm excretion and thus retention in the milk. On the other hand, the substances should only form residues in milk of low hygienic and toxicological interest and disappear within hours or a couple of days after treatment. Lindane was cancelled in certain countries from its use on the lactating animal, but proved to be very effective against most parasites. The successors are bromocyclene, coumaphos, trichlorphone and heptenophos, with the exception of bromocyclene organophosphates, they have waiting times of 'zero' or up to 1 day.

At present, these substances are only available by veterinary prescription as concentrates. It could be advantageous for low concentrated pulverized formulations to be sold freely.

Environmental chemicals

The rich abundance of environmental chemicals, either of natural origin or from human sources, can be discussed only with a few typical representatives from different groups.

Heavy metals[6]

Amongst the heavy metals, lead, cadmium, mercury and arsenic are of special toxicological and food hygiene interest. They belong to the normal mineralogical components of any site in the environment, so that life has time enough for physiological adoption of the typical concentrations in the environment. Only when this tolerated concentration is dramatically exceeded by emissions or other distribution in the biosphere the toxicological threshold will be passed with the well-known fatal phenomena of 'Minamata-' and 'Itai'-disease as two examples.

For milk, the bovine organism acts as a filter, which is capable of buffering very high concentrations from environmental sources, before milk is markedly affected. This, of course, is only valid for the inorganic forms of the metals under discussion. In the food chain, these elements are markedly diminished from the precursing to the final links.

A few typical concentrations found in milk and dairy products are featured in Table 52.5. The daily consumption of 1 l milk will contribute only a small percentage to the tolerated daily intake of lead, cadmium and mercury.

Table 52.5 Toxic trace elements in milk and dairy products (mg/kg wet weight, medians (ranges))

Product	*Lead*	*Cadmium*	*Mercury*	*Arsenic*
Market milk	0.02 (0.001–0.09)	0.0015 (0.0005–0.07)	0.0005 (0.0–0.025)	0.004 (0.0–0.018)
Condensed milk	0.18 (0.001–2.8)	0.018 (0.001–0.086)		
Butter	0.121 (0.01–0.45)	0.025 (0.0004–0.12)	(0.002–23)	0.009 (0.0–0.04)
Cheese	0.080 (0.001–0.610)	0.046 (0.006–0.104)	(0.009–0.03)	0.003 (0.0–0.015)

Polychlorinated biphenyls[9]

Other types of typical 'modern' environmental chemicals are the polyhalogenated biphenyls, especially the polychlorinated form, the PCBs. As they withstand nearly any environmental impact, including digestion (valid for the higher chlorinated molecules), and behave lipophilically, they accumulate in the natural food chain and food webs. In cow's milk there is a moderate contamination of 0.2 parts/10^6 in fat base, but in human milk these residues are magnified by at least one power of ten. As PCBs are a mixture of approximately 200 isomers, the toxicological evaluation is difficult. A worldwide ban on PCB in so-called open systems could help to stop further pollution of the global environment, as done in the EEC in 1978.

Mycotoxins[10, 12]

Twenty years ago the potent carcinogen aflatoxin M was discovered in milk. Continued studies revealed that approximately 1–3% of the orally administered dose of aflatoxin B appeared as the hydroxylated metabolite in milk. The main source of aflatoxin B is peanut meal from the oil seed industry, which is high energy feed concentrate for lactating animals. Beside peanuts, cottonseed linters are frequently contaminated with aflatoxin B.

As aflatoxin M residues in milk are exclusively secretory residues from a rather constant carry over, any measures for diminishing the contamination in the fodder will lead to less contamination of milk. Recent proposals for a tolerance level for aflatoxin M in market milk focus on the 50 ng/l limit, which would allow no more than 5–10 μg of aflatoxin B/kg in feed concentrates or half of this amount in the total ration, when high amounts of concentrates are fed. Normally, roughage is not contaminated with aflatoxin B. The following table shows some concentration figures in Germany 3 years ago (Table 52.6).

Table 52.6 Aflatoxin M_1 in milk and milk powder in the Federal Republic of Germany (ng/kg) (parts/10^{12}) November 1978–March 1980

Product	*Number of samples*	*Min.*	*Max.*	*Mean*
Market milk	279	0.2	67.5	13.7
Raw milk (road tanker)	46	0.6	37.8	8.3
Raw milk* (herds bulk)	53	3.3	333.3	50.3
UHT milk	28	2.4	28.1	9.1
Milk powder (10% reconstituted)	28	2.3	31.1	12.4

*All samples from winter period

Pesticides[13]

The most classic agrochemicals in connection with chemical residues in food are the pesticides. Whilst plant material is directly impacted with pesticidal agents, food of animal origin is normally indirectly contaminated with residues via the carry over mechanism in the food chain.

Lipophilic organochlorine pesticides are still of great public and food hygiene interest. Beginning in the 1940s with a climax in the mid 1960s, they are now almost banned from the pattern of insecticidal compounds in agriculture, due to their undesired persistence in the environment and their occurrence in nearly every food of animal origin.

In many industrial countries, the contamination of milk, meat and eggs with chlorinated hydrocarbons was carefully observed over years and reflected in legislation, with the establishment of tolerances or maximum residue limits for the consumer's protection. Meanwhile, the residues have markedly declined in these countries and only traces will be found. Most of the pesticides used in agriculture in industrial countries are herbicides. Under the insecticidal compounds, the organophosphates and carbamates, which bear no significant risk for residues in food when used in accordance with good agricultural practice, are favoured more and more and the lipophilic organochlorines have been abandoned.

In the following sections the organochlorine situation in Germany and the regional hot spot occurrence of HCH will be discussed.

Chlorinated hydrocarbons

As mentioned above, the organochlorines accumulate during their passage through the food chain from link to link. Despite this biological phenomenon, only traces in the range of a few hundreds of parts/10^6 in fat base are found in milk, meat and eggs. Figure 52.3 shows the relation of the average values in market milk to the legal tolerances over a period of 8 years in the Federal Republic of Germany.

As can be seen, the trend for the cyclodienes, HCB and DDT, is stable towards less than 10% contribution to the limit, whereas this movement in the case of the HCH isomers is irregular and still remains on rather high levels. Compared to the ADI, the consumption of 1 l of market milk per day will fill up this marginal dose to a maximum of 3% in the case of dieldrin.

The HCH problem[6]

Despite the nationwide decrease in the residues of organochlorines, except for HCH, these substances show sporadic and regional hot spots, which gave rise to further research work, especially in reconnaissance of the contamination sources.

The problem was characterized by rather frequent violations of the common tolerance for α- and β-HCH, with the climax in the winter months and extraordinary high concentrations in herds or individual lactating animals, which could not be explained from the present state of knowledge.

Under the HCH isomers, the γ-isomer is the most unstable configuration, due to the axial and equatorial position of the chlorines to the carbon skeleton, which favours ring fission and dechlorination in the environment. So γ-HCH is not the problematic compound in residue research. Far more stable is the β-configuration with all six chlorines in the equatorial or axial position. Such a molecule is extraordinarily stable and withstands even

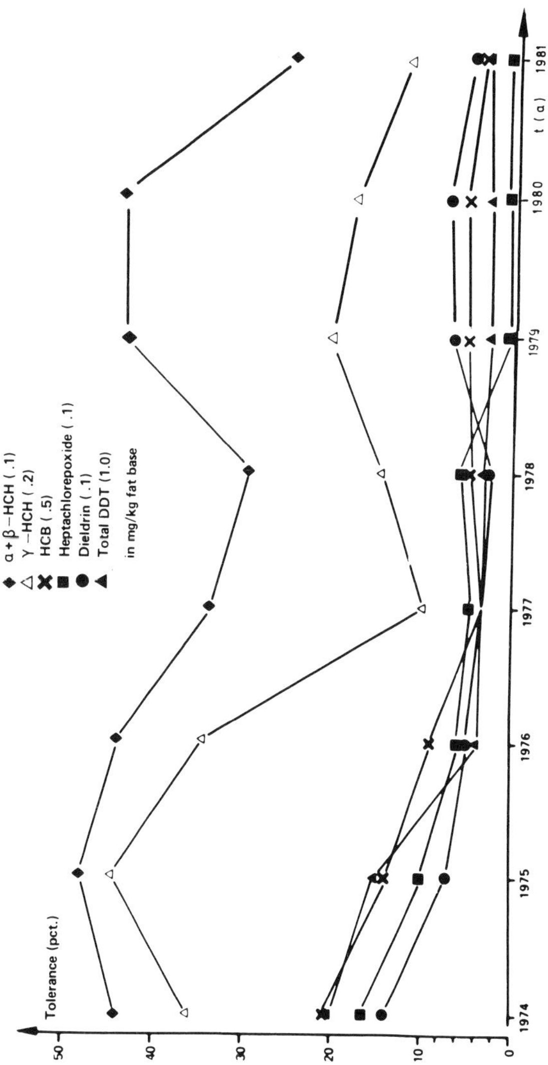

Figure 52.3 Residues of chlorinated hydrocarbons in market milk (in % of legal tolerances)

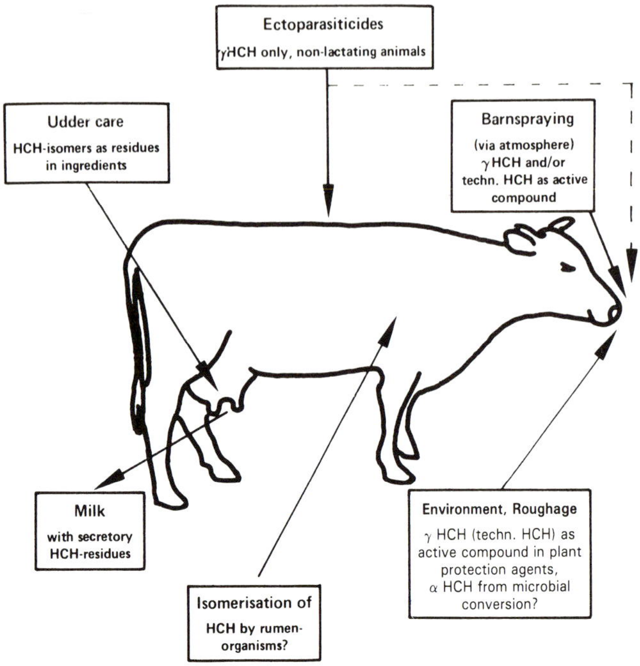

Figure 52.4 Pathways of contamination in the lactating cow with HCH-isomers

stronger alkaline media for a considerably long time. This chemical feature makes β-HCH the residue of the most toxicological interest due to its high chronic toxicity.

The occurrence of β-HCH in milk is always a signal for a long chronic exposure, whereas α-HCH points to a more recent event of contamination. For the bovine, the contamination pathways in Figure 52.4 are relevant. From the possibilities outlined, the ectoparasiticides, udder ointments and feed concentrates are the main causes of contamination, when containing HCH-isomers as the active agent or residue.

The use of technical HCH (α-, β-, γ-isomers and others) is forbidden in agriculture and veterinary medicine in Germany and many other countries. Only lindane (pure γ-isomer) may be used on non-lactating animals. Feed concentrates containing even traces of β-HCH in the parts/10^{12} range still become relevant, as the observed carry-over rate for β-HCH is 30–100%, which leads to appreciable contamination even with low contaminated forage. Here it is necessary to establish a tolerance for β-HCH in forage in the range of 2–5 parts/10^{12} on dry matter base to prevent excessive milk contamination over the 0.05 parts/10^6 level. The actual German tolerance in milk is 0.1 parts/10^6 for α- and β-HCH.

The fatal results of the treatment of a lactating cow with technical HCH are shown in Figure 52.5. The animal was powdered with 16 g (2 tablespoons) of a talc powder containing 4 g of technical HCH in the above given distribution.

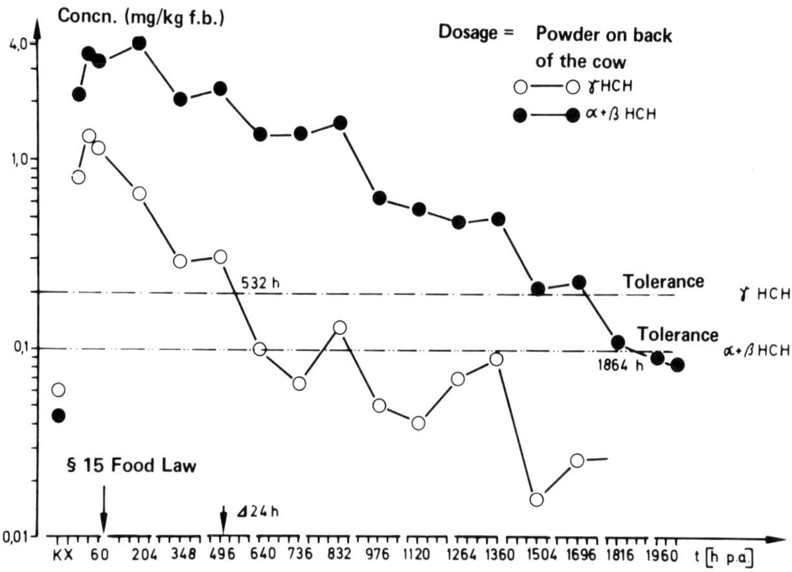

Figure 52.5 Excretion of HCH-isomers with milk after a single treatment with 16 g of talc powder, containing 4 g of technical HCH

The contamination for γ-HCH declined rather rapidly and reached the tolerance level after 3 weeks. On the other hand, the excretion of α- and β-HCH took more than three times longer to come to the 0.1 parts/10^6 level. This example points out the high persistence of β-HCH in lactating animals and the residue problems in milk associated with this isomer.

RESIDUES IN HUMAN MILK

Survey

It is a well-known fact that human milk is highly contaminated with organohalogenated compounds due to its final position in the food chain and to maternal lactation. The comparison of national monitoring data is problematic as the persons under study differ in nearly all parameters affecting the formation of residues in mother's milk. Table 52.7 shows the concentration figures of organochlorines in a rather small, but carefully selected, cohort of a small town in the middlewest of Germany.

The four major residues in human milk are HCB, β-HCH, *p,p'*-DDE and PCB. The right column gives the frequency of violations of the legal tolerances as established for cow's milk and applied to human milk. From the HCH-isomers, here also γ-HCH reveals no problem, whereas the β-isomer shows a very high frequency of samples above 0.1 parts/10^6.

Table 52.7 Residues of chlorinated hydrocarbons in human milk from a town in the middle west of Germany (mg/kg on fat base) (1981)

Compound	*Number of samples*	*Min.*	*Max.*	*Mean*	*Range factor*	*% of samples above tolerance**
HCB	102	0.015	2.209	1.011	146	82.4
α-HCH	100	0.001	0.208	0.030	521	3.0
β-HCH	102	0.023	5.319	0.553	230	92.2
α+β-HCH	100	0.023	5.383	0.593	228	95.0
γ-HCH	101	0.005	0.413	0.094	75	12.9
HepE	100	0.001	0.173	0.030	193	1.0
Dieldrin	91	0.001	0.438	0.054	389	12.1
DDT total	102	0.196	7.058	1.761	36	70.6
PCB	102	0.237	13.754	2.608	58	—

*As compared to the tolerances for cows milk

Tentative evaluation and toxicology

Though it is incorrect to compare the daily intake of a breastfed infant with the ADI parameters established for the adult, Figure 52.6 reveals one aspect of breast feeding. It is obvious that for some compounds the ADI is far exceeded, so that the two powers of ten safety distance to the no-effect level is shrinking to approximately 1 power of ten in the case of HCB. Unfortunately, β-HCH is not ranged in the ADI scale, so that this interesting and toxicologically relevant isomer cannot be evaluated this way.

As derived from assays with sensitive laboratory animals, the tumourigenic threshold for HCH-isomers *in toto* comes short of one power of ten, when a daily ration of highly contaminated mother's milk is drunk by the infant. The tumourigenic risk is enlarged, when all organohalogenic residues, present in the breast milk, are taken together. Nevertheless, despite the residues in human milk, the advantages of breast feeding must be estimated higher than the potential risk of toxic chemicals in concentrations between ADI and no-effect level.

SUMMARY

The impact of chemicals, either drugs and/or environmental chemicals on milk or the lactating animal respectively, is a phenomenon of our times, which is very complex in its estimation and evaluation. Use of chemicals in agriculture is a necessity of undoubted certainty to produce food of high quality and enough quantity. This area, however, seems to be governable by legislation and related administration to ensure a complete protection of the consumer's health. The latter should be the absolute aim in all efforts to increase agricultural production.

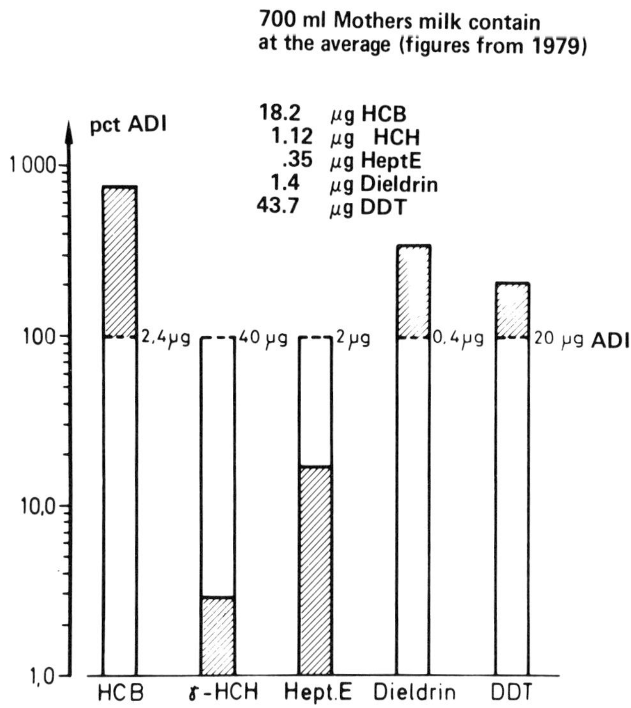

Figure 52.6 Percentage of the ADI for a breastfed infant drinking 700 ml of mother's milk daily

In the case of drugs for the treatment of farm animals, these efforts should be rather successful. *Antibiotics* should only be used with strict prescription by the veterinarian. After treatment, a withholding period is obligatory before the milk is delivered to the dairy. This seems to be sufficient to prevent residues in milk, which on one hand may affect the consumer by promoting resistant strains or sensitizing allergy processes. On the other hand, antibiotic residues may disturb microbial fermentation processes in the dairy, which lead to high financial losses, if large bulks are affected. The control of such inhibitory residues after the 3 day period is simple and reliable, so that there is hardly a risk of violation of the legal claim.

Parasiticides against parasites in or on the animal compile a widespread pattern of compounds and indication. Generally, the lactating animal should be treated with drugs,.which show no significant carry-over into the milk or, if impossible, the duration of excretion should be only in the order of a few days. Lipophilic compounds should be used in no case on the lactating animal. The latter problem became evident in the HCH hot spots in several regions of Germany. The organophosphates and carbamates, as well as natural or synthetic pyrethrins, are the compounds of choice due to their effectiveness, rapid metabolization and non-persistent residues, which bear no risk for the consumer. The waiting time for these compounds may be reduced to 0 hours.

The use of *pesticides* is always connected with the residue problem for different reasons. These substances necessarily hit their targets as well as the environment of man and farm animals. Some of them must be persistent to ensure effectiveness, few are of higher toxicity, in some cases health hazards are not yet known. In recent years in this field, a worldwide ban on the high persistent organochlorines was made and proved to be effective. In addition, registration of new formulations and compounds includes more and more the interest of consumer's health and food hygiene, so that residue problems become more transparent and resolvable, if not avoidable.

Under the organochlorines, the *HCH-isomers* α and especially β still cause some problems arising from their presence in feed concentrates, in addition to the high carry-over rate for β-HCH into milk. Far more difficult is the complex abundance of so-called environmental chemicals from human and non-human origin. As an approach to a short description of the problem, it can be stated that in all cases, where the natural balance and concentration is heavily disturbed by an human activity, toxicologically relevant sources and residues may arise. This can clearly be observed in the case of *heavy metals* in the biosphere. *Mycotoxins*, though belonging to the evolutionary process, has become of high interest in the last decades with a change in farm management and feeding of high amounts of concentrates.

Human milk is undoubtedly one of the highest contaminated foods of mammalian origin. An increase of the content of the lipophilic organochlorines in the last decade could not be observed, but there is a shift to slightly lower residues.

Though milk is a target for a great number of residue-forming chemicals from the natural and man-formed environment, it can be said that it is one of the best investigated foods for human consumption.

References

1. DVG, Deutsche Veterinärmedizinische Gesellschaft (1981). *Die subklinische Mastitis des Rindes und Vorschläge für bundeseinheitliche Richtlinien zu ihrer Bekämpfung*. Deutsche Veterinärmedizinische Gesellschaft, Frankfurter Straße, D-63 Gießen
2. Hamann, J., Tolle, A. and Heeschen, W. (1979). Antibiotics and sulfonamides. In *Chemical Residues in Milk and Milk Products*. pp. 43–56. IDF Bulletin Document 113
3. Heeschen, W. (1979). Fasciolicides. In *Chemical Residues in Milk and Milk Products*. pp. 30–9. IDF Bulletin Document 113
4. Heeschen, W. (1979). *Residues of Drugs, Anthelmintics and Teat Dips in Milk and Milk Products*. IDF A-Doc 46
5. Heeschen, W. (1980). Pestizide und Milchhygiene. *Dtsch. Tierärztl. Wschr.*, **87**, 209–48
6. Heeschen, W. (1982). Rückstände von Arzneimitteln, Pestiziden und Umweltchemikalien in der Milch – Ein Überblick zur gegenwärtigen Situation. *Tierärztl. Umschau.*, **37**, 538–45
7. IDF – International Dairy Federation (1970). *Detection of Penicillin in Milk by Disk Assay Technique*. IDF Standard 57
8. IDF – International Dairy Federation (1979). *Chemical Residues in Milk and Milk Products*. Bulletin Document 113

9. Kadis, V. W. (1969). Polychlorinated biphenyls (PCBs) and their occurrence in milk and milk products. In *Chemical Residues in Milk and Milk Products.* IDF Bulletin Document 113
10. Kiermeier, F. (1981). Mykotoxine in Milch und Milchprodukten. In Reiss, J: (ed.) *Mykotoxine in Lebensmitteln*. pp. 245–71. (Stuttgart and New York: Gustav Fischer Verlag)
11. Marek, B. (1979). Organophosphates (organic phosphoric acid esters) and carbamates. In *Chemical Residues in Milk and Milk Products.* pp. 17–22. IDF Bulletin Document 113
12. Reiss, J. (ed.) (1981). *Mykotoxine in Lebensmitteln*. (Stuttgart and New York: Gustav Fischer Verlag)
13. Snelson, J. T. and Tuinstra, L. G. M. Th. (1979). Chlorinated insecticides. In *Chemical Residues in Milk and Milk Products*. pp. 6–16. IDF Bulletin Document 113
14. Sommerville, J. M. and Rose, I. D. (1978). Control of bovine teat skin with glycerinated iodophor teat dips. *Vet. Rec.*, **102**, 262–3

53
Mycotoxin residue problem and human health hazard

P. Galtier and J. Le Bars

The word mycotoxin is used to designate a toxic secondary metabolite synthetized by fungi when moisture and temperature are suitable. These metabolites may be retained within the fungus or incorporated into an alimentary substrate. In this case, mycotoxicosis corresponds to poisoning of the host.

Mycotoxins have affected the health of man or animals for centuries: gangrenous and nervous ergotism caused by ingestion of ergot toxic alkaloids in European countries, deaths among horses which had eaten hay infested with *Stachybotrys atra* in the Soviet Union during the Second World War or facial eczema of sheep and cattle on pasture in New Zealand containing spores of the fungus *Pithomyces chartarum*. However, mycotoxins have definitely attracted the interest of an increasing number of scientists since the discovery of natural occurrence in foods and the carcinogenic power of aflatoxin B_1 elaborated by *Aspergillus flavus*.

Beside direct toxicological effects, edible tissues of food-producing animals may represent a toxicological food hazard for humans. Thus, the mycotoxin may occur specifically in edible tissues such as meat, fat and giblets or may be eliminated in milk and eggs. On the other hand, the toxin may be effectively transformed as a more or an equally toxic derivative which can exert its own deleterious effect, another possible pathway for the mycotoxic contamination of human alimentation. The purposes of this report are to summarize the sources and occurrence of the more significant mycotoxins in animal feed and to describe the fate and residue problems of mycotoxins in edible animal tissues, hence the human health risk related to mycotoxin-contaminated food consumption.

NATURAL OCCURRENCE OF MYCOTOXINS IN ANIMAL FEEDS

Toxigenic fungi have an ubiquitous geographic distribution. But their critical development and mycotoxin production depend on:

(1) Climatic conditions.
(2) Cultivation, harvesting and storage techniques.
(3) Method of livestock production (extensive or intensive).

Table 53.1 Origin of main mycotoxins

Toxins	*Fungi*	*Plant or feedstuffs*	*Promoting conditions and geographical distribution*
Mycotoxins produced in pasture			
Sporidesmins	*Pithomyces chartarum*	Ray grass	Wet autumn after dry summer, short grass (NZ, Australia)
Slaframine	*Rhizoctonia leguminicola*	Red clover	Second cutting, wet autumn, acid soils
Ergot alkaloids	*Claviceps purpurea, paspali*	Graminaceous plants (inflorescences)	Extensive grazing summer, autumn
Tremorgen toxins	*Claviceps paspali Penicillium* sp.	Paspalum, ray grass	Dry summer short grass (NZ, GB)
Phomopsin A & B	*Phomopsis leptostromiformis*	Lupin	After first rainfall in autumn (Australia, S. Africa)
Myrothecium toxins	*Myrothecium roridum verrucaria*	Ray grass, white clover	Summer, autumn (wet and warm
Coumestrol	*Pseudopeziza Leptosphoerulina*	Clover, alfalfa	Autumn
Toxins primarily produced in storage			
Aflatoxins	*Aspergillus flavus parasiticus*	Peanut, cotton, corn, sorghum, oats, barley, soya	Moist and warm conditions 1°/tropical countries, 2°/all over the world in bad storage conditions
Zearalenone	*Fusarium* spp.	Corn, hay, sorghum, barley	Sequence of cool and mild weather; temperate climates
Ochratoxin A	*P. viridicatum A. ochraceus*	Barley, oats corn, wheat	Wet and cool climates humid harvesting and storage conditions
Patulin	*Byssochlamys nivea P. granulatum*	Silages (corn, sugar, beet pulp, grass)	Anaerobiosis defect after first 3 months storage
Trichothecenes T_2, nivalenol, deoxynivalenol	*Fusarium tricinctum*	Cereals, hay, straw	Sequence of frost and thaw cool climates
Stachybotrys toxins	*St. atra*	Straw, hay (cereals)	Long time of wet storage
Dicoumarol	*Humicola, Mucor Penicillium* spp.	Sweet clover	Humid self-heated forage

It follows that these toxins occur primarily in particular feeds and regions. Moreover, for toxins from phytopathogenic fungi (which are often parasitic for only one plant species) and for toxins arising by fungal bioconversion of vegetal compounds (such as dicoumarol in mouldy sweet clover), the occurrence is closely linked to the plant species. The leading origins of the main mycotoxins harmful to animals are presented in Table 53.1.

Investigations on the mycotoxins produced in pasture lack analytical techniques for quantitative and epidemiologic studies, except for a few metabolites like coumestrol. Statements such as 'photosensitive pasture' and 'oestrogenic forage', give very little information. For storage toxins, international exchanges contribute to spread particular toxins into countries unfavourable for toxinogenesis (i.e. aflatoxins in peanut cakes). Surveys have concentrated on aflatoxins, ochratoxin A and zearalenone; natural occurrence of other mycotoxins has been described for patulin, sterigmatocystin, penicillic acid[72], citrinin and trichothecenes[65]. It is important to distinguish between unbiased surveys (usually on grains in commercial channels) and surveys or even single analyses biased because the samples are associated with mycotoxicoses in farm animals and are obviously moulded or improperly stored. In the first case, levels are low but widespread and main hazards for health result from toxins showing cumulative toxic effects. The second situation is concerned with undiluted feedstuffs where toxin yields may be high. In both cases, sampling is hazardous, because major contamination may occur in only a few of the kernels.

Aflatoxins

Since the discovery of aflatoxins in peanut cake, groundnut has been surveyed in many countries because of its harmful effect on human and animal health. Its occurrence, resulting from invasion by *Aspergillus flavus*, is comparatively high in subtropical regions and depends on numerous factors such as weak plants after drought stress, insect or mechanical damage, delay and climatic conditions before drying and improper storage conditions. In USA for the 1967–1972 period, the percentage of lots with more than 100 μg/kg aflatoxin B_1 varied from 0 to 3%. On the contrary, frequencies of 49 and 17% and mean levels of 1530 and 363 μg/kg were found in Thailand and Ouganda respectively[70]. Aflatoxin yield sometimes may exceed 10 mg/kg.

Aflatoxins may be formed on other grains like corn, cottonseed and soyabean, sometimes before harvest. Insect damage appears as a critical factor in field infection, which leads to moderate toxin levels. High contents result from bad harvesting and storage conditions. In an unbiased survey on 924 samples of corn in France, during the 1973–1974 period, only one was contaminated (42 μg/kg)[24]. In a biased study (mouldy samples of corn stored in cribs), aflatoxins were present in 2.6% of the 75 samples tested (10 μg/kg)[10]. During the last decade of our survey on feedstuffs associated with animal disorders, the most frequently contaminated grain was self-heated barley (up to 600 μg/kg AFB_1). In spite of a high *A. flavus* frequency in hay, a part of the thermopreferent mycoflora, AFB_1 is rare and levels are low; this substrate, like soya[40,71] is unfavourable for biogenesis of polyketide mycotoxins[38,69].

Zearalenone

Zearalenone, an oestrogenic factor formed by various species of *Fusarium*, particularly by *F. roseum graminearum*, is found in corn and to a lesser extent in other grains and in hay[48]. These organisms invade developing corn at the silking stage in periods of heavy rainfall and proliferate on mature grains that have not dried because of wet weather before and at harvest[7] or on prestored grains before drying[29]. But the main source of zearalenone is corn on cobs stored in cribs in regions where climatic conditions do not allow a sufficient initial drying rate, especially in humid autumns which are conducive to *Fusarium* ear rot in epidemic proportions. In a survey organized by CNEEMA in a mountainous zone, toxin yield varied from 2.8 to 6 mg/kg when cribs were discarded. In contrast, in Haute-Garonne (around Toulouse), a similar investigation on well-devised cribs revealed a maximal yield of 0.1 mg/kg in zones with 'Autan' wind and 1 mg/kg in the southern part (without this wind). We found a toxin level as high as 80 mg/kg in corn on cobs from a farm, with reproductive disorders in cows, in the central part of France. In USA, as a result of the bad year 1972, zearalenone was found in 17% of the 223 samples assayed, at an average level of 0.9 mg/kg (range 0.1–5 mg/kg) with no relation to grade or intended use including food use[14].

The concentration of zearalenone within the corn kernel is distributed in the same fashion as aflatoxin; on dry milling of contaminated corn, the highest concentrations of zearalenone were in the high fat fractions usually used for oil and feed.

Ochratoxin A

Ochratoxin A (OA) originally isolated from *Aspergillus ochraceus* strains, is more frequently concomitant with *Penicillium viridicatum*[66]. Because of reports from Denmark, showing contents as high as 27 500 μg/kg in barley associated with porcine nephropathy[36], FDA undertook a survey of domestic barley; OA was found in 14% of 159 samples (range 10–29 μg/kg) with no relation to grade. In a Canadian survey of mouldy feedstuffs, 18 of 29 samples of heated grains (wheat, oats, rye) were contaminated with OA at 30–27 000 μg/kg[66]. In a survey, on corn from commercial channels in France, 1.9% of samples presented OA content in the range 15–200 μg/kg[24].

Citrinin

Citrinin is often a co-contaminant with OA levels as high as 80 000 μg/kg found in mouldy grains in Canada[66]. In the Danish survey previously mentioned[36], citrinin was detected in the range 160–2000 μg/kg. We found this toxin at the 5000 μg/kg level in germinated barley associated with nephropathic and other disorders in goats.

Patulin

Natural occurrence of patulin, originally proved in rotten apples invaded with *Penicillium expansum*[6], appears at significant toxin levels in hydrated foods and feeds. Silages are the major source of this toxin: in a local survey it was found in 50% of samples (range 1.5–40 mg/kg)[15]. This contaminant is also highly probable in immature cereals, where the toxigenic agents *Byssochlamys nivea* and *Paecilomyces varioti* are frequent.

Trichothecenes

Out of more than 30 chemically known trichothecenes, only four have been identified as natural contaminants[31] (T_2, diacetoxyscipenol, nivalenol and deoxynivalenol) associated with haemorrhagic disorders or feed refusal. Practical detection is based on the dermonecrotic action of the extracts[27]. Several toxins from *Stachybotrys atra* are trichothecenes[13]. As a result of its ecological features, this fungi and its highly toxic metabolites primarily occur in old wet straws[39].

Other mycotoxins

Sterigmatocystin, formed by *Aspergillus versicolor* which is frequent in hay[38] and in hot spot grains, is seldom at a high level. Penicillic acid, produced by numerous *Penicillium* and *Aspergillus* species, is unstable at moderate temperatures, depending on water activity; it may occur and accumulate at significant concentrations in feeds stored at low temperatures.

FATE AND RESIDUES OF MYCOTOXINS IN EDIBLE ANIMAL TISSUES

The fate of a mycotoxin in an animal body depends upon the extent and rate of its absorption from gastrointestinal tract, its distribution, its binding or localization in tissues, its biotransformation and its excretion processes. The rate of each of these events, which contribute to both pharmacokinetics and pharmacodynamics of a drug or a toxin, is determined by the chemical and physical properties of the compound and by its interaction with tissues responsible for elimination.

It has been known that toxic chemical substances such as mycotoxins can alter normal physiological functions of animal and man, but it was recognized only relatively recently that contact with biological material could also affect the structure of a chemical compound. Considerable study of this latter process, especially during the past 20 years, has provided a great wealth of information and has led to the introduction of drug metabolism as a subdiscipline of pharmacology and toxicology. Strictly speaking, drug biotransformation refers exclusively to the chemical alteration of a drug – or a mycotoxin – produced by the biological environment and this represents one aspect of the physiological disposition, or fate of the toxic substance. One of the major natural functions of drug metabolism consists of the formation of more polar and water soluble derivatives which results in an increased rate of excretion of the toxin related to a reduction or an enhancement of the toxicological activity of the product.

Certain biotransformation pathways of toxins reaction could lead to less toxic derivatives than parent mycotoxin. *In vitro* transformation assay of ochratoxin A by animal microbial flora has demonstrated that toxin was mainly hydrolysed to ochratoxin α[19]. A similar result[19] was obtained with rumen fluids of cows and sheep obtained from the slaughter house. This hydrolytic reaction of a mycotoxin, ochratoxin A, leads in this case to the formation of ochratoxin α which is a non-toxic derivative since intravenous doses as great as 100 mg/kg did not induce any damages in adult rats. *In vivo*, this detoxifying conversion occurs principally in the caecum and large intestine of the rat and the rumen of cow as recently demonstrated by Ribelin[59]. So, although ochratoxin A is known to accumulate in the tissues of monogastric species such as swine, ochratoxicosis can be considered as an unlikely problem in ruminants (cow, ewe, goat) because of hydrolysis of the toxin within the rumen.

In other cases, biotransformation pathways lead to more or equally toxic derivatives. The metabolic fate of the well-known mycotoxin aflatoxin B_1, has been investigated in many species. More specifically the hepatic disposition of the toxin might consist of:

(1) A reversible cytoplasmic bioconversion in aflatoxicol which is considered as a 'metabolic reservoir' of aflatoxin.

(2) A microsomal formation of the hemiacetal metabolite, aflatoxin B_2A, which would be responsible for the acute toxicity attributed to the mycotoxin through non-specific inhibition of liver enzymes.

(3) A microsomal oxidation leading to a 2:3 epoxide proposed by Schoental[64] to be the 'active form' of the toxin, particularly in relation to its chronic effects, namely the carcinogenic activity. It had generally been thought probable that epoxide would be a short-lived metabolite particularly difficult to isolate from biological material which might contain dihydrodiol, the stable derivative of epoxide. In this particular case, the chronic toxicity of aflatoxin B_1 would be due to a biological process of animal organism which would so determine its own lethal consequences.

Another mycotoxin which is transformed in a toxic metabolite is T_2 toxin, an epoxytrichotecen elaborated by *Fusarium sp.* Disposition of this toxic compound has been studied by means of *in vitro* tests using bovine and human liver homogenates[12] so desacetylation of T_2 toxin in H-T_2 toxin is observed. This derivative would be one of major metabolites in animal organism as described by Matsumoto *et al.*[46] who detected considerable amounts from excreta of rats orally administered with $[^3H]T_2$ toxin; however, H-T_2 toxin is marked by a toxicity as high as T_2 toxin (9 vs. 5.2 mg/kg) for LD_{50} in mice following intraperitoneal administration; here again, biotransformation of the mycotoxin does not correspond to a true detoxification.

Such data demonstrate the importance of metabolic studies for a better understanding of the mode of toxic activity of mycotoxin; experiments in this field of action are needed, particularly about the fate of toxins in domestic animals, especially in ruminants in which bacterial floras should reduce the toxic action of natural contaminants of feedstuffs.

Residue problems of mycotoxins in non-ruminant species

Such problems result in the presence and residue of toxic residues in dairy products such as meat, fat and eggs. A toxin residue has to be determined not only as the residue of the mycotoxin itself but also as the residue of a possible toxic metabolite, aflatoxin B_2A, aflatoxin M_1 or HT_2 toxin, for instance. These studies are generally carried out in experimentally administered animals. However, the natural occurrence of mycotoxins and/or biological toxic derivatives has been also investigated in meat and eggs. Some studies led to relationships between the mycotoxin levels in animal feeds and the residual concentrations in edible tissues. In any case, data concerning toxin contamination did not correspond to the result of fungi development on dairy products, due to bad conservation but really to a contamination in the animal feed intake. Occurrence of mycotoxin residues in meat products from pigs, poultry and rabbits, naturally or experimentally fed with mycotoxin-containing feedstuffs, is given in Table 53.2. Most of the aflatoxin data have been reported from Rodricks *et al.*[61]. These authors tabulated ratios of aflatoxin levels in feed to levels in edible tissues of animals receiving the contaminated feed. However, such calculations appeared difficult to generalize because of considerable variation in experimental design of assay and execution of analytical procedure. In liver, kidneys and muscle of swine, aflatoxin B_1 was generally carried over as both unchanged form and aflatoxin M_1. On the other hand, residues of ochratoxin A were found as natural contaminants of kidneys and other tissues investigated in slaughter house cases of mycotoxic porcine nephropathy in Scandinavia, probably because of the cumulative effect of this mycotoxin[18] related to the *in vivo* binding to plasma protein[17]. In contrast, experimental data suggested that the zearalenone residue problem would be minimal in swine. In poultry, mycotoxin residues have been shown in liver and muscle of animals receiving diets containing aflatoxin B_1 or ochratoxin A. In case of administration of tritiated T_2 toxin to chicken, some radioactivity has been recovered in both liver and muscle. In rabbit, unchanged zearalenone has been carried over in liver of orally administered animals (Table 53.2).

On the other hand, egg contamination has been investigated because of the possible absorption of mycotoxins from contaminated feed by farm poultry. In this connection, experimental data generally demonstrated a lack in transfer of mycotoxin within yolk or white of eggs. Only low residue levels in eggs have been demonstrated following experimental intoxication of hen or quail

Table 53.2 Occurrence of mycotoxin residues in edible tissues (liver and muscle) from poultry and rabbit, in milk of dairy cattle and in eggs (ND: not detectable)

Ingested toxin	*Dose in feedstuff*	*Recovered form*	*Residue level* ($\mu g/kg$)	*Ref.*
Poultry				
Aflatoxin B_1	280–1600 $\mu g/kg$	AF B_1	<1	28
	4300 $\mu g/kg$	AF B_1	2	73
	100 $\mu g/kg$	AF B_1	0.35/0.23	47
	1000 $\mu g/kg$	AF B_1	3.70/0.19	47
	5000 $\mu g/kg$	AF B_1	18.35/6.47	47
	15 000 $\mu g/kg$	AF B_1	21.10/24.20	47
	1170 $\mu g/kg$	AF B_1	22	44
		AF M_1	198	44
Ochratoxin A	natural intake	OTA	/29	11
	1 mg kg^{-1} day^{-1}	OTA	<16	66
	5–20 mg/kg	OTA	+	57
^3H T_2 toxin	800 $\mu g/kg$	^3H	+	8
Rabbit				
Zearalenone	10 $\mu g/kg$	Zea	+	37
Milk				
Aflatoxin B_1	9690 $\mu g/kg$	AF M_1	15	2
	23 $\mu g/kg$	AF M_1	ND	1
	128 $\mu g/kg$	AF M_1	0.65	1
	367 $\mu g/kg$	AF M_1	2.8	1
	40–557 $\mu g/kg$	AF M_1	0.7–4.7	43
	3–466 $\mu g/kg$	AF M_1	ND–0.84	55
	356–1089 $\mu g/kg$	AF M_1	9.1–20.2	45
	540 $\mu g/kg$	AF M_1	0.92	50
	10 $\mu g/kg$	AF M_1	0.01–0.33	51
Ochratoxin A	1.66 mg/kg	OTA, α	+	59
	317–1125 $\mu g/kg$	OTA, α	ND	67
Zearalenone	385–1925 $\mu g/kg$	Zea	ND	67
	10 mg/kg	Zea	+	25
	25 mg/kg	Zea 35%	1300	49
T_2 toxin	50 mg/kg	T_2	10–160	49
Eggs				
Aflatoxin B_1	100 $\mu g/kg$	AF B_1	0.23	28
	400 $\mu g/kg$	AF B_1	1.40	28
	13 $\mu g/kg$	AF B_1	0.05	56
	84 $\mu g/kg$	AF B_1	0.33	56
	5000 $\mu g/kg$	AF B_1	0.09	42
	100 $\mu g/kg$	AF B_1	0.09	42
	8000 $\mu g/kg$	AF B_1	1.88	42
^{14}C Aflatoxin B_1	11–26 mg	^{14}C	+	63
Ochratoxin A	300–1000 $\mu g/kg$	OTA	ND	34
	5–20 mg	OTA	ND	54
^3H T_2 toxin	2000 $\mu g/kg$	^3H	white > yolk	9
^{14}C Patuline	50 mg/day	^{14}C	+	41

with aflatoxin B_1 or ochratoxin A. Some researchers described the carry-over of radioactivity in eggs following experimental administration of labelled (^{3}H of ^{14}C) toxins in laying hens[9,41,63]. Such studies should be related to the structural determination of the so-measured radioactivity because it can be due to toxin itself or toxic derivatives but also to non-toxic metabolites. This remark is particularly relevant in case of patulin which is known for its rapid *in vivo* inactivation, due to its high reactivity for sulphhydryl groups contained in amino acids or proteins.

Table 53.3 Occurence of mycotoxin residues in edible tissues from pigs and ruminants (ND: not detectable; nat. int.: natural intake)

Ingested toxin	*Dose in feedstuff*	*Recovered form*	*Residue level* (parts/10^9) *liver*	*kidneys*	*muscle*	*Ref.*
Pigs						
Aflatoxin B_1	100–400 μg/kg	AF B_1	0.3–2.7	0.3–0.3	0.2–0.2	28
		AF M_1	0.2–2.0	0.1–0.2	0.04–0.4	28
B_1	250–417 μg/kg	AF B_1	51–92	10–50		35
		AF M_1	3–4	3–6		35
B_1	4000 μg/kg	AF B_1	6	0.2	0.1	30
		AF M_1	3	1.0	0.05	30
B_1	662 μg/kg	AF B_1	0.07	0.27	0.07	16
B_2	273 μg/kg	AF B_1	0.04	0.17	0.01	16
G_1	300 μg/kg	AF M_1	0.12		0.12	16
G_2	285 μg/kg					
B_1	nat. int.	AF B_1	+0.1			5
Ochratoxin A	nat. int.	OTA	38	67	+[23]	32
	nat. int.	OTA		0–104		62
	1000 μg/kg	OTA	12	36	9[3]	32, 33
	0.38 mg/kg b.w.	OTA	0.34	0.70	0.13	53
Zearalenone	50 μg/kg	Zea	+			37
	2.2 μg/kg		ND			68
Ruminants						
Bovine						
Aflatoxin B_1	3750 μg/kg	ND	+			4
B_1	nat. int.	ND			+	58
B_1	1050 μg/kg	AF B_1	5	1–2	1–2	55
		AF M_1	5	ND	ND	55
B_1	693 μg/kg	AF B_1	0.05	ND	ND	43
		AF M_1	0.1	0.2	ND	43
Sheep						
Aflatoxin B_1	0.36 mg/kg b.w.	AF B_1	+	+		3
Calves						
Aflatoxin B_1	12–13 μg/kg	AF B_1	+	ND	ND	52
		AF M_1	+	0.03	ND	52
Ochratoxin A	320–540 μg/kg	OTA	ND	5	+	52
		OTA	ND	10	+	52
Cows						
Ochratoxin A	317–1125 μg/kg	OTA	ND	5	ND	67
Zearalenone	385–1925 μg/kg	Zea	ND	ND	ND	67
^{3}H T_2 toxin	180 mg	^{3}H	+		+	75

Except for the classic distribution and fate studies, the tissue residue of any xenobiotic can be investigated by means of pharmacokinetic modelling of the animal body. Thus, after a preliminary study concerning the fate of labelled ochratoxin A in the rat[23], the pharmacokinetic profiles of this toxin in pigs, rabbit and chicken[20] have been determined following both oral and intravenous administration of the toxin. Concentrations of the mycotoxin in the plasma were measured for up to 120 h following treatment. Pharmacokinetic parameters indicated a two-compartment open model. Following oral administration, the biological halflife of ochratoxin A was 88.8, 8.2 and 4.1 h in pigs, rabbits and chickens, respectively, and 65.7, 55.6 and 40.0% respectively of the administered dose was absorbed. These results indicated that ochratoxin A persists in the body of the pig (see Table 53.3). The large apparent volumes of distribution calculated for the rabbit and chicken indicated a wide distribution of the toxin in these organisms. Physiological processes such as serum albumin binding, digestive flow rate, or biotransformation pathways, are suggested as explanations for the observed species differences in the pharmacokinetics of ochratoxin A. In this respect, curves of toxin amounts contained in the two compartments and predicted plasma concentrations following one, two or three daily administrations, have been simulated by use of mathematical expressions programmed in a digital computer. These studies clearly showed the residue of ochratoxin A in deep compartment tissues such as muscle, fate or skin[20,23].

Residue problem of mycotoxins in ruminants

Table 53.3 illustrates some data concerning the occurrence of mycotoxin residues in edible tissues from ruminants. As in pig, both aflatoxins B_1 and M_1 were generally recovered in liver and kidneys, whereas the derivative M_1 appeared less frequently than the unchanged mycotoxin in muscle of cow, calves or sheep. It has been recognized that average ratios of aflatoxin B_1 concentration in the feed to the aflatoxin level in liver appeared greater in beef than in swine or broiler chicken[61]. On the other hand, the withdrawal time, calculated from available studies about aflatoxin residues in liver and muscle, varied in a range of 6–26 h and 18–72 h, respectively[61].

In spite of the hydrolysing action of ruminal microflora on ochratoxin A, this toxin has been recovered in kidneys of calves and cows receiving 300–1100 parts/10^9 ochratoxin A containing diets. Residues of zearalenone were not detected in muscle liver and kidneys of cow fed with concentrate rations containing about 400–2000 parts/10^9 of the mycotoxin.

Several data deal with the excretion of aflatoxins in the milk of farm animals (Table 53.2). The recovered form is aflatoxin M_1 which develops a similar toxic character to aflatoxin B_1. Patterson[51] described a linear relationship between the amount of aflatoxin B_1 ingested daily and the level of aflatoxin M_1 in cow milk. In this respect, about 1.5% of aflatoxin B_1 is excreted as the derivative M_1 and the concentration of the metabolite in milk is approximately 1/300 of the level of mycotoxin in the dairy ration. The possible occurrence of aflatoxin M_1 residues in milk is actually considered as an important econominal problem in Europe because of the possibility of both contamination from imported concentrate feeds and residue of carcinogenic derivatives in cheese. In current conditions of feedstuff contamination by ochratoxin A (300–1000 parts/10^9), the toxin was not recovered in bovine milk. However, the administration of larger doses led to the presence of ochratoxin A in cow milk. During an experimental study[21], the excretion of ochratoxin A in rabbit female was examined after a single intravenous administration of toxin. For the highest dose (4 mg/kg), the level in milk reached 1 parts/10^6. The mammary excretion was also studied while plasma concentration of ochratoxin A was constant; the percentage of protein-bound toxin in plasma and milk was determined. The similarity of the theoretical and experimental ratios between mycotoxin levels in milk and plasma ultrafiltrates led to the conclusion in favour of the passage through the blood–milk barrier by non-ionic passive diffusion of the free toxin. Such a result could, therefore, be representative for monogastric species only. Fusarium mycotoxins have been investigated for their milk excretion. Thus for Shreeve *et al.*[68], a balanced diet, which included 385–1925 parts/10^9 of zearalenone, did not result in the presence of detectable residues in milk of cows. In contrast, with higher dietary intake, Mirocha *et al.*[49] found zearalenone was transmitted into the milk of a cow as free toxin (45–64 parts/10^9), conjugate (31–182 parts/10^9 and zearalenol. Lastly T_2 toxin was carried over in cow (10–160 parts/10^9) and sow (76 parts/10^9) milk following daily consumption of contaminated feed, corresponding to 50 and 12 parts/10^6 respectively[60].

HUMAN HEALTH RISK

Two pathways of human dietary exposure have been described: the direct ingestion of toxins in contaminated foods of plant origin (cereals, nuts, coffee, flour) and the ingestion of toxin residues in edible tissues from breeding animals. Whereas exposure by the first pathway is likely to be greater than the second, these two possibilities lead to similar human health risks.

Such risks have already been reviewed[64,74]. Reasonable evidence to associate a mycotoxin to human disease exist only for some mycotoxicosis: ergotism, liver cancer or alimentary toxic aleukia. Such diseases originate generally from chronic effects of dietary mycotoxins exposure.

Ergotism is the oldest and best known human mycotoxicosis. This disease, occurring centuries ago in Central Europe, reached epidemic proportions in the Middle Age and was popularly known as St. Anthony's fire. It became associated with the consumption of bread made from flours invaded by *Claviceps purpurea*. It was recognized that alkaloids produced by the ergot were responsible for the disease that was characterized by a sensation of cold hands and feet which progressed to an intense burning sensation and possibly to gangrene and necrosis of extremities. Concerning liver cancer, correlations between aflatoxin intake and human liver cancer incidence have been established in surveys that included areas with high estimated aflatoxin exposure and high liver cancer incidence: Kenya, Mozambique, Swaziland or

Thailand. On the other hand, a diet deficient in lipotropes (choline, methionine, folate) enhanced liver cancer induction by aflatoxin B_1 in rats, whereas alimentary deficiency in protein also increased liver cancer incidence. In summary, aflatoxin ingestion may increase the risk of liver cancer and this risk depends on the amount of ingested aflatoxin and the reduction in daily aflatoxin exposure could be expected to reduce the liver cancer risk. In contrast, the involvement of aflatoxins in the aetiology of juvenile cirrhosis in India was not supported by later studies of aflatoxin exposure and analytical examination of urine and liver specimens. Alimentary toxic aleukia (ATA) was a disease encountered in Russian people in the period around 1940. An association was established with the ingestion of grain contaminated by *Fusarium poae* and *Fusarium sporotrichioides*. Necrotic lesions of the oral cavity, oesophagus and stomach were dominant pathological signs associated with a pronounced leukopenia. Some years ago, T_2 toxin and trichothecenes were identified in submerged cultures of *F. sporotrichioides*. Recently, occurrence of trichothecenes would have been demonstrated in samples associated with human haemorrhagic disease in South East Asia known as 'Yellow Rain' disease. Another possible incidence of mycotoxin in human health risk corresponds to Balkan endemic nephropathy. This is a chronic disease that is more common around 40 years of age and then progresses slowly up to death in rural populations of the Danube plain in Yugoslavia, Bulgaria and Romania. In the past 20 years, aetiological studies covering viruses, toxic metals and genetic factors have been conducted without convincing results. Attention has been called to the similarities in the changes of renal structure and function (tubular degeneration, intestinal fibrosis and decreased Tm PAH) found in this disease and in ochratoxin A-induced porcine nephropathy, suggesting common causal relationships. Results of surveys of foodstuffs indicate effectively that exposure to foodborne ochratoxin A seems to be higher in the Yugoslavia area with a higher prevalence of human endemic nephropathy than in non-endemic areas. However, the hypothesis, that ochratoxin A may be one of the causal determinants in this disease, needs further support.

Besides much suspected implications of mycotoxins for inducing well-determined human diseases, the occurrence of toxins in dietary intake of man could lead to both the participation of these poisons in other diseases and the interaction with other xenobiotics such as drugs, resulting in a toxic combined effect. In this respect, a toxicological study[22] demonstrated an increase in ochratoxin A toxicity when the toxin was administered with ethylbiscoumacetate or phenylbutazone in rats. This finding may reflect an *in vivo* displacement of the toxin from binding sites on the plasma proteins, although some additive or synergistic action of the toxin and the associated drug is another possibility.

On the other hand, some naturally occurring mycotoxins other than aflatoxins have been recognized as carcinogenic substances, namely penicillic acid, patulin or sterigmatocystin. Certain toxins have also been described as mutagens or teratogens. Thus in a recent monograph[26] Hayes reviewed the involvement of mycotoxins in animal and human health, the implication of mycotoxins in abnormal fetal development and the mutagenicity of these metabolites. Such toxicological properties have led the WHO task group on environmental health criteria for mycotoxins to express as general recommendation for further studies, the need for a 'better understanding of the role of mycotoxins in human disease'. This conclusion emphasizes the importance of studies concerning all pathways of human dietary exposure, particularly the problem concerning the transfer of mycotoxin residues from the contaminated animal feedstuffs into the edible tissue, especially for toxins as important and widely spread as patuline, zearalenone or tichothecenes. On the other hand, a better study of biotransformation pathways of such mycotoxins will lead to the discovery of toxic derivatives and the elaboration of their own analytical methods of carry-over in tissues and excreta. In addition to advantages in the fields of residue study or mycotoxicose diagnosis, the determination of their biotransformation pathways may lead to an explanation of the mode of toxic activity of some mycotoxins and to the determination of a specific treatment for reducing acute or chronic effects of these food contaminants in man and animals.

References

1. Allcroft, R. and Roberts, B. A. (1968). Toxic groundnut meal: the relationship between aflatoxin B_1 intake by cows and excretion of aflatoxin M_1 in milk. *Vet. Rec.*, **82,** 116–18
2. Allcroft, R., Roberts, B. A. and Lloyd, M. K. (1968). Excretion of aflatoxin in a cow. *Food Cosmet. Toxicol.*, **6,** 619–25
3. Armbrecht, B. H. (1971). Aflatoxin residues in food and feed derived from plant and animal sources. *Res. Rev.*, **41,** 13–54
4. Armbrecht, B. H., Shalkop, W. T., Rollins, L. D. *et al.* (1970). Acute toxicity of aflatoxin B_1 in wethers. *Nature (London)*, **225,** 1062–4
5. Bartos, J. and Matyas, Z. (1978). Research on the contingent presence of aflatoxin B_1 in the liver and muscle of slaughter animals. *Vet. Med. Praha*, **23,** 541–8
6. Brian, P. W., Elson, G. W. and Lowe, D. (1956). Production of patulin in apple fruits by *Penicillium expansum. Nature (London)*, **178,** 263–4
7. Caldwell, R. W. and Tuite, J. (1970). Zearalenone production in field corn in Indiana. *Phytopathology*, **60,** 1696–7
8. Chi, M. S., Robison, T. S., Mirocha, C. J. *et al.* (1978). Excretion and tissue distribution of radioactivity from tritium-labeled T2 toxin in chicks. *Toxicol. Appl. Pharmacol.*, **45,** 391–402
9. Chi, M. S., Robison, T. S., Mirocha, C. J. *et al.* (1978). Transmission of radioactivity into eggs from laying hens administered tritium labeled T2 toxin. *Poultry Sci.*, **57,** 1234–8
10. Collet, J. C. and Regnier, J. M. (1977). Contamination par mycotoxines de maïs conservés en cribs et visiblement altérés. *Ann. Nutr. Alim.*, **31,** 447–57
11. Elling, F., Hald, B., Jacobsen, C. *et al.* (1975). Spontaneous toxic nephropathy in poultry associated with ochratoxin A. *Acta Pathol. Microbiol. Scand.*, **83,** 739–41
12. Ellison, R. A. and Kotsonis, F. N. (1974). *In vitro* metabolism of T2 toxin. *Appl. Microbiol.*, **27,** 423–4
13. Eppley, M. and Bailey, W. J. (1973). 12–13 epoxytrichocenes as the probable mycotoxins responsible for stachybotryotoxicosis. *Science*, **181,** 758–60
14. Eppley, M., Stoloff, L., Trucksess, M. W. *et al.* (1974). Survey of corn for Fusarium toxins. *J. Assoc. Offic. Anal. Chem.*, **57,** 632–5
15. Escoula, L. (1974). Moisissures toxinogènes des fourrages ensilés. *Ann. Rech. Vét.*, **5,** 423–32; Ibid., 1975, **6,** 219–26
16. Furtado, R. M., Pearson, A. M., Hogberg, M. G. *et al.* (1979). Aflatoxin residues in the tissues of pigs fed a contaminated diet. *J. Agric. Food Chem.*, **27,** 1351–4
17. Galtier, P. (1974). Devenir de l'ochratoxine A dans l'organisme animal. *Ann. Rech. Vét.*, **5,** 311–28

18. Galtier, P., Bodin, G. and More, J. (1975). Toxicité de l'ochratoxine A par administration orale prolongée chez le rat. *Ann. Rech. Vét.*, **6**, 207–18
19. Galtier, P. and Alvinerie, M. (1976). *In vitro* transformation of ochratoxin A by animal microbial floras. *Ann. Rech. Vét.*, **7**, 91–8
20. Galtier, P., Alvinerie, M. and Charpenteau, J. L. (1981). The pharmacokinetic profiles of ochratoxin A in pig, rabbit and chicken. *Food Cosmet. Toxicol.*, **19**, 735–8
21. Galtier, P., Baradat, C. and Alvinerie, M. (1977). Etude de l'élimination d'ochratoxine A par le lait chez la lapine. *Ann. Nutr. Alim.*, **31**, 911–18
22. Galtier, P., Camguilhem, R. and Bodin, G. (1980). Evidence for *in vitro* and *in vivo* interaction between ochratoxin A and three acidic drugs. *Food Cosmet. Toxicol.*, **18**, 493–6
23. Galtier, P., Charpenteau, J. L., Alvinerie, M. *et al.* (1979). The pharmacokinetic profile of ochratoxin A in the rat after oral and intravenous administration. *Drug Metab. Dispos.*, **7**, 429–34
24. Galtier, P., Jemmali, M. and Larrieu, G. (1977). Enquête sur la présence éventuelle d'aflatoxines et d'ochratoxine A dans le maïs récolté en France en 1973 et 1974. *Ann. Nutr. Alim.*, **31**, 381–9
25. Hagler, W. H., Danko, G., Horvath, L. *et al.* (1980). Transmission of zearalenone and its metabolite into ruminant milk. *Acta Vet. Acad. Sci. Hung.*, **28**, 209–16
26. Hayes, A. W. (1981). *Mycotoxin Teratogenicity and Mutagenicity.* (Boca Raton: CRC Press)
27. Hsu, I. C., Smalley, E. B., Strong, F. M. *et al.* (1972). Identification of T2 toxin in moldy corn associated with lethal toxicosis in dairy cattle. *Appl. Microbiol.*, **24**, 684–90
28. Jacobson, W. C. and Wiseman, H. G. (1974). Transmission of aflatoxin B_1 into eggs. *Poult. Sci.*, **53**, 1743–5
29. Jemmali, M. (1973). Presence d'un facteur oestrogénique d'origine fongique, la zéaralénone ou F2 comme contaminant naturel dans du maïs. *Ann. Microbiol. (Inst. Pasteur)*, **124B**, 109–14
30. Jemmali, M. and Murthy, R. R. K. (1977). In Rodricks *et al.* (eds.) *Mycotoxins in Human and Animal Health.* p. 78. (Park Forest South: Pathotox.)
31. Jemmali, M., Ueno, Y., Ishii, K. *et al.* (1978). Natural occurrence of tichothecenes (Nivalenol deoxynivalenol, T2) and zearalenone in corn. *Experientia*, **34**, 1333–4
32. Krogh, P., Axelsen, N. H., Elling, F. *et al.* (1974). Experimental porcine nephropathy: changes of renal function and structure induced by ochratoxin A contaminated feed. *Acta Pathol. Microbiol. Scand.*, Suppl. 236
33. Krogh, P., Elling, F., Gyrd-Hansen, N. *et al.* (1976). Experimental porcine nephropathy changes of renal function and structure perorally induced by cristalline ochratoxin A. *Acta Pathol. Microbiol. Scand.*, **84**, 429–34
34. Krogh, P., Elling, F., Hald, B. *et al.* (1976). Experimental avian nephropathy: changes of renal function and structure induced by ochratoxin A contaminated feed. *Acta Pathol. Microbiol. Scand.*, **84**, 215–21
35. Krogh, P., Hald, B., Hasselager, E. *et al.* (1973). Aflatoxin residues in bacon pigs. *Pure Appl. Chem.*, **35**, 275–81
36. Krogh, P., Hald, B. and Pedersen, J. (1973). Occurrence of ochratoxin A and citrinin in cereals associated with mycotoxic porcine nephropathy. *Acta Pathol. Microbiol. Scand.*, **81**, 689–95
37. Lasztity, R. and Woller, L. (1975). Effects of zearalenone and some derivatives on animal feed or contaminated fodder. *Acta Aliment. Acad. Sci. Hung.*, **4**, 189–97
38. Le Bars, J. (1977). Bioproduction de stérigmatocystine par l'Aspergillus versicolor dans les fourrages secs. *Ann. Nutr. Alim.*, **31**, 575–81
39. Le Bars, J. (1977). La stachybotryotoxicose: une mycotoxicose fatale due à Stachybotrys atra. *Rev. Méd. Vét.*, **128**, 51–69
40. Le Bars, J. (1980). Facteurs favorisant la production d'acide pénicillique par Penicillium verrucosum var. cyclopium dans les denrées alimentaires. *Ann. Rech. Vét.*, **11**, 321–6
41. Lovett, J. (1972). Distribution of C^{14} in eggs from patulin-C^{14} fed hens. *Bacteriol. Proc. Abstr.*, E99
42. Lotzsch, R. and Leistner, L. (1977). Transmission of aflatoxins into eggs and egg products. *Ann. Nutr. Alim.*, **31**, 499–508

43. MacKinney, J. D., Canavagh, G. C., Bell, J. L. *et al.* (1973). Effects of ammoniation of aflatoxins in rations fed lactating cows. *J. Am. Oil Chem. Soc.*, **50**, 79 81
44. Mabee, M. (1972). *PhD Dissertation*, Ohio State University, USDA, Albany, California
45. Masri, M. S., Garcia, V. C. and Page, J. R. (1969). The aflatoxin M content of milk from cows fed known amounts of aflatoxins. *Vet. Rec.*, **84**, 146–7
46. Matsumoto, H., Ito, T. and Ueno, Y. (1978). Toxicological approaches to the metabolites of fusaria. XII. Fate and distribution of T2 toxin in mice. *Jap. J. Exp. Med.*, **48**, 393–9
47. Mintzlaff, H. J., Lotzsch, R., Tauchmann, F. *et al.* (1974). Aflatoxin-ruck stande in der Leber und in der Muskulatur von Masthanchen nach Verabreichung von Aflatoxin haltingen Fulttermitteln. *Fleisch Wirschaft*, **54**, 774–8
48. Mirocha, C. J., Harrison, J., Nichols, A. A. *et al.* (1968). Detection of a fungal estrogen in hay associated with infertility in dairy cattle. *Appl. Microbiol.*, **16**, 797–8
49. Mirocha, C. J., Pathre, S. V. and Robison, T. S. (1981). Comparative metabolism of zearalenone and transmission into bovine milk. *Food Cosmet. Toxicol.*, **19**, 25–30
50. Mucke, W. (1974). *PhD Dissertation*, München Technical University, Germany
51. Patterson, D. S. P., Glancy, E. M. and Roberts, B. A. (1980). The carry over of aflatoxin M_1 into the milk of cows fed rations containing a low concentration of aflatoxin B_1. *Food Cosmet. Toxicol.*, **18**, 35–7
52. Patterson, D. S. P., Shreeve, B. J. and Roberts, B. A. (1981). Effect on calves of barley naturally contaminated with ochratoxin A and groundnut meal contaminated with low concentrations of aflatoxins B_1. *Res. Vet. Sci.*, **31**, 213–18
53. Patterson, D. S. P., Roberts, B. A. and Small, B. J. (1976). Metabolism of ochratoxins A and B in the pig during early pregnancy and the accumulation in body tissues of ochratoxin A only. *Food Cosmet. Toxicol.*, **14**, 439–42
54. Piskorska-Pliszczynska, J. and Juskiewicz, T. (1979). Tissue deposition and passage into eggs of ochratoxin A in Japanese quail. Presented at *4th IUPAC Symposium, Lausanne*
55. Polan, C. E., Hayes, J. R. and Campbell, T. C. (1974). Consumption and fate of aflatoxin B_1 by lactating cows. *J. Agr. Food Chem.*, **22**, 635–8
56. Pons, W. A., Goldblatt, L. A., Cucullu, A. F. *et al.* (1977). In Rodricks *et al.* (eds.) *Mycotoxins in Human and Animal Health*. p. 78. (Park Forest South: Pathotox)
57. Prior, M. G. and Sisodia, C. S. (1978). Ochratoxicosis in white Leghorn hens. *Poult. Sci.*, **57**, 619–23
58. Purchase, I. F. H. (1973). The control of aflatoxin residues in food of animal origin. *Pure Appl. Chem.*, **35**, 283–9
59. Ribelin, W. E., Fukuschima, K. and Still, P. E. (1978). The toxicity of ochratoxin to ruminants. *Can. J. Comp. Med.*, **42**, 172–6
60. Robison, T. S., Mirocha, C. J., Kurtz, H. J. *et al.* (1979). Transmission of T2 toxin into bovine and porcine milk. *J. Dairy Sci.*, **62**, 637–41
61. Rodricks, J. V., Hesseltine, C. W. and Mehlman, M. A. (1977). In Rodricks *et al.* (eds.) *Mycotoxins in Human and Animal Health*. p. 67. (Park Forest South: Pathotox)
62. Rutqvist, L., Bjorklund, N. E., Hult, K. *et al.* (1977). Spontaneous occurrence of ochratoxin residues in kidneys of fattening pigs. *Zbl. Vet. Med.*, **24**, 402–8
63. Sawhney, D. S., Vadehra, D. V. and Baker, R. C. (1973). The metabolism of ^{14}C aflatoxin in laying hens. *Poult. Sci.*, **52**, 1302–9
64. Schoental, R. (1970). Hepatotoxic activity of retrorsine, senkirkine and hydroxysenkirkine in newborn rats and the role of epoxides in carcinogenesis by pyrrolizidine alkaloids and aflatoxins. *Nature (London)*, **227**, 401–2
65. Scott, P. M. (1978). Mycotoxins in feeds and ingredients and their origin. *J. Food Prot.*, **41**, 385–98
66. Scott, P. M., van Walbeek, W., Kennedy, B. *et al.* (1972). Mycotoxins (ochratoxin A, citrinin, sterigmatocystin) and toxigenic fungi in grains and other agricultural products. *J. Agr. Food Chem.*, **20**, 1103–9
67. Shreeve, B. J., Patterson, D. S. P. and Roberts, B. A. (1979). The carry over of aflatoxin, ochratoxin and zearalenone from naturally contaminated feed to tissues, urine and milk of dairy cows. *Food Cosmet. Toxicol.*, **17**, 151–2
68. Shreeve, B. J., Patterson, D. S. P., Roberts, B. A. *et al.* (1978). Effects of mouldy feed containing zearalenone on pregnant sows. *Br. Vet. J.*, **134**, 421–7

69. Smalley, E. B., Marasas, W. F. O. and Daugherty, S. (1972). Development of *Aspergillus flavus* and aflatoxins in harvested forage. *Res. Bull.* no. R 2412, Madison, Wisconsin
70. Stoloff, L. (1976). In Rodricks *et al.* (eds.) *Mycotoxins and other Fungal Related Food Problems.* Adv. in Chemistry Series, **149** Washington
71. Stoloff, L. (1977). In Rodricks *et al.* (eds.) *Mycotoxins in Human and Animal Health.* (Park Forest South: Pathotox)
72. Thorpe, C. W. and Johnson, R. L. (1974). Analysis of penicillic acid by gas-liquid chromatography. *J. Assoc. Off. Anal. Chem.*, **57**, 861–5
73. van Zytveld, W. A., Kelley, L. J. and Dennis, S. M. (1970). Aflatoxicosis: the presence of aflatoxins or their metabolites in livers and skeletal muscles of chickens. *Poult. Sci.*, **49**, 1350–3
74. Wyllie, T. D. and Morehouse, L. G. (1978). *Mycotoxic Fungi, Mycotoxins, Mycotoxicosis.* (3 Vols.). (New York: Marcel Dekker)
75. Yoshizawa, T., Mirocha, C. J., Behrens, J. C. *et al.* (1981). Metabolic fate of T2 toxin in a lactating cow. *Food Cosmet. Toxicol.*, **19**, 31–9

54 Residues of xenobiotics in animals, milk, and environment in the light of a 13 year surveillance

T. Juszkiewicz

Most of the potentially toxic chemicals contaminating the environment may penetrate animal organisms. They can manifest themselves with disease symptoms of various intensity and character or produce subclinical effects, which can be observed only as a drop in productivity of the animals, e.g. inhibition in growth, drop in milking yield or laying capacity. A considerable number of xenobiotics that pollute animals are excreted from the organism via milk or eggs or are accumulated in various tissues and organs, being thus transferred to the human body. It should be emphasized that the veterinary profession, due to its everyday life with animals, may play the important role in preventing environmental pollution and protecting human health.

MATERIAL AND METHODS

According to the system of national surveillance, sampling and analysis, which was developed for Poland in 1968[1,2], in the period from 1969 to 1981, samples of animal tissues from about 26 000 animals (cattle, horses, swine and poultry), 3000 pooled milk samples from over 250 000 cows and 25 000 eggs, were received for analysis of xenobiotic content (pesticides, polychlorinated biphenyls (PCBs) and potentially toxic elements). In addition, over 25 000 samples of animals slaughtered for export purposes (cattle, pigs, geese, ducks, rabbits, and game animals) were also analysed. Similar analyses were performed at the same time with occasional samples of human fat and human milk.

Determinations of organochlorine and organophosphorous pesticides and PCBs were conducted mainly by gas chromatography; for other xenobiotics various techniques of spectrophotometry, including atmoic absorption, were used[3,9,10,12–16].

RESULTS AND DISCUSSION

Results of the analysis are summarized and presented in Table 54.1–4 and in Figure 54.1. The sum of DDT (S-DDT = *p,p'*-DDE + *p,p'*-DDT + *p,p'*-DDD + *o,p'*-DDT) was found to be a prevailing pesticide, particularly within the first years of surveillance, although its levels of residues in animal tissues, milk, and in the environment, as well, have significantly declined, by approximately 75–85% during the 13 y since the initiation of this regular study in 1969 (Figure 54.1). As could be expected, the highest concentrations and the most persistent levels of DDT and PCB residues were found in human adipose tissues and in breast milk (Table 54.1). In consequence, in 1971 a moratorium on the use of DDT began in agriculture, followed in 1973–74 by its complete ban in Poland.

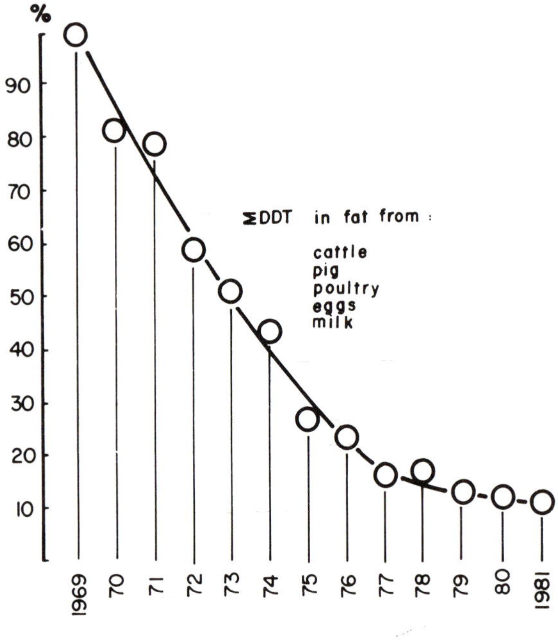

Figure 54.1 Decline of DDT residues, presented as calculated mean values expressed in percentages of the concentrations found in 1969

Other organochlorine pesticides were found in rather low concentrations and only in a percentage of the samples tested. There were mainly isomers α, β and γ of HCH, HCB, dieldrin, and methoxychlor.

During the latter years, occurrence of PCB was recorded quite frequently in animal tissues, eggs, and milk, human adipose tissues and human milk (Table 54.2). However, the concentrations of PCBs in animal samples were much lower than those in humans.

Table 54.1 Average residues of S-DDT, S-HCH and HCB in animal fat, milk, and eggs; values found from 1979 to 1981 expressed as mg/kg

Commodity	*Number of analyses*	*S-DDT* mean	*S-DDT* range	*S-HCH* mean	*S-HCH* range	*HCB* range (%)*
Pigs, fat	3036	0.18	0.01– 1.91	0.01	0.00–1.16	0.01–0.03 (6)
Cattle, fat	2074	0.14	0.01– 2.11	0.01	0.00–0.33	0.01–0.08 (9)
Horses, fat	35	0.10	0.03– 0.30	0.03	0.01–0.06	0.01 (20)
Chickens, fat	1082	0.74	0.01– 3.05	0.01	0.00–0.22	0.01–0.35 (6)
Geese, fat	915	0.35	0.01– 3.08	0.01	0.00–0.17	0.01–0.03 (6)
Ducks, fat	819	0.12	0.01– 2.10	0.01	0.00–0.11	0.01–0.02 (7)
Rabbits, fat	602	0.14	0.01– 2.80	0.01	0.00–0.23	0.01–0.13 (13)
Game, fat	1463	0.35	0.01– 3.12	0.01	0.00–0.22	0.01–0.07 (21)
Eggs, yolks	470	0.25	0.02– 1.83	0.01	0.00–0.05	0.01–0.02 (3)
Cow's milk, fat	579†	0.16	0.05– 0.39	0.05	0.04–0.13	0.01–0.05 (2)
Human milk, fat	161	6.70	0.70–16.31	0.09	0.00–0.25	0.02–0.85 (100)

*Percentage of positive samples
†Pooled samples from 300 cows each

Table 54.2 Average PCB concentrations in animal fat, milk, eggs, and human milk and fat; values found from 1979 to 1981 expressed as mg/kg

Commodity	*Number of analyses*	*Mean*	*Range*	*Positive samples* (%)
Pigs, fat	515	0.01	0.00–0.08	53
Horses, fat	35	0.09	0.02–0.45	100
Poultry, fat	625	0.05	0.01–0.30	95
Eggs, yolks	94*	0.02	0.00–0.15	70
Cow's milk, fat	473†	0.04	0.00–0.14	99
Human milk, fat	285	0.40	0.10–3.08	100
Human fat	118	0.56	0.08–3.21	100

*Pooled samples of five eggs each
†Pooled samples from 300 cows each

Average concentrations of some potentially toxic elements in bovine tissues and milk are given in Table 54.3. The levels of PCB and investigated elements were found to be dependent upon both incidental and environmental (industrial) exposures[6–8,11]. As an example, concentrations of cadmium and lead, determined in biological samples taken from agricultural areas (Bialystok and Lublin provinces) and heavy industrial areas (Krakow and Katowice provinces), were compared in Table 54.4.

Organophosphorous insecticides were not detected in the samples received for routine analyses, in spite of the fact that, in experimental conditions, residues of the compounds used for warble fly control were found in milk and tissues of cattle during the withdrawal period of time[4,5]. Practical implications of the results seem to be evident if they are evaluated from the point of view of animal health and human safety.

Table 54.3 Average concentrations of some potentially toxic elements in bovine tissues and milk; values found from 1979 to 1981 expressed as mg/kg

	Kidneys		*Meat*		*Milk**	
Elements	*mean (n)*	*range*	*mean (n)*	*range*	*mean (n)*	*range*
Hg	0.017 (875)	0.005–1.800	0.007 (565)	0.004–0.080	0.002 (290)	0.0005–0.003
Pb	0.62 (332)	0.14–3.48	0.09 (1265)	0.00–3.2	0.019 (376)	0.010–0.061
Cd	2.10 (332)	0.18–8.43	0.02 (655)	0.00–0.12	0.004 (376)	0.001–0.027
As	NA		0.05 (1052)	0.00–0.22	NA	
Zn	25.3 (250)	14.2–49.3	34.3 (607)	10.0–78.5	4.4 (376)	2.96–6.94
Cu	4.08 (250)	2.10–6.96	0.98 (577)	0.20–3.49	0.06 (376)	0.03–0.18
Fe	67.2 (250)	31.3–158	38.2 (250)	17.1–79.2	1.05 (376)	0.54–3.32

*Pooled samples from 300 cows each
NA: not analysed; *n*: number of samples

Table 54.4 Comparison between concentrations of cadmium and lead found in agricultural and industrial areas; all values given in mg/kg are means ± SD of over 150 samples each

	Agricultural area		*Industrial area*	
Samples	*Cd*	*Pb*	*Cd*	*Pb*
Bovine kidney	0.68 ± 0.41*	0.31 ± 0.10*	4.08 ± 1.57	1.42 ± 0.65
Bovine liver	0.13 ± 0.07*	0.14 ± 0.05*	0.88 ± 0.54	0.71 ± 0.34
Bovine muscles	0.01 ± 0.01*	0.06 ± 0.02	0.06 ± 0.03	0.08 ± 0.04
Bovine hair	0.26 ± 0.13*	1.12 ± 0.48*	0.54 ± 0.27	7.05 ± 3.35
Bovine milk	0.003 ± 0.002	0.017 ± 0.007	0.018 ± 0.009	0.029 ± 0.009
Human milk	0.004 ± 0.002*	0.014 ± 0.005*	0.007 ± 0.004	0.020 ± 0.007

*Denotes a significant difference ($p < 0.05$) between areas

References

1. Juszkiewicz, T. (1968). Pesticide residues control (in Polish). *Biul. Inst. Ochr. Rośl.*, **41**, 21–31
2. Juszkiewicz, T. (1973). Veterinary monitoring system of pesticide residues in the environment (in Polish). *Bromat. Chem. Toksykol.*, **6**, 471–6
3. Juskiewicz, T. (1974). Methods of pesticide analysis in foods of an animal origin (in Polish). *Bromat. Chem. Toksykol.*, **7**, 254–8
4. Juszkiewicz, T., Kosmala, K. and Żmudzki, J. (1974). Trichlorfon residues in milk following dermal application of Neguvon (Bayer) against *Hypoderma bovis*. *Bull. Vet. Inst. Pulawy*, **18**, 93–106
5. Juszkiewicz, T., Kosmala, K. and Żmudzki, J. (1975). Bromfenvinphos residues in bovine tissues following dermal application against ectoparasites (in Polish). *Medycyna Wet.*, **31**, 415–18
6. Juszkiewicz, T. and Szprengier, T. (1978). Fate of mercury in environment, animals and man (in Polish). *Post. Nauk Rol.*, **25**, 99–118
7. Juszkiewicz, T., Sikorski, R., Niewiadowska, A *et al.* (1979). Polychlorinated biphenyls in human adipose tissue and breast milk (in Polish). *Gin. Pol.*, **50**, 917–22
8. Juszkiewicz, T. (1979). Environmental toxicology and perinatal threats (in Polish). *Gin. Pol.* Suppl., 14–19
9. Juszkiewicz, T. (1983). The veterinary problems of pesticide monitoring and analysis. In *Proccedings of 2nd International Conference on Veterinary Pharmacology, Toxicology and Therapeutics.* (Amsterdam: Elsevier Science) (In press)
10. Niewiadowska, A. (1977). Determination of polychlorinated biphenyl residues in the presence of organochlorine insecticides in biological material (in Polish). *Pol. Arch. Wet.*, **20**, 71–8
11. Niewiadowska, A. and Juszkiewicz, T. (1978). Residues of polychlorinated biphenyls in milk. *Bull. Vet. Inst. Pulawy*, **22**, 80–5
12. *Official Methods of Analysis of the AOAC.* (Washington: Current Editions)
13. *Pesticide Analytical Manual* (1977). Vols. 1, 2, 3. (Washington: FDA)
14. Szprengier, T. (1977). A modified method for the determination of mercury in biological material using atomic absorption spectrometry (in Polish). *Medycyna Wet.*, **33**, 182–4
15. Żmudzki, J. (1977). Determination of lead in biological material by atomic absorption spectrometry (in Polish). *Medycyna Wet.*, **33**, 179–81
16. Żmudzki, J. (1980). Determination of cadmium in biological material by atomic absorption spectrometry (in Polish). *Bromat. Chem. Toksykol.*, **13**, 77–81

55
Persistence in milk of active antimicrobial intramammary substances

Ph. Archimbault

Milk, an essential foodstuff, is widely consumed as such or in the form of various milk derivatives. Like most agricultural products, because of the therapeutical treatment administered to dairy cows, milk is subject to a risk of contamination, especially in the case of antibiotically active substances.

The first attempts at reducing the antibiotic contamination of milk were not made to protect the consumer, but solely so as to limit the number of incidents during the production of milk derivatives obtained by fermentation. To this economic objective could be added the desire to offer a product which would be healthier and more hygienic, and not contaminated by antibiotics, the possible influence being unknown for the consumer's health.

At present, many teams of research workers are interested in this problem. It seems that the arguments which are most often used against antibiotic residues in food of animal origin for human consumption are:

(1) Possible occurrence of allergic symptoms (a well-known incident due to the penicillins).

(2) Disorders of the intestinal flora.

(3) Possible occurrence of strain-resistance to the antibiotics administered in human therapy.

However, it is necessary to mention that the acute toxic effects from these residues are not founded regarding milk. As a matter of fact, the quantity of antibiotics inferred is very low.

On the other hand, in most of the industrial countries, the manufacturer of a veterinary product is compelled to give a withdrawal time to be followed after the last administration of the product – whether the latter contains antibiotics or not. Consequently, it appears that the authorities do take or have already enforced the necessary regulations in order to avoid the proliferation regarding the effectiveness of this type of measure, thus making it necessary to reinforce the means of control.

ANTIBIOTICS USED IN VETERINARY MEDICINE

A classification of antibiotic substances can be made according to the number of times the drug is being used in dairy cows. The first group of drugs, which is the most widely distributed, is that of the β-lactams and their derivatives:

(1) Penicillins and their various salts (sodium, potassium, benzathine),
(2) Cloxacillin, oxacillin, dicloxacillin, ampicillin, amoxicillin, etc.,
(3) Cephalosporins: cefalexin, cephaloridine, cefapirin, cefacetrile.

Other groups of antibiotics are utilized almost as frequently:

(1) Aminoglycoside antibiotics: streptomycin and dihydrostreptomycin, neomycin, kanamycin, gentamicin;
(2) Chloramphenicol;
(3) Antibiotics of the tetracycline group, especially oxytetracycline and tetracycline;
(4) Antibiotics of the macrolide group: erythromycin, tylosin, spiramycin, etc.;
(5) Sulphonamides and sulphones and trimethoprim;
(6) Antibiotics of the polypeptide group with colistin and polymyxin B especially;
(7) Antibiotics of nitrofuran group: furazolidone, nitrofurazone, nitrofurantoin, etc.;
(8) Various antibiotics: novobiocin, rifamycin SV, lincomycin.

These different substances can be administered by several routes:

(1) Parenteral,
(2) Oral (seldom used in the dairy cow),
(3) Local (intramammary, intrauterine).

Therefore, it appears that the problem of the contamination of milk is extremely complex. Firstly, because of the number of substances presenting an antibiotic activity susceptible to be administered to dairy cows, secondly because of the multiple administration routes. Also, one must not forget that concomitant administration of several antibiotics according to two administration routes (i.e. intravenous and intramammary) are used routinely in veterinary therapy.

The major part of milk contamination should be the result of a local treatment, i.e. by intramammary route. The facts show that, usually, the intramammary route is not the chief element. As a matter of fact, the producer is well aware of the consequences of using this type of local administration, and it seems logical to him to discard the milk of several milkings after treatment has ceased. However, the mammary gland cannot be considered as an isolated and an hermetically sealed reservoir. The drugs cross the mammary epithelium either in the blood→udder direction, or just the opposite.

This phenomenon has been particularly well described[20]. The transfer mechanism is governed by the physicochemical characteristics of the drug and by those of the milk and blood.

The diffusion phenomena concern the portions which are unionized and non-protein-bound. The influence of the lipid solubility of the unionized portion is quite extensive also in this process.

Therefore, in the case of a mastitis, the increase of the milk pH of approximately 6.4–6.8 to 7.0–7.4, according to the pK_a of the drug contained in the udder, can modify the proportion of the unionized fraction. This is the only fraction that crosses the mammary epithelium and which is excreted in the blood circulation. Thus, according to the physicochemical criteria of the drug and of the pH of the milk, it is possible to foresee if the elimination of the drug contained in the udder will take place in the systemic circulation, and to what extent. The passage may modify the rate of the milk contamination which is later detected.

For all signs other than mastitis, milk contamination is also a corollary regarding the use of some antibiotic preparations, pharmacokinetic characteristics of which produce a high level of excretion by the intramammary route. This is the case, especially, of the antibiotics of the macrolide and tetracycline groups, chloramphenicol, and trimethoprim.

It is also necessary to observe that the galenical form of the product, and especially the nature of the excipient, have as much importance as the nature of the drug on the process of elimination of the antibiotic residues in the milk. Without prejudging the clinical effectiveness of the drugs, it is well-known that excipients of the 'slow-release' type for the intramammary or parenteral products, or the oil parenteral ones, can produce a prolonged mammary elimination of the antibiotic.

ELIMINATION IN THE MILK OF THE ANTIBIOTICS ADMINISTERED BY INTRAMAMMARY ROUTE

This mode of administration has been the subject matter of few studies[1–6]. In fact, in most cases, the veterinary drugs used are specifically adapted in their galenical form to intramammary therapy. The elimination characteristics of the antibiotic – or antibiotics – then depend upon the nature of the excipient.

It is also necessary to make a distinction between two type of treatment: (1) treatment in the lactation period, and (2) treatment in the dry period.

Treatment in the lactation period

The various studies published[16,22,27] show a great heterogenicity regarding the detection limits of the assay methods used, as well as in the number of quarters treated. The volume of the milk production is only seldom mentioned.

For penicillin G, which is one of the most commonly studied antibiotics, the various results available have been summarized in Table 55.1. The residue persistence spreads from 48 h to 18 days according to the administered dose, the excipient used, the number of treated quarters and the detection limit of

Table 55.1 Maximal time for elimination (hours: h and days: d) and detection limits of penicillin G alone or combined with dihydrostreptomycin (DHS) in relation with the excipient and the number of treated quarters

Product	*Dose* (IU)	*Excipient*	*Ref.*	*Treated No.*	*Elimination Time*	*Elimination Limits* (IU/ml)
Procaine pencillin	300 000	Mineral oil + Al. monostearate (3%)	28	4	18 d	0.02
Proc. Pen. + *D.H.S.*	100 000	Mineral oil + Al. monostearate (3%)	28	4	7 d	0.6
Proc. Pen. G	100 000	Oil suspension	2	1	>96 h	0.5
Proc. Pen. G	100 000	Aqueous suspension	2	1	60 h	0.5
Pen.	100 000	Ointment	9	1	6 d	0.01–0.02
Pen.	100 000	Water–oil emulsion	9	1	5 d	0.01–0.02
Pen. + *other antibiotics*	100 000	Water–oil emulsion	9	1	4 d	0.01–0.02
Pen.	100 000	Water	9	1	2 d	0.01–0.02
Sodium Pen. G	1 500 000	Water	14	4	60 h	0.005
Sodium Pen. G	3 000 000	Water	14	4	60 h	0.005
Proc. Pen. G + *D.H.S. 300 mg*	300 000	Diffusing medium	14	4	60 h	0.005
Proc. Pen. G + *Neo. 300 mg*	500 000	Diffusing medium	4	4	72 h	0.005
Proc. Pen. G + *Streptom. 300 mg* + *Neo. 300 mg*	300 000	Oil + Al. monostearate	14	4	>6.5 d	0.005
Proc. Pen. G + *D.H.S. 1000 mg*	300 000	Oil	31	1	>4 d	<0.005
Proc. Pen. G + *D.H.S. 1000 mg* + *Furazol. 142 mg*	300 000	Oil	31	1	>64 h	<0.005
Sodium Pen. G	500 000	Water	31	1	>72 h	<0.005
Proc. Pen. G + *D.H.S. 1000 mg*	1 500 000	—	31	-	—	—
Sod. Pen. G	1 000 000	—	31	-	—	—
Proc. Pen G + *D.H.S. 500 mg*	3 000 000	Water	31	1	>64 h	<0.005
Proc. Pen. G	400 000	Peanut oil + silica gel 0.5%	18	4	48 h	0.01
Proc. Pen. G	400 000	Peanut oil + Al. monostearate (3%)	18	4	120 h	0.01
Proc. Pen. G	400 000	Water	18	4	56 h	0.01
Proc. Pen. G	100 000	Peanut oil	19	4	56 h	0.01

the microbiological method applied. The residue of antibiotic which is tolerated is generally lower or equal to 0.01 IU of penicillin G per ml of milk.

A study[8] performed on 17 products with a penicillin acid in association with other antibiotics shows an elimination of penicillin in milk at times varying from 72 to 200 h after the end of the treatment. It is unquestionable that the influence of the nature of the excipient plays an important role, especially with the incorporation of aluminium monostearate presenting a definite slow-release effect.

A comparison carried out on various studies also confirms the fact that the elimination of penicillin residues is slower in animals suffering from mastitis than in healthy ones (more than approximately 12–24 h). The disappearance speed of the antibiotic is also lower in dairy cows with a limited milk production[24,26].

Regarding other β-lactam antibiotics, the information is more fragmentary, with the exception of cloxacillin (Table 55.2). Antibiotics of the aminoglycoside group, and dihydrostreptomycin and neomycin especially, are often incorporated into intramammary drugs. Since in association with the β-lactam antibiotics it is possible to enlarge the antibacterial spectrum of the drugs, the combination of these two types of antibiotics is used frequently. Our studies performed on neomycin should be compared with the results obtained for cloxacillin. With the same type of excipient, it does not always follow that, under the same conditions, the rate of elimination of both antibiotics will be similar.

According to therapeutical imperatives (rating of the products as either 'quick release' or 'long-acting'), the galenical study makes it possible to obtain either a fast or a slow elimination of the antibiotic from the udder. In the case of a mixture of antibiotics belonging to different groups, a compromise between them is necessary.

It is also necessary to consider the results[8] obtained when dihydrostreptomycin and neomycin are combined with penicillin in a very great number of intramammary drugs. The doses administered are from 100 to 300 mg for dihydrostreptomycin, and from 50 to 350 mg for neomycin. Elimination times are extremely variable according to the nature of the excipients and range from 72 to 200 h.

Although chloramphenicol is quite often used by the veterinary practitioner, only a restricted number of studies regarding its intramammary application are reported. The maximal time for elimination of chloramphenicol (10% in propylene glycol) which is 24 h[30] reaches 32 h in the case of 1 g as sodium succinate in water and more than 64 h for 0.5 g in water/oil excipient[31].

In the tetracycline group, only oxytetracycline, and in a slight proportion chlortetracycline and tetracycline, are administered by intramammary route.

Antibiotics of the macrolide group are represented by erythromycin especially. (Table 55.3). In most cases, its elimination is extremely rapid since 1–2 days following the application, the residue concentration in the milk is lower than 0.02 μg/ml.

Regarding the sulphonamides and sulphones administered by the intramammary route, studies conducted on the elimination of residues in milk

Table 55.2 Maximal time for elimination (d, h or milkings-m) of cloxacillin (clox) associated with colistin (col), neomycin (neo) and of dihydrostreptomycin (DHS) and neomycin

Product	*Dose*	*Excipient*	*Ref.*	*Treated*	*Elimination*	
Cloxacillin	200 mg	Peanut oil + OH stearin	3	4	> 6 m	0.015 μg/ml
+ *Neo.*	*200 mg*					
Clox.	400 mg	,, ,, ,, ,,	3	4	> 8 m	0.015 μg/ml
+ *Neo.*	*400 mg*					
Clox.	200 mg	,, ,, ,, ,,	4	2	10 m	0.015 μg/ml
+ *Col.*	*200 000 IU*					
Clox.	200 mg	,, ,, ,, ,,	6	1	7 m	0.015 μg/ml
+ *Neo.*	*200 mg*	Water PVP 1%		1	> 10 m	0.015 μg/ml
Na Ampicil.	2 g	Aqueous solution	33	2	> 48 h	0.01 μg/ml
Cefalexin	100 mg	Peanut oil	15	2	8 m	0.01 μg/ml
+ *Neo.*	*100 mg*					
Cefoxazole	250 mg	Oil	12	4	2 d	0.8 μg/ml
+ *Proc. Pen. G*	*250 mg*					
DHS	250 mg	Oil 3% + Monostearate Al.	28	4	48–72 h	0.3 μg/ml
DHS	100 mg	Oil 3% + Monostearate Al.	28	4	7 d	0.3 μg/ml
+ *Proc. Pen. G*	*100 000 IU*					
Neo.	100/500 mg	Water	25	1	84/ > 108 h	0.5 μg/ml
DHS	1 g	Oil	31	1	> 88 h	0.1 μg/ml
+ *Proc. Pen. G*	*300 000 IU*					

Table 55.3 Persistence in milk of active antimicrobial substances of the group of tetracyclines (oxytetracycline: OXY; chlortetracycline: CHLOR; tetracycline: TETRA) vs. macrolides (erythromycin: ERYTH) and polypeptides. Associated substances are prednisolone (PRED), hydrocortisone (HYDRO); the nitrofuran group is represented by nitrofurazone (NITRO), furaltadone (FURAL) and furazolidone (FURAZ)

Product	*Dose*	*Excipient*	*Ref.*	*Treated*	*Elimination*	
Tetracyclines						
Oxytetracycline	400 mg	Ointment	21	1–4	72 h	0.3 μg/ml
Oxy.	400 mg	Water	7	1–4	60 h	0.3 μg/ml
Oxy.	420 mg	Solution	9	1	60 h	0.5 μg/ml
Oxy.	420 mg	Ointment	9	1	48 h	0.5 μg/ml
Chlor.	426–852 mg	Ointment	9	1	180 h	0.5 μg/ml
Chlor.	200 mg	Unknown	17	4	>72 h	0.5 μg/ml
+ Neo.	*100 mg*					
Tetra.	500 mg	Water/oil	31	1	>40 h	0.02 μg/ml
Tetra.	500 mg	Water/oil	31	1	>56 h	0.02 μg/ml
+ Hydro.	*50 mg*					
Chlor.	426 mg	Oil	31	1	>40 h	0.02 μg/ml
Tetra.	100 mg	Aqueous sol.	32	2	>88 h	0.02 μg/ml
Macrolides						
Eryth.	300 mg	Oil	31	1	24 h	0.02 μg/ml
Spir.	600 mg	Water/oil	31	1	>144 h	0.02 μg/ml
Eryth.	1800 mg	Aqueous sol.	33	2	48 h	0.02 μg/ml
(as Estolate)						
Eryth.	250 mg	Peanut oil and	4	2	>10 m	0.04 μg/ml
+ DHS	*250 mg*	hydrogenated				
+ Pred.	*10 mg*	peanut oil				
Polypeptide + Nitrofuran						
Polymixin B	50 000 IU	Aqueous sol.	25	2	>84 h	
Col.	200 000 IU	Peanut oil + monost.	4	2	24 h	10 IU/ml
+ Clox.	*200 mg*					
Nitro.	60 mg	Unknown	13	1	>24 h	0.03 μg/ml
Fural.	500 mg	Peanut oil + monost.	8	4	32 h	0.01 μg/ml
Furaz.	150 mg	Mineral oil	23	2	23 h	3 μg/ml
+ Nitro.	*150 mg*					
Fural.	500 mg	Water/oil	31	1	>40 h	
Furaz.	355 mg	Oil	31	1	40 h	
Nitro.	200 mg	Unknown	29	1	72 h	0.005 μg/ml
Novobiocin	250 000 IU	Oil + 3% monost.	28	4	4 days	
Rifamycin SV	50 mg	Not mentioned	29		36 h	0.125 μg/ml

have not established the maximal time of elimination in relation to the determination of the withdrawal period.

Furthermore, in earlier published work, excessive doses were being used at the time (i.e. several grams per quarter), thus making them of no avail to us.

In the antibiotics of the polypeptide group, only colistin and polymyxin B have been used by the intramammary route. Both antibiotics are mainly used in the treatment of mastitis due to *Escherichia coli*.

Other substances with antibacterial activity which have been administered by the intramammary route, and whose elimination in the milk has been studied, are presented with the polypeptide antibiotics. These concern, especially, the nitrofuran derivatives which are very seldom applied in France.

Among all the antibiotics which have been utilized in intramammary therapy, it should be noted that the ones which have been studied regarding elimination from the milk, are the penicillins and their semisynthetic derivatives, the aminoglycosides, and the tetracyclines to a certain extent. The results given by the various authors are significant and very heterogenous, not only when a comparison is made between the various groups but also within the same group. Beside the dose administered, the nature of the intramammary excipient is one of the preponderant factors regarding the time of elimination of antibiotic residues from the milk.

Treatment in the dry period

Intramammary therapy in the dry period has progressed considerably in the last 10 years. As a matter of fact, at a time where immediate rentability of the dairy cow is not the main purpose, this makes it possible to undertake a prevention and/or curative therapy which is a determining factor for the good condition of the udder after calving.

Therapy in the dry period is obtained by introducing, in each of the previously dried-up quarters of the animal, some intramammary preparations characterized by a high dose of antibiotic and at the same time by a high retention of the latter. In theory, the administration is performed 4 or 5 weeks, at least, prior to the expected date of calving. In practice, a precise diagnosis of calving is more hazardous, thus resulting in a detrimental variability for the determination of a withdrawal period for this type of veterinary preparation. However, the production of colostrum, and the need to wait a few days before the excretion of a milk perfectly appropriate for market consumption, do reduce, in some way, the consequences of the practice of the intramammary treatment in the dry period.

A problem to be solved regarding the protection of the consumer's health and of the dairy processing industries can be summarized as the need for the manufacturing laboratory to produce an intramammary preparation during the non-lactating period, whose retention in the milk does not exceed 4–5 days after calving, whatever the application time. However, this requirement must be compatible with the persistence of the antibiotic activity in the treated quarters during an average drying-up time, i.e. 4 weeks.

Again, a certain ambiguity appears between the therapeutic action and the demand for the quality of the milk production after calving. This can be solved only by a better estimation of the calving date or the elimination of the milk several days following calving.

For the time being, intramammary preparations, to be used in the dry period, are composed first of antibiotics whose half-life in the mammary gland is long (i.e. a few days), and secondly of a drug-vehicle whose main property resides in the slow release of the active ingredient (incorporation of magnesium stearate for instance)[11,15,31]. Increasing the dose of antibiotic only is not judged as being satisfactory[25]. The use of a slow-release salt of the benzathine type is also widespread in the case of the penicillins and semi-synthetic penicillins[10, 11, 31].

The determination of a long and persistent antibiotic activity, a corollary of the true effectiveness of the drugs available, has consequently obliged the manufacturers to propose products whose safety can be fully warranted only in the case of a normal utilization a few weeks before calving. The major problem of the elimination of antibiotics in the milk of dairy cows treated too early prior to calving can be solved only by withdrawing the dairy production several days after calving, and by a determination establishing the absence of antibiotic activity.

CONCLUSIONS

The problem of milk contamination with active antimicrobial agents is genuine. Pressure from the milk processing industries, from the medical profession, and then from consumer's associations, have required that most countries enforce standards of milk quality, taking into account the absence of residues of therapeutically active substances, of pesticides, of heavy metals, etc. As far as the problem of contamination by active antibiotic agents is concerned, it is for the laboratory, which is responsible for the authorization of the product on the market, to offer a withdrawal period following administration of the drug which is susceptible to ensure the innocuousness and the quality of the milk. However, the criteria of such an appreciation do vary from one country to another, especially regarding the residue tolerance in the milk, and also the conditions of application of an experimental procedure making it possible to determine the level of contamination. Yet it should be noted that the WHO, the FDA and other national or international organizations have published the tolerance values concerning the residues of various substances in the milk (i.e. according to the WHO the tolerance for chloramphenicol should be equal to zero).

The actual trend seems, in theory, to reduce the contamination of the milk product. However, above all, the quality of the milk seems to rest entirely on the producer.

References

1. Abo-Elnaga, I. G., Abdel-Mottaleb, L. and Mahmoud, M. (1973). Excretion and incidence of antibiotics in milk. *Ind. J. Dairy Sci.*, **9**, 203–5
2. Albright, J. L., Ormiston, E. E., Brodie, B. O. *et al.* (1961). Penicillin in milk following intramuscular and intramammary administration of penicillin in normal and mastitic cows. *J. Am. Vet. Med. Assoc.*, **138**, 70–1
3. Archimbault, Ph., Aubert, A. and Haas, P. (1978). Résidus de cloxacilline et de néomycine dans le lait après leur administration, en association, par voie galactophore. *Rec. Méd. Vét.*, **154**, 951–6
4. Archimbault, Ph., Boutier, C., Fellous, R. *et al.* (1979). Concentration et élimination dans le lait de quelques antibiotiques après leur administration intramammaire. *Bull. Soc. Vét. Pract. France*, **63**, 2–16

5. Archimbault, Ph., Fellous, R. and Haas, P. (1979). Elimination d'antibiotiques dans le lait après injection intramammaire d'une association céphalexine–néomycine–prednisolone. *Rev. Méd. Vét.*, **5**, 721–34
6. Archimbault, Ph., Boutier, C., Fellous, R. *et al.* (1980). Influence de la nature de l'excipient sur l'élimination des antibiotiques administrés par voie intramammaire. *Rev. Méd. Vét.*, **131**, 209–22
7. Blobel, H. and Burch, C. W. (1960). Oxytetracycline concentrations in blood serum and milk secretions of cows following intravenous or intramammary treatment. *J. Am. Vet. Med. Assoc.*, **137**, 701–4
8. Cox, P. L. and Heotis, J. P. (1963). Determination of furaltadone in milk. *Agr. Food. Chem.*, **11**, 499–501
9. Fincher, M. G., Kosikowski, F. V., Guthrie, R. S. *et al.* (1962). Relative importance of persistence, transfer, and milking technique to antibiotic residue contamination of milk. *J. Am. Vet. Med. Assoc.*, **141**, 223–8
10. Gedek, W. and Richter, O. (1972). Arzneimittel-Hemmstoffe in der Milch nach intramammärer Behandlung in der Trockenzeit. *Zbl. Vet. Med. B.*, **19**, 40–4
11. Gedek, W., Matzke, P. and Baath, Chr. (1976). Verweildauer von Antibiotika im Trockensekret, Blutserum und Harn vom Rind nach Euterbehandlung beim Trockenstellen. *Tierärztl. Umsch.*, **31**, 383–6
12. Harris, A. M., Davies, A. M., Marshall, M. J. *et al.* (1977). The treatment of clinical mastitis with cephoxazole and penicillin. *Vet. Rec.*, **101**, 4–7
13. Henningson, R. W. (1961). Furacin residues in milk. *J. Dairy Sci.*, **44**, 1765–6
14. Jacobs, J. and Hanselaar, J. (1966). Antibiotic concentrations in milk of cows following intramammary administration. *Tijdschr. Diergeneesk*, **91**, 896–905
15. Johnson, M. E., Martin, J. H., Baker, R. J. *et al.* (1977). Persistence of antibiotics in milk from cows treated late in the dry period. *J. Dairy Sci.*, **60**, 1655–61
16. Katz, S. E., Fassbender, C. A., Ackrett, A. J. *et al.* (1973). Oxytetracycline residues in milk following intramammary infusion. *J. Assoc. Off. Anal. Chem.*, **56**, 706–12
17. Mercer, H. D., Geleta, J. N., Schultz, E. J. *et al.* (1970). Milk-out rates for antibiotics in intramammary infusion products used in the treatment of bovine mastitis: relationship of somatic cell counts, milk production level and drug vehicle. *Am. J. Vet. Res.*, **31**, 1549–60
18. Mercer, H. D., Geleta, J. N. and Carter, G. G. (1974). Absorption and excretion of penicillin G from the mastitic bovine udder. *J. Am. Vet. Med. Assoc.*, **164**, 613–17
19. Mercer, H. D., Geleta, J. N., Porteous, L. A. *et al.* (1974). Excretion of penicillin G and dihydrostreptomycin from quarters of cows with experimentally induced staphylococcal mastitis. *Am. J. Vet. Res.*, **35**, 1191–6
20. Rasmussen, F. (1966). In Mortensen, C. Fr. (ed.) *Studies on the Mammary Excretion and Absorption of Drugs*. pp. 1–87. (Copenhagen: Kandrup and Wunsch)
21. Schipper, I. A. and Petersen, W. E. (1953). Milk, blood and urine concentrations of terramycin following intravenous intramammary and intramuscular administration. *Vet. Med.*, **48**, 315–18
22. Schluep, J., Rosselet, A. and Heim, H. (1979). Comparative evaluation of cephacetrile in experimentally induced bovine mastitis. *Zbl. Vet. Med. B.*, **26**, 304–24
23. Shone, D. K. (1965). Residues in milk following the infusion of the udder with a nitrofuran preparation. *J.S. Afr. Vet. Med. Assoc.*, **36**, 115–17
24. Siddique, I. H., Loken, K. I. and Hoyt, H. H. (1965). Antibiotic residues in milk transferred from treated to untreated quarters in dairy cattle. *J. Am. Vet. Med. Assoc.*, **146**, 589–93
25. Siddique, I. H., Loken, K. I. and Hoyt, H. H. (1965). Concentrations of neomycin, dihydrostreptomycin and polymyxin in milk after intramuscular or intramammary administration. *J. Am. Vet. Med. Assoc.*, **146**, 594–9
26. Smith, A., Neave, F. K. and Jones, A. (1967). The persistence of penicillin G in the mammary gland when infused immediately after the last milking of lactation. *J. Dairy Res.*, **34**, 59–64
27. Terplan, G., Zaadhof, K. J. and Emde, H. (1971). Zur Ausscheidung von Antibiotika nach intrazisternaler Verabreichung unter besonderer Berücksichtigung des Erythromycins. *Dtsch. Milchwirtschaft, Hildesheim*, **38**, 1745–7
28. Uvarov, O. (1960). The concentration of some antibiotics in the milk after intramammary infusion. *Vet. Rec.*, **72**, 1228–31

29. Vilim, A. B. and MacIntosh, A. I. (1979). High pressure liquid chromatographic determination of nitrofurazone in milk. *J. Assoc. Off. Anal. Chem.*, **62,** 19–22
30. Wal, J. M., Peleran, J. C. and Bories, G. F. (1980). High performance liquid chromatographic determination of chloramphenicol in milk. *J. Assoc. Off. Anal. Chem.*, **63,** 1044–8
31. Ziv, G., Gordin, S., Bachar, G. *et al.* (1973). Concentration and persistence of antibiotics in milk following intramammary infusion in cows. *Refuah Vet.*, **30,** 85–100
32. Ziv, G., Saran-Rosenzuaig, A. and Risenberg, R. (1973). Retention of antibiotics in dry-udder secretions after the infusion of several 'dry cow' antibiotic products. *Zbl. Vet. Med. B.*, **20,** 415–24
33. Ziv, G., Gordin, S. and Bechar, G. (1974). Mode of transfer of antibiotics from treated to nontreated quarters in dairy cows. *Am. J. Vet. Res.*, **35,** 643–7

56
Evaluation of drug residues in animal tissues

P. Delatour

When one speaks about residues, everybody usually thinks of a legal definition such as that proposed by some national or supranational authority (EEC, FAO–WHO). Actually, the chemical nature of residues is diversified because of the complexity of the metabolic feature of drugs in the animal organism. Consequently, different residue fractions ultimately result which correspond to different risks and require different methods of investigation.

One intends first to correlate the main metabolic pathways of drugs in target animals with the chemical nature of the different residual fractions in edible tissues; secondly, to recall their biological significance to the animal itself; and finally, to try to determine their different possible hazards to the human.

METABOLISM-TOXICITY RELATIONSHIP

The biotransformation that drugs can undergo are numerous and, according to different cases, they lead either to metabolites which do not possess the activity of the parent compound or possibly to molecules responsible for the activity. The theoretical general Figure 56.1 illustrates the diversity of the possible pathways and the nature of the residues produced.

Following experimental administration of a labelled drug, animal metabolism produces three families of derivatives:

Products incorporated into endogenous metabolism

The drastic biodegradation of xenobiotics can lead to compounds which are identical to normal substrates of normal enzymic reactions. This has been reported with dichlorvos[21], trinitrine[9], parbendazole[10], carbaryl[11], DMAB[2], cambendazole[1], nihydrazone[19], dimetridazole, furazolidone[40], ronidazole[35], and even with inhaled carbonic anhydride[39] and carbonate[37]. The diversity of the incriminated molecules and animal species (rat, poultry, pig, ruminants) shows that this is a general phenomenon.

A comment should be made concerning the biochemical mechanisms of incorporation which is related to the position of labelling in the molecule; yet, the radioactivity of ^{14}C-ring labelled cambendazole is incorporated while the one of albendazole with the same labelling is not.

Production of inactive drug-related metabolites

A transformation of less toxicologic importance results in metabolites which possess no activity. This is the detoxication pathway. These metabolites appearing in the liver are often finally eliminated through urine, possibly as conjugates.

Production of toxic metabolites

Finally, studies of the metabolism–toxicity relationship enable us to define mechanisms responsible for the activity and the toxicity of drugs.

The most classical and frequent mechanism consists of reversible non-covalent binding of the parent compound or a similar stable metabolite on cellular structures by solubilization into membrane and lipids binding to

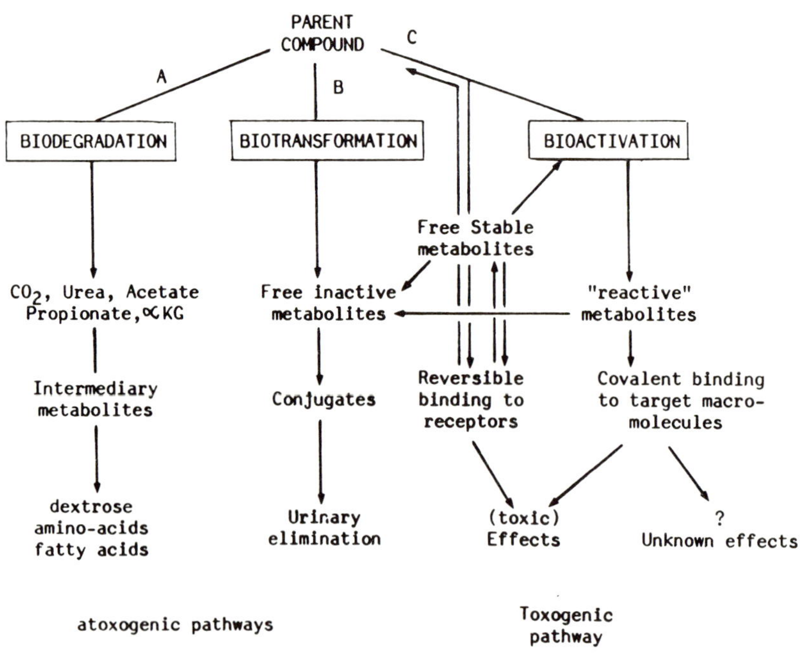

Figure 56.1 General metabolism of drugs in animal organism

receptors through hydrogen bonds, Vander Waal's forces, hydrophobic associations, etc. This mechanism explains reversible effects.

Since 1971, after the pioneer works of Brodie[4] and Mitchell[28], growing interest has been focussed on toxic mechanisms which involve covalent binding of metabolites on macromolecules.

This mode of action is similar to the one reported in 1947 by Miller and Miller for the carcinogen DMAB. This mechanism implies the appearance of a 'reactive metabolite' or 'ultimate toxin' which is highly electrophilic and able to react according to the following schema (Figure 56.1) (1) conversion into a free inactive metabolite through isomerization or hydration, (2) coupling with a soluble small molecule, and (3) finally, covalent binding to structural or informational target macromolecules, such as proteins or nucleic acids.

Toxicological significance for the animal

The distinction of the different residual fractions among the 'total residues' (arbitrarily expressed by global radioactivity) in target animals is founded on methodological criteria:

(1) Extractable residues: free parent compound and unconjugated metabolites, plus compounds which are reversibly bound.

(2) Intractable non-drug related residues: radioactivity corresponding to incorporation into intermediary metabolism.

(3) Intractable drug-related soluble residues: conjugated to sulphuric and glucuronic acids and glutathione.

(4) Intractable drug-related covalently-bound residues.

The biological activity of a chemical can, in most cases, involve either an extractable metabolite (parent compound or stable metabolite) or a covalent-bound metabolite. Today, this last group is incriminated in a growing number of circumstances such as carcinogenicity, necrogenicity, teratogenicity and allergenicity.

Carcinogenic effect

This process is accepted as the primary molecular mechanism for tumour inducers. For example, dimethyl nitrosamine leads to a methonium carbocathion binding to guanine of DNA in N-7 and O-6 positions[25]. Aflatoxin B_1 is oxidized by a cytochrome P-450 dependent mixed-function oxidase MFO into the ultimate carcinogen the 2-3, epoxide[38] which binds to DNA, RNA and proteins[17].

Necrogenic effect

Many hepatotoxins act this way including bromobenzene[45], acetaminophen[24], furosemide[33] and isoniazid[34]. In all cases, the electrophilic ultimate necrogen is produced by an enzymatic reaction. Enzyme inducers and inhibitors, as well as glutathione precursors and competitors, are modulation agents of this type of toxicity. The final binding of the reactive metabolite to its target is a non-enzymatic process. A threshold dose is necessary for this toxicity below which no reactive metabolite seems to appear. This has been demonstrated in the human and experimentally in animals. The pulmonary toxicity of ipomeanol is founded on a similar mechanism[3].

Teratogenic effect

Hypothesized for a long time, reactive metabolites have recently been demonstrated to be responsible for the toxicity of two major teratogens in the human, i.e. phenytoin and thalidomide.

In the mouse, diphenylhydantoin is teratogenic but none of its metabolites are[18]. Combination with TCPO, an inhibitor of epoxide-hydrase, increased significantly the incidence of embryotoxic manifestations and doubled the level of bound radioactivity in placental and fetal tissues[26]. These results are in favour of an electrophilic arene oxide as the ultimate teratogen.

Thalidomide is teratogenic in the rabbit but the rat is refractive. The hydrolytic metabolites are identical and non-teratogenic in both species. In the rabbit, but not in the rat, two additional phenol metabolites have been reported. The *in vitro* toxicity of thalidomide for human lymphocytes occurs in the presence of liver microsomal enzymes from the rabbit, but not from the rat. The cytotoxicity is enhanced by TCPO and decreased by the addition of purified hydrase to the culture medium. These facts support the transitory existence of an arene oxide metabolite which yields the two previously discovered phenols. As for phenytoin, the bimolecular target has not been identified to date.

Allergenic effect

Allergenic substances are haptens which have the capability to bind directly or indirectly to a protein that results in the final antigen. In the well-known example of penicillin, this compound or its metabolite penicillenic acid[32] are able to bind to lysine in proteins creating penicilloyl–protein conjugates which are the actual allergens.

Cross immune-reactions are numerous between penicillin and different degradation products which are also able to produce identical conjugates[31]. The specific quantitation of penicilloyl groups is possible, however[41].

Unknown effects

Frequently, one observes high levels of protein bound radioactivity without being able to correlate it with any biological effects to the animal. For example, although *p*-toluoyl-chloro-phenylhydrazone (TCPH) greatly binds to the haem and protein of sheep haemoglobin[23], no harmful consequence has been observed.

This also seems to be the rule with benzimidazol-anthelmintics. In the case of cambendazole, in addition to metabolic incorporation and glutathione coupling[42], a part of the radioactivity is bound to proteins through a product in which the carbamate group is not dissociated from the aromatic ring and which may be quantified in meat by non-radioactive methods[27]. With mebendazole and albendazole, similar findings have been reported; radioactivity is bound to blood, cytosol and microsomal proteins but not to nucleic acids[5].

Treatment of rats with [^{14}C]oxfendazole, the ultimate teratogen of febantel, and combination with proadiphen seems to result in disagreement between toxicity and bound radioactivity (Table 56.1). In this example, it seems that binding of reactive metabolites to macromolecules has no apparent toxicological significance in respect to embryotoxicity.

Table 56.1 Embryotoxicity and bound labelled metabolites of [^{14}C]oxfendazole in the rat

	Embryo lethality (%)	*Anomalies* *External* (%)	*Skeletal* (%)	*Total* *Plasma* (dpm/ml)	*Liver* (dpm/g)	*Bound* (dpm/mg)
Oxfendazole*	11.5	0	22	38 213†	70 998	28.5
Oxfendazole + proadiphen‡	34.4	16.3	59	40 927	58 856	2.4

*Oxfendazole (OFZ) = 15.75 mg/kg oral daily dose from day 8 to day 15 of pregnancy
†[^{14}C]Oxfendazole = 15.75 mg/kg (10.10^{6} dpm/rat) oral single dose
‡Proadiphen (SKF-525A) = 120 mg/kg p.o. 1 h before OFZ dosage and 60 mg/kg p.o. 4 h after OFZ dosage

The above experimental results show that covalent binding to macromolecules may or may not explain the toxic effects in the animal. Unfortunately, this results in poor predictability of the possible harm of covalently bound residues to the human.

TOXICOLOGICAL EVALUATION OF RESIDUES

The previous information suggests that the evaluation of different residual fractions will be methodologically different.

Incorporated radioactivity

This fraction is an artefact according to the definitions of residues. The innocuousness of this fraction is unanimously accepted, yet from the analytical point of view, it represents a complication[36], Its accurate quantitation is quite impossible because of the diversity of the compounds concerned. Nevertheless, it seems relatively simple to demonstrate the absence of this pathway by determining the specific activity of some principal intermediary metabolites such as CO_2, urinary urea, liver glycogen, lipid fatty acids, and protein glutamic acid in liver cytosol.

Extractible residues

Figure 56.1 points out that some free metabolites have maintained their toxic potential whereas others following irreversible enzymic reactions have definitely lost the capability to be turned into toxic compounds. The great interest in this fraction is related to its precocity and relative abundance; it also has a short halflife. Some authors[12,29,43] have discussed toxicological studies in order to determine whether the toxic effects are due entirely to the parent compound or due mainly to one of its metabolites. Such studies have been performed with human drugs. In the area of veterinary drugs, similar investigations have been conducted with anthelmintics. A recent example is that of Febantel. Figure 56.2 represents the main steps in the metabolism of this

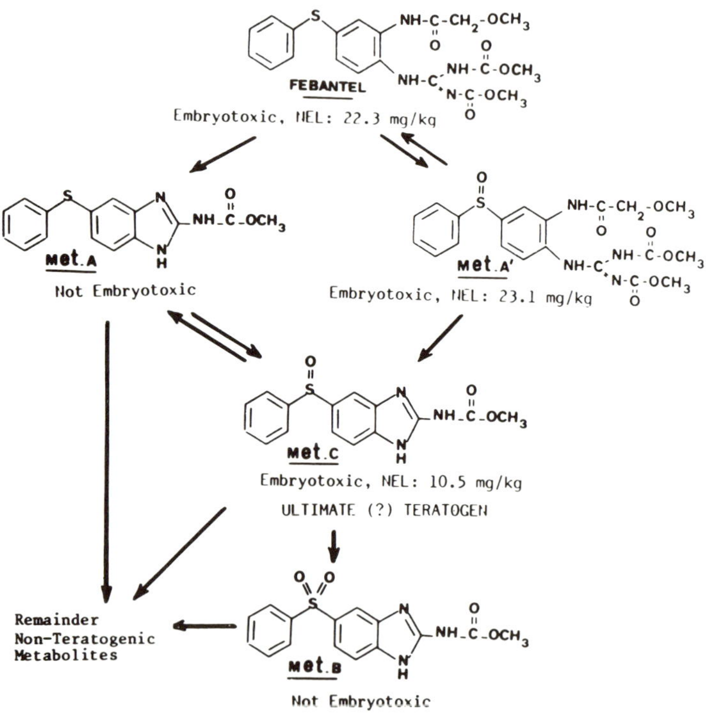

Figure 56.2 Main steps in metabolism of febantel

drug. The existence of reversible (double arrows) and irreversible (single arrow) enzymatic reactions enables us to suggest that in the series of ten metabolites, only four are actually or potentially toxic: parent compound plus metabolites A, A′, and C. All later derivatives which have been produced by oxidation (phenols) or hydrolysis (amines) are deprived of embryotoxicity (Table 56.2). Similar findings have been made with other anthelmintics which can be distinguised as follows:

Table 56.2 Some anthelmintics and their putative corresponding teratogenic metabolites

Parbendazole	methyl(5(1′-hydroxy,butyl)-1H, benzimidazol-2-yl) carbamate
Oxibendazole Thiabendazole	none
Albendazole	methyl(5-propylsulfinyl)-1H, benzimidazol-2-yl), carbamate
Fenbendazole Oxfendazole Febantel	methyl(5-phenylsulfinyl)-1H-benzimidazol-2-yl) carbamate
Ethyl-thiophanate	Ethyl, benzimidazol-2-yl-carbamate
Thiophanate Benomyl Carbendazim	Methyl, benzimidazol-2-yl-carbamate
Ciclobendazole	Methyl (5-cyclopropyl-carbonyl)-1H-benzimiazol-2-yl, carbamate and/or Methyl (5-cyclopropylhydroxymethyl)-1H-benzimidazol-2-yl, carbamate
Oncodazole	Methyl (5-(2-thenoyl)-1H-benzimidazol-2-yl) carbamate and/or Methyl(5-(2-thienylhydroxymethyl)-1H-benzimidazol-2-yl)carbamate
Mebendazole	Methyl(5-benzoyl,1H-benzimidazol-2-yl)carbamate and/or Methyl(5-phenylhydroxymethyl-1H-benzimidazol-2-yl) carbamate
Cambendazole	Unknown (not investigated)

(1) Those which are not teratogenic *per se* and have no teratogenic metabolite, e.g. oxibendazole.

(2) Those which are not teratogenic but give rise to a teratogenic metabolite, e.g. fenbendazole.

(3) Those which seem to be teratogenic *per se* but have no teratogenic metabolite, e.g. oxfendazole.

(4) Those which are possibly teratogenic *per se* and in addition have a metabolite which seems to be more toxic than the parent compound, e.g. mebendazole.

This approach is fruitful in that it provides for the identification of extractable metabolites, their synthesis, their toxicological study, the knowledge of the enzymes responsible for their appearance, and the use of enzyme inducers and inhibitors. It enables us to consider that the total extractable metabolites do not present the same toxicity as the parent compound. In addition, it can demonstrate the toxicity of some metabolites present in edible tissues whose effects had remained undetected in the animal after administration of the original compound (e.g. fenbendazole and thiophanates).

Intractable residues

Residues covalently bound to macromolecules are of great concern because of their long persistence in organs. As their accurate identification and isolation would require long and analytical methods, the literature today offers alternate imperfect indirect methods of evaluation.

Relay toxicity

The principles of this method have been described, especially by Truhaut and Ferrando[13]. It consists of spiking the standard diet of the consumer-like animal with tissues collected from the target-species that has received the drug. The possible effects of these residues are then investigated by the appropriate methodology.

To date, such trials have been directed to research such as the 90 day toxicity of TCPH residues in the sheep[23]; subacute tolerance of the duck to milk from goats fed a diet containing a high level of aflatoxin[14]; longterm tolerance to residues of natural or synthetic hormones including oestradiol, diethylstilboestrol, trenbolone; longterm tolerance of the dog (60 months) and rat 25 months, three generations) to carbadox residues[15]; and embryotoxicity of residues of cambendazole and albendazole[7]. Ferrando's DES-trail excepted, the following experiments did not demonstrate deleterious effects in spite of the well-known toxicity of the active principles: toxicity of aflatoxin B_1 in the duck, teratogenicity of cambendazole and albendazole[7] in the rat, and tumourigenicity and mutagenicity of carbadox[44]. This methodology is attractive because it experimentally reproduces the natural circumstances. Nevertheless, some criticisms have been made: (1) the safety coefficient is too low in some protocols, (2) the biological relay material often comes, for practical reasons, from a limited number of animals, and (3) the addition of the lyophillisat to a standard diet leads to an inappropriate diet. As a consequence, the authors generally mention biological variations which cannot be interpreted as residues-related or diet-related. The preparation of semi-synthetic diets attempted to avoid this problem.

Relay bioavailability

This assay tries to provide information about the intestinal absorption of residues by establishing the ratio between the absorbed and inabsorbed proportions. It requires a sophisticated method such as the one described by Gallo-Torres[16] who studied tocopherol, other sterols and triglycerides in the rat. A general review of this method has been presented by Huber *et al.*[20]. Identical studies have been performed with halofuginone, cambendazole, TCPH, and albendazole. These studies support the concept of very low availability of total residues compared to the parent drug incorporated into the diet as, for instance, is the case for albendazole (4.2% and 77.2%, respectively).

This method provides no information concerning the toxicity of the available fraction because we ignore it if the latter comes partly from free or only from bound residues. It would be of interest to perform identical feeding trials with the single intractable radioactivity previously isolated.

Target impact relay assay

Since relay toxicity often seems to lack sensitivity and relay availability provides no information about the fate of the absorbed fraction in the organism, it seems appropriate to investigate what happens to the potential target-molecules in the consumer-like animal. Some experiments have provided interesting results in this respect.

The main adduct of dimethylnitrosamine is 7-methylguanine which is found in the DNA from liver and kidney. The administration of [7-^{14}C]-methylguanine to rats showed that 95% of the total radioactivity was excreted unchanged, *N*-demethylation was responsible for incorporation of ^{14}C into intermediary metabolism and no adduct seems to be present on nucleic acids from the liver, intestine and fetus[6]. The lack of carcinogenicity of 7-methylguanine in the rat has been subsequently confirmed.

Six hours following administration ^{14}C- or ^{3}H-labelled aflatoxin B_1 to rats, a macromolecular and a conjugate fraction are found in the liver. These were then individually administered to other rats[22]; 9–12 h after dosage, no radioactivity was detected in DNA[22]. Calculations suggest that, in comparison to free aflatoxin, the ability of conjugated and macromolecular fractions to bind to DNA is at least 100 and 4000 times lower, respectively. The authors conclude that the carcinogenic risks of aflatoxin residues to humans are 'negligible'.

It is difficult to draw conclusions from the studies. There is general agreement in regard to the innocuousness of radioactivity incorporated into endogenous metabolism. Unfortunately, its quantitation is practically unrealizable; one can only hope to prove that this phenomenon has not occurred.

The investigation of individual extractable metabolites is a multidisciplinary, arduous work which can be fruitful only if some conditions have been met such as the simplicity of compounds and the possibility of screening with short-term or subacute tests. Outside these conditions, this methodology can be unrealistic. As Weiner and Newberne discussed[43], one must recall that effects observed after oral administration of a given metabolite may be different from those produced when the same compound appears spontaneously inside cells. These notions are limitations to the experimental analysis of toxicological potentials. In addition, some metabolic steps are absent in Figure 56.1. Phenols are generally turned into conjugates; however, the phenolic metabolites of benzene, bromobenzene, naphthalene and 2-2′-dichlorobiphenyl may become reactive metabolites. Aslo, all ester conjugates are not inactive forms destined for direct urinary excretion, since some are potential reactive metabolites, e.g. *N*-acetoxy-AAF, sulphate-esters of 3′-methyl-*N*, *N*-dimethyl-4-aminoazobenzene and of *N*-hydroxy-AAF, benzoyl-ester of methylaminoazobenzene and glucuronide of *N*-hydroxy-phenacetin[30].

Numerous uncertainties impede the evaluation of bound residues. We know that the main parameter for the efficacy of reactive metabolites in the organism is electrophilicity. The highly unstable reactive metabolites, with an ultra-short halflife are produced by the so-called 'suicide enzymes' and bound to the very place of their production. Those with a longer half-life are able to cause damage at locations removed from their site of production. Can the bound metabolites in animal tissues ingested by the human produce second generation reactive metabolites or, can we assume that, for thermodynamic reasons, the dangers of bound residues are definitively abolished as soon as they bind to the animal tissues? Concerning the last possibility, it would not be paradoxical to assume that the more instable, electrophilic and possibly toxic a reactive metabolite is in the target-animal, the safer it is for the human. Unfortunately, the accuracy of this 'teleological interpretation' has not been demonstrated by our present, too global, biological methods, such as relay toxicity. Probably, a better approach for the evaluation of drug residues will arise from a combination of relay-bioavailability and target impact relay assay, even if the evidence for the target molecules seems sometimes to be similar to 'searching for a needle in a haystack'. Only the future improving of our biological and analytical methods will enable us to answer these questions and to refute the famous sentence 'The analyst is creating the poison'. Yet, from now on, we can assume that it is probably exaggerated to look at bound residues *a priori* as carcinogens.

Finally, we are faced with a methodological three steps problem: the highest threshold is the one of the biological sensitivity of the methods, the intermediate one is that of analytical sensitivity, and the lowest one is the threshold of our suspicion. An accurate toxicological evaluation of drug residues in animal products will be performed only when these three thresholds are at the same level.

References

1. Baer, J. E., Jacob, T. A. and Wolf, F. J. (1977). Cambendazole and non-drug macromolecules in tissue residues. *J. Toxicol. Environ. Health*, **2**, 895–903
2. Berenbom, M. (1962). Studies on the utilisation of the carbon of *p*-dimethyl-azobenzene for rat liver nucleic acid synthesis. *Cancer Res.*, **22**, 1343–8
3. Boyd, M. R. and Burka, L. T. (1978). *In vivo* studies on the relationship between target organ alkylation and the pulmonary toxicity of a chemically reactive metabolite of 4-ipomeanol. *J. Pharmacol. Exp. Ther.*, **207**, 687–97
4. Brodie, B. B., Reid, W. D., Cho, A. K. *et al.* (1971). Possible mechanism of liver necrosis caused by aromat organic compounds. *Proc. Nat. Acad. Sci. USA*, **68**, 160–4
5. Burgat-Sacaze, V., Delatour, P. and Rico, A. (1981). Bound residues of veterinary drugs: bioavailability and toxicological implications. *Ann. Rech. Vét.*, **13**, 277–89
6. Craddock, V. M., Mattocks, A. R. and Magee, P. N. (1968). The fate of 7-(14-C)-methylguanine after administration to the rat. *Biochem. J.*, **109**, 75–8
7. Delatour, P., Parish, R. C. and Gyurik, R. J. (1981). Albendazole: a comparison of relay embryotoxicity with embryotoxicity of individual metabolites. *Ann. Rech. Vét.*, **12**, 159–67
8. Delatour, P., Lorgue, G., Lapras, M. *et al.* (1974). Propriétés embryotoxiques et résidus de trois anthelminthiques dérivés du benzimidazole. *Bull. Soc. Sci. Vet. Med. Comp. Lyon*, **76**, 147–54
9. Di Carlo, F. J., Viau, J. P. and Melgar, M. D. (1969). Incorporation of radioactivity from 14-C-nitroglycerine into rat liver glycogen, lipid, ribonucleic acid, and DNA. *Biochem. Pharmacol.*, **18**, 965–8
10. Di Cuollo, C. J., Miller, J. A., Mendelson, W. L. *et al.* (1974). Metabolic and tissue residue studies on parbendazole in sheep. *J. Agric. Food Chem.*, **22**, 948–53
11. Dorough, H. W. and Ivie, G. W. (1968). Carbon 14-C milk constituents resulting from feeding carbonyl-14-C carbamate to cows. *Science*, **159**, 732–3
12. Farber, T. M. (1980). Problems in the safety evaluation of tissue residues. *J. Environ. Pathol. Toxicol.*, **3**, 73–9

13. Ferrando, R. and Truhaut, R. (1972). La toxicité de relais. Nouvelle approche pour la méthodologie d'evaluation toxicologique des additifs aux aliments des animaux d'élevage. *C.R. Acad. Sci. Paris*, **275**, 279–83
14. Ferrando, R., Parodi, A., Henry, N. *et al.* (1977). Milk aflatoxine et toxicité de relais. *C.R. Acad. Sci. Paris*, **284**, 855–8
15. Ferrando, R., Truhaut, R., Raynaud, J. P. *et al.* (1975). La toxicité de relais. Applications de la méthodologie à l'évaluation de la sécurité d'emploi pour les consommateurs humains de carbadox. *Toxicology*, **3**, 369–98
16. Gallo-Torres, H. (1977). Methodology for the determination of bioavailability of labelled residues. *J. Toxicol. Environ. Health*, **2**, 827–45
17. Garner, R. C., Miller, E. C. and Miller, J. A. (1972). Liver microsomal metabolism of aflatoxin B1 to a reactive derivative toxic to *Salmonella typhimurium* TA530. *Cancer Res.*, **32**, 2058–66
18. Harbison, R. D. and Becker, B. A. (1974). Comparative embryotoxicity of diphenylhydantoin and some of its metabolites in mice. *Teratology*, **10**, 237–41
19. Herrett, R. J., Williams, C. W., Heotis, J. P. *et al.* (1967). Metabolism of 5-nitro-2-furaldehyde acetylhydrazone-C^{14} (Nihydrazone) in the chick. *J. Agric. Food Chem.*, **15**, 433–8
20. Huber, W. G., Becker, S. R. and Archer, B. P. (1980). Bioavailability of residues current status. *J. Environ. Pathol. Toxicol.*, **3**, 45–63
21. Hutson, D. H., Blair, D., Hoodley, E. C. *et al.* (1971). The metabolism of 14-C-Vapona in rats after administration by oral and inhalation routes. *Toxicol. Appl. Pharmacol.*, **19**, 378–9
22. Jaggi, W., Lutz, W. K., Luthy, J. *et al.* (1980). *In vivo* covalent binding of aflatoxin metabolites isolated from animal tissue to rat liver DNA. *Food Cosmet. Toxicol.*, **18**, 257–60
23. Jaglan, P. S., Glenn, M. W. and Neff, A. W. (1977). Experiences in dealing with drug-related bound residues. *J. Toxicol. Environ. Health*, **2**, 815–26
24. Jollow, D. J., Mitchell, J. R., Potter, W. Z. *et al.* (1973). Acetaminophen-induced hepatic necrosis. Role of covalent binding *in vivo*. *J. Pharmacol. Exp. Ther.*, **187**, 195–202
25. Loveless, A. (1969). Possible relevance of 0-6-alkylation of deoxyguanosine to the mutagenicity and carcinogenicity of nitrosamines and nitrosamides. *Nature (London)*, **223**, 206–7
26. Martz, F., Failinger, C. and Blake, D. A. (1977). Phenytoin teratogenesis: correlation between embryopathic effect and covalent binding of putative arene oxide metabolite in gestational tissue. *J. Pharmacol. Exp. Ther.*, **203**, 231–9
27. Milhaud, G., Pinault, L. and Bouchez, N. (1978). Résidus de cambendazole dans la viande et les abats d'animaux traités. *Rec. Méd. Vét.*, **154**, 43–7
28. Mitchell, J. R., Reid, W. D., Christie, B. *et al.* (1971). Bromobenzene-induced hepatic necrosis: species differences and protection by SKF-525A. *Res. Comm. Chem. Pathol. Pharmacol.*, **2**, 877–8
29. Morton, D. M. (1980). The toxicological evaluation of drug residues. *J. Environ. Pathol. Toxicol.*, **3**, 65–72
30. Mulder, C. J., Hinson, J. A. and Gillette, J. R. (1978). Conversion of the *N-O*-glucuronide and *N-O*-sulfate conjugates of *N*-hydroxyphenacetin to reactive intermediates. *Biochem. Pharmacol.*, **27**, 1641–50
31. Parker, C. W. (1982). Allergic reaction in man. *Pharmacol. Rev.*, **34**, 85–104
32. Parker, C. W., Shapiro, J., Kern, M. *et al.* (1962). Hypersensitivity to penicillenic acid derivatives in human with penicillin allergy. *J. Exp. Med.*, **115**, 821–38
33. Potter, W. Z., Nelson, W. L. and Thorgeirsson, S. S. (1973). Furosemide-induced hepatic necrosis. Comparison of necrosis with covalent binding of furosemide. *Fed. Proc.*, **32**, 305–7
34. Reid, W. D., Ilet, K. F., Grick, J. M. *et al.* (1973). Metabolism and binding of aromatic hydrocarbons in the lung. *Am. Rev. Resp. Dis.*, **107**, 539–51
35. Rosenblum, C., Trenner, N. R., Buhs, R. P. *et al.* (1972). Metabolism of ronidazole (1-methyl-5-nitroimidazole-yl methyl carbamate). *J. Agric. Food Chem.*, **20**, 360–71
36. Rosenblum, C., Trenner, N. R. and Wolf, D. E. (1971). The non-metabolite residue. A limitation to the tracer method. *J. Labelled Comp.*, **3**, 225–32

37. Schach von Wittenau, M. (1967). Long-term residues arising from 14-CO_2 fixation in swine tissues. *J. Sci. Food Agric.*, **18,** 608–9
38. Swenson, D. H., Miller, E. C. and Miller, J. A. (1974). Aflatoxin B1-2,3-oxide: evidence for its formation in rat liver *in vivo* and by human liver microsomes *in vitro*. *Biochem. Biophys. Res. Comm.*, **60,** 1036–43
39. Swick, R. W., Buchanan, D. L. and Nako, A. (1953). The normal content of fixed carbon in amino acids. *J. Biol. Chem.*, **203,** 55–61
40. Tennent, D. M. and Ray, W. H. (1963). Urinary metabolites of furazolidone. *Fed. Proc.*, **22,** 367–8
41. Wahl, J. M., Bories, C., Mamas, S. *et al.* (1975). RIA of penicilloyl groups in biological fluids. *FEBS Letters*, **57,** 1
42. Wolf, D. E., Van den Heuvel, W. J. A., Tyler, J. R. *et al.* (1980). Identification of a glutathione conjugate of cambendazole formed in the presence of liver microsomes. *Drug Met. Disp.*, **8,** 131–8
43. Weiner, M. and Newberne, J. W. (1977). Drug metabolites in the toxicologic evaluation of drug safety. *Toxicol. Appl. Pharmacol.*, **41,** 231–2
44. Yoshimura, H., Nakamura, M., Koeda, T. *et al.* (1981). Mutagenicities of carbadox and olaquindox, growth promoters for pigs. *Mut. Res.*, **90,** 49–55
45. Zampaglione, N., Jollow, D. J. and Mitchell, J. R. (1973). Role of detoxifying enzymes in bromobenzene-induced liver necrosis. *J. Pharmacol. Exp. Ther.*, **187,** 218–27

57
Photosensitization in ruminants: porphyrins and phylloerythrin

B. J. Blaauboer and M. van Graft

INTRODUCTION

Dermatitis in animals is often caused by the action of a phototoxic compound. The parts of the skin that are more exposed to light are affected especially (in sheep the head and the ears; in cattle the eyes, the udder and white or lightly pigmented areas of the skin). Many compounds have the ability to produce photosensitivity in animals, i.e. the condition in which animals become hypersensitive to light owing to the presence of a phototoxic compound in the peripheral circulation[7]. A distinction can be made between phototoxic and photoallergic activity. In the latter case the immune system is involved: light may promote a photochemical reaction with resultant formation of an antigen[2].

Phototoxicity *per se* can be defined as the process by which chemicals are toxic in the presence of light. The action spectrum for most photosensitivity reactions is generally in the long-wave UV range (320–420 nm). This allows distinction between phototoxicity and sunburn; the latter condition is a normal reaction of unprotected skin when exposed to excess sunlight. Here UV light of wavelengths shorter than 320 nm is involved.

COMPOUNDS INVOLVED IN PHOTOTOXICITY

Phototoxic compounds usually have a low molecular weight (200–500 dalton) and have a planar, tricyclic or polycyclic configuration with resonating structure; most of them are fluorescent. Many of these compounds are of vegetable origin[7] but some drugs and industrial chemicals are included as well. Phototoxicants from vegetable origin with identified structures are: hypericin (from *Hypericum* spp.), fagopyrin (from *Fagopyrum esculentum* (buckwheat)) and furocoumarins (psoralens) (from several plants in the Umbelliferae and Graminae families). Among drugs and industrial chemicals

Table 57.1 Compounds known to produce photosensitivity

A. Primary phototoxicity	
Drugs and industrial compounds	
some sulphonamides	
tetracyclins	
phenothiazines	
compounds in coal tars	
Of vegetable origin	
phylloerythrin	from all chlorophyll-containing plant parts
hypericin	from *Hypericum* spp. (e.g. St. John's Wort)
furocoumarins (psoralens)	from many plants (Umbelliferae, Graminae)
Porphyrins	
protoporphyrin	from endogenous haem synthesis
B. Secondary phototoxicity	
Compounds causing phylloerythrin accumulation due to liver damage	
icterogenin	
deoxiicterogenin	from many plants
(and probably other terpenes)	
sporidesmin	from the mould *Pithomyces chartarum* (saprophytic on *Lolium perenne*)
Porphyrogenic chemicals	
e.g. lead compounds?	
griseofulvin	
hexabromebenzene	
polychlorobiphenyls	

with a phototoxic action are: some sulphonamides, tetracyclins, phenothiazine and derivatives, hydroquinone, some polycyclic hydrocarbons in coal tars, etc. (Table 57.1).

Of special interest is a group of compounds with a porphyrin-like structure. Porphyrins are intermediates of haem synthesis or products of side-reactions in this process[19]. Another compound in this group is phylloerythrin. This is a breakdown product of chlorophyll, formed by microbes in the

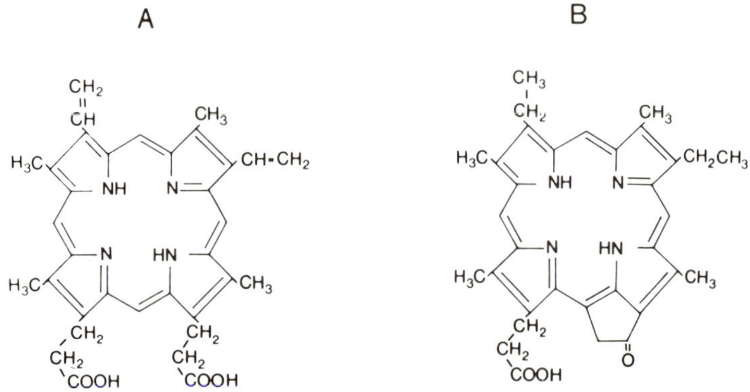

Figure 57.1 Structure of protoporphyrin (A) and phylloerythrin (B)

intestine. In ruminants, especially, considerable amounts of phylloerythrin are formed by protozoa in the rumen. Some of the phylloerythrin is normally absorbed and subsequently excreted by the liver[6] (Figure 57.1).

CLASSIFICATION

According to Clare[6], phototoxicity may be classified as congenital, primary or secondary.

Congenital photoxicity

In congenital phototoxicity, porphyrins (uro-, copro- and/or protoporphyrin) accumulate in the organism due to disturbances in the haem synthesis. Several forms of porphyria exist, some of them resulting in photodermatitis. These congential porphyrias are known in man as well as in the cat, the swine and in cattle and seems to be a 'normal' condition in the fox squirrel. Whether porphyria is accompanied by phototoxicity depends on the presence of higher concentrations of porphyrins in the skin.

Primary phototoxicity

In primary phototoxicity uptake of a compound directly responsible for the phototoxic reaction has occurred. Ingestion of hypericin (hexahydroxy-2,2-dimethylnaphthodianthrone), present in *Hypericum* spp. (e.g. St. John's Wort) is well known to result in phototoxicity. Buckwheat (*Fagopyrum esculentum*) contains fagopyrin, a phototoxicant with similar action and structure[6]. Other examples in this class are phenothiazines (where the sulphoxide metabolites cause the phototoxic reaction), furocoumarins (psoralens), tetracyclins, some sulphonamides and a number of polycyclic aromatic hydrocarbons like anthracene and acridine[8].

Secondary phototoxicity

Secondary phototoxicity is the condition in which a phototoxic compound accumulates due to the disturbance of its excretion. There appear to be many compounds giving liver damage and/or bile duct obstruction resulting in accumulation of phylloerythrin. This condition is commonly known as 'Geeldikkop' or Yellow Thick Head in sheep but is also known to occur in cattle. Structures responsible for this liver dysfunctioning are identified as icterogen, deoxyicterogen and related terpenes (Figure 57.2). These terpenes are present in many plants belonging to different families. High concentrations of hepatotoxic terpenes are present in *Tribulus terrestris*, *Lippia rehmanni* and *Lantana camara*. However, many other species are able to induce a similar condition. Toxicity of the plants is dependent on growing conditions and this results in the occurrence of intoxications in

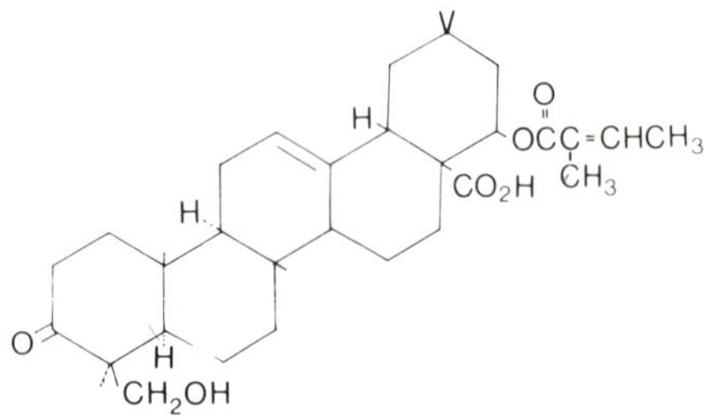

Figure 57.2 Structure of icterogen

certain regions or periods of the year. Another hepatotoxin causing phylloerythrin accumulation is sporidesmin, a product of the mould *Pithomyces chartarum* that lives saprophytically on roots of *Lolium perenne* pastures. Other mycotoxins with similar action are produced by moulds growing on rotting grass after it has been frosted or flooded.

Porphyrinogenic compounds (e.g. lead-containing compounds, hexachlorobenzene, polyhalogenated biphenyls, griseofulvin) may lead to accumulation of porphyrins in the skin and thus may be considered as secondary phototoxic. In some cases this is a result of liver damage and obstructed bile flow due to excessive (proto-)porphyrin production in the liver. As a result, porphyrins are not excreted by the liver, will reach the skin and thus cause phototoxicity. If this condition occurs in ruminants, it may also result in phylloerythrin accumulation. Some porphyrinogenic compounds (e.g. lead) do not impair liver function but disturb the erythropoietic system. As a result, porphyrins reach the circulation in red blood cells[19].

MECHANISMS OF ACTION OF PHOTOTOXIC COMPOUNDS

In all phototoxic reactions the first step is a change of transition state of the phototoxicant caused by light. This may result in a highly reactive intermediate which is able to bind to a cellular constituent (DNA, proteins, etc.). This type of reaction mechanism is involved in photoallergy and probably in the case of psoralens.

However, the majority of phototoxic reactions require oxygen. This type of reaction is referred to as photodynamic[8]. Here, energy absorbed by the phototoxic compound is transferred to molecular oxygen, resulting in singlet oxygen ($'O_2$) and superoxide anion ($O_2^{\cdot-}$) as shown in Figure 57.3A(a). They also may be produced by reactions between the different species of oxygen radicals (Figure 57.3A(b, c, d))[13]. The fate of $O_2^{\cdot-}$ in aqueous solutions will be the dismutation reaction. This process may be represented by the next overall equation (Figure 57.3A(b))

$$2\,O_2^{\cdot-} + 2H^+ \rightarrow H_2O_2 + O_2 \qquad \text{I}$$

Nevertheless, the spontaneous dismutation of superoxide radicals will be slow in biological systems as it needs acidic pH values. As a result, $O_2^{\cdot-}$

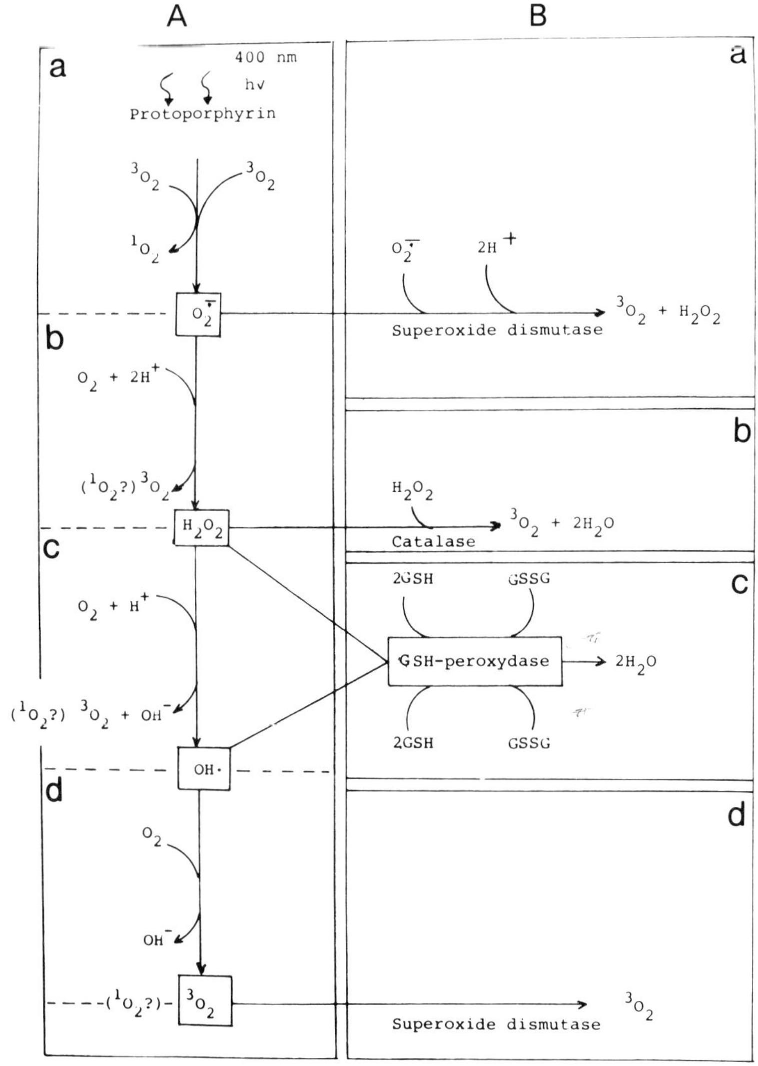

Figure 57.3 Scheme of the formation of different species of active oxygen after irradiation of protoporphyrin (A) and the relationship with the 'natural scavengers' (B)

radicals produced *in vivo* will have a significant lifetime, which allows them to diffuse away from their site of formation. In comparison with other active oxygen species, $O_2^{\overline{\cdot}}$ is a poorly reactive species. Deleterious effects which occur *in vivo* will be the result of other active species of oxygen like singlet oxygen or the hydroxyl radical (.OH). The formation of the hydroxyl radical may be the result of the reaction of H_2O_2 (formed in Equation (I)) and $O_2^{\overline{\cdot}}$ (Figure 57.3A(c)). However, traces of iron, either in complexed form or as iron salts, would be necessary for this reaction[12]:

$$Fe^{3+}-\text{chelate} + O_2^{\cdot -} \rightarrow Fe^{2+}-\text{chelate} + O_2 \qquad \text{II}$$

$$Fe^{2+}-\text{chelate} + H_2O_2 \rightarrow Fe^{3+}-\text{chelate} + .OH + OH^- \qquad \text{III}$$

$$\text{Net:} \quad H_2O_2 + O_2^{\cdot -} \rightarrow .OH + OH^- + O_2 \qquad \text{IV}$$

Equations III and IV are often referred to as the Fenton-type reaction and the Haber–Weiss reaction (Figure 57.3A(c)) respectively. Reports concerning the involvement of singlet oxygen in oxygen toxicity are confusing because of the lack of (a) specific scavenger(s) of this excited oxygen molecule. There is some evidence that part of the oxygen produced in the dismutation of $O_2^{\cdot -}$ (Equation I) will be in the singlet state[11]. Recently, Singh *et al.*[16] have described a method for the discrimination between $'O_2$, $O_2^{\cdot -}$ and .OH *in vitro* and *in vivo*, by using tryptophan as monitor. This system probably can elucidate the involvement of $'O_2$ in biochemical systems. In the last step in Figure 57.3A(d) singlet oxygen is generated by electron transfer from $O_2^{\cdot -}$ to .OH, as is suggested by Arneson[1]. In Figure 57.3B a scheme is given for mechanisms known to detoxify active oxygen species in biological systems. These mechanisms have the ability to act as 'natural scavengers'. Superoxide dismutase (SOD)[14] (Figure 57.3B(a)) detoxifies the superoxide anion to give oxygen and hydrogen peroxide (H_2O_2). In eukaryotic cells, different forms of this metalloprotein exist. The cytoplasmic SOD contains Cu/Zn ions, whereas the mitochondrial form is a Mn^{2+}-containing enzyme. Finally, the nucleus contains SOD, distinct from the cytoplasmic form (for a review, see ref. 9). SOD is inhibited by the end-product of the dismutation reaction: hydrogen peroxide. So, for an active dismutation-reaction, a second 'natural scavenger', the enzyme catalase, is of great importance in protecting cells against oxygen radicals. Catalase detoxifies H_2O_2 by oxidizing it to H_2O (Figure 57.3B(b)). H_2O_2 can also be decomposed by glutathione peroxidase, by using reduced glutathione as a cofactor (Figure 57.3B(c)). The oxidized glutathione is reduced by reaction with $NADPH + H^+$ catalysed by glutathione reductase. The detoxification of .OH-radicals by the glutathione system is hypothetic. Beside these enzymatic detoxifying mechanisms (or in other words, protective mechanisms against active oxygen species), cells and micro-organisms contain other compounds known to act as scavengers, e.g. β-carotene/vitamin A, ascorbic acid, mannitol, α-tocopherol, transferrin, caeruloplasmin and selenium.

PHOTOTOXICITY OF PROTOPORPHYRIN

There is some evidence that the photodynamic properties of porphyrins are the result of the photosensitized production of active oxygen species. In EPR studies, Cannistraro *et al.*[5] showed, for porphyrins with different side-chains after irradiation in ethanolic solutions, their ability to generate singlet oxygen with haematoporphyrin as the most effective singlet oxygen generator. In the haematoporphyrin-5,5-dimethyl pyrroline-1-oxide spin trapping system, Buettner and Oberley[4] observed the production of superoxide ions after irradiation in aqueous solutions, eventually resulting in hydroxyl radical formation. Although there is no direct evidence for protoporphyrin and phylloerythrin to form oxygen radicals, the similarity in structure with haematoporphyrin suggests a similarity in photodynamic action, i.e. by active oxygen species. Active species of oxygen are responsible for several *in vitro* damaging effects. The most studied effect is lipid peroxidation[11], but other effects are known as well, for instance oxidation/denaturation of proteins, degradation of biological important molecules (tryptophan, riboflavine), degradation/depolymerization of DNA, hydroxylation of aromatic substances, and depolymerization of polysaccharides[18]. Lipid peroxidation can be detected in several ways: by measuring diene conjugation[3], malondialdehyde, alkanes (ethane, pentane), chemiluminescence and fluorescence products[17]. In studies with hepatocytes, either incubated in a protoporphyrin solution or loaded with porphyrins by addition of δ-aminolevulinic acid to the culture medium, we could not detect malondialdehyde production or diene conjugation at protoporphyrin concentrations responsible for membrane damage. However, both degradation products of polyunsaturated fatty acids may be metabolized by the hepatocytes. Thus, lipid peroxidation cannot be ruled out as a phototoxic action of protoporphyrin. In studies with human foreskin fibroblasts cultured in a medium containing protoporphyrin, only traces of oxidized unsaturated fatty acids were found[15]. In studies with erythrocyte ghosts incubated with a relatively high protoporphyrin concentration, a remarkable lipid peroxidation was found. At low protoporphyrin concentrations, it was shown that lipid peroxidation was preceded by cross-linking of membrane proteins[10].

In our studies with primary cultures of hepatocytes incubated with protoporphyrin, we found membrane damage after irradiation which was measured by LDH-leakage into the culture medium. It was observed by varying the incubation conditions that only protoporphyrin absorbed in or at the cell membrane was responsible for the damaging effect. The damaging effect of protoporphyrin to hepatocytes increased with increasing culturing time of the primary cultures, which could be the result of loss(es) in the protecting mechanism(s) against active oxygen species.

Preliminary results suggesting this showed diminishing glutathione (reduced form) levels within hepatocytes incubated with protoporphyrin within 15 min after irradiation.

PHOTOHAEMOLYTIC ACTION OF PHYLLOERYTHRIN *IN VITRO*

In order to study the mechanism of phototoxic action of phylloerythrin, we measured the haemolysis of goat red blood cells caused by phylloerythrin after UV irradiation. Phylloerythrin was isolated from sheep faeces by ether extraction, followed by methylation of the carboxyl group and recrystallization from methanol–chloroform (3/1, v/v). Before use the ester was hydrolyzed and free phylloerythrin was dissolved in ethanol and added to washed goat erythrocytes (maximum ethanol concentration 5%).

Incubation with red cells was performed in tubes placed nearly horizontally in a rotating rack under an UV light source with a maximum emission between 360 and 390 nm. Haemolysis was determined by centrifuging a sample and measuring the haemoglobin concentration in the supernatant spectrophotometrically at 540 nm.

A typical result is shown in Figure 57.4. After a lag phase, the length of which is dependent on the phylloerythrin concentration, the haemolysis proceeds quickly. From these results the time needed to reach 50% haemolysis (HT_{50}) can be calculated (Figure 57.5), showing a linear relationship between the HT_{50} and the logarithm of the phylloerythrin concentration over the range 5–20 μmol/l. Addition of 11 mmol/l glucose resulted in inhibition of haemolysis. Dark controls never showed any haemolysis.

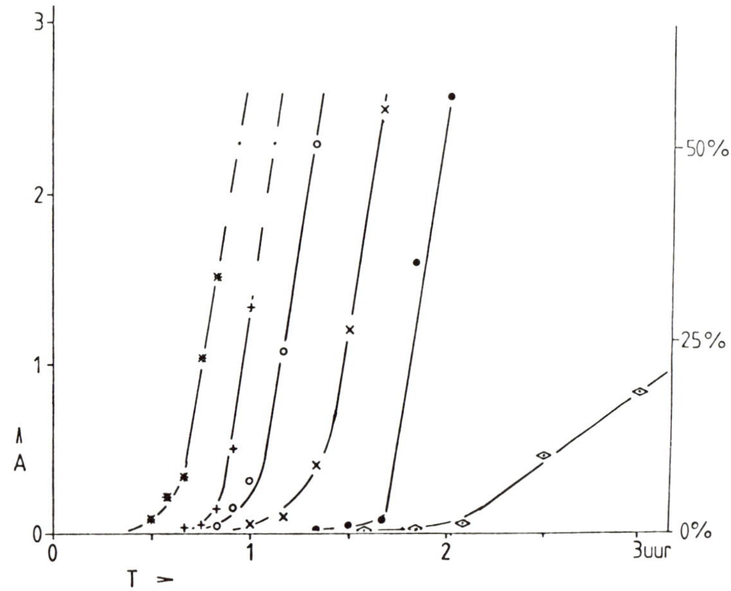

Figure 57.4 Effect of different concentrations of phylloerythrin on haemolysis after irradiation: ◇ = 2.7 μmol/l PE; • = 5.4 μmol/l PE; × = 8.1 μmol/l PE; ○ = 10.8 μmol/l PE; + = 13.5 μmol/l PE; * = 16.2 μmol/l PE

These results are compatible with the hypothesis that phylloerythrin causes membrane damage in red blood cells by producing radical intermediates after irradiation. The cells are able to defend themselves against these radicals only to a certain point, after which the haemolysis proceeds rapidly. This is reflected by the relationship between phylloerythrin concentration and the lag time, implicating a role for a natural radical scavenger within the cells with a finite capacity (e.g. catalase, superoxide dismutase). Preliminary results with the oxygen radical scavengers tiron and β-carotene suggest the involvement of singlet oxygen[19]. Further experiments will be carried out to elucidate the role of oxygen radicals in the mechanism.

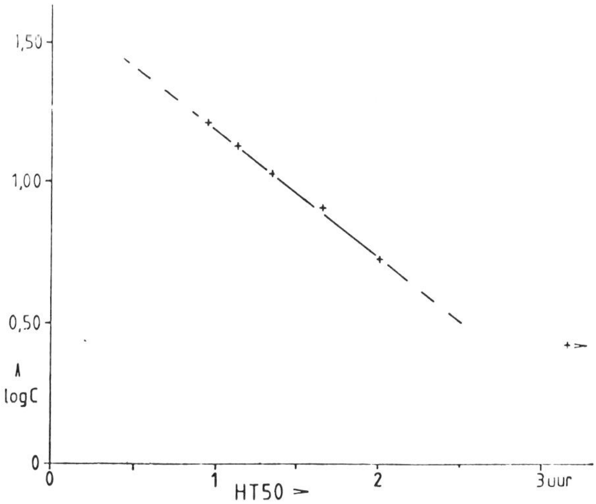

Figure 57.5 Relationship between phylloerythrin concentration and the time needed for 50% haemolysis (HT_{50})

CONCLUSION

Photosensitization in ruminants is brought on by various phototoxic compounds reaching the skin in distinct ways.

In primary phototoxicity phototoxic compounds (drugs, food additives, food components) reach the skin by a direct uptake from the food or drug into the bloodflow.

In congenital phototoxicity or secondary phototoxicity, phototoxic compounds mainly accumulate in the liver followed by an overflowing into the blood.

Many causes of the processes which lead to photosensitization are elucidated. However, the mechanisms of action of phototoxic compounds have yet to be elucidated. In many *in vitro* studies with phototoxic compounds evidence has been found that oxygen radicals play an important role.

References

1. Arneson, R. M. (1970). Substrate-induced chemiluminescence of xanthine oxidase and aldehyde oxidase. *Arch. Biochem. Biophys.*, **136**, 352–60
2. Bauer, R. L. and Bickers, D. R. (1981). Allergic contact dermatitis, photoallergic contact dermatitis and phototoxic dermatitis. *Compr. Immunol. (Immunoderm.)*, **7**, 259–71
3. Buege, J. A. and Aust, S. D. (1978). Microsomal lipid peroxidation. *Meth. Enzymol.*, **52**, 302–10
4. Buettner, G. R. and Oberley, L. W. (1980). The apparent production of superoxide and hydroxyl radicals by hematoporphyrin and light as seen by spin-trapping. *FEBS Letters*, **121**, 161–4
5. Cannistraro, S., van de Vorst, A. and Jori, G. (1978). EPR studies on singlet oxygen production by porphyrins. *Photochem. Photobiol.*, **28**, 257–9

6. Clare, N. T. (1952). *Photosensitization in Domestic Animals.* (Farnham Royal: Commonwealth Agricultural Bureaux)
7. Clarke, M. L., Harvey, D. G. and Humphreys, D. J. (1981). *Veterinary Toxicology.* pp. 191–2. (London: Ballière Tindall)
8. Emmett, E. A. (1979). Phototoxicity from exogenous agents. *Photochem. Photobiol.*, **30,** 429–36
9. Fridovich, I. (1974). Superoxide dismutases. *Adv. Enzymol.*, **41,** 35–97
10. Girotti, A. W. (1979). Protoporphyrin-sensitized photodamage in isolated membranes of human erythrocytes. *Biochemistry,* **18,** 4403–11
11. Halliwell, B. (1979). Oxygen-free-radicals in living systems: dangerous but useful? In Shilo, M. (ed.) *Strategies of Microbial Life in Extreme Environments.* pp. 195–221. (Berlin: Verlag Chemie)
12. Halliwell, B. (1981). The biological effects of the superoxide radical and its products. *Clin. Resp. Physiol.*, **17** (Suppl.), 21–8
13. Krinsky, N. I. (1977). Singlet oxygen in biological systems. *Trends Biol. Sci.*, **2,** 35–8
14. McCord, J. M. and Fridovich, I. (1969). Superoxide dismutase. *J. Biol. Chem.*, **244,** 6049–55
15. Schothorst, A. A., De Haas, C. A. C. and Suurmond, D. (1980). Photochemical damage to skin fibroblasts caused by protoporphyrin and violet light. *Arch. Dermatol. Res.*, **268,** 31–42
16. Singh, A., Singh, H., Kremers, W. *et al.* (1981). Involvement of singlet oxygen in biological systems. *Clin. Resp. Physiol.*, **17** (Suppl.), 31–41
17. Smith, M. T., Thor, H., Hartzell, P. *et al.* (1982). The measurement of lipid peroxidation in isolated hepatocytes. *Biochem. Pharmacol.*, **31,** 19–26
18. Spikes, J. D. (1977). Photosensitization. In Smith, K. C. (ed.) *The Science of Photobiology.* pp. 87–112. (London and New York: Plenum Press)
19. Woutersen, R. A. and Wit, J. G. (1980). Experimental protoporphyria in hairless mice: an animal model for photochemically induced dermatitis. *Vet. Res. Commun.*, **4,** 183–94

58
Fluorosis in the sheep: new data

G. Milhaud, B. Enriquez and F. Rivière

INTRODUCTION

In 1932, it was shown that the Darmous, that affected sheep in phosphate-rich areas in Morocco, is spontaneous fluorosis. Dental lesions and other clinical signs of the affection have been described[19]. The main source is fodder (hay, straw, barley), whereas water plays only a secondary role. A discrepancy, existing between the periods of ingestion of fluoride and the appearance of lesions on the incisors, has led to an experiment to study the relation between these phenomena[20]. Several experimental studies have been conducted in cattle[2, 15, 16, 18] and fewer experiments in sheep.

With 8–12 months old sheep receiving a concentrate mixture containing 25, 50, 75, 100 or 200 parts/10^6 fluorine over a period of 140 days, the growth rate is significantly reduced only in the animals receiving 200 parts/10^6 fluorine. With animals of the same age receiving up to 100 parts/10^6 fluorine over a period of 3 years, the weights of ewes and their lambs have been normal[3].

For 3½ years sodium fluoride was added to the drinking water, at 0, 2.5, 5, 10, and 20 parts/10^6, of merino sheep aged 13–14 months at the beginning of the experiment. Consumption varied greatly with the seasons. With the highest dosing, the fluorine ingestion was from 0.66 mg kg^{-1} day^{-1} during the winter to 1.45 mg kg^{-1} day^{-1} during the summer months[11]. Adult sheep aged from 2½ to 3½ years receiving water containing 10 or 20 parts/10^6 fluorine consumed less water than the previous sheep with fluorine ingestion (estimated) at 0.1 mg kg^{-1} day^{-1} during winter and 0.8 mg kg^{-1} day^{-1} during summer[12]. Lambs from treated mothers, when given water containing 0.3, 10 or 20 parts/10^6 fluorine have ingested (estimated) 0.3–0.8 mg kg^{-1} day^{-1} with the water at 10 parts/10^6 and 0.5–1.6 mg kg^{-1} day^{-1} with the water at[13] 20 parts/10^6.

Dental lesions have appeared in the young sheep with the highest fluorine intake[11, 13]. In the yearlings, the third and the fourth incisors are mostly affected[11], whereas the first incisors are most affected in the lambs[13].

Effects on growth rate are very slight, since only in the yearlings has weight decreased slightly prior to the third shearing. Reproduction is normal. Wool production is slightly reduced in the lambs receiving the water containing 20 parts/10^6 fluorine.

During 14 weeks, a fattening ration was given to lambs of about 32.3 kg and contributed 0.48, 0.62, 1.10, 2.05, and 3.90 mg of fluorine/body weight. Feed consumption, gain in weight, carcass weight and grade and wool weight have remained normal[1].

Experiments on 9 month old wethers given water containing 30 parts/10^6 fluorine during 25 months have resulted in adverse effects on growth after 32 weeks and sings of fluorosis after 72 weeks[14]. This paper briefly reviews the main results obtained in experiments conducted on fluorosis in goat and adult sheep.

FLUOROSIS IN GOAT

Experiments were conducted on three groups of four goats aged from 7 to 8 months, during 1, 2, and 3 years. Each lot contained one control and three animals receiving 2.5 mg kg^{-1} day^{-1} fluorine as sodium fluoride, orally in 10 ml water. Fluorine in the daily intake of feed ranged from 0.3 to 0.75 mg kg^{-1} day^{-1}. Weight variations were not observed, the average weight of controls remaining higher than that of the treated animals[9].

The mean plasma fluorine was 0.85 mg/l in the dosed goats and 0.15 mg/l in the controls. Animals with values above average (+35%) always had the most acute signs of fluorosis. Others, with low fluorine (−35%) had very slight dental lesions.

One of the treated goats (2 y group) died of chronic peritonitis after only 14 months in the experiment. Serious locomotion troubles occurred in a goat during the third year, following a traumatic dislocation of L4–L5 lumbar vertebrae.

The goats, mated every year, had normal fecondity, and number of gemellar gestations. Weight of kids were normal and similar at birth, but slightly lower in the treated group after 2 months.

Characteristic lesions of fluorosis occurred at the base of the first incisors (six out of nine) (pitting; rough, chalky enamel), on the other incisors (five out of six), and molars after 18 months of administration of fluorine. After 3 y, the irregularities of wear were marked and symmetrical and sometimes several lobes were eroded. One of the treated goats exhibited an osteitis of the mandible due to the presence of hay between the teeth and the gums.

On X-rays and postmortem examinations, the presence of pseudoarthrosis and bone exostoses on the ribs were clearly visible in five treated goats. The rather heavy and strong males used for mating were probably responsible for such lesions. On X-ray examination no other major change was noticed. Most treated animals showed a more irregular and slighter opacification of limb extremities and of mandibles. Two animals showed a thinning of metacarpal- and metatarsal–phalangeal joint spaces[10]. A scintigraphic examination with [^{99}technetium m]pyrophosphate on all goats failed to show inflammatory lesions of bones and joints, and abnormal remodelling of bone tissue.

Histological, haematological and biochemical results were normal.

Fluorine concentrations were measured in bones, teeth, and tissues. Levels were high initially in the mandibles and the ribs, but values were very similar after 2 and 3 y of treatment (Table 58.1). The teeth erupting during fluorine ingestion (adult corners, 2nd and 3rd molars) were richer in this element (5000–6000 parts/10^6). Teeth already present got impregnated too (lacteal incisors, premolars, first molar), together with premolars and first molar (3000–4000 parts/10^6) which go on developing and evolving long after their eruption. Fluorine levels were below 0.5 parts/10^6 in muscle, liver and milk, but higher in kidneys (2.6 parts/10^6) and brain (7.9 parts/10^6).

Table 58.1 Fluorine levels (p.p.m./fat free dry matter) in goat bone samples

		Mandible	*Ribs*	*Coxal*	*Metatarsus*	*Metacarpus*
Treated	1 year	4 600 ± 610	3 050 ± 790	2 680 ± 220	2 110 ± 180	2 500 ± 550
	2 years	6 860 ± 900	6 320 ± 200	5 520 ± 370	4 870 ± 80	5 210 ± 450
	3 years	6 610 ± 860	5 840 ± 1 400	4 990 ± 300	4 400 ± 450	4 700 ± 160
Controls	1 year	750	650	540	660	680
	2 years	1 580	1 410	1 090	1 600	1 660
	3 years	1 750	1 370	1 210	1 240	1 310

FLUOROSIS IN ADULT SHEEP

Sheep coming from a polluted area were used in experiments and to record signs of fluorosis.

The experimental design was meant to determine with accuracy the effects of fluorine in relation to the period of life when it is ingested. The experiment is still under way, and the final results are to be published. It can be noted already that dental lesions are less marked than those obtained in cattle[17] with a similar experimental procedure.

Observations were made, during 6 consecutive years from 1977 to 1982, on over 300 animals, coming from a valley where an aluminium plant is located. The first observations were meant to give a good knowledge of the chronic effects of fluorosis in that area and to interpret them in the light of the results of fluorine analyses in the plasma, the mandible and the teeth. These first observations concerning the animals reared in the vicinity of the plant were published[8] in 1978.

Then it proved necessary to find the elements for differential diagnosis between fluorosis and suppurant osteomyelitis of the mandible which were due often to the presence of hard, rough hay between the gum and the molars. This differential diagnosis is of major interest in the vicinity of the plant and at some distance around. Yearly examinations were conducted on about 50 sheep chosen from a rather extended area around the plant. Blood samples were taken from most animals before slaughtering, postmortem examinations were carried out, and mandibles were collected for macroscopic examination and fluorine determination.

In absolute values, fluorine levels in the plasma varied greatly from group to group according to feeding and rearing conditions. In relative values, the sheep reared in the closer vicinity of the plant always had the highest levels of fluorine.

After examination, the mandibles were classified in three groups according to:

(1) Characteristic fluorosis lesions. Lesions in the most acute cases were: very uneven wear of molars, symmetrical on the two branches of the mandible, with 1–2 cm peaks and cavities resulting from the complete

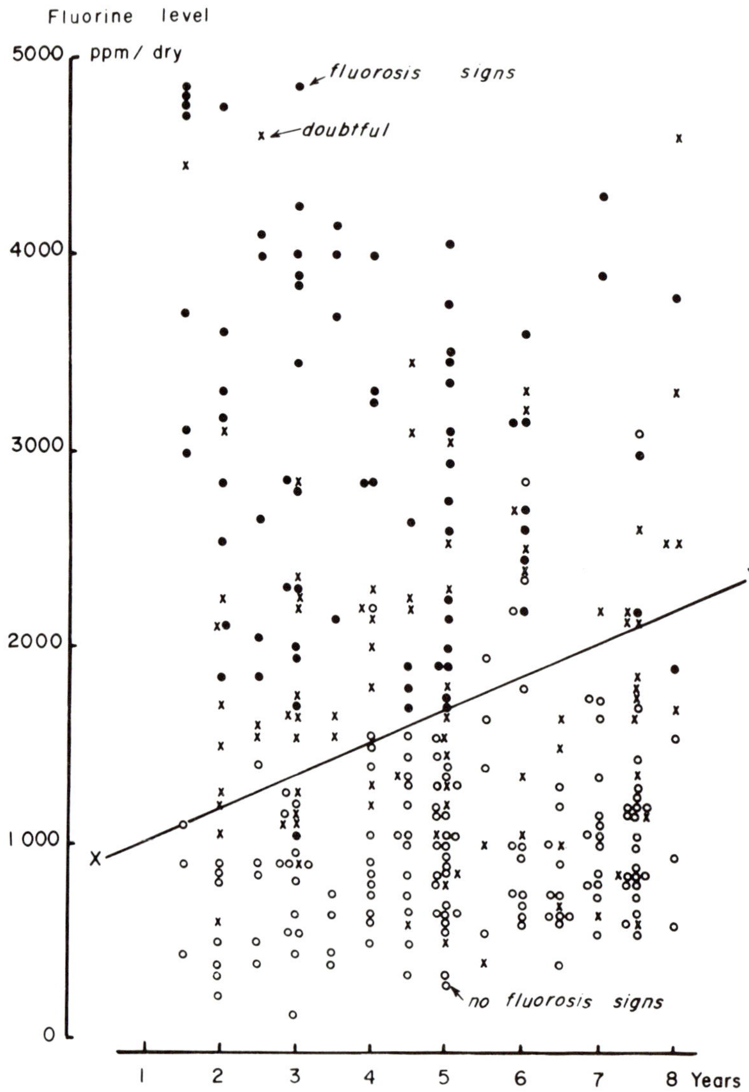

Figure 58.1 Fluorine levels in the mandible in relation to age and signs (positive: •, negative: ○, doubtful: ×)

disappearance of dental lobes. Nearly always, more lesions were accompanied by lesions of the incisors which were clearly visible only after removal of a brownish organic deposit. The enamel on the buccal face exhibited either pitting or a rough surface with cupuliform cavities. It was chalky, opaque, sometimes rough and brownish. In acute cases thickening of the mandible with exostoses were even observed (Figure 58.1). Also included in this group were mandibles which presented unilateral suppurant reaction at the level of molars, but fluorosis lesions on the other molar arcade and/or on incisors.

(2) Infectious reactions limited to the mandible. These reactions may be at different stages of evolution. Sometimes, there is only hypertrophia of one branch of the maxillar, with hay between the molars and the premolars. The latter may show more or less marked defects in wear that account for the presence of a long, eroded, and oblique surface. Loosening occurred in molars or premolars which then moved towards the buccal or jaw side. When these teeth fell, spaces on the mandibles allowed neighbouring teeth to slant forward, and teeth of the opposite dental table to grow for lack of wear.

The suppurant osteomyelitis of the maxillar causes an important hypertrophia with occasional fistulization of the external face. After the fall of one tooth or several teeth, the suppurant process receded, empty teeth-alveoles were filled, and as teeth corresponding to the empty spaces get longer, a very uneven profile of the two inferior and superior molar arcades may be established. Usually such an infectious process concerned only one side of the mandible. When bilateral, the fall of teeth and irregularities were rarely symmetrical.

This group includes sheep without any signs of fluorosis (Figure 58.1).

(3) Doubtful cases. Incisor lesions are very mild in sheep. When enamel of incisors exhibited vertical striations, and when the defects in the wear of molars could not be explained by the presence of an infectious process, it was clinically impossible to say whether the osteomyelitis reaction was complicated with fluorosis or not. Such rather numerous cases have been classified as 'doubtful' (Figure 58.1).

Out of the 330 mandibles examined, only 12 coming from young, deeply affected animals had fluorine levels ranging from 5000 to 8000 parts/10^6. They are not recorded in Figure 58.1, for easier reading. With two exceptions, the points corresponding to the mandibles with lesions characteristic of fluorosis are above a X Y axis which passes by the points corresponding to 2 y: 1200 parts/10^6; 5 y: 1700 parts/10^6; 8 y: 2200 parts/10^6. Most of the mandibles from animals free from fluorosis are below this line; only six, mainly from old animals are above the line. The points corresponding to the doubtful cases are scattered throughout the graph, rather similarly on either side of axis X Y. Thus it can be said that the axis determines two areas: the first one corresponding to animals presenting no sign of fluorosis, the second one corresponding to animals presenting signs of fluorosis. Some animals designated by the sign •, and in particular the 3 y old one located below the axis, presented very mild signs, which, at that stage, were not harmful. A diet deficient in phosphorus and vitamin D results in lesions of the molars similar to those of fluorosis[4,5]. In the present case phosphorus and calcium metabolism were not explored.

FLUOROSIS IN LAMBS

Experimental studies were conducted in sucking lambs and in lambs weaned at birth still receiving artificial feed. The results obtained with the sucking lambs have already been reported[6,7]. The investigations on the lambs weaned at birth are not over yet, but some of the results can be used for comparison.

The sucking lambs, 15 controls and 17 treated, were reared on a farm located not far from an aluminium plant but the mothers were given a feed free from fluorine contamination. The lambs weaned at birth (three groups of 28 animals) were reared on an experimental farm and fluorine was incremently given from the 3rd to 8th week, to stimulate what happens when alfafa is given to young lambs *ad libitum*.

The administration of fluorine to sucking lambs was based on an alfafa containing 150 parts/10^6 fluorine. The amount of fluorine brought by such fodder was estimated to be: 0.5 mg kg^{-1} day^{-1} in the 3rd week, 0.8 mg kg^{-1} day^{-1} in the 4th and the 5th week, 1 mg kg^{-1} day^{-1} in the 6th week, 1.5 mg kg^{-1} day^{-1} in the 7th week, and 2.5 mg kg^{-1} day^{-1} from the 8th week onwards. Fluorine, administered orally, every morning in the form of sodium fluoride, was diluted in 10 ml of water. These lambs were exclusively fed on their mothers' milk to avoid fluorine intake through the feed. They were slaughtered from the age of 13 weeks.

The lambs weaned at birth were allotted to one control group and two treated groups of 28 animals. The fluorine administration in the treated groups simulated alfafa containing 120 and 240 parts/10^6: 0.4 mg kg^{-1} day^{-1} in the 3rd week, 0.6 mg kg^{-1} day^{-1} in the 4th week, 0.7 mg kg^{-1} day^{-1} in the 7th week, 2 mg kg^{-1} day^{-1} after the 8th week for the first group and twice these amounts for the second. The diet comprised: artificial milk, mineral mixture, feed supplement, cereals and dehydrated alfafa mixture, straw and alfafa hay. This feed brought important quantities of fluorine estimated at 0.7–0.8 mg kg^{-1} day^{-1} from the 18th to the 42nd day, 1.2 mg kg^{-1} day^{-1} from the 43rd to the 66th day, 0.5 mg kg^{-1} day^{-1} from the 67th day to slaughtering, at 15 weeks.

Figure 58.2 lists fluorine levels in the plasma. The control group had levels of 0.1 mg/l. In the group of weaned lambs, the levels were higher. From a comparative analysis of the feed, greater differences were expected. The fluorine contained in the feed supplement and the mineral mixture (fluoroapatite) seemed to be hardly bioavailable.

As far as the treated animals are concerned, the evolutions of plasma levels varied greatly in the two experimental studies. In the two groups of weaned lambs, the plasma levels rose rapidly. The maxima values were reached by the 9th week; they were nearly twice higher in the group receiving 4 mg kg^{-1} day^{-1} (approx. 0.75 mg/l) than in the group receiving 2 mg kg^{-1} day^{-1}

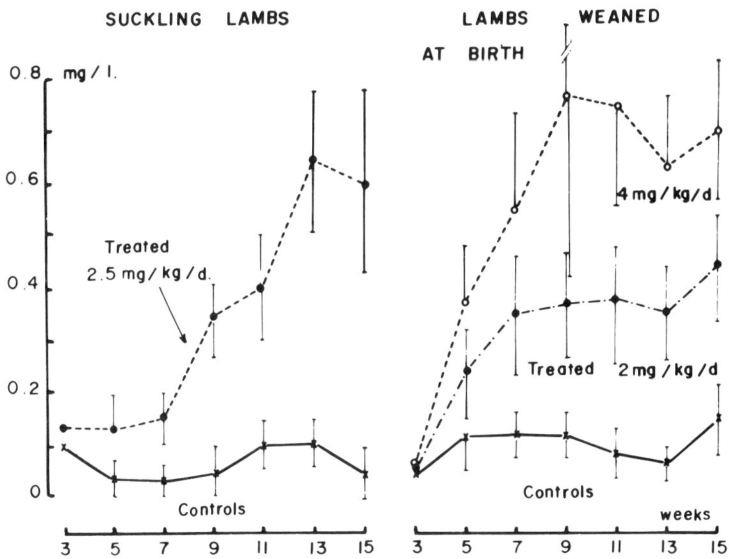

Figure 58.2 Fluorine plasma levels in suckling lambs (SL) treated and controls, and in lambs weaned at birth (WL) and treated: 2 mg/kg (●– –●) and 4 mg/kg: (○– –○)

(approx. 0.4 mg/l). In the sucking lambs, the fluorine levels in the plasma increased more slowly: maxima values, not reached before the 13th week, were high, around 0.65 mg/l.

Such differences may be partly accounted for by the different breeds: an alpine breed for sucking lambs, a more evolved breed for weaned lambs. Yet it seems that the nature of the feed played a more important role than the breed. The early withdrawal of artificial milk, the administration of dry feed (cereals and forage) that modified the flora and the pH of the digestive tract were certainly responsible for this more rapid absorption of fluorine in the form of sodium fluoride.

Figure 58.3 sets out the average body weight of the animals in relation to age. Although markedly lighter at 1 week (4.9 kg vs. 6.2) lambs weaned at birth reached, at 15 weeks, a body weight notably heavier than sucking ones (28.3 kg vs. 24.2). Throughout the experiment, the mean body weight of the control group remained higher than that of the treated group.

In the lambs weaned at birth the growth curves could practically be superimposed. The surprising drop recorded at week 6 corresponds to withdrawal of artificial milk. Considering previous performances, the first dose administered, with a maximum of 2.5 mg kg^{-1} day^{-1}, was close and perhaps slightly higher than the no-effect level on growth. For this was the reason, in the second experiment, that maxima doses of 2 and 4 mg kg^{-1} day^{-1} were chosen hoping for no effect with 2 mg kg^{-1} day^{-1} and a marked effect with 4 mg kg^{-1} day^{-1}. In spite of the differences between plasma concentration, no effect on growth is obvious during the first 15 weeks of life.

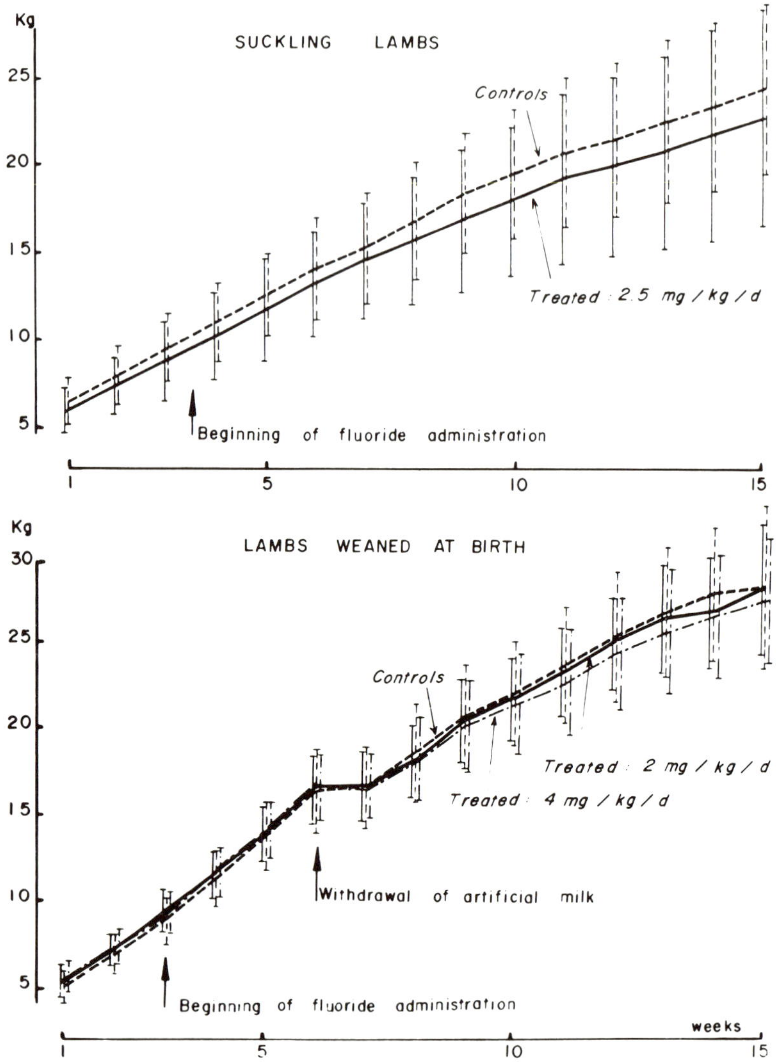

Figure 58.3 Average body weight of the animals in relation to age

Finally, it is interesting to compare fluorine concentrations in the mandible as expressed in parts/10^6 of fat free dry matter (Figure 58.4).

Fluorine concentrations in the mandible of controls weaned at birth were markedly higher than those in controls fed their mother' milk. In the treated sucking animals fluorine concentrations in the mandible were higher than in the animals weaned at birth.

For all the groups, the range of fluorine levels in the mandible was within limits comparable to plasma fluorine concentrations at week 15.

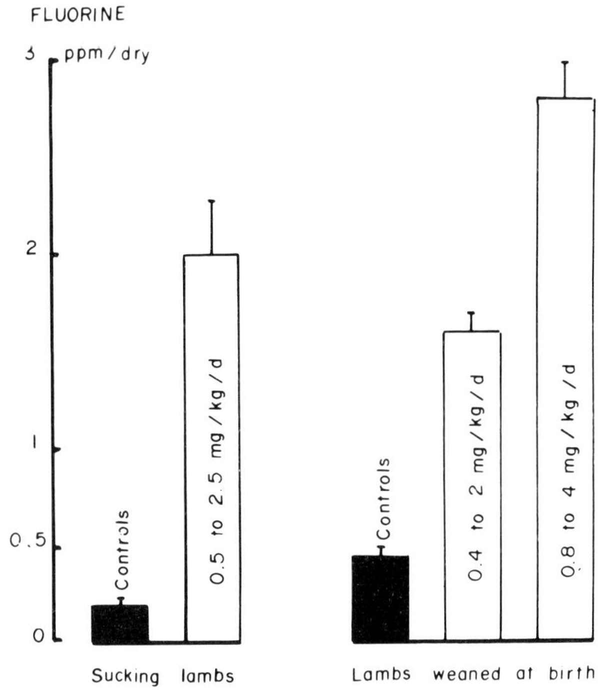

Figure 58.4 Fluorine mandible levels in suckling lambs and in lambs weaned at birth

CONCLUSION

The results obtained provide rather precise information as to the risks that small ruminants run at various ages.

Goat sensitivity to fluorine was quite comparable to that of sheep. Fluorine concentrations in plasma, bones, and anatomoclinical signs were identical. On the basis of these three parameters, a diagnosis of fluorosis may always be made, and fluorosis may be clearly distinguished from any infectious process of the maxillar.

Lamb proved comparatively resistant to fluorine. Doses rising steadily up to 4 mg kg^{-1} day^{-1} from the 3rd to the 8th week, followed by a dose of 4 mg kg^{-1} day^{-1} from the 8th to the 15th week, had no effect on growth rate in spite of high plasma fluorine levels and fast accumulation of fluorine in bones.

Yet, it remains obvious that further administration of such doses of fluorine would result in severe fluorosis before the eruption of all the permanent teeth.

References

1. Harris, L. E., Madsen, M. A., Greenwood, D. A. *et al.* (1958). Effect of various levels and sources of fluorine in the fattening ration of Columbia, Rambouillet and Targhee lambs. *J. Agric. Food Chem.*, **6**, 365–8

2. Hobbs, C. S. and Merriman, G. M. (1962). *Fluorosis in Beef Cattle*. Bull. 351. (Tennessee Agric. Exp. Stat., Knoxville: Univ. of Tennessee)
3. Hobbs, C. S., Moorman, R. P., Griffith, J. M. Jr. *et al.* (1954). *Fluorosis in Sheep. Experiments 10, 11*. Bull. 235. (Knoxville: Univ. of Tennessee)
4. McRoberts, M. R., Hill, R. and Dalgorno, A. C. (1965). The effects of diets deficient in phosphorus and vitamin D, or calcium on the skeleton and teeth of the growing sheep. I. The mineral status and clinical appearance of the teeth. *J. Agric. Sci.*, **65**, 1–10
5. McRoberts, M. R., Hill, R. and Dalgorno, A. C. (1965). The effects of diets deficient in phosphorus and vitamin D, or calcium on the skeleton and teeth of the growing sheep. II. Malocclusion of the teeth. *J. Agric. Sci.*, **65**, 11–14
6. Milhaud, G. and Cazieux, A. (1980). Preliminary studies on lamb fluorosis. *Vet. Human Toxicol.*, **22**, 81–3
7. Milhaud, G., Cazieux, A. and Enriquez, B. (1983). Experimental studies on fluorosis in the suckling lamb. *Fluoride* (in press)
8. Milhaud, G. and Gras, N. (1978). Dental lesions caused by fluorosis in sheep. Presented at *C.R. Symp. Cemo "Fluoride and Bone"*, Genève. Edn. Médicine et Hygiène. pp. 194–200
9. Milhaud, G., Zundel, E. and Crombet, M. (1980). Etude expérimentale de la fluorose caprine. I. Protocole expérimental, comportement des animaux, lésions dentaires. *Rec. Méd. Vét.*, **156**, 37–46
10. Milhaud, G., Mathieu, E., Chary, J. F. *et al.* (1980). Etude expérimentale de la fluorose caprine. II. Etude du squelette, discussion générale. *Rec. Méd. Vét.*, **156**, 211–18
11. Peirce, A. W. (1952). Studies on fluorosis of sheep. I. The toxicity of waterborne fluoride for sheep maintained in pens. *Aust. J. Agric. Res.*, **3**, 326–40
12. Peirce, A. W. (1954). Studies on fluorosis of sheep. II. The toxicity of waterborne fluoride for nature grazing sheep. *Aust. J. Agric. Res.*, **5**, 543–54
13. Peirce, A. W. (1959). Studies on fluorosis of sheep. III. The toxicity of waterborne fluoride for the grazing sheep throughout its life. *Aust. J. Agric. Res.*, **10**, 186–98
14. Said, A. N., Slagsvold, P., Bergh, H. *et al.* (1977). High fluorine water to wether sheep maintained in pens. Aluminium chloride as a possible alleviator of fluorosis. *Nord. Vet. Med.*, **29**, 172–80
15. Shuppe, J. L., Miner, M. L., Harris, L. E. *et al.* (1963). The effect of fluorine on dairy cattle. I. Clinical and pathologic effects. *Am. J. Vet. Res.*, **24**, 964–84
16. Suttie, J. W. (1969). Air quality standards for the protection of farm animals from fluorides. *J. Air Pollut. Control Assoc.*, **19**, 239–42
17. Suttie, J. W. and Faltin, E. C. (1971). Effect of a short period of fluoride ingestion on dental fluorosis in cattle. *Am. J. Vet. Res.*, **32**, 217–22
18. Suttie, J. W. and Phillips, P. H. (1959). Studies of the effects of dietary sodium fluoride on dairy cows. V. A three year study on mature animals. *J. Dairy Sci.*, **42**, 1063–9
19. Velu, H. (1932). Le Darmous, fluorose spontanée des zones phosphatées. *Arch. Inst. Pasteur, Alger*, **10**, 41–118
20. Velu, H. and Charnot, A. (1938). Données nouvelles sur l'étiologie et la pathogénie du darmous. *Bull. Inst. Hyg. du Maroc*, pp. 5–26

59
Chloramphenicol–propylene glycol toxicity following constant intravenous infusion in horses

S. L. Spurlock, T. E. Powers, K. J. Varma and J. D. Powers

A *Strep. zooepidemicus* disease model in young horses (3–6 months old) was used to examine the efficacy of penicillin therapy in treating this bacterial infection [16]. The disease model produced consistent clinical signs of disease and had acute and chronic phases. Acutely, the horses were febrile and depressed and chronically, the horses developed lameness associated with localization of the infection in joints.

Constant intravenous administration of chloramphenicol in propylene glycol over a 5 day period resulted in the death of 11 of 30 horses. Data suggest that propylene glycol may have been responsible for the deaths as well as other signs observed which were not related to the disease model.

MATERIALS AND METHODS

Thirty horses were divided into five groups of six horses each. Four of these groups were infected with *Strep. zooepidemicus*. One group of infected horses received only the diluent (propylene glycol) and the other three groups of infected horses received chloramphenicol dissolved in propylene glycol to maintain blood levels of 0.25 × MIC, 1 × MIC and 4 × MIC. The fifth group (healthy control) received chloramphenicol to maintain blood concentrations of 4 × MIC. All horses were to receive 2.1 l of diluent over the 5 day period at a rate of 17.5 ml/h. The diluent* used had the following constituents per ml: benzyl alcohol 0.9%, dimethylacetamide 15%, sodium succinate as a buffer, q.s. propylene glycol to 1 ml. During the experimental period, the animals were observed for clinical signs of the disease and the serum protein electrophoresis were performed to evaluate the changes in disease state. All animals were necropsied, either immediately after death or on the thirteenth postinfection day.

*Rachelle Laboratories, Inc., Long Beach, California, USA.

RESULTS

Some horses from each chloramphenicol treatment group, the diluent group and the uninfected group died during the experiment. Out of six animals in each group, three horses in the group receiving diluent, two in the 0.25 × MIC group, three in the 1 × MIC group, and two in the 4 × MIC group died and one of the uninfected control animals receiving drug to maintain 4 × MIC also died during the experimental period.

Beside the 11 animals that died, 13 other horses demonstrated signs not attributable to the disease model. These included alterations in gastrointestinal motility, foul-smelling diarrhoea, anorexia and depression. In two horses, ataxia was also observed.

The most consistent findings on necropsy were moderate to severe inflammation along the entire intestinal tract and ecchymotic haemorrhages on the serosal surface of the small intestine. Furthermore, five of the 11 animals that died before the planned termination date were found to have jejunal intussusceptions with resulting necrosis.

DISCUSSION

There was a statistically significant correlation between death and the weight of the horse. Most of the horses which died weighed under 152 kg. This fact combined with the fact that all groups had only the administration of propylene glycol in common suggest toxic effects of propylene glycol. Toxic effects similar to ones reported in this study have been reported in horses following oral administration of 3.4–9.1 l of propylene glycol[11].

Jejunal intussusceptions were found in five out of 30 horses used in this study. Tennant *et al.*[15] reported that 12 out of 75 cases of small intestinal strangulation involved intussusception and only one was a jejunal. Intussusceptions are considered to be rare in occurrence and, when present, the ileum and ileo-caecal junction are most commonly involved[18]. With the high incidence of jejunal intussusceptions in this study, the mechanism, by which this lesion occurs, could provide insight into the toxic effects of propylene glycol. It has been suggested that intussusceptions are the result of peristaltic waves striking a dilated, atonic segment of bowel. Rather than passing over this atonic area, it results in an inward loop[12]. Since gastrointestinal motility depends on the balance of the inherent electrical rhythm of intestinal smooth muscle and the modulating effect of the autonomic nervous system, endocrine and prostaglandin systems[10], anyone of these areas may be involved in alteration of motility.

Interestingly, propylene glycol has been incriminated in changes in bloodflow, smooth muscle contractility and autonomic control. Changes in bloodflow and involvement of the autonomic nervous system have been addressed by Goss *et al.*[5] in a study in calves. Intravenous administration of a propylene glycol bolus to conscious calves produced a decrease in renal and pulmonary bloodflow and an increase in blood pressure. Alterations in blood pressure and flow as well as associated alterations in cardiac function could be moderated with various autonomic blocking agents. In contrast, femoral artery instrumentation recorded systemic hypotension in anaesthetized cats given a rapid intravenous bolus of propylene glycol[7]. Similar hypotensive effects have been noted in humans receiving propylene glycol[6,7].

Haemolysis as a result of propylene glycol administration was seen in many of the samples taken from horses in this study. This may also be responsible or contribute in part to alterations in blood pressure. It has been shown that haemolyzed blood can alter pulmonary and systemic blood pressure. A study in dogs demonstrated an increase in pulmonary blood pressure and decrease in systemic blood pressure[9].

While the exact mechanism of vascular smooth muscle response to propylene glycol remains undefined, attempts have been made with gastrointestinal and uterine preparations to determine whether the propylene glycol affects membrane activity, the contractile mechanisms, or metabolism[1]. The mechanism of action on a cellular level has not been determined, but the statistically significant reduction of both frequency and amplitude of smooth muscle contraction with varying concentrations of propylene glycol seems to be due to a direct depression exerted on metabolism.

The ataxia reported in two of the horses in this study has also been seen in other species[13,19] after propylene glycol administration. A weak but significant CNS depressant activity was observed with propylene glycol volumes larger than would be included in therapeutic dosage of drugs in this solvent[19]. The horses in this study which lived up to postinfection day 13 received 2.1 l of the diluent. Strong evidence exists that propylene glycol is not an inert substance[19].

Aside from propylene glycol, chloramphenicol is also capable of producing toxic signs. Direct cardiovascular depression has been studied *in vivo* and with *in vitro* preparations in several animal species[2,14]. Bone marrow depression, either reversible or irreversible, has been reported in man, dog, cat, duck and other species with a range of daily dose and duration of therapy[8]. Chloramphenicol may also inhibit the function of messenger RNA formed in response to antigenic stimulus[17]. A lack of immune response to homograft plus transplantation was observed in rabbits with mean chloramphenicol serum levels as low as 5.9 μg/ml. Administration of therapeutic levels of chloramphenicol to humans has been shown to suppress the anamnestic response to tetanus toxoid[4].

Table 59.1 γ-Globulin (g/dl) in untreated *Strep. zooepidemicus* challenged horses

Horse No.	*Preinfection day*	*Postinfection day* 1	3	5	7	10	13
37	0.96	0.96	0.92	0.83	0.99	1.35	2.17
39	0.94	0.77	0.84	0.80	0.81	1.18	1.31
47	1.11	1.01	1.04	1.13	1.22	1.87	3.00
58	1.57	1.54	1.40	1.40	1.55	2.11	2.70
64	0.71	0.87	0.99	1.12	1.16	1.65	2.65
65	1.15	1.14	1.09	0.99	1.32	2.11	3.14
66	1.25	1.08	1.06	1.07	1.21	1.57	2.14

In all infected groups, albumin had a tendency to decrease. A decrease in albumin, along with an increase in γ globulins usually accompanies an immune response[3]. An increase in the γ fraction was observed between postinfection days 10–13 in horses used in the development of the disease model (Table 59.1). This same response was not observed in all of the chloramphenicol treatment groups.

Due to the death of animals in the chloramphenicol–propylene glycol study, results are limited. Those results available from the infected horses receiving chloramphenicol to maintain 4×MIC (approximately 6 μg/ml), demonstrate a failure of the γ fraction of the serum protein electrophoresis to increase (Table 59.2). This suggests that a constant serum level of 6 μg/ml may be capable of interfering with the ability of the horse to respond to antigenic stimulus. However another explanation would be that the antigenic

Table 59.2 2γ-Globulin (g/dl) in *Strep. zooepidemicus* challenged and unchallenged horses which received different doses of chloramphenicol

Horse No.	*Group*	*PRE*	*Postinfection day* 0	3	7	11	13
100	Diluent	0.60	0.69	0.73	0.98	0.83	0.93
111	Diluent	1.12	0.92	0.84			
113	Diluent	0.98	0.96	0.80	0.73		
129	Diluent	0.66	0.75	0.75	0.72		
133	Diluent	0.62	1.05	1.06	1.00	1.16	1.53
137	Diluent	0.86	0.77	0.90	0.89	0.87	1.14
103	4-MIC Cont.	0.68	0.77	0.71	0.67	0.60	0.50
114	4-MIC Cont.	0.84	0.91	0.81	0.61	0.73	0.61
116	4-MIC Cont.	0.46	0.63	0.66	0.54		
125	4-MIC Cont.	0.70	0.87	0.91	0.67		
130	4-MIC Cont.	1.08	1.23	1.25	1.05	0.89	0.86
140	4-MIC Cont.	0.84	0.88	0.79	0.83	0.64	0.60
105	0.25-MIC	0.78	0.82	0.79	0.86	0.70	0.67
118	0.25-MIC		0.72	0.94	0.86		
119	0.25-MIC	0.99	0.94	0.81	0.76		
122	0.25-MIC	1.25	0.30	1.11	1.03	1.31	1.67
128	0.25-MIC	0.92	1.21	0.95	1.01	1.08	1.12
138	0.25-MIC	0.50	0.49	0.61	0.74	0.76	0.89
104	1-MIC	0.72	0.70	0.60	0.68	0.67	0.79
115	1-MIC	0.86	1.18	1.09	1.19		
121	1-MIC	0.66	0.86	0.76	0.89	0.76	
123	1-MIC	1.24	0.99	1.16	0.93		
127	1-MIC	0.71	0.73	0.77	0.88	1.20	1.36
135	1-MIC	0.46	0.66	1.50	0.65	0.60	1.72
107	4-MIC	0.56	0.71	0.60	0.65	0.63	0.59
117	4-MIC	0.40	0.91	0.96	0.90		
120	4-MIC	0.74	1.03	1.03	0.73	0.88	0.81
124	4-MIC	0.76	0.78	0.67	0.82		
132	4-MIC	0.42	0.42	0.58	0.56	0.46	0.42
136	4-MIC	0.71	0.69	0.74	0.78	0.52	0.59

PRE = Preinfection day

stimulus of the *Strep. zoo.* organism was eliminated with the maintenance of this level of chloramphenicol.

CONCLUSION

The results of this study suggested two important points. First, propylene glycol can have toxic effects. Therefore, its use in pharmacological studies should include a control group to illustrate effects of the solvent alone. Secondly, when therapeutic blood levels of chloramphenicol are maintained at a constant level for a period of time, it may have an effect on the mammalian cells and the normal immune response.

ACKNOWLEDGMENT

This work was supported by the Food and Drug Administration Contract No. 223-79-7054.

References

1. Bonnardeaux, J. L. (1971). A comparison of the effects of 3 organic solvents: dimethyl sulfoxide, formamide, and propylene glycol on spontaneous activity of isolated smooth muscle. *Can. J. Physiol. Pharm.*, **49**, 632–41
2. Clark, C. H. (1978). Metabolic effects and toxicities of chloramphenicol. *Mod. Vet. Pract.*, **59**, 663–7.
3. Coffman, J. R. (1968). Clinical application of serum protein electrophoresis in the horse. In *Proceedings of 14th Annual Meeting of American Association of Equine Practitioners*. pp. 265–79
4. Daniel, T. M., Suhrland, L. G. and Weisberger, A. S. (1965). Suppression of anamnestic response to tetanus toxoid in man by chloramphenicol. *N. Engl. J. Med.*, **273**, 367–9
5. Goss, D. R., Kitzmann, J. V. and Adams, H. R. (1979). Cardiovascular effects of intravenous administration of propylene glycol and of oxytetracycline in propylene glycol in calves. *J. Am. Vet. Med. Assoc.*, **40**, 783–91
6. Kirman, C. S. (1976). Cardiac effects of diphenylhydantoin, isoniazid and propylene glycol. *Am. Heart J.*, **92**, 409
7. Leaders, F., Pettinger, C. B. and Long, J. P. (1960). Some pharmacological properties of selected antibiotics. *Antibiot. Chemother.*, **10**, 503–7
8. Louis, S., Kutt, H. and McDowell, F. (1967). The cardiovascular changes caused by intravenous dilantin and its solvent. *Am. Heart J.*, **74**, 523–9
9. McCrady, J. D., Pendery, G. B., Camp, B. J. *et al.* (1978). The effect of hemolyzed blood on pulmonary and systemic arterial pressure and heart rate of the dog. *J. Comp. Med.*, **42**, 69–72
10. Moore, J. N. and White, N. A. (1982). Acute abdominal disease, pathophysiology and preoperative management. *Vet. Clin. N. Am.*, **4**, 61–78
11. Myer, V. S. and Usenik, E. A. (1969). Propylene glycol intoxication of horses. *J. Am. Vet. Med. Assoc.*, **155**, 1841
12. Rooney, J. R. (1965). Volvulus, strangulation and intussusception in the horse. *Cornell Vet.*, **55**, 644–53
13. Ruddick, J. A. (1972). Toxicology, metabolism and biochemistry of 1,2-propanediol. *Toxicol. Appl. Pharmacol.*, **21**, 102–11
14. Swain, H. W., Kiplinger, G. F. and Brody, T. M. (1956). Actions of certain antibiotics on the isolated dog heart. *J. Pharmacol. Exp. Ther.*, **117**, 151–9

15. Tennant, B., Wheat, J. D. and Meagher, D. M. (1972). Observation of the causes and incidence of acute intestinal obstruction in the horse. In *Proceedings of 18th Annual Meeting of American Association of Equine Practitioners*. pp. 265–8
16. Varma, K. J., Powers, T. E., Garg, R. C. *et al.* (1982). Characterization of a therapeutic model of *Streptococcus Zooepidemicus* infection in the horse. Congress of the European Association for Veterinary Pharmacology and Toxicology, Toulouse, France, Sept. 13–17. *I.N.R.A. Publ.*, **8**, 485–6
17. Weisberger, A. S., Daniel, T. M. and Hoffman, A. (1964). Suppression of antibody synthesis and prolongation of homograft survival by chloramphenicol. *J. Exp. Med.*, **120**, 183–96
18. Wheat, J. D. (1972). Diseases of the small intestine: diagnosis and treatment. In *Proceedings of 18th Annual Meeting of American Association of Equine Practitioners*. pp. 265–8
19. Zaroslinsky, J. F., Browne, R. K. and Possley, L. H. (1971). Propylene glycol as a drug solvent in pharmacologic studies. *Toxicol. Appl. Pharmacol.*, **19**, 573–8

60
Heavy metal intoxications in horses

A. A. Seawright, J. Hrdlicka and J. C. Ng

Intoxication of horses by heavy metals is of comparatively uncommon occurrence, and mostly the diseases are chronic in type. Usually, poisoning is associated with the normal ingestion of intrinsically toxic (selenium) or secondarily contaminated pasture (lead, zinc, arsenic, copper), grain (mercury) or drinking water (cadmium). Of the few definitive reports in the literature, most concentrate on epizootological aspects of the conditions while experimental studies are few in number and tend to describe few or single intoxicated animals.

LEAD

In a recent review of historical aspects of lead toxicosis in the United States, Burrows[6] draws attention to the part played by lead mining and smelting in the high incidence of poisoning of both man and domestic animals about 100 years ago. Notwithstanding the universal recognition of this kind of industrial pollution of the environment and the steps taken to reduce toxic smelter emissions, sporadic outbreaks of lead poisoning in horses in such areas continue to occur in these and other parts of the developed world to the present day. In effect, the horses in lead mining and smelting regions may be regarded as sentinels to portend the likely hazard of the general environmental contamination.

In many respects the lead poisoning syndrome in the horse, as with other species, has a variety of manifestations[12,49] and it seems to be generally agreed that the syndrome is a chronic disease, often with acute onset and short duration of clinical signs, but most often characterized mainly by laryngeal hemiplegia and/or pharyngeal dysfunction due to neuropathy affecting the recurrent laryngeal and other regional motor nerves. The latter dysfunction, a segmental demyelination of the appropriate nerves leading to reduced conduction velocity[19], frequently gives rise to difficulty of swallowing and aspiration pneumonia. Acute lead poisoning in the horse is not well defined but, in a recent case brought to the attention of the authors, a stallion given to the wind-sucking habit died a few weeks after having been placed in a small yard, the fence of which was liberally painted with used engine oil. Sickness occurred suddenly and was characterized by muscle tremors, posterior ataxia and intermittent but violent convulsions lasting some 24 h before death occurred. The terminal blood lead level was 0.4 parts/10^6 while the liver and kidney contained 8 and 4.5 parts/10^6 wet weight, respectively.

Confusion has always existed concerning the daily dose of lead required to precipitate typical lead poisoning in the horse and the correlations between apparent metal intake, tissue concentrations and incidence and severity of clinical signs are poor. The most convincing experimental study is that by Willoughby *et al.*[46] in which 3 week old foals were given 3.5 mg/kg lead daily initially for 8 weeks, with regular weekly increase in the dose rate up to 108.5 mg/kg. Clinical signs did not appear until the daily intake reached 86 mg/kg and blood lead levels exceeded 0.6 parts/10^6 for at least 3 weeks. The latter dose rate was equivalent to 3400 parts/10^6 lead in the feed. An experimental design of this type does not indicate, however, what the required mean daily dose rate should be in order for poisoning to be produced in say the 6 month period of the study. It was of interest that the initial clinical signs were those of pharyngeal and/or laryngeal dysfunction; lameness, stiffness and signs of anaemia being completely absent. The liver and kidney cortical lead concentrations were 26.5 and 70 parts/10^6, respectively.

In a later study by Dollahite *et al.*[13] in older ponies, in which groups of two animals were dosed daily with 6.25, 7.8, 9.8 and 12.2 mg/kg lead acetate for 105 days, no significant toxic effect occurred, even though the final blood lead levels were between 0.35 and 0.75 parts/10^6. Groups of four cattle dosed similarly were mostly all dead of lead poisoning within 24 days of the start of the experiment, thus providing unequivocal evidence of the comparative tolerance of horses to lead ingestion. In the latter trial the lead doses were increased respectively to 15.3, 19.1, 23.8 and 29.8 mg/kg for a further 190 days. Apart from one animal given the lowest dose rate, the remaining horses died between 18 and 190 days after the start of the latter dose rates. The response of the horses was individual and apparently not related to the dose rate of lead. Animals in which blood lead levels rose fastest tended to die earliest and in no animal was the terminal blood lead level less than 1 part/10^6. Individual susceptibility to lead intoxication, other factors being equal, appeared to be related to the efficiency of absorption of the metal from the alimentary tract and/or retention of the element in the animal, since affected horses had higher tissue levels than unaffected animals, irrespective of the dose rate. It was significant that no horses exhibited signs of laryngeal or pharyngeal dysfunction, although clinical signs recorded included anorexia, weight loss, laboured breathing, convulsions, incoordination, laminitis and mild anaemia. Typical acid fast nuclear inclusions were present in the liver and kidney.

Similar results were later achieved with a single adult Shetland pony to which lead acetate was given in the feed at the mean daily rate of 41.24 mg/kg over 111 days[49]. Again, no laryngeal hemiplegia occurred although there was anorexia, depression, muscle tremors, transient jaundice, and anaemia characterized by typical basophilic stippling of erythrocytes and presence of reticulocytes when blood Pb levels reached 2.42 parts/10^6. The animal died suddenly some 6 days after apparent recovery, renal tubular epithelial intranuclear inclusions being the only relevant pathological finding.

The dose rate of lead required to induce lead poisoning experimentally in the horse seems, therefore, far higher than that estimated to occur under natural conditions of poisoning. Hammond and Aronson[21], for example, measured lead concentrations on pastures in the vicinity of a lead smelter where outbreaks of lead poisoning were occurring in both cattle and horses and concluded that the minimal daily intake of the metal required to cause cumulative poisoning in cattle within a few months was some 6–7 mg/kg, while that for horses was only 2.4 mg/kg. Knight and Burau[25] calculated that the mean daily intake of Pb for their affected horses on contaminated pasture was 6.4 mg/kg body weight.

Aronson[2], however, allowed that horses had different feeding habits from cattle and notes that horses will frequently pull out forage by the roots and eat the roots and attendant soil along with the remainder of the plant. Since soil in the vicinity of smelters is likely to contain very high concentrations of lead, it can be concluded that the actual lead intake by grazing horses is likely to be far higher than that estimated when only forage contamination is considered alone. This is also suggested from the study of equine lead intoxications by Schmidtt *et al.*[39] in which the forage of affected pastures at 400, 800 and 22 500 m north respectively from the smelter contained 264, 177 and 18 parts/10^6 Pb while the lead present in the top 2.5 cm of the soil in which the plants grew contained some 4200, 2900 and 280 parts/10^6 of the metal. In contrast, cattle were unaffected. With each pair of samples there was about 16 times more lead in the top soil than on the associated herbage. With the outbreaks recorded by Egan and O'Cuill[15] and Hammond and Aronson[21] the mean forage Pb levels in the affected pastures were 570 and 580 parts/10^6 DM respectively. If associated top soil Pb levels were in any way comparable to those recorded by Schmidtt *et al.*[39] it would not be difficult to visualize horses grazing such pastures consuming Pb in amounts of the order of 3400 parts/10^6 in their diet at least part of the time, as was apparently needed to precipitate typical lead poisoning in experimental foals[46]. Moreover, in a recent survey of top soil lead levels in paddocks near a smelter on which lead poisoning in horses had previously occurred, the lead concentrations reached 7000 parts/10^6 at 1.6 km from the plant while associated forage[7] contained 800 parts/10^6. The younger the exposed horses are, the more likely they are to present with a syndrome characterized by peripheral neuropathy[27].

A further factor which may be of importance in predisposing horses to lead intoxication is suboptimal dietary calcium and/or phosphorus which leads to enhanced absorption and retention of lead in the tissues[47]. Pasture grasses which lead to severe negative calcium balance in the horse are well known in various parts of the world[45] and may be relevant in some outbreaks of equine lead poisoning.

In relation to clinical diagnosis of lead intoxication, blood lead levels in excess of 0.35 parts/10^6 are normally regarded as of diagnostic significance, although in some poisoned animals blood lead concentrations within the normal range are not uncommonly recorded[21,25]. Useful diagnostic procedures include determination of urinary Pb concentration before and immediately after an intravenous dose of 75 mg/kg of Ca EDTA in which there will be a substantial increase in the post injection Pb level in poisoned horses[25] and more recently, determination of the erythrocyte zinc protoporphyrin level which indicates the degree of previous lead exposure and is independent of the blood lead level[27].

ZINC

As pointed out by Willoughby *et al.*[46], lead and zinc coexist in many areas and, in the mining and smelting of such ores, environmental contamination with toxic amounts of zinc may well occur as happens with lead. Although the possibility of participation by zinc in equine toxicity outbreaks associated with mainly lead smelting had been suspected[24,39] and poisoning of horses had earlier been reported in the vicinity of mainly zinc smelters[20], the first definitive experimental study of zinc toxicity in the horse is that of Willoughby *et al.*[46]. Natural chronic zinc intoxication of horses has also occurred after top dressing of pastures with zinc oxide[29,48].

In the latter experimental investigation, zinc oxide was incorporated in the diet of three newly weaned foals of 3–4 weeks old. The initial dose rate of zinc was about 25 mg/kg and this was increased periodically until the daily dose rate after some 20 weeks was 184 mg/kg. Clinical signs of poisoning marked by weight loss without depression of appetite occurred at about 17 weeks when the dose rate was 90 mg/kg, corresponding to about 3600 parts/10^6 zinc in the diet, and associated with a whole blood zinc level of about 6 parts/10^6. Death occurred in two of the foals at 23 weeks after 10 days of illness, and at 31 weeks in the other animal after 8 weeks of illness. The progress of clinical signs included initial non-painful epiphyseal enlargements of the limb joints with lameness apparent some 1–3 weeks later. As the pain increased the animals were reluctant to rise from lateral recumbency and assumed a stiff gait with disinclination to curve the spine laterally. The joints became swollen due to increased amounts of sterile joint fluid, and degenerative arthrosis[48], a condition subsequently described as an osteochondritis dessicans[29]. In the animal which lasted 31 weeks, there was also severe, progressive anaemia. Serum Ca, Mg and P values remained within normal limits but whole blood zinc values increased when the daily intake exceeded 60 mg/kg of the element. This juvenile osteodystrophy is typical of chronic zinc toxicity in other species such as the pig[4] and appeares to be due to a detrimental effect of high zinc levels on bone mineral metabolism[43]. It would not be unexpected that in-contact adult horses failed to develop such a syndrome[20,39]. Mean zinc concentrations in the liver, renal cortex, metacarpal epiphysis and lumbar vertebrae were 1523, 528, 180 and 255 parts/10^6 respectively, compared with values from control animals of about 35, 21, 83 and 78 parts/10^6 wet weight. Pasture and top soil zinc concentrations rarely appear to have been measured in outbreaks of suspected heavy metal poisoning round smelters but the level of 3500 parts/10^6 zinc recorded in overwintered grass in the outbreak described by Schmidtt *et al.*[39] would help confirm that the condition in their young horses was in fact zinc intoxication rather than lead poisoning, as was proposed.

The experimental study of Willoughby *et al.*[46] also confirmed the existence of a Pb and Zn interaction in intoxication of foals with these metals ingested together. When toxic amounts of lead and zinc were dosed simultaneously, typical zinc poisoning occurred while signs of lead poisoning were completely absent. The effect of the Zn was to increase the amount of lead stored in the kidney and liver, decrease the deposition in bone and uptake by brain and promote lower blood Pb concentrations than occurred in animals fed Pb alone and in which typical lead poisoning occurred. Mean Zn concentrations in the liver and renal cortex were 696 and 210 parts/10^6 respectively, compared with 1523 and 528 parts/10^6 wet weight in the foals supplemented with the same amount of Zn alone.

A factor that needs to be considered in the diagnosis of zinc poisoning is that, unlike many heavy metals after absorption, Zn is rapidly excreted and with cessation of intake, due either to inappetance or change in diet, blood and tissue Zn concentrations tend to fall quickly to control levels, notwithstanding the persistence of the typical skeletal lesions. The best samples for analysis are reported to be faecal samples collected from affected horses and unaffected in-contact animals while they are consuming feed and water from the area suspected of containing excessive amounts of zinc[48].

CADMIUM

Cadmium occurs in nature with lead and zinc but there is little definite implication of Cd in heavy metal intoxication in the horse. The acute oral toxicity of Cd compounds for animals generally varies from about 100 mg/kg for soluble salts to several thousand mg/kg for the metal itself and other insoluble forms. At acutely toxic doses Cd compounds are locally irritant[22] and in a horse, clinical signs such as colic and diarrhoea, salivation and death from shock and dehydration might reasonably be expected to occur. Should death be delayed, other systemic effects due possibly to renal injury and cardiopulmonary failure may be predicted. A single case report titled 'Probable cadmium poisoning in a group of ponies'[38] records death in three of four ponies on a farm on which the animals had access to yellow paint which almost certainly contained a $CdSO_4$ pigment. Clinical signs exhibited by affected animals included disorientation, staggering, colic and prostration. Necropsy findings included cyanosis of mucous membranes, hyperaemia of the lungs with froth in the bronchi, streaky subendocardial haemorrhages, and granularity of the renal cortical surface in one animal. Microscopic renal lesions included glomerulonephritis, tubular nephritis and associated interstitial changes, lymphocytic depletion in the spleen, and oedema, congestion and haemorrhage in the lungs. Cd levels recorded were 15 parts/10^6 in the kidney of a yearling filly and 81 and 91 parts/10^6 in the kidney and liver respectively of a 7 year old mare, its dam.

The critical target organ in chronic Cd exposure is generally held to be the kidney. After absorption into the body, Cd tends to accumulate in this organ and when the concentration of the metal becomes critical, pathological changes occur. In man, this level is put at some 200 parts/10^6 in the renal cortex, resulting in both glomerular and tubular damage, which leads initially to proteinuria and later to glucosuria and aminoaciduria.

In a recent survey of vascular, cardiac and renal pathology as well as renal cortical Cd concentration, in 50 horses slaughtered for meat in Sweden[16], it was shown that Cd concentrations ranged from 12 to 186 parts/10^6 with a mean value of 61 parts/10^6, and 10 to 12 animals respectively had myocardial fibrosis and arteriosclerosis. There was about 50% incidence of microscopic renal lesions which tended to be more marked the higher the Cd level. The latter, in turn, was directly related to the hardness of the water which the animals had been consuming throughout their lives. Lifetime consumption of soft water, therefore, predisposed to enhanced Cd uptake and accumulation in the kidney with pathological consequences for the latter organ as well as for various cardiovascular tissues. The mean renal Cd level at 61 parts/10^6 was, however, far below the 200 parts/10^6 critical level for renal dysfunction in man and the validity of conclusions concerning the relevance of the Cd levels in the equine kidneys to the pathology observed, remains to be confirmed.

COPPER

While copper poisoning of horses appears to be rare, some 30 cases of the condition are claimed to have been diagnosed at the Veterinary Faculty Clinic at Zagreb University in Yugoslavia[3], due possibly to contamination of their rations with Bordeaux mixture. This prompted experimental studies of copper sulphate poisoning in this species. The acute single oral dose of $CuSO_4$ was found to be 125 mg/kg, causing mainly acute gastroenteritis, as well as intravascular haemolysis, jaundice and haemoglobinuria with deaths occurring up to 2 weeks later. Chronic $CuSO_4$ intoxication occurred following contamination of the food with the compound for 2 or more months. Clinical signs included colic and weight loss as well as multiple haemolytic crises with deaths occurring after 6 months or so of the Cu supplementation. The actual concentration of the copper in the diet was not reported but, in animals dying from poisoning, the copper levels in the liver were stated to be 10 times normal.

ARSENIC

Arsenic poisoning of horses has been reported following consumption of grass treated with a weedicide containing 47% arsenic trioxide and 3.5% lead arsenate[5]. Clarke and Clarke[9] gave the acute single oral toxic dose of the insoluble arsenic trioxide as 10–45 g, while that for the soluble sodium arsenite as 1–3 g. In parts of the world such as tropical Australia where the latter compound as an 0.2% solution was used as an acaricide against the cattle tick, poisoning of horses was common. Horses, as well as cattle and other species, became infested with this parasite and control of the latter demanded that horses undergo regular treatment[41].

After ingestion of a fatally toxic dose of As_2O_3, death usually occurs within 4 days. The clinical signs of affected horses include weakness, depression, profuse diarrhoea, mild icterus, extreme dehydration, extensive subserous petechial haemorrhages, cyanotic mucous membranes and marked hyperaemia of the gastric and small intestinal mucosa. In severely poisoned animals there may be patchy diphtheritic inflammation of the small intestinal mucosa with blood-stained contents. The large intestines are usually filled with fluid contents and greatly distended. In contaminated grass containing in excess of 60 000 parts/10^6 arsenic fed to horses which resulted in fatal intoxication, about 20 parts/10^6 As was found in the liver and kidneys while more than 2000 parts/10^6 As was found in the stomach contents[5].

While similar clinical signs are reported in horses suffering from poisoning due to excessive percutaneous absorption, excessive epidermal exfoliation also occurs in animals treated in wet weather or else when animals' skins are re-wetted with sweat, following drying after spraying or dipping. Thirsty animals have also succumbed to As intoxication after drinking the dipping fluid and horses appear significantly more susceptible to poisoning than cattle under natural conditions of exposure[41].

Since absorbed As tends to clear rapidly and efficiently from the animal body and cumulation of the element in the body tissues is relatively low, chronic As intoxication tends to be uncommon[1]. However, Seddon[41] reported an encephalopathy in horses, which was attributed to the acaricide, after they had been subjected to some 30 inorganic arsenical treatments over 14 months in a specially intensive tick control programme. Clinical signs usually began within 3–13 days of treatment and included circling movements, depression, hyperexcitability, mania and death. The exact nature of the condition was not determined but such episodes no longer occurred when use of As was discontinued in this area.

SELENIUM

The acute single oral toxic dose of selenium given as sodium selenite for the horse lies between 3.3 and 6 mg/kg[30,44]. Clinical signs include profuse sweating, diarrhoea, tachycardia, tachypnoea, mild pyrexia, lethargy, mild to severe colic and death within 24 h. Head pressing just prior to death is considered a classical sign[44]. Serum Se levels in acute fatal selenosis reach just over 1 part/10^6.

When horses are dosed daily with small amounts of sodium selenite incorporated in the feed, 115 parts/10^6 Se was sufficient to cause death within 5 weeks. At substantially lower dose levels horses survived for about 17 months before death occurred. Clinical signs of such chronic inorganic Se poisoning include emaciation despite a good appetite, listlessness, looseness of hair in mane and tail and softening and scaling of the horny wall of the hoof. Blood Se levels at point of death were in excess of 6 parts/10^6 after a precipitate rise within the last few days from a plateau of about 3 parts/10^6 due, apparently, to terminal failure of renal Se excreting mechanisms. Chronic Se intake appears also to induce progressive tolerance to further dosing with the element[31]. Terminal tissue Se concentrations were 2–5 parts/10^6 in the kidneys, 1.5–5 parts/10^6 in the liver and about 5 parts/10^6 in the hair.

Chronic Se poisoning (alkali disease) occurs far more readily in horses when they obtain the element from plant sources, mostly in the organic form[9]. In fact, selenosis may occur when soil Se content is from 1 to 6 parts/10^6 and levels in the feed are in excess of 5 parts/10^6. Selenosis tends to develop on farms with seleniferous soils, particularly in times of drought[10]. Clinical signs may be present in horses within 3 weeks. Initially, there is lameness, particularly of the hind limbs, followed by loss of appetite and pain and swelling of the coronary bands and laminitis[17]. Within a further 7–10 days, there is exudation from the coronary bands, beginning at the heels, followed in 3–5 days by transverse cracking of the hoof wall distal to the coronary band. This is soon accompanied by loss of hair from mane and tail. Tail hair samples may have as much as 28 parts/10^6 Se[23], while Se levels in hair in excess of 5 parts/10^6 can be considered diagnostic of selenosis.

Selenosis often occurs following consumption of specific selenium accumulator plants. One such plant in Australia, *Morinda reticulata*, which is responsible for causing the disease in that country, contains from 1.5 to 1141 parts/10^6 Se in the leaves. Feeding 62.6 kg of the plant containing 13.3 g Se to a horse over 82 days caused typical selenosis with levels of Se in the liver, hair, mane and tail of 9.8, 11.2, 19.4 and 45.4 parts/10^6, respectively. The form of Se in this plant is the non-protein amino acid selenocystathionine[26].

The recommendation for the prevention of selenosis in endemic areas is the inclusion of 5 parts/10^6 sodium arsenite in the drinking water[9], and the proposed treatment of affected horses is oral dosing of 4.5 g naphthalene daily for 5 days followed by a similar course after a further 5 days[23].

MERCURY

While mercury as a metal and its salts are commonly available in the environment for a variety of purposes and are generally known to be toxic, there are few actual definitive descriptions of any form of mercurialism in the horse. The acute toxic oral dose of mercuric chloride, one of the more toxic mercury salts, is 5–10 g or 10–20 mg/kg, while that for mercurous chloride[9] is 12–16 g. No detailed clinical descriptions of such acute intoxication in this species appear to be available, although for all species colic, gastroenteritis often with haemorrhagic diarrhoea, tubular nephrosis characterized by oliguria and anuria, uraemia and death within 5 or 6 days, would appear to be the likely manifestation of the condition[11]. A description of an acute fatal illness in a horse, which was attributed to mercurialism following consumption some 3–4 days previously of fungicide-treated grain, included anorexia, salivation, diarrhoea, depression, unsteady gait, rapid respiration and pulse, pyrexia, foetid breath and a bloody bronchopurulent nasal discharge, the latter considered to be associated with gangrene of the lungs[14]. No reference was made to clinical signs of renal injury or colic, although the animal was regarded as a 'textbook description of advanced mercury poisoning', nor were pathological or toxicological findings reported.

Other syndromes of a more subacute or chronic nature following topical treatment of skin wounds and various musculoskeletal injuries with mercury containing ointments, include transient alopecia and dermatitis in some individuals[28], and destructive, haemorrhagic lesions of bones, liver and kidney of a horse within 3 weeks[33]. In the latter animal, a large quantity of the ointment was rubbed into a skin wound on the fetlock and it was proposed that microemboli containing irritant mercury compounds were carried from this site to the scapula, liver and kidney, causing severe local injury in these tissues. No histological studies of the lesions were reported nor were analyses of the tissues for mercury carried out.

Although short-chain monoalkyl mercurials are nowadays generally discouraged for use as fungicides on grain and have accordingly become less likely in recent times to be causes of poisoning of livestock fed fungicide treated grain, both organic and inorganic forms of mercury still have many uses which can result in contamination of horse fodder and may lead to suspected mercurial poisoning in this species. Following an outbreak several years ago of such a suspected mercurial poisoning in some thoroughbreds in Queensland, Australia, following consumption of oats that contained 2–20 parts/10^6 of mercury, detailed studies of various forms of mercurialism in individual horses were carried out.

Experimental chronic mercurialism

Four adult horses were used in the study. Of these animals two were dosed daily with either phenylmercuric acetate or mercuric chloride at 0.4 mg Hg/kg body weight. One was given 0.8 mg Hg/kg daily as mercuric chloride, and the other dosed with 0.43 mg Hg/kg of methylmercury (MeHg) chloride for 5 days out of 7. In each animal the mercury compound was given by the oral route. The syndromes which developed were different in each animal and will be briefly described and compared.

Methylmercurialism

The horse was dosed continuously with the MeHg for almost 10 weeks[40]. For the first 5 weeks or so the animal appeared unaffected after which it developed a progressive bilaterally symmetrical exudative dermatitis on the thoracolumbar region and flanks, extending to the head and neck, lasting for some 5 weeks. By day 50 the animal was lethargic and developed a mild, persistent laminitis. Appetite and body weight gradually declined after this period and by the 9th week the gait was slow and incoordinate although there was no longer evidence of laminitis. By the 10th week the horse was reluctant to move and there was incoordination, ataxia, dysmetria and hypermetria, continuous vertical head nodding both when in motion and at rest, hyperaesthesia, licking and chewing movements of the jaws, and apparently reduced field of vision. Fore and hind limb crossing without loss of balance when walking and turning was prominent. Visual placing reflexes, involving mainly the hind limbs, were exaggerated. The animal was profoundly depressed and emaciated and was destroyed on day 85.

Blood non-protein nitrogen levels increased from normal (9.9 mmol/l) on day 57 to about twice this level by day 84. Glucosuria appeared on day 70 and remained for the remaining period of the illness. Terminally, there was an increase in serum proteins and haematocrit with moderate leukocytosis and neutrophilia. Whole blood MeHg levels rose steadily to 2000 ng/ml by day 57, after which there was a precipitate rise to 6200 ng/ml by day 85. Inorganic Hg levels in blood rose steadily to 400 ng/ml by day 57, increasing to some 600–700 ng/ml during the terminal phase of the intoxication. Brain levels of MeHg and inorganic Hg were 10.8–12.9 parts/10^6 and 0.3–0.4 parts/10^6, respectively. Most mercury was found in the liver which contained 63 and 28 parts/10^6 of inorganic Hg and MeHg, respectively. The kidneys contained 21.5 and 18 parts/10^6 of inorganic Hg and MeHg respectively. MeHg levels in other tissues ranged from 4 to 14 parts/10^6 and inorganic Hg levels ranged from 0.3 to 4.3 parts/10^6.

Significant gross pathological changes were confined to the kidneys which were enlarged, pale and of tough consistency. Microscopically, there was marked interstitial fibrosis with infiltration by mononuclear inflammatory cells, extensive atrophy of nephrons and dystrophy of residual tubular epithelium, dilation of the lumens and numerous proteinaceous casts containing cellular debris. In the brain, there was sporadic eosinophilic necrosis of neurons in the cerebrum with perivascular lymphocytic cuffing, focal atrophy of the granular cell layer of the cerebellar cortex with vacuolation of the associated molecular layer, and Wallerian degeneration of the dorsal funiculus, particularly in the fasiculus gracilis, and of the dorsal nerve roots in the cervical spinal cord. In the dorsal root ganglia there was marked loss of large ganglion cells with proliferation of the associated satellite cells.

In effect, the terminal syndrome was one of progressive clinical deterioration characterized by anorexia, cachexia, marked disturbance of renal function, and neurological dysfunction mainly affecting proprioception.

Phenylmercurialism

Following daily oral dosing with phenylmercuric acetate, the horse remained normal for 11 weeks[36]. After this time feed intake was reduced and there developed a severe progressive chemical stomatis characterized by ulceration of the buccal mucosa, gingival atrophy and inflammation with periodontitis, loosening of the premolar teeth, oedema of the cheek tissues, and regional thickening of the ramus of the mandibles with marked atrophy of the masseter muscles. The animal gradually lost weight, became very weak and dehydrated and was finally destroyed on day 191. There was a mild terminal elevation of blood urea nitrogen with intermittent glucosuria in evidence from day 56. Proteinuria occurred from day 106. The animal became anaemic, hypoproteinaemic and leukopaenic throughout the period of intoxication. Dehydration, starvation due to pain of prehension and mastication of food, as well as mild renal dysfunction were considered to be the causes of the erratic changes in the plasma and urinary electrolyte levels that characterized this toxic condition.

Blood organic Hg levels rarely rose above 200 ng/ml throughout the intoxication period and occasionally were virtually zero, while blood inorganic Hg levels remained between 200 and 400 ng/ml with occasional levels reaching up to about 1000 ng/ml, most of which was carried in the plasma. There was substantial but intermittent excretion of inorganic Hg in the urine with only occasional traces of the organic form. The liver held the highest concentration of organic Hg at 12.5 parts/10^6 while no organic mercury was detectable in the kidney and negligible amounts were present in all other organs, including the nervous system. The concentration of inorganic Hg in the kidney, however, was 187 parts/10^6 while in the liver the concentration was 120 parts/10^6. In the alimentary tract, substantial amounts of inorganic mercury were found in the wall of the caecum (124 parts/10^6) while terminally, the faeces contained 275 parts/10^6. The amount of inorganic Hg in the buccal tissues was comparatively low at 7–8 parts/10^6.

Apart from the oral cavity in which there was severe atrophy and local ulceration of the gums, degenerative changes in the osseous alveoli of the mandibles and the periodontal membranes of the premolars, the most significant changes were observed in the kidneys. The latter organs were enlarged, pale and slightly firmer than normal. Microscopically, there was mild atrophy and degeneration of the nephrons with focal interstitial fibrosis and focal dystrophy, mineralization and dilation of the proximal convoluted tubules.

Subgingival proliferative periostitis of the mandibular rami associated with the areas of ulceration was marked. There was no clinical evidence of diarrhoea and changes in the lower alimentary tract were negligible. The rapid final deterioration in the condition of this animal was almost certainly the indirect result of the extensive, painful, oral lesions causing cachexia and dehydration, with some contribution from the mild chronic renal injuries.

Inorganic mercurialism

This horse was put down after having been dosed daily with 0.4 mg Hg/kg for 23½ weeks[35]. The animal appeared unaffected for the first 8 weeks of dosing, after which it experienced transient hyperaesthesia lasting some 3 weeks. By this time the appetite had become capricious and gradual weight loss began to occur. By 14 weeks the animal was depressed, inappetent and spent long periods each day in sternal recumbancy. There were episodes of transient diarrhoea from the 15th week and persistent polydipsia. There was also progressive weakness and apparent ataxia. After a short period of clinical improvement with return of appetite and consequent gain in weight at about 20 weeks, the horse developed generalized circulatory failure and progressive weakness and was destroyed 3½ weeks later.

Glucosuria and proteinuria were detected by the 12th and 15th weeks respectively and there were terminal elevations of blood urea nitrogen and white cell count with a sharp fall in the plasma protein concentrations. Blood mercury levels rose gradually to reach a plateau of about 250 ng/ml within some 30 days. Urinary excretion of the element was highly variable with mean concentration of mercury of about 2000 ng/ml throughout the whole dosing period. The terminal mercury concentrations in the kidney and liver were 318 and 32 parts/10^6 respectively and 4.6 and 2.0 parts/10^6 were found respectively in the walls of the ileum and large colon. There was negligible mercury in the brain.

Gross pathological findings were most marked in the large colon, the wall of which was markedly oedematous. The kidneys were pale and enlarged but of normal consistency. Macroscopically, there was extensive fatty infiltration of the urinary tubular epithelium and dystrophic changes in the tubular epithelium of various nephrons with presence of hyaline casts and foci of interstitial fibrosis and mononuclear inflammatory infiltration. The mucosa of the oedematous large intestine was dystrophic but not necrotic nor ulcerated and neutrophils and protein coagula were plentiful in distended submucosal lymphatics. There were no lesions in the oral cavity.

The main cause of the clinical deterioration of the animal appeared to be the persistent diarrhoea and possibly intestinal malabsorption, although the persistent but mild renal tubular injury could well have contributed significantly to sudden terminal circulatory failure.

Comparative aspects

The blood organic and inorganic mercury levels, as the case may be, of the three horses given comparable daily doses of methyl-, phenyl- and inorganic Hg respectively, are set out in Figure 60.1. It can be assumed that both the organic forms of mercury were virtually completely absorbed from the upper portion of the lower alimentary tract[32]. The simultaneous appearance of inorganic mercury in the blood indicates that with both types of organomercurial, breakdown of the C–Hg bond rapidly occurs after absorption but to a very much greater degree with the aryl Hg than with the short-chain alkyl compound. The latter compound tends to persist and accumulate in the animal, associated at the same time with a gradual increase in the blood inorganic Hg levels.

Although in the horse dosed with phenyl Hg signs of renal injury were present somewhat sooner and the terminal kidney inorganic mercury levels were 187–339 parts/10^6 as compared with 21 parts/10^6 in the methyl Hg horse, the renal lesions in the latter animal were much more severe and chronic in character than with the former animal. This suggests that for a given dose rate of Hg, methyl Hg itself appears much more toxic for the kidney of the horse for reasons that are not clear than does inorganic mercury. Substantial concentrations of methyl Hg (18 parts/10^6) were found in the kidney of the methyl Hg-dosed horse while in the aryl Hg-dosed animal no organic Hg at all was found. Both the pathological changes and the

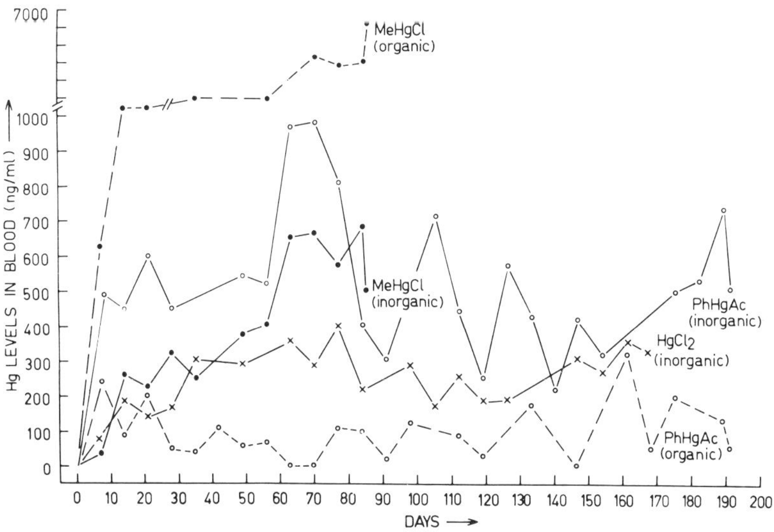

Figure 60.1 Blood levels of organic and inorganic mercury in three horses dosed orally with ≈ 0.4 mg Hg/kg body weight daily of methylmercury (MeHgCl), phenylmercury (PhHgAc) and mercuric chloride ($HgCl_2$)

terminal concentrations of mercury (about 300 parts/10^6) in the kidneys in both the $HgCl_2$- and aryl Hg-dosed horses were similar indicating that inorganic and aryl mercurialism are essentially the same form of mercurialism from the viewpoint of renal injury. In other respects, however, the form of mercurialism in the aryl Hg-dosed horse (chemical stomatitis and ptyalism) was severe. This lesion might well have been due to a direct effect of inorganic Hg formed from the aryl Hg in the mouth on the oral tissues but such lesions can occur whatever the route of intake of Hg compounds, and circulating blood inorganic Hg levels in the latter horse were persistently much higher than those in the $HgCl_2$-dosed animal (Figure 60.1) in which such lesions were absent.

Notwithstanding the severity of the lesions due to aryl Hg in the upper alimentary tract, there were no significant injurious effects in either structure or function of the lower alimentary tract, in spite of the relatively high levels of inorganic Hg found in the tissues of the caecum and colon (26–124 parts/10^6).

In the $HgCl_2$-dosed horse on the other hand, there were comparatively marked lesions in the large intestine while in the colon wall there was only 2 parts/10^6 of Hg. If the latter lesions were due, in fact, directly to the daily Hg dose, then possibly this was the result of a directly irritant effect of the unabsorbed part of the dose still present in the luminal contents on the large intestinal mucosa.

It has been suggested that injury caused by methyl Hg to neurons of the central nervous system and dorsal root ganglia might be due to intracellular dealkylation of organomercurial absorbed into the cell to inorganic mercury which then exerts a toxic effect on the cytoplasmic components[8]. For example, in the horse of the present series dosed with methyl Hg, the terminal feature of the intoxication was mainly peripheral sensory neuropathy. The levels of methyl- and inorganic Hg in the dorsal root ganglia were 8000 and 1600 mg/g, respectively, while in the cerebellum, for example, the respective levels of organic and inorganic Hg were 10 000 and 300 parts/10^6. This suggested that the apparent greater degree of dealkylation of methyl Hg to inorganic Hg in the dorsal root ganglia explained the greater degree of injury in the latter tissues as compared with that which occurred in the vulnerable areas of the central nervous system.

The inorganic Hg levels in the dorsal root ganglia of the horses dosed with aryl Hg and $HgCl_2$, however, were 3000 and 4000 ng/g respectively. Neither animal had any sign of peripheral neuropathy nor other neurological condition, nor were there any histopathological changes in the latter tissues. It appears therefore, that substantial levels of inorganic Hg can be deposited in the dorsal root ganglia simply by the process of perfusion, these tissues being without the blood–brain barrier, and that the comparatively high concentrations of inorganic Hg found there in methylmercurialism simply reflected high circulating inorganic Hg levels. It seems reasonable to presume, therefore, that changes found in CNS neurons and dorsal root ganglia cells are due to direct toxic effects of the alkyl Hg itself.

Inorganic mercurialism with respiratory complications

Considering the differing syndromes which resulted from dosing horses with 0.4 mg Hg $kg^{-1} day^{-1}$ both as inorganic $HgCl_2$ and phenyl Hg acetate, a further study was carried out using a single animal given the higher oral dose rate of 0.8 mg Hg $kg^{-1} day^{-1}$ as $HgCl_2$. The stated objective of the study was, in particular, to determine if the renal changes due to prolonged dosing with the compound were in fact reversible upon withdrawing of the compound[37].

The $HgCl_2$ dose was administered daily for 98 days and then withdrawn. During the first week of dosing the respiratory rate increased. Respiratory difficulty progressed until by 7 weeks there was marked reduction in excercise tolerance, wheezing and abdominal breathing without cough or nasal discharge. A symmetrical alopecia with skin encrustations appeared, extending from the thoracolumbar region caudally, down the flanks towards the stifles. Appetite became reduced.

After withdrawal of the $HgCl_2$ the clinical condition progressed with the appearance of transient lower limb oedema. By day 126 there was profound dyspnoea and hyperpnoea even at rest, muscular weakness, distended jugular veins and increased pulse rate. The animal became dull, anorexic, dehydrated and unwilling to move but there was no diarrhoea, nor oral or dental lesions.

The horse showed proteinuria from days 84 to 112 and glucosuria from days 42 to 133, with a normocytic, normochronic anaemia from day 70. Terminally, there was an increase of blood urea nitrogen. At necropsy the lungs were enlarged and congested and contained numerous, pale, tumour-like foci. The latter were also present in the liver and kidneys, which were enlarged, pale and more friable than normal. Histologically, the tumour-like nodules consisted of granulation tissue containing foci of caseation, giant cells, epithelioid cells, lymphocytes and neutrophils. In the lungs there was a diffuse granulomatous reaction, with interstitial fibrosis and alveolar epithelialization and desquamation of swollen pneumocytes, and emphysema. In the kidneys there was an interstitial granulomatous reaction similar to that seen in the lungs and tubular epithelial dystrophy, nephronal atrophy, casts, tubular necrosis, calcification and interstitial fibrosis. Foci of typical granulation tissue were seen in the bone marrow. No micro-organisms could be detected in these lesions.

The animal had a disseminated granulomatous disease very similar to that reported in cattle fed grain treated with the alkoxyalkylmercurial fungicide 'ceresan'[18]. The condition continued to be progressive, notwithstanding cessation of daily $HgCl_2$ dosing.

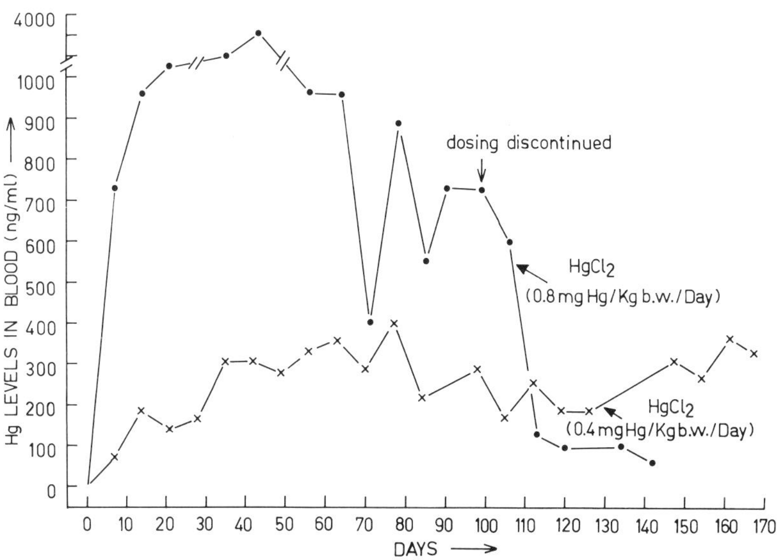

Figure 60.2 Blood levels of mercury in two horses dosed orally with 0.8 and 0.4 mg Hg/kg body weight daily as mercuric chloride. The lower dose rate animal is the same as in Figure 60.1

The progressive mercury levels for this animal compared with the earlier animal dosed with 0.4 mg Hg $kg^{-1}day^{-1}$ are shown in Figure 60.2. The concentration of Hg rose to very high levels within the first week, suggesting that, compared with the other horses given $HgCl_2$ as well as those given organomercurials, absorption of the Hg was exceptionally high. Possibly there were gastrointestinal lesions due to parasites present which might have facilitated absorption of Hg in such large amounts and perhaps even in particulate form, to account for the widespread foreign body-type granulomatous reactions. The Hg levels in the kidney were 93 parts/10^6, notwithstanding an elapse of 44 days since the last $HgCl_2$ dose. Hg levels in the lungs were negligible at 0.5 parts/10^6 and in the liver the concentration was 12 parts/10^6. A satisfactory explanation of the mechanism of the latter syndrome is not available but it is possible that the condition had an immunological basis, and that the reaction in this animal was individual, initiated by an unusually enhanced Hg absorption. Mercury is well known to give rise to immunopathological reactions in some individuals[42] and hypersensitivity in some strains of animals[34].

CONCLUSION

This review of equine heavy metal intoxications reveals that almost all of these diseases are far from completely understood. Given the sporadic nature of these intoxications, it is unlikely that large scale comprehensive studies designed to give clear and detailed pictures of their epidemiology and clinicopathological features will ever be justified. Detailed studies, however, of experimental intoxications of individual animals, as were carried out with mercurials above, should always be possible and will continue to play a valuable role in furthering our knowledge of naturally occurring episodes of heavy metal-induced diseases in horses as they arise. Metal–metal and various nutritional interactions will, of course, also continue to complicate these intoxications such that appreciation of all the factors involved in any particular outbreak of poisoning may often be difficult, if not impossible to attain.

References

1. Ammerman, C. B., Miller, S. M., Fick, K. R. *et al.* (1977). Contaminating elements in mineral supplements and their potential toxicity: a review. *J. Anim. Sci.*, **44,** 485–508
2. Aronson, A. L. (1972). Lead poisoning in cattle and horses following long-term exposure to lead. *Am. J. Vet. Res.*, **33,** 627–9
3. Bauer, M. (1975). Copper sulphate poisoning in horses. *Veterinarski Arhiv*, **45,** 257–8
4. Brink, M. F., Becker, D. E., Terrill, S. W. *et al.* (1959). Zinc toxicity in the weanling pig. *J. Anim. Sci.*, **18,** 836–42
5. Buck, W. B., Osweiler, G. D. and van Gelder, G. A. (1976). In *Clinical and Diagnostic Veterinary Toxicology*. 2nd Edn., p. 287. (Dubuque, Iowa: Kendall Hunt Publishing Co)
6. Burrows, G. E. (1981). Lead toxicosis in domestic animals: a review of the role of lead mining and primary lead smelters in the United States. *Vet. Hum. Toxicol.*, **23,** 337–43
7. Burrows, G. E., Sharp, J. W. and Root, R. G. (1981). A survey of blood lead concentrations in horses in the North Idaho lead/silver belt area. *Vet. Hum. Toxicol.*, **23,** 328–30
8. Cavanagh, J. B. (1973). Peripheral neuropathy caused by chemical agents. *Crit. Rev. Toxicol.*, **2,** 365–417
9. Clarke, E. G. C. and Clarke, M. L. (1975). In *Veterinary Toxicology*. pp. 37, 81–5 and 95–100. (London: Bailliere, Tindall)
10. Crinion, R. A. P. and O'Connor, J. P. (1978). Selenium intoxication in horses. *Irish Vet. J.*, **32,** 81–6
11. Derivaux, J. and Liégeois, F. (1962). In *Toxicologie Vétérinaire*. pp. 131–5. (Liege: Desoer)
12. Dollahite, J. W., Rowe, L. D. and Reagor, J. C. (1975). Experimental lead poisoning in horses and Spanish goats. *Southwest Vet.*, **28,** 40–5

13. Dollahite, J. W., Younger, R. L., Crookshank, H. R. *et al.* (1978). Chronic lead poisoning in horses. *Am. J. Vet. Res.*, **39,** 961–4
14. Edwards, C. M. (1942). Mercurial poisoning in a horse as a result of eating treated oats. *Vet. Rec.*, **54,** 5
15. Egan, D. A. and O'Cuill, T. (1970). Cumulative lead poisoning in horses in a mining area contaminated with galena. *Vet. Rec.*, **86,** 736–8
16. Elinder, C. G., Stenstrom, T., Piscator, M. *et al.* (1980). Water hardness in relation to cadmium accumulation and microscopic signs of cardiovascular disease in horses. *Arch. Environ. Health*, **35,** 81–4
17. Fitzgerald, W. J. (1979). Selenium toxicosis. *Equine Pract.*, **1,** 3, 6
18. Fujimoto, Y., Ohshima, K., Satoh, H. *et al.* (1956). Pathological studies on mercury poisoning in cattle. *Jap. J. Vet. Res.*, **4,** 17–31
19. Fullerton, P. M. (1966). Chronic peripheral neuropathy produced by lead poisoning in guinea pigs. *J. Neuropath. Exp. Neurol.*, **25,** 214–36
20. Graham, R., Sampson, J. and Hester, H. R. (1940). Results of feeding zinc to pregnant mares and to mares nursing foals. *J. Am. Vet. Med. Assoc.*, **97,** 41–7
21. Hammond, P. B. and Aronson, A. L. (1964). Lead poisoning in cattle and horses in the vicinity of a smelter. *Ann. N.Y. Acad. Sci.*, **3,** 595–611
22. Hammond, P. B. and Beliles, R. P. (1980). In Doull, J., Klassen, C. D. and Amdur, M. O. (eds.) *Toxicology, the Basic Science of Poisons.* 2nd Edn., pp. 428–35. (New York: Macmillan)
23. Hultine, J. D., Mount, M. E., Easley, K. H. *et al.* (1979). Selenium toxicosis in the horse. *Equine Pract.*, **1,** 57–60
24. Hupka, E. (1955). Über Flugstaubvergiftigungen in der Umbegung von Metallhütten. *Wein. Tierärztl. Wschr.*, **42,** 763–75
25. Knight, H. D. and Burau, R. G. (1973). Chronic lead poisoning in horses. *J. Am. Vet. Med. Assoc.*, **162,** 781–6
26. Knott, S. G., McCray, C. W. R. and Hall, W. T. K. (1958). Selenium poisoning in horses in North Queensland. *Queensland J. Agric. Sci.*, **15,** 43–58
27. Kowalczyk, D. F., Naylor, J. M. and Gunson, D. (1981). Thc valuc of zinc protoporphyrin in equine lead poisoning. A case report. *Vet. Hum. Toxicol.*, **23,** 12–15
28. Leuthold, A. (1963). Zur Kenntnis der Quecksilbervergiftung beim Pferd. *Schweiz. Arch. Tierheilk.*, **105,** 668–72
29. Messer, N. T. (1981). Tibiotarsal effusion associated with chronic zinc intoxication in 3 horses. *J. Am. Vet. Med. Assoc.*, **178,** 294–7
30. Miller, W. T. and Williams, K. T. (1940). Minimal lethal dose of selenium as sodium selenite for horses, mules, cattle and swine. *J. Agric. Res.*, **60,** 163–73
31. Miller, W. T. and Williams, K. T. (1940). Effect of feeding repeated small doses of selenium as sodium selenite to equines. *J. Agric. Res.*, **61,** 353–68
32. Nordberg, G. F. and Skerfving, S. (1972). In Friberg, L. and Vorstal, J. (eds.) *Mercury in the Environment. An Epidemiological and Toxicological Appraisal.* pp. 29–91. (C.R.C. Press)
33. Pico, R. (1936). Intossicazione di Mercurio. *Clin. Vet. (Milano)*, **59,** 401–4
34. Polák, L., Barnes, J. M. and Turk, J. L. (1968). The genetic control of contact sensitization to inorganic metal compounds in guinea pigs. *Immunology*, **14,** 707–11
35. Roberts, M. C., Ng, J. C. and Seawright, A. A. (1978). The effects of prolonged daily low level mercuric chloride dosing in a horse. *Vet. Hum. Toxicol.*, **20,** 410–15
36. Roberts, M. C., Seawright, A. A. and Ng, J. C. (1979). Chronic phenylmercuric acetate toxicity in a horse. *Vet. Hum. Toxicol.*, **21,** 321–7
37. Roberts, M. C., Seawright, A. A., Ng, J. C. *et al.* (1983). Some effects of chronic mercuric chloride intoxication on renal function in a horse. *Vet. Hum. Toxicol.*, **24,** 415–20
38. Sass, B., Hatziolos, B. C. and Hayes, J. E. (1972). Probable cadmium poisoning in a group of ponies. *Vet. Med./Small Anim. Clin.*, **67,** 745–6
39. Schmidtt, N., Brown, G., Devlin, E. L. *et al.* (1971). Lead poisoning in horses. An environmental health hazard. *Arch. Environ. Health*, **23,** 185–95
40. Seawright, A. A., Roberts, M. C. and Costigan, P. (1978). Chronic methylmercurialism in a horse. *Vet. Hum. Toxicol.*, **20,** 6–9

41. Seddon, H. R. (1951). In *Diseases of Domestic Animals in Australia, Tick and Mite Infestations.* Part 3, pp. 35–50. (Canberra: Commonwealth Department of Health)
42. Shull, R. M., Stowe, C. M., Osborne, C. A. *et al.* (1981). Membranous glomerulonephropathy and nephrotic syndrome associated with iatrogenic metallic mercury poisoning in a cat. *Vet. Hum. Toxicol.*, **23,** 1–5
43. Stewart, A. K. and Magee, A. C. (1964). Effect of zinc toxicity on calcium, phosphorus and magnesium metabolism of young rats. *J. Nutr.*, **82,** 287–95
44. Stowe, H. D. (1980). Effects of copper pretreatment upon the toxicity of selenium for ponies. *Am. J. Vet. Res.*, **41,** 1925–8
45. Walthall, J. C. and McKenzie, R. A. (1976). Osteodystrophia fibrosa in horses at pasture in Queensland: field and laboratory observations. *Aust. Vet. J.*, **52,** 11–16
46. Willoughby, R. A., McDonald, I., McSherry, B. J. *et al.* (1972). Lead and zinc poisoning and the interaction between Pb and Zn poisoning in the foal. *Can. J. Comp. Med.*, **36,** 348–59
47. Willoughby, R. A., Thirapatsakun, T. and McSherry, B. J. (1972). Influence of rations low in calcium and phosphorus on blood and tissue lead in the horse. *Am. J. Vet. Res.*, **33,** 1165–73
48. Willoughby, R. A. and Oyaert, W. (1973). Zinc poisoning in foals. *Vlaams Diergeneesk. Tijdschr.*, **42,** 134–43
49. Wilson, G. L., Osweiler, G. D. and Garner, H. E. (1979). Experimental induction and review of lead toxicity in a Shetland pony. *J. Eq. Med. Surg.*, **3,** 386–90

61
Evaluation of subclinical lead poisoning in dairy cattle

L. Pinault and G. Milhaud

Numerous reports dealing with cattle poisoning by lead are evidence that this element is widely spread in the environment and reveal the predisposition of such animals to be affected due both to the composition of their diet and feeding.

Increasing awareness over the last decades of the danger presented by this heavy metal to all species, including man, has enabled both its use and release in the environment to be progressively reduced. However, its elimination from contaminated areas has been prevented by its high environmental stability.

The development of lead pollution has been followed in the vicinity of an important lead-ore processing factory in an agricultural region of northern France. At first, acute, often lethal intoxications predominated. Then, as the polluting emissions of the factory decreased, chronic intoxications became more common and more difficult to diagnose[19]. Over recent years, release of lead into the atmosphere has practically ceased following the installation of efficient emission–retention systems (in 1977, the average atmospheric concentration in the surroundings was 1.3 mg lead/m^3 of air). However, lead deposited upon and accumulated in the soil constitutes a permanent source of contamination of plants harvested in such areas. This justifies the regular measurement of plant lead concentrations in order to divert from animal feeds all plants containing excessive lead.

Control of polluting discharges and surveillance of lead concentrations in vegetation have contributed to the disappearance of conventional forms of bovine lead poisoning from the region. Nevertheless, certain cattle breeders still suspect lead intoxication in animals with either poor zootechnical performances or obscure outbreaks of nervous disorders, especially in the period following calving, for which the aetiology could not be sufficiently clarified. As lead involvement cannot be disregarded *a priori* because of its ubiquity, there is a need to experimentally evaluate the effects of small doses of lead on the health of animals bred in such an environment in order to predict the economic prospects of cattle breeding in this region.

A series of surveys were first conducted on the affected farms to evaluate as precisely as possible the actual exposure of the animals to lead[21] and to appraise the wholesomeness of their products, especially of milk[22]. Experimental studies followed, one to measure the effects of lead on meat[20] and the other on milk production. The results of the latter study which is currently under progress and planned to encompass a period of 2 y is the subject of this report.

MATERIALS AND METHODS

Animals

Studies were carried out on 34 Holstein cows weighing about 620 kg each and allotted in two series, A of 24 cows and B of 10 cows. In each series the cows were divided into two equal groups of experimental (E) and control healthy (C) animals. The experimental animals from series A were fed lead for 24 weeks from the 7th month of gestation to the 3rd month of lactation; cows from series B received lead for 13 weeks in the period of lactation.

As it has been well demonstrated that the various lead compounds are not absorbed through the digestive mucosa with the same efficiency and therefore feature different toxicity levels[1], we elected, as in a previous study[20], to administer a mixture approaching that of industrial spoils of purified lead products of well-defined composition. Lead was administered at 1.5 g/cow daily as a mixture of PbO, $PbCl_2$, $PbSO_4$ (30/30/40) incorporated in a concentrated feed. Both experimental and control animals were fed mainly grass or corn-silage.

Experimental design and sample collection

Cows were weighed weekly, while food intake and milk production were recorded daily.

Samples of feeds and milk were collected periodically for determination of their lead content. Blood samples were also collected periodically with sodium heparin for determination of lead and haematological variables.

Lead concentrations in feeds and milk were determined by atomic absorption spectrophotometry after dry ashing at 500 °C. Blood lead concentrations were determined by an amperometric anodic stripping method (ESA 3010 A). The European standardized method[4] was used to assay blood Δ-aminolevulinic acid dehydratase (ALAD) activities. Blood samples were cooled at + 4 °C immediately after collection and stored at − 20 °C when the assay was conducted with a delay exceeding 24 h but always shorter than 7 days). Zinc protoporphyrin concentration was measured with a haematofluorometer (ESA ZnP 4 000). Packed cell volume was determined by centrifugation of blood in microtubes; reticulocyte counts and haemoglobin concentrations were determined with a Coulter counter.

RESULTS - COMMENTS

Exposure level

At the end of the 24 week experiment, animals E of the A series had received a total dose of 232.5 g of lead given at a rate of 1.6 mg/kg over the first 6 weeks and then at 2.4 mg/kg the following weeks. The dose corresponded to the ingestion of a ration containing 100 parts/10^6 of lead while that of the reference animals contained only 1–2 parts/10^6.

This contamination level of 100 parts/10^6 is definitely higher than that of the maximum lead content present in simple animal food and fixed by the EEC[9] and French[3] rules at 10 parts/10^6 (in food brought to a moisture content of 12%) with an exception for green fodder for which the tolerance is 40 parts/10^6. This value is close to that measured during the preliminary enquiry conducted on the cattle breeding farms of the northern France region referred to in the foregoing[21] and is also close to that measured in fodders harvested in the vicinity of highways[6]. It is lower than the 300 parts/10^6 usually considered as likely to cause clinical bovine lead poisoning after a few weeks. As expected, no animal displayed any pathological signs attributed to lead poisoning in these studies.

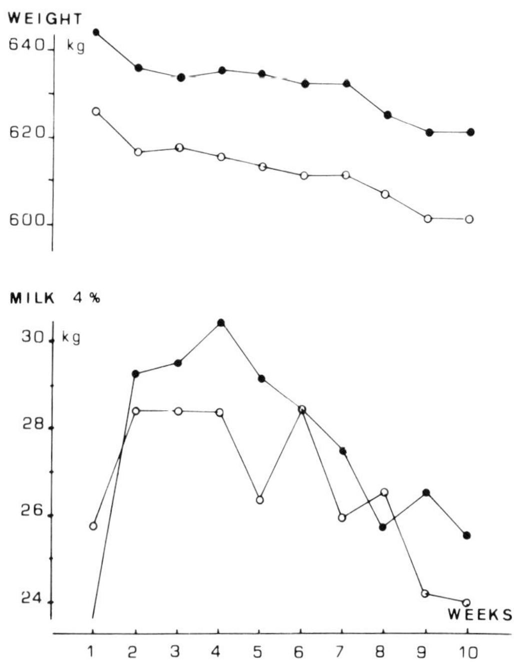

Figure 61.1 Variations in body weight and milk production from cows in series A during the first weeks of lactation. Each point represents the average value for the group of E lead-fed (•) and C control (○) animals

Production results

Examination of the results for cows of the A series (Figure 61.1), during the 10 weeks following the beginning of the lactation process, shows that no significant difference existed between groups E and C, as far as body weight and milk production were concerned. Similarly, no significant differences were found in the B series between groups E and C. Thus, a ration containing 100 parts/10^6 of lead fed over a period of 24 weeks to dairy cows did not modify their food consumption nor their weight gain or milk production rates. This dose was approximately five times greater than that administered by other authors, also without effect[31].

Contamination of the milk

The average lead concentration of the milk samples taken weekly from the combined production of the cow herd was 32.6 ± 18.3 parts/10^9 (standard deviation). Account was taken of the dilution factor of 2 due to the milk of the reference animals which contained a quantity of lead generally lower than the detection threshold of the applied technique (10 parts/10^9). The lead concentration in milk was close to that mentioned in other studies, i.e. 70 parts/10^9 from cows fed for 4 weeks with fodder containing 100 parts/10^6 of lead[6], 10–70 parts/10^9 from a ration containing 9–30 parts/10^6 of lead fed over a time period of 2 weeks[29], and 30–200 parts/10^9 in the milk of animals whose blood lead content reached 87 μg/100 ml[22]. In the latter study, it was concluded that no risks were presented to the consumers, as the maximal acceptable dose determined by the WHO (3 μg/week) cannot be attained with consumption of normal amounts of such milk.

Blood lead concentrations

The increase in the blood lead content in both the A and B cows occurred early in the studies (Figure 61.2 (a)). The maximum average value reached, but did not exceed, the 'critical' threshold of 35 μg/100 ml. This maximum value was reached in the 13th week for group B, and in the 19th week for group A. The extreme individual values measured beyond the lactation period reached 50 μg/100 ml in some animals. After a rapid increase over the first 4 weeks, a plateau can be noted at the period corresponding to calving for animals of the A series.

Systematic blood sampling around calving of seven pairs of E and C animals of the A series showed a transient increase in lead concentrations with a maximum around the 4th day (Figure 61.2 (b)). This variation is evidence of mobilization of lead stored in the organism and can be attributed to the beginning of lactation. In fact, it coincides with the expansion phase of milk secretion and resulting important calcium demands. Initially, this increased calcium demand is essentially covered by an endogenous source, the skeleton. The increase in intestinal calcium absorption occurs later. This observation is in full agreement with others performed on mice showing the

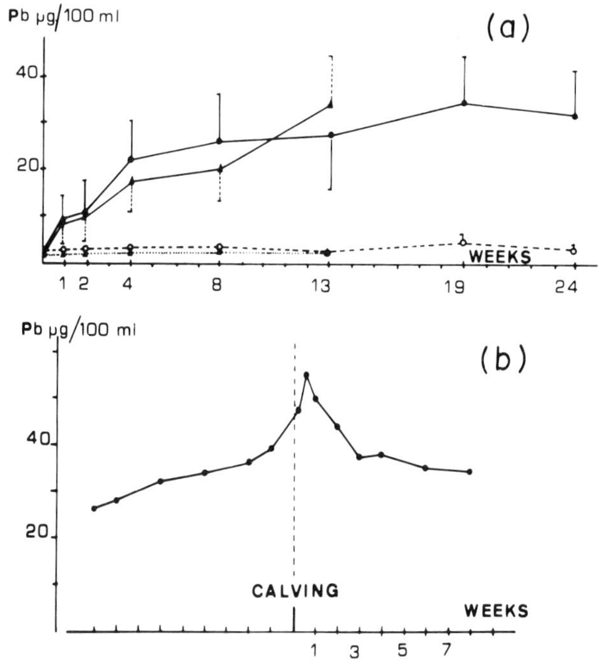

Figure 61.2 (a) Blood lead concentrations. Each point represents the average value ±sd for the group of lead-fed cows from series A (•) and B (▲) and control animals from series A (○) and B (△). (b) Blood lead concentrations around calving. Each point represents the average value of lead concentrations measured in seven cows from series A fed with the 100 parts/10^6 lead contaminated ration

mobilization of lead from the skeleton during the lactation phase and its transfer into the milk[15]. One may wonder, then, about the extent of this transfer and its consequences on animals subjected to greater lead exposure. Perhaps this phenomenon is the source of nervous clinical signs similar to certain symptoms of the hypocalcaemic puerperal syndrome.

The analysis of calf blood at birth has confirmed previous observations of lead transplacental transfer in this species. The lead content for cows of lot E at calving was $36.6 \pm 15.9\,\mu g/100$ ml and that of their calves of 6.5 ± 4.2 $\mu g/100$ ml while that of the reference animals was 3.25 ± 2.9 and 1.15 ± 0.36 $\mu g/100$ ml, respectively in cows and calves. The relationship between these pairs of values is described by the regression line shown in Figure 61.3 (a), the regression coefficient $r = 0.65$ being significant at the 1% level.

ALA dehydratase (ALAD)

The activity of blood ALAD, measured under optimum conditions for human blood, was low, similarly to what has already been reported in bovines[8,20]. Its value in unexposed animals ranged around 6 nmol ALA (ml erythrocyte)$^{-1}$ min^{-1}. This decrease in activity has been observed as early as

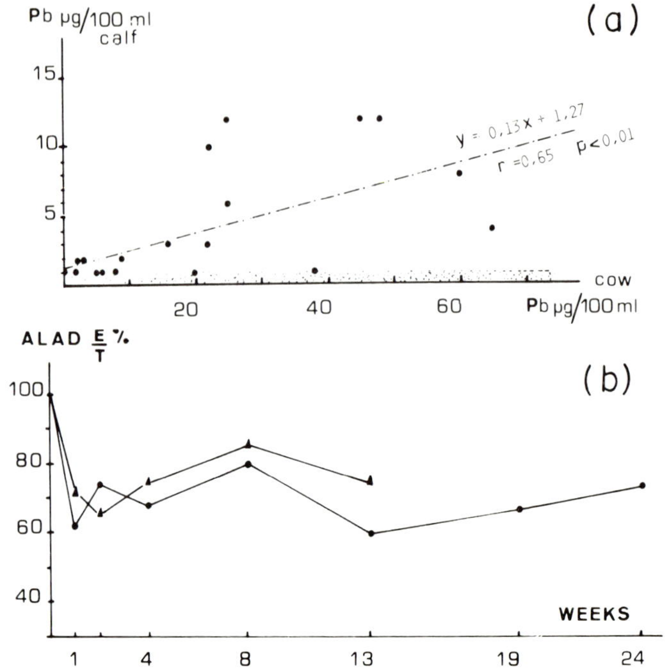

Figure 61.3 (a) Relationship between blood–lead concentrations of cows and of their offspring. The detection limit of the method (1 μg/100 ml) is indicated by the stippled zone. (b) Blood ALA dehydratase activities. Each point represents the average % activities of bloods from lead-fed cows (E) in series (A) (●) and B (▲) in comparison to controls at the same time

the first week[31]. It accompanies the increase in blood lead concentration, evidence of its direct action on this erythrocyte enzyme (Figure 61.3 (b)). The degree of suppression of ALAD activity was moderate, the blood of exposed animals maintaining 60–80% of the activity of that of the reference animals. This is of a magnitude which has previously been reported, i.e. 70% for higher blood lead concentrations (70 μg/100 ml)[23], 50–70% for practically sound bovines[27], and 66% for calves chronically intoxicated over a period of 3 months and exhibiting blood lead concentrations between 20 and 100 μg/100 ml[11]. Contrary to what has been reported in sheep exposed to small quantities of lead for a period of 15 weeks[10], no tendency for the recovery of partial activity was noted.

Zinc-protoporphyrin (ZPP)

The average ZPP concentrations in the blood of each E and C lot (Figure 61.4 (a)) became significantly different only after the 13th week. A significant increase in ZPP rate of production was observed after an average lead content of 30 μg/100 ml was attained, which is in conformity with observations

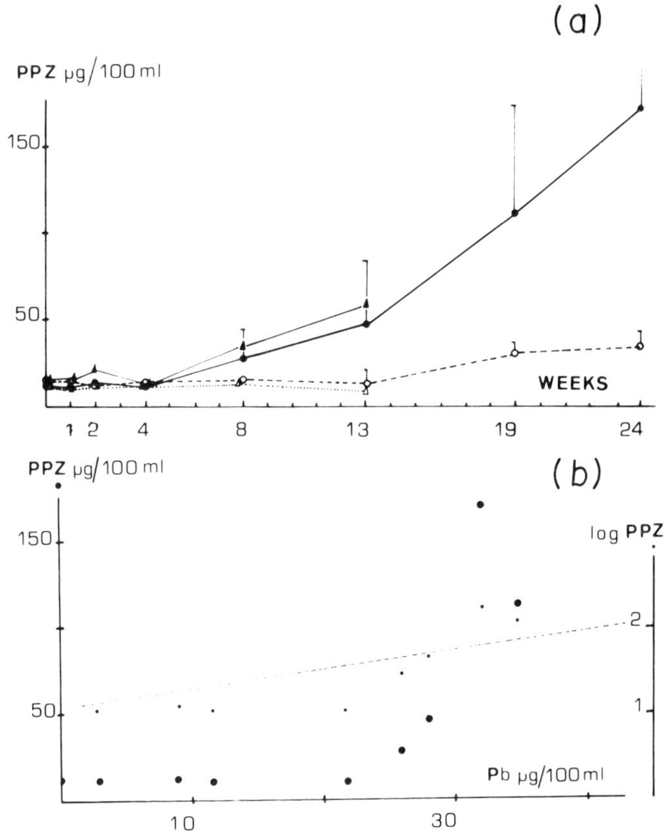

Figure 61.4 (a) Zinc-protoporphyrin (ZPP) concentrations. Each point represents the average value ± sd for lead-fed cows in series A (●) and B (▲) and for control cows in series A (○) and B (△). (b) Relations between blood ZPP concentrations and blood lead levels. Each point figures a pair of average values measured at different sample-collection times over the 24 weeks of lead intake in blood of lead-fed cows from the series A

made on man[7,18]. In the A series, it continued to increase until the end of the exposure period (24th week). Great variation in the results was observed, as shown by the standard deviations indicated on the curve. The maximum individual value was 330 μg/100 ml.

Several studies have been devoted to the measurement of total protoporphyrin in animals and to the appraisal of its diagnostic value[11,25,26,31]. However, only a few authors have used the ZPP test to trace lead poisoning in animals[16,27], while many publications have demonstrated an interest in this method in man as a means of estimating the rate of production of erythrocyte protoporphyrins[17,27]. Their increased concentration in blood results essentially from the inhibition by lead of ferrochelatase, a mitochondrial enzyme which, in the immature erythrocyte prior to its passage from the bone marrow to blood, enables iron-fixing into IX protoporphyrin to forme haem. A minimum time of 1 week is therefore necessary to observe the consequences of this medullary action of lead in peripheral blood. Free erythrocyte protoporphyrin combines to the greatest extent with zinc to form a stable ZPP complex bound to globin for the lifetime of the erythrocyte. It displays a fluorescence different from that of other porphyrins, thus enabling its direct analysis in diluted blood by spectrofluorimetry[16] or, more simply, in a drop of blood with a haematofluorimeter[5,13]. In man, where more than 90% of the protoporphyrins appear as ZPP, the measurement of the concentration of the latter constitutes a valid estimation of the former. This test has now been used for several years in various countries as a mean of tracing lead poisoning. In animals and especially in cattle, the proportion of ZPP appears to be smaller and was initially qualified as minor[24]. It has subsequently been determined to be between 50 and 70%. This poorer representation is a drawback but is off-set by the great simplicity of measurement with a haematofluorimeter, as long as the proportion of protoporphyrin complexes as ZPP is constant. Appraisal of this question by high performance liquid chromatography[12,28,30] is currently under study.

Other blood values

No significant differences were observed between the E and C lots in either reticulocyte count (5.5–6.5 millions/mm^3) or haematocrit (33–38%), which were within the ranges of normal variation. These results are in agreement with the established fact of an absence of haematologic changes due to blood lead concentrations lower than 35 μg/100 ml[15].

CONCLUSION

The preliminary results of this study, which is still in progress, show that a rate of 100 parts/10^6 of lead administered for a period of 24 weeks in the diet of dairy cows does not alter their health or production. The initiation of the lactation process, however, appears to be accompanied by mobilization of the previously stored lead. The effect of this on postpartum pathology would be worthy of study.

The change in lead and blood ALA dehydratase concentrations occurs early, the amplitude of the latter remains small in bovines. The increase in blood ZPP is delayed at this level of exposure. It appears only when the blood lead concentration reaches a value near 30 μg/100 ml. The measurement of ZPP, made very easy by the use of a haematofluorimeter and definitely well suited to measurement of many individuals, is a test whose validity needs to be better evaluated in animals.

References

1. Allcroft, R. (1951). Lead poisoning in cattle and sheep. *Vet. Rec.*, **63**, 583–90
2. Aronson, A. L. (1971). Biologic effects of lead in domestic animals. *J. Wash. Acad. Sci.*, **61**, 110–13

3. Arrêté Ministériel of 29 May, 1980. J.O. Rep. Française of 26 June, 1980 p. N.C. 5515
4. Berlin, A. and Schaller, K. H. (1974). European standardised method for the determination of δ-aminolaevulinic acid dehydratase activity in blood. *Z. Klin. Chem. Klin. Biochem.*, **12**, 389–90
5. Blumberg, W. E., Eisinger, J., Lamola, A. A. *et al.* (1977). The hematofluorometer. *Clin. Chem.*, **23**, 270–4
6. Bovay, E. (1970). Le dépôt de plomb sur la végétation le long des autoroutes. Essai d'affouragement des vaches laitières avec du foin souillé par du plomb. *Travaux de Chimie alimentaire et d'Hygiène*, **61**, 303–21
7. Chisolm, J. J. (1978). Heme metabolites in blood and urine in relation to lead toxicity and their determination. *Adv. Clin. Chem.*, **20**, 225–65
8. Dion, A. (1982). Etude de l'activité de l'acide δ-aminolévulinique dehydratase chez les bovins: son application dans le dépistage du saturnisme. *Thèse Doct. Vét.*, Créteil
9. Directive 76/934 C.E.E. of 1 December, 1972. J.O. COMM. n° L/364/20 of 31 December, 1972
10. Fassbender, C. P. and Rang, H. (1975). Experimentelle subklinische Bleivergiftung bei Schafen enzymatische, chemische und morphologische Untersuchungen. *Zbl. Vet. Med.*, **22A**, 533–48
11. George, J. W. and Ducan, J. R. (1981). Erythrocyte protoporphyrin in experimental chronic lead poisoning in calves. *Am. J. Vet. Res.*, **42**, 1630–7
12. Gotelli, G. R., Wall, J. H., Kabra, P. M. *et al.* (1980). Simultaneous liquid chromatographic determination of zinc protoporphyrin IX, protoporphyrin IX and coproporphyrin in whole blood. *Clin. Chem.*, **26**, 205–8
13. Grandjean, P. (1979). Occupational lead exposure in Denmark: screening with the haematofluorometer. *Br. J. Med.*, **36**, 52–8
14. Hammond, P. B. (1977). Exposure of humans to lead. *Ann. Rev. Pharmacol. Toxicol.*, **17**, 197–214
15. Keller, C. A. and Doherty, R. A. (1980). Bone lead mobilisation in lactating mice and lead transfer to suckling offspring. *Toxicol. Appl. Pharmacol.*, **55**, 220–8
16. Kowalczyk, D. F., Naylor, J. M. and Gunson, D. (1981). The value of zinc protoporphyrin in equine lead poisoning: a case report. *Vet. Hum. Toxicol.*, **23**, 12–15
17. Lamola, A. A., Joselon, M. and Yamane, T. (1975). Zinc protoporphyrin (ZPP): a simple sentitive fluorometric screening test for lead poisoning. *Clin. Chem.*, **12**, 93–7
18. Meredith, P. A., Morre, M. R. and Goldberg, A. (1979). Erythrocyte δ-amino levulinic acid dehydratase activity and blood porphyrin concentrations as indices of lead exposure and altered heme biosynthesis. *Clin. Sci.*, **56**, 61–9
19. Milhaud, G. and Pinault, L. (1977). Le saturnisme animal. *Symbiose*, **9**, 45–55
20. Milhaud, G., Mialot, M., Pinault, L. *et al.* (1978). Evaluation expérimentale de la toxicité du plomb pour les bovins. *Rec. Méd. Vét.*, **154**, 943–9
21. Milhaud, G., Pinault, L. and Parent, B. (1979). Résultats d'observations effectuées sur des bovins élevés dans une zone polluée par des émissions industrielles de plomb, zinc et cadmium. *Rec. Méd. Vét.*, **155**, 955–62
22. Milhaud, G. and Enriquez, B. (1981). Elimination du plomb par le lait chez les bovins. *Rec. Méd. Vét.*, **157**, 291–6
23. Osweiler, G. D. and Ruhr, L. P. (1978). Lead poisoning in feeder calves. *J. Am. Vet. Med. Assoc.*, **172**, 498–500
24. Penton, Z. and Bissell, G. (1978). Some factors affecting the utility of bovine blood as a control material in lead screening programs. *Clin. Chem.*, **24**, 504–6
25. Rolton, Ch. E., Horton, B. J. and Pass, D. A. (1978). Evaluation of tests for the diagnosis of lead exposure in sheep. *Austr. Vet. J.*, **54**, 393–7
26. Roscoe, D. E., Nielsen, S. W., Eaton, H. D. *et al.* (1975). Chronic plumbism in rabbits: a comparison of three diagnostic tests. *Am. J. Vet. Res.*, **36**, 1225–9
27. Schwartz, S., Stephenson, B., Sarkar, D. *et al.* (1980). Quantitative assay of erythrocyte "free" and zinc-protoporphyrin: clinical and genetic studies. *Int. J. Biochem.*, **12**, 1053–7
28. Scoble, H. A., McKeag, M., Brown, Ph. R. *et al.* (1981). The rapid determination of erythrocyte porphyrins using reversed-phase high performance liquid chromatography. *Clin. Chim. Acta*, **113**, 253–65

29. Sharma, R. P. and Street, J. C. (1980). Public health aspects of toxic heavy metals in animal feeds. *J. Am. Vet. Med. Assoc.*, **177**, 149–53

30. Smith, R. M., Doran, D., Mazur, M. *et al.* (1980). High performance liquid chromatographic determination of protoporphyrin and zinc protoporphyrin in blood. *J. Chromatogr. Biomed. Applic.*, **181**, 319–27

31. Street, J. C., Raghib, M. H., Sharma, R. P. *et al.* (1977). The influence of low level lead exposures on free erythrocytic porphyrin and blood and liver δ-amino levulinic acid dehydratase in three species of food-producing animals (summary). *Toxicol. Appl. Pharmacol.*, **41**, 151–2

62
Poisoning of animals in the Los Angeles area with pesticides (1981)

K. T. Maddy, S. Edmiston and J. Wellings

The Los Angeles County Medical Association Regional Poison Information Center (LACPIC) receives more than 45 000 telephone calls each year concerning exposure to many different type of chemicals, including pesticides. The majority of these calls are from physicians providing treatment to exposed persons. A small number of calls involve animals; most of these calls are from veterinarians trying to identify active ingredients when they have only been told of a trade name by an animal owner. It is not always clear from the poison centre reports whether serious poisoning actually occurred or whether the incident involved a low level exposure warranting concern and/or precautionary measures.

A study was conducted of 268 pesticide exposure incidents involving animals reported to the LACPIC in 1981. Most of the reported exposure incidents involved dogs (83%) with ingestion being the major route of exposure. It is thought that cats are exposed less frequently because of their selective eating habits. It was apparent that anticoagulants (25%), *N*-methyl carbamates (15.3%), organophosphates (11.9%) and a combination of *N*-methyl carbamates and organophosphates (2.2%) were the main single sources of reported poisonings. This has been the trend for the last several years.

The active ingredients involved in most of the anticoagulant exposures were diphacinone, warfarin, and pival. All products involved were used as rat and mouse baits.

The majority of exposures to the *N*-methyl carbamates involved carbaryl, propoxur and methiocarb, used to kill insects, slugs and snails in the home and garden situation. The organophosphates involved in these exposure incidents were primarily diazinon, DDVP, disulphoton and malathion. Most of these exposures also occurred in the home and garden setting.

Other pesticides were involved in a low incidence of exposure/poisonings; these included arsenicals (mostly ant poisons, 4.5%), metaldehyde (5.6%),

Table 62.1 Pesticides commonly involved in dog poisoning incidents in California with signs and suggested treatment

Pesticides	*Signs*	*Treatment*
Anticoagulants Coumarin types, Warfarin and Coumafuryl	Haemorrhage; sudden death without warning. In subacute cases, anaemia, weakness, pale mucous membranes; dyspnoea; moist rales; bloody faeces; scleral, conjunctival and intraocular haemorrhage; staggering, ataxia, blood tinged froth around mouth and nose; CNS signs appear if haemorrhage is in brain or spinal cord.	Sedation or light anaesthesia to prevent trauma; oxygen therapy, citrated whole blood i.v., thoracentesis to remove blood (if present), vitamin K, i.v. in dextrose. Keep animal warm and free from physical trauma for at least 24 h. Oral vitamin K for 4–6 days is indicated.
1,3 indandione types, Diphacinone and Pindone	Signs similar to coumarin effects plus signs of cardiopulmonary and neurologic damage.	Same as for coumarins.
Arsenic	Acute: Intense abdominal pain, staggering, extreme weakness, trembling, salivation, vomiting, diarrhoea fast-feeble pulse, normal to subnormal temperature, collapse and death. Subacute: Anorexia, depression, watery diarrhoea, increased urination followed by aurea, partial paralysis of hind limbs, stupor; subnormal temperature and eventual death.	Treatment must be administered early. Give emetics, epigastric lavage only if symptoms are not yet present. If signs are present, give BAL (dimercaprol) at the rate of 6–7 mg/kg body weight i.m. 3 times daily until recovery. Give supportive therapy for additional signs such as dehydration and uraemia. May also need antibiotics and meperidine if need is indicated.
N-Methyl Carbamates (i.e. carbaryl, propoxur, and methiocarb)	Acetylcholinesterase depression, hypermotility, abdominal cramping, vomiting, diarrhoea, sweating, dyspnoea, cyanosis, miosis, muscle twitching (in extreme cases, tetany followed by weakness and paralysis) and convulsive seizures. Death is usually a result of hypoxia due to bronchoconstriction.	Atropine sulphate (approximately 2 mg for an average dog). 2-PAM is supportive for most *N*-methyl carbamates; it is contraindicated only for treatment of carbaryl poisoning.
Metaldehyde	Muscle weakness, frothing at the mouth, hypersalivation, incoordination, tachycardia, loss of consciousness, cyanosis, and often convulsion. Death usually follows respiratory failure.	Emetics, gastric lavage, supportive treatment for respiratory stimulation, glucose and calcium gluconate for treatment of possible liver damage. It is often necessary to anaesthetize the animal to control convulsions.
Organochlorines (i.e. methoxychlor, lindane, toxaphene)	Apprehension, hypersensitivity, as spasms of the eyelids and front quarters progressing to the hind quarters; these may be continuous to intermittent/chlonotonic seizures, loss of coordination, circling frontwards or backwards and abnormal posturing. Animal may become comatose.	Convulsions should be controlled by anaesthetizing with chloral hydrate, or a long-lasting barbiturate. If exposure was oral, administer a gastric lavage and saline cathartic. Tranquillizing agents are often successful in controlling violent neuromuscular activity.
Organophosphates (i.e. malathion, diazinon, DDVP)	Hypersalivation; gastrointestinal hypermotility, abdominal cramping, vomiting, diarrhoea; sweating, dyspnoea; cyanosis; miosis, muscle twitching (in extreme cases, tetany, followed by weakness and paralysis), convulsive seizures. Death is usually a result of hypoxia due to bronchoconstriction.	Atropine sulphate (approximately 2 mg for an average dog); 2-PAM is useful as supportive treatment.

pyrethrins/pyrethroids (5.6%), and organochlorines (methoxychlor, dicofol, lindane, and toxaphene, 2.2%). In previous years (prior to 1980) there had been many reported poisonings of dogs involving the rodenticide Vacor. However, in 1981 none were reported; California suspended the registration of Vacor for home use in 1979 because of its hazard to man.

More than 75% of the incidents were reported during the period of June through September. Presumably this is the period when more pesticides are applied in the home and garden situation and/or the period of time when domestic animals spend more time outdoors. Table 62.1 gives signs and recommended treatment for pesticide poisonings in animals.

DISCUSSION

As recently as 15 y ago arsenic, strychnine and phosphorus were major causes of domestic animal poisonings in California. Since then, most of the urban uses of these three pesticides have been phased out; they are rarely involved in poisoning incidents now. Less than 10 y ago thousands of dogs were being poisoned in California by ingesting slug and snail baits containing metaldehyde. Regulatory action, initiated by the California Department of Food and Agriculture (CDFA) and later adopted by the US Environmental Protection Agency, required the reformulation of these baits to be less attractive to dogs. Changing from pellets to meals and the use of less palatable inert ingredients was followed by a significant reduction in the number of poisonings. Because of carelessness of some home gardeners (leaving bait containers where pets can get into them and applying baits in piles where dogs frequent) and the non-selective eating habits of some dogs, some serious metaldehyde poisoning cases still occur. Carefully complying with the precautionary statements on the labels and the use of child-proof and thus dog-proof containers could further reduce the number of poisonings of dogs. A summary of the pesticide exposure cases in animals reported to the LACPIC in 1981 is provided in Table 62.2.

Recently some snail baits have been formulated with *N*-methyl carbamates (methiocarb, carbaryl) as the active ingredients. The *N*-methyl carbamates (esters of *N*-methyl carbamic acid) are a fairly new entity as a cause of large numbers of poisonings in dogs. These *N*-methyl carbamates are now widely used in home and garden type pesticides. However, in comparing the 1981 exposure incidence with that in 1977, a possible downward trend is observed. In 1977, there were 79 cases reported while only 52 cases involving *N*-methyl carbamates (alone or in combination with other pesticides) were reported in 1981. Follow-up summaries in the next few years should reveal whether there is an actual decline in *N*-methyl carbamate poisonings. In 1981, products containing propoxur (Baygon) accounted for approximately 71% of the cases involving *N*-methyl carbamates. Exposure to the more toxic *N*-methyl carbamates can be serious and should be treated quickly with adequate amounts of atropine. *N*-methyl carbamate poisonings may be mistakenly attributed to organophosphate exposure due to the similarity of signs and symptoms and the response to treatment. Both types of pesticides are

Table 62.2 Poison exposure incidents involving 268 animals classified according to toxic ingredient responsible for the poisoning. In brackets, total number of cases

Anticoagulants (60 dogs, 4 cats, 2 rabbits, 1 cow)
- Crown Rat and Mouse Killer with (Diphacinone)
- D-Con rodenticides (warfarin and/or dicoumarol): 16 dogs
- Dicumarol (brand not specified)
- Diphacinone (brand not specified)
- Eaton's A-C Formula 50 Ready-To-Use Rodenticide (pival)
- Eaton's All Weather Bait Blocks Rodenticide (diphacinone)
- Fumarim (coumafuryl) (brand not specified)
- PC-2 Rodenticide (diphacinone)
- Pival (brand not specified)
- Ramik Green Rat Poison (diphacinone)
- Rodenticides (ingredient not specified): ten dogs
- Rodeth Throw Pack Mouse Killer
- Rozol Product (chlorophacinone)
- Strike Rat and Mouse Killer (warfarin and sulphaquinoxline)
- Talon rodenticide (brodifacoum)
- Warfarin (unknown brand)

Arsenicals (11 dogs, 1 cat)
- Antrol Ant Killer
- Ant stakes (brand not specified): five dogs
- Arsenic (brand not specified)
- Grant's Ant Stakes: four dogs

Metaldehyde (14 dogs, 1 horse)
- Corry's Slug and Snail Death
- Snail and Slug bait (brand not specified)
- Snarol Pellets: ten dogs, one horse

N-*Methyl carbamates* (34 dogs, 4 cats, 1 rabbit)
- Antrol Ant Traps with Baygon: eight dogs
- Baygon (brand not specified): two cats
- Black Flag Liquid Ant and Roach Killer (propoxur)
- Chacon Ant Poison (carbaryl)
- Echol's Roach, Ant and Waterbug Killer (propoxur)
- Ficam (bendiocarb)
- Flea powder (carbamate)
- Fly bait (methomyl)
- Mesurol (methiocarb)
- Methomyl (brand not specified)
- *N*-methylcarbamate (brand not specified)
- Ortho Earwig, Roach & Sowbug Bait (propoxur)
- Ortho Slug-geta Snail and Slug Bait (methiocarb)
- Sevin (carbaryl)
- Sergents Pump Dog Flea & Tick Spray (carbaryl)
- Slug and snail bait (mesurol)
- TAT Ant Trap (propoxur)

Organochlorines (6 dogs)
- Black Flag Insect Spray (methoxychlor, lethane 384-R)
- Dexol Red Spider Mite Spray (dicofol)
- Dieldrin
- Last Bite (lindale, toxaphene)
- Methoxychlor (brand not specified)
- Roach Away (paradichlorobenzene)

Table 62.2 (continued)

Organophosphates (20 dogs, 10 cats, 1 goat, 1 turtle)
DDVP (dichlorvos)
Diazinon (brand not specified): three dogs, five cats
Di-Syston (disulphoton)
Dursban 4E (chlorpyrifos)
Germain's Rose Guard (disulphoton)
Hartz 2-in-1 Flea Powder (tetrachlorovinphos)
Malathion (brand not specified): five dogs
Mr. Scott's Do It Yourself Pest Control (diazinon)
Ortho Dibrom Fly & Mosquito Spray (naled)
Ortho Lawn Insect Spray (chlorpyrifos): one turtle
No-Pest Strip Insecticide (DDVP)
Spectracide (diazinon): two dogs, one goat
Zodiac Pro-Dip II (Imidan)

N-*Methyl carbamates and organophosphates* (5 dogs, 1 cat)
Holiday Fogger (propoxur, DDVP): two dogs
Lannate, Nudrin, parathion (brands not specified)
Raid Ant and Roach Killer (propoxur, DDVP)
Starbar Super Golden Malrin Fly Bait (propoxur, DDVP)

Phenoxy herbicides (2 dogs, 1 cat)
Scott's Turf Builder Plus 2 (2,4-D): one cat
Scott's Weed Control (2,4-D, dicamba)
Trimec (2,4-D, MCPP, dicamba)

Pyrethrins and pyrethroids (9 dogs, 4 cats, 1 rabbit, 1 mouse)
Black Flag House and Garden Insect Killer (cismethrin, allethrin)
Hartz Mountain Flea Soap for Dogs
Hartz Mountain RID Flea Dog Shampoo
Holiday Puppy and Kitten Spray
Pyrenone 606
Pyrethrins: three dogs, one cat, one rabbit
Raid House and Garden Bug Killer: one mouse
R and C Spray Insecticide

Miscellaneous (46 dogs, 9 cats, 2 cows)
Ant Trap
Big Stinky Fly Trap
Black Flag product
Boric acid
Calico Weed Killer (petroleum hydrocarbons)
Cyanide
Liquid Lawn Disease Control (tetrachloroisophthalonitrile and chlorothalonil)
Dexol Contact Week Killer (petroleum hydrocarbons)
D-trans Allran P-68 insecticide
Dodecadienoate
Echol's Flea and Tick Spray
Eptam
Ezell's Sheep Dip (cresol)
Fly bait
Flea dip (brand not specified)
Fumigant (brand not specified)
Hartz Flea and Tick Spray
Holiday Fly Repellant
Methyl bromide
Ortho Funginex (triforine)
Ortho Isotox

Table 62.2 (continued)

Miscellaneous (continued)
Ortho Kleen-Up (glyphosate)
Ortho Vegetable Dust (captan)
Paramite (benzylbenzoate, rotenone, lindane)
Paraquat
Penguin-Down Dri-Die (ammonium fluosilicate)
Petro Sheep Dip
Piperine
Rotenone
Roundup (glyphosate)
Sheep dip (cresylic acid)
Simazine (atrazine): two cows
Sodium fluosilicate (brand not specified)
Strychnine (brand not specified)
Triox (prometon, PCP)
Unknown pesticide
Vikane (sulphuryl fluoride)
Weed Out

Multiple pesticides (16 dogs)
Antrol Ant Syrup and Antrol Ant Trap (propoxur)
Chlordane and Sevin
Diazinon, Dursban, malathion, pyrethrins, Sevin
Dinoseb and petroleum hydrocarbons
Dursban and Kill Master
Earwig bait and sodium fluosilicate
Malathion and ant stake product
Ortho flea product and kennel product
Ortho Rose & Flower Care (carbaryl, malathion, folpet, dicofol)
Raid Yard Guard (methoxychlor, tetramethrin)
Roundup and H_2SO_4
Snail Jail Snail & Slug Bait (metaldehyde, carbaryl)

acetylcholinesterase inhibitors. Both types respond well to treatment with atropine and oximes such as 2-PAM, except carbaryl for which oximes are contraindicted. Exposure to organophosphates (alone or in combination with other pesticides) numbered 43 in 1981 as compared to 42 in 1977. Most of these involved dogs; however, nearly one third of the incidents involved cats. This relatively high proportion of feline poisonings may be due to the fact that some organophosphates are readily absorbed through the skin. Dermal contact with recently treated foliage can accumulate enough pesticide residue on the hair and skin to result in poisoning. Organophosphates are widely used in agriculture. In rural and suburban areas organophosphates can be a major source of pesticide poisonings in animals.

The anticoagulant exposure/poisonings were due entirely to ingestion of rodenticides. Large quantities of these products in the form of rodent baits are used in California. However, poisoning usually occurs only after multiple sequential ingestions. For this reason, serious domestic animal poisonings occur less frequently than the statistics of exposure indicate. Many of the reported anticoagulant ingestion incidents appear to be calls for precautionary first aid measures following a single observed ingestion. Dogs, and less often cats, have occasionally become ill from eating a poisoned rodent.

Pyrethrins and pyrethroids (alone or in combination with other pesticides) were involved in 19 reported exposures and/or poisonings. (There were only two reported cases in 1977.) Domestic animal poisonings due to these products are a fairly new phenomena due to the recent introduction and rapidly increasing usage of these insecticides. The pyrethrins and pyrethroids were developed in response to increasing insect resistance to the more toxic organophosphates. As a group these products are relatively low toxicity pesticides and have a low potential for adverse health effects in most mammals.

Some of the ant control products used today still contain arsenicals; these account for most of the reported arsenical-related exposures and poisonings. (The arsenicals in ant poisons are gradually being replaced by other pesticides.) Ant stake products, in particular, seem to be attractive to dogs, probably because of their stick-like form and being put in areas accessible to the dog.

The phenoxy herbicides accounted for five reported exposure incidents in 1981. In 1977, six phenoxy herbicide cases were reported. It was not reported whether any of these cases developed symptoms of overexposure.

As of 1977, the incidence of domestic animal poisonings due to organochlorine exposure appeared to be declining. This is probably due to a decreased use in urban areas. The 1981 data shows a continuance of this trend with six cases compared to 12 in 1977. Exposure to these chemicals can be fatal if not adequately treated.

Not all poisonings were due to accidental exposure. Flea control products for use on cats and dogs accounted for eight cases of poisoning or approximately 3% of the total pesticide cases reported to the LACPIC. Puppies, kittens and weak or diseased animals are most susceptible. Directions on the label should be carefully followed for all pesticide products.

When a pesticide exposure is suspected, the pesticide container or label should be made available to the veterinarian as the toxic ingredients are listed. Also, treatment information for humans required on the labels of the more toxic pesticides, is often helpful in the treatment of animal poisonings.

63
Toxicological field data in ruminants

G. Keck, G. Lorgue and P. Jaussaud

The following informations are derived from (1) incoming calls received by the Centre of Veterinary Toxicology: 1410 telephone calls and 116 written inquiries for 1981, and (2) toxicological analysis completed by the laboratory, including epidemiological surveys, e.g. in acorn intoxication of cattle.

Since January 1980, a specific computer progam allows more efficient utilization and a statistical use of the data. Depending upon the information given, the degree of confidence in the intoxication suspected is measured using a scale from 1 to 6 (0 to 100%).

The species involved in 1980 were ruminants for nearly 40% of the calls (see Figure 63.1). Calves or adults (although the toxics involved are different) largely outnumber sheep and goats. The factors involved are the size of the corresponding herds and the tendency of cattle to eat whatever is 'on hand'.

Main species involved (1980)

	n	%
Bovine	183	29.23
Ovine	53	8.47
Swine	23	3.67
Equine	24	3.83
Goat	13	2.08
Dogs	209	33.39
Cats	28	4.47
Rabbit	5	0.80
Poultry	10	1.60
Other	18	11

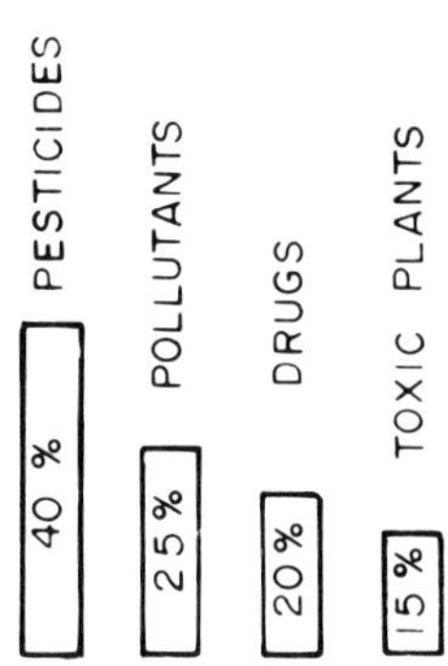

Figure 63.1 Species involved for the incoming calls in 1980 and distribution of the origin of substances during 1981

The severity of intoxications is reflected by the high number of animals involved: 69 calls dealt with more than six cows affected simultaneously and 20 calls for more than six sheep.

The annual distribution of the calls shows a slight drop in January and February when the animals are stabled and a rise in May when they are turned out at pasture. A peak recorded in December corresponds to incidents related to the prophylaxis against cattle grub.

The substances incriminated can be regrouped in four categories: pesticides, pollutants, drugs and plants (Figure 63.1).

PESTICIDES

The circumstances of intoxication for pesticides in 98 cattle, 19 sheep and 13 goats can be regrouped as (1) criminal intoxications (often implied by the farmer, they are rare in stock animals); (2) accidental intoxications (direct ingestion of pesticides, in powder or following dilution, account for the most frequent cause of intoxication, especially in cattle: improperly stocked bags, confusion with mineral additives, distribution of treated seed). The exposure of grazing animals to a pesticidal treatment of nearby fields especially by aerial crop-dusting, or ingestion of contaminated plants or water represent a source of intoxication (highly toxic pesticides such as parathion and other organophosphates, dinitrophenols, paraquat); (3) therapeutically-induced intoxication (after treatment by insecticides like organophosphates, carbamates or pyrethrinoids).

Acaricides-insecticides represent about one third of calls for pesticides in ruminants. Those concerning organochlorines are as important as those for organophosphates and carbamates. Recent photostable derivatives of pyrethroids, such as decamethrin, can be responsible for intoxications in calves because of a toxicity higher than that of pyrethrins.

Herbicides are also frequently implicated, due to a rather large use of these products for all types of culture including artificial pastures. In many cases, suspicions were not confirmed, due to the low toxicity of the implied agents (aryloxyacids, triazines). However, ruminants in field conditions are more susceptible to such intoxications than are laboratory animals. Unfortunately, clinical symptoms are not very characteristic and verification by analyses is difficult to carry out, contrarily to characteristic intoxications by dinitrophenols and paraquat.

Indirect toxicity of phytohormones due to the ingestion of treated plants seems linked to the increase in the amount of toxic substances (nitrates). A rise in appetence for toxic plants (fern, buttercups) and the abundant outcrop of plants resistant to herbicides (pig-weed, black night-shade), especially in feeding-corn, are to be considered.

Fungicides are rarely involved, except for colloidal sulphur; its ingestion in great amount (100 or 200 g per cow) is followed by tetanic symptoms.

Among other pesticides, coumarinic raticides are not frequently implicated in ruminants. Collective intoxications after the consumption of metaldehyde contained in mollucide bags were recorded. Finally, many questions concerning pesticides deal with the possibility of longterm effects of residues found in hay, forage and animal feed, in order to explain chronic disturbances. Knowledge in this area is poor as far as domestic animals are concerned.

POLLUTANTS

Copper (mineral complements overly charged in copper or ingestion of copper sulphate) and lead (lead paint ingestion) dominate this heterogenous group: lead (211 calls for cattle) and copper for sheep (17 calls, 24 positive analyses) and to a lesser extent, young cattle.

Intoxications caused by petrol derivatives and by the ingestion of fertilizers are sometimes seen in cattle. Nitrates in drinking water seem also of importance. Epidemiological data indicate that replacing drinking water by tap water largely improves the health, thus suggesting some longterm effects of nitrates and nitrites on the reproduction of domestic animals in the field.

DRUGS

Internal anthelmintics are frequently implied, especially in cattle; they represented 44.6% of the calls in 1980 and 28.8% in 1981. Among them, tetramisole, largely used for the treatment of strongyloses, is responsible for the greatest proportion of accidents in both cattle and sheep. In contrast, levamisole is rarely implied (only one call in 1980 and 1981).

Among the accidents observed with the 'pour-on' method of treatment against cattle-grub, immediate or late effects seem to be of allergic nature. The use of avermectin since 1981 is responsible for similar reactions.

Antimicrobial drugs represent another group for which intoxications are recorded. Nervous disorders and haemorrhagic lesions are recorded in calves with nitrofurans, especially furazolidone. In a recent case among 2400 intoxicated animals, 600 died as a result of the drug in feed. Dapsone can be also responsible for nervous disorders in calves.

Antibiotics were implied in 85 cases of allergic reactions within 3 y in cattle in the centre of France.

TOXIC PLANTS

Vegetal intoxications exhibited a regional as well as a seasonal origin in ruminants, especially during the periods of drought as in 1976.

The following plants are found: *Mercurialis*; *Taxus* (trimmings left on pastures); fern (*Pteridis aquilina*, especially when pastures derive from forest land); oenanthe (after tilling of ditches which exposes the toxic rhizomes); and acorn (especially in the central region of France).

Mycotoxins seem frequently implied for poorly observed feed but confirmation remains difficult, even in the case of hepatic fibrosis and ascites.

This overview of some intoxications in ruminants is not intended to be exhaustive but reflects fairly well the relative importance of different toxic sources in the field (pesticides, pollutants, drugs, etc.). Experimental data do not take into account the possible influence of the behaviour of the animals, the interaction of different chemical agents, and the indirect toxicity. Comparison between experimental data and field observation thus appears of paramount importance to elucidate the relevance of such environmental factors.

64
Adverse drug reactions and interactions (1979–1981)

Y. Ruckebusch

The 1200 adverse reactions to antibiotics reported in cattle by Brisbane in Alberta[2] referred to anaphylaxis with dispnoea, slobbering, staggering and collapse (90%), urticaria with swelling of the eyelids (5%) and pain at the injection site (3%). Stowe[11] also described anaphylactoid reactions to parenteral injection of antibiotics (University of Minnesota). Ndiritu and Enos[9] reviewed 130 cases of suspected adverse drug reactions (Veterinary Medical Teaching Hospital of Davis) and attributed 31.8% of the reactions to anti-infective agents, e.g. dyspnoea after a repeated dose of oxytetracycline hydrochloride intramuscularly in 15 of 150 calves and fatal toxicosis in a cow following an overdose of 25 mg/kg.

The complaints received from practitioners at the INRA Pharmacology–Toxicology Research Centre of Toulouse involved unpredicted reactions produced in animals by drugs used at the recommended dose, unpredicted modification of the effect of one drug by the presence of another, or clinical accidents. The information given by the practitioners included: (1) clinical diagnosis and drug used; (2) circumstances surrounding the adverse effect; and (3) comments on subsequent clinical experience in order to distinguish intolerance and effects related to overdosage from increased responsiveness due to age and/or disease.

CLASSIFICATION OF REACTIONS

The percentage of reactions of all types was 18.6 in the bovine ($n = 1085$) in 1979. No fundamental changes were recorded in 1980 and 1981. Local response and anaphylaxis seemed to be the most commonly encountered reactions in large animals. As described by Franciosi[5], they concern antibiotics, parasiticides to a lesser degree, and corticosteroids. In companion animals, anaesthetics were frequently involved, the percentage of death being 12% in dogs as compared to 3.8% in cattle (Figure 64.1).

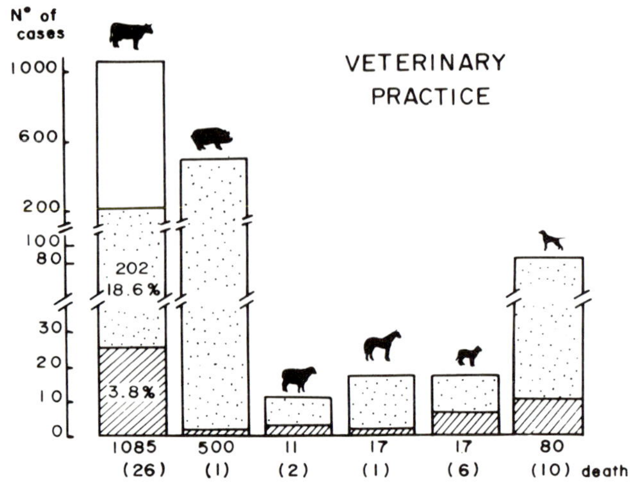

Figure 64.1 Percentages of adverse reactions (dotted area) and death (hatched area) which were reported in 1979 by practitioners, relative to 17 horses, 97 dogs or cats, 500 pigs and 1085 dairy cows or heifers and 11 sheep

Antibiotics

Intolerance consisted of abcesses (15–20 days after i.m. administration in calves), signs of local pain (after i.p. spiramycine in pigs, i.m. chloramphenicol in horses) and dyspnoea and recumbency following intrauterine administration of polymixin and oxytetracycline 15 days after calving. Two lactating cows suffering from mastitis in one quarter of the udder showed signs of mammary pain following an i.m. injection of spiramycin.

Anaphylactic shock was manifested in cows by pruritus and oedema of the udder, vulva and eyelids (after intramammary administration of colistin, spiramycin and prednisone), in heifers by ptyalism and bloating (for 6 h, 30 min following i.v. chlortetracycline), and in bullocks by dyspnoea and pulmonary oedema (within 2 min following i.v. oxytetracycline; within 10 min following i.m. oxytetracycline and phenylbutazone). Oedema and fatal shock were reported after a second injection of neomycin, oxytetracycline, trimethoprim and sulphadimethoxine 3–6 days following a similar dosage.

Adverse reactions were observed in horses (diarrhoea) and in cats (prostration) on the third day of oral administration of oxytetracycline; depression and dehydration were also reported with daily administration of 60 mg/kg of chloramphenicol for 10 days in cats. Interactions of antibiotics with barbiturates were prolongation of anaesthesia in dogs of about 6 h following an i.v. administration of doxycycline and an increase in anaesthesia duration of 30% after chloramphenicol.

Diarrhoea, apathy and anorexia were the predominant features before death within 48 h of 14 horses and within 3 months of 21 horses which had received a premix containing oxytetracycline, sulphadimethoxine and furazolidone and of 13 horses (five within 48 h and nine within 1.5 month) which had received a premix containing oxytetracycline and sulphadiazine. As already described by Andersson *et al.*[1], the prominent autopsy findings in horses that died spontaneously were acute catarrhal to haemorrhagic typhlitis and colitis, acute necrotizing nephrosis, and degenerative changes in the myocardium. It is also probable that the biliary excretion of oxytetracycline was involved in the long-lasting effect[3], including abnormal bacterial flora (e.g. *Clostridium perfringens* liberation of toxins from these microbes).

Parasiticides

In cattle, dyspnoea is a common side-effect following the administration of s.c. anapirin or i.m. berenil used for the treatment of tick-born diseases. Two injections of anapirin at 48 h intervals in the pregnant cow are used for the prevention of neonatal diseases, of placental retention and metritis. The second injection is always followed within 2–3 h by transient abdominal pain and by a yellow colour of the neonate. This effect is prevented by diluting anapirin 7–8 times with saline. Among the reactions following i.m. injection of lomidine or s.c. injection of oxopirvedine in dogs, paralysis of the mandible and glaucoma during 8–10 days were recorded. They were possibly associated with the use of corticosteroids, antihistamines and penicillin–streptomycin in an attempt to correct these side-effects of the antiparasiticides.

Fatalities and anaphylactic shock with sublingual oedema and rhinitis lasting 3–4 days were observed after the administration of the combination of tetramisole bithionol in cattle. Dyspnoea, ptyalism and oculopalpebral oedema (and bloating in sheep) occurred for 1 h after levamisole administration in heifers. Fatal cases were observed when chloramphenicol and a fluke vaccine were concomitantly administered. The side-effects of levamisole observed in young calves recently turned out to pasture were never found after a second injection 1 month later.

Anti-inflammatory agents

In dogs, aggressiveness was an unexpected interaction of metoclopramide and corticosteroid. The i.v. injection of chloramphenicol + prednisolone in heifers was followed by dyspnoea and respiratory distress which lasted from 30 min to 2–3 h. Anaphylactic reactions were reported in cattle receiving dexamethasone for joint diseases. The use of an antibiotics–corticosteroid mixture in calves suffering from (coccidiosis) diarrhoea is highly detrimental.

In a 6-year-old lactating cow, i.m. phenylbutazone resulted in abomasal ulcer within 48 h. Gastric ulcer was observed after longterm treatment with indomethacin, keratoconjunctivitis after noramidopyrine in dogs.

Anaesthetics

Ketamine hydrochloride, at a dosage in cats of 20 mg/kg body weight, may be accompanied by hyperkinesis and convulsions; the concomitant administration of ether was found to be detrimental. In dogs and horses, i.v. xylazine at a dosage of 1 mg/kg was associated with cardiac irregularities, apnoea and muscular rigidity. Increased susceptibility to penthiobarbitone was observed in horses undergoing phenylbutazone treatment. Susceptible pigs succumbed 2–3 h after an halothane-induced hyperthermia syndrome. The hyperthermic response to inhalation of the anaesthetic was greater during the springtime than in autumn in 3-month-old pig. An acaricide containing a local anaesthetic induced ataxia and circling for 2–3 h after being inserted in the auricular canal.

Miscellaneous

Four types of adverse reactions were reported on at least three occasions: (1) anaphylactic shock in cattle and horses after i.m. injection of vitamins A, D_3 and E, and sodium selenite + vitamins, and in bitches after the second injection of gonadotrophin for metritis; (2) haemolytic anaemia in calves after 5 days treatment with sulphadimethoxine; (3) haematuria after hydroxyquinoline was administered to dogs; and (4) abortion following the parenteral administration of prostaglandin $F_{2\alpha}$ to cows or by calcium in combination with methionine and vitamins or sodium lactate in 8-day-old calves.

MECHANISM OF ACTION

Many factors might be involved in an unexpected reaction to drug administration. It is essential to list them all to minimize their occurrence and for the resulting increased knowledge in the pharmacology of altered functions. The reactions may be (1) of an allergic type, i.e. the drug or a metabolite of the drug was combined with a body protein to form an antigen; (2) side-effects not sufficiently deleterious in a healthy animal but enhanced for different reasons during disease; (3) an abnormal susceptibility related to individuals or to interactions of drugs; and (4) misuse of the drugs by overdosage or obsolescence leading to toxicity (Figure 64.2).

Local or systemic anaphylactic reaction

Hypersensitivity can occur to the drug or an excipient such as carboxymethylcellulose; procaine and potassium ion for penicillins have been studied in cattle[6] and discussed by Marshall[7]. Reactions to procaine benzyl penicillinate were seen in cows after intramammary administration[8].

Reaction to levamisole was confirmed by skin tests in allergic and non-allergic sheep, the urticarial weal diameters being made readily visible by

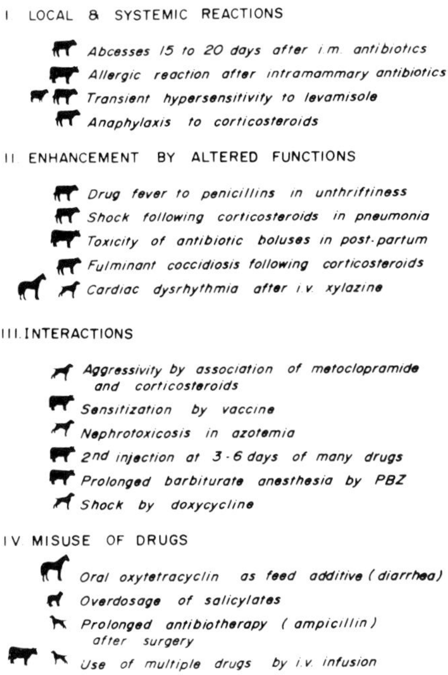

Figure 64.2 Mechanism of adverse drug reactions in veterinary medicine

previous injections of about 5 ml of 2% Evans blue. Reticular contractions stopped for 2–3 h after intradermal injection in susceptible sheep (unpublished observation). For corticosteroids, allergic reactions observed in cattle, 20–90 min after an injection of a suspension of prednisolone, were not linked to the carboxymethylcellulose carrier[10]. Calves and adults suffering from adrenocortical insufficiency were never involved, indicating the importance of age in such reactions.

One of the most detailed observations was the absence of a levamisole reaction in calves during August, whereas these animals always exhibited shock when receiving levamisole in June just after being turned out to pasture. This seasonal reaction is interesting when compared to the high susceptibility of pigs to halothane during the springtime.

Finally, sensitization to drugs was enhanced following treatment with vaccine and by administration at weekly intervals. The concomitant use of serum and antibiotics like colistin or chloramphenicol should be avoided.

Enhancement by altered functions

Nitrofuran derivatives were found detrimental in calves suffering from diarrhoea, even with a low dosage (5 mg/kg body weight). Higher dosages caused additional problems: anorexia (10 mg/kg), hyperirritability and convulsions (20 mg/kg) and hind-limb paralysis (25 mg/kg). Ampicillin and other antibiotics are only accompanied by drug fever in animals suffering from unthriftiness. Infusion of prednisolone and chloramphenicol caused a shock lasting only 10–15 min in calves suffering from pneumonia. Various types of antibiotic boluses may be toxic following calving due to an increased absorption of toxins from the uterus. Routine postpartum treatment of cows with antibiotics following calving resulted in a high incidence of pyometra due to *Corynebacterium pyogenes*[12]. A direct toxic effect of oxytetracycline is unlikely at a normal dosage of 5 g intravenously in ruminants. Doses above 7 mg/kg i.v. and 20 mg/kg per os cause reversible nephrotoxicosis in dogs and a Fanconi-like syndrome characterized by nausea, acidosis, proteinuria, glucosuria, and aminoaciduria may be associated with the oral administration of an overdosage or in patients with pre-existing azotemia. Increase in blood urea nitrogen, development of acidosis, electrolyte imbalance, and death may be considered as a direct toxic effect. Disorders of the haemopoietic system due to sulphamides are varied but the incidence seems as high as renal problems in dehydrated calves. Mild haemolytic anaemia may occur after only 5 days of treatment. The severity increases with further drug administrations and return to health is impeded due to aggravation of the original insult. Coccidiosis in calves which is self-limiting can quickly become a disaster with disruption corticosteroids. The bradydysrhythmia potential of xylazine may add to the oculocardiac reflex phenomenon in horses. Ruminants are the most sensitive to the effects of xylazine, requiring only about one tenth the dose to produce the equivalent state of sedation in horses and dogs; however, pre-existing atrioventricular block contraindicates its use for all species (see Appendix).

Interactions

The possibilities for drug interaction are numerous and it is frequently a problem to determine which drug is the culprit when several are being used in one patient. However, one should opt against the use of antibiotics or parasiticides at the time of vaccination and avoid repetitious infusion of many drugs at 6 day intervals. Other interactions are due to the displacement of drugs like barbiturates from plasma proteins by other drugs, such as phenylbutazone and doxycycline. A problem is to differentiate disease effects from drug effect, e.g. in nephrotoxicosis by oxytetracycline during azotemia or to identify the drug involved in behavioural reactions, e.g. aggressiveness due to prednisolone and metoclopramide.

Misuse of drugs

This is self-explanatory but becomes more and more important where several drugs are in use. For example, the use of feed additives containing oxytetracycline for horses is based on tolerance information for rabbits and on misleading labelling, e.g. all species except ruminants. The extrapolation of the canine dose of salicylate results in overdosage in cats.

SIGNIFICANCE OF DRUG REACTIONS

The counterpart of drug effectiveness is the incidence of clinical accidents. The factors contributing to the reports of side-effects and interactions as well as adverse drug reactions are (1) the great number of potent drugs available to practitioners and the practice of administering more than one drug to a patient; (2) lack of knowledge concerning the pharmacology of drug used and failure to set a therapeutic end-point, producing overdose effects; and (3) administration of useless drugs and ignorance of predisposing factors in both health and disease[4].

Difficulties in recognizing adverse drug reactions are numerous in practice, especially for the longterm effect of some drugs. The reluctance to consider that treatment may aggravate the patient's condition and the irrational use of multiple drugs in states of emergency are other reasons. On the other hand, some adverse non-drug reactions may be misinterpreted as drug effects, especially for the interactions between drugs like hormones and the nutritional state, e.g. lack of trace elements like copper. Any type of adverse effect, including direct toxicity, overdosage, allergy as the result of antigen–antibody combination, side-effects, and interactions between drugs should be avoided. Acute observation of unusual drug effects by alert clinicians is a crucial component of the process of tracking down the cause of adverse reactions (see References 13–20).

To summarize, in weighing the risk–benefit balance before prescribing, the following approach to therapeutics should be a professional obligation.

(1) Avoid multiple drug therapy and be aware of any previous drug administration by the owner.

(2) Limit intravenous infusions to the drugs you are thoroughly familiar with and after careful clinical examination.

(3) Have on hand appropriate single drugs like antihistamines, corticosteroids and aspirin-like drugs with which to treat acute allergic reactions.

References

1. Andersson, G., Ekman, L., Mansson, I. *et al.* (1971). Lethal complications following administration of oxytetracycline in the horse. *Nord. Vet. Med.*, **23**, 9–22
2. Brisbane, W. P. (1963). Antibiotic reactions in cattle. *Can. Vet. J.*, **4**, 234–5
3. Cook, W. R. (1973). Diarrhoea in the horse associated with stress and tetracycline therapy. *Vet. Rec.*, **75**, 15–17
4. Dunlop, R. H. (1978). Iatrogenic disease versus effective therapeutics. In *The Therapeutic Jungle, The Postgraduate Committee in Vet. Sci., Univ. Sydney, Proc.*, **2**, 1045–75
5. Franciosi, C. (1970). Allergic reactions in adult cattle following treatment with corticosterols. *Vet. Ital.*, **21**, 554–68
6. Leemann, W., de Weck, A. L. and Schneider, C. H. (1969). Hypersensitivity to carboxymethyl-cellulose as a cause of anaphylactic reactions to drugs in cattle. *Nature (London)*, **223**, 621–3
7. Marshall, A. B. (1980). Penicillin: suspected adverse reactions. *Vet. Rec.*, **106**, 207–8
8. Mayr, A. and Bibrack, C. (1980). Drug allergies in cattle. *Berl. Münch. Tierärztl. Wsch.*, **83**, 439–46

9. Ndiritu, C. G. and Enos, L. R. (1977). Adverse reactions to drugs in a veterinary hospital. *J. Am. Vet. Med. Assoc.*, **171**, 335–9
10. Signorini, G. (1969). Anaphylactic reactions in cattle treated with prednisolone. *Nuova Vet.*, **45**, 96–100
11. Stowe, C. M. (1975). Guest editorial: adverse drug reactions. *J. Am. Vet. Med. Assoc.*, **166**, 980–1
12. Whitmore, H. L., Mather, E. C., Hurtjen, J. P. *et al.* (1977). Evaluation of reproductive efficiency in dairy herds on a fertility program. *Proc. Soc. Theriogenol.*, 160–2
13. Eckhoff, G. A. (1980). Mechanisms of adverse drug reactions and interactions in veterinary Medicine. *J. Am. Vet. Med. Assoc.*, **176**, 1131–3
14. Glade, M. J. and Krook, L. (1982). Glucocorticoid-induced inhibition of osteolysis and the development of osteopetrosis, osteonecrosis and osteoporosis. *Cornell Vet.*, **72**, 76–91
15. Griffin, D. D., Morter, R. L., Amstutz, H. E. *et al.* (1979). Experimental oxytetracycline toxicity in feedlot heifers. *The Bovine Pract.*, **14**, 37–40
16. Hoskins, J. D., Hubbert, W. T. and Selig, J. O. (1982). A questionnaire for the clinical assessment of veterinary adverse drug reactions. *Cornell Vet.*, **72**, 3–15
17. Polzin, D. J., Stowe, C. M., O'Leary, T. P. *et al.* (1981). Acute hepatic necrosis associated with the administration of mebendazole to dogs. *J. Am. Vet. Med. Assoc.*, **179**, 1013–6
18. Snow, D. H. (1979). Phenylbutazone toxicity in ponies. *Vet. Rec.*, **105**, 26–30
19. Roberts, M. C. (1982). Adverse effects of indomethacine in the horse. *J. Vet. Pharm. Therap.*, **5**, 83–6
20. Swanson, J. F. and Breider, M. A. (1982). Hepatic failure following mebendazole administration to a dog. *J. Am. Vet. Med. Assoc.*, **181**, 72–3

APPENDIX

Recumbency of 1–2 h duration can result from the i.m. injection of 0.2 mg of xylazine/kg of body weight and anorexia may persist for as long as 24 h in ruminants. An antagonist would be useful for treating accidental overdoses of xylazine and reducing recovery time, thereby eliminating the possibility of bloating, regurgitation.

The combination of 4-aminopyridine (0.3 mg/kg) and yohimbine (0.125 mg/kg) intravenously produces antagonism of xylazine sedation superior to that produced by either agent alone (Kitzman, V., Booth, H., Hatch, C. *et al.* Antagonism of xylazine sedation by 4-aminopyridine and yohimbine in cattle, *Am. J. Vet. Res.*, 1982, **43**, 2165–9). Among the α-adrenergic blocking agents able to antagonize xylazine-induced depression and the forestomach inhibition of central origin, tolazoline was found the most effective at doses of 0.4–1 mg/kg (Toutain, P. L., Zingoni, M. R. and Ruckebusch, Y., Assessment of alpha-2 adrenergic antagonists on the central nervous system using reticular contraction in sheep as a model, *J. Pharmacol. Exp. Therap.*, **223**, 215–8).

Workshop I
Medicated Feed

Chairmen: **M. Lobry**
A. S. J. P. A. M. van Miert

WORKSHOP I
Medicated feed

Chairmen: **M. Lobry and A. S. J. P. A. M. van Miert**

Since 1950, The use of medicated feeds has become an integral part of livestock production. The term *medicated feeds* is defined in the Official Journal of the European Communities n° C41/³–1982 as any mixture of one or more veterinary medicinal products and one or more feedingstuffs which is prepared prior to being put into circulation and which, because of its prophylactic or therapeutic properties . . . is intended to be fed to animals without alteration. In contrast, the *additives* are substances which, when incorporated in feedingstuffs are likely to affect their characteristics on livestock production. Antibiotics included in a feed at growth promotion and/or feed efficiency levels are drug additives, and feeds containing such antibiotics are not included in the definition of 'medicated feed' category.

low levels: to improve { growth rates in *healthy* animals
(5–15 parts/10^6) { feed efficiency

medium levels: to prevent { infectious disease in *healthy* animals
(50–150 parts/10^6) { stress-induced diseases

high levels: for treatment of *diseased* animals
(350–1000 parts/10^6)

Because of the potential health hazard resulting from incorrect inclusion of feed additives in the feed of animals grown for human consumption or from contamination of feeds with these compounds, it is essential that the additives be properly handled in the feed plant and that the products be adequately controlled and assayed.

In healthy animals feed intake, water consumption, the efficacy of the drug and the pharmacokinetic behaviour of the compound used can be studied, including the extent and the duration of residues in food products obtained from the animals under treatment, and the possible hazards to human health from these residues. From these data, withdrawal times can be calculated. Disease conditions may influence feed intake, water consumption, drug bioavailability and/or tissue uptake, biotransformation and excretion of drugs. Therefore, the registration of medicated feeds intended for the treatment of respiratory and/or gastrointestinal diseases in animals, is much more complicated.

The current good manufacturing practice (GMP) regulations are an attempt by Food and Drug Administration (FDA) to describe basic quality control procedures that are desired for the manufacture of medicated feeds. According to R. A. Wilcox (*Feed Additive Compendium*, 1979, p. 49), medicated feed includes (1) medicated complete feed which is intended to be the sole ration for an animal; (2) medicated supplements which are safe for direct consumption by the use animal and can be offered in a free-choice feeding plan, and (3) medicated concentrates which are mixed with other feed materials to make either a supplement or a complete feed before being offered to the animal. Medicated concentrates are used at levels from 44.6 to 446 kg/tonne of complete feed.

Medicated premixes which are defined as intended for further mixing using less 'than 44.6 kg of premix per tonne of complete feed, do not come under these GMPs'. The high level of drug(s) in premixes requires more rigorous measures*.

The following papers refer to the situation of medicated feeds in French and European legislation (Lobry), to the problems of their usage (van Miert) and manufacturing (Dumonteil); the evaluation of residues is considered (van der Kreek) and specific aspects of prevention and treatment of internal parasites in animal production are presented (Raynaud). Also are appended some reports on feed additives efficacy (virginiamycin, monensin, lasalocid and salinomycin).

*The Food and Drug Administration proposed definitions for *medicated feed articles* were published in the January 17, 1978 Federal register; the most concentrated article will be designated as *type A*.

This is a true drug premix for medicating animal feed. The article will be solely for use in the manufacture of other medicated animal feed articles (animal feed bearing or containing a new animal drug), and it will, of course, be limited to use solely in accordance with its approved labelling. It will consist principally of a new animal drug in a diluent (carrier substance), and it must be further diluted with nutrient material to produce either a type B, C, or D medicated feed article. The proposed type A medicated feed article is comparable to the present 'feed additive premix'.

A proposed *type B* medicated feed article will conform to the statutory definition of animal feed because it contains substantial source of nutrients and is intended for use as such in an animal's diet. Before the article can be used in the feed of animals, however, it must be substantially diluted with a nutrient substance to form a type C or D medicated feed article. The type B medicated feed article will be similar to the present 'feed concentrate'. The definition of the type B article, however, has been revised to encompass intermediate premixes.

A proposed *type C* medicated feed article is also a medicated animal feed bearing or containing a new animal drug. It will be produced by substantially diluting a type A or type B medicated feed article with other feed ingredients to a level for a use that is covered by an approved NADA. A type C article may be further diluted or mixed to produce type D medicated feed articles, i.e. a complete feed; or it may be fed top dressed, undiluted, or offered free-choice in conjunction with other animal feed to supplement the animal's total daily ration.

A *type D* medicated feed article will be essentially identical to the current 'complete feed'. It will be for administration as the sole ration to an animal.

Medicated feed in French Legislation and European Economic Community

M. Lobry

The definition of the medicated feed is based in France on the law 75-409 of 29th May 1975: 'A medicated feed is a medicinal product which has been made from a mixture prepared in advance of a medicinal product and a feed'. A premix is 'a medicinal product prepared in advance and exclusively intended to the subsequent manufacture of medicated feedingstuffs'. Both premix and medicated feedingstuffs are thus veterinary medicinal products. In addition, other indications based on the law of August 1905 (decrete of 1973 and *sq.* concerning repression and control of frauds) regulate the use of additives in animal feeds. These are substances introduced in the animal feed during a long part of the life of the animal and at a relatively low dosage (in the range of 30–100 parts/10^6) and authorization is given for the substance. A critical report about the French drug approval process has been published by M. Weintraub in *The Journal of Clinical Pharmacology*, (1982). **22,** 213–22. On the contrary, in the 'medicated feedingstuff' system, the authorization (marketing authorization = A.M.M., 'Autorisation de mise sur le marché') is given on the final premix (chemical substance + feed support).

Since some of the additives are given at a level which results in some preventive effects (this is the case for coccidiostats and for some antibiotics), the border line between an additive to be used in a supplemented feed and a medicinal product to be used in a medicated feed is sometimes uneasy to define.

These regulations result in constraints at different levels for medicated feedingstuffs.

(1) At the manufacture level, it is compulsory that the medicated feedingstuff be produced in an establishment with pharmaceutical status (article L. 615), i.e. with a chemist or a veterinary surgeon in its Directorate.

(2) The marketing authorization must be given at two levels: premix and medicated feedingstuffs.

(3) The distribution can only be carried out through the chemist or the veterinary surgeon with the exception of some agricultural organizations (co-operatives) which have a special agreement (article L. 612). The direct delivery from manufacturer to the stockfarmer is not allowed.

This system is recognized as not being realistic and, therefore, impossible to implement. The proposal for amending the law which has been put forward to the Parliament consists of three parts:

(1) At the manufacture level: the medicated feed could be prepared in a feed factory but still under the responsibility of a chemist or a veterinary.

(2) The marketing authorization would be given to the premix; the medicated feed, provided it is prepared according to the manufacturer's instructions, could be sold without authorization.

(3) At the retail level, the medicated feed could be delivered directly from the manufacturer to the cattle owner, with a veterinary prescription.

SITUATION AT EUROPEAN ECONOMIC COMMUNITY LEVEL

At the EEC level, two directives (one on veterinary medicinal products and the other on analytical, pharmacotoxicological and clinical standards and protocols in respect to the testing of veterinary medicinal products) have been issued in 1981 (*Official Journal of EEC*, 6th November, 1981).

The medicated premix (and not the medicated feedingstuff) is included in these directives. The medicated premix is therefore considered as a full medicinal product, submitted to the marketing authorization procedure.

A third directive (still in preparation) is being drafted in order to deal with preparation, manufacture, agreement and distribution of the medicated feedingstuff.

The main lines of this directive are going along with our national legislative amendment proposals: (1) manufacture of the medicated feedingstuff in an authorized feed factory; (2) waiving of marketing authorization if the medicated feedingstuff has been prepared from an authorized premix, or following a 'standard prescription'; and (3) distribution, on veterinary prescription, directly from the factory to the farmer.

COMMENTS

During years of discussion, two proposals were conflicting with each other. For some of the member states, the 'marketing authorization' procedure has to be applied for the premix, as for medicinal products. For others, the procedure of authorization has to be given on each chemical substance, as for the additives in our country. Finally, as a compromise, it was decided that the Directive 81/851/CEE (veterinary medicinal products) would include the premixes (art. 2) but the Commission, within 2 years, should prepare a list of 'pharmacological products which could be used in the fabrication of medicated premixes'.

Advantages and inconveniences of both systems have been largely debated by all concerned. However, the concomitant use of both procedures in the same country results in some difficulties, such as to define accurately what is an additive and what is a medicinal product, or what is the right limit between premix and medicinal powder to be given in top feeding.

As a conclusion, it might be questioned if it would not be better to adopt *a unique system of procedure* (which works satisfactorily in USA) and which could be anticipated as follows: the marketing authorization would be given on one premix (chemical + feed support), which could be used later at two different concentration rates: one lower level for the preparation of supplemented feed and one higher for the manufacture of medicated feedingstuff.

Medicated feed: problems and solutions

A. S. J. P. A. M. van Miert

In the Netherlands, two special committees give advice to the Minister of Agriculture concerning the registration of growth-promoting feed additives and feed additives intended for the prevention of diseases ('Veevoederovergorgaan') or for treatment of diseases of animals (Standard medicated feed: 'Receptuur' Committee). Most members of the latter committee are well trained in veterinary medicine.

STANDARD MEDICATED FEED

Today, 15 different standard medicated feeds have been preliminarily registrated: one for poultry, one for lambs and 13 for swine. Active ingredients in the standard medicated feeds are: lincomycin, spectinomycin, neomycin, oxytetracycline, sulphadimidine, furazolidone, ronidazole, dimitridazole, amprolium and Intagen®, a product which contains lipopolysaccharides from *E. coli*.

The feed manufacturer can obtain these drugs directly from the drug suppliers. The delivery of standard medicated feed, however, is only permitted on prescription by a veterinary practitioner. The law requires the listing of all drugs processed by a feed manufacturer. Furthermore, feed labels are required, which contain relevant information such as: product name and brand name under which the commercial feed is distributed, the net weight of each drug used (in grams per ton feed), the expiry date of the medicated feed, name and principal mailing address of the manufacturer and adequate directions for use such as animal species, age, treatment time and withdrawal time.

BIOAVAILABILITY

An administered antibacterial agent can elicit only the desired therapeutic response for which it was developed, provided that sufficient concentrations of the drug reach and are available to pathogenic bacteria. Drugs that are chemically equivalent may not be therapeutically equivalent because of differences in dosage form. Certainly, the more potent the pharmacologic action of the drug, the more imperative is the need for bioavailability testing. Bioavailability describes the extent to which and the rate at which the active drug reaches the systemic circulation, and ultimately the receptors or sites of action at concentrations that are effective, and thereby defines the efficiency of the dosage formulation. The bioavailability of a drug is characterized by two important parameters: the area under the blood concentration–time curve and the peak height of this curve together with its time of occurrence (Figure 1). Rates of bioavailability are likely to be important for drugs, which are actively absorbed, for sparingly soluble drugs, drugs with a low therapeutic index, such as furazolidone, and for drugs that are destroyed in the gastrointestinal tract, such as some penicillins.

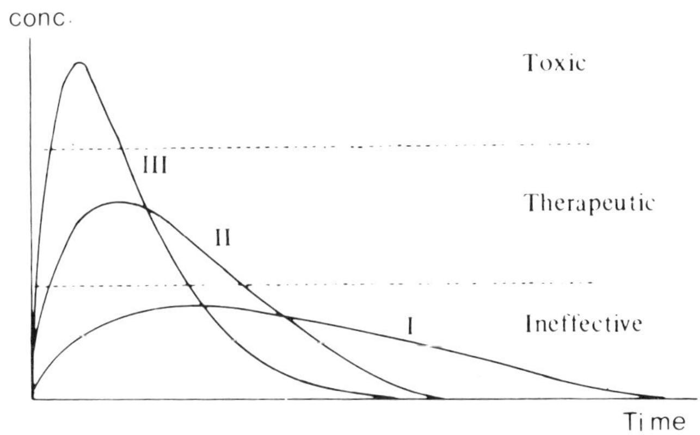

Figure 1 Plasma concentration–time curves for a hypothetical drug, which needs to attain a minimum concentration in the plasma to be pharmacologically active. Inspection of the relationships shows that a formulation producing curve I is *in*effective, that producing curve II is active and the preferred dosage form, and that producing curve III is active but also leads to toxicity. Similarity of the areas under all three curves does not necessarily indicate that the drug will be therapeutically effective in all cases

VARIATIONS IN BIOAVAILABILITY

A drug is subjected to tissue uptake, biotransformation and excretion and, therefore, much of an administered dose never reaches the receptors. So that patients are provided with drug formulations that are physically and chemically stable and pharmaceutically reliable, drugs are prepared in various physical forms with a number of other ingredients which may influence their bioavailability[5,20]. To be absorbed from the gastrointestinal tract, the drug must be presented in a soluble form to the site of absorption. Different dosage forms of drugs may thus provide varying amounts of the drug for absorption and thereby cause differences in the onset, extent, and duration of therapeutic effect. These differences may derive from modified bioavailability and be due to pathology of the patient and/or his genetic make-up, or alternatively from dosage-form modified bioavailability and be due to the physicochemical properties of the drug, interaction with feed components or other drugs, or to the methods of manufacture of the medicated feed[1,16,21,22]

DRUG

The greater the surface area of a drug in contact with the gastrointestinal fluids, the more rapid the dissolution rate (Table 1). Thus with the decrease in particle size, there is an increase in dissolution rate. However, particle size reduction provides more opportunity for particle interaction, which may sometimes lead to aggregation[21]. The rate of bioavailability is enhanced if the rate of diffusion from the dosage form is increased by the use of a more soluble drug form. Administration of soluble salts of penicillin V resulted in higher blood levels of antibiotic than were obtained with the less soluble free acid[9], while anhydrous ampicillin has a greater extent of bioavailability than the less soluble trihydrate[19]. Some drugs exist in several crystalline forms of differing solubilities and other physical properties with resultant differences in bioavailability[10]. Moreover, some of the agents added to drug formulations can influence the bioavailability of the active ingredient.

Table 1 Factors affecting bioavailability of a drug

Factors
Particle size, weight and form
Chemical form
Hydration, solvation
Formulation adjuvants
Manufacturing method

FEED

Feed generally impairs the absorption of drugs[11,24] (Table 2). The rate, and partly also, the extent of drug absorption depends mainly on the rate of gastric emptying. Feed affects drug absorption negatively because of its slowing of gastric emptying rate. Several antimicrobial agents have been shown to have an impaired bioavailability when given with feed or food. This has been reported for drugs such as ampicillin[26], oxacillin, dicloxacillin, lincomycin, rifampicin, some erythromycin preparations, isoniazid and the first generation tetracyclines[16]. It seems well established that non-absorbable chelates are formed between metal-ions – such as iron and calcium – and the tetracyclines by concominant intake of calcium/iron-containing feed[18]. The antifungal drug griseofulvin shows a special interaction with fat: ingestion of feed with a high fat content markedly increases griseofulvin absorption. This is most probably explained by fat-induced enhancement of the dissolution of griseofulvin, which is very lipophilic[4]. Moreover, protein-rich feeds enhance, while carbohydrate-rich feeds reduce the rate of oxidation

Table 2 Factors of the feed affecting bioavailability

Energy content
Fats, proteins, carbohydrates
Vitamins, minerals, pH
Presence of mould spores
Presence of adjuvants and other drugs
Manufacturing method (mixer, humidity, temperature, mixing time, pelleted feed, etc.)

of certain drugs such as theophylline[25]. However, feed does not seem to affect the bioavailability of amoxycillin[26], metronidazole, sulphadimidine and spiramycin[16]. In addition, some human studies indicate that food improves rather than impairs the absorption of certain drugs such as erythromycin stearate, nitrofurantoine, hydrallazine and propranolol[16]. The food-induced enhancement of bioavailability of propranolol and hydrallazine is probably due to reduced first pass metabolism of these drugs[15]. It follows from the above mentioned observations that feed–drug interactions are very complex and that valid conclusions pertinent to this problem must be derived from direct studies on the specific drug in question.

We often assume that medicated feeds are completely and uniformly mixed. It should be, of course, but is it? Electrostatic properties of a drug can prevent adequate blending of the ingredients. Furthermore, the weight and form of drug particles can promote 'unmixing'. This has been demonstrated, for instance, for some sulphonamides[21]. During the process of manufacturing, a loss of drug activity can occur (Table 3).

Table 3 Standard medicated feeds with oxytetracycline (400 parts/10⁶) or sulphadimidine (400 parts/10⁶)

	*Loss of drug activity**			
	Oxytetracycline		*Sulphadimidine*	
Type of feed	*detected* (parts/10⁶)	*deviation* (%)	*detected* (parts/10⁶)	*deviation* (%)
Baby pigs	230	−42	270	−32
	250	−37		
	220	−45		
Growing swine	320	−20	275	−31
	312	−22		
Sows	430	+8	290	−27
	270	−33	340	−15
	240	−40	295	−26
	225	−44	220	−45

*From P. vah de Kerk, CLO Institute 'De Schothorst', The Netherlands, with permission

Underdosing can also be caused by concurrent administration of other feed products. Another problem is the possibility of drug interaction. Drug interaction refers to the reaction between two or more therapeutic agents administered concurrently or in a close sequence, resulting in an altered response. The total effect may be increased (addition or potentiation) or weakened (antagonism) but an unforeseen side-effect may also occur. Such an unforeseen toxic reaction has been reported in poultry when tiamulin was administered concurrently with monensin[8]. Tiamulin was given for the treatment of a respiratory infection in the form of medicated drinking water, while monensin – mixed in the feed – was administered for the prevention of coccidiosis.

HOST

Absorption of drugs may be affected by the physiological status of the gastrointestinal tract, but also is influenced by the age and the species of animal undergoing therapy[1,17] (Table 4). Furthermore, drug absorption may be influenced by gastrointestinal diseases. Rasková *et al.*[13] found faster absorption of sulphadimidine in diarrhoeic calves whereas the elimination halflife of the drug was significantly shortened. In human studies, normal absorption of chloramphenicol was found, whereas sulphafurazole showed retarded uptake during atrophy of the intestinal villi[14]. In Crohn's disease, normal bioavailability has been found for cephalexin, erythromycin succinate, rifamycin and trimethoprim. Increased absorption has been found for clindamycin, sulphamethoxazole, metronidazole and possibly reduced absorption for lincomycin[3]. Furthermore, the rates of drug absorption after oral administration to veal-calves[6,7] and pigs[12] were reduced during pyrogen-induced fever. It has been demonstrated that pyrogens are strong inhibitors of both gastric emptying rate and gastric secretion[23]. The pH raising, during pyrogen-induced fever or due to feed intake, is important, as the solubility of some drugs – such as tetracycline – is reduced with increasing pH[2]. Despite the frequent use of antibacterial agents in animals suffering from infectious diseases, little is known of the effects of pathophysiologic states upon the pharmacokinetic behaviour of these drugs. It follows from the above-mentioned observations that the influence of pathophysiologic states, on bioavailability, biotransformation and excretion of drugs, is very complex and that valid conclusions pertinent to this problem must be derived from direct studies with patients and the specific drugs in question.

Disease states may have a negative influence on feed intake, but not on water consumption. For these reasons, it has been suggested that medicated drinking water is an attractive alternative way to treat diseases of animals. However, there are some restrictions concerning medicated drinking water such as taste, solubility and stability of the drug and – last but not least – a suitable drinking water system. Finally, since large variations in feed intake

Table 4 Factors of the host affecting bioavailability

Factors
Species (intestinal and bacterial enzymes)
Breed
Age
Time of administration
Diseases (fever, gastric emptying rate, intestinal secretion and motility)
Other drugs (water medication)

and water consumption commonly occur among diseased animals from one flock, only drugs with high therapeutic indices should be used in medicated feed and drinking water to treat pathological conditions.

References

1. Baggot, J. D. (1977). *Principles of Drug Disposition in Domestic Animals.* (Philadelphia and London: Saunders Corp.)
2. Barr, W. H., Adir, J. and Garrettson, L. (1971). *Clin. Pharmacol. Ther.*, **12**, 779–84
3. Bergan, T., Bjerke, E. M. and Fausa, O. (1981). *Chemotherapy*, **27**, 233–8
4. Crounse, R. G. (1963). *Arch. Dermatol.*, **87**, 176–80
5. Gibaldi, M. and Feldman, S. J. (1970). *Pharm. Sci.*, **59**, 579–89
6. Groothuis, D. G., van Miert, A. S. J. P. A. M., Ziv, G. *et al.* (1978). *J. Vet. Pharmacol. Ther.*, **1**, 81–4
7. Groothuis, D. G., van Gogh, H. and van Miert, A. S. J. P. A. M. (1980). In van Miert, A. S. J. P. A. M., Frens, J. and van der Kreek, F. W. (eds.) *Trends in Veterinary Pharmacology and Toxicology. Proc. 1st EAVPT Congr.*, Zeist, 1979. pp. 77–86. (Amsterdam and New York: Elsevier)
8. Horrox, N. E. (1980). *Vet. Rec.*, **106**, 278
9. Kaipainen, W. J. and Härkönen, P. (1956). *Scand J. Clin. Lab. Invest.*, **8**, 18–20
10. Khalil, S. A., Moustafa, M. A., Eiban, A. R. *et al.* (1972). *J. Pharm. Sci.*, **61**, 1615–17
11. Koch-Weser, J. (1974). *N. Engl. J. Med.*, **291**, 233–7 and 503–6
12. Ladefoged, O. (1979). *J. Vet. Pharmacol. Ther.*, **2**, 209–14
13. Lapka, R., Urbanova, Z., Kobylka, B. *et al.* (1978). *Drug Metab. Disp.*, **6**, 637–9
14. Mantilla, M. J., Jussila, J. and Takki, S. (1973). *Arzneim. Forsch.*, **23**, 583–5
15. Melander, A., Danielson, K., Schersten, B. *et al.* (1977). *Clin. Pharmacol. Ther.*, **22**, 108–112
16. Melander, A. (1978). *Clin. Pharmacokin.*, **3**, 337–51
17. Morselli, P. L., Franco-Morselli, R. and Bossi, L. (1980). *Clin. Pharmacokin.*, **5**, 485–527
18. Neuvonen, P. J. (1976). *Drugs*, **11**, 45–54
19. Poole, J. W., Owen, G., Silverio, J. *et al.* (1968). *Curr. Ther. Res.*, **10**, 292–303
20. Prescott, L. F., Steele, R. F. and Ferrier, W. R. (1970). *Clin. Pharmacol. Ther.*, **11**, 496–504
21. Telser, E. (1978). *Dtsch. Tierärztl. Wschr.*, **85**, 483–8
22. Telser, E. (1979). *Dtsch. Tierärztl. Wschr.*, **86**, 69–73
23. van Miert, A. S. J. P. A. M. (1980). In Lipton, J. M. (ed.) *Fever*. pp. 57–70. (New York: Raven Press)
24. Welling, P. G. (1977). *Postgraduate Med.*, **62**, 73–82
25. Welling, P. G., Lyons, L. L., Craig, W. A. *et al.* (1975). *Pharmacol. Ther.*, **17**, 475–80
26. Ziv, G., Nouws. J. F. M., Groothuis, D. G. *et al.* (1977). *Am. J. Vet. Res.*, **38**, 1007–13

Medicated feed manufacturing

C. Dumonteil

The position of feed manufacturers is that feed conveys medicaments as water do. On the other hand, the medicated feed is, according to the Law 75-409 on Pharmacy (1975), a drug without taking in account any specificity of such a pharmaceutical form for manufacturing, prescription and delivery. The law project Sordel and the EEC Directive proposal try to take out the deadlock, in France named 'amendment', of this pharmaceutical form.

MEDICATED FEED MANUFACTURING

Medicated feeds are generally prepared by a feed manufacturer rather than by a pharmaceutical company. The reason is that the pharmaceutical industry is evidently not able to manufacture and deliver great quantities of medicated feed. In contrast, the medicated feed manufacturers are in possession of a good controlled technology that permits the homogeneous incorporations of microingredients.

These different conditions, foreseen in the project of EEC Directive 'medicated feed', are

(1) Buildings and adapted technical equipments.

(2) A qualified personnel having sufficient knowledge in mixing techniques.

(3) Laboratory controls.

(4) Records on nature and quantities of premixes and medicated feeds that are manufactured, stored and delivered.

(5) A particular stock of premixes and medicated feeds in buildings provided for this purpose.

MEDICATED COMPONENTS

In both the law project 'amendment Sordel' and the EEC Directive proposal, only approved premix could be utilized in manufacturing a medicated feed. Incorporation rate of premix should be such that the posology in weight of prescribed active substances by the veterinarian is respected. Therefore, it is necessary to take into account the daily quantity of feed that is consumed by animals. On the other hand, a good homogeneity for the incorporation of active substances in the feed is necessary. Therefore, a minimal rate of 1% for final mixing was retained as a result of a consultation of concerned professionals. This rate corresponds to routine practices for mixing and to the usual equipment of feed manufacturers. In particular other cases, only the use of lower rates (0.5% or 0.25%) could be possible.

COMMENTS

The choice of a minimal rate for incorporation of premix in the feed obliges the manufacturers to consider two categories of medicated premix:

(1) The final premix, incorporated at 1% and directly utilized for manufacturing medicated feed (the final premix is itself prepared either from an active substance or from a primary premix);

(2) The primary premix, which generally presents an active substance diluted and will be prepared for use at a level in the final premix of 0.5–1% incorporation. This premix (and also the final premix in France) are subject to a request of delivery authorization but are not directly utilizable for manufacturing medicated feed.

The proper use of premix is of importance as a guarantee of the quality of medicated feed. In fact, appropriate control of the 'finished product' is not feasible in conditions similar to those for drugs. The two major reasons are

(1) The absence of store room as the manufacturing is only a day-to-day production.

(2) The assays which are not easy to monitor routinely with low levels of highly diluted substances in feeds and drugs. The EEC Directive project recommends a continuous control for which precise details are still lacking but they will be probably only slightly different from those required for the use and manufacturing of feed additives.

Animal drugs and the evaluation of residues in milk and meat

F. W. van der Kreek

Animal drugs can be categorized according to (1) pharmacological action (antibiotics, anthelmintics, ectoparasiticides, etc.), (2) animal species (dairy cattle, pigs, poultry, etc.), (3) application (oral, parenteral, intramammary), and (4) purpose (growth improvement, prophylactic action and therapy).

Diseases and treatments are generally not specific for the species. For example, oxytetracycline is an antibiotic used for the treatment of all kinds of infection in cattle, pigs, poultry, etc. applied as a feed- or drinking water-additive or via an injection, provided for long or short periods of the entire life or injected once or for a number of times. Residues of oxytetracycline may therefore be expected at any time in milk, milk products, meat, meat products of cattle, pigs and poultry, and in eggs.

With the help of pharmacokinetic research in target animals and toxicological investigations, it is possible to establish (1) (qualitatively and quantitatively) what residues are present in milk and meat after several intervals of time, and (2) what amount of residue is acceptable regarding the health of the consumer of milk and meat.

The toxicological investigations include a long list of toxicity tests, acute and chronic toxicity tests for the establishment of the quantitative toxicity and specific tests like biotransformation, mutagenicity, neurotoxicity, etc. for the establishment of the qualitative toxicity. Essential investigations for the establishment of acceptable drug residues in milk and meat involve pharmacokinetic, teratogenicity and mutagenicity tests.

The pharmacokinetic research will give the information with respect to the interval needed for a non-detectable residue and the required information about the profile of the metabolites. The teratogenicity tests will appoint the non-toxic effect level which is the most sensitive toxicological criterium.

The results of mutagenicity tests which give an insight into the carcinogenic potential of the compound are at the most a qualitative indication. These types of toxicological investigations will be carried out for any active substance, independent of the application of the drug.

The quantitative toxic profile of a substance makes it possible to establish an acceptable daily intake for the consumer through the food products of animal origin. It is assumed that the non-toxic effect level in the target or experimental animal with a safety or uncertainty factor applied, is also non-toxic for human beings. Some authorities apply a safety factor of 100, others think it necessary to apply a safety factor of 1000 for teratogenic effects. The calculated acceptable amount of the substance, the first-order health-based limit, may be present as a total residue in the food basket. Accordingly, it is necessary to know (1) the food pattern of the human population, presented as an average diet of an average adult on a total base or based on the fat fractions or presented as an average intake of sucklings, and (2) the use pattern of the substance involved.

Then various situations are possible: (1) The substance may be used as a fungicide in agriculture and as a fungicide in animal hygiene. In this case, the total amount of acceptable residue should be spread over the whole diet (e.g. thiabendazol). (2) When a substance is lipophylic, the allotting should be carried out over the lipid fractions of the food basket (e.g. lindane). (3) When a substance is lipophilic and exclusively used as an animal drug, the allotting should be done over the fat fractions of food of animal origin, the fat of milk, meat of cattle, pigs and poultry, eggs and fish (vegetable oils and fats, 40 g; milk fat, 26 g; other animal fat, 39 g). (4) When a substance is hydrophilic and exclusively used as an animal drug, the allotting can be carried out over the food products of animal origin on a total base. Residues of this kind of animal drug will be found in the 500 g milk and milk products and in the 130 g meat and meat products (e.g. foxim and benzimidazoles).

The food pattern of an adult shows that milk and milk products are much more important in the risk evaluation of residues of animal drugs than meat and meat products. The paramount importance is even greater for the suckling and the toddler. The meat consumption of man per kg body weight is the same during his whole life, namely 2 g per kg body weight. Against that, the milk consumption starts for a suckling with 150 ml per kg body weight, and drops to 8 ml per kg body weight for an adult: the milk consumption is a factor of 4–75 times higher than the meat consumption.

The allotment of residues of animal drugs over the total food basket is not yet carried out in authorizing committees: the current procedure is that the residue will be kept as low as possible and preferably not detectable by establishing safety intervals between application and milk delivery and/or slaughter.

This approach is the best one, but not always feasible. Besides, an interval between application and slaughter is a practical and applicable method to prevent intake of residues, but on the other hand, an interval between application and milk delivery is not realistic for the farmer.

A minimum residue will be achieved only after optimum therapeutic applications. This ideal situation appears far from that resulting from medicated feed as shown by comparison of the Italian and Dutch lists for anti-infective compounds in medicated feed: oxytetracycline: 500–1000 parts/10^6 in Italy vs. 300–400 parts/10^6 in Netherlands; sulphadimidine: 3750–5000 parts/10^6 vs. 200–400 parts/10^6; furazolidone: 400–500 parts/10^6 vs. 300–400 parts/10^6; dimetridazol: 1000–2500 parts/10^6 vs. 450 parts/10^6.

The following drugs will be given as examples of risk calculation.

(1) *Bromophenofos* (Acedist) is used as a prophylactic and therapeutic treatment for the control of liver fluke in sheep and cattle at the effective dose of 6 mg and 12 mg per kg body weight, respectively. The no-effect level in rat toxicity studies is also 6 mg per kg body weight and no residues are detected in meat for a slaughter interval of 7 days. In the case of dairy cows, pharmacokinetic studies have found that the maximum residue is 0.15 mg per kg of milk (third day). The total maximum residue in a daily diet, therefore, may be 0.08 mg, i.e. an average of 0.0015 mg per kg body weight. For the safety factor of 4000 between rat and man, it may be concluded that no risk is involved.

(2) *Thiabendazole* is a broad spectrum anthelmintic for sheep, cattle, pigs, etc. used at a dosage of 44–100 mg/kg body weight. It is also used as a fungicide pre- and post-harvest treatment on bananas, citrus and pome fruit at the dose of 100–5000 parts/10^6. Thiabendazole is also used as a fumigant in glass houses and as a spray to protect stored potatoes. The thiabendazole concentration in a 2700 Kcal diet may be calculated as being between 1620 and 4000 μg. The toxicological evaluations are no-effect level for 10 mg/kg body weight daily in rats and 20 mg/kg body weight daily in dogs or no effects in volunteers with a dose of 250 mg/day. The acceptable daily intake is thus 0.3 mg/kg body weight with a safety factor of 10. The actual, potential and acceptable intakes are 1.6 mg, 4 mg and 20 mg, respectively. The conclusion is that no risk is involved with the consumption of food that may contain residues of thiabendazole.

(3) *Lindane* is used in preharvest treatments of fruits, vegetables and other edible crops and for the protection of cereals, pulses, etc. Lindane is also involved in the treatment of livestock for control of flies, ticks and mites and in applications on forage crops. The lindane concentration in a 2700 Kcal diet is between 107 and 591 μg. The toxicological evaluations are no-effect level for 1.25 mg/kg body weight in rats and 1.6 mg/kg body weight for dogs. The acceptable daily intake is thus 0.01 mg/kg body weight with a safety factor of 100. The actual, average, potential and acceptable daily intakes are 9–19 μg, 107 μg, 591 μg and 700 μg respectively. No risk is involved with the consumption of food that may contain residues of lindane. However, since lindane is carcinogenic in mice and haemotoxic in man, it remains a prudent policy to minimize lindane applications and residues as much as possible.

(4) *Foxim* (Sebacil) is an insecticide applied early into the soil to control soil insects, used in and around the house to control ants, and to control mange mites in cattle and sheep by dermal application (2.5 g). The maximal concentration in milk is 0.21 parts/10^6; the no-effect level in rat is 0.04 mg/kg body weight with an acceptable daily intake of 0.4 μg/kg body weight. Dutch authorities have authorized the application on dairy cattle on the basis that milk delivered in tanks concerns the production of 3 days, with a maximum residue in milk of 0.1 parts/10^6 as the

average of six milkings after the application. It must be stated also that mange treatments of cattle are exceptional situations and that foxim is a good alternative for lindane

(5) *Benzimidazoles* are used to control nematodes and other helminths with a system of intervals to minimize residues. These intervals (slaughter and milkings) differ in a very unusual way: albendazole (Valbazen): 10 mg/kg body weight, no intervals given; fenbendazole (Panacur): 5–50 mg/kg body weight, 7–14 days, 0–6 milkings; febantel (Rintal): 5–7.5 mg/kg body weight, 7–14 days, 0–4 milkings; oxfendazole (Synanthic): 4.5 mg/kg body weight, 8–10 days, 6–10 milkings; oxfendazole (Systamex): 4.5 mg/kg body weight, 10 days, 0–10 milkings; mebendazole (Ovitelmin): 10–15 mg/kg body weight, 7 days, two milkings.

It is therefore necessary to estimate the average residue of the different benzimidazoles over the first six milkings after application and the potential intake should be assessed against the acceptable daily intake, derived from the teratogenic studies and with the application of a safety factor.

In conclusion, a general consensus in the European countries is needed not only for the acceptable daily intakes but also with respect to the development of the second-order health-based limits: the residues in meat and milk.

Drugs for prevention or treatment of internal parasites in farm animals. Particular cases of medicated feed

J. P. Raynaud and P. Gorse

In the actual farm practices in France, pathological risks were identified where internal parasites are the main causative factor and classified in categories, i.e. permanent, frequent or occasional risks.

Some are controversial: for example, Balantidiosis in swine. In this country, *Balantidium* is frequently seen in postmortem examinations during intestinal problems associated with diarrhoea. The frequent use of dimetridazole or other nitroimidazoles, as additive or in medicated feeds, is known and justified by routine practice more than true demonstration of aetiological relationship.

Taking into account the known reputation of pathological agents and the rationale of drug usage (Table 1), the permanent risks are coccidia for poultry and rabbits, and gastrointestinal worms for swine and ruminants. The occasional risks are gastrointestinal worms for rabbits, ascaris and coccidia for veal calves, tapeworms and coccidia for pasture cattle, and liver fluke and coccidia for sheep and goats.

The economics, as cost to the farmers of drugs to prevent or treat the known internal parasites are presented in Table 2 and allocated in the sections:

(1) Feed additives section.

(2) Veterinary drugs section (under veterinary prescription) divided, according to the physical presentation, in:
   (a) medicated feeds,
   (b) other veterinary products.

COSTS BY PARASITIC INFECTIONS

Coccidiosis costs about 86 000 000 Francs, i.e. 31% of the total. In this disease, 82% of the expenses are for poultry, 13% for rabbits and 5% for sheep and goats. The main market: poultry is 71 000 000 F with 88%

Table 1 Pathological risks due to internal parasites in farm practice (France). Protozoa (*Coccidia, Trichomonas, Histomonas, Balantidium*); worms (gastrointestinal: GI, tape worms, liver fluke, lung worms, *Dicrocoelium* fluke, *Prostostrongylinae* lung worms, *Capillaria, Ascaridia, Ascaris*); others (yeast-like fungi)

Risks frequency	*Permanent*	*Frequent*	*Occasional*
Poultry			
Broilers	*Coccidia*		
Pullets	*Coccidia*	Worms: *Capillaria* + *Ascaridia*	
Layers		*Coccidia* + worms (*Capillaria*)	
Turkeys, guinea fowls	Coccidia + *Trichomonas* + *Histomonas*	Worms	
Wild fowls	*Coccidia*	*Trichomonas* + *Histomonas* + worms + others	
Rabbits	*Coccidia*		GI worms
Swine			
Sows + boars	GI worms*		
Piglets		*Balantidium* + GI worms	
Growing finish, swine	GI worms + *Balantidium**		
Cattle			
Veal calves			*Ascaris* + *Coccidia*
Calves, steers		GI worms + *coccidia*	
On pasture cattle	GI worms + lung worms lung worms**		Tape worms *Coccidia***
Sheep + goats	GI worms + tape worms *Dicrocoelium* fluke + *prostrongylinae* lung worms*		Lung worms + *Coccidia*

*In some periods of life; **In some geographical areas

(63 000 000 F), as feed additives and 11% (7 500 000 F) as drinking water treatments.

Helminths cost about 174 800 000 Francs, i.e. 63% of the total. In this disease, 72% of the expenses are for cattle, 20% for sheep and goats, 5% only (but 9 300 000 F) for swine and 3% for poultry. The main market: cattle represents 125 000 000 Francs, with 96% (120 000 000 F) as drenches or injections.

The protozoa except coccidia: *Histomonas, Trichomonas* and *Balantidium* are a small market: 5% (16 676 000 F) of the total, with 59% (8 640 000 F) for swine, 74% being used as feed additives and 24% as medicated feeds. The poultry market 41% (6 036 000 F) is mainly as feed additives.

Table 2 Cost to the stockfarmer (1980) in FF of internal parasites prevention or treatment. Values in thousand Francs (× 1000), when the drugs are available as additives, medicated feeds and other veterinary products

Species	*Additives*	*Medicated feeds*	*Other veterinary products*	*Total*
To prevent or treat coccidiosis				
Cattle	0	0	60	60
Sheep, goats	0	1 500	2 500	4 000
Rabbits	4 200	1 680	5 200	11 080
Poultry	63 000	840	7 500	71 340
	67 200	4 020	15 260	86 480
To prevent or treat helminths				
Rabbits	0	0	1 000	1 000
Poultry	0	1 800	2 500	4 300
Swine	0	6 000	3 300	9 300
Sheep, goats	0	200	35 000	35 200
Cattle	0	5 000	120 000	125 000
	0	13 000	161 800	174 800
To prevent or treat Histomonas, Trichomonas, Balantidium				
Poultry	5 000	36	1 000	6 036
Swine	6 400	2 040	200	8 640
	11 400	2 076	1 200	14 676
Total	78 600	19 096	178 260	275 956

COSTS BY FARM ANIMAL SPECIES

Prevention or treatment of internal parasitic diseases cost:

(1) 125 060 000 F in cattle, 120 060 000 F: 96% as drenches or injections, 5 000 000 F: 4% as medicated feeds.

(2) 81 676 000 F in poultry, 68 000 000 F: 83% as feed additives, 11 000 000 F: 13% in drinking water and 2 676 000 F: 3% in medicated feeds.

(3) 39 200 000 F in sheep and goats, 37 500 000 F: 96% as drenches (mainly) and 1 700 000 F: 4% in medicated feeds.

(4) 17 940 000 F in swine, 8 040 000 F: 45% as medicated feeds, 6 400 000 F: 36% as feed additives and 3 500 000 F: 20% as 'other vet. products'.

(5) 12 080 000 F in rabbits: 6 200 000 F: 51% as 'other vet. products', 4 200 000 F: 35% as feed additives, and 1 680 000 F: 14% as medicated feeds.

COSTS BY DISTRIBUTIVE METHOD

On an overall cost, the *medicated feeds* represent only 19 096 000 F, i.e. 7% of the total of the drugs used for prevention or treatment of internal parasites.

They count for 8 040 000 F in swine (45% in this species), 5 000 000 F in cattle (4%), 2 676 000 F in poultry (3%), 1 700 000 F in sheep and goats (4%) and 1 680 000 F in rabbits (14%).

The drugs used in *feed additives* represent 78 600 000 F (28% of the total) and as 'other vet. products' (drenches, injectables, drinking water treatments), they count for 178 260 000 F (65% of the total).

RATIONALE AND PRACTICAL USE OF DRUGS

In contradiction to the EEC Directives on feed additives, some antibiotics and growth promotants are approved at a dose which is preventive and it is probably for this reason that those products have a general use. According to Professor B. Gedek: 'For the best economical result, an additive should be used continuously in the feed at the right dose which prevents diseases as they play an important role at the early stage of breeding'*.

When a *risk* is identified as *permanent*, the only way to prevent the pathological troubles or the low performance, is continuous supplementation, i.e. an additive *at the right dose to prevent.*

But a dossier for the approval of an additive is long to complete, difficult and expensive. It is this reason why many companies prefer not to introduce such a dossier and propose the same drug at the 'level for prevention' in the veterinary channel, i.e. medicated feed or medicated drinking water.

When a risk is occasional, for a certain time during the breeding period, the prevention should be done through the medicated feed or medicated drinking water.

For therapy, the decision is taken on the number of sick animals.

- few animals, no extension of the disease: individual treatments with the right dose at the right time.
- few animals, but risks of extension: individual treatments and prevention for the animals at risk.
- large number of animals: treatment for all, via feed and/or drinking water.

*In Aumaitre, A. and Raynaud, J. P. (1978). Les additifs chez le Porc – Resultats techniques, intérêt pratique et limites de leur utilisation. *Dossiers de l'Elevage*, **5**, 73–83

Virginiamycin activity and safety in ruminants

R. D. Hedde, L. Shor and R. Quach

Virginiamycin, an antibiotic comprising two distinct chemical entities, has been used a a growth-enhancing agent in non-ruminating animals. Cocito[1] described virginiamycin as having primarily gram-positive activity with a unique synergism occurring between the two chemical components of the antibiotic complex.

Vervaeke *et al.*[3] described virginiamycin as an inhibitor of bacteria in the small intestine of the pig. Such inhibition produced energy sparing via reduced lactic acid formation in the gastrointestinal tract. In subsequent studies in our laboratories, we have found virginiamycin to be selectively active against small intestine organisms with little activity against fibre-digesting organisms of the caecal and large intestinal regions of the digestive tract[2].

Virginiamycin's selective inhibition of lactate-producing bacteria prompted study of its effect on rumen fermentation. Growth trials have also been conducted along with measures of virginiamycin safety in cattle.

PROCEDURES

Virginiamycin was compared with chlortetracycline, monensin (sodium salt), and lasalocid (sodium salt) for effect against rumen organisms involved with lactic acid metabolism. *Streptococcus bovis* (ATCC 15351) and *Lactobacillus ruminis* (ATCC 27780) were considered as examples of lactate producers while *Megasphera elsdenii* was considered to be a lactate utilizer. Incubations of organisms with test chemical were done for 24 h at 39 °C under anaerobic conditions in media appropriate to each organism. Antibiotics were tested at concentrations ranging from 0.05 to 9 parts/10^6 in the incubate. Growth was measured in terms of optical density (600 nm).

Growth and feed utilization efficiency measures were obtained using 74 Normande bullocks. Starting weight was 200 kg and slaughter weight was approximately 550 kg. The diet consisted of 3 kg of concentrate fed to each animal daily throughout the study. Maize silage was fed *ad libitum*. Cattle were weighed at 28 day intervals. Virginiamycin was fed in the concentrate at levels of 120 mg/animal daily when cattle were 200–350 kg body weight and 240 mg/animal daily when cattle were 350–550 kg body weight. Carcass measurements were taken at slaughter.

Safety was determined with feed inclusion levels of approximately 20 times the average inclusion level studied in efficacy trials. Zero, 100 and 500 parts/10^6 dietary levels were fed for 6 months to both male and female cattle (three of each/treatment). Beet pulp and concentrate were the basal dietary ingredients. Cattle started on test weighing 280 kg and finished at 470 kg. Feed consumption, weight gains, and clinical observations were taken at 4 week intervals. At study completion, all animals were necropsied and rumen pH and volatile fatty acid (VFA) levels measured.

RESULTS

Virginiamycin, monensin, and lasalocid were all found to manipulate rumen fermentation *in vitro* toward increased propionic acid production[2].

The ionophores, monensin, and lasalocid produced the greatest shift in VFA formation, while virginiamycin appeared to produce initial manipulation at lower concentrations (0.15–0.5 parts/10^6) than the ionophores. VFA production was not inhibited by monensin, lasalocid or virginiamycin.

D- and L-lactic acid production was inhibited by virginiamycin at concentrations of 0.05 parts/10^6 or greater. Ionophores were less effective than virginiamycin in blocking lactic acid production.

Virginiamycin produced increased growth and feed utilization efficiency in bullocks. The major response to virginiamycin occurred early in the fattening period.

During the growing phase, virginiamycin improved growth rate by 6.25% and feed utilization by 3.3%. Response to virginiamycin was smaller during the fattening phase, leaving an overall virginiamycin response of 2–3% for both growth and feed utilization efficiency. Virginiamycin inclusion levels were approximately 20 parts/10^6 during the growing phase and 30 parts/10^6 during the fattening phase. Virginiamycin inclusion levels in the diet were different during different phases in an attempt to obtain comparable virginiamycin dosing on a body weight basis. It is probable that dosing based on feed concentration is superior to dosing based on body weight for rumen target chemicals.

When virginiamycin was included at 100 and 500 parts/10^6 in the diet of cattle, an initial reduction in feed intake occurred; however, over the 6 month study, no detrimental effect was observed for growth rate or feed utilization.

No clinical effects due to virginiamycin were noted during the study. Unplanned pregnancies in two females were not affected by virginiamycin. In the 100 parts/10^6 virginiamycin group, the pregnancy had progressed to within 3 weeks of parturition at the time of necropsy. No lesions were noted in the fetus. A pregnancy in the 500 parts/10^6 group resulted in the birth of a live bull calf at day 140 of the study. Rumen pH was higher in 100 and 500 parts/10^6 virginiamycin treatments. This effect has been noted in other

Table 1 Effects of virginiamycin in the diet of cattle (safety study)

	Control	*Virginiamycin* 100 parts/10^6	*Virginiamycin* 500 parts/10^6
Beginning weight (kg)	290.2	289.6	285.4
Average daily gain (kg)	0.99	0.98	0.97
Feed/gain	8.66	8.87	9.29
Rumen pH	5.71	6.05	6.01

studies with less virginiamycin feed inclusion levels (e.g. 30 and 60 parts/10^6). The reducing of rumen lactate levels by virginiamycin is a probable factor in the virginiamycin rumen pH effect. Rumen content analysis indicated reduced volatile fatty acid concentrations from virginiamycin treatments; however, differences were not statistically significant.

CONCLUSIONS

Virginiamycin affects rumen fermentation by inhibiting D- and L-lactic acid-producing organisms while not inhibiting lactic acid utilizers. Under *in vitro* conditions, virginiamycin alters the volatile fatty acid profile much like monensin and lasalocid; however, the degree of response is not as great with virginiamycin as with the ionophores. In a feeding trial, virginiamycin improved average daily gain and feed utilization efficiency with greatest incremental responses developing during the first 3–5 months of feeding. Although feed inclusion levels have not yet been identified, measurable growth promotion has been observed at 20–30 parts/10^6 of total daily ration dry matter. Safety studies with feed inclusion levels up to 500 parts/10^6 for 168 days revealed no adverse effects of virginiamycin on animal health, growth rate or feed utilization efficiency.

References

1. Cocito, C. (1979). Antibiotics of the virginiamycin family, inhibitors which contain synergistic components. *Microbiol. Rev.*, **43**, 145
2. Hedde, R. D., Shor, L., Quach, R. *et al.* (1982). Virginiamycin activity and safety in ruminants. *Les Colloques de l'INRA*, **8**, 391–6
3. Vervaeke, I. J., Decuypere, J. A., Dierick, N. A. *et al.* (1979). Quantitative *in vitro* evaluation of the energy metabolism influenced by virginiamycin and spiramycin used as growth promoters in pig nutrition. *J. Anim. Sci.*, **49**, 346–56

The use of monensin in cattle: effectiveness and safety to the consumer

J. I. D. Wilkinson

Monensin is a polyether antibiotic produced by the fermentation of *Streptomyces cinnamonensis*. It was the first of this class of compounds to be identified as a promoter of zootechnical efficiency in ruminant animals. The discovery of this attribute of the polyethers arose from a systematic application of *in vitro* rumen fermentation techniques in a search for compounds capable of shifting the balance of volatile fatty acids produced in the rumen towards increased propionic acid production. Monensin is able to effect this change and to sustain it over extended periods of time, regardless of whether rations are forage-based or contain a high proportion of readily fermented carbohydrate. The research leading to the development of monensin as a feed additive for beef cattle has been summarized by Raun[3].

GROWTH PERFORMANCE RESPONSES

The effect of monensin on the growth performance of grain-fed cattle in the American feedlot system was studied in 19 experiments. A further 12 experiments demonstrated the compound's effects in cattle fed rations composed almost entirely of freshly-harvested or conserved forage and, in 24 trials, effects in pastured cattle were studied. In grain-fed cattle the rate of average daily liveweight gain (ADG) was not altered, while feed intake was reduced. The optimal dosage of monensin was 33 parts/10^6 in the ration on a 90% dry matter basis. This inclusion level resulted in an improvement of feed conversion efficiency (FCE) of 10.6%. In contrast, when cattle were fed high-roughage rations, feed intake was little altered while ADG was increased by 14.7% and FCE improved by 15.3%. In pastured cattle the addition of 200 mg of monensin to the daily pasture supplement increased ADG by 16.3%.

This well-demonstrated effect of monensin on the growth performance of cattle has led to its inclusion in the rations of over 95% of cattle being finished in large US feedlots.

In Europe, the effect of monensin on the growth performance of confined growing beef cattle was studied in 35 trials carried out in nine countries under typical local management and rationing conditions. A total of 2371 cattle of ten different beef and dual purpose breeds was involved in the series of experiments. Of the 35 trials, 12 employed rations substantially composed of maize silage and in eight studies rations were based on barley concentrate. A further 12 trials involving 434 cattle were carried out in four European countries to study the effect of the addition of 200 mg of monensin to the daily pasture supplement. In the 35-trial pooled analysis the inclusion of 37–40 parts/10^6 monensin in the ration (90% dry matter basis) resulted in an improvement of FCE of 10.3%. In those trials in which maize silage was fed, 30 parts/10^6 monensin improved FCE by 8.3% and in trials with rations based on barley grain the FCE improvement was 9.7% at 30–40 parts/10^6. For pastured cattle, 200 mg monensin per head per day increased the rate of ADG by 13.7% above that of control cattle fed unmedicated supplements.

Details of these European trials have been given by Hawkridge[2] and by Wilkinson *et al.*[4]. Numerous independent publications from Eastern and Western Europe have also confirmed the ability of monensin to improve the efficiency of beef production under widely diverse management conditions.

METABOLISM AND TISSUE RESIDUES

Balance studies have been carried out using radio-labelled monensin in cattle. 300 mg of [^{14}C]monensin were given orally. The animals also received 300 mg per day of unlabelled monensin for 2 weeks prior to, and for 2 weeks following the labelled dosage. The administered dosage was recovered quantitatively in the faeces. The urine contained no detectable radio-activity over the background counts measured during the predosage period.

Column and thin-layer chromatographic separation of extracts from the faeces of orally-dosed cattle showed that 40–50% of the total radioactivity was recovered in the faeces as unchanged monensin and 50–60% as metabolites[1].

Monensin was fed to cattle at levels of 100 and 500 mg per head per day for 148 days and at 750 mg per head per day for 106 days. Animals were slaughtered at various times after withdrawal of monensin from the ration according to the schedule shown in Table 1. Samples of fat, lean meat, liver and kidney were removed at each sampling time and submitted for microbiological assay of monensin. No monensin residues above the test sensitivity

Table 1 Slaughter schedule for a monensin residue study in cattle

Monensin dosage		
mg/head daily	*Average concentration in ration* (parts/10^6)	*Withdrawal time* (h)
100	15	0, 48, 120, 240
500	80	0, 48, 120, 240
750	130	0, 48

of 0.05 μg/g were detectable in any tissues of animals receiving 100 or 500 mg per head per day at any withdrawal time. Only one liver sample from one animal receiving 750 mg per head per day at zero withdrawal time contained a residue which was estimated to be at the test sensitivity of 0.05 μg/g. This level of monensin feeding is approximately twice the maximum recommended and permitted amount.

CONCLUSION

Very extensive research programmes conducted in the USA and throughout Europe have clearly demonstrated the ability of monensin to improve the efficiency with which cattle convert feedstuffs to meat. At the effective levels of use, the inclusion of monensin in the feed produces no detectable residue in any edible tissue. The use of this compound and the benefits it offers to animal production present no hazard to the consumer.

References

1. Donoho, A., Manthey, J., Occolowitz, J. *et al.* (1978). Metabolism of monensin in the steer and rat. *Agric. Food Chem.*, **26,** 1090
2. Hawkridge, J. (1978). Monensin dose–response relationship under European conditions. Presented at *Eur. Congress for Improved Beef Productivity.* (Paris: Eli Lilly and Co.)
3. Raun, A. P. (1978). Monensin. Effect on energy efficiency. Presented at *Eur. Congress for Improved Beef Productivity.* (Paris: Eli Lilly and Co.)
4. Wilkinson, J. I. D., Shaw, C. J., Appleby, W. G. C. *et al.* (1980). The use of monensin in European pasture cattle. *Anim. Prod.*, **31,** 159

Effect of lasalocid sodium on digestion in sheep

P. Thivend, J. P. Jouany and J. Senaud

Lasalocid, like other ionophore antibiotics (monensin), has been shown to bring on increased propionic acid production and reduced methane formation in the rumen[3, 13]. These effects would be due to a selection of bacteria that produce succinate and which ferment lactate, and also to an inhibition of bacteria that produce acetate, butyrate, and lactate as end products, and formiate and hydrogen as intermediary precursors to methane[2, 5].

The extent of digestion in different parts of the digestive tract, and the nature of the end products of the digestion in the rumen as a function of the amount of lasalocid given in sheep have been determined to quantify the changes in microbial digestion.

MATERIALS AND METHODS

Four adult Texel sheep, fitted with a rumen cannula and with simple cannulae at the duodenum and ileum, were fed four different feeds successively according to a latin-square design. The four diets studied contained 0 (LO), 21 (L1), 43 (L2) and 64 (L3) parts/10^6 of lasalocid sodium, respectively. The feed was made up of highly pressed and ensiled sugar beet pulp (56.2%), cereal (barley and maize 27.6%), urea (1.5%) and chopped wheat straw (14.1%). The feed rations were prepared daily and given in two equal meals. Animals were fed *ad libitum* for the first 3 weeks. Then they were given an amount of feed that corresponded to the intake of the animal with the lowest feed consumption during the *ad libitum* period[9].

The determination of the diet digestibility was based on quantitative faeces collection over a period of 1 week. Rumen content samples and duodenum and ileum samples were taken during a 2 day period at 6 h intervals and immediately frozen at $-20\,°C$.

To measure the protozoa population, samples were taken 1 h after feeding in the morning for 5 consecutive days[10]. The cellulolytic activity of rumen bacteria was measured by the nylon bag method[10].

Ruminal digestion and total digestion coefficients for organic matter and nitrogen based on nutrient-indicator ratios were corrected to represent 100% recovery of chromic oxide. Data were analysed as a latin-square design by analysis of variance.

RESULTS

End products of fermentation

The presence of lasalocid in the feed resulted in an increased amount of propionic acid in the volatile fatty acid (VFA) mixture, when sheep were fed 43 and 64 parts/10^6 of lasalocid (Table 1). The proportions of acetic to butyric acids decreased. The concentrations to other volatile fatty acids tended to decrease, particularly when the amount of lasalocid given exceeded 21 parts/10^6, but the differences were only significant for valerianic and caproic acids. The total amount of VFA of rumen fluid was also decreased when animals were given 43 or 64 parts/10^6 of lasalocid.

Table 1 Effect of lasalocid sodium on rumen fermentation (means of 10 measurements and standard deviations)

	Lasalocid sodium (parts/10^6)			
	0 (L0)	21 (L1)	43 (L2)	64 (L3)
Total VFA (mmol/l)	74.2 ± 4.0*	73.6 ± 15.0*†	71.2 ± 14.3†‡	70.4 ± 10.5‡
Acetic (mol/100 mol)	60.6 ± 6.1*	59.0 ± 1.7*†	56.6 ± 2.9†	55.7 ± 2.0†
Propionic (mol/100 mol)	23.2 ± 4.4**	26.6 ± 3.9**	32.3 ± 5.7††	32.5 ± 4.5††
Butyric (mol/100 mol)	11.3 ± 0.9*	10.0 ± 1.9*†	8.2 ± 2.5†	8.6 ± 2.4†
Isobutyric (mol/100 mol)	0.45 ± 0.06*	0.57 ± 0.07*	0.32 ± 0.04*	0.32 ± 0.05*
Valeric (mol/100 mol)	2.92 ± 0.73*	2.20 ± 0.55*†	2.00 ± 0.49†‡	2.05 ± 0.45‡
Isovaleric (mol/100 mol)	1.45 ± 0.81*	1.25 ± 0.76*	0.50 ± 0.31*	0.45 ± 0.43*
Caproic (mol/100 mol)	0.67 ± 0.09**	0.26 ± 0.03††	0.22 ± 0.04††	0.17 ± 0.02††
pH	5.88 ± 0.17*	5.86 ± 0.16*†	5.95 ± 0.22*†	6.00 ± 0.22†
rH (mV)	− 392 ± 55*	− 414 ± 37*	− 402 ± 27*	− 419 ± 32*
CO_2/CH_4	2.23 ± 0.44**	2.75 ± 0.32†	2.88 ± 0.38††	2.55 ± 0.41**††
Ammonia nitrogen (mg/l)	154 ± 58*	187 ± 65*	152 ± 50*	150 ± 45*

Means with different superscripts are significantly different (**, ††: $p<0.01$; *, †, ‡: $p<0.05$)

The gas composition[9] was considerably altered when 21 and 43 parts/10^6 lasalocid were fed. The methane fraction dropped by 20% and the CO_2/CH_4 ratio increased significantly.

Finally, lasalocid did not alter the mean value of rumen fluid ammonia nitrogen content[11]. The drastic increase in ammoniogenesis after feeding can be attributed to fermentation of the ureic nitrogen in the feed. After that, the decrease noted with the control diet was quicker than with the experimental diets, which probably indicated a greater bacterial synthesis when the sheep did not receive any lasalocid.

Organic matter digestion

Lasalocid modified the extent and sites of organic matter (OM) digestion (Table 2). The overall digestibility was lower with feeds which contained 43 and 64 parts/10^6 lasalocid. Values were only significantly different from control values with the higher lasalocid diet (L3). This influence of lasalocid takes place mainly in forestomachs. On average the decrease in the amount of organic matter truly digested in the rumen is about 12%, whatever the diet concentration of lasalocid.

Table 2 Effect of lasalocid sodium on site and extent of organic matter (OM) digestion (means and standard deviations)

	Lasalocid sodium (parts/10^6)			
	0 (L0)	21 (L1)	43 (L2)	64 (L3)
Intake (g/day)	823 ± 17*	824 ± 17*	827 ± 21*	785 ± 60‡
Ruminal digestion (% intake)				
OM apparently digested	59.5 ± 6.2**	52.4 ± 4.4††	55.8 ± 4.8†	50.8 ± 3.9††
OM truly digested	79.2 ± 6.5**	69.4 ± 4.8††	71.2 ± 4.3††	68.1 ± 4.8††
Ruminal and small intestinal digestion (% intake)	81.6 ± 3.8*	75.9 ± 5.6*	74.2 ± 6.8*†	72.3 ± 3.1††
Total digestion (% intake)	82.8 ± 0.8*	82.8 ± 0.1*	80.7 ± 3.9*†	78.5 ± 2.5†
Ruminal digestion (% digest. OM)				
OM apparently digested	71.9 ± 7.8*	64.4 ± 5.3†	69.7 ± 4.1*	63.1 ± 4.5†
OM truly digested	95.3 ± 8.0**	85.2 ± 5.7††	89.1 ± 3.8†	84.7 ± 6.3††
Small intestinal digestion (% OM, entering duodenum)	54.8 ± 2.6*	49.0 ± 12.8*	45.9 ± 8.2†	43.9 ± 1.9†

Means with different superscripts are significantly different, (**, ††: $p<0.01$; *, †, ‡: $p<0.05$)

Due to the lower digestibility of organic matter in the forestomach, the quantity of organic matter entering the small intestine increases. OM was poorly hydrolysed by the intestinal enzymes, because the used diets were rich in structural carbohydrates (36% dry matter (DM)) and relatively poor in starch (18% DM). At the ileum, organic matter digestibility was also lower (75.9, 74.2, and 72.3% in lasalocid-fed animals vs. 81.6% in control animals). In the large intestine, a part of the OM was fermented by the microflora, but in high lasalocid diets the breakdown was insufficient to compensate the decrease in rumen digestion.

Nitrogen digestion

Lasalocid, given at a concentration of 21 and 43 parts/10^6 in the feed had no effect on nitrogen digestibility. But the dosage of 64 parts/10^6 depressed significantly the nitrogen digestibility (70.4% vs. 76.8%). Lasalocid significantly lowered bacterial synthesis in the rumen. As a consequence, the amount of undegraded dietary nitrogen in the rumen increased (43 and 64 parts/10^6). Finally, the efficiency of microbial synthesis (g bacterial nitrogen per 100 g OM truly fermented in the rumen) was not significantly modified by lasalocid.

DISCUSSION

Lasalocid, like other ionophorous antibiotics, modifies microbial activity in the rumen. By selecting specific bacteria, it alters rumen fermentation towards higher production of propionic acid and smaller production of methane. When inhibiting the development of other bacteria, it reduces the intensity of microbial synthesis and consequently has a limiting effect on the degradation of feed protein.

The results obtained confirm previously published data[4,6,7,11,12], although the animals were fed quite a different type of diet which was rich in structural carbohydrates. A drastic effect of lasalocid on the ciliate protozoa in the rumen, as already observed with monensin[8], could be demonstrated. It has also been shown that lasalocid, dependent on the dosage, can alter the bacteria population quantitatively as well as qualitatively. These observations are in good agreement with other results[2] which showed that lasalocid or monensin select resistant strains, such as *Bacteroides* which produce succinate and *Selenomonas* which decarboxylize succinate to propionate. The effect of lasalocid on the microbial population in the rumen, expressed as a decrease in the amount of organic matter fermented and of bacterial protein synthesized in the rumen, are similar to those obtained in cattle which were fed cereal-rich diets (90% corn) supplemented with 33 parts/10^6 monensin. However, the decrease in fermented organic matter in the rumen was independent of the dose of lasalocid, whereas an effect of lasalocid on the microbial population was significant with doses equal to or higher than 43 parts/10^6. Other mechanisms may be involved in this decrease in rumen digestion, e.g. an increased consumption of water which in turn increased the passage of digesta towards the small intestine.

The reduced digestion of organic matter in the rumen can be compensated by higher digestion in the small intestine and/or in the large intestine. As already mentioned, the high carbohydrate portion in the experimental diet, which was not degraded in the rumen, could not be hydrolysed to full extent in the small intestine. Dependent on the lasalocid concentration, the digestion of the remaining carbohydrates takes place in the large intestine. However, it seems that there is no negative effect of lasalocid up to a dosage[1,7] of 50 parts/10^6.

CONCLUSION

In the ruminant, lasalocid has, in general, a favourable effect on feed efficiency[4] by modifying energy and nitrogen digestion. The increased propionic acid and the decreased methane production in the rumen, as well as the increase in the portion of starch digested as glucose in the small intestine, result in an improved diet energy utilization. The amount of non-degraded dietary nitrogen in the rumen increases, which could be of particular interest in case of protein compounds in the feed which are well balanced in essential amino acids. The slight decrease of bacterial synthesis could limit the use of lasalocid in diets with a high content of soluble nitrogen (more than 40–50% total nitrogen).

References

1. Berger, L. L., Ricke, S. C. and Fahey, G. C. (1981). Comparison of two forms and two levels of lasalocid with monensin on feedlot cattle performance. *J. Anim. Sci.*, **53**, 1440–5
2. Chen, M. and Wolin, M. J. (1979). Effect of monensin and lasalocid sodium on the growth of methanogenic and rumen saccharolytic bacteria. *Appl. Environ. Microbiol.*, **38**, 72–7
3. Durand, M. (1982). Orientation du métabolisme du rumen au moyen des additifs. *Ann. Zootech.*, **31**, 47–76
4. Foreyt, J., Parish, S. M. and Foreyt, K. M. (1981). Lasalocid for improved weight gains and control of coccidia in lambs. *Am. J. Vet. Res.*, **42**, 57–60
5. Fuller, J. R. and Johnson, D. E. (1981). Monensin and lasalocid effects on fermentation *in vitro*. *J. Anim. Sci.*, **53**, 1574–80
6. Gutierrez, G. G., Schake, L. M. and Byers, F. M. (1982). Whole plant grain sorghum silage processing and lasalocid effects on stocker calf performance and rumen fermentation. *J. Anim. Sci.*, **54**, 863–8
7. Horton, G. M. J. and Stockdale, P. H. G. (1981). Lasalocid and monensin in finishing diets for early weaned lambs with naturally occurring coccidiosis. *Am. J. Vet. Res.*, **42**, 433–6
8. Jouany, J. P. and Senaud, J. (1978). Utilisation du monensin dans la ration des ruminants. II. Effets sur les fermentations et la population microbienne du rumen. *Ann. Zootech.*, **27**, 61–74
9. Jouany, J. P. and Senaud, J. (1979). Description d'une technique permettant d'effectuer des prélèvements répétés de gaz dans le rumen. *Ann. Biol. Anim. Biochim. Biophys.*, **19**, 1007–10
10. Jouany, J. P. and Senaud, J. (1982). Influence des ciliés du rumen sur la digestion de différents glucides chez le mouton. I. Utilisation des glucides pariétaux (cellulose et hémicellulose) et de l'amidon. *Reprod. Nutr. Develop.*, **22**, 735–52
11. Nagaraja, T. G., Avery, T. B., Bartley, E. E. *et al.* (1982). Effect of lasalocid, monensin or thiopeptin on lactic acidosis in cattle. *J. Anim. Sci.*, **54**, 649–58
12. Thonney, M. L., Heide, E. K., Duhaime, D. J. *et al.* (1981). Growth, feed efficiency and metabolite concentrations of cattle fed high forage diets with lasalocid or monensin supplements. *J. Anim. Sci.*, **52**, 427–33
13. van Nevel, C. J. and Demeyer, D. I. (1977). Effect of monensin on rumen metabolism *in vitro*. *Appl. Environ. Microbiol.*, **34**, 251–7

Evaluation of the efficacy of lasalocid sodium on the fattening of steers

D. Droumev, D. Jourbinev and D. Pashov

Lasalocid sodium (Bovatec®) is a polyether antibiotic produced by the fermentation of *Streptomyces lasaliensis* and is similar to monensin and salinomycin[1–] . It is used for the prevention of coccidiosis of broiler chicken (Avatec®) and is also an effective coccidiostat in ruminants[6–8]. In ruminants, however, lasalocid (LSC) reveals a positive influence on rumen fermentation and feed efficiency by altering the proportion of volatile fatty acids in rumen contents towards higher propionate and lower acetate, while methane production is reduced at the same time[8,9]. The addition of LSC to feedlot diets improves feed efficiency by reducing feed intake without adversely affecting growth rate. In most of the investigations the antibiotic has an additional positive influence on the performance of feedlot animals[2,8,9].

The aim of the present trial was to study the ergotropic action of LSC on fattening steers and to determine the optimal period of treating.

MATERIAL AND METHODS

The trial was carried out with 20 steers of the 'Black Spot Cattle' breed, with an average initial weight of about 240 kg. The animals were uniformly allotted to two treatment groups of ten each, chained up in a fattening beef cattle barn, equipped for individual feeding. The steers were fed once daily during the whole experimental period of 214 days. During the fattening and finishing period of the trial the animals were put on different diets given as a blend containing all the ingredients of the ration including the crude components. Lasalocid sodium was given to the animals of the test group in daily individual doses as a 15% Bovatec premix (Hofmann-La Roche & Co), which was mixed by hand into the daily ration. The daily dose was calculated as 0.84 mg lasalocid sodium per kg body weight and was altered according to the weight once a month.

The following parameters, such as body weight, average weight gain, feed intake, feed efficiency of the fattening steers as well as the carcass quality of the slaughtered animals (five of each group) were measured. While the steers were weighed individually at monthly intervals, the feed consumption was recorded daily and the general appearance and the state of health of the animals were observed every day. Statistical analyses of the data were performed using Wilcoxon's signed-rank test (for slaughter data - Student-Fischer's method).

Before starting the test the animals were treated with levamisole hydrochloride (Nilverm, ICI) and with tylosin preventively (Tylan-200, Elanco Products Co.). They were vaccinated against foot and mouth disease.

RESULTS AND DISCUSSION

The results of the trial summarized in Table 1 show a beneficial effect of LSC fed to the experimental animals. The antibiotic in doses ranging from 206 mg/animal per day, at the beginning, to 372 mg/animal per day, at the end of the trial, resulted in a significant increase in the average daily body weight gain of 8.8% in comparison to the control group. The general nutritive effect was well manifested throughout the test period of 214 days, whereas the relatively highest increase in weight gain was recorded during the initial 2 months of the experiment (up to +25.8%). During the subsequent period, the ergotropic influence of LSC persisted with some fluctuations of average daily gain between 8.5 and 16.7%.

The average amount of the daily feed consumption of the treated steers decreased by 5%. The feed conversion was improved - the feed intake per kg body weight gain was lowered by 12% compared to the control group during the whole experimental period. For the initial 4 months the feed efficiency was improved by 17 to 24%. Feeding LSC to the fattening steers did not result in any considerable changes of the slaughter data and the meat quality.

The obtained results show that LSC in a dose of 0.84 mg/kg body weight daily reveals a nutritive action on steers. The dose calculated according to the daily feed intake was in the range of 32 and 43 parts/10^6 for the 1st and

Table 1 Effects of lasalocid (0.84 mg/kg body weight) on steer performance in a 214 day trial

Group	*Control* ($n = 9$)	*Lasalocid* ($n = 10$)
Initial body weight (kg)	239.8 ± 18.8	243.7 ± 14.3
Final body weight (kg)	454.1 ± 22.4	477.0 ± 11.8
Weight gain (kg)	214.3 ± 10.0	233.3 ± 10.3
Av. daily weight gain (g)	1001.8 ± 47.0	1090.2 ± 48.0
daily weight gain rel.	100.0	108.8*
Av. feed intake (kg)	1922.1 ± 80.5	1826.2 ± 53.4
feed intake rel.	100.0	95.0
Feed to gain ratio, feed	9.07 ± 0.46	7.97 ± 0.46
dry matter	7.98 ± 0.40	7.01 ± 0.40
rel.	100.0	87.8**

*$p < 0.02$; **$p < 0.01$

the 7th months, respectively. The effect of LSC in respect of average daily gain was manifested best during the first 2 months when the concentration of LSC in the feed was 32 and 34 parts/10^6.

References

1. Bartley, E. E., Herod, E., Bechtle, R. *et al.* (1979). Effects of rumensin and lasalocid on rumen fermentation *in vitro. Cattlemen's Day*, **350,** 73–5
2. Berger, L. L. and Ricke, S. C. (1980). Comparison of lasalocid and monensin for feedlot cattle. *J. Anim. Sci.*, **49** (Suppl. 1), 357–8
3. Berger, L. L., Ricke, S. C. and Fahey, G. C. Jr. (1981). Comparison of two forms and two levels of lasalocid with monensin on feedlot cattle performance. *J. Anim. Sci.*, **51** (Suppl. 1), 345–6
4. Droumev, D., Pahov, D., Jourbinev, D. *et al.* (1981). The effect of salinomycin (K-364) on calves for fattening. *Vet. Sci. (Bulg.)*, 10, **18,** 34–40
5. Gutierrez, G., Schake, L. M. and Byers, F. M. (1981). Effect of whole plant grain sorghum silage processing methods and lasalocid sodium on stocker calf performance. *J. Anim. Sci.*, **54,** 863–8
6. Foreyt, W. J., Parish, S. M. and Foreyt, K. M. (1981). Lasalocid for improved weight gains and control of coccidia in lambs. *Am. J. Vet. Res.*, **42,** 57–60
7. Horton, G. M. J. and Stockdale, P. H. G. (1981). Lasalocid and monensin in finishing diets for early weaned lambs with naturally occurring coccidiosis. *Am. J. Vet. Res.*, **42,** 433–6
8. Lomas, L. W. (1982). Lasalocid for ruminants – application. In Proceedings of *37th Annual Kansas Formula Feed Conference*
9. Mies, W. L., Sherrod, L. B. and Summers, C. G. (1979). Evaluation of lasalocid sodium for growth promotion and feed efficiency improvement in finishing heifers. *Beef Research Report.* pp. 45–7. (Texas: Tech. Univ. Publ.)
10. Thonney, M. L., Heide, E. K., Duhaime, D. J. *et al.* (1981). Growth, feed efficiency and metabolite concentrations of cattle fed high forage diets with lasalocid or monensin supplements. *J. Anim. Sci.*, **52,** 427–33

Salinomycin, a new polyether antibiotic for fattening cattle and lambs

W. Sambeth and G. Dost

Due to its structure and mode of action, salinomycin belongs to the group of polyether antibiotics[3,6]. It exerts its ionophorous properties on the cation transport through the cell walls of animal tissues, of bacteria and of protozoa[5]. This effect within the gastrointestinal tract influences growth and feed efficiency as well as coccidial infections in ruminants and non-ruminants.

GROWTH-PROMOTING ACTIVITY

Based on the dose–response curve, calculated by computer from many feeding experiments, salinomycin can be recommended for fattening cattle at a dose of 100–200 mg/head daily (Figure 1). At the optimum level, weight gain and feed conversion are improved by around 11%, compared with the unmedicated control groups. This level corresponds to approximately 0.6 mg/kg body weight daily. Much higher doses lead to reduced feed intake, lower weight gains and impaired feed efficiency. The maximum tolerable dose tested in bulls was 8 mg salinomycin/kg body weight, applied in a single drench.

For fattening lambs, the recommended dosage of 10–20 parts/10^6 in the total feed allows an improvement of about 12–13% in weight gain and feed efficiency (Figure 1). The negative effect after high concentrations of salinomycin in the feed looks similar in lambs as in cattle.

MODE OF ACTION IN RUMINANTS

As for other polyether antibiotics, salinomycin markedly increases the propionic acid concentration in the ruminal fluid, while molar proportions of butyric acid and acetic acid, methane gas production[2,8] as well as cellulose catabolism[1] are reduced (Table 1). Thus, the feed energy is better utilized in

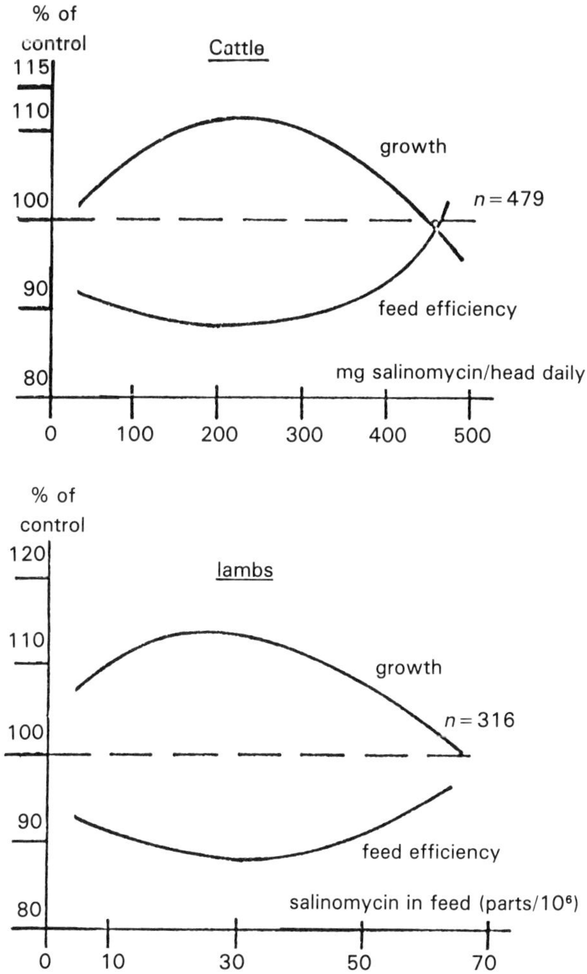

Figure 1 Dose–response relation when feeding salinomycin

terms of economics. On the other hand, salinomycin reduces the catabolism of feed protein in the rumen, as indicated by lowered ammonia concentrations[8] and retarded microbial protein synthesis[1]. These observations have been made partially *in vitro*, but most of them *in vivo*.

BLOOD PARAMETERS, PATHOLOGY

The blood parameters showed an increase of serum urea with increasing salinomycin doses in cattle. However, other biochemical and haematology parameters (i.e. Ca, P, Mg and total protein in serum, haemoglobin, leukocyte and erythrocyte counts) remained normal also under salinomycin at a

Table 1 Changes in ruminal production by feeding salinomycin

	Salinomycin intake (mg/head daily) 0	121	242
Ammonia-*N* in ruminal fluid (mg/l)	32.4	2.2	1.1
Total VFA (μmol/ml)	91.3	98.6	101.2
Moles fatty acid/100 moles total VFA			
acetic acid	60.0	44.3	47.5
propionic acid	21.8	41.5	41.6
isobutyric acid	0.94	1.01	0.69
butyric acid	14.0	9.1	7.0
isovaleric acid	1.94	1.53	0.51
valeric acid	1.34	2.53	2.64
Methane production (ml/h)	48.9	27.9	18.3

According to Webb, K. E., Fontenot, J. P. and Lucas, D. M. (1980)[8]

concentration twice higher than the recommended dosage[4]. At the fourfold dosage there was a non-significant increase in AP, SGPT and serum globulin level, indicating a changed liver metabolism. All other organs and tissues exhibited neither macroscopic nor histological changes.

CARCASS QUALITY, RESIDUES

Better growth of salinomycin-fed beef cattle yielded carcasses which were equal or slightly better than the control animals in terms of dressing percentage or visual scoring of the carcass quality[7].

After 3 days withdrawal time of the drug, only liver tissues in one experiment showed minute salinomycin residues, using a very specific and sensitive

Table 2 Residues of salinomycin

	Withdrawal days	*Expt. Bayerseich*	*Expt.* H 78/10*	*Expt. Sch 725*
Animals		bulls	steers	lambs
Salinomycin intake mg/head daily		200	286	40
Salinomycin residues in tissues (μg/g)				
liver	1	0.08–0.17	0.03–0.05	0.06–0.17
	3	0.03–0.07	0	0
	5	0	—	—
kidney, muscle, renal fat, back fat	1	0	0	0
	3	0	0	0

All salinomycin assays with 0.01 μg/g sensitivity limit
*According to Turnbull (1978)

microbiological assay method (Table 2). All other important tissues tested were without residues. After 5 days withdrawal time the liver had no detectable residues in all three experiments. In order to demonstrate the insignificance of the maximum salinomycin residue after 1 day withdrawal in relation to toxicological hazards for human beings, one would have to eat 160 kg liver within a single day to reach the maximum tolerable dose of salinomycin which was tested in pigs.

References

1. Cafantaris, B. (1981). Über die Wirkung von Antibiotika-Zusätzen auf die mikrobielle Gärung im Pansensaft *in vitro. Diss. Univ. Hohenheim*
2. Fontenot, J. P., Webb, K. E. Jr. and Lucas, D. M. (1980). Effect of salinomycin on *in vitro* and *in vivo* ruminal volatile fatty acids. *J. Anim. Sci.*, **51** (Suppl. 1), 360
3. Kinashi, H., Otake, N. and Yonechara, H. (1973). The structure of salinomycin - a new member of the polyether antibiotics. *Tetrahedron Letters*, **49**, 4955–8
4. McClure, W. N., Fontenot, J. P., Webb, K. E. Jr. *et al.* (1980). Feedlot performance of cattle fed different salinomycin levels. *J. Anim. Sci.*, **51** (Suppl. 1), 380
5. Mitani, M., Yamanishi, T. and Miyazaki, Y. (1975). Salinomycin: a new monovalent cation ionophore. *Biochem. Biophys. Res. Commun.*, **66**, 4
6. Miyazaki, Y. *et al.* (1974). Salinomycin, a new polyether antibiotic. *J. Antibiot.*, **27**, 814–21
7. Müller, W. and Wiedemann, R. (1980). Bullenmast auf der Basis von Maissilage mit dem Fütterungszusatz Salinomycin. *Der Tierzüchter*, **32**, 29–32
8. Webb, K. E. Jr., Fontenot, J. P. and Lucas, D. M. (1980). Metabolism studies in steers fed different levels of salinomycin. *J. Anim. Sci.*, **51** (Suppl. 1), 407

Salinomycin activity in ruminants

D. Droumev, V. Roussev, A. Petkov and D. Pashov

The polyether antibiotic salinomycin (SLM), supplemented in low concentrations to the feed, showed nutritive activity in ruminants. The increase of weight gain and of feed utilization of steers was due to an increase in the percentage of propionic acid, and a decrease in the percentage of acetic acid and butyric acid in the rumen[8]. The aim of the present investigation was to study the effect of SLM on the fattening of ruminants, partly described in References 12 and 13.

D. Jourbinev, S. Vangelov, I. Boshnakov, E. Enev, K. Sivkova, K. Krastanov, V. Drinkov, N. Lalov and O. Petkova also participated in this investigation.

MATERIALS AND METHODS

Four investigations were carried out on 180 uncastrated lambs of the stock 'Thracian Fine Fleece' weighing about 20 kg, and 40 young steers of the stock 'Black Spot Cattle' Breed weighing about 180 kg. Twenty young rams were operated on with chronic fistula of the dorsal sac of the rumen. Apart from SLM (Hoechst AG), monensin (Rumensin, Elanco Prod. Co.) (MON), and flavophospholipol (Flavomycin, Hoechst AG) (FPL) were included in some of the trials. The number of the animals, the scheme of application of the nutritive antibiotics in the individual investigations, the number and the composition of the groups and the duration are indicated in Table 1.

The lambs were fed in groups and the steers individually. The lambs were raised in covered premises, freely in separate boxes, on a concrete floor covered with sawdust. The basic ration, composed of soya groats 20%, barley 63%, wheat bran 12%, dry skim milk 2%, dicalcium phosphate 1.3%, salt 0.5% and vitamin premix (AD_3E) 0.5% in non-granulated form, was given twice a day.

The steers were kept in covered premises, tied and arranged in line on a brick floor. They received a ration composed of a blend of: whole maize plant meal 84%, lucerne meal 12%, urea 1%, dicalcium phosphate 1%, salt 1%, trace elements premix 0.5% and vitamin premix 0.5%.

The nutritive antibiotics for the lambs were mixed with the feed in advance. For the steers they were put in the feed by spreading over the individual daily ration and mixing by hand.

Table 1 Details of investigations using salinomycin, monensin and flavophospholipol

Trial	*Antibiotics*	*Dosage regimen*	*Duration* (days)
No. 1 Lambs 3 months 18.65 kg $n = 80$	SLM	Control SLM 6 parts/10^6 SLM 12 parts/10^6 SLM 24 parts/10^6	90
N. 2 Lambs 3 months 20 kg $n = 80$	FPL SLM	Control FPL 5 parts/10^6 SLM 5 parts/10^6 SLM 10 parts/10^6	90
No. 3 Lambs 3 months 21.25 kg $n = 20$	SLM	Control SLM 6 parts/10^6 SLM 12 parts/10^6 SLM 24 parts/10^6	90
No. 4 Steers 5 months 140 kg $n = 40$	SLM FPL Mon	Control MON 0.7 mg/kg SLM 0.5 mg/kg SLM 0.5 mg/kg FPL 0.1 mg/kg	269

The data were generally processed statistically by Student–Fisher tests and the differences in the average daily gain and the feed utilization in trial no. 4 were analyzed by means of Wilcoxon's signed-rank test.

RESULTS

Nutritive effect of SLM in lambs

At the end of the experimental period, animals that received SLM at the level of 6, 12 and 24 parts/10^6, had higher body weight and larger average daily gain in comparison with the control animals (by 12.2%, 16.7% and 19.4%, respectively) (Figure 1 (a)). Statistically significant ($p \leqslant 0.05$) differences were found between those that received SLM at the rate of 12 and 24 parts/10^6. The average daily feed consumption for those receiving SLM at 6 parts/10^6 was close to that of the control animals, but for those treated with 12 and 24 parts/10^6 less feed was consumed (by 2.3 and 6.5%, respectively). The average feed consumption for 1 kg of gain in the three groups of test animals was lower than that of the control animals (with 9.7, 16.6 and 22.2%, respectively). Measurement at intervals of 15 days showed that the favourable effect of SLM on the gain and the feed utilization manifested itself in the course of the whole 90 day experimental period. The data on consumption of starchy feed-units, dry matter, crude and digestible protein and Danish feed-units for 1 kg of gain correlated with the expected average feed consumption per 1 kg of gain.

The slaughter analysis done for 16 animals (four from each group) after the end of the 90 day experimental period showed that SLM did not bring

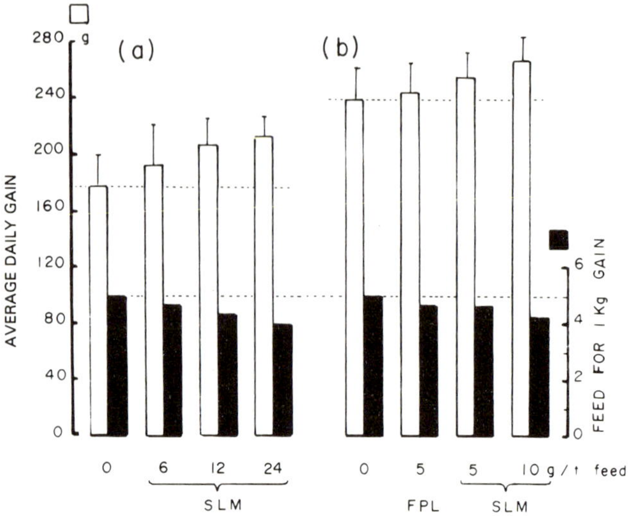

Figure 1 Nutritive effect of salinomycin (SLM) and flavophospholipol (FPL) in lambs

considerable changes in the yield at the slaughter, brought a certain decrease in water contents (by 2.2, 1.4 and 1.3%, respectively), and increased the amount of fat (by 2.8, 2.78 and 1.04%, respectively) (measured at initial moisture) – without statistical significance. No considerable changes were found in the content of nucleic acids in the meat, a relative decrease of DNA and RNA and of the RNA/DNA ratio in liver (statistically not significant). SLM had not a considerable influence upon the content of cyanocobalamin in meat and liver.

Investigating the development of the alimentary canal, there was a higher absolute weight of forestomach in the lambs that had received SLM (by 20–29%). The differences in the relative weights with respect to live body weight of the corresponding animals in relation to the control group were considerably lower (0.9–7%). An increase in the length of the small intestine was found in relation to the control group in parallel with the magnitude of the dose of SLM (by 2.3, 6.2 and 12.37%, respectively) at decrease of their relative weight (by 8.42, 11.58 and 12.63%, respectively) as well as of their absolute weight (SLM 12 and 24 parts/10^6). The indicated differences were not statistically significant. Differences in the weight of thc large intestine and length were negligible.

Antibiotic residues were not found in the meat and the internal organs of the lambs on the 5th day after withdrawal of SLM.

Study of the nutritive effect of SLM and FPL

Administration of SLM at the level of 5 and 10 parts/10^6 promoted the increase (in relation to the control group) of the live body weight (by 2.4% and 5.7%) and of the average daily gain (by 7% and 12.7%) at lower average daily consumption (by 2.7% and 2.5%, respectively). The average feed intake for 1 kg gain was smaller (by 8.9% and 13.6%, respectively) (Figure 1 (b)).

FPL used in identical experimental conditions, at a level of 5 parts/10^6 increased (in relation to the control animals) the body weight by 2.4%, the average daily gain by 4.5% with a lower average daily feed consumption by 4.2%, and decreased the average feed intake for 1 kg gain by 8.9%. This effect manifested itself in the course of the whole 90 day experimental period.

The data about the starchy feed units, dry matter, crude and digestible protein and Danish feed-units consumed for 1 kg gain of the lambs that received FPL and SLM corresponded to the data about the feed utilization.

The statistical significance of the differences in the body weight and the average daily gain in the three experimental groups in relation to the control group was established with respect to the average daily gain of the lambs which received SLM at a level of 10 parts/10^6 ($p \leqslant 0.05$).

Little difference was found in the yields of the animals slaughtered at the end of the trial (three from each group).

The chemical composition of the meat of the animals treated with FPL had a relatively higher fat content. The quantity of proteins, determined in absolutely dry state, was relatively lower in those that received SLM (5 parts/10^6) and relatively higher in those that were treated with SLM (10 parts/10^6). The differences in the chemical composition were not statistically significant.

SLM effect on rumen processes and blood components

After applying SLM for 90 days on lambs with chronic fistula of the dorsal sac of the rumen in doses 6, 12 and 24 parts/10^6, certain changes appeared in the rumen and in the blood of the test animals.

The total amount of the volatile fatty acids in the control group and the experimental groups fluctuated within the limits from 2.93 mmol/l to 3.9 mmol/l and did not change considerably under the influence of the three levels of SLM. In tracing the percentage correlation of the acetic, propionic and butyric acids on the 60th and the 90th day of the treatment, it was found that the increase of the propionic acid in all groups receiving SLM is significant. The molar percentage of the propionic acid in the control group was 19.6–21.6% and in the experimental groups reached 27.3–32.5%. The percentage of the butyric acid in the experimental groups was reduced (7.0–8.6%) in relation to the percentage in the control group (9.3–14.9%), without any statistical significance. In the greater part of the experiments a decrease in the content of the acetic acid was determined under the influence of SLM (62.4–60.0%) in comparison with the control animals (71.1–63.4%). The difference was statistically significant at the 60th day in groups receiving SLM 6 and 12 parts/10^6. The pH of the rumen liquid changed from 6.6 to 7.2 but without any definite regularity. The ammonia concentration was from 0.0085 to 0.019% in the four groups of lambs.

The total infusoria number of the control animals (Figure 2 (a)) until the 60th day was comparatively higher. Towards the 90th day of the trial it

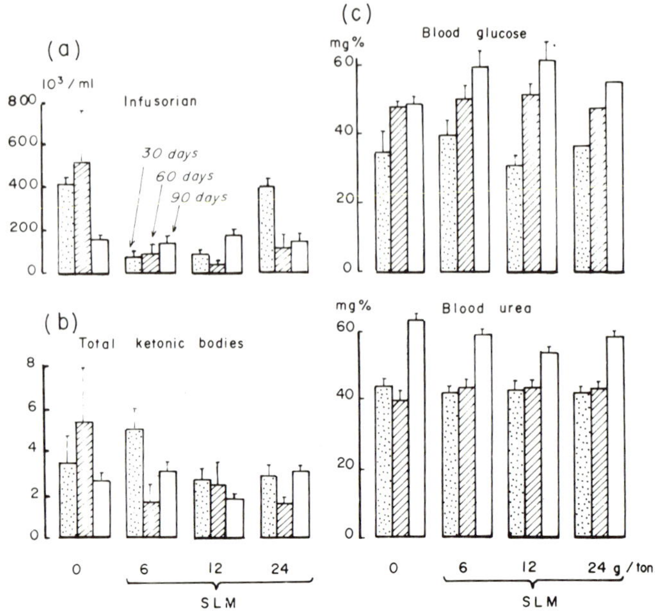

Figure 2 Changes induced by administration in lambs during 1, 2 and 3 months of SLM at 6, 12 and 24 parts/10^6

decreased in relation to the 30th and the 60th day. In the lambs which received SLM, the total infusoria number on the 30th day at levels of 6 and 12 parts/10^6, and on the 60th day at levels of 6, 12 and 24 parts/10^6, was lower in comparison to that of the control animals. The differences were statistically significant ($p \leqslant 0.001$ on the 30th day, and $p \leqslant 0.05$ on the 60th day for 12 parts/10^6). On the 90th day, considerable differences were not determined in the total infusoria number in the control group and the experimental groups.

In the lambs treated with SLM the predominating infusoria were from the *Ophryoscolecidae* family (80–90%) with genera *Entodinium* and *Diplodinium*. The rest of the infusoria were from the *Isotrichidae* family (10–20%) with genera *Isotricha* and *Dasytricha*.

The decrease of infusoria on the 30th day was mainly in the *Isotricha*, *Dasytricha* and *Diplodinium* in all experimental groups, on thc 60th day, to the *Isotricha* and *Dasytricha* (6 parts/10^6 SLM) and in the *Entodinium* and *Diplodinium* (12 and 24 parts/10^6 SLM).

The cellulolytic activity of the rumen content was relatively lower on the 60th day in the three experimental groups (7.40–8.58%) in comparison with the control group (11.60%). On the 90th day, it increased in relation to that of the control group (7.82%) in the lambs treated with 6 and 24 parts/10^6 SLM (12.21 and 9.06%, respectively). No statistically significant differences were found.

The blood sugar content (Figure 2 (c)) in lambs which received SLM was higher on the 60th and the 90th day after the treatment and this coincided with the increased percentage of the propionic acid in the rumen content. The rise in the blood sugar amount is statistically significant ($p \leqslant 0.05$) in the lambs which received 12 parts/10^6 SLM on the 90th day.

The content of urea in the blood decreased ($p \leqslant 0.05$) on the 30th day in the lambs treated with 24 parts/10^6 SLM and on the 90th day in case of 6 and 24 parts/10^6SLM ($p \leqslant 0.05$) and 12 parts/10^6 SLM ($p \leqslant 0.001$).

The amount of the ketonic bodies in the blood (Figure 2 (b)) showed a tendency to decrease, especially in the lambs from the groups which received 12 and 24 parts/10^6 SLM. This refers to the total amount of the ketonic bodies, and also to both acetone and aceto-acetic acid, and to β-hydroxybutyric acid. The decrease is significant for the content of acetone/aceto-acetic acid in the blood of the lambs which received 24 parts/10^6 SLM ($p \leqslant 0.05$) on the 60th day and for β-hydroxybutyric acid and the total amount of ketone bodies in the lambs treated with 12 parts/10^6 on the 90th day ($p \leqslant 0.05$).

The content of alkali reserves in the blood was increased in the experimental groups on the 60th day (151.5–166.7 mg/100 ml) in comparison with the control group (148.6 mg/100 ml). A statistically significant difference was found in the animals treated with SLM at the level of 24 parts/10^6 ($p \leqslant 0.001$).

The content of total protein, albumins and globulins in the blood showed similar changes in the control and the test animals.

Nutritive effect of SLM in steers

The average daily gain at the end of the 269 day experimental period (the body weight of the steers was about 460 kg) in the group treated with MON was 1083 g, i.e. 6% larger than that of the negative control group at 1022 g ($p \leqslant 0.01$). In the group treated with SLM it was 1066 g, and 1083 g in the group treated with SLM + FPL, respectively larger by 4.3 and 6% ($p \leqslant 0.02$ and $p \leqslant 0.01$, respectively). The average daily gain of the steers from the three experimental groups was more manifested during the first two quarters respectively for the group with MON (13.1 and 6.1%), for the group with SLM (9.2 and 14.4%), and for the group with SLM + FPL (12.4 and 5.7%) ($p \leqslant 0.05$). In the cumulative expression of the average daily gain up to the 6th month (the weight of the animals came to 370 kg), the values of the three experimental groups were 9.9%, 11.7% and 9.3%, respectively. In the final period of fattening (from the 7th to the 9th month), the average daily gain of the groups which received MON and SLM + FPL was close to that of the control group, but lower in the group treated with SLM only (Figure 3).

The average daily feed consumption per animal for the whole 269 day experimental period of the three groups which received nutritive antibiotics was lower than that of the control group by 4% for MON, by 2.7% for SLM, and by 3.6% for SLM + FPL.

The average feed consumption per kg gain for the 269 day experimental period in the experimental groups was lower in comparison with the control

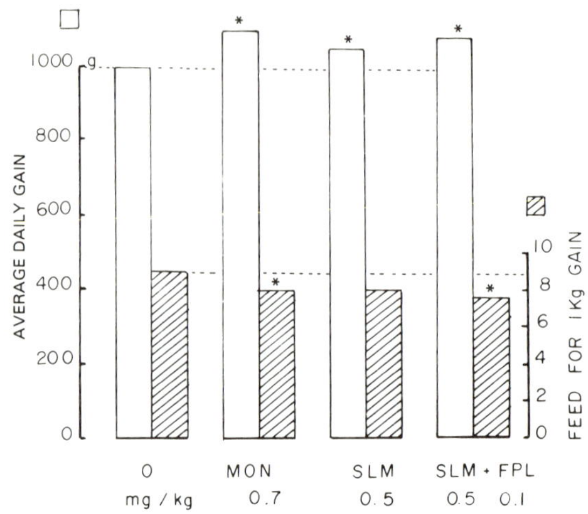

Figure 3 Average daily gain and feed efficiency of steers receiving monensin (MON), salinomycin (SLM) and SLM with flavophospholipol (FLP). * = significant

group: by 9.5% for MON, by 6.3% for SLM, and by 9.1% for SLM + FPL. Statistically significant differences were found for MON ($p \leqslant 0.01$) and for SLM + FPL ($p \leqslant 0.02$). For the first 6 months of the experiment the decreases were respectively by 12.1% for MON, by 10.8% for SLM, and by 10.8% for SLM + FPL.

The data concerning the consumption of starchy feed-units, dry matter, crude and digestible protein per kg gain were approximately parallel to the data about the feed utilization.

The slaughter analysis showed that the slaughter yield in the control group was somewhat higher than that of the experimental group: 1.63% for MON, 1.84% for SLM, and 2.46% for SLM + FPL. The differences were without statistical significance. With respect to the chemical composition of the meat in comparison with the control group, no practical difference was observed in the steers treated with SLM. In the groups receiving MON and SLM + FPL the content of proteins was relatively higher (by 2.88 and 3.64%, respectively) and the amount of fats was lower (by 2.91 and 4.51%, respectively), without statistical significance.

DISCUSSION

The results of the investigations show that SLM favours the increase of weight gain and the improvement of feed utilization in lambs and calves.

In the lambs, the nutritive effect of SLM manifests itself to a relatively larger degree in the whole range of the used doses (5–24 parts/10^6) and usually in the course of the whole period from the age of 2–6 months. Regardless of the differences in the rate of the average daily weight gain and average decrease in feed consumption per kg gain in trials no. 1 and no. 2, the existence of a dose–response relationship existed between the size of the applied dose and the degree of the nutritive effect (for each one of the two trials taken separately). The data show that SLM does not lead to considerable changes in the slaughter indices and in the chemical composition of the meat. It does not cause antibiotic residues to persist in the meat and the internal organs on the 5th day after SLM withdrawal.

The results from the investigations, concerning the indices of the rumen content and of the blood of the lambs, testify that SLM exerts influence on some of the processes in the forestomachs and on the development of the alimentary canal and improves the digestibility of the feed, facts also established in earlier experiments[11]. The observed coincidence in the increase of the propionic acid percentage, in the increase of the blood sugar, in the decrease of the blood urea and of the ketonic bodies can be ascribed to the positive effect of SLM on the carbohydrate metabolism in lambs. It can be considered as a sign of increased glucogenesis. The changes in the examined volatile fatty acids in the lambs show that SLM exerts influence on the fermentation processes in the rumen of lambs analogous to those observed in cattle. These facts were also established by other authors[2,3,7,8,10].

The decrease in the number and the changes in the proportion of genera of the different infusoria in the rumen liquid of the animals, treated with SLM during the first 2 months, must be accepted to be connected with the effect of the antibiotics. The established equalization of the total infusoria number in the control and the experimental group lambs on the 90th day from the SLM application is probably duc to the development of certain resistance.

The decrease of the cellulolytic activity in the rumen content can be explained to a certain extent with the decrease in the infusoria number from the *Ophryoscolecidae* family (hydrolysing the cellulose), with the pH of the rumen liquid (6.6–7.2 pH) which is not optimum for hydrolysis of cellulose from the infusoria (pH = 5)[4].

It is of interest that a tendency was found in the lambs treated with SLM toward an increase of the relative weight of the forestomach. Also, there is an increase in the length of the small intestines and a simultaneous decrease of their absolute and relative weight. The problem concerning the relation between these changes and the nutritive effect of SLM is worth further research.

The experimental data show that the ergotropic effect of FPL determined in the present comparative investigation is relatively lower than that of SLM in relation to the increase the average daily gain, and is equivalent in relation to the feed utilization.

The results from the SLM application in calves shows that the nutritive effect, at the doses used, manifests itself in the predominant part of the 269 day period, and is relatively best expressed in the period up to the 6th month, inclusive of the application.

The comparative examination with MON showed that its inclusion in the feed at a dose of 0.7 mg/kg body weight contributes to obtaining final values for gain and for feed utilization close to those of SLM. The favourable effect of SLM on the gain and the feed efficiency in the calves must be explained by an improvement of the fermentation processes.

From the data concerning the simultaneous application of SLM + FPL in calves, it can be seen that the combination does not increase significantly the nutritive effect of SLM.

The results about the independent application of SLM are close to those already published[9]. In comparison with other results[8] on the influence of SLM at a dose near to the one used in calves for fattening and based on maize silage administered for a shorter period (182 days), they are higher in relation to the increase of the gain (11.7% instead of 8.8%) and lower in relation to the feed utilization (10.8% instead of 15.6%) (for the corresponding interval). The final results differ also from those reporting [1,5] higher values for the average daily gain and for feed utilization and from those[6] stating the absence of a nutritive effect of SLM during 364 day application in calves. These differences are connected, most probably, with the differences in the experimental conditions.

In conclusion, it can be noticed that SLM manifests an ergotropic effect in lamb, as in cattle, that is related to an increase of the propionic acid content of the rumen, to a positive influence on the metabolism of carbohydrate, and to changes in the number and the correlation of the *infusoria genera* in the rumen. The combination SLM + FPL does not increase significantly the nutritive effect of SLM when it is used in calves. The ergotropic effect of MON in steers is close to that of SLM. FPL in lambs manifests a moderate nutritive effect.

References

1. Byers, F. M. (1981). Rumen research. The advent of monensin has triggered a great search for other compounds that may improve efficiency. *Feedlot Management*, **23,** 48 and 51–2
2. Cafantaris, B. and Menke, K. H. (1980). Über die Wirkung von Antibiotika-Zusätzen auf die mikrobielle Gärung im Pansensaft *in vitro. Z. Tierphysiol. Tierernähr. Futtermittelk.*, **44,** 19–20
3. Cafantaris, B. (1981). Über die Wirkung von Antibiotika-Zusätzen auf die mikrobielle Gärung im Pansensaft *in vitro. Diss. für Doktor der Agrarwissensch. Hohenheim*
4. Delfosse-Debussher, J., van Hoof, F., Hellings, P. *et al.* (1979). Hydrolytic activities of rumen ciliates. *Ann. Rech. Vét.*, **10,** 258–60
5. Gfrörer, F., Rutzmoser, K., Kartaly, A. *et al.* (1981). Ein Praxisver such mit dem Wachstumsförderer "Salinomycin" in der Bullenmast. *Bayerischer Landwirtsch. Jahrbuch*, **58,** 244–9
6. Leitgeb, K., Mader, H. and Lettner, F. (1981). The influence of rumensin, flavomycin and salinomycin on the performance of fattening bulls. *Proceedings of International Conference Feed Additives, Budapest*, **1,** 177
7. McClure, W. H., Fontenot, J. P. and Webb, K. E. Jr. (1980). Feedlot performance of cattle fed different salinomycin levels. *J. Anim. Sci.*, **51** (Suppl. 1), 380
8. Müller, W. and Wiedemann, R. (1980). Bullenmast auf der Basis von Maissilage mit dem Futterzusatz Salinomycin. *Der Tierzüchter*, **1,** 29–32
9. Oostendorpen, D. and Harmsen, H. E. (1981). Goede resultaten met antibiotica in krachtvoer voor vleesstieren. *Boerderij*, **66,** 18–19 VE
10. Webb, K. E. Jr., Fontenot, J. P. and Lucas, D. M. (1980). Metabolism studies in steers fed different levels of salinomycin. *J. Anim. Sci.*, **51** (Suppl. 1), 407
11. Wolf, I., Richter, G. and Flachowsky, G. (1981). Verdaulichkeit von mechanisch behandeltem Stroh nach Einsatz von Pansenfermoregulatoren. *Arch. Tierernähr.*, **31,** 254
12. Droumev, D., Roussev, V., Petkov, A. *et al.* (1981). Effect of salinomycin on lambs for fattening. *Vet. Sci. (Bulg.)*, **18,** 9, 60–4
13. Droumev, D., Pashov, D., Jourbiner, D. *et al.* (1981). The effect of salinomycin (IG364) on calves for fattening. *Vet. Sci. (Bulg)*, **18,** 10, 34–40

WORKSHOP II
Animal Anaesthesia

Chairmen: **P. Lees**
E. L. Gerring
E. P. Steffey

WORKSHOP II
Animal anaesthesia

Chairmen: **P. Lees, E. L. Gerring and E. P. Steffey**

Anaesthesia of both animals and man, whether undertaken for clinical or experimental purposes, is both an art and a science. It depends for its success on the skill and judgement of the individual anaesthetist no less than on his knowledge of the actions of drugs, their fate in the body and the ways in which they interact with each other. However, the art and the science of anaesthesia are not inseparable entities; they are closely interrelated. In this Workshop on Animal Anaesthesia, thirteen papers were presented which encompassed all the disciplines necessary to an understanding of the mechanisms of anaesthesia and to the application of anaesthetic techniques. The papers describe: (1) anaesthetic equipment and methodology for inhalation anaesthesia; (2) an appraisal of the clinical efficacy of the injectable anaesthetic etomidate used in conjunction with the narcotic-analgesic fentanyl; (3) the haemodynamic effects of methoxyflurane and halothane in the dog; (4) interactions between halothane and acepromazine on arterial blood pressure and pharmacokinetic interactions between chloramphenicol and injectable anaesthetics, leading to variable effects on duration of anaesthesia; (5) the clinical efficacy and clinical pharmacology of the dissociative anaesthetic ketamine in horses, calves and pigs; (6) the actions and uses in farm animals of a new sedative-analgesic, detomidine, and the actions in the dog of a new skeletal muscle relaxant, atracurium; (7) exciting new discoveries relating to the modes of action of barbiturates, dissociative anaesthetics and narcotic and non-narcotic analgesics; and (8) e.e.g. monitoring during anaesthesia.

Detomidine hydrochloride. A novel imidazole-type sedative analgesic

O. Vainio

During screening for sedative-analgesic effects of many imidazole-type compounds, detomidine proved to be potent sedative-analgesic agent for horses and cattle.

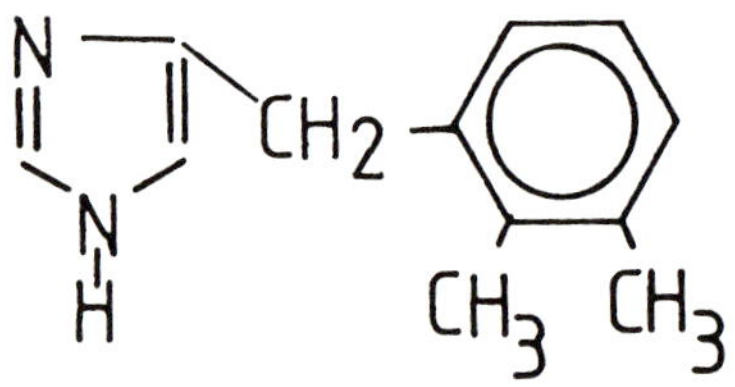

In the hot-plate test in mice, detomidine showed a clear dose-dependent analgesic effect at dose rates of 300–600 μg/kg and in the writhing test at doses of 150–600 μg/kg. These doses did not decrease the spontaneous motility of mice, therefore, a true analgesic effect occurred. In the hot-plate and writhing tests in mice, detomidine was superior to morphine in its analgesic effect. Detomidine did not exhibit any neuromuscular blocking effects in the isolated rat phrenic nerve-hemidiaphragm and chick m. biventer cervicis preparation.

The analgesic properties of detomidine may therefore be mediated by two mechanisms: (1) an anti-inflammatory action based on inhibition of prostaglandin synthesis, and (2) an effect in the CNS inhibiting transmission of pain impulses. Some of these effects may be mediated through an agonistic action on central α_2-receptors.

In screening studies, detomidine showed CNS depression in mice at oral doses of 1 mg/kg in the Irwin screen test. In the chicken, detomidine was hypnotic. However, in rats and mice, detomidine did not show true hypnotic properties (general anaesthesia was not obtained at any dose level). Sedation was accompanied by a decrease in spontaneous motility of mice at a dose rate of 1500 μg/kg. The prolongation of barbiturate sleeping time in mice at doses above 150 μg/kg also demonstrated the CNS depressant action of detomidine.

Detomidine showed sympathomimetic effects such as piloerection and exophthalmous in rats. The blood pressure of rats decreased after i.v. doses 10–300 μg/kg but increased at higher doses. Following cerebroventricular administration of small doses, the blood pressure decreased. Both hypotensive and hypertensive doses decreased the heart rate of rats, as did agents traditionally documented as α_2-adrenoceptor agonists (such as clonidine). The sedative effect of detomidine occurred at doses which increase blood pressure. Detomidine did not induce contractions in rat or cow isolated uterus preparations.

Detomidine was rapidly distributed after i.m., i.v. or s.c. administration. The maximal concentration in mouse brain (higher than in plasma) was found 0.16 h after i.v. injection. Detomidine was eliminated into urine and faeces mainly as three metabolites. The elimination $t_{1/2}$ in the rat was 12.7 h, in the dog 22.1 h and in the calf 20 h. Detomidine was well tolerated in all the species studied. In domestic species of animal, detomidine was an extremely good sedative in horses, cattle, sheep and goats but it was less effective in pigs, dogs and cats. Therefore, clinical pharmacological investigations were performed as double-blind studies against xylazine on three adult horses and three dairy cows. The doses of detomidine were 100–300 μg/kg in horses and 30–150 μg/kg in cows. The administration routes were i.m. and i.v. Xylazine was used at the recommended doses of 400–1200 μg/kg in the horse and 50–150 μg/kg in cattle.

A clinical study on 109 horses and 103 cows used dose levels of 8–250 μg/kg detomidine for horses and 18–120 μg/kg for cattle. Detomidine induced sedation in 5–15 min and this facilitated handling. The i.v. doses had a more rapid onset of action. The animals remained standing. The duration of action was dose-dependent, lasting between 1 and 5 h. Using the same dose rates as recommended for xylazine, detomidine had superior sedative and analgesic effects, especially in horses. On horses detomidine was particularly effective, only 1% of the dose of xylazine being required to obtain a similar effect. Detomidine at sedative doses induced a rapid and dose-dependent increase in arterial blood pressure and consistent bradycardia in both horses and cattle. The bradycardia was accompanied by SA and AV-blocks in horses. No serious arrhythmias were detected. Respiratory rate was increased slightly in horses and decreased slightly in cattle. No adverse side-effects such as abortions were seen during the studies.

The cardiovascular effects of ketamine, thiopentone and methohexitone after xylazine premedication in horses

G. J. Brouwer

In horses, the combination of xylazine with ketamine has been shown to produce short periods of surgical anaesthesia characterized by a smooth induction and a rapid, quiet recovery[2,5]. This paper describes the cardiovascular effects of this combination and compares them with the combination of xylazine and either thiopentone or methohexitone. Four ponies with clinical evidence of cardiopulmonary disease were anaesthetized in a random sequence with each drug combination. Arterial blood pressure was recorded from a previously raised carotid artery using a standard cannula/transducer/recorder system. A lead II electrocardiogram was recorded continuously from standard limb leads using subcutaneous needle electrodes. One pony had a surgically implanted Doppler-shift ultrasonic flow transducer around its main pulmonary artery and this animal was used for cardiac output and myocardial contractility determinations[3]. All parameters were measured at 10 and 2 min before the injection of xylazine and the averages taken as control values. Xylazine (1.1 mg/kg) was given intravenously over 2 min. After a 2 min pause, ketamine (2.2 mg/kg), thiopentone (5.5 mg/kg) or methohexitone (2.8 mg/kg) was given intravenously as a bolus injection.

The injection of xylazine was followed by 'dropped beats' so that heart rate decreased significantly (Figure 1), but the rate increased again on induction of anaesthesia by injection of the second drug. The dropped beats appeared to be due to atrioventricular block. Marked hypertension followed the injection of xylazine and this was probably due to increased sympatho-adrenal activity (Figure 2). Blood pressure fell after the induction of anaesthesia, but there were no significant differences between the effects of ketamine, thiopentone and methohexitone. Xylazine alone produced a decrease in cardiac output to about 75% of the control value, which agrees with previous reports[4,5], and xylazine apparently produced a decrease in myocardial contractility. Both cardiac output and myocardial contractility were further

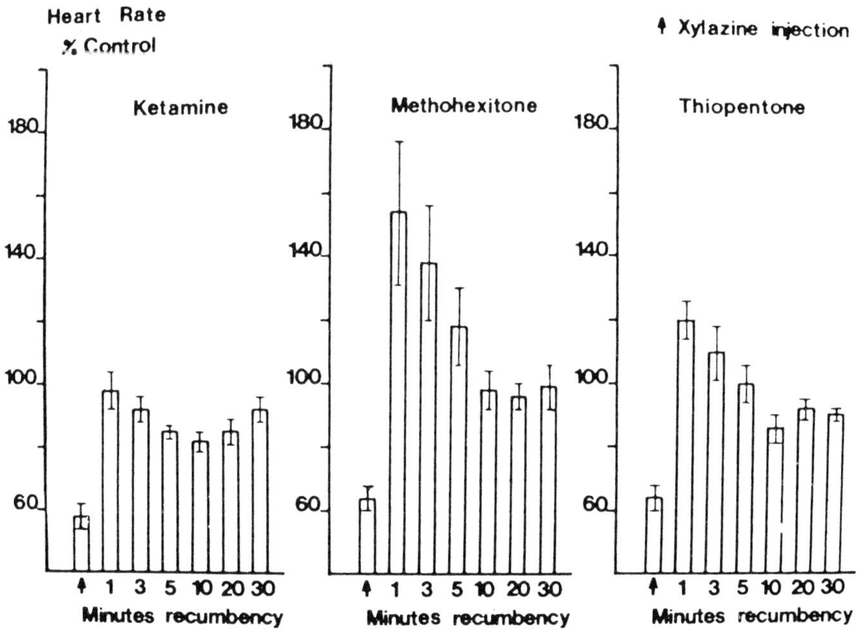

Figure 1 Changes in heart rate (shown as a percentage of the control value ± SEM) after each combination ($n = 4$)

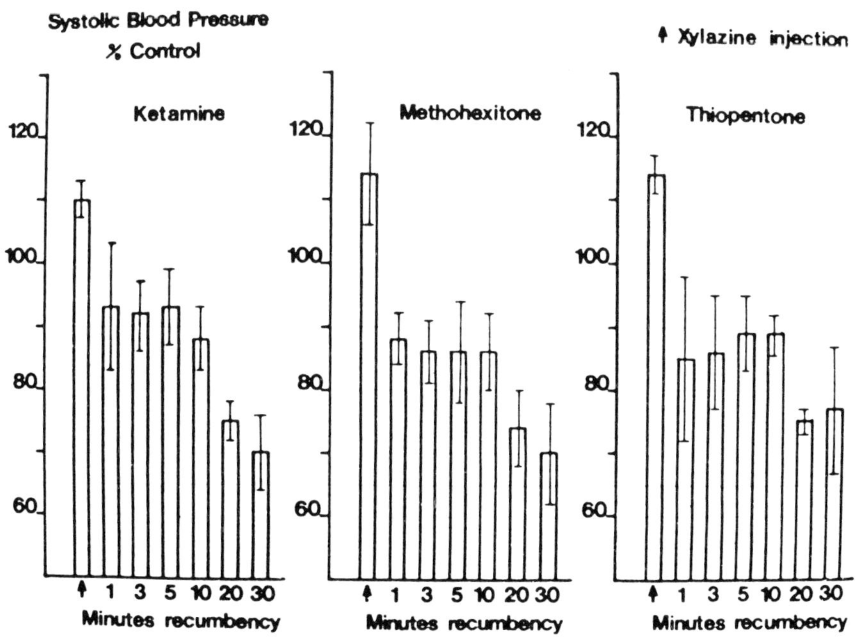

Figure 2 Changes in systolic blood pressure (shown as a percentage of the control values ± SEM) after each combination ($n = 4$)

depressed by each of the anaesthetic agents, but the effects are least with ketamine.

This study suggests that the xylazine/ketamine combination, in particular, may be a useful anaesthetic combination in horses where surgery is necessary and where cardiovascular function is already compromised.

During this study G. J. Brouwer was in receipt of a Horserace Betting Levy Board Research Training Scholarship. This report is based on a more detailed study[1].

References

1. Brouwer, G. J., Hall, L. W. and Kuchel, T. R. (1980). *Vet. Rec.*, **107**, 241
2. Ellis, R. G., Lowe, J. E., Schward, W. S. *et al.* (1977). *J. Equine Med. Surg.*, **1**, 259
3. Hall, L. W. and Clarke, K. W. (1974). *Cardiovasc. Res.*, **8**, 796
4. Kerr, D. D., Jones, E. W., Holbert, D. *et al.* (1972). *Am. J. Vet. Res.*, **33**, 777
5. Muir, W. W., Skarda, R. T. and Milne, D. W. (1977). *Am. J. Vet. Res.*, **38**, 195

Study on interactions between chloramphenicol and intravenous anaesthetics

H.-H. Frey and R. Reiche

Chloramphenicol has been reported to prolong the action of barbiturate hypnotics by an inhibition of liver mixed-function oxidases. We have studied the importance of this interaction for short-acting intravenous anaesthetics, the effect of which is terminated by distribution rather than metabolic inactivation. Mice were pretreated orally with 50 mg/kg chloramphenicol as the sodium succinate 1 h before the i.v. injection of the anaesthetics, and the sleeping times were compared to those of untreated controls. The duration of action of methohexitone was prolonged when doses of 15 and 20 mg/kg were injected, but not with the lowest dose of 10 mg/kg. After injection of thiopentone (30, 40 and 50 mg/kg), only the medium dose was prolonged significantly. Chloramphenicol prolonged the effect of etomidate (3 and 5 mg/kg), but not that of propanidid (60 mg/kg) or ketamine (30 and 40 mg/kg). The results show that the experimental finding of an interaction between chloramphenicol and barbiturates cannot be generalized: it will not play a major role with usual clinical induction doses, the effect of which is terminated by distribution, but may be of importance when higher doses are administered.

A full account of these findings has been published elsewhere[1].

Reference

1. Reiche, R. and Frey, H.-H. (1981). *Anaesthesist*, **30**, 504

The neuromuscular blocking action of a new muscle relaxant atracurium in the dog

R. S. Jones, J. M. Hunter and J. E. Utting

Atracurium besylate is a new non-depolarizing muscle relaxant, the elimination of which is independent of both the liver and the kidney. It was found that a dose of 0.25 mg/kg was required to produce total neuromuscular blockade in the dog, as assessed by single twitch and tetanic responses of the gastrocnemius muscle. The time to full recovery was 43 min for single twitch and 56 min for tetanic response.

The investigations were carried out in four mature labrador dogs using techniques employed previously. After premedication with acepromazine (0.1 mg/kg) and atropine (0.044 mg/kg), anaesthesia was induced with thiopentone (22 mg/kg) and the trachea intubated. Anaesthesia was maintained with nitrous oxide and oxygen (2:1) and ventilation was controlled using a type of Maplesen E circuit. The animals were maintained in a state of moderate hyperventilation with a $P\text{a}CO_2$ in the region of 35 mmHg. The $P\text{a}CO_2$ was controlled by adjusting the fresh gas flow to the circuit by reference to the arterial blood gas values. The dogs were placed in left lateral recumbency and the left foreleg was fixed in a padded wooden clamp. The left ulnar nerve was stimulated at the elbow using steel needle electrodes. Square wave stimuli of 0.3 ms duration were delivered from a Grass stimulator. The voltage was adjusted to 20% above that which was required to produce a supramaximal response. Train-of-four stimuli of frequency 2 Hz were applied and repeated at a frequency of 0.1 Hz. The mechanical response was monitored by attaching a Grass force displacement transducer (FT03) to the foot and recording the signal on a Devices 2 channel recorder.

A control recording was obtained before the administration of atracurium. The drug was administered into a rapidly running drip of normal saline inserted into the cephalic vein in the right forelimb. Doses of 0.2, 0.4 and 0.6 mg/kg of atracurium were employed. At the point when the twitch height of the first of the four stimuli returned to 50% of its original height atropine (0.6 mg) was administered. This was followed 1 min later by atropine (0.6 mg) plus neostigmine (2.5 mg) and again 1 min later by a second dose of neostigmine (2.5 mg). The observations were repeated once in each dog for each of the three doses at intervals of not less than 1 week.

The increase in dosage of atracurium was associated with a decreased time of onset of neuromuscular block, the times being 2.7 min (range 2.17–3.00) at 0.2 mg/kg, 1.6 min (range 1.33–2.66) at 0.4 mg/kg and 1.5 min (range 1.00–2.00) at 0.6 mg/kg, the difference between the first two times (but not between the second and third) being significant ($p < 0.0001$). Increase in dosage was associated also with an increased duration of action: the times to full reversal from the time of administration of atracurium were 20 min (range 14.0–32.4) at 0.2 mg/kg, 31 min (range 20.3–39.1) at 0.4 mg/kg and 47 min (range 34.5–66.7) at 0.6 mg/kg. The differences between the first and second times mentioned and between the second and third were statistically significant.

Haemodynamic effects of methoxyflurane in dogs

E. P. Steffey, T. B. Farver and M. Woliner

Despite its relatively widespread clinical veterinary usage, little objective information is available regarding the cardiovascular effects of methoxyflurane (MOF). Accordingly, studies were performed in dogs during controlled (CV) and spontaneous (SV) ventilation to supply missing data and to compare directly these results with data similarly derived while these same dogs were anaesthetized with halothane (Hal). Alveolar MOF and Hal dose vs. circulatory response relationships were defined in the absence of modifying factors such as variations in PaO_2, variations in end tidal anaesthetic concentration or body temperature, surgical stress and other anaesthetic or adjuvant drugs.

The circulatory effects of three different alveolar concentrations of MOF and Hal were studied in eight healthy, unmedicated, fasted, adult, mongrel dogs weighing 22.7 ± 1.1 kg. Anaesthesia was induced and maintained with the intended agent of study in oxygen. The minimum alveolar concentration which just prevented gross purposeful movement in response to a noxious stimulus (MAC) was previously determined for each agent in each intubated animal according to established techniques[1,2]. MAC in these dogs averaged $0.29 \pm 0.01\%$ for MOF and $0.89 \pm 0.02\%$ for Hal. Circulatory measurements were made at MAC multiples of 1.0, 1.5 and 2.0 according to previously described techniques[3]. Oesophageal temperature was maintained at 37.9 ± 0.1 °C and during CV $PaCO_2$ averaged 34–38 torr. The order of agent initially studied and whether increasing or decreasing concentrations were investigated were randomized to minimize effects of sequence and time. At least 7 days separated studies in each animal. Prior to each set of measurements during CV, a period of anaesthetic over pressure preceded at least 30 min of constant end tidal anaesthetic concentration. Immediately following completion of these measurements, CV was discontinued and measurements repeated at the same unvarying alveolar dose after at least 20 min of SV. CV was then reinstituted and the anaesthetic dose increased or decreased as circumstances dictated for succeeding measurements. A mean and standard error for the data was calculated. Data were analyzed with Student's paired and unpaired *t*-tests. A level of $p < 0.05$ (MOF vs. Hal at a given MAC multiple) or $p < 0.01$ (MAC × vs. MAC 1.0) was considered significant.

Table 1 Circulatory changes (X ± SE) with methoxyflurane (MOF) and halothane (Hal) anaesthesia during controlled (C) and spontaneous (S) ventilation

			MAC 1.0	*MAC 1.5*	*MAC 2.0*
Heart rate ($n=8$)	MOF	C	119 ± 5†	123 ± 3†	127 ± 5†
		S	132 ± 5†	125 ± 5†	130 ± 6†
	Hal	C	89 ± 6	98 ± 4	110 ± 5
		S	104 ± 4	111 ± 5	113 ± 5*
Stroke volume (ml/min) ($n=7$)	MOF	C	24.1 ± 2.1†	19.4 ± 1.1†	12.2 ± 1.6*†
		S	27.1 ± 1.9	25.0 ± 1.5	28.4 ± 1.7†
	Hal	C	29.4 ± 3.1	24.7 ± 1.9	16.1 ± 1.1*
		S	31.1 ± 2.4	25.9 ± 1.9	20.6 ± 1.5*
Cardiac output (l/min) ($n=7$)	MOF	C	2.80 ± 0.20	2.39 ± 0.18	1.51 ± 0.18*
		S	3.61 ± 0.32†	3.11 ± 0.24†	3.70 ± 0.40†
	Hal	C	2.58 ± 0.28	2.38 ± 0.18	1.73 ± 0.14*
		S	3.29 ± 0.33	2.40 ± 0.23	2.32 ± 0.25
Mean aortic pressure (torr) ($n=8$)	MOF	C	107 ± 5	87 ± 5*	61 ± 4*
		S	106 ± 4	91 ± 6	79 ± 4*
	Hal	C	100 ± 5	82 ± 5*	68 ± 5*
		S	104 ± 5	87 ± 5	71 ± 5*
Total peripheral resistance (dyn s cm^{-5}) ($n=7$)	MOF	C	3165 ± 214	3087 ± 241	3719 ± 582
		S	2406 ± 188†	2420 ± 197†	1776 ± 118†
	Hal	C	3240 ± 241†	2849 ± 178	3303 ± 117
		S	2611 ± 159	2486 ± 152	2536 ± 182
Left ventricular work (kg m min^{-1}) ($n=7$)	MOF	C	4.15 ± 0.42	2.92 ± 0.29	1.31 ± 0.21*
		S	5.14 ± 0.57	3.95 ± 0.54	4.09 ± 0.64
	Hal	C	3.56 ± 0.46	2.74 ± 0.32	1.70 ± 0.23*
		S	4.72 ± 0.61	3.51 ± 0.50	2.34 ± 0.41*
$PaCO_2$ (torr) ($n=8$)	MOF	C	33.9 ± 0.9	33.8 ± 1.3	38.1 ± 2.0
		S	40.1 ± 2.5	57.1 ± 5.5	70.2 ± 5.1*†
	Hal	C	33.8 ± 1.0	35.0 ± 1.5	37.7 ± 1.6
		S	39.5 ± 1.6	46.4 ± 1.7	54.9 ± 2.8*

*$p<0.01$ MAC × vs. MAC 1.0; †$p<0.05$ MOF vs. Hal at a given MAC multiple

Data are given in Table 1. PaO_2 was rarely below 450 torr in any dog, regardless of the anaesthetic depth or agent. When ventilation was controlled, MOF, like Hal, caused dose-related cardiovascular depression in unstimulated healthy dogs. Except for a greater heart rate and lesser stroke volume with MOF, little difference was noted between the anaesthetics at equipotent doses during CV. The cardiovascular depression observed with increasing doses of MOF and Hal with CV and stable $PaCO_2$ was attenuated during MOF anaesthesia when ventilation was spontaneous and $PaCO_2$ rose in response to increasing anaesthetic dose.

References

1. Eger, E. I. II, Saidman, L. J. and Brandstater, B. (1965). Minimum alveolar anesthetic concentration: a standard of anesthetic potency. *Anesthesiology*, **26**, 756–63
2. Steffey, E. P., Gillespie, J. R., Berry, J. D. *et al.* (1974). Anesthetic potency (MAC) of nitrous oxide in the dog, cat and stumptail monkey. *J. Appl. Physiol.*, **36**, 530–2
3. Steffey, E. P., Gillespie, J. R., Berry, J. D. *et al.* (1974). Circulatory effects of halothane and halothane–nitrous oxide anesthesia in the dog: controlled ventilation. *Am. J. Vet. Res.*, **35**, 1289–93

Afferent inputs to mammalian spinal neurons: studies with anaesthetic and analgesic agents

P. M. Headley, N. M. Honhold, D. C. West and D. Lodge

It is evident that anaesthetic and analgesic agents must interrupt afferent information at some site between the incoming stimulus and the centres of awareness in the forebrain, but it is still far from clear at which sites, and by what mechanisms, this may be achieved. We are interested in the mechanisms which may control the transfer of afferent nociceptive and other information through the spinal cord.

Experiments are performed on rats and cats. Cats are either anaesthetized throughout with α-chloralose, or are decerebrated at mid-collicular level under temporary anaesthesia; they are usually paralysed, end tidal CO_2 levels being maintained near 4%. The lumbar spinal cord is exposed by laminectomy and is sectioned at L1 level to isolate the lumbar recording area from descending supraspinal influences. Rats are decerebrated or are anaesthetized throughout with urethane or pentobarbitone.

Recordings are made using 7-barrel glass micropipettes of overall tip diameter 4–7 μm. The central barrel contains 3.5 mol/l NaCl and is used to record extracellularly the action potentials of individual neurons. The other six barrels contain solutions of drugs which can be administered to the cell under study by controlled electrical currents through the appropriate barrels (microelectrophoresis). Cells are identified on the bases of their peripheral receptive field, of their differential sensitivity to cutaneous stimuli and of their location in the spinal cord. The firing rate of the cell under study is displayed continuously on a pen recorder.

Neuronal responses are elicited both by electrophoretically-administered agents, and by natural stimuli applied to the appropriate receptive field. It is important that the duration, intensity and sequence of all stimuli are absolutely regular, and in our experiments these are always controlled electronically. Sensory stimuli which we can control in this way include non-noxious movements of hairs, skin or joints, and noxious radiant heat or mechanical pinch. The electrophoretic stimuli are ejections of the three agents currently considered to specify three classes of receptor for excitatory amino acids, which are probably the major excitatory neurotransmitters in the CNS; these characterizing amino acids are *N*-methyl-aspartate, quisqualate and kainate. In our experiments, we try to combine these various stimuli in tests designed to determine (1) whether the agent has a selective effect on one class of amino-acid receptor, (2) whether the agent has a selective effect on one type of sensory input, and (3) whether sensory synaptic inputs can be related to particular classes of amino-acid receptor.

In the original experiments of this type[1] we found that morphine and enkephalins, infused electrophoretically into the superficial substantia gelatinosa region of the spinal dorsal horn of cats, reduced the responses of deeper neurons (in Rexed's laminae IV–VI) to noxious radiant heat stimuli whilst having no effect on non-nociceptive responses to hair movement. These actions could be reversed by the opiate antagonist naloxone with intravenous doses (0.1–0.3 mg/kg) similar to those which are just adequate to reverse the behavioural analgesia elicited by systemic morphine. This site of antinociceptive activity correlates both with the high concentrations of opiate receptors subsequently defined in binding studies, and with the behavioural analgesia elicited by spinally-administered opiates[4]. Amino acids and substance P were inactive when ejected at the same site, but noradrenaline and 5HT had potent morphine-like actions[2].

More recently, it has been reported that the dissociative anaesthetic (±)-ketamine is a selective antagonist of the *N*-methyl-aspartate class of amino-acid receptor[3]. Although other antagonists of this receptor type have been described in recent years, none cross the blood-brain barrier. Ketamine on the other hand clearly does so; the effects of electrophoretic administration can, therefore, be compared with those of intravenous administration and so can perhaps be related to the behavioural actions of the drug. Ketamine has potent analgesic properties (in rodents, maybe, more than in cats) and so we have examined it for effects on nociceptive and other responses of dorsal horn neurons in decerebrate cats and rats and in pentobarbitone-anaesthetized rats. Figure 1 illustrates an experiment in which a cell was activated in a regular cycle by pinching skin and by electrophoretic administration of quisqualate and *N*-methyl-aspartate. (±)-ketamine was ejected concurrently with a dose sufficiently high to block entirely the responses to both amino acids, but the pinch response was unaffected. This lack of effect of ketamine, whether administered electrophoretically or intravenously (up to 24 mg/kg) has been consistent on all tests on nociceptive and non-nociceptive responses.

We are currently beginning to examine those non-steroidal anti-inflammatory drugs which have good analgesic properties. Paracetamol and acetanilide have shown a clear ability to reduce kainate responses whilst leaving *N*-methyl-aspartate and quisqualate responses relatively unaffected. To date, however, we have not found any consistent effect by electrophoretic or intravenous paracetamol on nociceptive or non-nociceptive synaptic responses.

These results therefore suggest (1) that opiates may exert significant analgesic actions in the dorsal horn, (2) that *N*-methyl-aspartate and kainate receptors are not important in mediating afferent inputs of the types tested

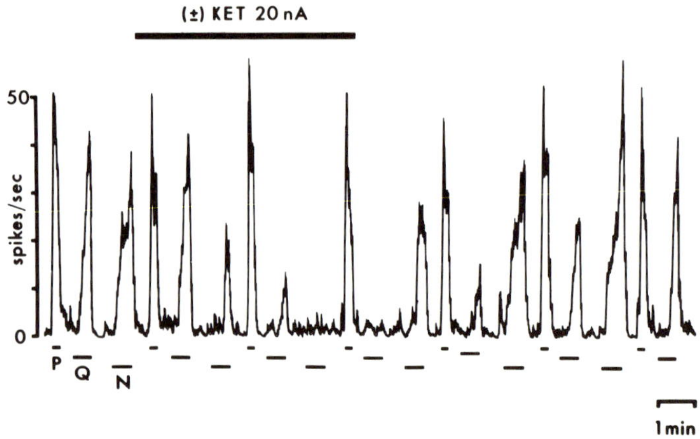

Figure 1 Pen recorder trace of the firing rate of a dorsal horn neuron (ordinate) against time. Excitatory responses were elicited in a regular cycle by pinching the skin over the gastrocnemius muscle (P) and by electrophoretic ejections of quisqualate (Q) and *N*-methyl-aspartate (N). During the period indicated by the horizontal bar, (±)-ketamine was ejected (20 nA ejecting current). On this cell this dose was sufficient to block responses to both amino acids, but the pinch responses were unaffected. Raising the ketamine current to 80 nA in a further test still left the pinch responses unaffected. Decerebrate spinalized cat, lamina IV neuron

on dorsal horn neurons, and (3) that a spinal site of action does not contribute significantly to the central analgesic effects of (±)-ketamine and of paracetamol.

References

1. Duggan, A. W., Hall, J. G. and Headley, P. M. (1976). Morphine, enkephalin and the substantia gelatinosa. *Nature (London)*, **264**, 456–8
2. Headley, P.M., Duggan, A. W. and Griersmith, B. T. (1978). Selective reduction by noradrenaline and 5-hydroxytryptamine of nociceptive responses of cat dorsal horn neurones. *Brain Res.*, **145**, 185–9
3. Lodge, D., Anis, N. A. and Burton, N. A. (1982). Effects of optical isomers of ketamine on excitation of rat and cat spinal neurones by amino-acids and acetylcholine. *Neurosci. Lett.*, **29**, 281–6
4. Yaksh, T. L. (1981). Spinal opiate analgesia: characteristics and principles of action. *Pain*, **11**, 293–346

Evaluation of etomidate and fentanyl in dog anaesthesia

O. Glardon

The usefulness of etomidate for short periods of anaesthesia (e.g. to perform biopsy, skin suture, radiography) is related both to its short duration of action and the absence of significant side-effects. The aim of this study has been to monitor the course of anaesthesia using a combination of etomidate and fentanyl.

109 apparently healthy dogs were studied. They were allocated to three groups. Dosage regimens for etomidate and fentanyl were respectively: group 1 ($n = 62$): 1 mg/kg plus 0.005 mg/kg; group 2 ($n = 24$): 1 mg/kg plus 0.010 mg/kg; group 3 ($n = 23$): 1.5 mg/kg plus 0.005 mg/kg. Doses were administered by the intravenous route. For 19 dogs in each group, the heart rate and respiratory frequency, the level and duration of muscle relaxation and analgesia were recorded. Assessment of muscle relaxation was made qualitatively. It was graded as deep when the animal was immobile and moderate when some spontaneous movements (tail, legs) were observed. Analgesia was considered to be marked when no response was evoked by a painful stimulus (prick with a needle) and when the interdigital reflex was absent. Analgesia was considered to be moderate when the interdigital reflex was again recorded. In addition, rotation of the eyeball and the times between administration and the first righting of the head and between administration and the first attempt to walk were measured.

Results for relaxation, analgesia and recovery parameters are summarized in Table 1. When the 109 anaesthetized dogs were considered, 11 cases of excitation were observed, which necessitated an additional ketamine administration (2.5–5 mg/kg). Most of the excitated dogs were very nervous prior the induction of anaesthesia as a result of prolonged travel. In all three groups, bradycardia occurred after the first minute postinjection: in the first group, return to control values occurred before the end of anaesthesia (13th minute). When marked bradycardia occurred, several dogs displayed arrhythmias such as bigeminism, trigeminism and extra beats. Other side-effects were: vomiting ($n = 1$), coprostasis ($n = 1$) and recovery excitation ($n = 2$).

This study confirms previously reported data. The normally recommended dosage regimen (group 1) is generally sufficient for most purposes. In 6.5%

Table 1 Responsę (duration in minutes or minutes after administration) of dogs to the administration of a combination of etomidate and fentanyl. Values are expressed as mean + SD

Groups	*I* ($n=19$)	*II* ($n=19$)	*III* ($n=19$)
Etomidate (mg/kg)	1.0	1.0	1.5
Fentanyl (mg/kg)	0.005	0.010	0.005
Muscle relaxation			
deep	7±3	6±3	8±4
moderate	10±3	11±3	15±4*
Analgesia			
marked or moderate	9±3	13±3*	14±5*
Eyeball rotation	4±3	6±3	7±4*
Awakening	10±5	9±3	
First righting of the head	12±3	14±4	18±5*
First attempt to stand	17±4	19±5	24±7*
Walking	22±5	23±5	32±7*

*Significant ($p<0.05$) with group I as control

of the cases, doses of etomidate had to be increased by 50%. This combination of drugs produces only slight cardiovascular effects and has the shortest duration of action. In contrast, when the dose of fentanyl is doubled, analgesia is prolonged by 4 min but the depressant effects on the cardiovascular system become a limiting factor. The dose levels used in the third group led also to undesirable side-effects (the depressant effect on the cardiovascular system is the most important and, in addition, awakening is delayed).

In conclusion, the main advantages of etomidate–fentanyl are the following: (1) a short duration of action, (2) sufficient analgesia for minor surgery, and (3) few side-effects on the cardiovascular system which makes this combination useful in cases of shock. The main disadvantages are: (1) excitation in about 10% of dogs which necessitates ketamine administration, (2) the occurrence of panting, which makes radiographic examination difficult especially in the large dogs, (3) the volume of the administered dose is important (6 ml/kg) and necessitates an intravenous catheter, (4) the presence of fentanyl prevents its use in some sensitive breeds such as chow-chow, Spitz, samoyède and toy-poodle, and (5) the combination is expensive.

Interactions between dissociative anaesthetics and neurotransmitter receptors in the mammalian central nervous system

D. Lodge, N. R. Burton, S. C. Berry and N. A. Anis

General anaesthetics depress the transfer of information within the central nervous system (CNS) by an action at the level of synaptic transmission[3]. Since the balance between the various pharmacological aspects of anaesthesia varies from agent to agent it seems likely that there is not a common mode of action. It is well established that barbiturates enhance particular inhibitory mechanisms, namely those mediated by the neurotransmitter, γ-aminobutyric acid (GABA). This effect of the barbiturates, which explains at least in part their central depressant properties, is brought about by an action at the GABA receptor–effector complex on the postsynaptic membrane[3]. The dissociative anaesthetics do not enhance GABA-mediated inhibitions but rather depress polysynaptic excitations[4]. Since the acidic amino acids, L-aspartate and L-glutamate, are thought to be neurotransmitters at many excitatory synapses in the brain and spinal cord[5], we have investigated the interaction between dissociative anaesthetics and excitatory amino-acid receptors on central neurons in the cat and the rat.

Experiments were performed on decerebrate cats or pentobarbitone-anaesthetized rats and cats using standard neurophysiological techniques. Extracellular action potentials from single neurons in the spinal cord were recorded via the centre barrel of seven barrel glass microelectrodes (overall tip diameter 4–10 μm). The outer barrels contained ionized solutions of drugs and neurotransmitter candidates and analogues which could be ejected, into the region of the neuron being studied, by passing a small electrical current of the appropriate polarity through the drug barrel. The microelectrophoretic currents, measured in nanoamperes, were monitored continuously on a pen recorder together with the action potential discharge rate of the neuron.

Initial experiments were performed to compare the effects of ketamine (a dissociative anaesthetic), methohexitone (a barbiturate anaesthetic) and alphaxalone/alphadolone (saffan; a steroid anaesthetic mixture) on spinal reflexes and inhibitions. While methohexitone and saffan enhanced prolonged inhibitions and dorsal root potentials, ketamine had no such effect at doses up to 10 mg/kg i.v. On the other hand, polysynaptic and not monosynaptic reflexes were reduced by ketamine more than by the other anaesthetics. The results with saffan and methohexitone suggest that these two anaesthetics enhance the postsynaptic action of GABA, whereas the results with ketamine suggest a selective action on excitatory interneurons which may use aspartate as their transmitter[5].

Using microelectrophoretic administration to study the interaction of ketamine and tiletamine with L-aspartate and L-glutamate on 13 cat spinal neurons, it was found that the postsynaptic actions of L-aspartate were depressed more than those of L-glutamate but the selectivity of this effect was not great. It is, however, known that, just as acetylcholine interacts with muscarinic and nicotinic receptors, so L-aspartate and L-glutamate interact with three classes of amino-acid receptor. The selective agonists for these three receptors are *N*-methyl-aspartate (NMA), quisqualate and kainate[5]. Accordingly, the actions of ketamine, tiletamine and phencyclidine have been investigated on the responses of neurons to these three agonists. All three dissociative anaesthetics reduced or abolished the action of NMA more than the actions of quisqualate and kainate. For example, on 82 cat spinal neurons, ketamine reduced responses to NMA by 33 to 100% (mean 78 ± 18%), those to quisqualate by 0 to 55% (mean 9 ± 11%) and those to kainate by 0 to 30% (mean 8 ± 10%).

Excitatory responses to acetylcholine (ACh) of spinal Renshaw cells were also reduced by the three dissociative agents, although to a smaller extent than those to NMA. For example on 25 cat Renshaw cells, during ketamine ejection (3–30 nA) responses to ACh were reduced by 0 to 80% (mean 37 ± 22%) whereas responses to NMA were reduced by 35 to 100% (mean 77 ± 18%). On 14 of these Renshaw cells, responses to kainate or quisqualate were reduced by 0 to 30% (mean 14 ± 9%). Results from a Renshaw cell are shown in Figure 1. Qualitatively and quantitatively similar results were obtained with tiletamine and phencyclidine, although the latter drug was an order of magnitude more potent (see Figure 1).

It is of particular relevance that the (+) isomer of ketamine, which is approximately three times more potent than the (−) isomer as an anaesthetic/analgesic, was also approximately three times more potent as an antagonist of NMA but only 1–1½ times as potent as an ACh antagonist[1].

In the cerebellum, the depressant effects of phencyclidine and ketamine are thought to be mediated via a noradrenergic mechanism[2]. We therefore compared the action of noradrenaline and ketamine on responses of spinal neurons to the excitatory amino acids. On both cat and rat spinal neurons noradrenaline did not mimic the action of ketamine but rather reduced the responses to quisqualate more than those to kainate and NMA. For example, on five cat spinal neurons, noradrenaline reduced responses to quisqualate by 20 to 70% whereas responses to NMA were reduced by 0 to 20%. Thus it appears that noradrenergic mechanisms are unlikely to explain the NMA-antagonism seen following local administration of the dissociative anaesthetics.

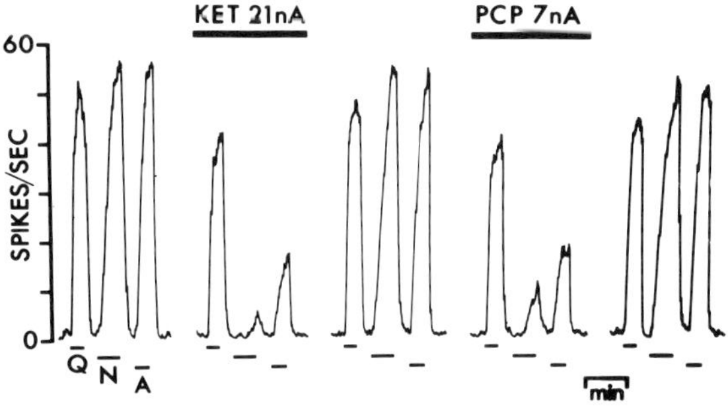

Figure 1. Effect of ketamine and phencyclidine on the responses of a Renshaw cell in a pentobarbitone-anaesthetized cat to quisqualate (Q), *N*-methyl-aspartate (N) and acetylcholine (A). The record shows the firing rate of a neuron in response to the electrophoretic ejection of the three agonists indicated by the bar below the record. Quisqualate (5 mmol/l in 200 mmol/l NaCl) was ejected with a current of 103 nA, *N*-methyl-DL-aspartate (200 mmol/l) with a current of 22 nA and acetylcholine (200 mmol/l) with a current of 10 nA. The concurrent ejection of ketamine (KET. 21 nA from a 50 mmol/l solution in 150 mmol/l NaCl) and of phencyclidine (PCP. 7 nA from a 10 mmol/l solution in 200 mmol/l NaCl) selectively depressed the response to NMA more than to ACh and to ACh more than to quisqualate. Recovery from ketamine (middle panel) and from phencyclidine (far right) was observed 3 and 15 min after stopping the ejection of the respective anaesthetic. Ordinate: firing rate in spikes/sec. Abscissa: time in min

It has been reported that ketamine analgesia may be reduced by administration of naloxone, suggesting that ketamine acts in part at central opiate receptors. In an initial series of experiments electrophoretically administered morphine and naloxone were without any clear effect on responses of spinal neurons to NMA, quisqualate and kainate nor did naloxone affect the NMA-blocking action of ketamine. Thus, it appears unlikely that an action at classical opiate receptors underlies the actions of ketamine described above, but in preliminary experiments we have found that cyclazocine, a sigma opiate receptor ligand, is a potent NMA antagonist.

Systemic administration of both ketamine (2.5–20 mg/kg i.v.) and phencyclidine (0.25–0.5 mg/kg i.v.) also selectively blocked responses of spinal neurons to electrophoretically administered NMA with relatively small effects on the actions of ACh, quisqualate and kainate. These highly selective effects on NMA receptors, which mediate information transfer throughout the central nervous system[5], probably contribute substantially to the clinical effects of the dissociative anaesthetics. The minimum systemic dose levels producing NMA antagonism are in the range of those producing analgesia rather than surgical anaesthesia, although full anaesthetic dose levels still show similar selective effects.

These results, together with the selective enhancement of GABA-mediated inhibitions by barbiturates and steroids, do not support unitary hypotheses of anaesthesia but rather suggest specific interactions with particular protein elements in the postjunctional membranes.

References

1. Lodge, D., Anis, N. A. and Burton, N. R. (1982). Effects of optical isomers of ketamine on excitation of cat and rat spinal neurones by acidic amino acids. *Neurosci. Lett.*, **29**, 281–6
2. Marwaha, J., Palmer, M. R., Woodward, D. J. *et al.* (1980). Electrophysiological evidence for presynaptic actions of phencyclidine on noradrenergic transmission in rat cerebellum. *J. Pharm. Exp. Ther.*, **215**, 606–13
3. Richards, C. D. (1980). The mechanism of general anaesthesia. In Norman, J. and Whitman, J. (eds.) *Topical Reviews of Anaesthesia.* Vol. 1, pp. 1–84. (Bristol: Wright)
4. Tang, A. H. and Schroeder, L. A. (1973). Spinal-cord depressant effects of ketamine and etoxadrol in the cat and the rat. *Anaesthesiology*, **39**, 37–43
5. Watkins, J. C. and Evans, R. H. (1981). Excitatory amino acid transmitters. *Ann. Rev. Pharmacol. Toxicol.*, **21**, 165–204

Clinical pharmacology of ketamine in the pig

P. Lees and M. J. Meredith

The pig is possibly the most difficult of all domesticated animal species to restrain and anaesthetize under field conditions. There is, therefore, a need for agents with wide safety margins, which can be injected intravenously and intramuscularly and which are compatible with other premedicants and with volatile anaesthetics. The dissociative anaesthetic, phencyclidine, filled this role for several years, but it is no longer available for general use. Ketamine, though less potent and with a shorter duration of action than phencyclidine, has replaced the latter drug for use in several species including man. Since azaperone is probably the most widely used tranquillizer–sedative agent in pigs, the present investigation of the actions of ketamine in the pig was carried out both with and without premedication with this agent.

The actions of ketamine were studied in two circumstances:

(1) The general clinical efficacy of ketamine given intravenously (i.v.) or intramuscularly (i.m.) at varying dose rates both alone and following azaperone premedication was investigated in approximately 200 pigs of differing breeds, ages and weights.

(2) The effects of premedication with azaperone (2 mg/kg i.m.) followed 15 min later by induction of anaesthesia with ketamine (15 mg/kg i.m.) on respiration and the cardiovascular system were investigated in one Large White and eight Göttingen miniature pigs. Measurements and blood samples were taken from previously implanted arterial and venous catheters. In control experiments the pigs received either azaperone or ketamine alone.

Azaperone/ketamine or ketamine alone produced a light plane of anaesthesia lasting for 10 to 30 min with doses of ketamine ranging from 10 to 20 mg/kg. No deaths occurred even in animals receiving doses of 60 mg/kg. The central depressant actions of ketamine were increased only slightly by azaperone premedication. Anal, laryngeal and pharyngeal reflexes were retained and the apneustic, jerky pattern of respiration was commonly accompanied by mild tremor. Muscle tone was decreased for

15–30 min, although occasional spontaneous movements occurred in this period. Responses to auditory stimuli were abolished for 30 min. Increased salivation occurred, although atropine was not administered. Analgesia was judged to be fair or poor and major surgery could not be performed. However, ketamine anaesthesia did allow the following procedures to be undertaken: endoscopy of the reproductive tract, ultrasonic examination of the fetus, electroejaculation, castration, hernia operations, laparoscopy of the abdomen, teeth cutting, examination of the feet and limbs, mange washing and sucking by piglets. Moreover, although endotracheal intubation was not possible with ketamine doses of less than 20 mg/kg, these doses did permit the administration of halothane by face-mask and the subsequent passage of an endotracheal tube. Recovery from ketamine anaesthesia was often quiet but myoclonic jerks and floundering sometimes occurred and animals were sensitive to tactile stimuli during recovery.

In one Large White and eight miniature pigs azaperone (2 mg/kg i.m.) and ketamine (15 mg/kg i.m.) produced a mild or moderate degree of bradycardia, while an initial small rise in pcv was followed by a small decrease

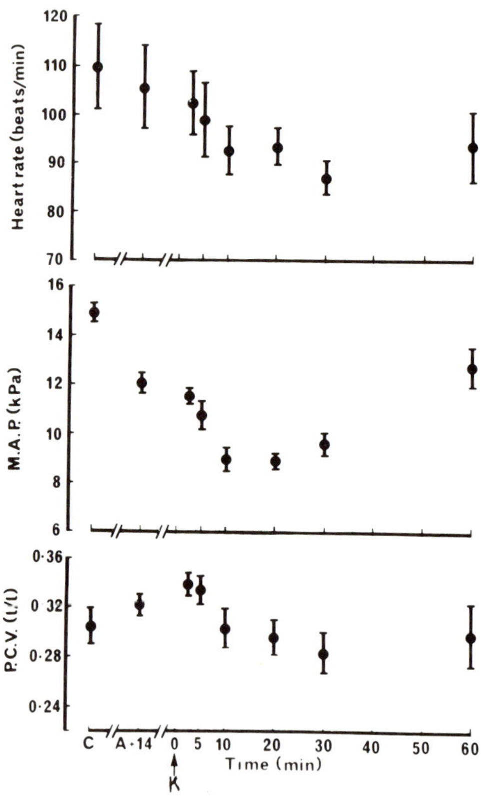

Figure 1 Cardiovascular effects of azaperone (A: 2 mg/kg i.m.) and ketamine (K: 15 mg/kg i.m.) in miniature pigs. Each point is the mean ± SE for 8 (heart rate), 7 (MAP), and 6 (PCV) determinations

(Figure 1). The principal cardiovascular effect, however, was a moderate degree of hypotension in all animals; in the eight miniature pigs MAP was reduced, on average, from 14.9 to 12.0 kPa 14 min after azaperone administration, with a further reduction to a minimum of 8.9 kPa 20 min after injecting ketamine (Figure 1). MAP was still reduced at 60 min (12.7 kPa) but had returned to normal by 90 min. The administration of azaperone alone also caused hypotension but ketamine alone, in contrast, increased MAP for periods ranging from 20 to 60 min.

The level of respiratory depression occurring during ketamine anaesthesia could not be readily assessed from direct observations of respiratory rate and depth because of the changed character of respiration (apneustic and jerky). However, from arterial blood gas measurements it became clear that breathing was stimulated by azaperone premedication; after 14 min mean PaO_2 was increased to 13.2 kPa from a control level of 12.4 kPa and mean $PaCO_2$ was reduced from 5.9 to 5.3 kPa. After inducing anaesthesia with ketamine respiratory depression, the magnitude of which varied considerably from animal to animal, usually occurred; it was severe in one pig, moderate in two, mild in two, unchanged in one and in a single animal stimulation occurred. For seven pigs, the mean value of oxygen tension was lowest at 5 min ($PaO_2 = 9.9$ kPa) and the respiratory acidosis which was usually slight was maximal at 20 min ($PaCO_2 = 6.5$ kPa).

It is concluded that the wide safety margin of ketamine in clinical use permits several experimental and clinical procedures to be performed. Anaesthesia and recovery were usually satisfactory and both i.v. and i.m. routes of administration were feasible. However, profound analgesia was not obtained and endotracheal intubation was not possible with moderate dose rates. For large pigs anaesthetic doses would be expensive and large volumes of solution would be required, but cost and injection volume are not excessive for smaller animals. The rise in blood pressure produced by ketamine was probably caused by the drug's well known sympathetic stimulant action. The hypotension which followed azaperone administration was probably due to this agent's α-adrenoceptor blocking properties. α-blockade by azaperone may also have accounted for reversal of the pressor action of ketamine. The apneustic respiratory pattern was accompanied by variable degrees of respiratory depression.

The use of a combination of xylazine and ketamine in calves

A. E. Waterman

Ketamine hydrochloride has been widely used for anaesthesia in many species. Although its use in adult cattle has been reported[1,2], there is no information regarding its use in calves. General anaesthesia often presents a problem in calves, especially if lack of equipment precludes the use of volatile anaesthetic agents. It seemed possible that a combination of xylazine and ketamine might offer a better alternative to barbiturates in such circumstances, and the following clinical study was therefore undertaken.

Thirty calves, ranging in age from 1 to 52 weeks and in weight from 30 to 360 kg were used in this study. The animals were allocated to one of three groups, details of which are given in Table 1.

Table 1

Group	*Ketamine dosage and route*	*No. of animals*	*Age* (weeks)	*Weight* (kg)	*Sex ratio (M/F)*
A	5 mg/kg i.v.	6	17.5 ± 7.2	86.7 ± 26.4	1/5
B	10 mg/kg i.m.	12	20.3 ± 4.2	118.3 ± 25.3	4/8
C	10 mg/kg i.m.	12	10.0 ± 2.8*	81.3 ± 16.4	8/4

*Significantly different from Group B, $p < 0.01$
Values are mean ± SEM

Following premedication with xylazine (0.2 mg/kg), which was given intramuscularly, anaesthesia was induced 10 min later by the intravenous (Group A) or intramuscular (Group B) administration of ketamine at a dose rate of 5 mg/kg and 10 mg/kg, respectively. In the third group (C), xylazine (0.2 mg/kg) and ketamine (10 mg/kg) were mixed together in the same syringe and administered simultaneously. Anaesthesia was maintained when necessary either by inhalation of halothane in oxygen (Group A) or by supplementary doses of ketamine at a dose rate of 5 mg/kg given intramuscularly (Groups B and C). The time to onset of anaesthesia, the duration of anaesthesia and the times taken for the calves to recover the ability to raise their heads, resume sternal recumbency and stand unaided were recorded. Respiratory and pulse rates were monitored and an attempt was made to assess the 'quality' of anaesthesia.

GROUP A

Following the intravenous administration of ketamine, anaesthesia was immediate. There was some initial respiratory depression but no apnoea. Bradycardia occurred following xylazine sedation but this was soon reversed by the ketamine. This dose of ketamine gave about 20 min anaesthesia and thereafter anaesthesia was maintained using halothane. As indicated in Table 2, all the calves recovered quickly at the end of anaesthesia.

Table 2 Results of anaesthesia using xylazine and ketamine. Values in minutes (mean ± SEM)

Group	*Route*	*Duration of anaesthesia*	*Time to head up*	*Time to sternal recumbency*	*Time to standing*
A	i.v.	19.0 ± 2.4	8.8 ± 1.4*	13.4 ± 1.8*	37.0 ± 7.5*
B	i.m.	23.5 ± 1.8	32.0 ± 7.5†	43.0 ± 8.6†	85.0 ± 10.8†
C	i.m.	37.0 ± 3.4	54.0 ± 4.6†	72.5 ± 7.1†	107.6 ± 10.5†

*Measured from cessation of halothane administration
†Measured from last injection of ketamine

GROUP B

All the calves became sedated within 3–5 min of xylazine administration and three became recumbent. The remainder were anaesthetized within 4 min of the injection of ketamine. This initial dose gave about 23 min anaesthesia; additional increments were required to prolong anaesthesia in seven animals for periods of 14–60 min. In these cases a mean total dose of 17.4 ± 1.6 mg/kg ketamine was given. As in Group A, the pulse rate fell after xylazine administration but soon returned to normal when the ketamine was given. Respiratory rates tended to be high (48 breaths/min) during anaesthesia.

GROUP C

The 12 animals in this group were anaesthetized by the intramuscular administration of xylazine and ketamine mixed together in the same syringe. The onset of incoordination and recumbency was extremely rapid; incoordination was apparent within 2 min (mean 1.6 ± 0.2 min) and all the calves were recumbent within 4 min (mean 3.2 ± 0.2 min). The duration of anaesthesia in this group, 37.0 min, was significantly longer than in Group B ($p<0.01$). Additional doses of ketamine were given to five calves in order to prolong anaesthesia for periods ranging from 10 to 30 min (mean 20.0 ± 3.4 min) and in these animals a mean total dose of 15.3 ± 0.4 mg/kg ketamine was used. Respiratory rates rose during anaesthesia but there was little change in pulse rates.

In all three groups, the calves appeared to be only lightly anaesthetized, palpebral and corneal reflexes remained brisk throughout except in the very youngest calves. There was pupillary dilatation and some animals exhibited nystagmus but muscle relaxation and analgesia were judged to be good, although there were occasional involuntary limb movements. Salivation and lachrymation were noted to a variable degree in all animals. No calf regurgitated and there were no complications in the recovery period. Comparison of Groups B and C revealed a significantly longer duration of action of ketamine in Group C. This was found to be related to the age of the calves. The duration of anaesthesia decreased with age for calves from 1 to 10 weeks of age, the linear relationship being described by the equation $y = 53.4 - 3.22x$ (correlation coefficient 0.74). In calves over 10 weeks of age the duration of action of the drug appeared to be almost constant at approximately 23 min.

This study has shown that ketamine in combination with xylazine produces satisfactory anaesthesia in calves. The unique state of anaesthesia produced by ketamine, however, was quite unlike that induced by other anaesthetic agents and this necessitated adjustment of the criteria normally used to judge the depth of anaesthesia. The greater sensitivity of the calves in Group C to the effects of ketamine seemed to be related to their age. This effect of age has previously been recorded in rats[4] and shown in this species to be related to the relative inability of young animals to metabolize the drug. In circumstances when facilities are not available for the administration of inhalational agents, it seems that a combination of ketamine and xylazine is effective both for the induction and maintenance of anaesthesia in calves, especially those under 10 weeks of age which are particularly sensitive to the effects of barbiturates[3].

References

1. Fuentes, V. O. and Tellez, E. (1974). *Vet. Rec.*, **94,** 482
2. Fuentes, V. O. and Tellez, E. (1976). *Vet. Rec.*, **99,** 338
3. Hall, L. W. (1971). *Wrights Veterinary Anaesthesia and Analgesia.* 7th Edn. (London: Baillière Tindall)
4. Waterman, A. E. and Livingston, A. (1978). *Br. J. Anaesth.*, **50,** 885

E.e.g. frequency analysis of barbiturate and ketamine anaesthesia

E. L. Gerring

The electro-encephalogram (e.e.g.) may be used to monitor the level of unconsciousness during anaesthesia and recovery as well as states of conscious awareness. The resting pattern of low frequency, large amplitude bursts of activity interspersed with high frequency, low amplitude waves can be instantly converted to the all high frequency arousal pattern by any mild stimulus, such as stroking the coat. Surgical anaesthesia is usually associated with a burst suppression pattern, in which short bursts of low frequency, high amplitude waves are superimposed on periods of electrical quiescence. A variety of patterns occur in recovery from anaesthesia but usually well-defined low frequency, large amplitude sleep spindles can be observed around the time of return of consciousness and soon after. The present study was undertaken to investigate the very different anaesthetic character observed between anaesthesia induced by barbiturates and that due to ketamine.

E.e.g. recordings were obtained from implanted bipolar gold electrodes in rabbits. The signal was passed through high gain a.c. amplifiers and displayed on a polygraph. The output signal was also fed into a gated e.e.g. analyser with bandwidths of 2–3 Hz, 3–6 Hz, 6–9 Hz, 12–18 Hz, 25–35 Hz and 52–70 Hz. The analyser recorded and displayed the percentage presence of e.e.g. waves in each band per 4 min unit of time. After a control period of recording, thiopentone (25 mg/kg) or ketamine (20 mg/kg) was injected into a marginal ear vein and recording continued until consciousness had been recovered. Following barbiturate injection a burst suppression level of anaesthesia was reached. This correlated well with activity in the 3–6 Hz band (Figure 1), surgical anaesthesia coinciding with low levels of activity. Activity increased with lightening of anaesthesia and then declined to coincide with recovery of consciousness at 42 min after injection. The high frequency band, 52–70 Hz, was predominant before injection as the arousal pattern and returned progressively during recovery.

The pattern with ketamine was markedly different. Slow waves in the 3–6 Hz band were present only in the first 6 min following injection. The 52–70 Hz band, however, was very prominent during this period (Figure 1)

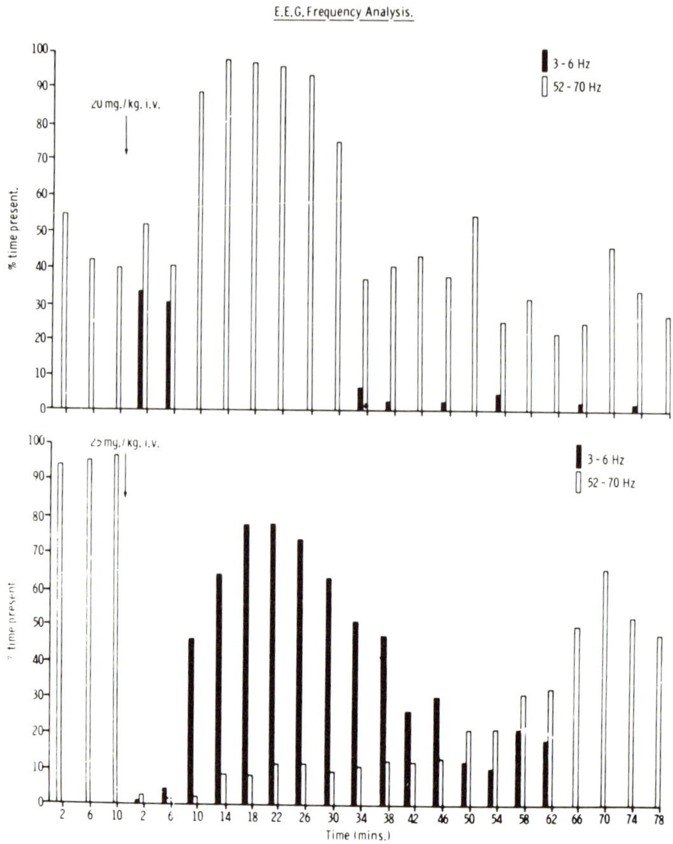

Figure 1 E.e.g. analysis of thiopentone and ketamine anaesthesia in the 3–6 Hz and 52–70 Hz bands. Upper panel ketamine, lower panel thiopentone

and throughout anaesthesia until recovery of consciousness at 54 min. Surface electrodes monitor the total resultant electrical activity from the brain and do not discriminate between activity centres. The effect of a barbiturate is almost completely to suppress all electrical activity in the brain, while ketamine produces only a transient decrease in electrical activity, quickly followed by high frequency waves.

Could this stimulation of high frequency activity be involved in blocking the lower frequency discharges, thereby producing the anaesthetic and cataleptic action of ketamine? Further study of this high frequency activity is required.

Index